Principles and Practice
of
Positron Emission Tomography

Principles and Practice
of
Positron Emission Tomography

Editor

Richard L. Wahl, M.D.

Henry N. Wagner, Jr. Professor of Nuclear Medicine
Professor of Radiology
Russell H. Morgan Department of Radiology and Radiological Science
Director, Division of Nuclear Medicine
The Johns Hopkins University School of Medicine
Baltimore, Maryland

Associate Editor

Julia W. Buchanan, B.S.

Associate in Research
Russell H. Morgan Department of Radiology and Radiological Science
Division of Nuclear Medicine
The Johns Hopkins University School of Medicine
Baltimore, Maryland

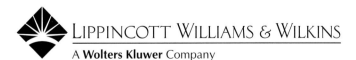

LIPPINCOTT WILLIAMS & WILKINS
A **Wolters Kluwer** Company
Philadelphia • Baltimore • New York • London
Buenos Aires • Hong Kong • Sydney • Tokyo

Acquisitions Editor: Joyce-Rachel John
Developmental Editor: Selina M. Bush
Production Editor: Jodi Borgenicht
Manufacturing Manager: Colin J. Warnock
Cover Designer: Mark Lerner
Compositor: Maryland Composition
Printer: Maple Press

© 2002 by LIPPINCOTT WILLIAMS & WILKINS
530 Walnut Street
Philadelphia, PA 19106 USA
LWW.com

Printed in the USA

Library of Congress Cataloging-in-Publication Data

Principles and practice of positron emission tomography / editor, Richard L. Wahl.
     p. ; cm.
   Includes bibliographical references and index.
   ISBN 0-7817-2904-1
     1. Tomography, Emission. I. Wahl, Richard L.
     [DNLM: 1. Tomography, Emission-Computed—methods. 2. Neoplasms—radionuclide imaging. WN 206 P957 2002]
   RC78.7.T62 P75 2002
   616.07′575—dc21

                                 2002016286

---

10 9 8 7 6 5 4 3 2 1

To my ever-patient and supportive wife Sandy, my children, my mother,
and to the many investigators, trainees, technologists, and study participants
whose efforts were essential to development of the discipline of PET.

RLW

To Henry N. Wagner, Jr., M.D., who has guided my career in nuclear medicine
for over 40 years and who has taught me so much.

JWB

Contents

Contributing Authors

Anissa Abi-Dargham, M.D.   *Associate Professor, Department of Clinical Psychobiology, Columbia University, New York State Psychiatric Institute, New York, New York*

Rob S.B. Beanlands, M.D.   *Professor of Medicine (Cardiology) / Radiology; Chief, Cardiac Imaging; and Director, Cardiac PET Centre, University of Ottawa Heart Institute, Ottawa, Ontario, Canada*

Nicolaas I. Bohnen, M.D., Ph.D.   *Assistant Professor of Neurology and Radiology, Departments of Neurology and Radiology, Division of Nuclear Medicine, University of Pittsburgh Medical School, Pittsburgh, Pennsylvania*

Inga Buchmann, M.D.   *Department of Nuclear Medicine, University Hospital of Ulm, Ulm, Germany*

Chuong Dac Huy Bui, M.D.   *Nuclear Medicine Fellow, Division of Nuclear Medicine, University of Michigan Medical Center, Ann Arbor, Michigan*

Jerry M. Collins, Ph.D.   *Director, Laboratory of Clinical Pharmacology, United States Food and Drug Administration, Rockville, Maryland*

Leonard P. Connolly, M.D.   *Assistant Professor, Department of Radiology, Division of Nuclear Medicine, Children's Hospital, Harvard Medical School, Boston, Massachusetts*

Gary J. R. Cook, M.D., F.R.C.P., M.B.B.S., F.R.C.R.   *Head, Department of Nuclear Medicine, The Royal Marsden Hospital and Institute of Cancer Research, London, United Kingdom*

Farrokh Dehdashti, M.D.   *Associate Professor of Radiology, Division of Nuclear Medicine, Edward Mallinckrodt Institute of Radiology, Washington University School of Medicine, St. Louis, Missouri*

Robert deKemp, Ph.D.   *Head of PET Physics and Assistant Professor of Medicine, University of Ottawa Heart Institute, Ottawa, Ontario, Canada*

Dominique Delbeke, M.D., Ph.D.   *Professor, Director of Nuclear Medicine and PET, Department of Radiology and Radiological Sciences, Vanderbilt University Medical Center, Nashville, Tennessee*

Yu-Shin Ding, Ph.D.   *Senior Scientist, Head of Radiotracer Development Neuroscience and Imaging Group, Chemistry Department, Brookhaven National Laboratory, Upton, New York*

Ronald D. Finn, Ph.D.   *Chief, Radiopharmaceutical Chemistry Service, and Director, Cyclotron Core Facility, Departments of Radiology and Medical Physics, Memorial Sloan-Kettering Cancer Center, New York, New York*

Joanna S. Fowler, Ph.D.   *Director, Brookhaven PET Program; and Senior Chemist, Chemistry Department, Brookhaven National Laboratory, Upton, New York*

Michael J. Fulham, F.R.A.C.P.   *Clinical Director of Medical Imaging; Senior Staff Neurologist and Director of the Department of PET and Nuclear Medicine; and Associate Professor, Department of Medicine, University of Sydney; Royal Prince Alfred Hospital, Sydney, Australia*

Uwe A. Haberkorn, M.D.   *Clinical Cooperation Unit Nuclear Medicine, German Cancer Research Center; and Department of Nuclear Medicine, University of Heidelberg, Heidelberg, Germany*

ix

Karl F. Hubner, M.D.   *Professor and Director of Research, Department of Radiology, The University of Tennessee Medical Center at Knoxville, Knoxville, Tennessee*

Ora Israel, M.D.   *Director of Nuclear Medicine, Rambam Medical Center; and Associate Professor, School of Medicine, Technion - Israel Institute of Technology, Haifa, Israel*

Hossein Jadvar, M.D., Ph.D.   *Assistant Professor of Radiology and Biomedical Engineering, Department of Radiology, Division of Nuclear Medicine, University of Southern California, Los Angeles, California; and Visiting Associate in Bioengineering, California Institute of Technology, Pasadena, California*

Robert A. Koeppe, Ph.D.   *Professor of Radiology, Director of PET Physics Section, Division of Nuclear Medicine, Department of Radiology, University of Michigan Medical School, Ann Arbor, Michigan*

Marc Laruelle, M.D.   *Associate Professor, Department of Psychiatry, Columbia University, New York State Psychiatric Institute, New York, New York*

Val J. Lowe, M.D.   *Associate Professor of Radiology, Mayo Medical School; and PET Imaging, Department of Radiology, Mayo Clinic, Rochester, Minnesota*

Homer A. Macapinlac, M.D.   *Associate Professor, Chief and Director of PET Section, Division of Diagnostic Imaging, University of Texas MD Anderson Cancer Center, Houston, Texas*

Jamshid Maddahi, M.D.   *Clinical Professor of Molecular and Medical Pharmacology and Radiological Science, UCLA School of Medicine, Los Angeles, California*

William H. Martin, M.D.   *Assistant Professor, Department of Radiology and Radiological Sciences, Division of Nuclear Medicine, Vanderbilt University Hospital, Nashville, Tennessee*

Diana Martinez   *Assistant Professor, Department of Clinical Psychobiology, Columbia University, New York State Psychiatric Institute, New York, New York*

Ichiro Matsunari, M.D.   *Chief Investigator, Clinical Research Section, The Medical and Pharmalogical Research Center Foundation, Hakui, Japan*

Sven N. Reske, M.D.   *Professor of Nuclear Medicine, and Head and Chief, Department of Nuclear Medicine, University of Ulm, Ulm, Germany*

Terrence D. Ruddy, M.D.   *Associate Professor of Medicine and Radiology, and Director, Nuclear Cardiology, University of Ottawa Heart Institute; Chief of Nuclear Medicine, The Ottawa Hospital, Ottawa, Ontario, Canada*

Martin P. Sandler, M.D.   *Professor and Chair, Department of Radiology and Radiological Sciences, Vanderbilt University Medical Center, Nashville, Tennessee*

David J. Schlyer, Ph.D.   *Chemist, Department of Chemistry, Brookhaven National Laboratory, Upton, New York*

Markus Schwaiger, M.D.   *Director, Technische Universitaet Muenchen, Nuklearmedizinische Klinik u. Poliklinik, Munich, Germany*

Anthony F. Shields, M.D., Ph.D.   *Professor, Department of Medicine, Wayne State University, Karmanos Cancer Institute, Detroit, Michigan*

Paul D. Shreve, M.D.   *Associate Professor, Radiology Department, University of Michigan, Ann Arbor, Michigan*

Barry L. Shulkin, M.D.   *Professor, Department of Radiology, Division of Nuclear Medicine, University of Michigan, Ann Arbor, Michigan*

Hans C. Steinert, M.D.   *Associate Professor, Division of Nuclear Medicine, Department of Medical Radiology, University Hospital of Zurich, Zurich, Switzerland*

Yoshifumi Sugawara, M.D.   *Assistant Professor, Department of Radiology, Ehime University School of Medicine, Shigenobu, Ehime, Japan*

Peter Talbot, M.D. *Post-Doctoral Resident Scientist, Department of Psychiatry, Columbia University, New York State Psychiatric Institute, New York, New York*

Nagara Tamaki, M.D., Ph.D. *Professor and Chairman, Department of Nuclear Medicine, Hokkaido University Graduate School of Medicine, Sapporo, Japan*

Christopher J. Thompson, D.Sc., F.C.C.P.M. *Professor, Montreal Neurological Institute, McGill University, Montreal, Quebec, Canada*

Heikki Ukkonen, M.D., Ph.D. *Department of Medicine, Turku University Hospital and Turku PET Centre, Turku, Finland; and Clinical Fellow, Cardiac PET, University of Ottawa Heart Institute, Ottawa, Ontario, Canada*

Richard L. Wahl, M.D. *Henry N. Wagner, Jr. Professor of Nuclear Medicine, Professor of Radiology, Russell H. Morgan Department of Radiology and Radiological Science; and Director, Division of Nuclear Medicine, The Johns Hopkins University School of Medicine, Baltimore, Maryland*

Foreword: Historical Outline

Positron emission tomography (PET) is the most important advance in biomedical science since the invention of the microscope. It became available just as it was needed to advance the new molecular orientation of biology. Its promise was foreseen in 1941 by the late William Myers, who received his Ph.D. degree (he also had a M.D. degree) with a thesis that described the potential of the cyclotron in producing radiotracers that emitted positrons and could revolutionize medicine. Half a century later, we can see the wisdom of his words. He told me that, "The worse thing that ever happened to nuclear medicine was the discovery of technetium-99m". Dr. Meyers spoke with tongue-in-cheek because he and all of us in the field of nuclear medicine recognized the importance of technetium-99m radiotracers. Technetium-99m radiotracers have a six-hour half-life, are available from a molybdenum generator, and emit 140 keV photons, an energy ideal for measurement with radiation detectors located outside of the body. This radionuclide was an essential ingredient for use with the scintillation camera, invented in the late 1950s by Hal Anger. Technetium-99m radiotracers and the Anger camera were responsible for the rapid growth of subspecialties of nuclear medicine, especially nuclear cardiology, which advanced rapidly in the 1970s and 1980s. In the 1990s, PET proved to be the means by which molecular medicine could be incorporated into medical practice, beginning with its use in the detection, treatment planning, and monitoring of patients with cancer.

When I was a medical student, pathology—the matching of the patient's symptoms to what one could see under the microscope—provided the dominant scientific foundation of medicine. Its derivative science was biochemistry, the elucidation of the chemical events occurring in the body. Carbon was the defining element of organic chemistry and biochemistry, and it brought an entirely new and exciting challenge to medical science. In Berlin, Otto Meyerhof had discovered the chemical pathway by which the cells turn glucose into energy, a process that would subsequently be the chemical process that would thrust PET into the mainstream of medical practice.

In 1953, when I was an intern in internal medicine at Johns Hopkins Hospital, Fritz Lipmann and Hans Krebs were awarded the Nobel Prize for their discovery of how glucose is oxidized. At the same Institution in Berlin, Otto Warburg had related glucose metabolism to cancer. In 1953, Watson and Crick published the structure of DNA, and the Society of Nuclear Medicine was founded. Using deuterium as a tracer, Schoenheimer and Rittenberg at the Rockefeller Institute in New York had discovered that the chemical constituents of the body were constantly turning over—the "dynamic state of body constituents", a principle second only to the "tracer" principle as the essence of the medical specialty of nuclear medicine.

The great science and technology that are the foundation of modern health care today did not just happen. People working together with the support of government, academia, and industry made things happen. Molecular nuclear medicine was the result of the joint efforts of the Atomic Energy Commission (now called the Department of Energy) and the National Institutes of Health, the AEC as the sponsor of technological developments, and the NIH as the sponsor of basic research. Pioneers, especially James Shannon and his colleagues at the NIH, were able to convince the government that only by understanding basic biological mechanisms could one learn how to intervene in disease processes. Shannon was able to relate molecular advances in basic science to their practical applications in the clinic. His vision was to use "quantitative concepts of biology. . .to understand the nature of disease and ultimately its management."

One hundred and fifty years ago, in his classic *Introduction to the Study of Experimental Medicine*, the father of physiology, Claude Bernard, wrote that physiologists make use of "instruments and procedures borrowed from physics and chemistry in order to study and measure the diverse vital phenomena whose laws they seek to discover." Bernard also wrote: "The grand principle is not to stop until one has reached, for the phenomenon one is studying, the physico-chemical explanation suitable to them." He and his followers incorporated the principal results of the discoveries of chemists into their attempts to understand physiological processes that they could examine in experimental animals. He argued that physiology must be the light in which the chemistry of the body should be viewed. The science and technology of nuclear medicine, using the tracer principle, extended biochemical and physiological studies to the examination of the living human body in health and disease. Just as were the early physiologists one hundred and fifty years ago, nuclear medicine physicians and scientists were particularly concerned with where in the living body chemical reactions occur. When Carl Lehmann published the first *Textbook of Physiological Chemistry* in 1842, he proposed that the first step for the investigator is to try to understand the chemical properties of body constituents in relation to the roles that they play in the entire organism. The next step is to determine the "topography" of these substances, that is, where the chemical processes are occurring in the body. The greatest contribution of nuclear medicine has been to make possible the measurement of regional function and biochemistry.

One of the most fundamental principles of physiology is that of the dynamic state of body constituents, which states that the apparent constancy of the biological constituents in the extracellular fluid, described first by Claude Bernard, is the result of a delicate balance between the rates of production and breakdown of biochemicals that are in a continual state of flux. The existence of electromagnetic radiation, including photons, that are ever present in the environment, and that are produced by radioactive substances, makes it possible to "trace" the movement and chemical behavior of substances taken into and existing in the body. Radiation detectors, which can identify and measure these photons, make it possible to examine the chemical processes going on in all parts of the body. Without their use, measurements can only be made of the concentrations of substances in blood, urine, or other collectible body fluids. Measurement of the rate of accumulation of radioactive materials, such as radioiodine by the thyroid gland, was among the first procedures widely developed after the end of World War II. Measurement of the radioactivity at multiple points in the neck after the administration of radioiodine made it possible to predict whether a nodule within the thyroid was likely to be cancer. The invention of the nuclear reactor as a result of wartime research made large quantities of inexpensive radioactive tracers available throughout the world soon after the war ended.

These reactor-produced radiotracers resulted in a diminution in the use of cyclotrons that had been developed during the 1930s. These early studies of the thyroid illustrated the principles that still underlie nuclear medicine: (1) measurement of regional biochemistry in the living body; (2) characterization of a disease (hyperthyroidism) by measurement of a regional biochemical process; (3) characterization of cancer by loss of normal biochemical processes (accumulation of iodine); and (4) therapy based on regional biochemical processes (radioiodine therapy of hyperthyroidism). The general applicability of these principles is what ensures the permanent position of nuclear medicine in healthcare.

About the same time that radioiodine was attracting worldwide attention as an alternative to thyroid surgery, George Moore at the University of Minnesota began to use radiotracers to help locate brain tumors at surgery, another fundamental principle that today is becoming more widely accepted.

Illustrating the historical fact that technology advances parallel conceptual advances, in 1951 Benedict Cassen invented the "rectilinear scanner", replacing hand-held Geiger-Muller detectors with motorized crystal scintillation detectors. The latter made possible differentiation of multiple radiotracers present in the body at the same time, and facilitated portrayal of the spatial distribution of radiotracers within the body. These images were called "scans" because the radiation detector moved back and forth, "scanning" the region of interest. Within a decade, Hal Anger replaced the moving detector with a large crystal "camera" that used electronic logic to localize the site of origin of photons emitted from the regions of interest. The invention of the "radionuclide generator" by Stang and Richards made the man-made radionuclide, technetium-99m, available for widespread use, and its greater photon yield made it possible to create interpretable "images" of regional function and biochemistry. The combination of a suitable radiotracer (^{99m}Tc) and a device (the Anger camera) that could examine an entire region simultaneously gave birth to a very important area of nuclear medicine today, namely, nuclear cardiology. Structure and function had been brought together, and "functional images" could be made of biological processes occurring anywhere in the body. It became possible to measure "what, where, and how fast" a biochemical or physiological process was occurring. Building these images was facilitated by the invention of computers, which were moving away from centralized "computer centers" to the bedside of the patient. Nuclear medicine was the first field of medicine to employ computers on a routine basis.

Interestingly, the newly created radionuclide images were used to examine organs of the body, such as the liver and spleen, that were not visualized by conventional x-rays. This can probably be explained by the pioneering work of radiologists, such as Merrill Bender and David Kuhl, in the growth of nuclear medicine. But in the background lay the positron-emitting radionuclides that had enormous potential for the study of body chemistry.

In 1925, in a feat difficult to understand by anyone who is not a physicist, the British physicist, Paul Dirac, had postulated the existence of the positron, or negative electron, because his mathematical analysis revealed a square root term. This eventually led to the conclusion that every type of elemental particle had an antiparticle of the same type. When a particle meets such an antiparticle, they annihilate, leaving behind only energy. In the case of a positron-emitting tracer, two 511 keV photons are released in opposite directions. In 1932, proof of the existence of positrons (positively-charged particles with the mass of a negatively-charged electron) in the real world was provided by Carl Anderson by photographic analysis of cosmic radiation. Subsequently, two other Nobel Prize winners, Irene Curie and her husband Frederick Joliot, in 1934 discovered it was possible to artificially make radioactive elements. They correctly identified the radionuclides that they produced in their early experiments as positron-emitters.

Irene Curie and Frederick Joliot had used alpha particle-emitting radionuclides to produce positron-emitting radionuclides, such as nitrogen-13. Their report in 1934 created great excitement in Berkeley, California, where Ernest Lawrence and his colleagues had several years before the invention of the cyclotron in order to bombard elements with positively charged particles. In their own experiments, the Berkeley scientists had been producing artificial radioactivity, but had not discovered its existence because the same power supply used to operate the cyclotron was also used to power their radiation detection devices. Both were shut off simultaneously. Today, the decommissioning of cyclotrons requires months for the radioactivity produced by the operation of the machine to decline to safe levels, which indicates the large amounts of induced radioactivity in the cyclotron itself.

With their cyclotrons (the fourth was called a "medical" cyclotron), the Berkeley group could produce large amounts of artificial radionuclides, among which were carbon-11, nitrogen-13, oxygen-15, and fluorine-18. Up until that time, the study of physiological processes was limited by the chemical and physical properties of naturally occurring radionuclides, such as radium. While these had led to the development of the "tracer principle", the most fundamental principle of nuclear medicine, by George Hevesy, the ability to "trace" all body constituents with a whole variety of artificial radionuclides caused great excitement in the scientific and medical world. People from all over the world flocked to Berkeley to apply radiotracer methodology to the study of biochemistry and physiology. Among the important investigations were studies of photosynthesis by Kamen and his colleagues.

Oxygen-15 was not used in these early studies because of its short (approximately two minutes) half-life. In 1957, Kamen stated, "No radioactive tracer of oxygen is sufficiently long-lived to be useful in tracer work." The discovery of carbon-14 in 1940 by Kamen and Ruben provided a far more readily available tracer of carbon because of its half-life and the ability to be produced in nuclear reactors, invented during World War II. Biochemists abandoned carbon-11 in favor of carbon-14, and produced biochemistry as we know it today. The nuclear medicine community turned to reactor-produced iodine-131 and phosphorus-32 because they were easy to produce and use, and could be used for therapy as well as for diagnosis and research. For all practical purposes, after the early experiments of Tobias and colleagues (1945), carbon-11, fluorine-18, and nitrogen-13 were all but forgotten. In the mid-1950s Ter-Pogossian at Washington University in St. Louis, began the renaissance of positron-emitting radiotracers, produced by the cyclotron or linear accelerators. He did so because of a strong desire to carry out studies with oxygen-15, which could only be produced by an accelerator. Their cyclotron installed in the physics department in the 1940s was built to carry out these studies. In 1955, the success of the oxygen-15 studies stimulated the group at Hammersmith Hospital in London to commission a cyclotron within a medical center itself, primarily for the study of radioactive gases of biological interest, including oxygen-15 and carbon-11 dioxide.

Their success led to the installation of a new cyclotron at Washington University, as well as at the Massachusetts General Hospital and Memorial Sloan-Kettering Medical Center. At Ohio State University and the University of California at Berkeley workers continued their studies with radiotracers produced by existing cyclotrons. Together they showed that the biological importance of carbon, hydrogen (fluorine is to some extent an analogue of hydrogen), nitrogen, and oxygen warranted the overcoming of the barriers to the production and synthesis of biologically-important tracers that could not be produced in a nuclear reactor. Initially there was considerable skepticism about the possibility of labeling complex molecules with such short-lived radionuclides, and PET imaging was considered an elitist, impractical device. Fortunately, the persistence and results of the pioneers proved that this was a misconception, and today PET is a major focus of biomedical research and medical practice.

Henry N. Wagner, Jr., M.D.
Director
Division of Radiation Health Sciences
Johns Hopkins Bloomberg School of Public Health
Baltimore, Maryland

Preface

Our purpose in writing this book is to present a comprehensive guide to how positron emission tomography (PET) works, but more critically, how to use PET to enhance the care of patients. The basic principles of the technique are presented first and discuss how PET radionuclides are produced and incorporated into useful compounds to measure a specific molecular process *in vivo*. Once in the human body, these compounds are detected with specialized and ever evolving equipment, such as PET/CT scanners. Quantification of PET data requires sophisticated processing of the data sets to produce the displayed images. While much of the focus of the book is clinical, research applications of PET across a wide range of organ systems are also presented.

For nearly twenty years PET was a potent research tool, but it was available only at select academic institutions. Large teams of investigators from diverse disciplines were needed to handle the complexities involved in the production of short-lived isotopes with balky cyclotrons, the performance of rapid radiochemistry to generate suitable human tracers, and to produce and analyze the often "fuzzy" images resulting from these efforts. Several scans a week represented a "busy" PET operation. The possibility that the "complex" PET technique could become a routine diagnostic method throughout the world by the turn of the century seemed exceedingly unlikely in the late 1970s and early 1980s. However, through the persistence of many investigators and advances in computer technology, cyclotrons and chemistry are now computer-controlled and substantially automated. Instead of an entire floor of computers that was required to process images, now a single small console sitting on a desk does the task. A single outpatient PET scanner can now perform 10 to 20 scans a day and scanners are becoming faster.

In the late 1980s it became apparent that the PET technique and 2-[^{18}F]-fluoro-2-deoxy-D-glucose (FDG) had huge clinical potential. Pilot studies in animals and humans showed FDG PET's ability to image lung, breast, and other cancers—in addition to its known ability to image function in the brain and heart. By the mid 1990s it became clear to those working with PET that it was clinically effective, but its dissemination was delayed largely due to concerns about health care costs and the prevailing enthusiasm for CT and magnetic resonance imaging (MRI) at that time. Compelling scientific data, reimbursement for PET, involvement of large medical equipment manufacturers in PET, and acceptance of PET by referring physicians due to the excellent clinical results have moved the field rapidly forward in the last few years.

Nearly five years before the publication of this book, we felt there was a very large gap in the PET literature and we saw a critical need for a textbook that would provide a comprehensive guide to the rapidly evolving field of PET, from the fundamental physics and chemistry, to details on how to implement and interpret clinical PET images.

PET is used to study most organ systems of the body and has contributed to our understanding of the basic physiology and pathophysiology of oncological disorders, the brain, the heart, and other organ systems. PET is also playing a major role in the development of new stable (nonradioactive) drugs and is an ideal tool to image phenotypic alterations resulting from the altered genotype. To date, the greatest application of PET in routine clinical studies has been in patients with cancer, where PET images functional alterations caused by molecular changes in contrast to the traditional anatomic methods of imaging cancer like CT.

The increased metabolism of malignant cells makes it possible to image a wide variety of tumors with the glucose analog, FDG. In this book we have chosen authors who have made major contributions in establishing FDG PET as an accurate, sensitive, and useful technique for evaluating and monitoring patients with numerous types of cancer. The validation of the clinical findings, combined with the current speed at which a study can be completed and the fact that third party payers will now provide reimbursement for many studies, has made FDG PET a modality that medical centers cannot be without. The recent addition of PET/CT is further adding to the refinement of these studies by combining precise fusion of anatomic information with the molecular image data as ''anatomolecular'' images. Referring physicians can quickly relate to images that fuse form and function, and they now routinely wish to have PET or PET/CT to enhance the care for their patients. A variety of other PET radiotracers are discussed, which will further expand the use of clinical PET beyond FDG.

At present, PET is the most rapidly growing area of medical imaging because of its considerable power, and it has now reached a new plateau of widespread, worldwide distribution. We hope this book, which reviews all aspects of PET, will serve as a useful starting point and reference tool to all who use PET in their clinical or research work.

Richard L. Wahl
Julia W. Buchanan

Acknowledgments

The support and encouragement of Joyce-Rachel John at Lippincott Williams & Wilkins over the nearly five-year period of development of this book is much appreciated.

Principles and Practice
of
Positron Emission Tomography

CHAPTER 1

Production of Radionuclides for PET

Ronald D. Finn and David J. Schlyer

Coupled with the advancement in noninvasive cross-sectional imaging techniques to identify structural alterations in diseased tissues, there have been significant advances in the development of *in vivo* methods to quantify functional metabolism in both normal and diseased tissues. Positron emission tomography (PET) is an imaging modality that yields physiologic information necessary for clinical diagnoses based on altered tissue metabolism.

One of the most widely recognized advantages of PET is the use of the positron-emitting biologic radiotracers (carbon-11 [^{11}C], oxygen-15 [^{15}O], nitrogen-13 [^{13}N], and fluorine-18 [^{18}F]) that mimic natural substrates. These radionuclides have well-documented nuclear reaction cross sections appropriate for "baby" cyclotron energies and the corresponding "hot atom" target chemistries are reasonably well understood. A disadvantage these biologic radionuclides possess is their relatively short half-lives, which means they cannot be transported to sites at great distances from the production facility.

Currently, there are four PET drugs officially recognized by the U.S. Food and Drug Administration (FDA) and approved for intravenous injection. They are sodium fluoride (^{18}F), rubidium-82-chloride (^{82}Rb), ^{13}N-ammonia and fluorodeoxyglucose (^{18}F-FDG). In 1972, sodium fluoride (^{18}F) (New Drug Application [NDA] 17-042) was approved as an NDA for bone imaging to define areas of altered osteogenic activity, but the manufacturer ceased marketing this product in 1975. Rubidium-82-chloride (NDA 19-414) was approved in 1989 and is indicated for assessment of regional myocardial perfusion in the diagnosis and localization of myocardial infarction. Most recently, ^{18}F-FDG (NDA 20-306) was recognized in 1994 for identification of regions of abnormal glucose metabolism initially associated with foci of epileptic seizures, but it is now mostly used and approved for its application to various primary and metastatic malignant diseases (1). Nitrogen-13-ammonia is approved for assessment of myocardial blood flow.

Over the past few decades, PET studies with radiolabeled drugs have provided new information on drug uptake, biodistribution, and various kinetic relationships. A critique on the design and development of PET radiopharmaceuticals has been published (2), as well as several articles involving the future of PET in drug research and development and the production targetry available from various manufacturers of cyclotrons (3). Growth in clinical PET applications has led to increased interest in and demand for new PET radiopharmaceuticals.

PRODUCTION

Definition of Nuclear Reaction Cross Section

A nuclear reaction is one in which a nuclear particle is absorbed into a target nucleus, resulting in a very short-lived compound nucleus. This excited nucleus will decompose along several pathways and produce various products. A wide variety of nuclear reactions are used in an accelerator to produce artificial radioactivity. The bombarding particles are usually protons, deuterons, or helium particles. The energies used range from a few million electron volts to hundreds of million electron volts. One of the most useful models for nuclear reactions is the compound nucleus model originally introduced by Bohr in 1936. In this model, the incident particle is absorbed into the nucleus of the target material and the energy is distributed throughout the compound nucleus. In essence, the nucleus comes to some form of equilibrium before decomposing and then emitting particles. These two steps are considered to be independent of each another. Regardless of how the compound nucleus got to the high-energy state, the decay of the radionuclide will be independent of the way in which it was formed. The total amount of excitation energy contained in the nucleus will be given by the following equation:

$$U = \frac{M_A}{M_A + M_a} T_a + S_a$$

where

U = excitation energy
M_A = mass of the target nucleus
M_a = mass of the incident particle

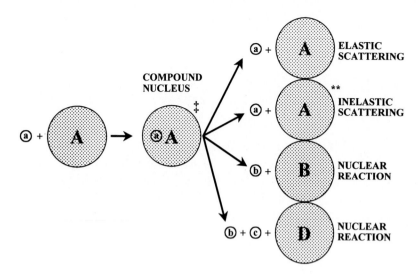

FIG. 1.1. Formation and disintegration of the compound nucleus.

T_a = kinetic energy of the incident particle
S_a = binding energy of the incident particle in the compound nucleus

The nucleus can decompose along several channels, as shown in Fig. 1.1.

When the compound nucleus decomposes, the kinetic energy of all the products may be either greater or less than the total kinetic energy of all the reactants. If the energy of the products is greater, then the reaction is said to be exoergic. If the kinetic energy of the products is less than that of the reactants, then the reaction is endoergic. The magnitude of this difference is called the Q value. If the reaction is exoergic, Q values are positive. An energy-level diagram of a typical reaction is shown in Fig. 1.2.

The nuclear reaction cross section represents the total probability that a compound nucleus will be formed and that it will decompose in a particular channel. There is a minimum energy below which a nuclear reaction will not occur except by tunneling effects. The incident particle energy must be sufficient to overcome the coulomb barrier and to overcome a negative Q value of the reaction. Particles with energies below this barrier have a very low probability of reacting. The energy required to induce a nuclear reaction increases as the Z of the target material increases. For many low Z materials, it is possible to use a low-energy accelerator, but for high Z materials it is necessary to increase the particle energy (4).

The following relationship (4) gives the number of reactions occurring in 1 second:

$$dn = I_0 N_A ds \sigma_{ab}$$

where

dn is the number of reactions occurring in 1 second
I_0 is the number of particles incident on the target in 1 second
N_A is the number of target nuclei per gram
ds is the thickness of the material in grams per centimeter squared
σ_{ab} is the parameter called the cross section expressed in units of centimeters squared

In practical applications, the thickness ds of the material can be represented by a slab of thickness Δs thin enough that the cross section can be considered as constant. N_A ds are then the number of target atoms in a 1-cm² area of thickness Δs. If the target material is a compound, rather than a pure element, then the number of nuclei per unit area is given by the following expression:

$$N_A = \frac{F_A C}{A_A}$$

where

N_A is the number of target nuclei per gram
F_A is the fractional isotopic abundance
C is the concentration in weight

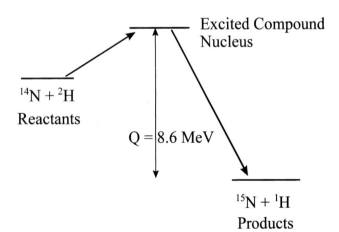

FIG. 1.2. Energy level diagram for a nuclear reaction. The Q value is the difference in the energy levels of the reactants and the products.

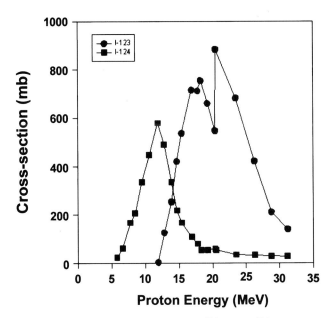

FIG. 1.3. Plot of yield from the $^{124}Te(p,n)^{124}I$ and the $^{124}Te(p,2n)^{123}I$ nuclear reactions as a function of energy on target.

$\mathfrak{I}$ is the Avogadro number

A_A is the atomic mass number of nucleus A

This leads to one of the basic facts of life in radioisotope production. It is not always possible to eliminate the radionuclidic impurities even with the highest isotopic enrichment and the widest energy selection. An example of this is given in Fig. 1.3 for the production of iodine-123 (^{123}I) with a minimum of iodine-124 (^{124}I) impurity (5–8).

As can be seen from Fig. 1.3, it is not possible to eliminate the ^{124}I impurity completely during the ^{123}I production since the ^{124}I is being concurrently formed at the same energy. To minimize the ^{124}I impurity irradiation of the target at an energy where the production of ^{124}I is near a minimum becomes an option. In this case, a proton energy higher than 20 MeV will give a minimum of ^{124}I impurity.

Enriched Targets

Although they generally play a supplementary role to the applications in the production of radionuclides, stable isotopically labeled compounds find widespread use in pharmacologic and toxicologic investigations. Their use as internal standards in such sensitive and specific analytical techniques as gas chromatography–mass spectroscopy and high-pressure liquid chromatography coupled with mass spectroscopy is of great benefit in the assay of body fluids. Paramagnetic stable nuclides such as carbon-13 (^{13}C) offer opportunities for nuclear magnetic resonance (NMR) analyses of biological samples and possibly whole-body NMR in metabolic studies (9–11).

Stable isotopes have for many years been the foundation for the production of radionuclides when pure radionuclides are necessary. Since the invention of the "cyclotron" by Professor E.O. Lawrence in 1929 and proof of acceleration by M.S. Livingston in 1931, the accelerators have provided unique radionuclides for numerous applications.

In the past decade, there has been a significant increase in the acquisition and use of "small" cyclotrons devoted principally to operation by chemists for the production of the biomedically useful radiolabeled compounds or radiopharmaceuticals. The primary impetus has been the acceptance of the potential of PET as a dynamic molecular imaging technique applicable to clinical diagnoses while providing the opportunity to evaluate novel radiotracers and radioligands for monitoring *in vivo* biochemical or physiologic processes with exquisite sensitivity.

Concurrent with the growth of PET/cyclotron facilities has been an emphasis on the production of larger amounts of the short-lived radionuclides in a chemical form suitable for efficient synthetic application. The radionuclidic purity of the final nuclide is an important concern. Targetry and target chemistry continue to be factors for the synthetic chemist's consideration and appreciation of material science and radiation chemistry effects.

With energy constraints imposed by the various accelerators chosen for installation in imaging facilities, the availability and the application of stable enriched target materials for the production of the biologically equivalent radionuclides is of paramount concern. The calutrons at Oak Ridge National Laboratory are no longer in service to prepare and provide the numerous stable enriched nuclides needed for the variety of radionuclides being evaluated for clinical applications. These concerns still plague many investigators who have experienced the lack of or shortages in availability of such important target materials. A current example involves $H_2^{18}O$ for ^{18}F production. The $H_2^{18}O$ target is the choice of most centers for the production of ^{18}F-labeled fluoride anion used in most ^{18}F-labeled radiopharmaceutical production (12,13).

TARGETS AND IRRADIATION

Traditional PET Radioisotopes

There are four positron-emitting radioisotopes that are considered the biologic tracers and their clinical and investigational uses are extensive. The radionuclides are ^{18}F, ^{11}C, ^{13}N, and ^{15}O. The reason these are so commonly used is that they can be easily substituted directly onto biomolecules. Carbon-11, ^{13}N, and ^{15}O are the "elements of life." Substitution of ^{11}C for carbon-12 (^{12}C) does not significantly alter the reaction time or mechanisms of a molecule. A similar situation exists for ^{13}N and ^{15}O. Fluorine-18 can often be substituted for a hydroxy group in a molecule or placed in a position where its presence does not significantly alter the biological behavior of the molecule. When the nucleus decays, the positron emitted will slow to thermal energies, annihilate upon interaction with an electron to produce two 511 keV gamma rays emitted at nearly 180 degrees to each other. The decay characteristics of the positron-emitting radionuclides allow the physiologic processes occurring *in vivo* to be quantitated by detectors outside the body. Physiologic modeling can be carried out using this information and quantitative assessments of the biologic function can be made.

Target Irradiation

The positron-emitting radionuclides are produced during the target irradiation and converted to a synthetic precursor, either in the target or immediately after exiting the target. The precursor is next converted into the molecule of interest. This chapter covers only the targetry and the formation in the target of the chemical compound. The formation of precursors outside the target and the conversion of these precursors to the desired radiotracer are covered in other chapters (see Chapter 2). Most of the targets for the production of the biologic radionuclides have been either gases or liquids, although several solid targets have been developed.

The number and type of products, which are obtained in a target, are a function of the irradiation conditions, the mixture of gases or liquids in the target, and the presence of any impurities in the target or gas mixture. Changing the chemical composition or physical state of the target during irradiation (14) can alter the chemical form of the final product. These are all results of the "hot atom" chemistry and radiolysis occurring in the target during the irradiation. "Hot atom" is the term used to identify atoms with excessive thermal or kinetic energy, or electronic excitation. When an atom undergoes a nuclear transformation, it usually has a great deal of excess energy imparted from the incident bombarding particle and perhaps from the nuclear reaction. This energy can be manifested in any or all of the normal modes of excitation including rotational, translational, or electronic. In nearly all cases, the amount of energy present is sufficient to break all the existing chemical bonds to the atom and to send the newly transformed atom off with high kinetic energy. This energy is called the recoil energy, and as the atom slows down, it imparts this energy to the surrounding environment. After the atom has transferred most of its excess energy to the surroundings and slowed to near thermal energies, it usually reacts chemically with the surroundings to form a compound. This compound may be stabilized or may undergo further reactions to form other chemical products.

Several distinguishing characteristics set these types of reactions apart from other chemical reactions. These are as follows: (a) The reactions are insensitive to the temperature of the surroundings, (b) they are independent of the phase of the reaction, (c) they are dependent on the radical scavengers present in the medium, and (d) they are dependent on moderators in the medium such as inert gases (15). There have

been several excellent reviews concerning the topic of hot atom chemistry (16–18).

Specific Activity

Another topic of importance in the preparation of radioisotopes is that of specific activity. It is important in several applications and particularly important in PET where the radionuclide is incorporated into a radiotracer that is used to probe some physiologic process in which very small amounts of the biomolecule are being used. PET is basically a tracer method and the goal of the PET experiment is to probe the physiologic process without perturbing that process. If the amount of radiotracer is very small in comparison to the amount of the native compound or its competitor, then the process will be perturbed very little. When carrying out studies such as probing the number of receptors or probing the concentration of an enzyme, these considerations become even more important (19).

The usual way to express the concept of specific activity is in terms of the amount of radioactivity per mole of compound. There is, of course, an ultimate limit, which occurs only when the radioactive atoms or radiolabeled molecules exist. Table 1.1 lists the characteristics of the PET radionuclides presented in this chapter (20).

As an example, typical specific activities for ^{11}C-labeled molecules being reported are on the order of 10 Ci/μmol (370 GBq/μmol). Therefore, it can be appreciated that only 1 in 1,000 of the radiotracer molecules is actually labeled with ^{11}C. The rest contain stable ^{12}C. The specific activity is important in probing areas such as receptor binding, enzyme reaction, gene expression, and in some settings antigen binding with radiolabeled monoclonal antibodies.

In the area of monoclonal antibody labeling, there is the problem of the incorporation of the label into the molecule. If there is excessive carrier, then a smaller amount of the radiolabel will be incorporated into the molecule. This means that a diagnostic radioisotope may be more difficult to visualize or the dose of a therapeutic radioisotope to the target organ may be less than could be achieved. The specific activity of other PET tracers has been explored extensively. Some recent issues are the specific activity of radiotracers produced from the stable species (21), bromine-76 (^{76}Br) (22), and ^{13}N-labeled ammonia (23).

The radionuclide on which more effort has been expended in attempts to control specific activity is ^{11}C, and we will use it as an example of the things that may be done to maximize the specific activity. Carbon-11 is a challenging radioisotope for achieving high specific activity because carbon is so ubiquitous in the environment. There can never be a truly carrier-free radiotracer labeled with ^{11}C, but only one in which no carrier carbon has been added and steps have been taken to minimize the amount of carbon that can enter the synthesis from outside sources. There can never be less carbon incorporated into the molecule than there is carbon

TABLE 1.1. *Decay characteristics for specific PET radionuclides*

Nuclide	Half-life (min)	Decay mode	Maximum energy	Mean energy	Maximum range in water	Maximum specific activity (theoretical)
Carbon-11	20.4	100% β^+	0.96 MeV	0.386 MeV	4.1 mm	9,220 Ci/μmol
Nitrogen-13	9.98	100% β^+	1.19 MeV	0.492 MeV	5.4 mm	18,900 Ci/μmol
Oxygen-15	2.03	100% β^+	1.7 MeV	0.735 MeV	8.0 mm	91,730 Ci/μmol
Fluorine-18	109.8	97% β^+	0.69 MeV	0.250 MeV	2.4 mm	1,710 Ci/μmol
Copper-62	9.74	99.7% β^+	2.93 MeV	1.314 MeV	14.3 mm	19,310 Ci/μmol
Gallium-68	68.0	89% β^+	1.9 MeV	0.829 MeV	9.0 mm	2,766 Ci/μmol
Bromide-75	96.0	75.5% β^+	1.74 MeV	0.750 MeV	8.2 mm	1,960 Ci/μmol
Rubidium-82	1.25	95.5% β^+	3.36 MeV	1.5 MeV	16.5 mm	150,400 Ci/μmol
Iodine-122	3.62	75.8% β^+	3.12 MeV	1.4 MeV	15.3 mm	51,950 Ci/μmol
Iodine-124	6019.2	23.3% β^+	2.13 MeV	0.8 MeV	10.2 mm	31 Ci/μmol

present in the target during the irradiation to produce ^{11}C. It is critical to use the highest possible purity of nitrogen gas in the target and to ensure that the target is absolutely as gas tight as possible.

The walls of the target can also influence the specific activity, because many alloys used to fabricate targets contain traces of carbon from the manufacturing process. During irradiation, these traces of carbon can make their way out of the target walls and into the gas phase where they will be incorporated into the final product. A correlation between the target surface area and the mass of carbon introduced into the synthesis has been observed and documented (24, 25). Solvents used to clean the metal surfaces or oils left over from the fabrication process can also serve as sources for carbon in the targets. The input and output lines can also have the same or similar contaminants, and such equipment as valves, connectors, insulators, regulators, and flow controllers all can contribute to the carrier carbon and care must be taken to minimize the carbon added from these sources.

All the chemical reagents used in the synthesis may also add carrier carbon and must be scrutinized to minimize this contribution.

Fluorine-18

Fluorine-18 has a 109.8-minute half-life and decays 97% by positron emission. The other 3% is by electron capture. It forms very strong covalent bonds with carbon compounds and can be incorporated into a wide variety of organic molecules. It can be substituted for a hydroxy group, as in the case of deoxyglucose or can be substituted for a hydrogen atom. The van der Waals radius of the fluorine atom is similar to that of the hydrogen atom; therefore, substitution of fluorine for hydrogen causes very little steric alteration of the molecule. The concern with the fluorine for hydrogen substitution is that the electronegative nature of fluorine can alter the electron distribution in a way that will alter the binding properties of a molecule. In some ways, however, fluorine is the most attractive of the four positron emitters commonly used in organic synthesis. The low energy of the positron gives the highest potential resolution for PET

imaging. The range of the positrons with average energy in water is much less than 2 mm. The nearly 2-hour half-life allows for a more complex synthesis to be carried out within the decay time of the radioisotope. The electronic perturbation has also sometimes resulted in a molecule that has more physiologically desirable properties than the original compound.

The most widely used radiotracer in PET by far is 2-[^{18}F]fluoro-2-deoxyglucose (^{18}FDG). It has proven to be of great utility in the measurement of the rate of metabolism in a wide variety of organs and disease states in humans.

Production Reactions for Fluorine-18

There are a number of nuclear reactions that can be used to produce ^{18}F. The major routes are the ^{18}O(p,n)^{18}F reaction (26) usually carried out on oxygen-18 (^{18}O)–enriched water or oxygen gas, and the ^{20}Ne(d,α)^{18}F reaction (27). A number of other reactions are being used, but these two are the principal routes to ^{18}F.

The cross sections for these reactions have been explored extensively and the values are well characterized. The most common reaction in routine applications is the proton reaction on enriched ^{18}O. The yield is significantly higher than the other reactions and the availability of low-energy proton accelerators has made this the reaction of choice even in the face of the cost of the enriched ^{18}O target material. The other common reaction, particularly for the production of electrophilic fluorine, is the ^{20}Ne(d,α)^{18}F reaction on natural neon. The yield from this reaction is substantially less, but the ability to add other chemical constituents and the natural abundance of the target material are advantages (28–30).

Targetry for Fluorine-18

The number and types of targets that have been designed and fabricated for the production of ^{18}F are very large. There have been several reviews of the types of targets (28,29,31, 32). For descriptive purposes, the targets can be divided into three basic categories. The first is the gas target primarily used for the production of electrophilic fluorine. The second is the liquid target, usually used for production of ^{18}F-fluoride and the third are the solid targets, which are not commonly used for the production of ^{18}F.

For gaseous targets, there are two basic considerations. The first is the neon gas target. This target was used for many years for the production of F_2^{18}F from the ^{20}Ne(d,α)^{18}F reaction (27,28). In this target, a small amount of fluorine gas, typically 0.1% to 0.2%, is added to the neon gas before irradiation. The design of the target has undergone significant changes from the first targets to the current design. Early targets were made of nickel or nickel alloys. The reason for this choice was that it was known that nickel parts would withstand a fluorine atmosphere and most fluorine handling systems were made from nickel or alloys such as Inconel or Monel, which have a high nickel content. It was later shown that any surface that could be passivated by fluorine could be used in the fluorine target (33). This discovery opened up the possibility of using aluminum target bodies for the production of elemental fluorine. The activation properties of aluminum are vastly superior to those of nickel or steel in terms of avoidance of the long-lived activities, which are produced within the target body during the bombardment. Target bodies constructed of aluminum significantly reduce the radiation dose received by the technical staff during the cleaning and maintenance of the target. A more extensive investigation of the properties of the surface has been made (30,34). It was shown that aluminum, copper, and nickel form fluoride layers and therefore passivate. The metal surfaces may also contain oxide layers. Only gold does not form a fluoride layer. Exposure to air after passivation does not alter the surface layer (33,34).

The direct addition of fluorine to the neon before irradiation was one method for the recovery of the fluorine in elemental form. The other method was developed by Nickles et al. (35) and is called the ''two shoot'' method. In this method, the fluorine is allowed to stick to the walls of the target during the irradiations and is then removed by creating a plasma containing elemental fluorine, which reacts with the ^{18}F on the walls and brings it into the gas phase. The usual gas for this target is the ^{18}O-enriched O_2 gas. Other methods for converting the ^{18}F in other chemical forms such as HF to F_2 outside the target have also been attempted, but with limited success (36,37). In this latter case, the neon or ^{18}O-enriched oxygen gas is irradiated and the fluorine allowed to stick to the walls. In some cases, hydrogen is added to the target gas during irradiation. After irradiation, the target gas is removed, and then the target is heated and flushed with hydrogen to bring the fluorine out in the form of HF (3). The production of other fluorinating intermediates has also been described by using in-target chemistry, but these are not currently in widespread use (38).

A high-energy reaction of protons on neon can also be used in the same way as the deuterons on neon (39,40). The fluorine can be brought out of the target in the form of fluoride ion if the target is washed after irradiation with an aqueous solution (29,31), or the glass liner of the target can be used directly as the reaction vessel (35). In all cases, the fluorine is recovered from the surface in relatively high yields (more than 70%). Whether the protons on ^{18}O or neon, or the deuterons on neon reaction is used, the result and methodology are essentially the same.

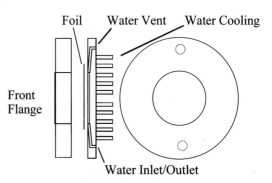

FIG. 1.4. Typical water target for the production of fluorine-18 from oxygen-18–enriched water.

By far the most commonly used target compound for the production of ^{18}F in the form of fluoride ion is the H_2^{18}O target. The basic design is relatively straightforward and similar to most of the targets being used routinely. There are wide variations, however, in the details of the design and the construction materials (41–53). The primary constraint is to use as little of the H_2^{18}O as possible while leaving enough volume to take maximum advantage of the cross section and to absorb or transfer the heat created by the passage of the beam. A typical target is shown in Fig. 1.4.

There are several considerations in the operation of the target. The first is the fact that the water would boil due to high temperatures generated by irradiation unless the pressure in the target is increased to diminish or inhibit the boiling (54–56). To reduce this problem, the target may be run under elevated pressure of helium, nitrogen, or some other inert gas, or the target may be valved off and allowed to find its own pressure level. In this case, pressure can exceed 40 atm, particularly if the water has not been completely degassed before use. Because a relatively thin foil contains the pressure, there is a limit to the beam current that can be applied in this situation.

The decision to operate at low or high pressure will also have an impact on the target fabrication and the materials chosen for the target. The radiolysis products of the water will have different effects depending on the conditions inside the target. The materials used to construct the target can also have an effect on the chemical reactivity of the fluoride obtained from the target (57–59). If the target is operated at low pressure, there will be some loss of the water out of the beam strike area due to bubble formation (45,54).

There have been some unique target designs for the water target using spherical targets (60) or flowing targets (46) or frozen ^{18}O-enriched carbon dioxide targets (61). The helium-3 or alpha reaction on natural water has also been used to produce ^{18}F for synthesis (8,62,63). These targets work exactly the same way as the proton on water targets, except that the level of heat deposition is higher with the heavier particles. These targets are not commonly used because the yields are substantially lower.

Radioisotope Separation for Fluorine-18

There are two separate scenarios for recovery of ^{18}F from the target, which depend on the mode of production. In the case of the gas target, the fluorine (with the carrier F_2) is removed from the target as a gas mixture and can be used in the synthesis from there. In the case of the water target, the activity is removed in the aqueous phase. There are two general methods after that. The first is to use the $H_2^{18}O$-containing ^{18}F-fluoride ion directly in the synthesis. This method is used by several investigators who have small-volume water targets and the cost of losing the $H_2^{18}O$ is minor compared with the cost of the cyclotron irradiation. The other method is to separate the fluoride from the $H_2^{18}O$, either by distillation or by using a resin column (64–66). When the resin is used, it also separates the metal ion impurities from the enriched fluoride solution. This resin purification generally increases the reactivity of the fluoride.

Carbon-11

Carbon-11 has a 20.4-minute half-life and decays 99.8% by positron emission and only 0.2% by electron capture. It decays to stable boron-11. Carbon-11 offers the greatest potential for the synthesis of radiotracers that track specific processes in the body. The short half-life of ^{11}C limits processes that can be adequately studied. The chemical form of ^{11}C can vary depending on the environment during irradiation. The usual chemical forms of ^{11}C obtained directly from the target are carbon dioxide and methane.

Production Reactions for Carbon-11

There are several reactions used to produce ^{11}C. By far the most common reaction is the $^{14}N(p,\alpha)^{11}C$ reaction on nitrogen gas (67,68). This reaction produces a high yield of ^{11}C, and with the addition of trace amounts of oxygen, ^{11}C is almost exclusively in the chemical form of carbon dioxide.

Targetry for Carbon-11

Carbon-11 targets can be either gases or solids. The basic design of the gas target has not changed a great deal since the first targets were developed (69,70). The basic body design is an aluminum cylinder, which can be held at a high enough pressure to stop the beam or at least degrade the

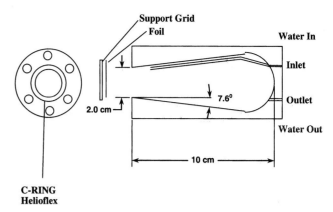

FIG. 1.5. Typical gas target for the production of radioisotopes from gaseous targets.

energy below the threshold of the reaction being used. A typical gas target is shown in Fig. 1.5.

The choice of aluminum for the target body is a result of its excellent activation properties. The activation products are produced in relatively small amounts or have a short half-life. This aids in the maintenance of the target because the radiation dose to the chemist handling the target is greatly reduced. The usual labeled products from the gas target are carbon dioxide (18,69,71,72) and methane, but other products have been attempted (71–73).

Some recent advances in the design of gaseous targets for the production of ^{11}C are the realization (a) that carrier carbon was being added by the surface of the aluminum (24), (b) that the target was more efficient if it was conical, taking into consideration the fact that the beam was undergoing multiple scattering through the foil window and in the gas (74,75), and (c) that the density of the gas was significantly reduced at high beam currents (76–78).

The foil material used on these targets is also important for several reasons. If the beam energy is high enough, a relatively thick aluminum foil may be used to contain the gas. If the beam energy is lower, then a thinner foil must be used and aluminum does not have sufficient tensile strength to withstand the pressures that are built up inside the target during irradiation. In this case, a thin foil of Havar or other high tensile strength material can be used to withstand the pressures. It is also possible to place grids across the foils to increase the burst pressure of the foils (79,80).

Some solid targets have been used for the production of ^{11}C. These are, for the most part, boron oxide either enriched or natural abundance. A typical target for this would be a stepped plate similar to the inclined plane target used for various isotopes. The difference is that here the powder is pressed into the groves of the target plate and irradiated (70). The difficulty of removing the carbon from the matrix in comparison to the ease of separation in the gas target has made the solid target less widely used.

Radioisotope Separation for Carbon-11

The separation of ^{11}C in the gas target is a simple matter, because the ^{11}C is usually in the form of carbon dioxide when it comes out of the target. The nitrogen gas used as the target material is usually inert in chemical reactions, so the target gas can be passed through a solution for reaction. The carbon dioxide can also be removed by trapping, either in a cold trap or on an adsorbent substrate such as molecular sieves. From there, the ^{11}C can be used to produce a wide variety of precursors.

The separation of the carbon dioxide from the solid matrix of the boron oxide is a more difficult problem but can be accomplished under the correct conditions. The target containing the boron oxide is contained in a gas-tight box (70). A sweep gas is passed through the box during irradiation. The beam heating is sufficient to cause the boron oxide to melt and the carbon dioxide is released into the sweep gas. The labeled gas is trapped downstream and the irradiation is continued until sufficient ^{11}C has been collected for use in the synthesis. The advantage of this type of target is that once made, it can be used repeatedly without further maintenance.

Nitrogen-13

Nitrogen-13 decays by pure positron emission (100%) to stable ^{13}C. As with ^{11}C, the short half-life of 9.98 minutes somewhat restricts the potential utility of this radionuclide. Several compounds incorporating ^{13}N have been made, but the time for accumulation in the body is short and the physiologic processes that may be studied must be rapid (81,82). By far the most widely used compound of ^{13}N for PET is in the chemical form of ammonia. It is used as a blood-flow tracer and has found utility in cardiac studies to determine areas of ischemic or infarcted tissue.

Production Reactions for Nitrogen-13

Several reactions lead to the production of ^{13}N. The reactions that are commonly used are the $^{13}C(p,n)^{13}N$ reaction (83,84), the $^{12}C(d,n)^{13}N$ reaction (83) and the $^{16}O(p,\alpha)^{13}N$ reaction (85,86).

The proton on ^{13}C reaction has an advantage in that it requires a low-incident proton energy but suffers from the disadvantage of requiring isotopically enriched material. The most common reaction is the $^{16}O(p,\alpha)^{13}N$ reaction on natural water (87–90).

Targetry for Nitrogen-13

The target for the production of ^{13}N can either be solids, liquids, or gases, depending on the chemical form of the nitrogen that is desired. The chemical form can also be changed by a number of other factors such as the dose and dose rate to the target, the pH level of the liquid targets and the physical state.

The first target for the production of ^{13}N was a solid target of boron that was bombarded by an alpha beam by Joliot and Curie (91). Solid targets have been used for the production of ^{13}N, particularly in the form of either nitrogen gas or ammonia (24,92,93). Solids mixed with liquids have also been used, particularly in the production of ammonia (34,94,95). Solid targets of frozen water have also been used to produce ammonia (14).

Liquid targets are by far the most popular and widely used. The reaction of protons on natural water produces nitrate and nitrite ions, which can be converted to ammonia by reduction (82,87–89,96). The water target can also be used to form ammonia directly with the addition of a reducing agent or with a radical inhibitor (90,97–101). The chemistry involved in the production of the final product distribution in the water target has been a topic of interest and debate (14,87,102, 103). It has been found that high-dose irradiation of liquid water results in the formation of oxidized species while the same irradiation of frozen water maintains the initial distribution of reduced products (14).

Gas targets have also been used, particularly in the production of nitrogen gas, and there have also been attempts to use the gas target for the production of ammonia (17,104, 105).

Radioisotope Separation for Nitrogen-13

The separation of the ^{13}N from the solid target is usually accomplished by burning or heating the solids (93,106,107). The water target with no additives usually produces ^{13}N in the chemical form of nitrates and nitrites. The conversion of the nitrogen, nitrates, or nitrites to other chemical forms requires rapid radiopharmaceutical synthesis techniques.

Oxygen-15

Oxygen-15 is the longest lived of the positron-emitting isotopes of oxygen. The half-life is 122 seconds and it decays 99.9% by positron emission. It decays to stable nitrogen-15 (^{15}N). It was one of the first artifical radioisotopes produced with low-energy deuterons using a cyclotron (108). Oxygen-15 is used to label gases for inhalation such as oxygen, carbon dioxide, and carbon monoxide, and it is used to label water for injection. The major purpose of these gases and liquids is to measure the blood flow, blood volume, and oxygen consumption in the body.

Production Reactions for Oxygen-15

There are several reactions for the production of ^{15}O. The most common are the $^{14}N(d,n)^{15}O$ reaction (109–111), the $^{15}N(p,n)^{15}O$ reaction (112), and the $^{16}O(p,pn)^{15}O$ reaction (113). Of these reactions, the ones that are used commonly are the deuterons on natural nitrogen gas, the protons on enriched ^{15}N nitrogen gas, and the protons on natural oxygen when specific activity is not an issue, as in the case of oxygen gas or labeled water.

Targetry for Oxygen-15

The targets for these compounds are, for the most part, gaseous targets. The ^{15}O-containing compound can be made either directly in the target (114–116) or outside the target in a separate recovery module. The gas targets are usually nitrogen gas bombarded with either protons or deuterons depending on the accelerator characteristics.

Solid targets have been explored as a source for producing ^{15}O-ozone (117). In this target, irradiating quartz microfibers and allowing the nucleogenic atoms that exit the fibers to react with the surrounding gas produces the ^{15}O.

Radioisotope Separation for Oxygen-15

The radioisotopes can be separated or, in some circumstances, the target gas can be used with a minimum of processing (113,118,119). An example of this is the production of $H_2{}^{15}O$. It can be made directly in the target by adding 5% hydrogen to the nitrogen gas in the target (114). In this case, the water is produced directly. Ammonia is concurrently produced in the target as a radiolytic product of the nitrogen and hydrogen, and it must be removed. The other option is to produce ^{15}O-labeled oxygen gas in the target and then process it to water outside the target. The water has also been produced by bombarding water using the $^{16}O(p,pn)^{15}O$ reaction with a final clean up on an ion-exchange column (120).

Novel Solid Targets for PET Radiopharmaceutical Preparation

The most well known medical application of cyclotrons is the production of radionuclides for diagnostic studies applied to nuclear medicine and the nuclear sciences. Yields of most of the medically used radionuclides produced with cyclotrons using various nuclear reactions and energies have been reported (32,121–123).

The increasing amount of clinically relevant data available from PET studies involving the biologic tracers has contributed to the expanding interest in additional positron-emitting radionuclides for both basic research studies and additional clinical applications. The spectrum of physiologic processes that could potentially be studied grows as the number of "alternative" positron-emitting radionuclides that can be prepared increases (121). With the introduction of the new generation of cyclotrons that are capable of delivering hundreds of microamperes of beam current, the potential for increased amounts of numerous radionuclides can no longer be considered limited by the beam fluence, but rather by the optimal thermal performance of the particular target materi-

als and target backings. This is particularly true in the case of the cooling-water/target-backing interface and beam profile considerations for solid target stations now becoming available on some of the "baby" cyclotrons.

Iodine-124, a radionuclide that has potential for both diagnostic and therapeutic applications, is an important example. This nuclide was often viewed as an unwanted radionuclidic impurity in the production of ^{123}I from the energetic proton irradiation of tellurium targets at cyclotron facilities engaged in the commercial production of ^{123}I. Iodine-124 has a half-life of 4.18 days and decays by positron emission (23.3%) and electron capture (76.7%). Although several nuclear reactions have been suggested for its production, the precise measurement of the excitation function for the $^{124}Te(p,n)^{124}I$ reaction indicates its suitability for use on low-energy cyclotrons (124,125). A detailed preparation of this radionuclide via the $^{124}Te(p,n)^{124}I$ nuclear reaction using low-energy cyclotrons has recently been published (126). It uses a reusable target composed of windowless aluminum oxide and an enriched tellurium-124 oxide solid solution matrix. The radioiodide is effectively recovered using a dry distillation process with the volatile iodine species being trapped on a thin Pyrex glass tube coated with a minute amount of sodium hydroxide. Although recovery of the radioiodine from the tube was nearly quantitative, the recovery of the radioiodine from the target was somewhat less (65% to 75%) and appears to be a function of the crystal structure of the tellurium oxide that was irradiated (126).

Another element within the halogen family that possesses several radioisotopes of potential clinical use is bromine. In particular, bromine-75 (^{75}Br) ($t_{1/2}$ = 1.6 hours, $I_{\beta+}$ = 75.5%, $E_{\beta+}$ = 1.74 MeV) has several nuclear reactions reported for its production, but only the proton irradiation processes appear suitable for medium-energy cyclotrons (more than 25 MeV) (i.e., $^{76}Se[p,2n]^{75}Br$). The major impurity associated with the proton process is ^{76}Br. The optimal production conditions for ^{75}Br proton irradiation of enriched selenium-76 (^{76}Se) targets used an incident energy of 30 MeV degraded within the target to 22 MeV and had a reported production rate of ^{75}Br of 100 mCi/μAh with an impurity level for the ^{76}Br reported at 0.9% (127). Several selenides such as those of silver or copper have been found as suitable targets for irradiation at low beam currents (128, 129), and an external rotating target system was reported for preparation of radiobromine from the low melting elemental selenium target (130). Losses of ^{76}Se were approximately 1% after a 1-hour irradiation period at 20υA for this target system.

As in the case of radioiodine, the separation of the radiobromine from the ^{76}Se-irradiated target material was effected by thermochromographic evolution at 300°C, followed by dissolution of the bromine in a small volume of hot water. The radiochemical yield for the overall process was not exceedingly high, and this as well as the difficulties associated with targetry using highly enriched selenium nuclides may be part of the reason that the application of this procedure for the preparation of ^{75}Br is not more widely employed.

The more widely used method for the production of ^{75}Br requires the acceleration of helium-3 particles of energies, nominally 36 MeV, onto arsenic target materials (131,132). Bromine positron emitters may become more important for PET imaging over the coming years.

Generator-produced Positron-emitting Radionuclides

The molybdenum-99/technetium-99m (^{99}Mo/^{99m}Tc) generator remains the dominant source for radionuclide availability in nuclear medicine departments and is usually applied to prepared commercially available kits for radiopharmaceutical formulation. However, the impetus for change caused by the expanded application of PET radiopharmaceutical agents, including the equipment fusion of PET with computed tomography or PET with magnetic resonance imaging tomographs, will ensure the continued growth and radiopharmaceutical development of short-lived positron-emitting diagnostic and potentially therapeutic agents. Generator systems for specific PET radionuclides remain a potential resource for further development of the role of PET.

Radionuclide generator systems consist of a parent radionuclide, usually a relatively long-lived nuclide that decays to a daughter nuclide, itself radioactive but with a shorter half-life. The system requires an efficient technique to separate the daughter nuclide from the parent. Conventionally, the parent is adsorbed onto a solid support and decays by particle emission. A solvent in which the daughter complex is soluble is employed to elute (i.e., separate) the desired radionuclide. Unlike the ^{99}Mo/^{99m}Tc generator developed at Brookhaven National Laboratory (133,134), which revolutionized the practice of nuclear medicine, the generator systems currently being applied to PET studies are still primarily research sources for radiopharmaceutical development.

For those research centers and clinical facilities without the luxury of a cyclotron, several generator systems for production of positron-emitting radionuclides have been proposed. Their production routes have been reviewed (135–140). Of the systems proposed, copper-62 (^{62}Cu), gallium-68 (^{68}Ga), and rubidium-82 (^{82}Rb) radionuclides continue to find applications. The decay characteristics of these three generator systems are included in Table 1.2. A great deal of effort has been expended on the production and construction of these generator systems, including investigations into solid support materials and elution characteristics.

The production routes for the parent radionuclide zinc-62 (^{62}Zn) include the irradiation of a copper disc or copper-electroplated alloy to use the ^{63}Cu(p,2n)^{62}Zn irradiation at an optimal proton energy of 26-21 MeV (141–144). The copper is dissolved in hydrochloric acid and the solution is transferred to an anion-exchange resin column (AG 1×8, 100-200 mesh, Cl$^-$ form). Copper is effectively eluted from the resin with 3 M HCl, and ^{62}Zn is eluted effectively with water. After evaporation to dryness, the zinc is dissolved in 2 M HCl and adsorbed onto an anion-exchange column for periodic elution of the ^{62}Cu. Alternative routes to the preparation of the ^{62}Zn via irradiation of enriched nickel targets or zinc targets have been proposed but have found only limited application (145–147).

Gallium-68 is used to assess blood–brain barrier integrity, as well as tumor localization. It is widely used as a source for the attenuation correction of most PET scanners. The parent germanium-68 is long-lived ($t_{1/2} = 271$ days) and its production is generally not attempted on medium-energy accelerators due to the low production yields (148,149). The primary sources for the parent radionuclide are the spallation processes available at large energy accelerators where parasitic position and operation are available (150,151). The recovery of the germanium-68 involves several multistep chemical processes.

The earlier generator systems provided the gallium product in a complexed form as a result of either using solvent/solvent extraction techniques or chromatographic supports of alumina or antimony oxide. Refinements made to elute the ^{68}Ga in an ionic form were compromised by solubility problems of the oxide in the eluant and therefore slowed the potential for direct clinical use. Many of the limitations of previous chromatographic systems were overcome with the report of a tin oxide/HCl generator (152). The negative pressure generator consisted of tin oxide (0.16 to 0.25 mm in diameter) contained in a glass column (10 mm in diameter) between glass wool plugs atop a sintered glass base. One normal HCl, with flow rate controlled by a valve at the base of the column, serves as eluant. Results indicate a radiochemical yield approaching 80% in roughly 2 minutes using 5 mL of eluant. The generator performance remains high in spite of accumulated dose delivered to the solid support.

There are two types of chromatographic nuclide generator

TABLE 1.2. *Examples of generators yielding positron-emitting daughter radionuclides of clinical interest*

Parent (half-life)	Decay mode (%)	Daughter (half-life)	Decay mode (%)	Characteristic gamma energy (%)
Strontium-82 (25 d)	EC (100)	Rubidium-82 (76 sec)	β$^+$(96), EC (4)	0.78 MeV (9)
Germanium-68(278 d)	EC (100)	Gallium-68 (68 min)	β$^+$(88), EC (12)	1.078 (3.5)
Zinc-62 (9.13 hr)	β$^+$ (18), EC (82)	Copper-62 (9.8 min)	β$^+$(98)	1.17 (0.5)
Xenon-122 (20.1 hr)	EC (100)	Iodine-122 (3.6 min)	β$^+$(77), EC (23)	0.56 (18.4)

systems: positive or negative pressure. As is customary in all systems, the parent is adsorbed onto a column support, commonly an organic exchanger or mineral exchanger, which is contained within a borosilicate glass cylinder. The ends of the cylinder are terminated with a filter to ensure that a minimum of particulate materials are eluted from the column and that terminal sterilization by filtration will be possible if the radionuclide is to be used without further modification.

As the half-lives of the daughter nuclides become shorter, the opportunity for chemical manipulation before clinical administration is reduced to such an extent that the eluant must be physiologically acceptable, and quality assurance for parent breakthrough or exchanger breakdown becomes increasingly important. The column is housed within a lead or tungsten shield for radiation protection of the personnel using the system. For efficient elution, attempts are made to minimize both the number of fittings and joints involved in preparing the system and the internal diameter and overall length of the cylindrical tubing.

Rubidium-82 is a myocardial blood-flow agent and has found clinical application. The application of ^{82}Rb-chloride in the diagnosis of ischemic heart disease and location of myocardial infarcts is an active area of application for this generator system (153). The short half-life (1.27 minutes) of ^{82}Rb and its similarity to potassium in biologic transport and distribution suggest that this generator-produced radionuclide might find a clinical role in thrombolytic therapy monitoring. The myocardial uptake of ^{82}Rb is flow limited, being linear up to 2.5 times normal flow rates, giving rise to underestimation and overestimation of values (154,155). The production methods for the preparation of the parent radionuclide strontium-82 have been studied quite extensively (156–159). For this nuclide also, the spallation of molybdenum with high-energy protons is the production route of choice (151,160).

The most commonly used generator system is the strontium/rubidium system for the production of ^{82}Rb. It consists of an alumina column and uses 2% saline as eluent to achieve 85% to 95% elution efficiency. The generator system has a life span of approximately 3 to 4 months and requires periodic quality assurance for sterility, apyrogenicity, and measurement of breakthrough concentrations. The generator is a positive pressure system with operating pressures of 50 to 100 psi, and it can function in both the bolus mode and the constant infusion mode. In the latter case, the activity yield is a function of the flow rate (161).

Radionuclide Generator Equations

A synopsis of the equations to allow the calculation of the maximal concentrations of daughter nuclide from a particular generator or the determination of the appropriate time to elute a generator is given through the following expressions (136).

Considering a simple radionuclide generator system of parent daughter in which the half-life of the parent is longer than that of the daughter, the pair will eventually enter a state of transient equilibrium. This can be represented schematically as

$$A \rightarrow B \rightarrow C$$

where A is the parent radionuclide, which decays to the radioactive daughter B, which in turn decays to the daughter nuclide C.

The ratio of decay of each radionuclide is described by the following equation:

$$\frac{dN}{dt} = \lambda N \qquad \text{or} \qquad N = N_0 e^{-\lambda t}$$

where N is the number of radioactive atoms at a specific time t and λ is the decay constant for the radionuclide and is equivalent to $(\ln(2)/t_{1/2})$.

Considering a generator system, the parent is generally adsorbed onto a solid support and serves as the sole source for the daughter radionuclide production. However, the number of daughter atoms present at any time t is described in a slightly more involved expression:

$$\frac{dN_B}{dt} = \lambda_A N_A - \lambda_B N_B$$

Because the daughter is decaying as well as being produced, the net rate of change on N_B with time is indicated by the decay of A to B minus the decay of B to C. Substitution of the integral of the expression for A yields the net rate of change for B as follows:

$$\frac{dN_B}{dt} = \lambda_A N_A^0 e^{-\lambda_A t} - \lambda_B N_B$$

Integrating this equation to calculate the number of atoms of B at time t gives the following expression:

$$N_B = \left(\frac{\lambda_A}{(\lambda_B - \lambda_A)}\right) N_A^0 (e^{-\lambda_A t} - e^{-\lambda_B t}) + N_B^0 e^{-\lambda_B t}$$

The first term on the right side of the equation represents the growth of the daughter nuclide B from the parent A decay and the loss of B through decay. The second term represents the decay of B atoms, but because the parent A is generally considered a pure parent radionuclide at the time the generator is manufactured, this term is zero. The equation can be rewritten in terms of activities and results as follows:

$$A_B = \left(\frac{\lambda_A}{(\lambda_B - \lambda_A)}\right) A_A^0 (e^{-\lambda_A t} - e^{-\lambda_B t})$$

There are two general conditions for parent–daughter pairs; transient equilibrium in which the parent half-life is greater than the daughter half-life, or secular equilibrium in which the parent half-life is much greater than the daughter half-life. Naturally if the decay should involve branching ratios, the equation above must be appropriately modified.

Further, in the case of the PET generators, it is often useful to calculate the time when the daughter activity is at the maximum value t_{max}. Differentiation of the equation with respect to time gives the following result:

$$t_{max} = \ln\left(\frac{\left(\frac{\lambda_A}{\lambda_B}\right)}{(\lambda_B - \lambda_A)}\right)$$

The role of generators for the future of clinical PET remains uncertain. The initial supposition that generators have potential for PET imaging at sites without a cyclotron or accelerator is being reevaluated due to the costs associated with the procurement and scheduled availability of the parent radionuclide. Further, any supplementary equipment, such as that of the infusion system required for the strontium/rubidium generator, may result in low demand or choice of alternative radionuclides (140). Nevertheless, the strontium/rubidium generator is in routine clinical use in various medical centers in the United States and elsewhere.

SUMMARY

During recent years, research efforts in nuclear medicine have concentrated on the decay characteristics of particular radionuclides and the design of unique radiolabeled tracers necessary to achieve time-dependent molecular images. The specialty is expanding with specific PET and single photon emission computed tomography radiopharmaceuticals, allowing for an extension from functional process imaging in tissue to pathologic processes and radionuclide-directed treatments. PET is an example of a technique that has been shown to yield the physiologic information necessary for multiple diagnoses including those in cancer based on altered tissue metabolism.

Most PET drugs are currently produced using a cyclotron at locations that are in close proximity to the hospital or academic center at which the radiopharmaceutical will be administered. In November 1997, a law was enacted in the United States called the Food and Drug Administration Modernization Act of 1997. It directed the FDA to establish appropriate procedures for the approval of PET drugs in accordance with section 505 of the Federal Food, Drug, and Cosmetic Act and to establish current good manufacturing practice requirements for such drugs. At this time, the FDA is considering adopting special approval procedures and cyclic guanosine monophosphate requirements for PET drugs. The evolution of PET radiopharmaceuticals has introduced a new class of ''drugs'' requiring production facilities and product formulations that must be closely aligned with the scheduled clinical utilization. The production of the radionuclide in the appropriate synthetic form is one of the critical components in the manufacturing of the finished positron-emitting radiopharmaceutical.

ACKNOWLEDGMENTS

This research was supported in part by grants at Memorial Sloan-Kettering Cancer Center from the U.S. Department of Energy (DE-F02-86-E60407) and the Cancer Center Support Grant (NCI-P30-CA08748) and at Brookhaven National Laboratory under contract DE-AC02-98CH10886 with the U.S. Department of Energy and its Office of Biological and Environmental Research, and by the National Institutes of Health (National Institutes of Neurological Diseases and Stroke grant no. NS-15380).

REFERENCES

1. Dotzel MM. PET drug products; safety and effectiveness of certain PET drugs for specific indications. *Federal Register* 2000;65: 12999–13010.
2. Crouzel C, Clark JC, Brihaye C, et al. Radiochemistry automation for PET. In: Stocklin G, Pike VW, eds. *Radiopharmaceuticals for positron emission tomography.* Dordrecht: Kluwer Academic Publishers, 1993:45–90.
3. Satyamurthy N, Phelps ME, Barrio JR. Electronic generators for the production of positron-emitter labeled radiopharmaceuticals: where would PET be without them? *Clin Positron Imaging* 1999;2:233–253.
4. Deconninick G. *Introduction to radioanalytical physics, nuclear methods monographs,* no 1. Amsterdam: Elsevier Scientific Publishing, 1978.
5. Guillaume M, Lambrecht RM, Wolf AP. Cyclotron production of ^{123}Xe and high purity ^{123}I: a comparison of tellurium targets. *Int J Appl Radiat Isot* 1975;26:703–707.
6. Lambrecht RM, Wolf AP. Cyclotron and short-lived halogen isotopes for radiopharmaceutical applications. In: *New developments in radiopharmaceuticals and labelled compounds,* vol 1. Vienna: IAEA, 1973: 275–290.
7. Clem RG, Lambrecht RM. Enriched ^{124}Te targets for production of ^{123}I and ^{124}I. *Nucl Instruments Methods* 1991;d03:115–118.
8. Qaim SM, Stocklin G. Production of some medically important short-lived neutron deficient radioisotopes of halogens. *Radiochimica Acta* 1983;34:25–40.
9. Newman E. Sources of separated isotopes for nuclear targetry. In: Jaklovsky J, ed. *Preparation of nuclear targets for particle accelerators.* New York: Plenum Publishing, 1981:229–234.
10. Meese CO, Eichelbaum M, Ebner T, et al. ^{13}C and ^{2}H NMR as exvivo probe for monitoring human drug metabolism. In: Buncel E, Kabalka GW, eds. *Synthesis and applications of isotopically labelled compounds 1991.* Amsterdam: Elsevier Science, 1992:291–296.
11. Browne TR, Szalio GK. Stable isotope tracer studies of pharmacokinetic drug interaction. In: Buncel E, Kabalka GW, eds. *Synthesis and applications of isotopically labelled compounds 1991.* Amsterdam: Elsevier, 1992:397–402.
12. Finn RD, Johnson R. The radionuclide: an endangered resource? In: Buncel E, Kabalka GW, eds. *Synthesis and applications of isotopically labelled compounds 1991.* Amsterdam: Elsevier Science, 1992: 291–296.
13. Finn RD. The search for consistency in the manufacture of PET radiopharmaceuticals. *Ann Nucl Med* 1999;13:379–382.
14. Firouzbakht ML, Schlyer DJ, Ferrieri RA, et al. Mechanisms involved in the production of nitrogen-13 labeled ammonia in a cryogenic target. *Nucl Med Biol* 1999;26:437–441.
15. Helus F, Colombetti, eds. *Radionuclide production.* Boca Raton, FL: CRC Press, 1983.
16. Wolf AP. The reactions of energetic tritium and carbon atoms with organic compounds. In: Gold V, ed. *Advances in physical organic chemistry,* vol 2. New York: Academic Press, 1964:201–277.
17. Welch MJ, Wolf AP. Reaction intermediates in the chemistry of recoil carbon atoms. *Chem Commun* 1968;3:117–118.
18. Ferrieri RA, Wolf AP. The chemistry of positron emitting nucleogenic (hot) atoms with regard to preparation of labelled compounds of practical utility. *Radiochimica Acta* 1983;34:69–83.
19. Dannals RF, Ravert HT, Wilson AA, et al. Special problems associated with the synthesis of high specific activity carbon-11 labeled radiotracers. In: Emran A, ed. *New trends in radiopharmaceutical synthesis, quality assurance, and regulatory control.* New York: Plenum Publishing, 1991.
20. Fowler JS, Wolf AP. *The synthesis of carbon-11, fluorine-18, and*

nitrogen-13 labeled radiotracers for biomedical applications. US Department of Energy; 1982. Washington DC: Nuclear Science Series National Technical Information Services NAS-NS-3201.

21. Link JM, Krohn KA, Weitkamp WG. In-target chemistry during the production of ^{15}O and ^{11}C using ^{3}He reactions. *Radiochimica Acta* 2000;88(03/04):193.

22. Forngren BH, Yngve U, Forngren T, et al. Determination of specific radioactivity for ^{76}Br-labeled compounds measuring the ratio between ^{76}Br and ^{79}Br using packed capillary liquid chromatography mass spectrometry. *Nucl Med Biol* 2000;27(8):851–853.

23. Suzuki K, Haradahira T, Sasaki M. Effect of dissolved gas on the specific activity of N-13 labeled ions generated in water by the ^{16}O(p,α)^{13}N reaction. *Radiochimica Acta* 2000;88(03/04):217.

24. Ferrieri RA, Alexoff DA, Schlyer DJ, et al. *Target design considerations for high specific activity [^{11}C]CO$_2$: proceedings of the Fifth Workshop on Targetry and Target Chemistry, September 19–23, 1993, Upton, NY.* 1993:140–149.

25. Suzuki K, Yamazaki I, Sasaki M, et al. Specific activity of [^{11}C]CO$_2$ generated in a N$_2$ gas target: effect of irradiation dose, irradiation history, oxygen content and beam energy. *Radiochimica Acta* 2000; 88(03/04):211.

26. Ruth TJ, Wolf AP. Absolute cross-section for the production of ^{18}F via the ^{18}O(p,n)^{18}F reaction. *Radiochimica Acta* 1979;26:21–24.

27. Casella V, Ido T, Wolf AP, et al. Anhydrous F-18 labeled elemental fluorine for radiopharmaceutical preparation. *J Nucl Med* 1980;21: 750–757.

28. Guillaume M, Luxen A, Nebeling B, et al. Recommendations for fluorine-18 production. *Appl Radiat Isot* 1991;42:749–762.

29. Helus F, Maier-Borst W, Sahm U, et al. F-18 Cyclotron production methods. *Radiochem Radioanalytical Lett* 1979;38:395–410.

30. Helus F, Uhlir V, Wolber G, et al. Contribution to cyclotron targetry, II: testing of target construction materials for ^{18}F production via ^{20}Ne(d,α)^{18}F, recovery of ^{18}F from various metal surfaces. *J Radioanalytical Nucl Chem* 1994;182:445–450.

31. Blessing G, Coenen HH, Franken K, et al. Production of [^{18}F]F$_2$, H^{18}F and ^{18}F$^{-}_{aq}$ using the ^{20}Ne(d,α)^{18}F process. *Appl Radiat Isot* 1986; 37:1135–1139.

32. Qaim SM. Target development for medical radioisotope production at a cyclotron. *Nucl Instruments Methods Phys Res* 1989;ƒ82:289–295.

33. Bishop A, Satyamurthy N, Bida GT, et al. Metals suitable for fluorine gas target bodies—first use of aluminum for the production of [^{18}F]F$_2$. *Nucl Med Biol* 1996;23:181–185.

34. Alvord CW, Cristy S, Meyer H, et al. *Surface-sensitive analysis of materials used in [F-18]electrophilic fluorine production, II: effects of post-passivation exposure: proceedings of the Seventh Workshop on Targetry and Target Chemistry, June 8–11, 1997, Heidelberg, Germany.* 1997:92–98.

35. Nickles RJ, Hichwa RD, Daube ME, et al. An ^{18}O-target for the high yield production of ^{18}F-fluoride. *Int J Appl Radiat Isot* 1983;34: 625–629.

36. Straatmann MG, Schlyer DJ, Chasko J. *Conversion of HF to F$_2$ from an O-18 O$_2$ Gas target: proceedings of the 4th International Symposium on Radiopharmaceutical Chemistry, 1982, Julich, West Germany.* 1982:103.

37. Clark JC, Oberdorfer F. Thermal characteristics of the release of fluorine-18 from an Inconel 600 gas target. *J Labelled Compounds Radiopharm* 1982;29:1337–1339.

38. Lambrecht RM, Neirinckx R, Wolf AP. Cyclotron isotopes and radiopharmaceuticals, XXIII: novel anhydrous ^{18}F-fluorinating intermediates. *Int J Radiat Isot* 1978;29:175–183.

39. Lagunas-Solar MC, Carvacho OF. Cyclotron production of PET radionuclides: no-carrier-added fluorine-18 with high energy protons on natural neon gas targets. *Appl Radiat Isot* 1995;46:833–838.

40. Ruth TJ. The production of ^{18}F-F$_2$ and ^{15}O-O$_2$ sequentially from the same target chamber. *Appl Radiat Isot* 1985;36:107–110.

41. Wieland BW, Wolf AP. Large scale production and recovery of aqueous [F-18]fluoride using proton bombardment of a small volume [O-18]water target. *J Nucl Med* 1983:122.

42. Kilbourn MJ, Hood JT, Welch MJ. A simple ^{18}O water target for ^{18}F production. *Int J Radiat Isot* 1985;36:327–328.

43. Kilbourn MJ, Jerabek PA, Welch MJ. An improved ^{18}O water target for ^{18}F production. *Int J Radiat Isot* 1985;35:599–602.

44. Keinonen J, Fontell A, Kairento A-L. Effective small volume water

45. Berridge MS, Tewson TJ. Effects of target design on the production and utilization of [F-18]-fluoride from [O-18]-water. *J Labelled Compounds Radiopharm* 1986;23:1177–1178.

46. Iwata R, Ido T, Brady F, et al. [^{18}F]Fluoride production with a circulating [^{18}O]water target. *Appl Radiat Isot* 1987;38:979–984.

47. Mulholland GK, Hichwa RD, Kilbourn MR, et al. A reliable pressurized water target for F-18 production at high beam currents. *J Labelled Compounds Radiopharm* 1989;26:192–193.

48. Huszar I, Weinreich R. Production of ^{18}F with an ^{18}O-enriched water target. *J Radioanalytical Nucl Chem* 1985;93:349–354.

49. Vogt M, Huzar I, Argentini M, et al. Improved production of [^{18}F]fluoride via the [^{18}O]H$_2$O(p,n)^{18}F reaction for no-carrier-added nucleophilic synthesis. *Appl Radiat Isot* 1986;37:448–449.

50. O'Neil JP, Hanarahan SM, VanBrocklin HF. *Experience with a high pressure silver water target system for [^{18}F]fluoride production using the CTI RDS-111 cyclotron: proceedings of the Seventh Workshop on Targetry and Target Chemistry, June 8–11, 1997, Heidelberg, Germany.* 1997:232.

51. Gonzales-Lepera CE. *Routine production of [^{18}F]fluoride with a high pressure disposable [^{18}O]water target: proceedings of the Seventh Workshop on Targetry and Target Chemistry, June 8–11, 1997, Heidelberg, Germany.* 1997:234.

52. Steel CJ, Dowsett K, Pike VW, et al. *Ten years experience with a heavily used target for the production of [^{18}F]fluoride by proton bombardment of [^{18}O]water: proceedings of the Seventh Workshop on Targetry and Target Chemistry, June 8–11, 1997, Heidelberg, Germany.* 1997:55.

53. Roberts AD, Daniel LC, Nickles RJ. A high power target for the production of [^{18}F]fluoride. *Nucl Instruments Methods* 1995ω9: 797–799.

54. Heselius S-J, Schlyer DJ, Wolf AP. A diagnostic study of proton-beam irradiated water targets. *Int J Appl Radiat Isot* 1989;40[pt A]: 663–669.

55. Pavan RA, Johnson RR, Cackette M. *A simple heat transfer model of a closed, small-volume, [^{18}O]water target: proceedings of the Seventh Workshop on Targetry and Target Chemistry, June 8–11, 1997, Heidelberg, Germany.* 1997:226.

56. Steinbach J, Guenther K, Loesel E, et al. Temperature course in small volume [^{18}O]water targets for [^{18}F]F^{-} production. *Appl Radiat Isot* 1990;41:753–756.

57. Schlyer DJ, Firouzbakht ML, Wolf AP. Impurities in the [^{18}O]water target and their effect on the yield of an aromatic displacement reaction with [^{18}F]fluoride. *Int J Appl Radiat Isot* 1993;44:1459–1465.

58. Solin O, Bergman J, Haaparanta M, et al. Production of ^{18}F from water targets: Specific radioactivity and anionic contaminants. *Appl Radiat Isot* 1988;39:1065–1071.

59. Zeisler SK, Helus F, Gaspar H. *Comparison of different target surface materials for the production of carrier-free [^{18}F]fluoride: proceedings of the Seventh Workshop on Targetry and Target Chemistry, June 8–11, 1997, Heidelberg, Germany.* 1997:223.

60. Becker DW, Erbe D. *A new high current spherical target design for ^{18}O(p,n)^{18}F with 18 MeV protons: proceedings of the Seventh Workshop on Targetry and Target Chemistry, June 8–11, 1997, Heidelberg, Germany.* 1997:268.

61. Firouzbakht ML, Schlyer DJ, Gately SJ, et al. A cryogenic solid target for the production of [^{18}F]fluoride from enriched [^{18}O]carbon dioxide, *Appl Radiat Isot* 1993;44:1081–1084.

62. Nozaki T, Iwamoto M, Ido T. Yield of ^{18}F for various reactions from oxygen and neon. *Int J Appl Radiat Isot* 1974;25:393–399.

63. Fitschen J, Beckmann R, Holm U, et al. Yield and production of ^{18}F by ^{3}He irradiation of water. *Int J Radiat Isot* 1977;28:781–784.

64. Schlyer DJ, Bastos MAV, Alexoff D, et al. Separation of F-18 fluoride from O-18 water using anion exchange resin. *Int J Appl Radiat Isot* 1990;41[pt A]:531–533.

65. Mock BH, Vavrek MT, Mulholland GK. Back-to-back "one-pot" [^{18}F]FDG syntheses in a single Siemens-CTI Chemistry Process Control Unit *Nucl Med Biol* 1996;23:497–501.

66. Pascali C, Bogni A, Remonti F, et al. *A convenient semi-automated system for optimizing the recovery of aqueous [^{18}F]fluoride from target: proceedings of the Seventh Workshop on Targetry and Target Chemistry, June 8–11, 1997, Heidelberg, Germany.* 1997:60.

67. Bida GT, Ruth TJ, Wolf AP. Experimentally determined thick target

yields for the $^{14}N(p,\alpha)^{11}C$ reaction. *Radiochimica Acta* 1980;27:181–185.

68. Casella VR, Christman DR, Ido T, et al. Excitation function for the $^{14}N(p,\alpha)^{11}C$ reaction up to 15 MeV. *Radiochimica Acta* 1978;25:17–20.

69. Christman DR, Finn RD, Karlstrom KI, et al. The production of ultra high activity ^{11}C-labelled hydrogen cyanide, carbon dioxide, carbon monoxide and methane via the $^{14}N(p,\alpha)^{11}C$ reaction. *Int J Appl Radiat Isot* 1975;26:435–442.

70. Clark JC, Buckingham PD. Carbon-11. In: *Short-lived radioactive gases for clinical use.* London: Butterworth, 1975:215–260.

71. Finn RD, Christman DR, Ache HJ, et al. The preparation of cyanide-^{11}C for use in the synthesis of organic radiopharmaceuticals. *Int J Appl Radiat Isot* 1971;22:735–744.

72. Helus F, Hanisch M, Layer K, et al. Yield ratio of [$^{11}C]CO_2$, [$^{11}C]CO$, [$^{11}C]CH_4$ from the irradiation of N_2/H_2 mixtures in the gas target. *J Labelled Compounds Radiopharm* 1986;23:1195–1198.

73. Buckley KR, Huser J, Jivan S, et al. ^{11}C-methane production in small volume, high pressure gas targets. *Radiochimica Acta* 2000:88:201–205.

74. Schlyer DJ, Plascjak PS. Small angle multiple scattering of charged particles in cyclotron target foils—a comparison of experiment with simple theory. *Nucl Instruments Methods* 1991ʻ6/57:464–468.

75. Helmeke HJ, Hundeshagen H. Design of gas targets for the production of medically used radionuclides with the help of Monte Carlo simulation of small angle multiple scattering of charged particles. *Appl Radiat Isot* 1995;46:751–757.

76. Wieland BW, Schlyer DJ, Wolf AP. Charged particle penetration in gas targets designed for accelerator production of radionuclides used in nuclear medicine. *Int J Appl Radiat Isot* 1984;35:387–396.

77. Heselius S-J, Lindblom P, Solin O. Optical studies of the influence of an intense ion beam on high pressure gas targets. *Int J Appl Radiat Isot* 1982;33:653–659.

78. Heselius S-J, Malmborg P, Solin O, et al. Studies of proton beam penetration in nitrogen gas targets with respect to production and specific radioactivity of carbon-11. *Int J Appl Radiat Isot* 1987;38:49–57.

79. Hughey BJ, Shefer RE, Klinkowstein RE, et al. *Design considerations for foil windows for PET radioisotope targets: proceedings of the Fourth Workshop on Targetry and Target Chemistry, September 9–12, 1991.* Villigen, Switzerland: PSI, 1991:12.

80. Schlyer DJ, Firouzbakht ML. *Correlation of hole size in support windows with calculated yield strengths: proceedings of the Sixth Workshop on Targetry and Target Chemistry, August 17–19, 1996, Vancouver, BC, Canada.* 1996:142–143.

81. Straatmann MG, Welch MJ. Enzymatic synthesis of nitrogen-13 labeled amino acids. *Radiat Res* 1973;56:48–56.

82. Tilbury RS, Emran AM. [^{13}N] Labeled tracers, synthesis and applications. In: Emran A, ed. *New trends in radiopharmaceutical synthesis, quality assurance, and regulatory control.* New York: Plenum Publishing, 1991:39–51.

83. Firouzbakht ML, Schlyer DJ, Wolf AP. Cross-section measurements for the $^{13}C(p,n)^{13}N$ and $^{12}C(d,n)^{13}N$ nuclear reactions. *Radiochimica Acta* 1991;55(1):1–5.

84. Austin SM, Galonsky A, Bortins J, et al. A batch process for the production of ^{13}N-labeled nitrogen gas. *Nucl Instruments Methods* 1975;126:373–379.

85. Sajjad M, Lambrecht RM, Wolf AP. Cyclotron isotopes and radiopharmaceuticals, XXXVII: excitation functions for the $^{16}O(p,\alpha)^{13}N$ and $^{14}N(p,pn)^{13}N$ reactions. *Radiochimica Acta* 1986;39:165–168.

86. Parks NJ, Krohn KA. The synthesis of ^{13}N labeled ammonia, dinitrogen, nitrite, nitrate using a single cyclotron target system. *Int J Appl Radiat Isot* 1978;29:754–757.

87. Tilbury RS, Dahl JR. ^{13}N Species formed by the proton irradiation of water. *Radiat Res* 1979;79:22–33.

88. Tilbury RS, Dahl JR, Marano SJ. N-13 species formed by proton irradiation of water. *J Labelled Compounds Radiopharm* 1977;13:208.

89. Helmeke HJ, Harms T, Knapp WH. *Home-made routinely used targets for the production of PET radionuclides: proceedings of the Seventh Workshop on Targetry and Target Chemistry, June 8–11, 1997, Heidelberg, Germany.* 1997:241.

90. Mulholland GK, Kilbourn MR, Moskwa JJ. Direct simultaneous production of [$^{15}O]$water and [$^{13}N]$ammonia or [$^{18}F]$fluoride ion by 26

MeV proton irradiation of a double chamber water target. *Appl Radiat Isot* 1990;41:1193–1199.

91. Joliot F, Curie I. Artificial production of a new kind of radio-element. *Nature* 1934;133:201–202.

92. Shefer RE, Hughey BJ, Klinkowstein RE, et al. A windowless ^{13}N production target for use with low energy deuteron accelerators. *Nucl Med Biol* 1994;21:977–986.

93. Dence CS, Welch MJ, Hughey BJ, et al. Production of [^{13}N] ammonia applicable to low energy accelerators. *Nucl Med Biol* 1994;21:987–996.

94. Bida G, Wieland BW, Ruth TJ, et al. An economical target for nitrogen-13 production by proton bombardment of a slurry of C-13 powder on ^{16}O water. *J Labelled Compounds Radiopharm* 1986;23:1217–1218.

95. Zippi EM, Valiulis MB, Grover J. *Synthesis of carbon-13 sulfonated poly(styrene/ divinylbenzene) for production of a nitrogen-13 target material: proceedings of the Sixth Workshop on Targetry and Target Chemistry, August 17–19, 1995, Vancouver, BC, Canada.* 1995:185–188.

96. Wieland BW, McKinney CJ, Coleman RE. *A tandem target system using $^{16}O(p,pn)^{15}O$ and $^{16}O(p,\alpha)^{13}N$ on natural water: proceedings of the Sixth Workshop on Targetry and Target Chemistry, August 17–19, 1995, Vancouver, BC, Canada.* 1995:173–179.

97. Berridge MS, Landmeier BJ. In-target production of [^{13}N]ammonia: target design, products and operating parameters. *Appl Radiat Isot* 1993;44:1433–1441.

98. Korsakov MV, Krasikova RN, Fedorova OS. Production of high yield [^{13}N]ammonia by proton irradiation from pressurized aqueous solutions. *J Radioanalytical Nucl Chem* 1996;204:231–239.

99. Medema J, Elsinga PH, Keizer H, et al. *Remote controlled in-target production of [^{13}N]ammonia using a circulating target: proceedings of the Seventh Workshop on Targetry and Target Chemistry, June 8–11, 1997, Heidelberg, Germany.* 1997:80–81.

100. Wieland BW, Bida G, Padgett H, et al. In-target production of [^{13}N] ammonia via proton irradiation of dilute aqueous ethanol and acetic acid mixtures. *Appl Radiat Isot* 1991;42:1095–1098.

101. Bida G, Satyamurthy N. *[^{13}N]Ammonia production via proton irradiation of CO_2/H_2O: a work in progress: proceedings of the Sixth Workshop on Targetry and Target Chemistry, August 17–19, 1995, Vancouver, British Columbia, Canada.* 1995:189–191.

102. Patt JT, Nebling B, Stocklin G. Water target chemistry of nitrogen-13 recoils revisited. *J Labelled Compounds Radiopahrm* 1991;30:122–123.

103. Sasaki M, Haradahira T, Suzuki K. Effect of dissolved gas on the specific activity of N-13 labeled ions generated in water by the $^{16}O(p,\alpha)^{13}N$ reaction. *Radiochimica Acta* 2000;88:217–220.

104. Mikecz P, Dood MG, Chaloner F, et al. *Glass target for production of [$^{13}N]NH_3$ from methane, revival of an old method: proceedings of the Seventh Workshop on Targetry and Target Chemistry, June 8–11, 1997, Heidelberg, Germany.* 1997:163–164.

105. Straatmann MG. A look at ^{13}N and ^{15}O in radiopharmaceuticals. *Int J Appl Radiat Isot* 1977;28:13–20.

106. McCarthy TJ, Gaehle GG, Margenau WH, et al. *Evaluation of a commercially available heater for the rapid combustion of graphite disks used in the production of [$^{13}N]NO$ and [$^{13}N]NO_2$: proceedings of the Seventh Workshop on Targetry and Target Chemistry, June 8–11, 1997, Heidelberg, Germany.* 1997:205.

107. Ferrieri RA, Schlyer DJ, Wieland BW, et al. On-line production of ^{13}N-nitrogen gas from a solid enriched ^{13}C-target and its application to ^{13}N-ammonia synthesis using microwave radiation. *Int J Appl Radiat Isot* 1983;34:897–900.

108. Livingston MS, McMillian E. The production of radioactive oxygen. *Phys Rev* 1934;46:439–440.

109. Del Fiore G, Depresseux JC, Bartsch P, et al. Production of oxygen-15, nitrogen-13 and carbon-11 and of their low molecular weight derivatives for biomedical applications. *Int J Appl Radiat Isot* 1979;30:543–549.

110. Retz-Schmidt T, Weil JL. Excitation curves and angular distributions for $^{14}N(d,n)^{15}O$. *Phys Rev* 1960;119:1079–1084.

111. Vera-Ruiz H, Wolf AP. Excitation function of ^{15}O production via the $^{14}N(d,n)^{15}O$ reaction. *Radiochimica Acta* 1977;24:65–67.

112. Sajjad M, Lambrecht RM, Wolf AP. Cyclotron isotopes and radiopharmaceuticals, XXXIV: excitation function for the $^{15}N(p,n)^{15}O$ reaction. *Radiochimica Acta* 1984;36:159–162.

113. Beaver JE, Finn RD, Hupf HB. A new method for the production of high concentration oxygen-15 labeled carbon dioxide with protons. *Int J Appl Radiat Isot* 1976;27:195–197.

114. Vera-Ruiz H, Wolf AP. Direct synthesis of oxygen-15 labeled water of high specific activity. *J Labelled Compounds Radiopharm* 1978; 15:186–189.

115. Votaw JR, Satter MR, Sunderland JJ, et al. The Edison lamp: O-15 carbon monoxide production in the target. *J Labelled Compounds Radiopharm* 1986;23:1211–1213.

116. Harper PV, Wickland T. Oxygen-15 labeled water for continuous intravenous administration. *J Labelled Compounds Radiopharm* 1981; 18:186.

117. Wieland BW, Russel ML, Dunn WL, et al. *Quartz micro-fiber target for the production of O-15 ozone for pulmonary applications—computer modeling and experiments: proceedings of the Seventh Workshop on Targetry and Target Chemistry, June 8–11, 1997, Heidelberg, Germany.* 1997:114–119.

118. Strijckmans K, VandeCasteele C, Sambre J. Production and quality control of $^{15}O_2$ and $C^{15}O_2$ for medical use. *Int J Appl Radiat Isot* 1985;36:279–283.

119. Wieland BW, Schmidt DG, Bida G, et al. Efficient, economical production of oxygen-15 labeled tracers with low energy protons. *J Labelled Compounds Radiopharm* 1986;23:1214–1216.

120. Van Naeman J, Monclus M, Damhaut P, et al. Production, automatic delivery and bolus injection of [^{15}O]water for positron emission tomography studies. *Nucl Med Biol* 1996;23:413–416.

121. Pagani M, Stone-Elander S, Larsson SA. Alternative positron emission tomography with non-conventional positron emitters: effects of their physical properties on image quality and potential clinical applications. *Eur J Nucl Med* 1997;24:1301–1327.

122. Chaudhir MA. Yields of cyclotron produced medical isotopes: a comparison of theoretical potential and experimental results. *IEEE Trans Nucl Sci* 1979#-26:2281–2286.

123. Qaim SM. Nuclear data relevant to cyclotron produced short-lived medical radioisotopes. *Radiochimica Acta* 1982;30:147–162.

124. Qaim SM, Hohn A, Nortier FM, et al. Production of ^{124}I at small and medium size cyclotrons. In: *Programs and abstracts of the 8th International Workshop on Targetry and Target Chemistry,* 1999; St. Louis, MO. Abstract.

125. Scholten B, Kovacs Z, Tarkanyi F, et al. Excitation functions of $^{124}Te(p,xn)^{124,123}I$ reactions from 6 to 31 MeV with special reference to the production of ^{124}I at a small cyclotron. *Appl Radiat Isot* 1995; 46:255–259.

126. Sheh Y, Koziorowski J, Balatoni J, et al. Low energy cyclotron production and chemical separation of "no carrier added" ^{124}I from a reusable, enriched tellurium-124 dioxide/aluminum oxide solid solution target. *Radiochimica Acta* 2000;88:169–173.

127. Qaim SM. Recent developments in the production of ^{18}F, $^{75,76,77}Br$ and ^{123}I. *Int J Appl Radiat Isot* 1986;37:803–810.

128. Paans AMJ, Welleweerd J, Vaalburg W, et al. Excitation functions for the production of ^{75}Br: a potential nuclide for the labeling of radiopharmaceuticals. *Int J Appl Radiat Isot* 1980;31:267–272.

129. Vaalburg W, Paans AMJ, Terpstra JW, et al. Fast recovery by dry distillation of ^{75}Br induced in reusable metal selenide targets via the $^{76}Se(p,2n)^{75}Br$ reaction. *Int J Appl Radiat Isot* 1985;36:961–964.

130. Kovacs Z, Blessing G, Qaim SM, et al. Production of ^{75}Br via the $^{76}Se(p,2n)^{75}Br$ reaction at a compact cyclotron. *Int J Appl Radiat Isot* 1985;36:635–642.

131. Blessing G, Qaim SM. An improved internal Cu_3As-alloy cyclotron target for the production of ^{75}Br and ^{77}Br and separation of the by-product ^{67}Ga from the matrix activity. *Int J Appl Radiat Isot* 1984; 35:927–931.

132. Blessing G, Weinreich R, Qaim SM, et al. Production of ^{75}Br and ^{76}Br via the $^{75}As(^{3}He,3n)^{75}Br$ and $^{75}As(\alpha,2n)^{77}Br$ reactions using Cu_3As-alloy as a high-current target material. *Int J Appl Radiat Isot* 1982;33:333–339.

133. Richards P. *Tc99m: production and chemistry.* Upton, NY: Brookhaven National Laboratory, 1965. Report no BNL-9032.

134. Richards P. *The Tc-99m generator.* Upton, NY: Brookhaven National Laboratory, 1965. Report no BNL-9061.

135. Lambrecht RM. Radionuclide generators. *Radiochimica Acta* 1983; 34:9–24.

136. Finn RD, Molinski VJ, Hupf HB, et al. *Radionuclide generators for biomedical applications.* Springfield: National Technical Information Service, 1983.

137. Knapp FF Jr, Butler TA, eds. *Radionuclide generators.* Washington, DC: American Chemical Society, 1984. ACS Symposium series 241.

138. Guillaume M, Brihaye C. Generators for short-lived gamma and positron emitting radionuclides: current status and prospects. *Nucl Med Biol* 1986;13:89–100.

139. Qaim SM. Cyclotron production of generator radionuclides. *Radiochimica Acta* 1987;41:111–117.

140. Welch MJ, McCarthy TJ. The potential role of generator-produced radiopharmaceuticals in clinical PET. *J Nucl Med* 2000;41:315–317.

141. Robinson GD Jr, Zielinski FW, Lee AW. The $^{62}Zn/^{62}Cu$-generator: a convenient source of ^{62}Cu for radiopharmaceuticals. *Int J Appl Radiat Isot* 1980;31:111–116.

142. Fujibayashi Y, Matsumoto K, Yonekura Y, et al. A new $^{62}Zn/^{62}Cu$ generator as a copper-62 source for PET radiopharmaceuticals. *J Nucl Med* 1989;30:1838–1842.

143. Green MA, Mathias CJ, Welch MJ, et al. Copper-62–labeled pyruvaldehyde bis(N^4-methylthiosemicarbazonato) copper, II: synthesis and evaluation as a positron emission tomography tracer for cerebral and myocardial perfusion. *J Nucl Med* 1990;31:1989–1996.

144. Zweit J, Goodall R, Cox M, et al. Development of a high performance zinc-62/copper-62 radionuclide generator for positron emission tomography. *Eur J Nucl Med* 1992;19:418–425.

145. Neirinckx RD. Excitation function for the $^{60}Ni(\alpha,2n)^{62}Zn$ reaction and production of ^{62}Zn bleomycin. *Int J Appl Radiat Isot* 1977;28: 808–809.

146. Yagi M, Kondo K. A ^{62}Cu generator. *Int J Appl Radiat Isot* 1979; 30:569–570.

147. Piel H, Qaim SM, Stocklin G. Excitation functions of (p,xn)-reactions on ^{nat}Ni and highly enriched ^{62}Ni: possibility of production of medically important radioisotope ^{62}Cu at a small cyclotron. *Radiochimica Acta* 1992;57:1–5.

148. Pao PJ, Silvester DJ, Waters SL. A new method for the preparation of ^{68}Ga-generators following proton bombardment of gallium oxide targets. *J Radioanalytical Chem* 1981;64:267–272.

149. Loc'h C, Maziere B, Comar D, et al. A new preparation of germanium-68. *Int J Appl Radiat Isot* 1982;33:267–270.

150. Grant PM, Miller DA, Gilmore JS, et al. Medium-energy spallation cross sections, I: RbBr irradiation with 800-MeV protons. *Int J Appl Radiat Isot* 1982;33:415–417.

151. Robertson R, Graham D, Trevena IC. Radioisotope production via 500 MeV proton-induced reactions. *J Labelled Compounds Radiopharm* 1982;19:1368(abst).

152. Loc'h C, Maziere B, Comar D. A new generator for ionic gallium-68. *J Nucl Med* 1980;21:171–173.

153. Gould KL. Clinical positron imaging of the heart with Rb-82. In: *PET/SPECT: instrumentation, radiopharmaceuticals, neurology and physiology measurement.* Washington, DC: American College of Nuclear Physicians, 1988:122–133.

154. Goldstein RA, Mullani NA, Fisher DJ, et al. Myocardial perfusion with rubidium-82, II: effects of metabolic and pharmaceutical interventions. *J Nucl Med* 1983;24:907–915.

155. Selwyn AP, Allan RM, L'abbate A, et al. Relation between regional myocardial uptake of rubidium-82 and perfusion: absolute reduction of cation uptake in ischemia. *Am J Cardiol* 1982;50:112–121.

156. Waters SL, Coursey BM, eds. The $^{82}Sr/^{82}Rb$ generator. *Appl Radiat Isot* 1987;38:171–240.

157. Tarkanyi F, Qaim SM, Stocklin G. Excitation functions of ^{3}He- and α-particle induced nuclear reactions on natural krypton: production of ^{82}Sr at a compact cyclotron. *Appl Radiat Isot* 1988;39:135–143.

158. Tarkanyi F, Qaim SM, Stocklin G. Excitation functions of high-energy ^{3}He- and α-particle induced nuclear reactions on natural krypton with special reference to the production of ^{82}Sr. *Appl Radiat Isot* 1990;41: 91–95.

159. Mausner LF, Prach T, Srivastava SC. Production of ^{82}Sr by proton irradiation of RbCl. *Appl Radiat Isot* 1987;38:181–184.

160. Thomas KE. Strontium-82 production at Los Alamos National Laboratory. *Appl Radiat Isot* 1987;38:175–180.

161. Yano Y, Cahoon JL, Budinger TF. A precision flow controlled Rb-82 generator for bolus or constant-infusion studies of the heart and brain. *J Nucl Med* 1981;22:1006–1010.

CHAPTER 2

Chemistry

Joanna S. Fowler and Yu-Shin Ding

Carbon-11 (^{11}C) and fluorine-18 (^{18}F), the most commonly used radionuclides for positron emission tomography (PET), were discovered more than 60 years ago. The discovery of ^{11}C preceded that of carbon-14 (^{14}C) by several years, so it became the first radioactive isotope of carbon to be used for chemical and biochemical tracer studies before and during World War II (1). Because of the extraordinary experimental limitations imposed by its 20.4-minute half-life, ^{11}C was largely replaced by ^{14}C ($t_{1/2} = 5,730$ years), which became available after World War II.

Interest in ^{11}C and three other short-lived positron emitters (^{18}F, nitrogen-13 [^{13}N], and oxygen-15 [^{15}O]) (Table 2.1) was rekindled two decades later when it was appreciated that their short half-lives and body-penetrating photons resulting from positron decay provided the potential to image biochemical transformations in the living human body with a low radiation dose (2). This stimulated the study of the chemistry of ^{11}C and the other short-lived positron emitters, as well as the development of PET, a medical imaging method for measuring the spatial and temporal distribution of the positron emitters in the human and animal body by coincidence detection of the annihilation photons resulting from positron decay (3). Over the past 30 years, advances in synthetic chemistry and PET instrumentation have merged to make PET a powerful scientific tool for studying biochemical transformations and the movement of drugs in the human brain and other organs in the body.

There have been many chapters, monographs, and review articles describing various aspects of radiotracer chemistry with the short-lived positron emitters (4–11). Of special significance is an up-to-date listing with references plus structures of most of the PET-labeled compounds ever made. They are classified according to compound type and it is available in PDF format (12).

The purpose of this chapter is to distill some of the essential contemporary considerations in the design and synthesis of PET tracers for modern applications and to site examples that illustrate general principles. This is followed by sections on three classes of labeled compounds: those that bind to synaptic elements involved in neurotransmission, those involved in amino acid transport and protein synthesis, and those involved in DNA synthesis. We focus on ^{11}C and ^{18}F because they are the two positron emitters that form the heart of PET chemistry and application.

RAPID RADIOTRACER CHEMISTRY

Time dominates all aspects of a PET study, particularly the synthesis of the radiotracer. In essence, PET radiotracers must be synthesized and imaged within a time frame compatible with the half-life of the isotope. Time is of the utmost importance when selecting a synthetic strategy (13). For ^{11}C, this typically amounts to about 10 minutes for isotope production (cyclotron bombardment), 40 minutes for radiotracer synthesis, and up to about 90 minutes for PET imaging. Thus, the entire study from the end of cyclotron bombardment to the end of an imaging session must be orchestrated and performed within about 2.5 hours. Large amounts of radioactivity must be used to compensate for radioactive decay and for the sometimes low synthetic yields. Shielding, remote operations, and automation are integrated into the experimental design (14,15). It is ideal to introduce the radioactivity at the last step in the synthesis, which may require multistep syntheses of suitably protected substrates into which ^{11}C or ^{18}F can be introduced. When protective groups are used, they must be stable to the labeling conditions and the de-protection conditions must be rapid. The crude reaction mixture is usually purified by high-pressure liquid chromatography (HPLC) or a combination of solid-phase extraction and HPLC. Because radiotracers are typically administered intravenously, procedures must be developed to yield radiotracers that are not only chemically and radiochemically pure but also sterile and free from pyrogens (16).

Carbon-11 and Fluorine-18 Production

Basic research in ''hot atom chemistry'' provided some of the knowledge to understand the chemistry that takes place during the production of the short-lived positron emitters and set the stage for producing the short-lived positron emitters in chemical forms that were useful for the synthesis of complex radiotracers (1). Because of the short half-lives

TABLE 2.1. *Physical properties of the short-lived positron emitters*

Isotope	Half-life (min)	Specific activity (Ci/mmol)[a]	Maximum energy (MeV)	Range (mm) in H_2O[b]	Decay product
Fluorine-18	110	1.71×10^6	0.635	2.4	Oxygen-18
Carbon-11	20.4	9.22×10^6	0.96	4.1	Boron-11
Oxygen-15	2.1	9.08×10^7	1.72	8.2	Nitrogen-15
Nitrogen-13	9.96	1.89×10^7	1.19	5.4	Carbon-13

[a]Theoretical maximum; in reality, the measured specific activities of carbon-11, fluorine-18, and nitrogen-13 are about 5,000 times lower because of unavoidable dilution with the stable element.
[b]Maximum linear range.

of ^{11}C and ^{18}F, each radiotracer synthesis requires the production of the isotope and its conversion to a useful labeled precursor molecule either directly or via some postirradiation synthesis. Production involves bombarding appropriate stable (and sometimes enriched) isotopes with charged particles such as protons and deuterons, which are most commonly and conveniently produced using a cyclotron. Three nuclear reactions, the $^{14}N(p,\alpha)^{11}C$, the $^{18}O(p,n)^{18}F$, and the $^{20}Ne(d,\alpha)^{18}F$ reactions are most commonly used for ^{11}C and ^{18}F production (Fig. 2.1) (5).

An important point is that the substrate that is used for the nuclear reaction (referred to as the "target") is usually a different element than the radioisotope produced. Carbon-11, for example, is usually produced from the cyclotron bombardment of stable nitrogen (nitrogen-14[p,α]^{11}C). In principle, at the end of cyclotron bombardment, the only isotope of carbon present would be ^{11}C. However, because stable carbon is ubiquitous in nature, it is not possible to remove it completely from the target and from the reagents used in the synthesis. Even with this unavoidable dilution, the specific activity (units of radioactivity per unit of mass) of PET radiotracers is quite high (Table 2.1). Thus, it is typical that the ratio of ^{12}C:^{11}C is about 5,000 : 1, which generally produces radiotracers of sufficiently high specific activity for tracer studies.

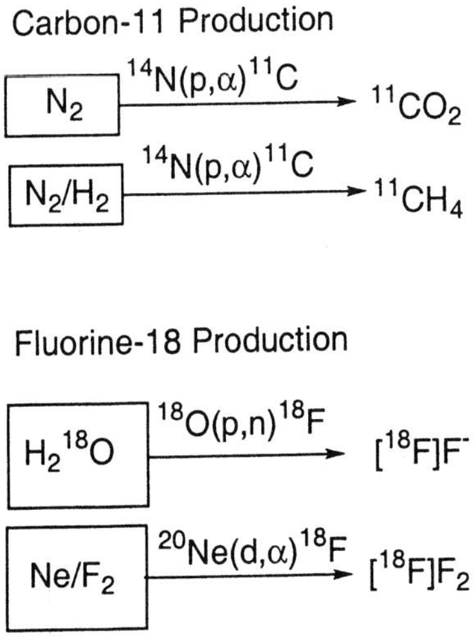

Fluorine-18 is most commonly produced by bombarding ^{18}O enriched water with protons to yield ^{18}F-fluoride (17). As is the case with ^{11}C, it is not possible to remove all stable fluoride ions from the target materials and from the reagents used in the synthesis, so the isotope is always diluted with stable fluoride. In contrast to ^{18}F-fluoride, which is always produced without the *intentional* addition of stable fluoride, ^{18}F-F_2 is always deliberately diluted with unlabeled F_2. In general, for equal amounts of radioactivity, the chemical mass associated with an F_2 ^{18}F-derived radiotracer (carrier added) exceeds that of an ^{18}F-fluoride ion derived radiotracer (no carrier added) by a factor of 1,000 (6). However, there has been progress in achieving high specific activity ^{18}F-labeled elemental fluorine by mixing no-carrier-added (NCA) ^{18}F-labeled methyl fluoride (synthesized from aqueous ^{18}F-fluoride ion) with a small amount of elemental fluorine in an inert neon matrix and subjecting it to an electrical discharge (18). The resulting labeled elemental fluorine has a specific activity of up to 55 GBq/μmol, which is sufficiently high for tracer studies of the dopamine transporter (19). Although ^{18}F-XeF_2 has been prepared and used in labeling, labeling required the use of ^{18}F-F_2 (6). It was recently reported that XeF_2 exchanges ^{18}F-fluoride under mild conditions (20). Specific activity has not been optimized.

High specific activity radiotracers provide the opportunity for imaging biologic substrates such as neurotransmitter receptors at tracer concentrations (21). However, the chemical mass that constitutes a tracer dose depends on the process being measured. For example, biologic targets such as neurotransmitter receptors occur at much lower concentrations than enzymes, so higher specific activities are required for neurotransmitter or steroid hormone receptor studies. Specific activity is typically expressed by one of the following terms (22,23):

Carrier free (CF) should mean that the radionuclide or stable nuclide is not contaminated with any other radionuclide or stable nuclide of the same element. This has probably never been achieved with ^{11}C or ^{18}F tracers.

No carrier added (NCA) should apply to an element or compound to which no carrier of the same element or

Carbon-11 Production

$$N_2 \xrightarrow{\,^{14}N(p,\alpha)^{11}C\,} \,^{11}CO_2$$

$$N_2/H_2 \xrightarrow{\,^{14}N(p,\alpha)^{11}C\,} \,^{11}CH_4$$

Fluorine-18 Production

$$H_2\,^{18}O \xrightarrow{\,^{18}O(p,n)^{18}F\,} [^{18}F]F^-$$

$$Ne/F_2 \xrightarrow{\,^{20}Ne(d,\alpha)^{18}F\,} [^{18}F]F_2$$

FIG. 2.1. Common nuclear reactions and target materials for carbon-11 and fluorine-18 production.

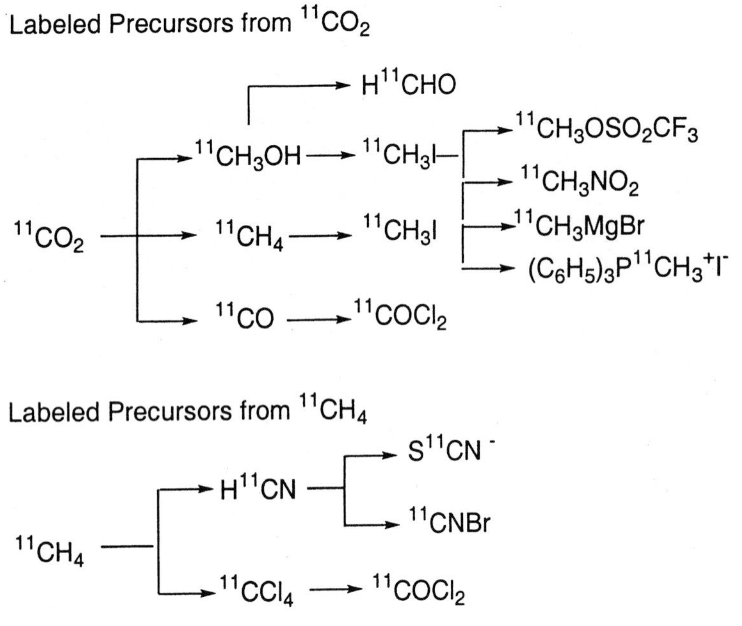

Labeled Precursors from $^{11}CO_2$

$$^{11}CO_2 \longrightarrow \begin{cases} ^{11}CH_3OH \longrightarrow H^{11}CHO \\ ^{11}CH_3OH \longrightarrow ^{11}CH_3I \\ ^{11}CH_4 \longrightarrow ^{11}CH_3I \\ ^{11}CO \longrightarrow ^{11}COCl_2 \end{cases}$$

$$^{11}CH_3I \longrightarrow \begin{cases} ^{11}CH_3OSO_2CF_3 \\ ^{11}CH_3NO_2 \\ ^{11}CH_3MgBr \\ (C_6H_5)_3P^{11}CH_3{}^+I^- \end{cases}$$

Labeled Precursors from $^{11}CH_4$

$$^{11}CH_4 \longrightarrow \begin{cases} H^{11}CN \longrightarrow \begin{cases} S^{11}CN^- \\ ^{11}CNBr \end{cases} \\ ^{11}CCl_4 \longrightarrow ^{11}COCl_2 \end{cases}$$

FIG. 2.2. Some carbon-11–labeled precursors synthesized from $^{11}CO_2$ and $^{11}CH_4$.

compound has been intentionally or otherwise added during its preparation. This applies to most radiotracers.

Carrier added (CA) should apply to any element or compound to which a known amount of carrier has been added.

Because the reporting of specific activities has ambiguities, particularly in the older literature, other descriptive terms have been introduced to describe radiotracer-specific activities (6). These include the term "effective specific activity," which refers to the value of specific activity that is measured by biologic or biochemical assay. This term takes into account the presence of species that have biological effects similar to the parent compound. The factors influencing the values of specific activities of compounds that are determined physicochemically and by radioreceptor techniques have been discussed (24).

The high specific activity of ^{11}C- and ^{18}F-labeled precursors influences the stoichiometry and the scale of the reaction. For example, in an NCA synthesis with $Na[^{11}C]N$ (specific activity: 2,000 Ci/mmol), the quantity of NaCN used if one starts with 100 mCi is 50 nmol. With this small quantity of $Na[^{11}C]N$, all other substrates or reactants used in the synthesis are necessarily in large excess, which is problematic when an excess of a given reagent cannot be tolerated. One must consider that the substrate that will undergo reaction with the label precursors must be in sufficient concentration to react both with the labeled precursors *and* with other competing reactants that may be present in the reaction mixture.

With such high specific activity ^{11}C- and ^{18}F-labeled precursors, syntheses are always carried out on a microscale or a semi-microscale and typical chemical masses associated with NCA PET radiotracers are a few micrograms or less. The small scale is advantageous in terms of the relative ease and speed with which one can handle small quantities of reagents and solvents, in minimizing the amounts of substances to be removed in the final purification and in avoid-

ing the unintentional introduction of impurities that may negatively influence the course of the reaction. However, losses caused by surface-to-volume effects and by adsorption properties of vessels and materials used for purification can heavily affect yields.

Carbon-11-labeled Compounds

The advantages of ^{11}C as a label are many, including the fact that it can be substituted for stable carbon in an organic compound without changing the properties of the molecule. In addition, PET studies can be repeated at 2-hour intervals with a ^{11}C-labeled tracer, allowing baseline and experimental studies to be performed in a single individual within a short time frame. However, there are large experimental hurdles imposed by the 20.4-minute half-life and the limited number of labeled precursors available for synthesis. More specifically, only $^{11}CO_2$ and $^{11}CH_4$ come directly from the cyclotron target using properly adjusted radiation conditions (Fig. 2.1). A number of other precursor molecules, some of which are shown in Fig. 2.2, are synthesized from labeled carbon dioxide or methane, but all require some synthetic manipulation during or after cyclotron bombardment (25).

Some of the earliest syntheses with ^{11}C depended directly on labeled carbon dioxide and hydrogen cyanide (26). Today, however, alkylation with ^{11}C-methyl iodide is the most widely used method for introducing ^{11}C into organic molecules (27). Alkylations are generally straightforward, as in the case of the synthesis of ^{11}C-raclopride, a widely used radiotracer for the dopamine D_2 receptor, which is synthesized by alkylating the nor compound with ^{11}C-methyl iodide (equation 2.1) (28). Frequently, however, reactive centers on the reaction substrate must be masked with protective groups that can be rapidly removed. This is illustrated by the synthesis of ^{11}C-*d-threo*- (or *l-threo*-) methylphenidate from labeled methyl iodide and a protected derivative of *d*- or *l-threo*-ritalinic acid (equation 2.2) (29). In the case of relatively sensitive compounds like deuterium-substituted ^{11}C-phenylephrine, alkylation can be carried out under milder conditions using ^{11}C-methyl triflate (equation 2.3) (30,31). The recent introduction of an on-line gas-phase synthesis to give high specific activity ^{11}C-methyl iodide from labeled methane is a major advance (32,33). Other precursors from ^{11}C-methyl iodide include ^{11}C-methyl magnesium iodide (34) and the Wittig reagent ^{11}C-methylenetriphenylphosphorane (35).

Carbon-11 synthesis is frequently complicated by the need for chiral-labeled products. In the case of radiotracers like [11]C-*d-threo*-methylphenidate described above, this is readily accomplished because the chiral center is present in the substrate (*d*-ritalinic acid) and the reaction conditions preserve the chirality, or by using chiral HPLC to separate the desired labeled enantiomer from a labeled racemic mixture. However, asymmetric syntheses have also been developed to directly obtain the desired enantiomer. For example, enantio-

merically enriched 3-^{11}C-L-alanine was synthesized from [11]CO$_2$ (via methyl iodide; equation 2.4) (36).

Labeled methane is also very useful in synthesis because it is available in large quantities and can be readily converted to H[11]N by passing the target gas (N$_2$/H$_2$ plus a small quantity of ammonia) over a hot platinum wool at 1,000°C (26). It has been used in the synthesis of labeled amines, ketones, aldehydes, acids, and amino acids (5).

A special problem in [11]C (and ^{18}F) synthesis is the need to design substrate molecules that are amenable to rapid labeling. Frequently, a new synthetic strategy must be developed for these molecules. The synthesis of carboxyl-^{11}C-γ-vinyl-γ-aminobutyric acid (^{11}C-GVG) is a good example. Because the synthetic methods for GVG reported previously were not suitable for the radiosynthesis of ^{11}C-GVG, a new five-step synthetic strategy was required to prepare a suitably protected molecule for the displacement reaction (equation 2.5) (37).

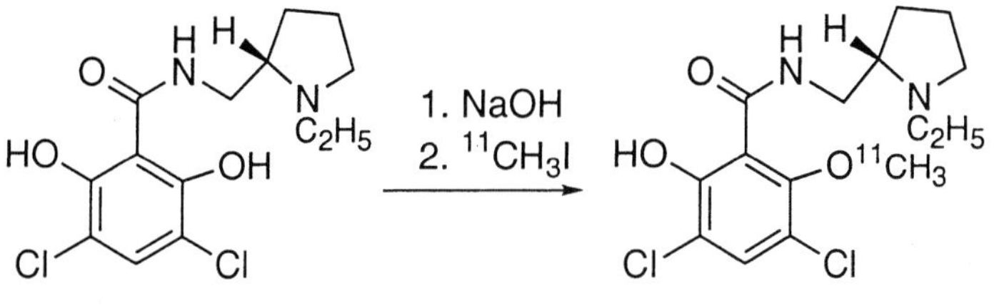

(eq. 2.1)

[11]C]raclopride

(eq. 2.2)

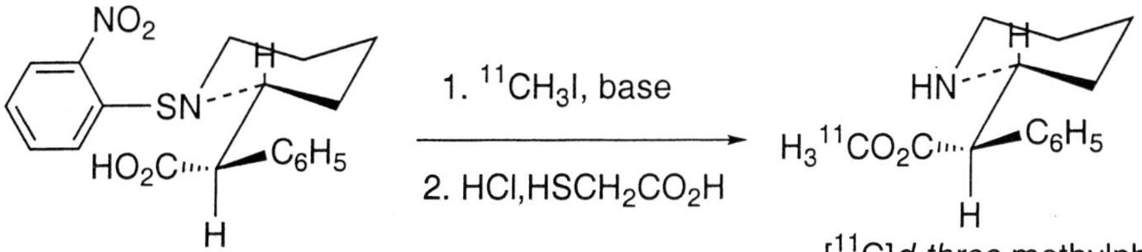

[11]C]*d-threo*-methylphenidate

(eq. 2.3)

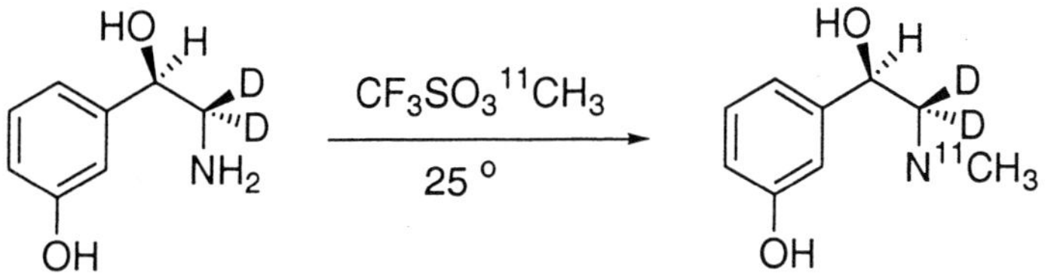

[11]C]-α,α–dideutero-phenylephrine

(eq. 2.4)

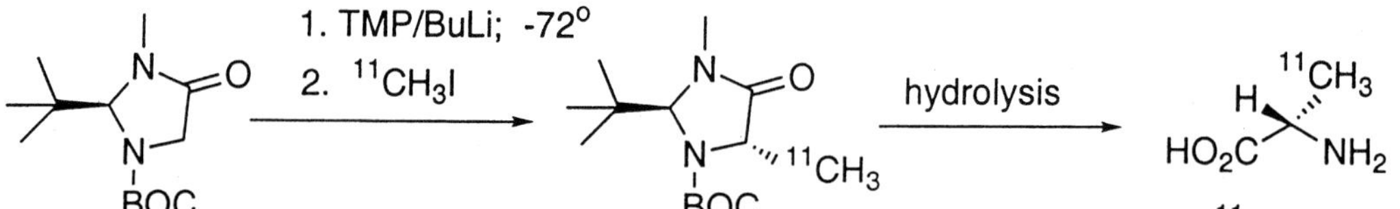

3-^{11}C]alanine

(eq. 2.5)

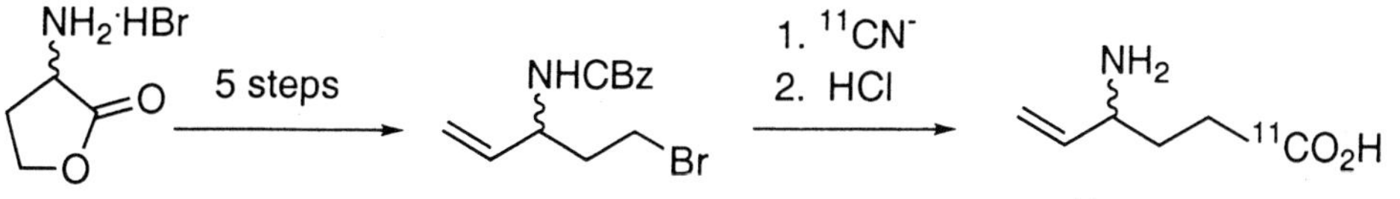

[11]C]GVG

In another example, the palladium catalyzed coupling of labeled cyanide to an aromatic ring was used in the synthesis of the radioligand ^{11}C-NAD-299, used for evaluation for binding to the 5-HT$_{1A}$ receptor (equation 2.6) (38).

Labeled methane has also been converted to ^{11}C-phosgene, which has been used in the synthesis of many compounds including a ring-labeled monoamine oxidase inhibitor (MAOI) befloxatone (equation 2.7) (39).

Problems in ^{11}C synthesis generally include rigorously excluding stable carbon to maximize the specific activity of the product, optimizing reaction rates, and developing chromatographic methods that separate the labeled product from starting materials and byproducts. Reaction times have been reduced and yields have been increased for many labeled compounds by applying microwave technology (40).

Fluorine-labeled Compounds

Whereas the 20-minute half-life of ^{11}C requires that the entire synthesis be accomplished in about 40 minutes, the 110-minute half-life of ^{18}F allows more time for relatively complex synthetic manipulations and for more lengthy biologic studies. An additional advantage of ^{18}F is its low positron energy and thus its maximum range (2.4 mm), which allows for the sharpest imaging with a high-resolution PET camera (Table 2.1). Disadvantages relative to ^{11}C include the fact that fluorine is not normally present in biologic molecules or drugs and the fact that the 110-minute half-life

precludes the performance of multiple studies on the same subject on the same day.

There are two simple labeled forms of ^{18}F (fluoride ion and elemental fluorine), which are directly available for radiotracer synthesis. Fluoride ion is the more desirable of the two because it can be produced in higher yield and without added carrier. In principle, 100% of the isotope can be incorporated into the tracer. An example is synthesis of 3′-deoxy-3′-^{18}F-fluorothymidine (^{18}F-FLT) based on the ^{18}F-fluoride displacement of a protected nosylate precursor (equation 2.8) (41).

In contrast, the maximum radiochemical yield when ^{18}F-F$_2$ is used as a precursor is usually only 50%, because only one of the fluorine atoms in the fluorine molecule is labeled and typically only one atom of fluorine is incorporated into the final product after electrophilic fluorination. This loss of 50% of the label also applies when labeled fluorine is converted to other precursors like labeled acetyl hypofluorite (6). 2-(^{18}F)fluoro-2-deoxy-D-glucose (^{18}F-FDG), which is used to measure glucose metabolism, exemplifies the evolution and improvement of a synthesis with the passage of time (Fig. 2.3). ^{18}F-FDG was first synthesized by electrophilic fluorination with ^{18}F-F$_2$ and an improved synthesis from ^{18}F-acetyl-hypofluorite was reported a few years later (42,43). However, the synthesis of ^{18}F-FDG via a nucleophilic substitution with ^{18}F-fluoride was a major breakthrough (44). It gave significantly higher yields and has largely replaced the

Nos = p-NO$_2$-C$_6$H$_5$-SO$_2$

DMTr = dimethoxy-trityl

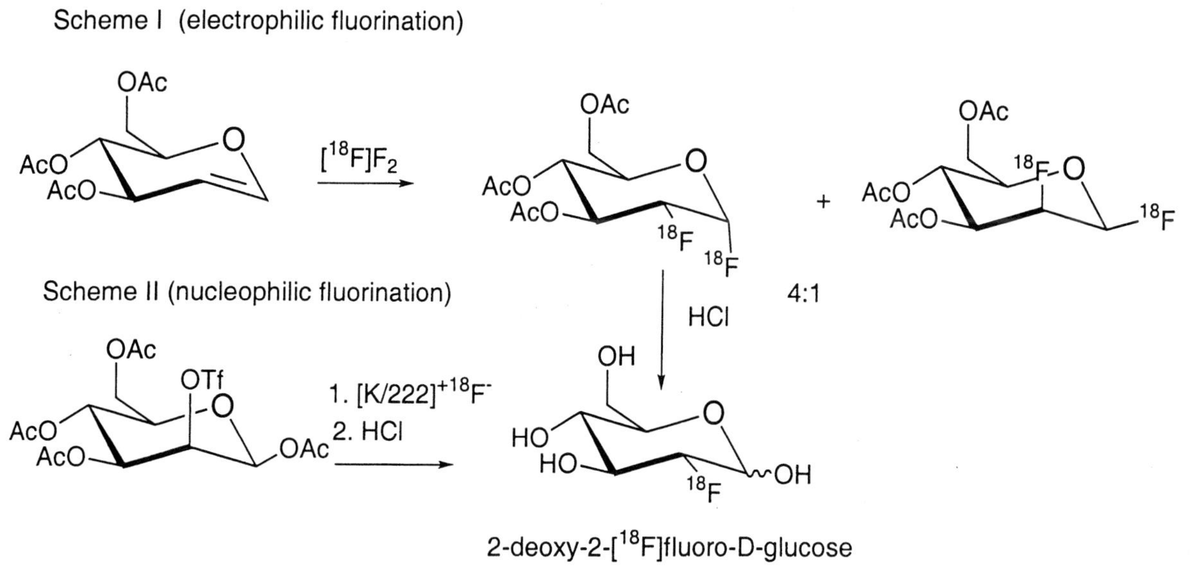

Scheme I (electrophilic fluorination)

Scheme II (nucleophilic fluorination)

2-deoxy-2-[^{18}F]fluoro-D-glucose

FIG. 2.3. Electrophilic and nucleophilic routes to fluorine-18-fluorodeoxyglucose.

electrophilic route. Although some radiotracers such as ^{18}F-fluoro-DOPA (6-[^{18}F]fluoro]-3,4-dihydroxyphenylalanine) (45) are still conveniently synthesized from ^{18}F-F$_2$ or ^{18}F-acetyl-hypofluorite (46), most ^{18}F-labeled radiotracers including ^{18}F-fluoro-DOPA can now be prepared from ^{18}F-fluoride ion (47,48).

The most successful approach for preparing high specific activity ^{18}F-substituted aromatic compounds is the nucleophilic aromatic substitution reaction (49). The minimal structural requirements for efficient nucleophilic aromatic substitution are the presence of an electron withdrawing, activating substituent such as RCO, CN, NO$_2$, and others, as well as a leaving group, such as nitro- or trimethylammonium. This approach is used for the high-yield one-pot, two-step synthesis of ^{18}F-fluoro-epibatidine, a radiotracer with high specificity for nicotinic acetylcholine (ACh) receptors (equation 2.9) (50).

In addition to simple fluorine-substituted aromatic compounds, there are important radiotracers with electron-donating substituents on the aromatic ring, which can impede the nucleophilic aromatic substitution reaction. Recent mechanistic studies have established that nucleophilic aromatic substitution can be carried out in the presence of suitably protected electron-donating groups, thus extending the utility of the nucleophilic aromatic substitution to the synthesis of 6-^{18}F-fluoro-DOPA and 6-^{18}F-fluorodopamine (51), (+)- and (−)-6-^{18}F-fluoro-norepinephrine (52) (equation 2.10). The use of the nucleophilic aromatic substitution reaction gave 6-^{18}F-fluorodopamine in sufficiently high specific activity for tracer studies without producing the hemodynamic effects (53) that are observed when low specific activity 6-^{18}F-fluorodopamine is used. Progress in the synthesis of chiral PET radiotracers has been recently reviewed (54).

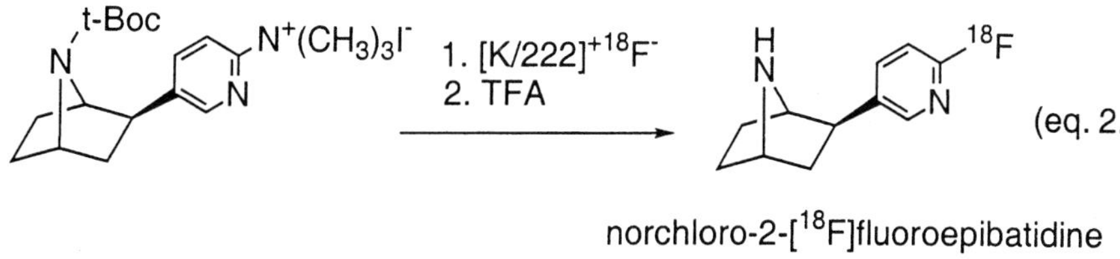

norchloro-2-[^{18}F]fluoroepibatidine (eq. 2.9)

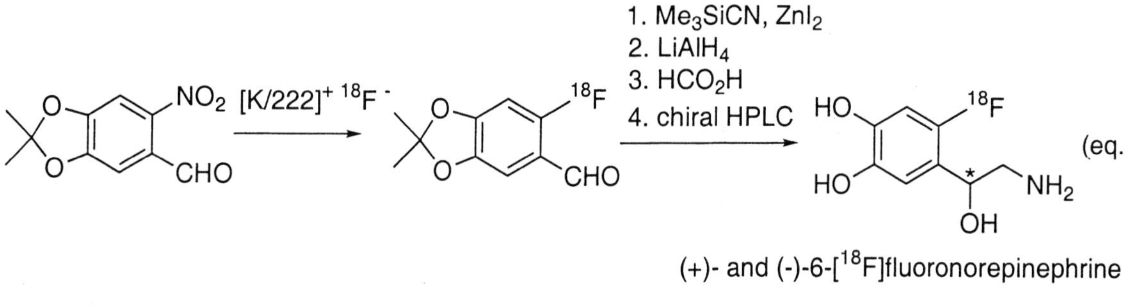

(+)- and (-)-6-[^{18}F]fluoronorepinephrine (eq. 2.10)

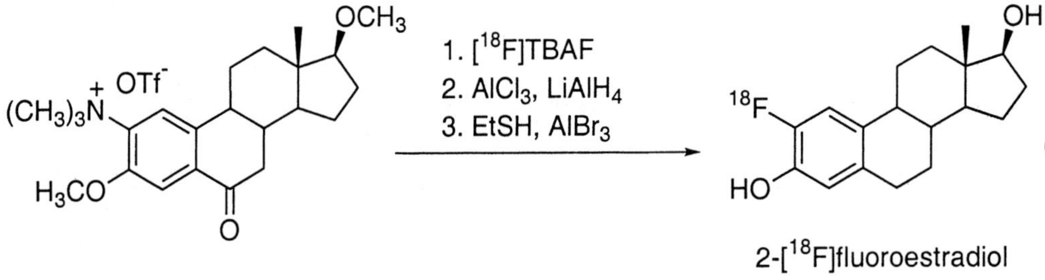

$$\text{(eq. 2.11)}$$

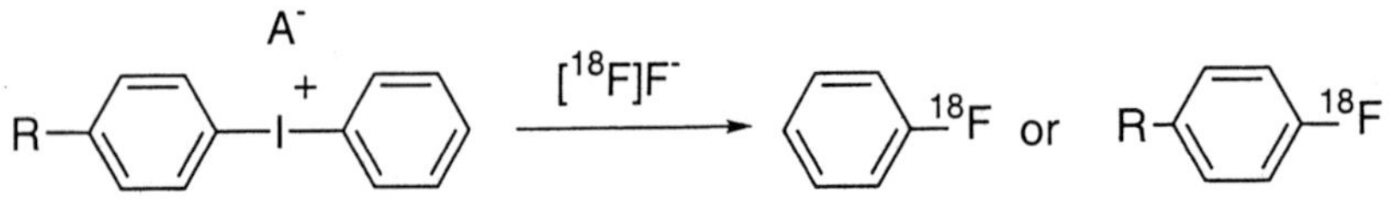

2-[^{18}F]fluoroestradiol

$$\text{(eq. 2.12)}$$

In another example of nucleophilic aromatic substitution on an electron-rich ring, 2-^{18}F-fluoroestradiol was synthesized by the displacement of a trimethylammonium group on the C_2 of an estrogen, with additional activation being provided by a 6-keto group, which was subsequently removed by reduction (equation 2.11) (55).

Simple, NCA ^{18}F-fluoroarenes have also been synthesized via the reaction of ^{18}F-fluoride with diaryliodonium salts (56) (equation 2.12).

RADIOTRACER DESIGN AND MECHANISMS

Radiotracer design refers to the process of choosing priority structures for synthesis. The process is complicated because it is not possible to predict the behavior of an organic compound in the human body. For most radiotracers, the physicochemical properties of the compounds such as their size, charge, solubility, and lipophilicity (57) also come into play and are particularly important in the design of tracers that penetrate the blood–brain barrier (58). In addition, factors such as rapid metabolism and binding to plasma proteins may be unanticipated pitfalls. However, studies in animals and isolated tissues can guide the process, and the literature of biochemistry and pharmacology are essential resources. In addition, some of the same issues that apply in drug development also apply in radiotracer development. In both cases information about the behavior of a chemical compound determined from *in vitro* studies and from measurements in animals must be combined with other interdependent factors to try to anticipate the behavior in a human. Thus, the phar-maceutical literature can be a valuable resource in the radiotracer design and evaluation process (59).

The design of ^{18}F-FDG is a good example of a radiotracer design that benefitted a great deal from information that was in the literature at the time. ^{18}F-FDG was modeled after ^{14}C-labeled 2-deoxy-glucose (^{11}C-2DG), a tracer used to measure brain glucose metabolism in animals using autoradiography (Fig. 2.4) (60). In the initial design of a positron emitter labeled version of 2-DG, there were the following requirements:

1. The resulting molecule must contain a positron emitter.
2. The resulting molecule must be a substrate for the glucose transporter that facilitates the transport of glucose from the blood to the brain.
3. The resulting molecule must be a substrate for hexokinase, the pivotal enzyme in glycolysis.
4. The resulting molecule must *not* undergo metabolism past the point of phosphorylation, allowing the phosphorylated product to be trapped at the site of phosphorylation.

As was reported in 1954, the hydroxyl group on carbon-2 (C-2) on the glucose skeleton is the only hydroxyl group on glucose that can be removed and still retain the ability of the molecule to be a substrate for hexokinase (the rate-limiting enzyme in glycolysis) (61). For this reason, C-2 was selected for fluorine substitution. Moreover, the glucose transporter is not sensitive to substitution on C-2, and the metabolism beyond the hexokinase step requires the hydroxyl group in C-2. Thus, ^{18}F-FDG, in which the ^{18}F is on C-2, undergoes carrier-mediated transport into the brain where

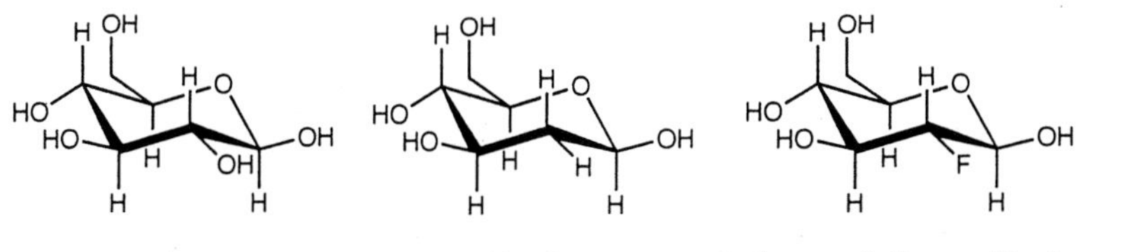

D-glucose   2-deoxy-D-glucose   2-deoxy-2-fluoro-D-glucose

FIG. 2.4. Structures of glucose, 2-deoxy-D-glucose and 2-deoxy-2-fluoro-D-glucose.

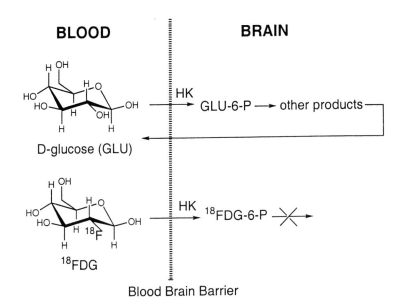

BLOOD | **BRAIN**

D-glucose (GLU)

HK
GLU-6-P → other products

^{18}FDG

HK
^{18}FDG-6-P ⇸

Blood Brain Barrier

FIG. 2.5. Simplified diagram comparing the behavior of glucose and 2-deoxy-2-fluoro-D-glucose in the brain. Glucose crosses the blood–brain barrier by facilitated transport and enters a cell. There, it enters the glycolytic cycle, where it is first phosphorylated by hexokinase *(HK)* and eventually produces adenosine triphosphate *(ATP)* and metabolites, which can leave the cell. Like glucose, fluorine-18-fluorodeoxyglucose (^{18}F-FDG) also undergoes facilitated transport into the brain and is phosphorylated by hexokinase to produce ^{18}F-FDG 6-phosphate. However ^{18}F-FDG 6-phosphate does not undergo further metabolism and is trapped in the cell.

it is phosphorylated to ^{18}F-FDG 6-phosphate by hexokinase. However, because the hydroxyl group in C-2 is missing, no further metabolism occurs and ^{18}F-FDG-6-phosphate is trapped in the cell where metabolism has occurred (Fig. 2.5). When imaged, metabolically trapped ^{18}F-FDG 6-phosphate provides a map of glucose metabolism in all brain regions (and throughout the body) simultaneously. 1-^{11}C-2-deoxy-D-glucose was also labeled with ^{11}C shortly after the development of ^{18}F-FDG and provided the opportunity to do multiple studies on the same subject in a single scanning session (62,63).

Although ^{18}F-FDG was initially developed for imaging brain metabolism, early studies showed that it was concentrated in animal tumors due to enhanced glycolysis in cancer cells (64,65). Consequently, ^{18}F-FDG has had a profound impact on the management of patients with cancer (66). The success of ^{18}F-FDG in the detection of human cancers also relates in part to the replacement of the hydroxyl on C-2, rather than on another carbon atom. Because the hydroxyl group on C-2 is required for active transport of glucose and because the active transport of glucose across the renal tubule is required for glucose resorption (67), ^{18}F-FDG, in contrast to glucose, is excreted. This, in effect, lowers the body background after the injection of ^{18}F-FDG, creating the high contrast for imaging metabolically active tumors.

A key step in the development of a new radiotracer is to characterize its binding *in vivo*. Because the PET image itself originates from the annihilation photons produced by positron decay, it provides no information on the chemical compound giving rise to the image or on the cellular or subcellular localization or binding site. One way to obtain this information is to compare the distribution and kinetics of the isotope before and after treatment with a pharmacologically specific drug or with a pharmacologic dose of the tracer molecule to assess specificity and saturation ability. Other

tools of mechanistic organic and biochemistry can also serve to interrogate the image. These include an examination of the behavior of the same compound labeled in different positions, the comparison of labeled stereoisomers and in limited cases, the use of deuterium isotope effects to probe specific reactions (68). Radiotracer kinetics can also be a limiting factor in quantitation and therefore must be critically examined and appropriate kinetic models developed to calculate parameters that can be related to receptor concentration, enzyme activity, or some other factors (69–74). Some examples are given for illustration.

Dual-tracer Studies of the Same Molecule Labeled in Different Positions

Frequently, the position of the label can be adjusted to simplify the profile of labeled metabolites contributing to the image or to determine the localization mechanism. For example, high pancreas uptake of ^{11}C was observed after the injection of ^{11}C-L-DOPA (75). To determine the mechanism by which ^{11}C concentrates in the pancreas, a comparison of the radiotracer labeled in the carboxyl group and in the β position was made in the same subject. Only the radiotracer labeled in the β position was retained in the pancreas. This demonstrated that aromatic amino acid decarboxylase (AAADC) (which would result in the loss of the ^{11}C in the carboxyl position, but not the β position) was responsible for the retention of ^{11}C-L-DOPA in pancreas and pancreatic tumors.

A similar comparative study of ^{11}C-5-hydroxytryptophan labeled in the β position and in the carboxyl position demonstrated tumor uptake and decarboxylation and provided the means for quantitating AAADC activity. A PET study of ^{11}C-dimethylphenethylamine labeled in two different positions (*N*-methyl versus α-methylene) also illustrates the profound difference in ^{11}C kinetics depending on the position of the label, illustrating the importance of label position for

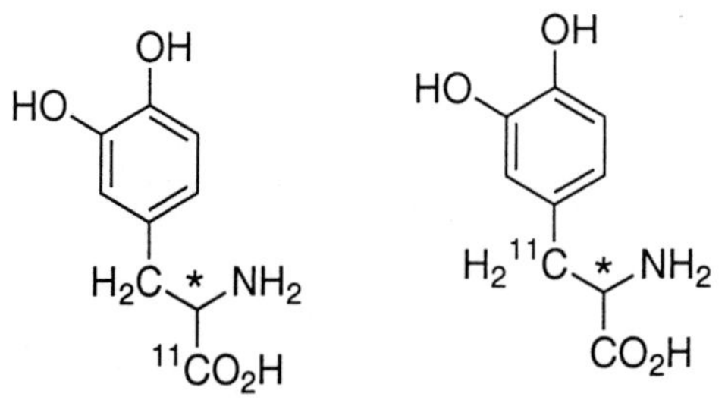

[11C-carboxyl]L-DOPA   [β-11C]L-DOPA

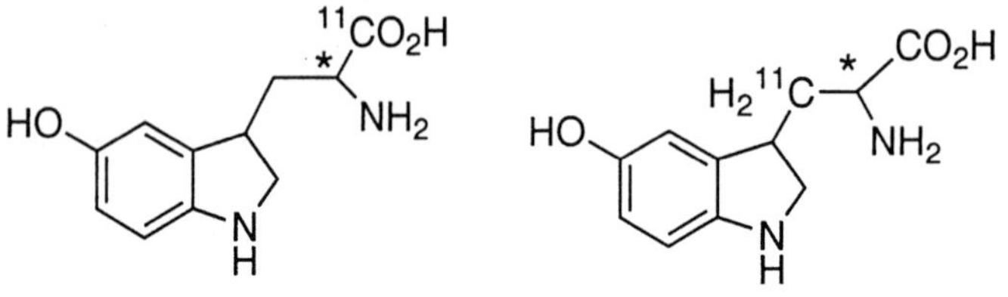

[11C-carboxyl]5-hydroxytryptophan and   [β-11C]5-hydroxytryptophan

[N-11C-methyl]dimethylphenethylamine   [α-11C-methylene]dimethylphenethylamine

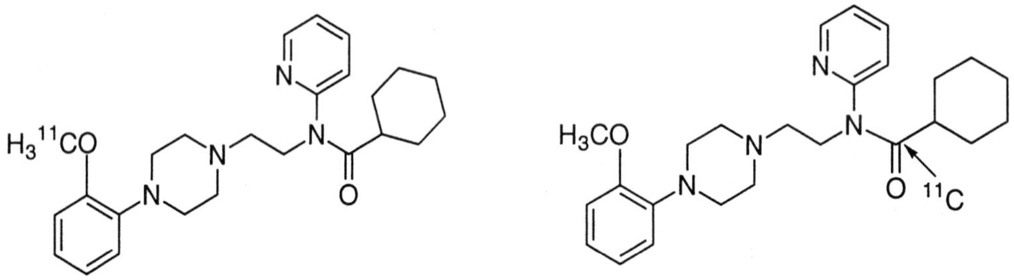

[O-11C-methyl] WAY-100, 635   [carbonyl-11C]WAY-100,635

FIG. 2.6. Structures of labeled compounds in which different label positions have been synthesized and compared either to obtain mechanistic information or to simplify the interpretation of the PET image.

probing enzyme activity (76). 11C-WAY-100635, which has been developed as a radiotracer for the 5-HT$_{1A}$ receptor was initially labeled in the methoxy position but was subsequently labeled in the carbonyl position to reduce the contribution of labeled metabolites (77). Structures of these labeled compounds are shown in Fig. 2.6.

Comparison of Labeled Stereoisomers

Biologic targets (enzymes, receptors, and others) are chiral molecules, and frequently chiral ligands and drugs show binding selectivity for one enantiomer over the other. In

some cases, this is useful in assessing binding specificity. For example, methylphenidate (Ritalin) is a racemic drug that binds to the dopamine transporter and that is used in the treatment of attention deficit hyperactivity disorder and narcolepsy. Comparative PET studies of two enantiomers, 11C-D-*threo*-methylphenidate and 11C-L-*threo*-methylphenidate provided confirmatory evidence that the pharmacologic activity of the drug resides in the D-*threo* enantiomer, which binds to the human striatum in contrast to 11C-L-*threo*-methylphenidate, which shows no specific retention (78). In addition, 11C-D-*threo*-methylphenidate proved to be an excellent radiotracer for measuring dopamine transporter availability in the human brain (79). A comparison of labeled enantiomers has also been applied in the study of radiotracers for the muscarinic cholinergic system, ^{11}C-dexetimide and ^{11}C-levetimide (80). Another example applies to the development of radiotracers for studies of the serotonin transporter. In one case, comparative studies of ^{11}C-(+)McN-5652 and ^{11}C-(−) McN-5662 in both mice and humans showed the expected retention of the (+) enantiomer and clearance of the (−) enantiomer (81).

Although the comparison of active and inactive enantiomers *in vivo* is potentially a powerful mechanistic tool, there are pitfalls. This was encountered in the comparison of the active and inactive enantiomers of cocaine ([−]- and [+]cocaine) to assess cocaine's binding specificity to the dopamine transporter. Instead of demonstrating stereoselective binding in the brain, as was anticipated, the comparison of ^{11}C-labeled (−)- and (+)-cocaine revealed an extraordinarily rapid metabolism of ^{11}C-(+)-cocaine by butyrylcholinesterase, which prevented its penetration into the brain (82). Thus, in this case, rapid peripheral metabolism, rather than stereospecific binding to the dopamine transporter, was responsible for the observed behavior *in vivo*.

Deuterium Isotope Effects

A carbon–hydrogen bond is more easily cleaved than a carbon–deuterium bond. Therefore, if a specific carbon–hydrogen bond in a radiotracer is cleaved in the rate-limiting or rate-contributing step of a chemical or biochemical reaction, its substitution with deuterium will reduce the rate of reaction and reduce the rate of accumulation in tissue.

Deuterium isotope effects have been used as a mechanistic tool in radiotracer studies of MAO, an enzyme known to exhibit strong isotope effects due to the cleavage of the C–H bond α to the nitrogen atom where oxidation is occurring (83). There are several examples in the radiotracer literature, including [^{11}C-L-deprenyl and deuterium-substituted ^{11}C-L-deprenyl; ^{13}N-phenethylamine and deuterium-substituted ^{13}N-phenethylamine; ^{11}C-phenylephrine and deuterium-substituted phenylephrine; 6-^{18}F-fluorodopamine and deuterium-substituted 6-^{18}F-fluorodopamine. The binding of these radiotracers in tissue (and the PET images) shows deuterium isotope effects consistent with MAO-catalyzed cleavage of a specific bond (84–87).

In the case of 6-^{18}F-fluorodopamine, a comparison of deuterium substitution in the α and β positions was used to determine that MAO and not dopamine-β-hydroxylase was responsible for the kinetic profile of 6-^{18}F-fluorodopamine in the heart (86). In the case of ^{11}C-L-deprenyl, the slower rate of trapping of the deuterium-substituted molecule in brain facilitated kinetic modeling in humans (88).

Although the deuterium isotope effect is dramatic in these cases, it is important to note that this only is useful in special cases such as MAO where C–H bond cleavage occurs in the *slow* (rate-limiting) step. Radiotracer structures are shown in Fig. 2.7.

Binding to Plasma Proteins

Organic compounds all bind to plasma proteins to some degree, and in some cases, this limits bioavailability. However, even highly bound compounds can display acceptable bioavailability if binding is rapidly reversible. Nonetheless, there are exceptions that need to be noted. For example, a comparative study of ^{11}C-cocaine and of ^{11}C-labeled iodinated derivatives of cocaine and its *o*-, *m*-, and *p*-isomers showed free fractions of 10%, 0.3%, 1.6%, and 6%. Peak brain uptakes in the baboon as determined with PET imaging corresponded to 0.06%, 0.01%, 0.03%, and 0.04% injected dose per milliliter. The negligible brain uptake for ^{11}C-*o*-iodococaine could be accounted for by a very small free fraction. Subsequent studies showed that binding of ^{11}C-*o*-iodococaine to α$_1$-acid glycoprotein accounted for the low free fraction and presumably for the low brain uptake (89). In another example, 3,4-dihydroxy-5-nitro-2'-fluorobenzophenone (Ro-41-0960), a "central" inhibitor of the enzyme catechol-*O*-methyltransferase (COMT) was labeled with ^{18}F to image COMT in the brain (90). Although Ro-41-0960 is similar to tolcapone, which is marketed for Parkinson therapy as a central COMT inhibitor, PET studies in the baboon with ^{18}F-Ro-41-0960 showed no brain uptake. Incubation of ^{18}F-Ro-41-0960 with whole baboon blood showed more than 99% of the tracer was associated with plasma proteins. This may account for its failure to enter the brain in spite of its partition coefficient of 4, which would normally suggest that it would readily enter the brain.

RADIOTRACERS FOR NEUROTRANSMITTER SYSTEMS

The development of radiotracers for imaging neurotransmitter systems (including their receptors, their plasma membrane and vesicular transporters, the enzymes that synthesize and degrade them, and the processes involved in signal transduction) has dominated radiotracer research. The reasons for this are obvious when one considers that mental processes are driven by the complex interplay of neurotransmitter systems and that their disruption underlies many diseases of the central nervous system (CNS) (91). Indeed PET has made it possible to visualize many different aspects of neurotransmitter activity in living systems. In the following sections, we highlight some of the major transmitter systems including the dopamine system, the opiate system, the serotonin system, the benzodiazepine system, and the cholinergic system. Where possible, we refer to review articles that summarize each area in more detail.

The Brain Dopamine System

Dopamine plays a pivotal role in the regulation of movement, motivation, and cognition. It is also closely linked

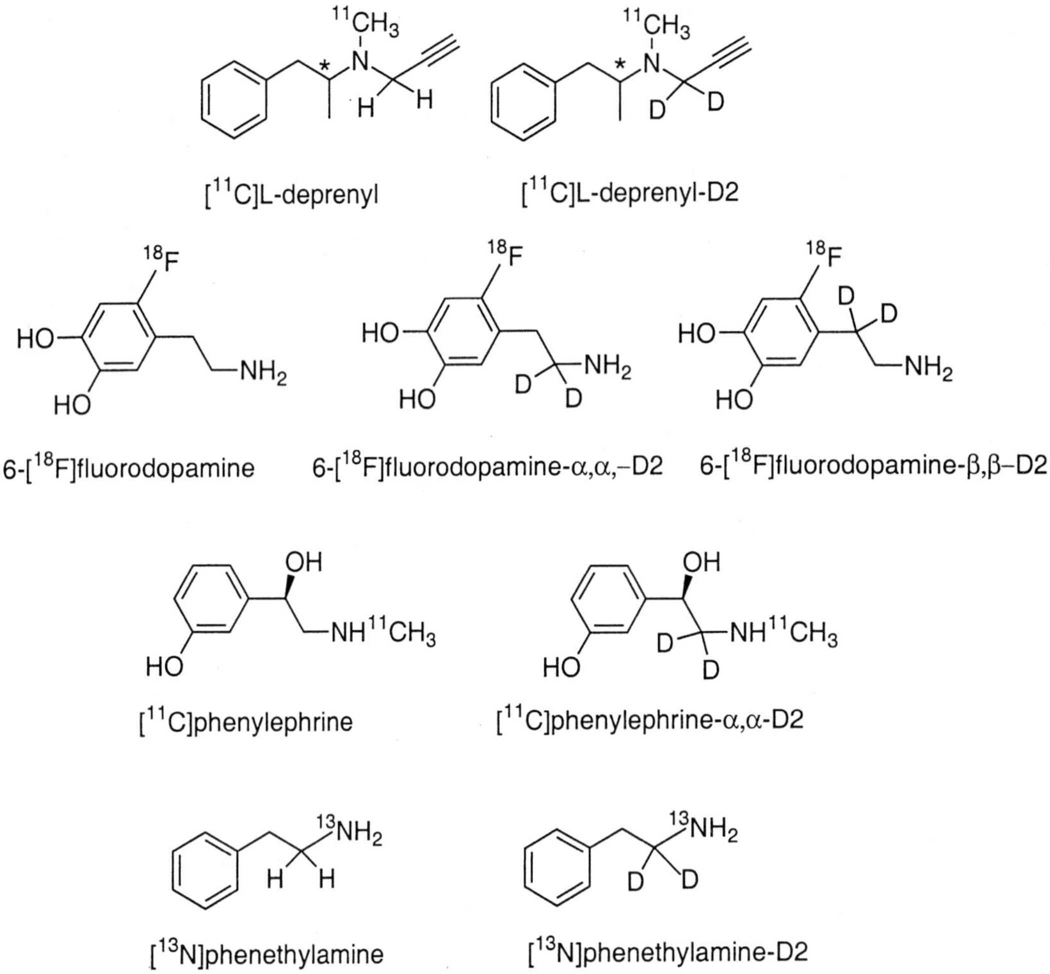

FIG. 2.7. Structures of labeled compounds substituted with deuterium to obtain mechanistic information and/or to improve radiotracer kinetics.

to reward, reinforcement, and addiction, and it is a major molecular target of drugs to treat Parkinson disease and schizophrenia. Drugs abused by humans also elevate brain dopamine, though by a variety of different mechanisms. Because of its importance, the study of the brain dopamine system has been a major focus in the basic and clinical neurosciences, and it is by far the most widely studied neurotransmitter system in PET research (92,93).

Dopamine is synthesized in the dopaminergic neurons in the substantia nigra, the ventral tegmental area, and the retrorubral area of the mesencephalon. It is stored within vesicles to protect it from oxidation by MAO. It is released into the synapse in response to an action potential and interacts with dopamine receptors that are present on both postsynaptic sites (where they function in cell-to-cell communication) and on presynaptic sites (where they regulate exocytotic release and dopamine synthesis). There are five subtypes of dopamine receptors, which are grouped in two major families, those that stimulate adenylate cyclase (D_1, D_5) and those that inhibit it (D_2, D_3, D_4) (94). The dopamine D_1 and D_2

receptors have significantly higher concentrations than the other subtypes and have the highest density in the striatum. Quantitative PET studies of the brain dopamine system are facilitated by the high concentration of dopamine receptors and dopamine transporters in the basal ganglia and an absence of these elements in the cerebellum.

The synaptic concentration of dopamine is regulated primarily by reuptake. Dopamine release is regulated by presynaptic autoreceptors and by other neuroanatomically distinct neurotransmitters through interactions with the dopamine neuron (95). Dopamine is also removed by oxidation by MAO and methylation by COMT.

Dopamine Metabolism

Dopamine does not cross the blood–brain barrier, so the investigation of brain dopamine metabolism with PET required a labeled derivative of L-DOPA, the amino acid precursor of dopamine that is transported into the brain via the large neutral amino acid carrier. ^{18}F-fluoro-DOPA was the first radiotracer developed to probe brain dopamine metabolism (96,97). 6-^{18}F-Fluoro-DOPA crosses the blood–brain barrier and is accumulated in dopamine terminals and converted to 6-^{18}F-fluorodopamine (98). Decreased ^{18}F-fluoro-DOPA accumulation is associated with the loss of dopaminergic neurons (99). Because the metabolism of ^{18}F-fluoro-DOPA is complex, ^{18}F-labeled *m*-tyrosine, which has simpler metabolism, has also been developed to improve quantitation (100). ^{11}C-L-DOPA has also been synthesized with the label in two different positions and represents a labeled version of the native amino acid (Fig. 2.6) (101).

Dopamine Receptors

Although there are five dopamine receptor subtypes, only radiotracers with specificity for dopamine D_2 and D_1 receptors have been developed. Dopamine D_1 and D_2 receptors are highly concentrated in the striatum, with lower concentrations occurring in extrastriatal regions. High-affinity radiotracers are required for imaging extrastriatal receptors because of their low density. Although most of the radiotracer development work has focused on labeled dopamine receptor antagonists, agonists are also of interest because of the potential to image the high-affinity state of the receptor.

Dopamine D_2 receptor availability has been examined with PET using ^{11}C- and ^{18}F-labeled antagonists to the D_2 receptor. For example, *N*-methylspiroperidol has been labeled with ^{11}C and with ^{18}F and used to measure dopamine receptor availability and absolute concentration in the healthy and diseased brain and to probe dopamine receptor occupancy by antipsychotic drugs (102–105). 3-(2′-^{18}F-fluoroethyl)spiperone has also been used for the quantitative estimation of D_2 receptor sites (106,107), including its expression as a marker/reporter gene (108). The irreversible or near-irreversible binding of the spiroperidol derivatives has been a limitation in terms of quantitation because the receptor-binding parameter may be influenced by radiotracer delivery.

^{11}C-Raclopride is the most widely used PET radiotracer for studies of dopamine D_2 receptor availability (109,110). Drug-induced changes in synaptic dopamine have also been measured with ^{11}C-raclopride because its moderate affinity for the dopamine D_2 receptor and reversible binding allow it to compete with dopamine in the synapse (111,112). Repeated measures with ^{11}C-raclopride with an intervening challenge with dopamine-enhancing drugs such as methylphenidate and amphetamine have been successfully used to assess dopaminergic function (113–115).

High-affinity reversibly binding benzamide radiotracers have also been developed to allow a longer scanning period and higher striatum : cerebellum ratios and to potentially image extrastriatal dopamine D_2 receptors, which are present in low concentration. There are a number of examples including the ^{18}F-fluoropropylbenzamines (116–119) such as ^{18}F-fallypride, as well as a ^{11}C tracer ^{11}C-FLB 457 (120). It has also been recently reported that extrastriatal ^{11}C-FLB 457 binding is sensitive to drug-induced increases in dopamine (121).

The development of radiotracers to label *in vivo* the high-affinity state of the dopamine D_2 receptor has been approached by a number of investigators (122–124). In particular, recent PET studies with ($-$)-*N*-(^{11}C)propyl-norapomorphine show a striatum : cerebellum ratio of 2.8 in the primate, so it is promising as a tracer for agonist affinity states of the D_2 receptor (125).

The D_1 receptor antagonists, SCH-23390 and SCH-39166, have also been labeled with ^{11}C and used to study the CNS D_1 receptor (126). More recently, a high-affinity ligand ^{11}C-labeled NNC-112 has been developed for imaging extrastriatal D_1 receptors in humans (127). The positive enantiomer of NNC-112 binds selectively and reversibly while the negative enantiomer did not show appreciable binding. Recent studies with ^{11}C-NNC-12 in humans have shown that kinetic analysis of uptake provides an appropriate method with which to derive dopamine D_1 receptor parameters in regions of both high and low receptor density (128). Dopamine D_1 agonist ligands ^{11}C-SKF-75670 and ^{11}C-SKF-82957 also show promise for PET studies of the functional high-affinity state of D_1 receptors (129). Structures of some of these compounds are shown in Fig. 2.8.

It is interesting that dopamine v receptor radioligands ^{11}C-NNC-756 and ^{11}C-SCH-23390 do not appear to compete with endogenous dopamine, possibly due to the predominantly extrasynaptic location of the D_1 receptor (130,131).

An attempt to visualize the D_4 receptor with ^{11}C-*N*-[2-[4-(4-chlorophenyl)piperazin-1-yl]ethyl]-3- methoxybenzamide (^{11}C-PB-12) was unsuccessful, probably due to the low concentration of dopamine D_4 receptors, insufficient binding affinity of the ligand, and high background nonspecific binding (132).

Dopamine Transporters

The plasma membrane dopamine transporter has been studied using ^{11}C-nomifensine (133), ^{11}C-cocaine (134), ^{11}C-D-*threo*-methylphenidate (135), cocaine analogues (136–143), and ^{18}F-GBR-13119 (144). These tracers and others have been applied in studies of neurodegeneration, aging, and dopamine transporter occupancy by drugs including cocaine and methylphenidate (136,145–149). ^{11}C-Cocaine is worthy of mention. Although it was initially developed to measure cocaine pharmacokinetics in the human brain, its rapid reversible kinetics have also served to measure dopamine transporter availability using a graphical analysis for reversible systems (150). The structures of some of these dopamine transporter radioligands are shown in Fig. 2.9.

Vesicular amine transporters (VMAT2) remove monamines like dopamine from the cytosol into intracellular vesicles, where they are protected from intracellular enzymes such as MAO and stored for eventual exocytotic release. Studies have shown that VMAT2 is not altered by regulatory

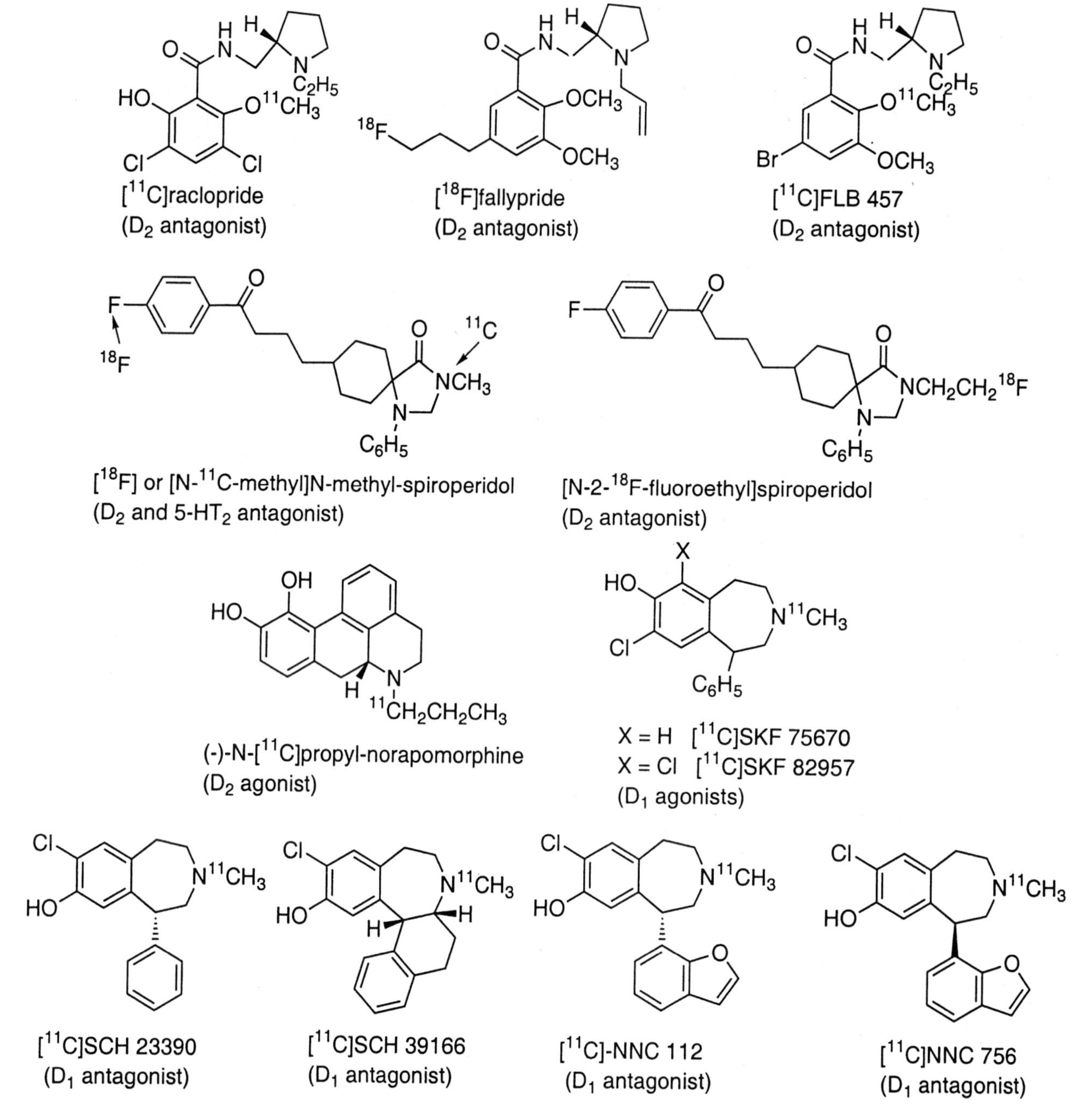

FIG. 2.8. Structures of some of the radioligands developed for studies of dopamine receptors (D_1 and D_2).

responses to nigrostriatal lesions or changes in dopamine synthesis or turnover (151,152). Thus, VMAT2 is a useful molecular target for dopamine terminal density. Accordingly, $\alpha(+)$-^{11}C-dihydrotetrabenazine (Fig. 2.10) has emerged as an excellent radiotracer, devoid of lipophilic metabolites and showing stereoselectivity and kinetics amenable to modeling (153–155). Studies in normal aging and Parkinson disease have been carried out, showing a small decline in normal aging and the expected marked decreased in Parkinson disease (156). It is noteworthy that even though

labeled tetrabenazine also binds to other vesicular monoamine transporters, most of the transporters in the striatum are dopamine transporters.

Monoamine Oxidase

Dopamine is also regulated by MAO, a flavin-containing enzyme that exists in two subtypes (MAO-A and MAO-B). MAO oxidizes amines including dopamine and other neurotransmitters (157). Medical interest in MAO stems

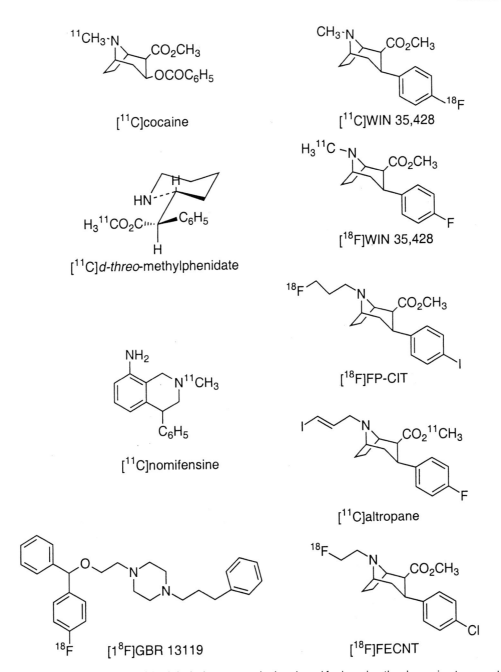

FIG. 2.9. Structures of some of the labeled compounds developed for imaging the dopamine transporter.

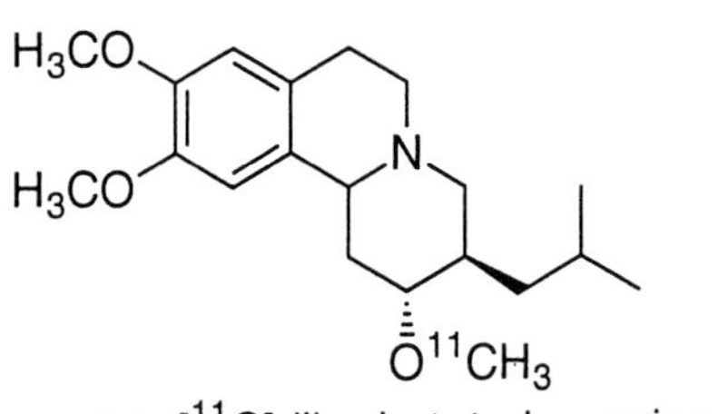

α–(+)–[¹¹C]dihydrotetrabenazine

FIG. 2.10. Structure of α(+)-carbon-11-dihydrotetrabenazine for studies of the vesicular monoamine transporter.

from the utility of MAO inhibitor drugs in the treatment of depression and Parkinson disease. The first images of functional MAO activity in the human brain were made with ^{11}C-labeled suicide enzyme inactivators (^{11}C-clorgyline and ^{11}C-L-deprenyl), which covalently label the enzyme *in vivo* (158). Mechanistic PET studies with deuterium-substituted ^{11}C-L-deprenyl demonstrated that the C–H bond in the propargyl group was involved in the rate-limiting step for the formation of the PET image and provided a means of selectively controlling the rate of trapping of tracer in brain to improve quantitation (88). ^{11}C-L-deprenyl and the deuterium-substituted derivative have been used to directly exam-

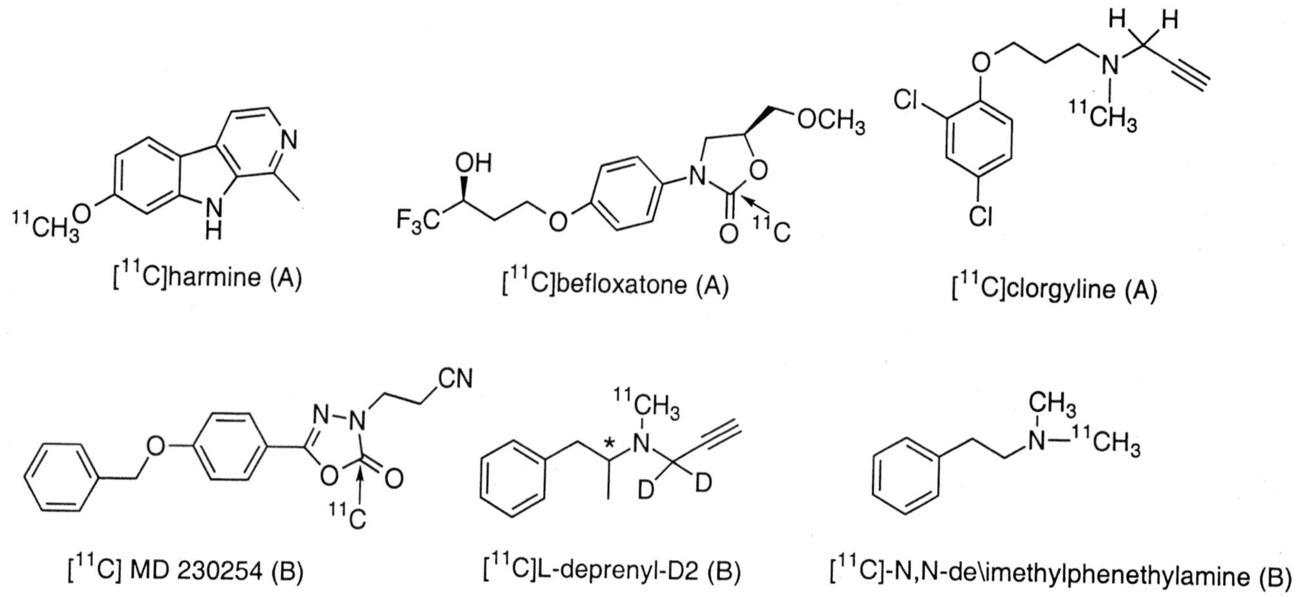

FIG. 2.11. Radiotracers for PET studies of monoamine oxidase (MAO). Subtype specificity (MAO type A or type B) is in parenthesis.

ine the effects of MAO-B inhibitor drugs, lazabemide and L-deprenyl in the human brain (159,160).

^{11}C-Clorgyline and ^{11}C-L-deprenyl-D$_2$ and PET have also revealed a reduction in MAO-A and MAO-B in smokers (161,162). This is a pharmacologic effect of smoke, because former smokers have normal MAO levels. Interestingly, the MAO-B inhibitory constituent in smoke is not nicotine. In fact, an MAO inhibitory compound was recently isolated from tobacco leaves (163). Reduced brain MAO in smokers may be an important neurochemical link to smoking epidemiology, including the documented decreased risk of Parkinson disease in smokers (164).

A number of labeled selective, reversible inhibitors of MAO-A including ^{11}C-harmine, ^{11}C-methylharmine, ^{11}C-harmaline, ^{11}C-MD 230254, and ^{11}C-blefoxatone have also been developed and evaluated for their specificity as MAO tracers *in vivo* (39,165,166). Structures of some of the labeled MAO tracers are shown in Fig. 2.11.

The Brain Serotonin System

The cells that produce serotonin are located in the dorsal raphe nucleus, which extensively innervates neocortical regions. Abnormalities in the brain serotonin system have been implicated in various neuropsychiatric disorders such as anxiety, depression, sleep disorders, eating disorders, and violence. Drugs that change serotonin levels have been widely used in the treatment of depression, anxiety, and obesity. The physiologic actions of serotonin are mediated through its interactions with serotonin receptors. These are now assigned to one of seven families, 5-HT$_{1-7}$, comprising a total

of 14 structurally and pharmacologically distinct mammalian 5-HT receptor subtypes (167). Thus far, most of the effort in PET radiotracer development has been focused on the 5-HT$_{2A}$ and the 5-HT$_{1A}$ receptor subtypes, as well as the serotonin transporter.

Progress in the development of radiotracers for the 5-HT$_{2A}$ receptors was reviewed in 1992 and 1996 (168,169). ^{11}C-N-Methylspiroperidol labeled with ^{11}C and with ^{18}F binds both to the dopamine D$_2$ receptor in the striatum and to the 5-HT$_{2A}$ receptor in the frontal cortex and has been used to image the 5-HT$_{2A}$ receptor (170,171). Other more selective 5-HT$_{2A}$ radiotracers including ^{18}F-altanserin (172), ^{18}F-setoperone (173), and ^{11}C-MDL-100907 (174,175) have been developed and applied in human studies. As with most PET radiotracers, none of these is perfect and each has problems with either lipophilic metabolites, nonspecific binding, binding to other neurotransmitter receptors, or slow kinetics, making their quantification susceptible to blood-flow artifacts. The quantification of 5-HT$_{2A}$ receptors with ^{18}F-altanserin in the human brain has been examined using a constant infusion paradigm to reduce the difficulties associated with lipophilic radiolabeled metabolites (176). Structures of some of these labeled compounds are shown in Fig. 2.12.

5-HT$_{1A}$ receptors are concentrated on cell bodies of the raphe nuclei and serve as autoreceptors mediating serotonin release. They occur both presynaptically and postsynaptically. There is a high density of 5-HT$_{1A}$ postsynaptic receptors in the neocortex. The presynaptic sites have been proposed to mediate drug treatment of anxiety and depression while postsynaptic sites have been found to be elevated in schizophrenic brains postmortem. Radiotracer studies of the

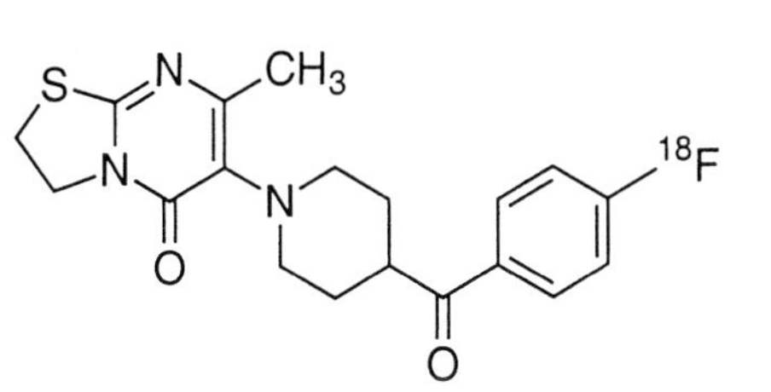

[^{18}F]setoperone
(5-HT_{2A} antagonist)

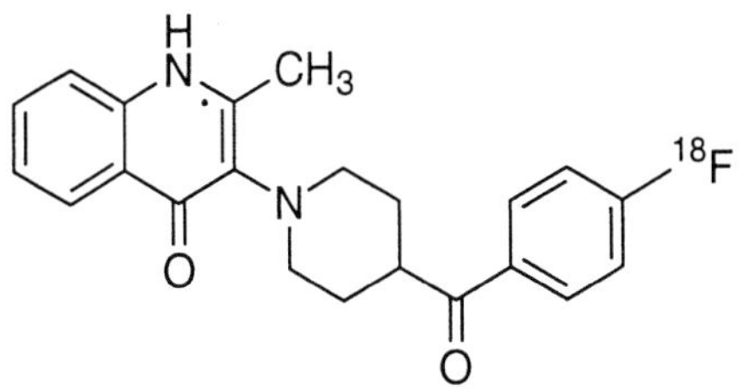

[^{18}F]altanserin
(5-HT_{2A} antagonist)

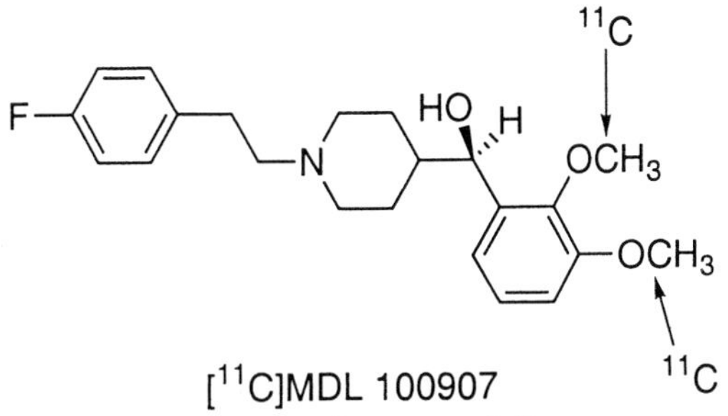

[^{11}C]MDL 100907
(5-HT_{2A} antagonist)

FIG. 2.12. Radiotracers for PET studies of the 5-HT_{2A} receptor.

5-v receptor have used the WAY-100635 structure as a template. WAY-100635 was first labeled with ^{11}C in the *O*-methyl group (177). This radiotracer was metabolized rapidly producing a lipophilic-labeled metabolite, WAY-100634, via loss of the cyclohexanecarbonyl group (178, 179). Unfortunately, this metabolite also has a high affinity for the 5-HT_{1A} receptor and crosses the blood–brain barrier, limiting quantitation. For this reason, WAY-100635 was later labeled in the carbonyl group (77) to avoid the formation of the ^{11}C-WAY-100634 (see Fig. 2.6). Human studies with both labeled versions of WAY-100635 have been carried out, with improved delineation of 5-HT_{1A} receptors being obtained with the ^{11}C-carbonyl compound (180).

Initial human studies have also been carried out with ^{11}C-CPC-222, a compound similar in structure to WAY-100635, with a bicyclooctyl group replacing the cyclohexyl group. This structurally modified compound is not metabolized to WAY-100634, so labeling in the *N*-methyl group (which is simpler) does not carry the disadvantage found with carbonyl-labeled WAY-100635 (181). The synthesis and *in vitro* evaluation of ^{11}C-(R)-3-*N,N*-dicyclobutylamino-8-fluoro-3,4-dihydro-2H-benzopyran-5-carboxamide (^{11}C-NAD-299; see equation 2.6) in human brain indicated that it is also a promising ligand for the 5-HT_{1A} receptor (182). An ^{18}F-labeled radiotracer (*p*-^{18}F-MPPF; ^{18}F-4-(2'-methoxyphenyl)-1-[2'-[*N*-(2''-pyridinyl)-*p*-^{18}F-fluorobenzamido]ethyl]-piperazine) for the 5-HT_{1A} receptor has also been prepared and human studies show promise (183–185). A special issue of *Nuclear Medicine and Biology* was recently dedicated to the imaging of 5-HT_{1A} receptors (186).

Radiotracers have also been developed to image the serotonin transporter, which removes serotonin from the synapse. The serotonin transporter is also the molecular target for the selective serotonin reuptake inhibitor class of antidepressant drugs. This is an important area in radiotracer development because of the need to assess toxicity to serotonergic neurons by compounds such as methylenedioxymethamphetamine. Accordingly, the pyrrolo isoquinoline McN-5652 was labeled with ^{11}C by S-methylation of the normethyl precursor (187). McN-5652 has a chiral center. The positive enantiomer is active while the negative enantiomer is inactive (Fig. 2.13). PET studies in humans have compared the two enantiomers using the negative enantiomer to assess nonspecific binding (188). Although the distribution of (+)-^{11}C-McN-5652 parallels the known distribution of serotonin transporters, there is evidence that it underestimates nonspecific binding in some brain regions (189,190). Another serotonin transporter ligand, ^{11}C-*N,N*-dimethyl-2-(2-amino-4-cyanophenylthio)benzylamine (^{11}C-DSAB) has been shown to have very attractive properties to image the serotonin transporter in recent human studies (191). ^{11}C-Citalopram, *N*-^{11}C-methylparoxetine, and ^{11}C-fluoxetine all have low target : nontarget ratios (144,192,193).

The possibility of measuring the serotonin synthesis rate has also been probed by ^{11}C-α-methyltryptophan (194,195), although recent PET studies in monkeys report that ^{11}C-

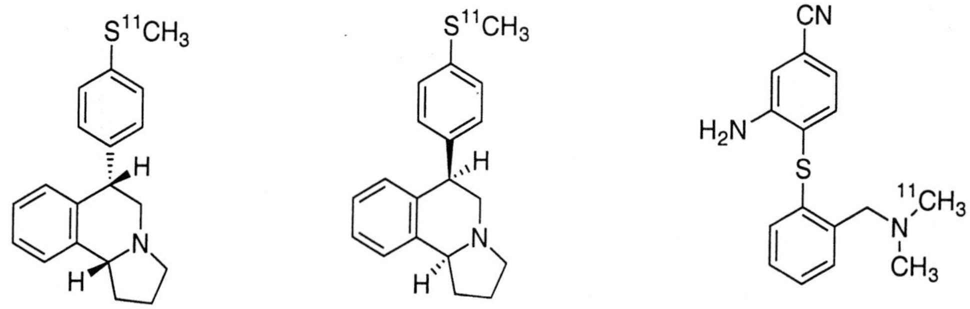

FIG. 2.13. Structures of radiotracers for studies of the serotonin transporter.

α-methyltryptophan is acting predominantly as a tracer of tryptophan uptake (196).

The Brain Opiate System

Opiate receptors mediate the effects of endogenous and exogenous opioids including respiratory depression, analgesia, reward, and sedation. There are three major opiate receptor subtypes, μ, δ, and κ with subclasses of these subtypes. The first PET tracer for the opiate receptor was ^{11}C-carfentanil, a high affinity μ opiate agonist (197). ^{11}C-Carfentanil localizes in opiate receptor–rich regions of the human brain such as the basal ganglia and the thalamus (198). Its uptake can be reduced by pretreatment with the opiate antagonist, naloxone. PET studies with ^{11}C-carfentanil suggest that both age and gender are variables to consider in the interpretation of measures of brain opioid function (199). Another nonsubtype-specific opiate agonist ^{11}C-diprenorphine has been synthesized using 1-^{11}C-cyclopropanecarbonyl chloride (200). Buprenorphine, a compound with a combination of agonist and antagonist properties, has been labeled with ^{11}C in two different positions, the O-methyl position (201–203) and the cyclopropylmethyl position (204). Comparison between ^{11}C-buprenorphine and ^{11}C-diprenorphine in the baboon shows that ^{11}C-diprenorphine may be superior for PET studies due to its more rapid clearance from the cerebellum. However, buprenorphine has low toxicity and it is an approved analgesic drug that could facilitate approval for human studies. The high-affinity opiate antagonist cyclofoxy binds to both μ and κ sites. It has been labeled with ^{18}F for opiate receptor imaging with PET (205,206). Recently a high-affinity κ-selective compound, GR89696 was labeled with ^{11}C and shows promise in mice for *in vivo* binding to κ sites (207). Delta opioid receptors have been imaged in the human brain with ^{11}C-naltrindol and PET (208). Structures of some of these labeled compounds are in Fig. 2.14.

The Benzodiazepine System

Benzodiazepines are a class of chemical compounds that are potent anxiolytics, anticonvulsants, and hypnotics. Binding sites for the benzodiazepines have been subdivided into "central" and "peripheral" types. Central types are thought to constitute one of the subunits on the γ-aminobutyric acid A (GABA$_A$) receptor complex and are responsible for the anxiolytic actions of this class of drugs through facilitation of the inhibitory actions of GABA (209). Peripheral binding sites are not associated with GABA and have very low affinity for the central type (210). However, they display high affinity for the benzodiazepine Ro-5-4864 and the isoquinoline derivative PK-11195, both of which are inactive at the central site. Peripheral binding sites occur in the kidneys, liver, and lungs, as well as mast cells and macrophages. However, they also occur in the CNS on nonneuronal elements such as glial and ependymal cells.

Radiotracers for PET imaging of both the central and the peripheral benzodiazepine receptors have been developed, and progress was reviewed in 1996 (211). For the central site, the most completely studied radiotracer is ^{11}C-Ro-15-1788 (^{11}C-flumazenil), a benzodiazepine antagonist. With ^{11}C-Ro-15-1788 and PET, a clear dose-dependent binding was demonstrated (212). ^{11}C-Ro-15-1788 also has excellent kinetic properties for the quantitative measurement of the central site, permitting parametric images of flow and benzodiazepine receptor availability from a single tracer injection (213). It has been applied in the study of epilepsy, in which it was shown that receptor binding was significantly lower in the area of the epileptic focus (214). Another benzodiazepine antagonist iomazenil, which was originally labeled with iodine-123 for single-photon emission computed tomography studies, has been labeled with ^{11}C in high specific activity and has been shown to provide a reliable measure of benzodiazepine receptor binding using a three-compartment model and more than 30-minute acquisition time (215).

Peripheral benzodiazepine receptors have been imaged with the isoquinoline ^{11}C-PK-11195 and ^{11}C-Ro-5-4864 with different results. Whereas ^{11}C-Ro-5-4864 showed a lower uptake in tumor than in normal brain tissue (216), ^{11}C-PK-11195 showed a high uptake in glioma relative to normal brain tissue (217). Moreover, tumor uptake was sat-

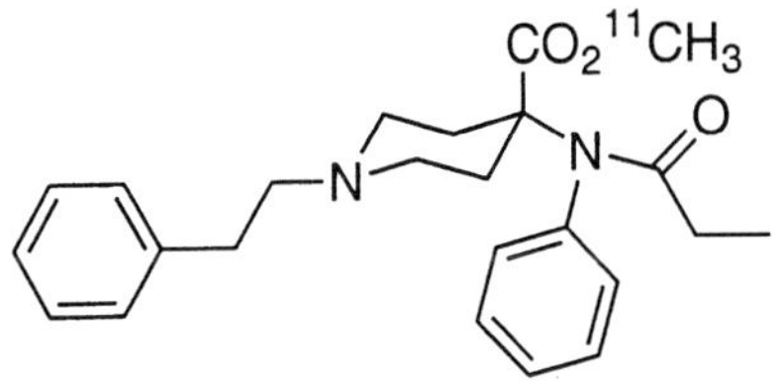

[11C]carfentanyl
(μ agonist)

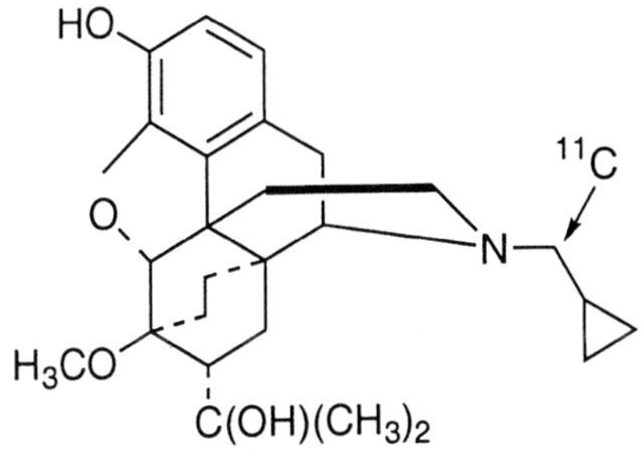

[11C]diprenorphine
(mixed; agonist)

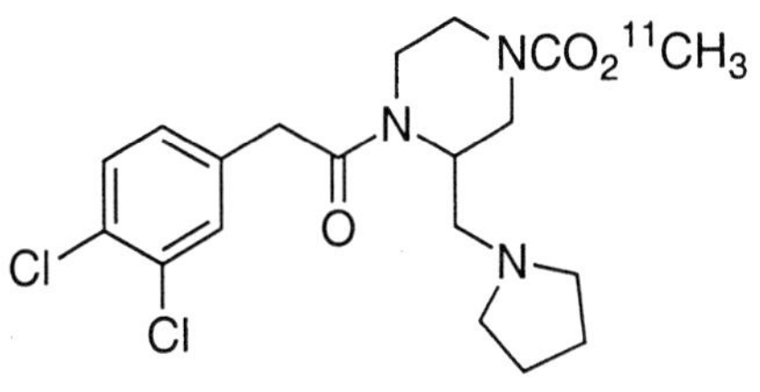

[11C]GR89696
(κ antagonist)

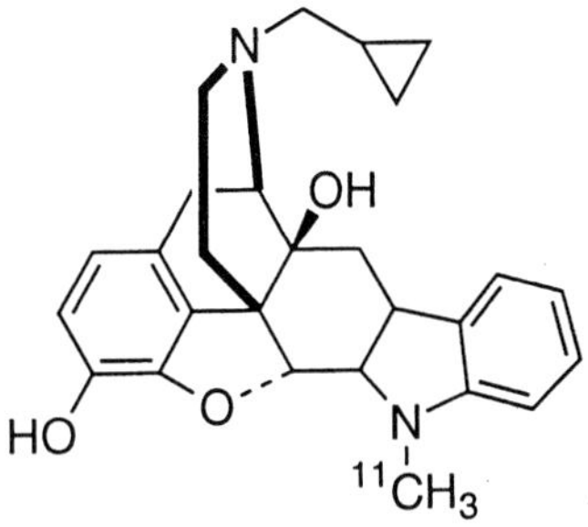

[11C]naltrindole
(δ antagonist)

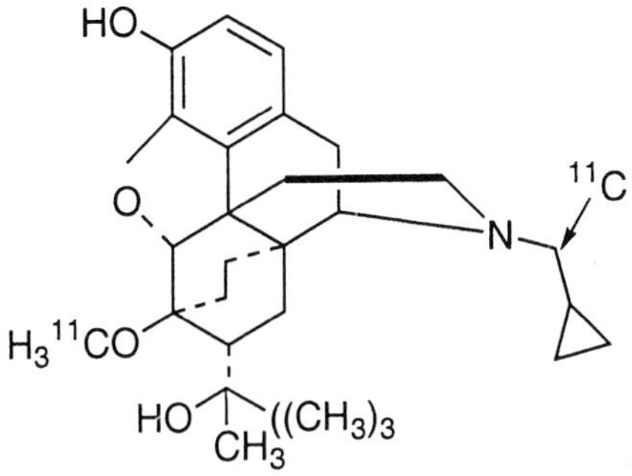

[11C]buprenorphine
(mixed; agonist/antagonist)

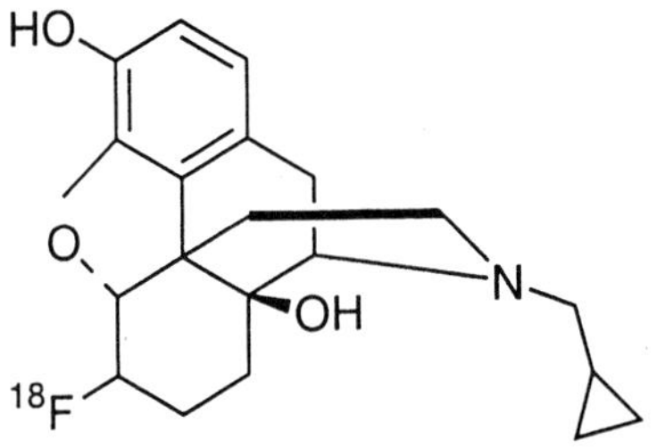

(-)-[18F]cyclofoxy
(mixed; antagonist)

FIG. 2.14. Structures of some of the radiotracers developed for PET studies of opioid receptors. Receptor subtype is indicated in parenthesis.

urable, indicating a receptor-mediated process. A high signal-to-noise ratio was obtained in non–contrast-enhancing gliomas, demonstrating that uptake was not related to blood–brain barrier breakdown. More recently, ^{11}C-PK-11195 was examined as a marker for activated microglia in the human brain in multiple sclerosis after *in vitro* radioligand studies that showed that microglial activation leads to an increase in the number of peripheral benzodiazepine binding sites. This study showed an increase in ^{11}C-PK-11195 binding in areas of focal pathology identified by magnetic resonance imaging and additional binding in areas of central gray matter, which delineated projection areas (218).

Structures of some of these compounds are shown in Fig. 2.15.

The Cholinergic System

There are two major classes of receptors for the neurotransmitter acethycholine (ACh), the muscarinic cholinergic

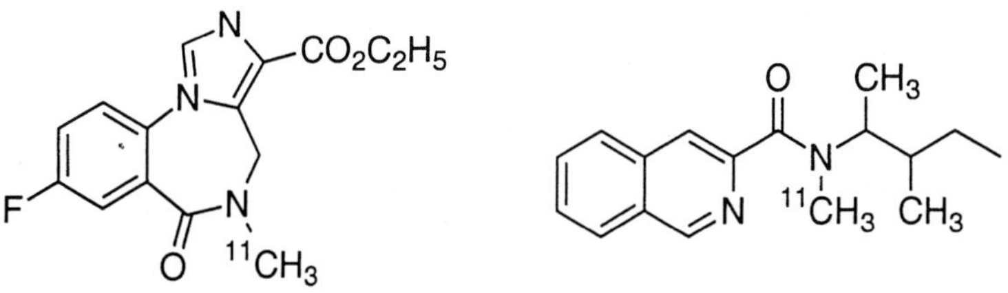

FIG. 2.15. Structures of labeled compounds for PET studies of central and peripheral benzodiazepine receptors.

[^11^C]Ro15 1788
(central)

[^11^C]PK-11195
(peripheral)

receptors (mAChRs) and the nicotinic acetylcholine receptors (nAChRs). Because of the importance of ACh in learning and memory and mounting evidence of cholinergic deficits in Alzheimer disease (219), the receptors mediating cholinergic neurotransmission, as well as enzymes such as choline acetyltransferase (ChAT) that mediate its synthesis, and acetylcholinesterase (AChE), which terminates its action, are of intense interest and prime targets for radiotracer development (220).

Muscarinic Cholinergic Receptors

The mAChRs can be divided into four pharmacologically distinct subtypes (M_1 through M_4) and into five genetically distinct subtypes (m1 through m5) (221). The development of radiotracers suitable for imaging this system, particularly the M_2 subtype, has been pursued for many years because this subtype is involved in Alzheimer disease (222). PET tracers ^{11}C-scopolamine (223), ^{11}C-tropanylbenzilate (224), and ^{11}C-N-methyl-4-piperidinyl benzilate (225) have been developed and evaluated. ^{11}C-Tropanyl benzilate has been applied in studies of normal aging, where it was reported that there is not a significant decline of these proteins in normal aging (226). A very recent study assessing muscarinic receptor concentration in normal aging and Alzheimer disease with ^{11}C-N-methyl-4-piperidinyl benzilate reported that aging is associated with a decrease in binding in neocortical regions and in thalamus, but that the quantitation of binding in patients with Alzheimer disease is limited by statistical uncertainty, requiring normalization to a reference region and therefore limiting its use in neurodegenerative processes (227). A previous study reported that binding is decreased in Alzheimer disease (228). In a recent PET study in monkeys, a positional isomer, ^{11}C-N-methyl-3-piperidinyl benzilate has been reported to be superior to the 4-isomer in terms of regional distribution and region-to-cerebellum ratios (229).

The anticholinergic drug benztropine mesylate (Cogentin) has been labeled with ^{11}C and its regional distribution in the human brain has been shown to parallel cholinergic receptors, and its uptake in the baboon brain can be reduced by blockade with both cholinergic antagonists such as scopolamine and agonists such as pilocarpine (230). ^{11}C-Benztropine also shows a reduction in specific binding in the human

brain with increasing age (231). ^{11}C-Dexetimide, a potent muscarinic cholinergic antagonist, and levetimide, its inactive enantiomer, have also been synthesized for studies of this receptor system (80).

In general, tracers for the muscarinic cholinergic receptors have been limited by low subtype selectivity, as well as very rapid binding and slow dissociation, limiting the resolution of blood-flow effects from receptor binding (232). In a recent development, an M_2 selective agonist 3-(3-(3-^{18}F-fluoropropyl)thio-1,2,5-thiadiazol-4-yl)-1,2,5,6-tetrahydro-1-methylpyridine (^{18}F-FP-TZTP) was synthesized (233). PET studies in six rhesus monkeys showed a binding pattern consistent with the distribution of M_2 sites. In addition, pretreatment with the AChE inhibitor physostigmine caused a reduction in ^{18}F-FP-TZTP binding, indicating that the tracer is sensitive to drug-induced changes in ACh. The degree of reduction is smallest in the striatum, which has high levels of AChE (234). Thus, this tracer shows promise for PET studies of the mAChRs (M_2 subtype) and for the measurement of drug-induced changes in ACh.

Acetylcholinesterase

AChE hydrolyzes ACh, so it is crucial for ACh regulation. The consequences of its inhibition are of great importance both in toxicology and in therapeutics. Because Alzheimer disease is characterized by a deficiency in cholinergic activity, cholinesterase inhibitors represent the most extensively developed class of compounds for its treatment. Similar to the mAChR, the development of radiotracers for quantitation of AChE offers the potential of gaining more insight into the pathophysiology of Alzheimer disease, as well as a tool for the design, development, and evaluation of cholinergic therapy.

There have been two approaches to radiotracer development for studies of AChE: the synthesis of labeled inhibitors of AChE such as ^{11}C-physostigmine (^{11}C-PHY), which measures the number of binding sites and the synthesis of labeled substrates of AChE such as []N-^{11}C-methyl]-4-piperidinyl acetate (^{11}C-AMP) and [N-^{11}C-methyl]4-piperidinyl propionate (^{11}C-PMP), which measures enzyme activity. Both of these classes of radiotracers have been evaluated in healthy human subjects with PET.

Physostigmine inhibits AChE by covalent attachment of

the carbamate moiety to the enzyme. ^{11}C-PHY has been synthesized from ^{11}C-methylisocyanate and eseroline (235). The label is on the carboxyl carbon atom. This ensures covalent binding of ^{11}C with the serine residue of the enzyme's active site, so the retention of ^{11}C after the injection of ^{11}C-PHY would, in principle, represent AChE activity. Human studies with ^{11}C-PHY showed a retention pattern of ^{11}C, typical of AChE activity with a striatum-to-cortex ratio of 2 (236).

Another approach to measuring the number of binding sites of AChE uses a ^{11}C-labeled substrate for AChE, such as ^{11}C-AMP or ^{11}C-PMP. These radiotracers are labeled in the *N*-methyl position such that when they are hydrolyzed by AChE, the labeled hydrophilic product (which has limited ability to diffuse out of the brain) is trapped at the site of AChE activity in proportion to AChE activity and cerebral blood flow (237). Because of the need to optimize the rate of trapping of radiotracer so the concentration of radioactivity in a volume element of tissue is not limited by radiotracer delivery into the brain, different esters have been evaluated. In a comparison of ^{11}C-AMP and ^{11}C-PMP, ^{11}C-PMP was found to have a slower rate of hydrolysis, which makes it a more favorable candidate (238). Accordingly, PET studies of AChE with ^{11}C-PMP in normal aging and Alzheimer disease revealed stable AChE levels in normal aging and deficits in Alzheimer disease. As predicted from monkey studies, the measures of AChE were independent of changes in brain blood flow (239). These radioligands can be used to assess the efficacy of the various anticholinesterases used therapeutically and to determine the doses required to achieve optimal inhibition. They can also help identify patients in whom the concentration of AChE may be too low for anticholinesterases to be effective.

Radiotracers have also been developed to image cholinergic terminals. One of these, ^{18}F-NEFA, an aminobenzovesamicol, was studied in primates with PET to probe striatal dopamine D_2/ACh interactions (240). The measurement of cholinergic terminal density through imaging of the vesicular ACh transporter with [18]F-(+)-4-fluorobenzyltrozamicol has recently been studied (241). One of the difficulties in radiotracer development in this area is the high toxicity of model compounds.

Structures of some of these compounds are shown in Fig. 2.16.

Nicotinic Cholinergic Receptors

nAChRs are excitatory ligand-gated cation channels. They are widely distributed in the CNS and the peripheral nervous system, the neuromuscular junction, and the adrenal glands. The nAChR is the major molecular target for nicotine and it is also emerging as an important molecular target for the development of drugs to treat neurodegenerative disorders and pain (242). nAChRs are associated with the axons and cell bodies of neurons that comprise several major neurotransmitter systems including the dopamine, norepinephrine, ACh, GABA, and glutamate neurons (243). Neuronal nAChRs are believed to mediate the CNS effects of nicotine on motor activity, alertness, emotional state, neuroendocrine function, reward, and pain (244). They exist as pentamers comprised of α and β subunits, leading to considerable diversity. The most abundant subtype in the mammalian brain is the $\alpha_4\beta_2$, which also has the highest affinity for nicotine. Studies with β_2 knockout mice suggest a role for the β_2-containing nicotinic receptors in nicotine reinforcement (245). Studies in human brain postmortem have documented losses in nAChR with normal aging, which is accentuated in Alzheimer disease (246). In contrast, nAChRs are *elevated* in smokers (247).

There have been three general classes of compounds developed as radiotracers for nAChRs: nicotine and its derivatives; epibatidine and its derivatives; and 3-pyridyl ether derivatives (248). Although ^{11}C-nicotine has been used in human studies, images are dominated by nonspecific binding, making ^{11}C-nicotine a poor tracer for nicotinic binding sites (249,250). Two other nicotinic agonists, (R,S)-1-[^{11}C]methyl-2-(3-pyridyl)azetidine (^{11}C-MPA) and (S)-3-methyl-5-(1-[^{11}C]methyl-2-pyrrolidinyl)isoxazole (^{11}C-ABT-418) were compared with (S)(−)-^{11}C-nicotine (251). Although ^{11}C-MPA showed a small degree of specific binding relative to ^{11}C-nicotine and ^{11}C-ABT-418, the magnitude was low.

A breakthrough in the development of nicotinic tracers with high specific binding *in vivo* came with the discovery of epibatidine, which was isolated from the Ecuadorian poison frog (252) and the demonstration of potent analgesic properties that are mediated through the nAChRs (253). The reported specificity of epibatidine for CNS nicotinic receptors stimulated the development of methods to label epibatidine with ^{18}F, where fluorine is substituted for the chlorine atom that is present in the natural product to produce ^{18}F-norchlorofluoroepibatidine (^{18}F-NFEP) (50,254). Although the ^{18}F-labeled epibatidine derivatives proved to be good radiotracers for the central nAChR and have been used in measuring nAChR occupancy by nicotine (255), as well as interactions between the nicotinic and dopamine systems (256), application in humans is not possible because of the high toxicity of epibatidine and it derivatives (257,258).

The development of 3-pyridyl ether derivatives, which had higher selectivity for the $\alpha_4\beta_2$ subtype and significantly lower toxicity, provided an attractive alternative for radiotracer development (259). Both 2-fluoro-A-85380 and 6-fluoro-A-85380 are nicotinic agonists that have a high affinity for neuronal nAChRs but do not elicit the pronounced toxicity of epibatidine (260). ^{18}F-Labeled analogues, 2-^{18}F-fluoro-A-85380 and 6-^{18}F-fluoro-A-85380 are therefore promising radioligands for PET studies. Several research groups have reported the radiosyntheses of 2-^{18}F-fluoro-A-85380 (261–263) and 6-^{18}F-fluoro-A-85380 (264,265) using either iodo or nitro as a leaving group, although the use of a trimethylammonium precursor to 6-^{18}F-fluoro-A-85380 offers an advantage over other leaving groups (266).

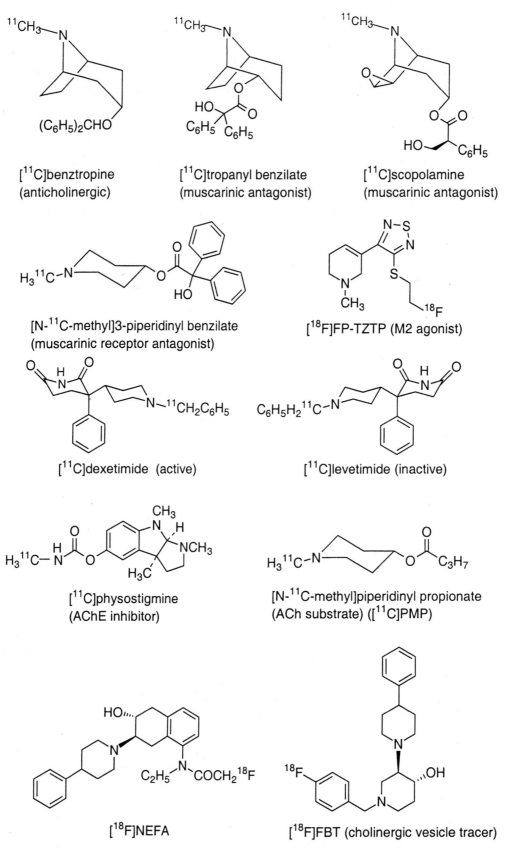

[¹¹C]benztropine
(anticholinergic)

[¹¹C]tropanyl benzilate
(muscarinic antagonist)

[¹¹C]scopolamine
(muscarinic antagonist)

[N-¹¹C-methyl]3-piperidinyl benzilate
(muscarinic receptor antagonist)

[¹⁸F]FP-TZTP (M2 agonist)

[¹¹C]dexetimide (active)

[¹¹C]levetimide (inactive)

[¹¹C]physostigmine
(AChE inhibitor)

[N-¹¹C-methyl]piperidinyl propionate
(ACh substrate) ([¹¹C]PMP)

[¹⁸F]NEFA

[¹⁸F]FBT (cholinergic vesicle tracer)

FIG. 2.16. Structures of labeled compounds for PET studies of muscarinic cholinergic receptors and for acetylcholinesterase.

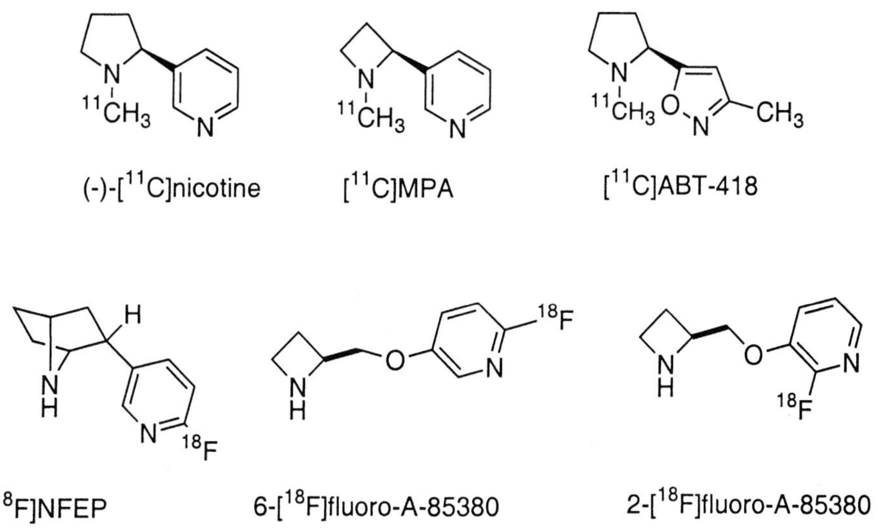

FIG. 2.17. Structures of labeled compounds for PET studies of nicotinic acetylcholine receptors.

Translation of these radiotracers from preclinical to the clinical application and the development of other subtype selective tracers for the nAChRs can be expected to add to our knowledge of the *in vivo* behavior of the nAChRs in the human brain.

Structures for some of these compounds are shown in Fig. 2.17.

Signal Transduction Pathways

The effects of neurotransmitter binding to monoamine receptors are mediated by intracellular signal transduction cascades. The second-messenger signal transduction pathways (cyclic adenosine monophosphate [cAMP], diacylglycerol, inositol triphosphate, Ca^{2+}) mediate the actions of many monoamine receptors. This regulation occurs via G proteins that couple receptors to effectors such as adenylate cyclase and phospholipase C that catalyze cAMP and inositol triphosphate formation, respectively. These second messengers regulate the action of second-messenger–dependent protein kinases. All aspects of neuronal functioning that are fundamental to the ability of the brain to respond and to adapt to pharmacologic and environmental input are controlled by these pathways (267).

Radiotracers for imaging different aspects of the signal transduction pathways are under development. For example ^{11}C-1,2-diacylglycerol and ^{11}C-forskolin have been synthesized and evaluated as probes for signal transduction in tumor cells and in a glioma patient with PET (268,269). After ^{11}C-1,2-diacylglycerol, ^{11}C was incorporated into the phosphoinositide pool and another phospholipid pool in the proliferative state. When the proliferative state was inhibited by (−)-3D-3-deoxy-3-fluoro-*myo*-inositol, incorporation into the phosphoinositide pool decreased selectively. A PET study in a human glioma patient showed promise for visual-

izing the proliferation signal. ^{18}F-Labeled diacylglycerols (1,2-^{18}F-FDAG) are also being investigated (270). The selective phosphodiesterase-IV inhibitor rolipram has also been labeled with ^{11}C and shown to have high uptake in brain regions (e.g., cortex and olfactory system) known to show high expression of phosphodiesterase-IV enzymes (271). It was concluded that these studies support further development of ^{11}C-rolipram as a promising radioligand for the *in vivo* study of the phosphodiesterase-IV family using PET.

Structures for some of these labeled compounds are shown in Fig. 2.18.

AMINO ACID TRANSPORT AND PROTEIN SYNTHESIS

Protein synthesis, like energy metabolism, is one of the fundamental processes supporting growth and development. Many positron emitter labeled amino acids and amino acid derivatives have been synthesized over the past 30 years (272–274). The major quest has been to develop a method to quantitatively measure the protein synthesis rate similar to the ^{18}F-FDG method for measurement of brain glucose metabolism. Such a method would offer the opportunity to assess how the protein synthesis rate changes with brain development, regeneration and repair, neurodegenerative disease, cancer, learning and memory, and in response to therapeutic drugs and drugs of abuse, as well as trace protein synthesis in tumors and other organs.

The essential processes involved in protein synthesis are the transport of the amino acid into the brain (a process that involves an amino acid carrier protein and that is subject to competition with endogenous amino acids) and the esterification of the amino acid to form the aminoacyl-t-RNA, which forms the polypeptide chain in the ribosome. Other

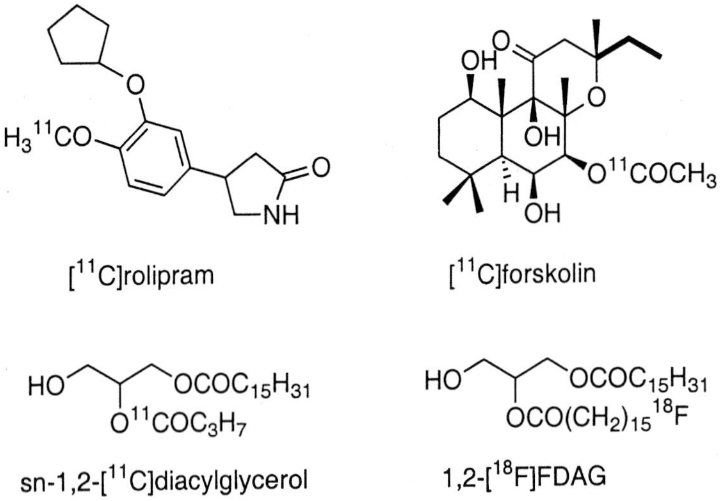

[^11^C]rolipram

[^11^C]forskolin

sn-1,2-[^11^C]diacylglycerol

1,2-[^18^F]FDAG

FIG. 2.18. Labeled compounds for PET studies of signal transduction.

processes can occur in addition to the formation of proteins including transamination and decarboxylation. One approach to the measurement of the protein synthesis rate uses ^{11}C-carboxyl-L-leucine, where the products of amino acid metabolism (loss of O_2 ^{11}C) are not labeled, but the proteins of interest are labeled (275,276). The quantification of the protein synthesis rate using this approach has been limited by recycling of amino acids derived from the degradation of proteins that must be taken into account in the estimation of the precursor pool-specific activity in tissue from measurements in plasma (277).

^{11}C-S-methyl-L-methionine and 1-^{11}C-L-methionine have also been examined as substrates for protein synthesis (278, 279). With ^{11}C-S-methyl-L-methionine, the behavior *in vivo* is complicated by the fact that it can undergo both protein synthesis and transmethylation, which would produce unwanted labeled metabolites. Labeled methionine has been used extensively to delineate tumor tissue, although the mechanism for sequestration has not been fully characterized. ^{11}C-D- and L-methionine have been compared to show that methionine transport into some tumors is nonselective (280). However, ^{11}C-L-methionine shows irreversible trapping in some tumors (281).

Because its longer half-life would be more compatible with the slow rate of incorporation of amino acids into proteins, ^{18}F has also been investigated as a label for tyrosine and phenylalanine for detecting and grading brain tumors (282). 2-^{18}F-Fluorotyrosine has been synthesized (283). Brain uptake in mice increased with time and ^{18}F was incorporated into protein without significant catabolism. However, a comparative revaluation of 2-^{18}F-fluorotyrosine, S-^{11}C-methyl-L-methionine and 1-^{11}C-leucine in mice bearing mammary carcinoma reported that these three amino acids are affected by alterations in the amino acid transport system in the brain and in tumor tissues but that only leucine incorporation is significantly reduced by cycloheximide, an inhibitor of protein synthesis (284). Nonetheless L-2-^{18}F-fluoro-

tyrosine was studied in brain tumor patients with PET and it showed high accumulation in tumor with little accumulation in healthy brain tissue. Kinetic analysis showed that the accumulation was associated with a twofold higher transport rate in tumor, although the rate constants for irreversible accumulation (which would reflect protein synthesis) were decreased in the tumor. L-2-^{18}F-fluorotyrosine transport rates clearly delineated tumor relative to healthy tissue and even low-grade tumors with an intact blood–brain barrier were detected (285). A similar study with L-2-^{18}F-fluorophenylalanine in cerebral glioma patients showed that the influx of ^{18}F into tumor tissue is mainly related to carrier-mediated active transport, and thus, its value is in tumor detection, rather than in assessing tumor malignancy (286).

Because most *in vivo* PET studies and kinetic modeling of labeled amino acid uptake in tumors indicate that the accumulation of radioactivity is dominated by transport rather than protein synthesis, the search for an amino acid whose uptake and retention reflects the protein synthesis rate has been largely replaced by the search for an amino acid that fulfills the following characteristics: (a) easy high-yield synthesis with ^{18}F; (b) high transport rate into tumors; (c) low uptake in healthy brain and peripheral tissues; and (d) high metabolic stability. Such a labeled compound would not have the disadvantage of uptake into healthy brain, and it would provide a low background for detection of tumors in the periphery. Providing that a high-yield synthesis could be developed, it could be widely distributed from a central radiopharmacy for tumor diagnosis.

Recently, a rapid high-yield synthesis of O-2-^{18}F-fluoroethyl-L-tyrosine was developed. This radiotracer was evaluated in mammary carcinoma–bearing mice and in a patient with a recurrent astrocytoma (287). PET imaging provided a clear delineation of the astrocytoma with a tumor-to-cortex ratio of 2.7 at 30 minutes after injection. There was no significant accumulation in peripheral organs at 40 minutes after injection. The ease of synthesis, the low healthy brain and peripheral tissue accumulation and rapid tumor uptake support further studies of this compound. L-3-^{18}F-fluoro-α-methyltyrosine (^{18}F-FMT) has also been synthesized (288). The brain uptake in healthy volunteers ranged from 2.8% to 4.9%. In patients with brain tumor, the tumor-to-normal brain ratios were higher than for those for ^{18}F-FDG (average, 2.53 ± 1.31 vs. 1.32 ± 1.46) (289,290). More recently the unnatural, nonmetabolized amino acid 1-amino-3-^{18}F-fluorocyclobutane-1-carboxylic acid was synthesized and studies were performed in mice and in one patient with a malignant brain tumor (291). There was low uptake in healthy brain, which contrasted to intense uptake in the brain tumor, with a tumor-to-normal brain ratio of 6 at 20 minutes.

In summary, the development of a PET method to quantitatively measure protein synthesis rates in the human brain has been largely unsuccessful, as labeled amino acid uptake and retention by healthy human brain and by tumors appears to be dominated by transport processes rather than protein synthesis. Nonetheless, there is promise in the development of ^{18}F-labeled amino acids, which will allow the detection of brain and other tumors with high signal-to-noise ratios because of enhanced amino acid transport in tumor and low uptake in healthy brain and many normal structures. Challenges are the development of high-yield syntheses that will allow distribution to remote clinical sites from a central distribution facility.

The structures of some of these labeled amino acids are shown in Fig. 2.19.

DNA SYNTHESIS

The incorporation of labeled thymidine (tritium or ^{14}C labeled) into cells has long been the gold standard for measuring tissue proliferation and growth kinetics (292). The extension of this approach to the measurement of DNA synthesis in humans using PET was explored in the early 1970s before the availability of modern PET instrumentation (293). ^{18}F-Fluorouridine was also synthesized early on. It is also taken up by proliferating cells, but it is incorporated into both DNA and RNA (294).

More recent research with labeled thymidine has focused on characterizing the biochemistry and kinetics of ^{11}C-thymidine in tumors (295,296), as well as imaging with PET (297,298,299,300). Although in principle ^{11}C-thymidine should be the gold standard for measuring cellular proliferation, its rapid metabolism, which leads to interference from labeled metabolites, has been a limiting factor. Labeling in both the methyl group and the C_2 positions has been examined to minimize the interference of labeled metabolites. With ^{11}C-methyl-thymidine, labeled metabolites thymine, dihydrothymine, β-ureidoisobutyric acid, and β-aminoisobutyric acid appear after intravenous injection (301). Labeled CO_2 is the most abundant radiolabeled metabolite after the administration of ring-labeled thymidine (302).

With both of these labeled thymidines, the calculation of proliferation rates, as well as image quality, is impaired by the presence of labeled metabolites and the short half-life

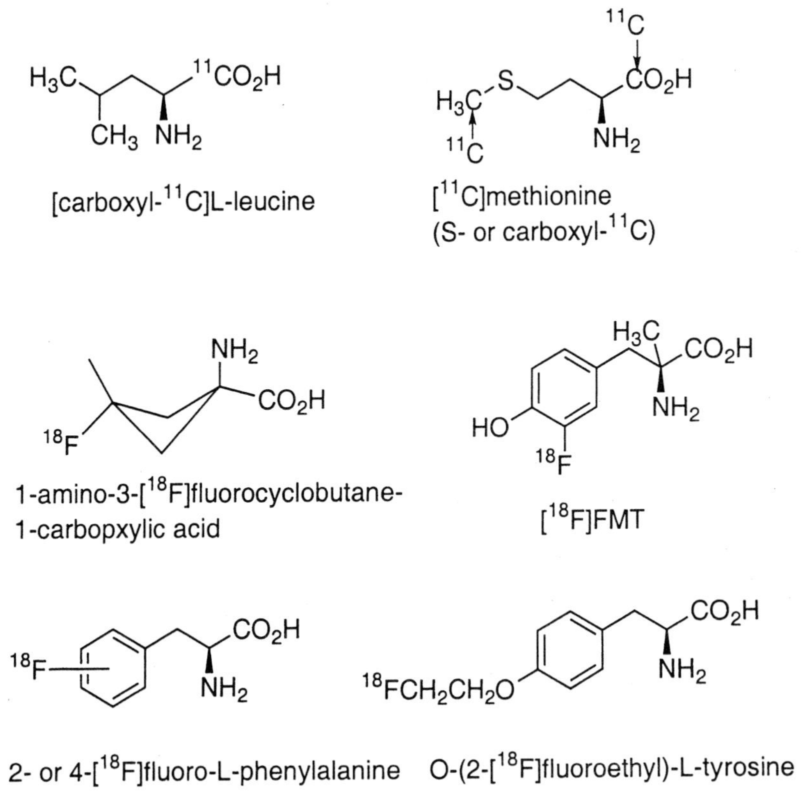

FIG. 2.19. Labeled amino acids for PET studies of protein synthesis and amino acid transport.

[carboxyl-^{11}C]L-leucine

[^{11}C]methionine (S- or carboxyl-^{11}C)

1-amino-3-[^{18}F]fluorocyclobutane-1-carbopxylic acid

[^{18}F]FMT

2- or 4-[^{18}F]fluoro-L-phenylalanine   O-(2-[^{18}F]fluoroethyl)-L-tyrosine

of ^{11}C. This has led to the search for a metabolically stable thymidine-like compound labeled with ^{11}C or ^{18}F, but preferably with ^{18}F (303). Ideally, such a tracer would share the following characteristics with thymidine: cellular transport, phosphorylation by thymidine kinase, incorporation into DNA, and limited *in vivo* catabolism. One recent approach has been the synthesis of 2'-fluoro-5-^{11}C-methyl-1-^{11}C-methyl-1-β-D-arabinofuranosyluracil (^{11}C-FMAU) (304). ^{11}C-FMAU, like thymidine, is transported into cells, phosphorylated by thymidine kinase, and incorporated into DNA. It also has limited catabolism, which could simplify kinetic modeling for the estimation of cellular proliferation rates.

Probably the most promising candidate to date is 3'-deoxy-3'-^{18}F-fluorothymidine (^{18}F-FLT) (41). Unlabeled FLT has been tested as an antiviral compound in patients with acquired immunodeficiency syndrome (305). It was shown to be taken up by cells and phosphorylated by thymidine kinase 1, leading to the 5'-phosphate, which is intracellularly trapped (306). ^{18}F-FLT is metabolically stable, with 90% to 97% of the plasma ^{18}F being in the parent compound at 50 minutes after injection. PET studies show high-contrast images of normal bone marrow and tumors in canine and human subjects (307). In humans, ^{18}F-FLT also shows high uptake in liver (possibly due to glucuronidation in hepatocytes), which would limit its use in imaging tumors within the liver and those near marrow. There is a need to develop a model for quantification and to further improve the synthetic yield.

Structures of some of these labeled compounds are shown in Fig. 2.20.

OTHER PET RADIOTRACERS

Fluorine-18 and ^{11}C radioisotopes are by far the most commonly used PET tracers. However, ^{15}O (t$\frac{1}{2}$ = 2.1 minutes) and ^{13}N (t$\frac{1}{2}$ = 9.96 minutes) both have important applications (Table 2.1). By virtue of their short half-lives, only limited chemistry can be performed with these agents. Oxygen-15 and its production method are described in detail in Chapter 1. The production of ^{13}N is also discussed in Chapter 1. Nitrogen-13 is used most commonly in the form of ^{13}N-ammonia, which is an excellent tracer for imaging myocardial blood flow. The Food and Drug Administration has approved this agent for blood-flow measurements as well. The requirements for producing sterile ^{13}N-ammonia for injection are described in detail in a recent United States Pharmacopeia monograph (308). Additional PET isotopes and their modes of production are also reviewed in Chapter 1.

SUMMARY

Modern day PET research is enriched and strengthened from the integration of many disciplines. However, it is advances in radiotracer chemistry that have played the pivotal role in driving the field in new directions in studies of human physiology. At the heart of this development is synthetic chemistry directed to the rapid incorporation of simple short-lived precursor molecules into organic compounds and drugs that can be used to map specific processes. Advances in organic synthesis can have a potentially important impact on neuroimaging and diagnosis in cancer and heart disease,

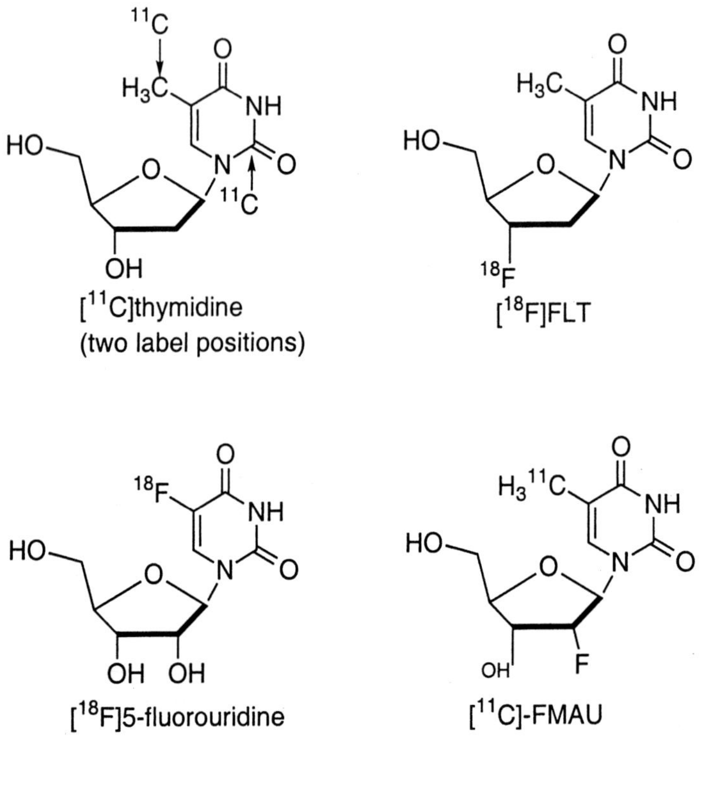

[^{11}C]thymidine
(two label positions)

[^{18}F]FLT

[^{18}F]5-fluorouridine

[^{11}C]-FMAU

FIG. 2.20. Labeled compounds for PET studies of DNA synthesis.

particularly advances in the rapid microscale, on-line conversion of simple single labeled carbon compounds such as methane and carbon dioxide to useful precursors for organic synthesis and in the development of simple methods for high specific activity electrophilic fluorination.

Perhaps the greatest challenge is to advance our understanding of the interactions between chemical compounds and living systems. This major challenge is at the heart of successful radiotracer design. For example, we are just scratching the surface relative to understanding the complexities in designing labeled molecules with biologic and kinetic properties that allow the visualization of a single biochemical process in a system in which all of the chemical reactions of life are occurring.

There is also a need to develop synthetic routes to the positron emitter labeled versions of important therapeutic drugs, both to understand drug mechanisms and to advance the development of new drugs. In this regard, PET is a sufficiently important tool in drug research and development to be considered in the actual drug design process to say nothing of drug development costs obviated by PET results. For example, the deliberate incorporation of a fluorine atom into a drug molecule for eventual ^{18}F labeling for PET studies, or design drug molecules with ^{11}C labeling in mind, would permit the determination of the short-term distribution and pharmacokinetics of the drug in the human body. One of the payoffs would be the ability to determine drug concentration and kinetics directly *in vivo*. In fact, PET is the only way to noninvasively determine whether and how much of a drug enters into the human brain. Because PET studies are possible in humans, the unique ability of humans to describe how they feel permits a new dimension to understand the link between brain chemistry and behavior.

ACKNOWLEDGMENTS

Much of this work was carried out at Brookhaven National Laboratory under contract DE-AC02-98CH10886, with the U.S. Department of Energy and supported by its Office of Biological and Environmental Research and by the National Institutes of Health (National Institutes of Neurological Diseases and Stroke (NS-15380). The authors thank John Gatley, Chester Mathis, and Michael Kilbourn for helpful discussions. Part of this chapter was excerpted with permission from Fowler and Wolf (11).

REFERENCES

1. Wolf AP, Redvanly CS. Carbon-11 and radiopharmaceuticals. *Int J Appl Radiat Isot* 1977;28:29–48.
2. McCarthy TJ, Schwarz SW, Welch MJ. Nuclear medicine and positron emission tomography: an overview. *J Chem Ed* 1994;71:830–836.
3. Phelps ME, Cherry SR. The changing design of positron imaging systems. *Clin Positron Imaging* 1998;1:31–45.
4. Fowler JS, Wolf AP. *The synthesis of carbon-11, fluorine-18 and nitrogen-13 labeled radiotracers for biomedical applications.* National Academy of Sciences, National Technical Information Service, 1982. Nuclear Science Series no. NAS-NS-3201.
5. Fowler JS, Wolf AP. Positron emitter-labeled compounds: priorities and problems. In: Phelps M, Mazziotta J, Schelbert H, eds. *Positron emission tomography and autoradiography: principles and applications for the brain and heart.* New York: Raven Press, 1986:391–450.
6. Kilbourn MR. *Fluorine-18 labeling of radiopharmaceuticals.* National Academy of Sciences, National Academy Press, 1990. Nuclear Science Series no. NAS-NS-3203.
7. Langstrom B, Antoni G, Bjurling P, et al. Synthesis of compounds of interest for positron emission tomography with particular reference to synthetic strategies for ^{11}C labeling. *Acta Radiol* 1990;374[Suppl]:147–151.
8. Firnau G, Chirakal R, Nahmias K. New ^{18}F tracers for the investigation of brain functions. *Acta Radiol* 1990;374[Suppl]:37–40.
9. Tewson TJ, Krohn KA. PET radiopharmaceuticals: state-of-the-art and future prospects. *Semin Nucl Med* 1998;28:221–234.
10. Ding Y-S, Fowler JS. ^{18}F-Labeled tracers for positron emission tomography studies in the neurosciences. In: Ojima I, McCarthy JR, Welch JT, eds. Biomedical frontiers of fluorine chemistry. Washington, DC: American Chemical Society, 1996:328–343. ACS Symposium Series no. 639.
11. Fowler JS, Wolf AP. Working against time. Rapid radiotracer synthesis and imaging the human brain. *Accounts Chem Res* 1997;30:181–188.
12. Iwata R. Reference book for PET radiopharmaceuticals. Available on-line at : http://kakuyaku.cyric.tohoku.ac.jp/.
13. Langstrom B, Kihlberg T, Bergstrom M et al. Compounds labelled with short-lived beta(+)-emitting radionuclides and some applications in life sciences. The importance of time as a parameter. *Acta Chimica Scand* 1999;53:651–669.
14. Brodack J, Kilbourn M, Welch M. Automated production of several positron-emitting radiopharmaceuticals using a single laboratory robot. *Appl Radiat Isot* 1988;39:689–698.
15. Alexoff DL. *New trends in radiopharmaceutical manufacturing for positron emission tomography.* New York: Plenum Publishing, 1991:339–353.
16. Vera-Ruiz H, Marcus CS, Pike VW, et al. Report of an international atomic energy agency's advisory group meeting on quality control of cyclotron-produced radiopharmaceuticals. *Int J Radiat Appl Instrum* 1990;17[Pt B]:445–456.
17. Guillaume M, Luxen A, Nebeling B, et al. Recommendations for fluorine-18 production. *Appl Radiat Isot* 1991;42:749–762.
18. Bergman J, Solin O. Fluorine-18 labeled fluorine gas for synthesis of tracer molecules. *Nucl Med Biol* 1997;24:677–683.
19. Laakso A, Bergman J, Haaparanta M, et al. [^{18}F]CFT([^{18}F]WIN 35,428), a radioligand to study the dopamine transporter with PET: characterization in human subjects. *Synapse* 1998;28:244–250.
20. Constantinou M, Aigbirhio FI, Smith RG, et al. Xenon difluoride exchanges fluoride under mild conditions: a simple preparation of [^{18}F]xenon difluoride for PET and mechanistic studies. *J Am Chem Soc* 2001;123:1780–1781.
21. Eckelman WC, Reba RC, Gibson RE, et al. Receptor-binding radiotracers: a class of potential radiopharmaceuticals. *J Nucl Med* 1979;20:350–357.
22. Wolf AP. Synthesis of organic compounds labeled with positron emitters and the carrier problem. *J Labelled Compounds Radiopharm* 1981;18:1–2(abst).
23. Wolf AP, Fowler JS. Organic radiopharmaceuticals—recent advances. *Radiopharmaceuticals II.* New York: Society of Nuclear Medicine, 1979:73–92.
24. Venturino A, Rivera ES, Bergoc RM, et al. A simplified competition data analysis for radioligand specific activity determination. *Nucl Med Biol* 1990;17:233–237.
25. Ferrieri RA, Wolf AP. The chemistry of positron emitting nucleogenic (hot) atoms with regards to the preparation of labeled compounds of practical utility. *Radiochim Acta* 1983;34:69–83.
26. Christman DR, Finn RD, Karlstrom KI, et al. The production of ultra high activity ^{11}C-labeled hydrogen cyanide, carbon dioxide, carbon monoxide, and methane via the 14N(p,α)^{11}C reaction. *Int J Appl Radiat Isot* 1975;26:435–442.
27. Langstrom B, Lundqvist H. The preparation of ^{11}C-methyl iodide and its use in the synthesis of ^{11}C-methyl-L-methionine. *Int J Appl Radiat Isot* 1976;27:357–363.

28. Ehrin E, Gawell L, Hogberg T, et al. Synthesis of [methoxy-3H]- and [methoxy-^{11}C]-labeled raclopride. Specific dopamine-D$_2$ receptor ligands. *J Labelled Compounds Radiopharm* 1987;24:931–940.

29. Ding Y-S, Sugano Y, Fowler JS, et al. Synthesis of the racemate and individual enantiomers of ^{11}C]methylphenidate for studying presynaptic dopaminergic neurons with positron emission tomography. *J Labelled Compounds Radiopharm* 1994;34:989–997.

30. Jewett DM. A simple synthesis of [^{11}C]methyl triflate. *Int J Radiat Appl Instrum A* 1992;43:1383–1385.

31. Del Rosario RB, Wieland DM. Synthesis of [^{11}C]-α,α-dideuterio-phenylephrine for *in vivo* kinetic isotope studies. *J Labelled Compounds Radiopharm* 1995;36:625–630.

32. Larsen P, Ulin J, Dahlstrom K, Jensen M. Synthesis of [^{11}C]iodomethane by iodination of [^{11}C]methane. *Appl Radiat Isot* 1997;48:153–157.

33. Link JM, Krohn KA, Clark JC. Production of [^{11}C]CH$_3$I by single pass reaction of [^{11}C]CH$_4$ with I$_2$. *Nucl Med Biol* 1997;24:93–97.

34. Elsinga PH, Keller E, De Groot TJ, et al. Synthesis of [^{11}C]methyl magnesium iodide and its application to the introduction of [^{11}C]-*N*-tert-butyl groups and [^{11}C]-sec-alcohols. *Appl Radiat Isot* 1995;46:227–231.

35. Kihlberg T, Gullberg P, Langstrom B. [^{11}C]Methylenetriphenylphosphorane, a new ^{11}C-precursor used in a one-pot Wittig synthesis of [(-^{11}C]styrene. *J Labelled Compounds Radiopharm* 1990;28:1116–1120.

36. Fasth KJ, Hörnfeldt K, Langström B. Asymmetric synthesis of ^{11}C-labelled L- and D-amino acids by alkylation of imidazolidinone derivatives. *Acta Chem Scand* 1995;49:301–304.

37. Ding Y-S, Studenoff AR, Zhang Z, et al. Novel synthesis of [^{11}C]GVG (vigabatrin) for pharmacokinetics studies of addiction treatment. Paper presented at: *International Symposium on Radiopharmaceutical Chemistry*; 2001; Interlaken, Switzerland.

38. Sandell J, Halldin C, Hall H, et al. Radiosynthesis and autoradiographic evaluation of [^{11}C]NAD-299, a radioligand for visualization of the 5-HT$_{1A}$ receptor. *Nucl Med Biol* 1999;26:159–164.

39. Dolle F, Bramoulle Y, Bottlaender M, et al. [^{11}C]Befloxatone, a novel highly potent radioligand for *in vivo* imaging monoamine oxidase A. *J Labelled Compounds Radiopharm* 1999;42[Suppl 1]:S608–S609.

40. Stone-Elander SA, Elander N, Thorell J-O, et al. *J Labelled Compounds Radiopharm* 1994;34:949–960.

41. Grierson JR, Shields AF, Early JF. Radiosynthesis of 3'-[^{18}F]fluoro-3'-deoxynucleosides. *J Labelled Compounds Radiopharm* 1997;40:60–62.

42. Ido T, Wan C-N, Casella V, et al. Labeled 2-deoxy-D-glucose analogs. ^{18}F-labeled 2-deoxy-2-fluoro-D-glucose, 2-deoxy-2-fluoro-D-mannose and ^{14}C-2-deoxy-2-fluoro-D-glucose. *J Labelled Compounds Radiopharm* 1978;14:175–183.

43. Fowler JS, Wolf AP. 2-Deoxy-2-[^{18}F]fluoro-D-glucose for metabolic studies: current status. *Int J Appl Radiat Isot* 1986;37:663–668.

44. Hamacher K, Coenen HH, Stocklin G. Efficient stereospecific synthesis of no-carrier-added 2-[^{18}F]-fluoro-2-deoxy-D-glucose using amino polyether supported nucleophilic substitution. *J Nucl Med* 1986;27:235–238.

45. Firnau G, Garnett ES, Chirakal R, et al. [^{18}F]fluoro-L-dopa for the *in vivo* study of intracerebral dopamine. *Appl Radiat Isot* 1986;37:669–675.

46. Luxen A, Guillaume M, Melega WP, et al. Production of 6-[^{18}F]fluoro-L-dopa and its metabolism *in vivo*—a critical review. *Nucl Med Biol* 1992;19:149–158.

47. Ding Y-S, Shiue C-Y, Fowler JS, et al. No-carrier-added (NCA) aryl[-^{18}F]fluorides via the nucleophilic aromatic substitution of electron rich aromatic rings. *J Fluorine Chem* 1990;48:189–205.

48. Lemaire C, Damhaut P, Plenevaux A, et al. Enantioselective synthesis of 6-[fluorine-18]-fluoro-L-dopa from no-carrier-added fluorine-18-fluoride. *J Nucl Med* 1994;35:1996–2002.

49. Attina M, Cacace F, Wolf AP. Displacement of nitro group by ^{18}F-fluoride ion. A new route to high specific activity aryl fluorides. *J Chem Soc Chem Commun* 1983;107–109.

50. Ding Y-S, Gatley SJ, Fowler JS, et al. Mapping nicotinic acetylcholine receptors with PET. *Synapse* 1996;24:403–407.

51. Ding Y-S, Fowler JS, Gatley SJ, et al. Synthesis of high specific activity 6-[^{18}F]fluorodopamine for positron emission tomography studies of sympathetic nervous tissue. *J Med Chem* 1991;34:861–863.

52. Ding Y-S, Fowler JS, Gatley SJ, et al. Synthesis of high specific activity (+) and (−)-6-[^{18}F]fluoro-norepinephrine via the nucleophilic aromatic substitution reaction. *J Med Chem* 1991;34:767–771.

53. Ding Y-S, Fowler JS, Dewey SL, et al. Comparison of high specific activity (−) and (+)-6-[^{18}F]fluoro-norepinephrine and 6-[^{18}F]fluorodopamine in baboons: heart uptake, metabolism and the effect of desipramine. *J Nucl Med* 1993;34:619–629.

54. Ding Y-S, Fowler JS. Highlights of PET studies on chiral radiotracers and drugs at Brookhaven. *J Drug Dev Res* 2000 *(in press)*.

55. Hostetler ED, Jonson SD, Welch MJ, et al. Synthesis of 2-[^{18}F]fluoro-estradiol, a potential diagnostic imaging agent for breast cancer: strategies to achieve nucleophilic substitution of an electron-rich aromatic ring with [^{18}F]F$^-$. *J Organ Chem* 1999;64:178–185.

56. Shah A, Widdowson DA, Pike V. Synthesis of substituted diaryliodonium salts and investigation of their reactions with no-carrier-added [^{18}F]fluoride. *J Labelled Compounds Radiopharm* 1997;40:65–67.

57. Dischino DD, Welch MJ, Kilbourn MJ, et al. Relationship between lipophilicity and brain extraction of C-11 labeled radiopharmaceuticals. *J Nucl Med* 1983;24:1030–1038.

58. Abbott NJ, Chugani DC, Zaharchuk G, et al. Delivery of imaging agents into brain. *Adv Drug Delivery Rev* 1999;37:253–277.

59. Lin JH. Applications and limitations of interspecies scaling and *in vitro* extrapolation in pharmacokinetics. *Drug Metab Dispos* 1998;26:1202–1212.

60. Sokoloff L. Mapping of local cerebral functional activity by measurement of local cerebral glucose utilization with [^{14}C]deoxyglucose. *Brain* 1979;102:653–668.

61. Sols A, Crane RA. Substrate specificity of brain hexokinase. *J Biol Chem* 1954;210:581–595.

62. MacGregor RR, Fowler JS, Wolf AP, et al. A synthesis of ^{11}C-2-deoxy-D-glucose for regional metabolic studies. *J Nucl Med* 1981;22:800–803.

63. Volkow ND, Brodie JD, Wolf AP, et al. Brain organization in schizophrenics. *J Cereb Blood Flow Metab* 1986;6:441–446.

64. Weber G. Enzymology of cancer cells. *N Engl J Med* 1977;296:541–551.

65. Som P, Atkins HL, Bandoypadhyay D, et al. A fluorinated glucose analog, 2-fluoro-2-deoxy-D-glucose (F-18): nontoxic tracer for rapid tumor detection. *J Nucl Med* 1980;21:670–675.

66. Coleman RE. FDG imaging. *Nucl Med Biol* 2000;27:689–690.

67. Silverman M. Specificity of monosaccharide transport in the dog kidney. *Am J Physiol* 1970;218:743–750.

68. Langstrom B, Andersson Y, Antoni G, et al. Design of tracer molecules with emphasis on stereochemistry, position of label and multiple isotopic labeling. An important aspect in studies of biologic function using positron emission tomography. *Acta Radiol* 1991;376[Suppl]:31–35.

69. Mintun MA, Raichle ME, Kilbourn MR, et al. A quantitative model for the *in vivo* assessment of drug binding sites with positron emission tomography. *Ann Neurol* 1984;15:217–227.

70. Wong DF, Gjedde A, Wagner HN, et. al. Quantification of neuroreceptors in the living human brain, II: inhibition studies of receptor density and affinity. *J Cereb Blood Flow Metab* 1986;6:147–153.

71. Logan J, Wolf AP, Shiue C-Y, et al. Kinetic modeling a receptor-ligand binding applied to positron emission tomographic studies with neuroleptic tracers. *J Neurochem* 1987;48:73–83.

72. Carson RE. Parameter estimation in positron emission tomography. In: Phelps M, Mazziotta J, Schelbert H, eds. *Positron emission tomography and autoradiography: principles and applications for the brain and heart*. New York: Raven Press, 1986:347–390.

73. Patlak CS, Blasberg RG, Fenstermacher JD. Graphical evaluation of blood-to-brain transfer constants from multiple-time uptake data. *J Cereb Blood Flow Metab* 1983;3:1–7.

74. Logan J, Fowler JS, Volkow ND, et. al. Graphical analysis of reversible radioligand binding from time-activity measurements applied to [*N*-^{11}C-methyl]-(−)-cocaine PET studies in human subjects. *J Cereb Blood Flow Metab* 1990;10:740–747.

75. Bergstrom MJ, Eriksson B, Oberg K, et al. *In vivo* demonstration of enzyme activity in endocrine pancreatic tumors. Decarboxylation of carbon-11 DOPA to carbon-11 dopamine. *J Nucl Med* 1996;37:32–37.

76. Halldin C, Burling P, Stalnacke C-G, et al. ^{11}C-Labeling of dimethyl phenethylamine in two different positions and biodistribution studies. *Appl Radiat Isot* 1989;40:557–560.

77. Pike VW, McCarron JA, Lammertsma AA, et al., Exquisite delinea-

tion of 5-HT$_{1A}$ receptors in human brain with PET and [carbonyl-^{11}C]WAY-100635. *Eur J Pharmacol* 1996;301:R5–R7.

78. Ding YS, Fowler JS, Volkow ND, et al. Chiral drugs: comparison of the pharmacokinetics of [^{11}C]D-*threo* and L-*threo*-methylphenidate in the human and baboon brain. *Psychopharmacology* 1997;131:71–78.

79. Volkow ND, Ding Y-S, Fowler JS, et al. A new PET ligand for the dopamine transporter: studies in the human brain. *J Nucl Med* 1995;36:2162–2168.

80. Dannals RF, Langstrom B, Ravert HT, et al. Synthesis of radiotracers for studying muscarinic cholinergic receptors in the living human brain using positron emission tomography [^{11}C]dexetimide and [^{11}C]levetimide. *Int J Radiat Appl Instrum A* 1988;39:291–295.

81. Szabo Z, Kao PF, Scheffel U, et al. Positron emission tomography imaging of serotonin transporters in the human brain using [^{11}C](+)McN5652. *Synapse* 1995;20:37–43.

82. Gatley SJ, MacGregor RR, Fowler JS, et al. Rapid stereoselective hydrolysis of (+) cocaine in baboon plasma prevents its uptake in the brain: implications for behavioral studies. *J Neurochem* 1990;54:720–723.

83. Belleau B, Moran J. Deuterium isotope effects in relation to the chemical mechanisms of monoamine oxidase. *Ann N Y Acad Sci* 1963;107:822–839.

84. Fowler JS, Wolf AP, MacGregor RR, et al. Mechanistic positron emission tomography studies. Demonstration of a deuterium isotope effect in the MAO catalyzed binding of [^{11}C]L-deprenyl in living baboon brain. *J Neurochem* 1988;51:1524–1534.

85. Tominaga T, Inoue O, Suzuki K, et al. [^{13}N]β-phenethylamine ([^{13}N]PEA): a prototype tracer for measurement of MAO B activity in heart. *Biochem Pharmacol* 1987;36:3671–3675.

86. Ding Y-S, Fowler JS, Gatley SJ, et al. Mechanistic PET studies of 6-[^{18}F]fluorodopamine in living baboon heart: selective imaging and control of radiotracer metabolism using the deuterium isotope effect. *J Neurochem* 1995;65:682–690.

87. Raffel DM, Corbett JR, del Rosario RB, et al. Sensitivity of [^{11}C]phenylephrine kinetics to monoamine oxidase activity in normal human heart. *J Nucl Med* 1999;40:232–238.

88. Fowler JS, Wang G-J, Logan J, et al. Selective reduction of radiotracer trapping by deuterium substitution: comparison of [^{11}C]L-deprenyl and [^{11}C]L-deprenyl-D$_2$ for MAO B mapping. *J Nucl Med* 1995;36:1255–1262.

89. Yu DW, Gatley SJ, Wolf AP, et al. Synthesis of carbon-11 labeled iodinated cocaine derivatives and their distribution in baboon brain measured using positron emission tomography. *J Med Chem* 1992;35:2178–2183.

90. Ding Y-S, Sugano Y, Koomen J, et al. Synthesis of [^{18}F]RO41-0960, a potent catechol-*O*-methyltransferase inhibitor, for PET studies. *J Labelled Compounds Radiopharm* 1997;39:303–318.

91. Deutsch A, Roth RH. Neurochemical systems in the central nervous system. In: Charney DS, Nestler EJ, Bunney BS, eds. *Neurobiology of mental illness.* New York: Oxford University Press, 1999:10–25.

92. Volkow ND, Fowler JS, Gatley SJ, et al. PET evaluation of the dopamine system of the human brain. *J Nucl Med* 1996;37:1242–1256.

93. Stoessl J, Ruth T. Neuroreceptor imaging: new developments in PET and SPECT imaging of neuroreceptor binding (including dopamine transporters, vesicle transporters and postsynaptic receptor sites). *Curr Opinion Neurol* 1998;11:327–333.

94. Sibley DR. Molecular biology of dopamine receptors. *Trends Pharmacol Sci* 1992;13:61–69.

95. Jackson DM, Westlind-Danielsson A. Dopamine receptors: molecular biology,, biochemistry and behavioral aspects. *Pharmacol Ther* 1994;64:291–369.

96. Garnett ES, Firnau G, Nahmias C. Dopamine visualized in the basal ganglia in living man. *Nature* 1983;305:137–138.

97. Firnau G, Garnett ES, Chirakal R, et al. [^{18}F]Fluoro-L-dopa for the *in vivo* study of intracerebral dopamine. *Int J Radiat Appl Radiat* 1986;37[Pt A]:669–675.

98. Firnau G, Sood S, Chirakal R, et al. Cerebral metabolism of 6-^{18}F-fluoro-L-3,4-dihydroxy-phenylalanine in the primate. *J Neurochem* 1987;48:1077–1082.

99. Perlmutter JS. New insights into a pathophysiology of Parkinson's disease: the challenge of positron emission tomography. *TINS* 1988;11:203–208.

100. DeJesus OT, Endres CJ, Shelton SE, et al. Evaluation of fluorinated M-

101. Bjurling P, Antoni G, Watanabe Y, et al. Enzymatic synthesis of carboxy-^{11}C-labeled L-tyrosine, L-DOPA, L-tryptophan and 5-hydroxy-L-tryptophan. *Acta Chem Scand* 1990;44:178.

102. Arnett CD, Wolf AP, Shiue C-Y, et al. Improved delineation of human dopamine receptors using [^{18}F]-*N*-methylspiroperidol in PET. *J Nucl Med* 1986;27:1878–1882.

103. Smith M, Wolf AP, Brodie JD, et al. Serial [^{18}F]-*N*-methylspiroperidol PET studies to measure changes in antipsychotic drug D$_2$ receptor occupancy in schizophrenic patients. *Biol Psychiatry* 1988;23:653–663.

104. Wagner HN Jr, Burns HD, Dannals RF, et al. Assessment of dopamine receptor densities in the human brain with carbon-11–labeled N-methylspiperone. *Ann Neurol* 1984;15[Suppl]S79–S84.

105. Wong DF, Wagner HN Jr, Tune LE, et al. Positron emission tomography reveals elevated D$_2$ dopamine receptors in drug-naive schizophrenics. *Science* 1986;234:1558–1563.

106. Satyamurthy N, Barrio JR, Bida G, et al. 3-(2'-[^{18}F]Fluoroethyl)spiperone, a potent dopamine antagonist: synthesis, structural analysis and *in vivo* utilization in humans. *Appl Radiat Isot* 1990;41:113–129.

107. Welch MJ, Katzenellenbogen JA, Mathias CJ, et al. *N*-(3-[^{18}F]fluoropropyl)-spiperone: the preferred ^{18}F labeled spiperone analog for PET studies of the dopamine receptor. *Nucl Med Biol* 1988;15:83–97.

108. Gambhir SS, Barrio JR, Herschman HR, et al. Assays for noninvasive imaging of reporter gene expression. *Nucl Med Biol* 1999;26:481–490.

109. Farde L, Ehrin E, Eriksson L, et al. Substituted benzamides as ligands for visualization of dopamine receptor binding in the human brain by positron emission tomography. *Proc Natl Acad Sci U S A* 1985;82:3863–3867.

110. Moerlein S, Perlmutter JS, Welch MJ. USP standards for raclopride C 11 injection. *Pharmacopeial Forum* 1995;21:172–176.

111. Dewey SL, Smith GS, Logan J, et al. Striatal binding of the PET ligand ^{11}C-raclopride is altered by drugs that modify synaptic dopamine levels. *Synapse* 1993;13:350–356.

112. Volkow ND, Wang G-J, Fowler JS, et al. Imaging endogenous dopamine competition with [^{11}C]raclopride in the human brain. *Synapse* 1994;16:255–262.

113. Volkow ND, Wang G-J, Fowler JS, et al. Decreased striatal dopaminergic responsiveness in detoxified cocaine-dependent subjects. *Nature* 1997;386:830–833.

114. Breier A, Su TP, Saunders R, et al. Schizophrenia is associated with elevated amphetamine-induced synaptic dopamine concentrations: evidence from a novel positron emission tomography method. *Proc Natl Acad Sci U S A* 1997;94:2569–2574.

115. Laruelle M. Imaging synaptic neurotransmission with *in vivo* binding competition techniques: a critical review. *J Cereb Blood Flow Metab* 2000;20:423–451.

116. Mathis CA, Bishop JE, Gerdes JM, et al. Synthesis and evaluation of high affinity aryl substituted [^{18}F]fluoropropylbenzamides for dopamine D$_2$ receptor studies. *Nucl Med Biol* 1992;19:571–588.

117. Mach RH, Nader MA, Ehrenkaufer RLE, et al. Comparison of two fluorine-18 labeled benzamide derivatives that bind reversibly to dopamine D$_2$ receptors: *in vitro* binding studies and positron emission tomography. *Synapse* 1996;24:322–333.

118. Christian BT, Narayanan TK, Shi B, et al. Quantitation of striatal and extrastriatal D-2 dopamine receptors using PET imaging of [^{18}F]fallypride in nonhuman primates. *Synapse* Oct 2000;38(1):71–79.

119. Kessler RM, Votaw JR, dePaulis T, et al. Evaluation of 5-[^{18}F]fluoropropylepidepride as a potential PET radioligand for imaging dopamine D$_2$ receptors. *Synapse* 1993;15:169–176.

120. Halldin C, Farde L, Hogberg T, et al. Carbon-11-FLB 457: a radioligand for extrastriatal D$_2$ dopamine receptors. *J Nucl Med* 1995;36:1275–1281.

121. Chou YH, Halldin C, Farde L. Effect of amphetamine on extrastriatal D$_2$ dopamine receptor binding in the primate brain: a PET study. *Synapse* 2000;38:138–143.

122. Halldin CJ, Swahn C-G, Neumeyer JL, et al. Preparation of two potent and selective dopamine D$_2$ receptor agonists: R-[propyl-^{11}C]-2-OH-NPA and R-[methyl-^{11}C]-2-OCH$_3$-NPA. *J Labelled Compounds Radiopharm* 1993;32:S265–S266.

123. Zilstra S. Synthesis and *in vivo* distribution in the rat of several fluo-

rine-18 labeled *N*-fluoroalkylporphines. *Appl Radiat Isot* 1993;44: 651–658.

124. Shi B, Narayanan TK, Yang ZY, et al. Radiosynthesis and in vitro evaluation of 2-(*N*-alkyl-*N*-1-^{11}C-propyl)amino-5-hydroxytetralin analogs as high affinity agonists for dopamine D_2 receptors. *Nucl Med Biol* 1999;26:725–735.

125. Hwang D-R, Kegeles LS, Laruelle M. (−)-*N*-^{11}C]Propyl-Noraporphine: a positron-labeled dopamine agonist for PET imaging of D_2 receptors. *Nucl Med Biol* 2000;27:533–539.

126. Kung HF. SPECT and PET ligands for CNS imaging. *Neurotransmissions* 1993;9:1.

127. Halldin C, Foged C, Chou Y-H, et al. Carbon-11-NNC 112: a radioligand for PET examination of striatal and neocortical D_1-dopamine receptors. *J Nucl Med* 1998;39:2061–2068.

128. Abi-Dargham A, Martinez D, Mawlawi O, et al. Measurement of striatal and extrastriatal dopamine D_1 receptor binding potential with ^{11}C]NNC 112 in humans: validation and reproducibility. *J Cereb Blood Flow Metab* 2000;20:225–243.

129. DaSilva JN, Wilson AA, Nobrega JN, et al. Synthesis and autoradiographic localization of the dopamine D-1 agonists ^{11}C]SKF 75670 and ^{11}C]SKF 82957 as potential PET radioligands. *Appl Radiat Isot* 1996;47:279–284.

130. Abi-Dargham A, Simpson N, Kegeles L, et al. PET studies of binding competition between endogenous dopamine and the D_1 radiotracer ^{11}C]NNC 756. *Synapse* 1999;32:93–109.

131. Chou YH, Karlsson P, Halldin C, et al. A PET study of D_1 like dopamine receptor ligand binding during altered endogenous dopamine levels in the primate brain. *Psychopharmacology* 1999;146: 220–227.

132. Langer O, Halldin C, Chou Y-H, et al. Carbon-11 PB-12: an attempt to visualize the dopamine D_4 receptor in the primate brain with positron emission tomography. *Nucl Med Biol* 2000;27:707–714.

133. Salmon E, Brooks DJ, Leenders KL, et al. A two compartment description and kinetic procedure for measuring regional cerebral ^{11}C]nomifensine uptake using positron emission tomography. *J Cereb Blood Flow Metab* 1990;10:307–316.

134. Fowler JS, Volkow ND, Wolf AP, et al. Mapping cocaine binding in human and baboon brain in vivo. *Synapse* 1989;4:371–377.

135. Ding Y-S, Fowler JS, Volkow ND, et al. Pharmacokinetics and *in vivo* specificity of ^{11}C]DL-*threo*-methylphenidate for the presynaptic dopaminergic neuron. *Synapse* 1994;18:152–160.

136. Frost JJ, Rosier AJ, Reich SG, et al. Positron emission tomographic imaging of the dopamine transporter with ^{11}C-WIN 35,428 reveals marked declines in mild Parkinson's disease. *Ann Neurol* 1993;34: 423–431.

137. Wong DF, Yung B, Dannals RF, et al. *In vivo* imaging of baboon and human dopamine transporters by positron emission tomography using ^{11}C-WIN 35,428. *Synapse* 1993;15:130–142.

138. Madras BK. ^{11}C-WIN 35, 428 for detecting dopamine depletion in mild Parkinson's disease. *Ann Neurol* 1993;34:423–431.

139. Brownell AL, Elmaleh DR, Meltzer PC, et al. Cocaine congeners as PET imaging probes for dopamine terminals. *J Nucl Med* 1996;37: 1186–1192.

140. Chaly T, Dhawan V, Kazumata K, et al. Radiosynthesis of ^{18}F]*N*-3-fluoropropyl-2-β-carbomethoxy-3-β-(4-iodophenyl)nortropane and the first human study with positron emission tomography. *Nucl Med Biol* 1996;23:999–1004.

141. Deterding TA, Votaw JR, Wang CK, et al. Biodistribution and radiation dosimetry of the dopamine transporter ligand ^{18}F]FECNT. *J Nucl Med* 2001;42:376–381.

142. Fischman AJ, Bonab AA, Babich JW, et al. [11]C, 127]I]Altropane: a highly selective ligand for PET imaging of dopamine transporter sites. *Synapse* 2001;39:332–342.

143. Halldin C, Chou Y-H, Guilloteau D, et al. [11]C]PE21—a highly selective radioligand for PET-examination of the dopamine transporter in human brain. *Neuroimage* 2000;11:S37.

144. Kilbourn MR, Haka MS, Mulholland GK, et al. Synthesis of radiolabeled inhibitors or presynaptic monoamine uptake systems: [18]F]GBR 13119 (DA), ^{11}C]nisoxetine (NE), and ^{11}C]fluoxetine (5-HT). *J Labelled Compounds Radiopharm* 1989;26:412–414.

145. Volkow ND, Fowler JS, Wang G-J, et al. Decreased dopamine transporters with age in healthy human subjects. *Ann Neurol* 1994;36: 237–239.

146. Tedroff J, Aquilonius S-M, Hartvig P, et al. Monoamine reuptake sites in the human brain evaluated in vivo by means of ^{11}C nomifensine and positron emission tomography: the effect of age and Parkinson's disease. *Acta Neurol Scand* 1988;77:92–101.

147. Volkow ND, Wang G-J, Fischman M, et al. Relationship between subjective effects of cocaine and dopamine transporter occupancy. *Nature* 1997;386:827–830.

148. Volkow ND, Wang G-J, Fowler JS, et al. Dopamine transporter occupancies in the human brain induced by therapeutic doses of oral methylphenidate. *Am J Psychiatry* 1998;155:1325–1331.

149. Volkow ND, Wang G, Fowler JS, et al. Therapeutic doses of oral methylphenidate significantly increase extracellular dopamine in the human brain. *J Neurosci* 2001;21:RC21.

150. Logan J, Fowler JS, Volkow ND, et al. Graphical analysis of reversible radioligand binding from time activity measurements applied to [*N*-^{11}C-methyl]-(−)cocaine PET studies in human subjects. *J Cereb Blood Flow Metab* 1990;10:740–747.

151. Kilbourn MR, Frey KA, Vander Borght T, et al. Effects of dopaminergic drug treatments on *in vivo* radioligand binding to brain vesicular monoamine transporters. *Nucl Med Biol* 1996;23:467–471.

152. Vander Borght T, Kilbourn M, Desmond T, et al. the vesicular monoamine transporter is not regulated by dopaminergic drug treatments. *Eur J Pharmacol* 1995;294:577–583.

153. Kilbourn MR. *In vivo* tracers for vesicular neurotransmitter transporters. *Nucl Med Biol* 1997;24:615–619.

154. Kilbourn MR, Lee L, Vender Borght T, et al. Binding of α- dihydrotetrabenazine to the vesicular monoamine transporter is stereospecific. *Eur J Pharmacol* 1995;278:249–252.

155. Koeppe RA, Frey KA, Kume A, et al. Equilibrium versus compartmental analysis for assessment of the vesicular monoamine transporter using (+)-α-^{11}C]dihydrotetrabenazine (DTBZ) and positron emission tomography. *J Cereb Blood Flow Metab* 1997;17:919–931.

156. Frey KA, Koeppe RA, Kilbourn MR, et al. Presynaptic monoaminergic vesicles in Parkinson's disease and normal aging. *Ann Neurol* 1996;40:873–884.

157. Singer T. Monoamine oxidases: old friends hold many surprises. *FASEB J* 1995;9:605–610.

158. Fowler JS, MacGregor RR, Wolf AP, et al. Mapping human brain monoamine oxidase A and B with ^{11}C-suicide inactivators and positron emission tomography. *Science* 1987;235:481–485.

159. Fowler JS, Volkow ND, Logan J, et al. Monoamine oxidase B (MAO B) inhibitor therapy in Parkinson's disease: the degree and reversibility of human brain MAO B inhibition by Ro 19 6327. *Neurology* 1993;43:1984–1992.

160. Fowler JS, Volkow ND, Logan J, et al. Slow recovery of human brain MAO B after L-deprenyl withdrawal. *Synapse* 1994;18:86–93.

161. Fowler JS, Volkow ND, Wang G-J, et al. Inhibition of monoamine oxidase B in the brains of smokers. *Nature* 1996;379:733–736.

162. Fowler JS, Volkow ND, Wang G-J, et al. Brain monoamine oxidase A inhibition in cigarette smokers. *Proc Natl Acad Sci U S A* 1996; 93:14065–14069.

163. Khalil AA, Steyn S, Castagnoli N. Isolation and characterization of a monoamine oxidase inhibitor from tobacco leaves. *Chem Res Toxicol* 2000;13:31–35.

164. Morens DM, Grandinetti A, Reed D, et al. Cigarette smoking and protection from Parkinson's disease: false association or etiological clue. *Neurology* 1995;45:1041–1051.

165. Bergstrom M, Westerberg G, Kihberg T, et al. Synthesis of some ^{11}C-labeled MAO A inhibitors and their *in vivo* uptake kinetics. *Nucl Med Biol* 1997;24:381–388.

166. Bernard S, Fuseau C, Schmid L, et al. Synthesis and *in vivo* studies of a specific monoamine oxidase B inhibitor 5-[4-benzyloxy)phenyl]-3-(2-cyanoethyl)-1,3,4-oxadiazo-^{11}C]-2-(3H)-1. *Eur J Nucl Med* 1996;23:150–156.

167. Barnes NM, Sharp T. A review of central 5-HT receptors and their function. *Neuropharmacology* 1999;38:1083–1152.

168. Crouzel C, Guillaume M, Barre L, et al. Ligands and tracers for PET studies of the 5-HT system—current status. *Nucl Med Biol* 1992;19: 857–870.

169. Pike VW. Radioligands for PET studies of central 5-HT receptors and re-uptake sites—current status. *Nucl Med Biol* 1995;22:1011–1018.

170. Wong DF, Wagner HN, Dannals RF, et al. Effects of age on dopamine and serotonin receptors measured by positron tomography in the living human brain. *Science* 1984;226:1393–1396.

171. Wang G-J, Volkow ND, Logan J, et al. Evaluation of age-related changes in serotonin 5-HT$_2$ and dopamine D$_2$ receptor availability in healthy human subjects. *Life Sci* 1995;56:249–253.

172. Biver F, Goldman S, Luxen A, et al. Multicompartmental study of fluorine-18 altanserin binding to brain 5-HT$_2$ receptors in humans using positron emission tomography. *Eur J Nucl Med* 1994;21:937–946.

173. Blin J, Sette G, Fiorelli M, et al. A method for the *in vivo* investigation of the serotonergic 5-HT$_2$ receptors in the human cerebral cortex using positron emission tomography and ^{18}F-labeled setoperone. *J Neurochem* 1990;54:1744–1754.

174. Ito H, Nyberg S, Halldin C, et al. PET imaging of central 5-HT$_{2A}$ receptors with carbon-11-MDL 100,907. *J Nucl Med* 1998;39:208–214.

175. Mathis CA, Mahmood K, Simpson NR, et al. Synthesis and preliminary *in vivo* evaluation of [^{11}C]MDL 100907: a potent and selective radioligand for the 5-HT$_{2A}$ receptor system. *Med Chem Res* 1996;6:1–10.

176. Van Dyck CH, Tan PZ, Baldwin RM, et al. PET quantification of 5-HT$_{2A}$ receptors in the human brain; a constant infusion paradigm with [^{18}F]altanserin. *J Nucl Med* 2000;41:234–241.

177. Mathis CA, Simpson NR, Mahmood K, et al. [^{11}C]WAY 100635: a radioligand for imaging 5-HT$_{1A}$ receptors with positron emission tomography. *Life Sci* 1994;55:PL403–PL407.

178. Osman S, Lundkvist C, Pike VW. Characterization of the radioactive metabolites of the 5-HT$_{1A}$ receptor radioligand, [*O*-methyl-^{11}C]WAY-100635, in monkey and human plasma by HPLC: comparison of the behavior of an identified radioactive metabolite with parent radioligand in monkey using PET. *Nucl Med Biol* 1996;23:627–634.

179. Osman S, Lundkvist C, Pike VW, et al. Characterization of the appearance of radioactive metabolites in monkey and human plasma from the 5-HT$_{1A}$ receptor radioligand, [carbonyl-^{11}C]WAY-100635—exploration of high signal contrast in PET and an aid to biomathematical modeling. *Nucl Med Biol* 1998;25:215–223.

180. Farde L, Ito H, Swahn C-G, et al. Quantitative analyses of carbonyl-carbon-11-WAY-100635 binding to central 5-hydroxytryptamine-1A receptors in man. *J Nucl Med* 1998;39:1965–1971.

181. Houle S, Wilson AA, Inaba T, et al. Imaging 5-HT$_{1A}$ receptors with positron emission tomography: initial human studies with [^{11}C]CPC-222. *Nucl Med Commun* 1997;18:1130–1134.

182. Sandell H, Halldin C, Hall H, et al. Radiosynthesis and autoradiographic evaluation of [^{11}C]NAD-299, a radioligand for visualization of the 5-HT$_{1A}$ receptor. *Nucl Med Biol* 1999;26:159–164.

183. Shiue C-Y, Shiue GG, Mozley PD, et al. P-[^{18}F]-MPPF: a potential radioligand for PET studies of 5-HT$_{1A}$ receptors in humans. *Synapse* 1997;25:147–154.

184. Plenevaux A, Lemaire C, Aerts J, et al. [^{18}F]p-MPPF: a radiolabeled antagonist for the study of 5HT$_{1A}$ receptors with PET. *Nucl Med Biol* 2000;27:467–471.

185. Plenevaux A, Weissmann D, Aerts J, et al. Tissue distribution, autoradiography, and metabolism of 4-(2'-methoxyphenyl)-1-[2'-[N-2'-pyridinyl)-p-[(18)F]fluorobenzamido-ethyl]piperazine (p-[(18)F]MPPF), a new serotonin 5-HT(1A) antagonist for positron emission tomography: an *in vivo* study in rats. *J Neurochem* 2000;75:803–811.

186. Entire issue. *Nucl Med Biol* 2000;27(5).

187. Suehiro M, Ravert HT, Dannals RF, et al. Synthesis of a radiotracer for studying serotonin uptake sites with positron emission tomography: [^{11}C]McN-5652-Z. *J Labelled Compounds Radiopharm* 1992;31:841–848.

188. Szabo Z, Kao PF, Scheffel U, et al. Positron emission tomography imaging of serotonin transporters in the human brain using [^{11}C](+)McN5652. *Synapse* 1995;20:37–43.

189. Suehiro M, Scheffel U, Ravert HT, et al. [^{11}C](+)McN5652 as a radiotracer for imaging serotonin uptake sites with PET. *Life Sci* 1993;53:883–892.

190. Buck A, Gucker PM, Schönbächler RD, et al. Evaluation of serotonergic transporters using PET and [^{11}C](+)McN-5652: assessment of methods. *J Cereb Blood Flow Metab* 2000;20:253–62.

191. Houle S, Ginovart N, Hussey D, et al. Imaging the serotonin transporter with positron emission tomography: initial human studies with [^{11}C]DAPP and [^{11}C]DASB. *Eur J Nucl Med* 2000;11:1719–1722.

192. Scheffel U, Dannals RF, Suehiro M, et al. Evaluation of ^{11}C-citalopram and ^{11}C-fluoxetine as *in vivo* ligands for the serotonin uptake site. *J Nucl Med* 1990;31:883–884.

193. Dannals RF, Ravert HT, Wilson AA, et al. Synthesis of a radiotracer for studying serotonin-2 receptors: carbon-11 labelled *N*-methylparoxetine. *J Labelled Compounds Radiopharm* 1989;26:205–206.

194. Diksic M, Tohyama Y, Takada A. Brain net unidirectional uptake of α-methyltryptophan. *Neurochem Res* 2000;25:1537–1546.

195. Diksic M, Nagahiro S, Sources TL, et al. A new method to measure brain serotonin synthesis *in vivo*. Theory and basis data for a biological model. *J Cereb Blood Flow Metab* 1990;10:1–12.

196. Shoaf SE, Carson RE, Hommer D, et al. The suitability of [^{11}C]-α-methy-L-tryptophan as a tracer for serotonin synthesis: studies with dual administration of [^{11}C] and [^{14}C] labeled tracer. *J Cereb Blood Flow Metab* 2000;20:244–252(and references therein).

197. Dannals RF, Ravert HT, Frost JJ, et al. Radiosynthesis of an opiate receptor binding radiotracer: [^{11}C]carfentanil. *Int J Appl Radiat Isot* 1985;36:303–306.

198. Frost JJ, Wagner HN Jr, Dannals RF, et al. Imaging opiate receptors in the human brain by positron tomography. *J Comput Assisted Tomogr* 1985;9:231–236.

199. Zubieta JK, Dannals RF, Frost JJ. Gender and age influences on human brain mu-opioid receptor binding measured by PET. *Am J Psychiatry* 1999;156:842.

200. Luthra AK, Pike VW, Brady F. The preparation of carbon-11 labelled diprenorphine: a new radioligand for the study of the opiate receptor system *in vivo*. *J Chem Soc Chem Commun* 1985;1423–1425.

201. Luthra SK, Pike VW, Brady F, et al. Preparation of [^{11}C]buprenorphine—a potential radioligand for the study of opiate receptor system *in vivo*. *Appl Radiat Isot* 1987;38:65–66.

202. Lever JR, Mazza SM, Dannals RF, et al. Facile synthesis of [^{11}C]buprenorphine for positron emission tomographic studies. *Appl Radiat Isot* 1990;41:745–752.

203. Galynker I, Schlyer DJ, Dewey SL, et al. Opioid receptor imaging and displacement studies with [6-*O*-[^{11}C]methyl]buprenorphine in baboon brain. *Nucl Med Biol* 1996;23:325–331.

204. Shiue CY, Bai LQ, Teng RR, et al. A comparison of the brain uptake of *N*-(cyclopropyl [^{11}C]methyl)norbuprenorphine ([^{11}C]buprenorphine) and *N*-(cyclopropyl[^{11}C]methyl) nordiprenorphine ([^{11}C]diprenorphine) in baboon using PET. *Nucl Med Biol* 1991;18:281–288.

205. Channing M, Eckelman WC, Bennett JM, et al. Radiosynthesis of [^{18}F] 3-acetylcyclofoxy: a high affinity opiate antagonist. *Int J Appl Radiat Isot* 1985;36:429–433.

206. Carson RE, Basberg RG, Channing MA, et al. Tracer infusion for equilibrium measurements: applications to ^{18}F-cyclofoxy opiate receptor imaging with PET. *J Cereb Blood Flow Metab* 1989;9[Suppl 1]:S203.

207. Ravert HT, Mathews WB, Musachio JL, et al. [^{11}C]-Methyl 4-[(3,4-dichlorophenyl)acetyl]-3-[(1-pyrrolidinyl)-methyl]-1-piperazinecarboxylate ([^{11}C]GR89696): synthesis and *in vivo* binding to kappa opiate receptors. *Nucl Med Biol* 1999;26:737–741.

208. Madar I, Lever JR, Kinter CM, et al. Imaging of delta opioid receptors in human brain by N1'-[^{11}C]methylnaltrindol and PET. *Synapse* 1996;24:19–28.

209. Barnard EA, Skolnick P, Olsen RW, et al. International Union of Pharmacology, XV: subtypes of gamma-aminobutyric acid A receptors: classification on the basis of subunit structure and receptor function. *Pharmacol Rev* 1998;50:291–313.

210. Gavish M, Bachman I, Shoukrun R, et al. Enigma of the peripheral benzodiazepine receptor. *Pharm Rev* 1999;51:630–646.

211. Pike VW, Halldin C, Crouzel C, et al. Radioligands for PET studies of central benzodiazepine receptors and PK (peripheral benzodiazepine) binding sites—current status [Review]. *Nucl Med Biol* 1993;20:503–525.

212. Persson A, Ehrin E, Eriksson L, et al. Imaging of [^{11}C]-labeled Ro 15-1788 binding to benzodiazepine receptors in the human brain by positron emission tomography. *J Psychiatry Res* 1985;19:609–622.

213. Koeppe RA, Holthof VA, Frey KA, et al. Compartmental analysis of [^{11}C]flumazenil kinetics for the estimation of ligand transport rate and receptor distribution using positron emission tomography. *J Cereb Blood Flow Metab* 1991;11:735–744.

214. Savic I, Roland P, Sedvall G, et al. *In vivo* demonstration of reduced benzodiazepine receptor binding in human epileptic foci. *Lancet* 15 Oct 1988:863–866.

215. Bremner JD, Horti A, Staib LH, et al. Kinetic modeling of benzodiazepine receptor binding with PET and high specific activity [^{11}C]iomazenil in healthy human subjects. *Synapse* 2000;35:68–77.

216. Bergstrom M, Mosskin M, Ericson K, et al. Peripheral benzodiazepine binding sites in human gliomas evaluated with positron emission tomography. *Acta Radiol* 1986;369[Suppl]:409–411.

217. Junck L, Olson JMM, Cilliax BJ, et al. PET imaging of human gliomas with ligands for the peripheral benzodiazepine binding site. *Ann Neurol* 1989;26:752–758.

218. Banati RB, Newcombe J, Gunn RN. The peripheral benzodiazepine binding site in the brain in multiple sclerosis: quantitative *in vivo* imaging of microglia as a measure of disease activity. *Brain* 2000; 123:2321–2337.

219. Coyle JT, Price DL, DeLong MR. Alzheimer's disease: a disorder of cortical cholinergic innervation. *Science* 1983;219:1184–1190.

220. Volkow ND, Ding Y-S, Fowler JS, et al. Imaging brain cholinergic activity with positron emission tomography: its role in the evaluation of cholinergic treatments in Alzheimer's dementia. *Biol Psychiatry* 2001;49:211–220.

221. Schliebs R, Robner S. Distribution of muscarinic acetylcholine receptors in the CNS. In: Stone TW, ed. *CNS neurotransmitters and neuromodulators: acetylcholine.* Boca Raton, FL: CRC Press, 1994;67–83.

222. Flynn DD, Farrari-DiLeo G, Mash DC, et al. Differential regulation of molecular subtypes of muscarinic receptors in Alzheimer's disease. *J Neurochem* 1995;64;1881–1891.

223. Frey KA, Koeppe RA, Mulholland GK. *In vivo* muscarinic cholinergic receptor imaging in human brain with [^{11}C]scopolamine and positron emission tomography. *J Cereb Blood Flow Metab* 1992;12:147–154.

224. Mulholland GK, Otto CA, Jewett DM, et al. Radiosynthesis and comparisons in the biodistribution of carbon-11 labeled muscarinic antagonists: (+)2U-tropanyl benzilate and *N*-methyl-4-piperidyl benzilate. *J Labelled Compounds Radiopharm* 1989;26:202.

225. Mulholland GK, Kilbourn MR, Sherman P, et al. Synthesis, *in vivo* biodistribution and dosimetry of [^{11}C]*N*-methylpiperidyl benzilate ([^{11}C]NMPB), a muscarinic acetylcholine receptor antagonist. *Nucl Med Biol* 1995;22:13–17.

226. Lee KS, Frey KA, Koeppe RA, et al. *In vivo* quantification of cerebral muscarinic receptors in normal human aging using positron emission tomography and [^{11}C]tropanyl benzilate. *J Cereb Blood Flow Metab* 1996;16:303–310.

227. Zubieta JK, Koeppe RA, Frey KA, et al. Assessment of muscarinic receptor concentrations in aging and Alzheimer disease with [^{11}C]NMPB and PET. *Synapse* 2001;39:275–287.

228. Yoshida T, Kuwabara Y, Ichiya Y, et al. Cerebral muscarinic acetylcholinergic receptor measurement in Alzheimer's disease patients on [^{11}C]-*N*-methyl-4-piperidinyl benzilate—comparison with cerebral blood flow and cerebral glucose metabolism. *Ann Nucl Med* 1998; 12:35–42.

229. Tsukada H, Takahashi K, Miura S, et al. Evaluation of novel PET ligands (+)*N*-[^{11}C]methyl-3-piperidinyl benzilate ([^{11}C](+)3-MPB) and its stereoisomer [^{11}C](−)3-MPB for muscarinic cholinergic receptors in the conscious monkey brain: a PET study in comparison with [^{11}C]4-MPB. *Synapse* 2001;39:182–192.

230. Dewey SL, MacGregor RR, Bendreim B, et al. Mapping muscarine receptors in human and baboon brain using [N-^{11}C-methyl]benztropine. *Synapse* 1990;5:213–223.

231. Dewey SL, Volkow ND, Logan J, et al. Age-related decreases in muscarinic cholinergic receptor binding in the human brain measured with positron emission tomography (PET). *J Neurosci Res* 1990;27: 569–575.

232. Buck A, Mulholland GK, Papadopoulos SM, et al. Kinetic evaluation of positron-emitting muscarinic ligands employing direct carotid injection. *J Cereb Blood Flow Metab* 1996;16:1280–1287.

233. Kiesewetter DO, Lee J, Lang L, et al. Preparation of ^{18}F-labeled muscarinic agonist with M2 selectivity. *J Med Chem* 1995;38:5–8.

234. Carson RE, Kiesewetter DO, Jagoda E, et al. Muscarinic cholinergic receptor measurements with [^{18}F]FP-TZTP: control and competition studies. *J Cereb Blood Flow Metab* 1998;18:1130–1142.

235. Bonnot-Lours S, Crouzel C, Prenant C, et al. Carbon-11 labelling of an inhibitor of acetylcholinesterase. *J Labelled Compounds Radiopharm* 1993;33:277–284.

236. Pappata S, Tavitian B, Traykov L, et al. *In vivo* imaging of human cerebral acetylcholinesterase. *J Neurochem* 1996;67:876–879.

237. Irie T, Fukushi K, Akimoto Y, et al. Design and evaluation of radioactive acetylcholine analogs for mapping brain acetylcholinesterase (AChE) *in vivo*. *Nucl Med Biol* 1994;21:801–808.

238. Kilbourn MR, Snyder SF, Sherman PS, et al. *In vivo* studies of acetyl-

239. Kuhl DE, Koeppe RA, Minoshima A, et al. *In vivo* mapping of cerebral acetylcholinesterase in aging and Alzheimer's disease. *Neurology* 1999;52:691–699.

240. Ingvar M, Stone-Elander S, Rogers GA, et al. Striatal D$_2$/acetylcholine interactions: PET studies of the vesamicol receptor. *Neuroreport* 1993;4:1311–1314.

241. Gage HD, Voytko ML, Ehrenkaufer RL, et al. Reproducibility of repeated measures of cholinergic terminal density using [^{18}F](+)-4-fluorobenzyltrozamicol and PET in rhesus monkey brain. *J Nucl Med* 2000;41:2069–2076.

242. Gopalakrishnan M, Donnelly-Roberts DL. Nicotine: therapeutic prospects? *Pharm News* 1998;5:16–20.

243. Domino EF. Tobacco smoking and nicotine neuropsychopharmacology: some future research directions. *Neuropsychopharmacology* 1998;18:456–468.

244. Arneric SP, Sullivan JP, Williams M. Neuronal nicotinic acetylcholine receptors—novel targets for central nervous system therapeutics. In: Bloom FE, Kupfer DJ, eds. *Psychopharmacology: the fourth generation of progress.* New York: Raven Press, 1995:95–110.

245. Picciotto MR, Zoli M, Rimondini R, et al. Acetylcholine receptors containing the beta2 subunit are involved in the reinforcing properties of nicotine. *Nature* 1998;391:173–177.

246. Nordberg A. Human nicotinic receptors—their role in aging and dementia. *Neurochem Int* 1994;25:93–97.

247. Perry DC, Davila-Garcia MI, Stockmeier CA, et al. Increased nicotinic receptors in brains from smokers: membrane binding and autoradiography studies. *J Pharm Exp Ther* 1999;289:1545–1552.

248. Sihver W, Nordberg A, Langstrom B, et al. Development of ligands for *in vivo* imaging of cerebral nicotinic receptors. *Behav Brain Res* 2000;113:143–157.

249. Nyback H, Nordberg A, von Holst H, et al. Attempts to visualize nicotinic receptors in the brain of monkey and man by positron emission tomography. *Prog Brain Res* 1989;79:313–319.

250. Muzik RF, Berridge MS, Friedland RF, et al. PET quantification of specific binding of carbon-11-nicotine in human brain. *J Nucl Med* 1998;39:2048–2054.

251. Sihver W, Fasth J, Ogren M, et al. *In vivo* positron emission tomography studies on the novel nicotinic receptor agonist [^{11}C]MPA compared with [^{11}C]ABT-418 and (S)-(−)[^{11}C] nicotine in rhesus monkeys. *Nucl Med Biol* 1999;26:633–642.

252. Spande TF, Garraffo HM, Edwards MW, et al. Epibatidine: a novel (chloropyridyl)azabicycloheptane with potent analgesic activity from the Ecuadorian poison frog. *J Am Chem Soc* 1992;114:3475–3478.

253. Qian C, Li T, Shen TY, et al. Epibatidine is a nicotinic analgesic. *Eur J Pharmacol* 1993;250:R13–R14.

254. Horti A, Ravert HT, London ED, et al. Synthesis of a radiotracer for studying nicotinic acetylcholine receptors: (±)-*exo*-2-(2-[^{18}F]fluoro-5-pyridyl)-7-azabicyclo[2.2.1]heptane. *J Labelled Compounds Radiopharm* 1996;38:355–365.

255. Ding Y-S, Volkow ND, Logan J, et al. Occupancy of brain nicotinic acetylcholine receptors by nicotine doses equivalent to those obtained when smoking a cigarette. *Synapse* 2000;35:234–237.

256. Ding Y-S, Logan J, Bermel R, et al. Dopamine receptor-mediated regulation of striatal cholinergic activity: PET studies with [^{18}F]norchlorofluoroepibatidine. *J Neurochem* 2000;74:1514–1521.

257. Ding Y-S, Molina PE, Fowler JS, et al. Comparative studies of epibatidine derivatives [^{18}F]NFEP and [^{18}F]*N*-methyl-NFEP: kinetics, nicotine effect and toxicity. *Nucl Med Biol* 1999;26:139–148.

258. Molina PE, Ding Y-S, Carroll FI, et al. Fluoro-norchloroepibatidine: preclinical assessment of acute toxicity. *Nucl Med Biol* 1997;24: 743–747.

259. Abreo MA, Lin N-H, Garvey DS, et al. Novel 3-pyridyl ethers with subnanomolar affinity for central neuronal nicotinic acetylcholine receptors. *J Med Chem* 1996;39:817–825.

260. Valette H, Bottlaender M, Dolle F, et al. Imaging central nicotinic acetylcholine receptors in baboons with [^{18}F]fluoro-A-85380. *J Nucl Med* 1999;40:1374–1380.

261. Horti AG, Koren AO, Ravert HT, et al. Synthesis of a radiotracer for studying nicotinic acetylcholine receptors: 2-[^{18}F]fluoro-3-(2(S)-azetidinylmethoxy)pyridine (2-[^{18}F]A-85380). *J Labelled Compounds Radiopharm* 1998;XLI:309–318.

262. Dolle F, Valette H, Bottlaender M, et al. Synthesis of 2-[^{18}F]fluoro-

3-[2(S)-2-azetidinylmethoxy]pyridine a highly potent radioligand for in vivo imaging central nicotinic acetylcholine receptors. *J Labelled Compounds Radiopharm* 1998;XLI:451–463.

263. Dolle F, Dolci L, Valette H, et al. Synthesis and nicotinic acetylcholine receptor *in vivo* binding properties of 2-fluoro-3-[2(S)-2-azetidinyl-methoxy]pyridine: a new positron emission tomography ligand for nicotinic receptors. *J Med Chem* 1999;42:2251–2259.

264. Koren AO, Horti AG, Mukhin AG, et al. Synthesis and *in vitro* characterization of 6-[^{18}F]fluoro-3-(2(S)-azetidinylmethoxy)pyridine, a high-affinity radioligand for central nicotinic acetylcholine receptors. *J Labelled Compounds Radiopharm* 1999;42:S409.

265. Scheffel U, Horti AG, Koren AO, et al. 6-[^{18}F]Fluoro-A-85380: an *in vivo* tracer for the nicotinic acetylcholine receptor. *Nucl Med Biol* 2000;27:51–56.

266. Ding Y-S, Liu N, Wang T, et al. Synthesis of 6-[^{18}F]fluoro-3-(S)-azetidinylmethoxy) pyridine for PET studies of nicotine acetylcholine receptors. *Nucl Med Biol* 2000;27:381–389.

267. Duman RS, Nestler EJ. Signal transduction pathways for catecholamine receptors. In: Meltzer H, ed. *Psychopharmacology: the fourth generation.* New York: Raven Press, 1995:303–320.

268. Imahori Y, Ohmori Y, Fujii R, et al. Rapid incorporation of carbon-11 labeled diacylglycerol as a probe of signal transduction in glioma. *Cancer Res* 1995;55:4225–4229.

269. Sasaki T, Enta A, Nozaki T, et al. Carbon-11-forskolin: a ligand for visualization of the adenylate cyclase-related second messenger. *J Nucl Med* 1993;34:1944–1948.

270. Takahashi T, Ootake A. [^{18}F]Labeled 1,2-diacylglycerols: a new tracer for imaging second messenger system. *J Labelled Compounds Radiopharm* 1994;35:517–519.

271. Lourenco CM, DaSilva J, Warsh JJ, et al. Imaging of cAMP-specific phosphodiesterase-IV: comparison of [^{11}C]rolipram and [^{11}C]Ro 20-1724 in rats. *Synapse* 1999;31:41–50.

272. Vaalburg W, Coenen HH, Crouzel C, et al. Amino acids for the measurement of protein synthesis *in vivo* by PET. *Nucl Med Biol* 1992; 19:227–237.

273. Jager PL, Vaalburg W, Pruim J, et al. Radiolabeled amino acids: basic aspects and clinical applications in oncology. *J Nucl Med* 2001;42: 432–445.

274. Jager PL, de Vries EG, Piers DA, et al. Uptake mechanisms of L-3-[125I] iodo-alpha-methyl-tyrosine in a human small-cell lung cancer cell line: comparison with L-1. *Nucl Med Commun* 2001;22:87–96.

275. Hawkins RA, Huang S-C, Barrio JR, et al. Estimation of local cerebral protein synthesis rates with L-[1-^{11}C]leucine and PET: methods, model, and results in animals and humans. *J Cereb Blood Flow Metab* 1989;9:446–460.

276. Smith CB, Davidsen L, Deibler G, et al. A method for the determination of local rates of protein synthesis in man. *Trans Am Soc Neurochem* 1980;11:94.

277. Smith CB, Deibler GE, Eng N, et al. Measurement of local cerebral protein synthesis *in vivo:* influence of recycling of amino acids derived from protein degradation. *Proc Natl Acad Sci U S A* 1988;85: 9341–9345.

278. Ishiwata K, Vaalburg W, Elsing PH, et al. Comparison of L-[1-^{11}C]methionine and L-methyl-[^{11}C]methionine for measuring *in vivo* protein synthesis rates with PET. *J Nucl Med* 1988;29:1419–1427.

279. Bolster JM, Vaalburg W, Elsinga PH, et al. The preparation of ^{11}C-carboxyl labeled L-methionine for measuring protein synthesis. *J Labelled Compounds Radiopharm* 1986;23:1081–1082.

280. Schober O, Duden C, Meyer G-J, et al. Nonselective transport of [^{11}C]methyl]-L- and D-methionine into a malignant glioma. *Eur J Nucl Med* 1987;13:103–105.

281. Bergstrom M, Muhr C, Lundberg PO, et al. Amino acid distribution and metabolism in pituitary adenomas using positron emission tomography with D-[^{11}C]methionine and L-[^{11}C]methionine. *J Comput Assisted Tomogr* 1987;11:384–389.

282. Bodsch W, Coenen HH, Stocklin G, et al. Biochemical and autoradiographic study of cerebral protein synthesis with [^{18}F]- and [14C]fluorophenylalanine. *J Neurochem* 1988;50:979–983.

283. Coenen HH, Kling P, Stocklin G. Cerebral metabolism of L-2-[^{18}F]fluorotyrosine, a new PET tracer for protein synthesis. *J Nucl Med* 1989; 30:1367–1372.

284. Ishiwata K, Kubota K, Murakami M, et al. Re-evaluation of amino acid PET studies: can the protein synthesis rates in brain and tumor tissues be measured *in vivo?* *J Nucl Med* 1993;34:1936–1943.

285. Weinhard K, Herholz K, Coenen HH, et al. Increased amino acid transport into brain tumors measured by PET of L-(2-^{18}F)fluorotyrosine. *J Nucl Med* 1991;32:1338–1346.

286. Ogawa T, Miura S, Murakami M, et al. Quantitative evaluation of neutral amino acid transport in cerebral gliomas using positron emission tomography and fluorine-18 fluorophenylalanine. *Eur J Nucl Med* 1996;23:889–895.

287. Wester HJ, Herz M, Weber W, et al. Synthesis and radiopharmacology of O-(2-[^{18}F]fluoroethyl)-L-tyrosine for tumor imaging. *J Nucl Med* 1999;40:205–212.

288. Tomiyoshi K, Amed K, Muhammed S, et al. Synthesis of a new fluorine-18 labeled amino acid radiopharmaceutical: L-^{18}F-alpha-methyl tyrosine using separation and purification system. *Nucl Med Commun* 1997;18:169–175.

289. Inoue TJ, Shibasaki T, Oriuchi N, et al. ^{18}F-α-methyl tyrosine PET studies in patients with brain tumors. *J Nucl Med* 1999;40:399–405.

290. Inoue TJ, Tomiyoshi K, Higuchi T, et al. Biodistribution studies on L-3-[fluorine-18]fluoro-α-methyl tyrosine: a potential tumor-detecting agent. *J Nucl Med* 1998;39:663–667.

291. Shoup TM, Olson JMH, Votaw J, et al. Synthesis and evaluation of [^{18}F]1-amino-3-fluorocyclobutane-1-carboxylic acid to image brain tumors. *J Nucl Med* 1999;40:331–338.

292. Cronkite EP, Fliedner TM, Bond VP, et al. Dynamics of hemopoietic proliferation in man and mice studied by 3H-thymidine incorporation into DNA. *Ann N Y Acad Sci* 1959;77:803.

293. Christman DR, Crawford EJ, Friedkin M, et al. Detection of DNA synthesis in intact organisms with positron-emitting methyl ^{11}C-thymidine. *Proc Natl Acad Sci U S A* 1971;69:988–989.

294. Crawford EJ, Friedkin M, Wolf AP, et al. ^{18}F-5-fluorouridine, a new probe for measuring the proliferation of tissue *in vivo. Adv Enz Regul* 1982;20:3–22.

295. Shields AF, Coonrod DV, Quackenbush RC, et al. Cellular sources of thymidine nucleotides: studies for PET. *J Nucl Med* 1987;28: 1435–1440.

296. Shields AF, Larson SM, Grunbaum Z, et al. Short-term thymidine uptake in normal and neoplastic tissues: studies for PET. *J Nucl Med* 1984;25:759–764.

297. Mankoff DA, Dehdashti F, Shields AF. Characterizing tumors using metabolic imaging: PET imaging of cellular proliferation and steroid receptors. *Neoplasia* 2000;2:71–88.

298. Shields AF, Mankoff DA, Link JM, et al. Carbon-11-thymidine and FDG to measure therapy response. *J Nucl Med* 1998;39:1757–1762.

299. Mankoff DA, Shields AF, Link JM, et al. Kinetic analysis of 2-[^{11}C]thymidine PET imaging studies: validation studies. *J Nucl Med* 1999;40:614–624.

300. Eary JF, Mankoff DA, Spence AM, et al. 2-[C-11]thymidine imaging of malignant brain tumors. *Cancer Res* 1999;5:615–621.

301. Conti PS, Hilton J, Magee CA, et al. Analysis of nucleoside metabolism during positron emission tomography (PET) imaging studies of brain tumors with carbon-11 labeled thymidine (TdR). *Paper presented at: 199th Meeting of the American Chemical Society*; April 22–27, 1999; Boston, Massachusetts.

302. Shields AF, Lim K, Grierson J, et al. Utilization of labeled thymidine in DNA synthesis: studies for PET. *J Nucl Med* 1990;31:337–342.

303. Shields AF, Grierson JR, Kozawa SM, et al. Development of labeled thymidine analogs for imaging tumor proliferation. *Nucl Med Biol* 1996;23:17–22.

304. Conti PS, Alauddin MM, Fissekis JR, et al. Synthesis of 2'-fluoro-5-[^{11}C]-methyl-1-beta-D-arabinofuranosyluracil ([^{11}C]-FMAU): a potential nucleoside analog for *in vivo* study of cellular proliferation with PET. *Nucl Med Biol* 1995;22:783–789.

305. Flexner C, van der Horst C, Jacobson MA, et al. Relationship between plasma concentrations of 3'-deoxy-3'-fluorothymidine (alovudine) and antiretroviral activity in two concentration-controlled trails. *J Infect Dis* 1994;170:1394–1403.

306. Kong XB, Zhu QY, Vidal PM, et al. Comparisons of anti-human immunodeficiency virus activities, cellular transport, and plasma and intracellular pharmacokinetics of 3'-fluoro-3'-deoxythymidine and 3'-azido-3'-deoxythymidine. *Antimicrob Agents Chemother* 1992;36: 808–818.

307. Shields AF, Grierson JR, Dohmen BM, et al. Imaging proliferation *in vivo* with [F-18]FLT and positron emission tomography. *Nat Med* 1998;4:1334–1336.

308. *The United States Pharmacopeia: The National Formulary: 2000.* Rockville, MD: United States Pharmacopeial Convention, 2000.

CHAPTER 3

Instrumentation

Christopher J. Thompson

FORMATION OF PET IMAGES

Radioactive Decay By Positron Emission

Unlike other instruments used in nuclear medicine, dedicated positron emission tomography (PET) scanners use electronic, as opposed to lead, collimators. Modern dedicated PET cameras preferentially detect radioisotopes that decay by positron emission. PET scanners can also detect high-energy gamma rays such as those emitted by cesium-137 (^{137}Cs), which is used in some PET scanners for performing transmission scans. The most common PET radioisotopes (and their properties) used in clinical practice are given in Table 3.1.

A schematic diagram showing what happens after positron decay is shown in Fig. 3.1. When a radioisotope emits a positron, the mass difference between the parent and daughter isotopes becomes energy, which is shared unevenly between the daughter nucleus and the positron. The positron is therefore ejected with enough kinetic energy to travel some distance from the parent nucleus. It must lose this energy before combining with an electron and eventually annihilating. It does this by making collisions in the medium in which it is traveling. An important part of Table 3.1 is the "mean positron range," which imposes a lower limit on the spatial resolution of any PET system. The mean range values in Table 3.1 are given for water. The values are smaller in bones but are much larger in the lungs, and several meters in air! The blurring associated with this process is known as positron range blurring, and it depends on the isotope and the medium in which the radioactive decay occurs.

Annihilation of Positrons and Electrons

The fundamental signal in PET results from the mutual annihilation of the positron and an electron. This results in the production of two annihilation photons, each having the energy corresponding to the mass of an electron (i.e., 511 keV) and a neutrino.

Production of Two Annihilation Photons

The two photons are emitted exactly 180 degrees apart with respect to the electron–positron pair (Fig. 3.1). However, because both the electron and the positron are moving when this happens, the apparent angle is not quite 180 degrees but has a random variation of about 0.5 degrees. Because this angle is unpredictable and cannot be measured, PET scanner software assumes that the angle is 180 degrees, and this causes additional blurring of the image. The magnitude of this error depends on the distance separating the two detectors, so it can be reduced in scanners designed for brain-only studies or in small-animal PET scanners. The blurring associated with this process is known as non-colinearity blurring, and it depends on the energy of the electron involved in the annihilation and the separation of the detectors.

Both Annihilation Photons Must Escape the Patient and be Detected

Both of the annihilation photons must escape from the patient to be detected. If neither is scattered, then the line joining the two detectors will intersect the point of annihilation (apart from the error due to non-colinearity referred to in the previous section). Only unscattered photon pairs contribute useful information to the process of image formation. Unscattered photon pairs are referred as true counts, to distinguish them from scattered counts.

Coincident Detection of Annihilation Photons Constitutes One "Count"

The near-simultaneous detection of a pair of annihilation photons represents one event or count in the image. The line joining the two detectors is referred to as a line of response (LOR) (the dashed line in Fig. 3.1). Images are formed from millions of these counts. Even though both photons are emitted simultaneously, they may not be detected at exactly the same time. The point of annihilation is not confined to the center of the image field, and during transmission scans it

TABLE 3.1. *Properties of radioisotopes commonly used with PET*

Isotope	Half-life (units)	Positron range (mm)	Production	Applications
Carbon-11	20.4 (min)	1.7	Cyclotron	Various
Nitrogen-13	10.0 (min)	2.0	Cyclotron	Cardiac blood flow
Oxygen-15	2.07 (min)	2.7	Cyclotron	Cerebral blood flow
Fluorine-18	110 (min)	1.4	Cyclotron	Glucose metabolism
Rubidium-82	1.2 (min)	4.0	Generator	Cardiac blood flow
Germanium-68	260 (d)	3.0	Purchase	Transmission scan
Cesium-137	5 (yr)	NA	Purchase	Transmission scan

is beyond the edge of the image field. Because the photons travel at the speed of light (about 30 cm/ns), the detection times can be different by more than 2 ns for a typical PET scanner with an aperture of 60 cm. For this reason, and due to errors in timing, a short time window is set, during which pairs of annihilation photons are considered to be "in coincidence." This window is typically in the range of 8 to 16 ns for body scanners with relatively "slow" scintillation crystals.

It is possible, and at high count rates quite likely, that two photons that did not originate in the same annihilation can be detected within this time window. Such events are referred to as random counts.

Counts Recorded in Sinogram for Image Reconstruction

During a PET scan, all of these counts must be collected and stored. An array of memory is allocated for this purpose, and all the memory locations are set to zero before the scan starts. Memory locations associated with each LOR are in-

cremented during the scan so each event is "counted" as it comes in. Modern PET scanners have thousands of detectors, resulting in millions of LORs. The storage matrix representing all the LORs can be made more compact by recognizing symmetries in PET scanners and by combining counts from very close LORs into one memory location.

The memory arrays used for data storage are often referred to as "sinograms" and are derived from the pattern associated with counting events from an off-center point source in one of these arrays. The horizontal coordinate is derived from the difference of the detector numbers in a ring scanner, and the vertical coordinate is the average of the detector numbers. This format of data storage is both compact and in a suitable form for direct use by the image-reconstruction program. Figures 3.2 and 3.3 illustrate the relationship between the detectors on the circumference of a circle and a sinogram. Consider that there is activity in only one location in the scanner's field of view. The point of annihilation (represented by A in Fig. 3.2) is a distance d from the center, and the two photons are detected by crystals at positions A and B. The chord PQ is a distance s from the center of the

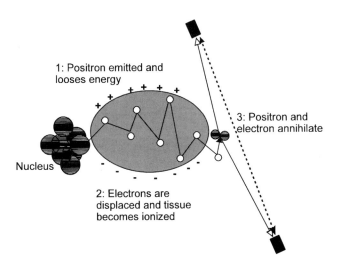

FIG. 3.1. A nucleus undergoes positron decay. Subsequent annihilation of a positron and an electron produces two photons that travel away from the site at almost 180 degrees and are then detected. This is not to scale; the positron range is typically a few millimeters, but the detectors (three) are often separated by more than 60 cm.

1: Positron emitted and looses energy

Nucleus

2: Electrons are displaced and tissue becomes ionized

3: Positron and electron annihilate

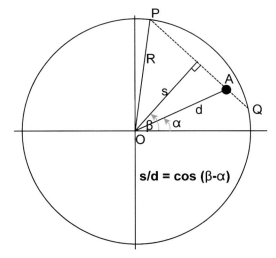

$$s/d = \cos(\beta - \alpha)$$

FIG. 3.2. *A* is the point of annihilation, *P* and *Q* are the detectors involved. The distance from *A* to the origin is represented by *d*. The distance from the line of response (LOR) (*dashed line*) to the origin is represented by *s*. The angle α is measured to the line joining the point of annihilation to the origin, and angle β is measured to the normal of the LOR.

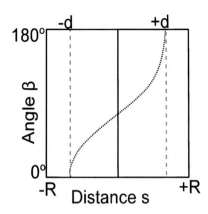

FIG. 3.3. Sinogram for a point source at distance *d* from the origin of a PET detector ring of radius R. The angle β is the average angle of the two detectors defining the line of response.

ring. The line from A to the origin makes and angle α and the line from the chord AB to the center makes an angle beta or (P + Q)/2. All annihilation photon pairs emanating from the source pass through A but will interact with other detectors so although *d* and α are constant for this point, β and *s* will vary (Fig. 3.3). The relationship is given by

$$s = d\cos(\beta - \alpha)$$

This one point source will cause counts to be accumulated along the cosine curve (dotted line in Fig. 3.3). The points in one horizontal row of a sinogram make up a "projection."

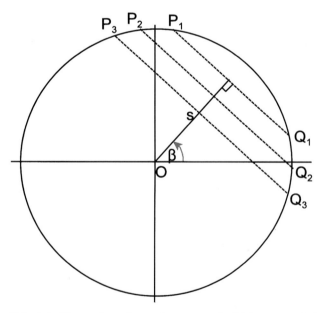

FIG. 3.4. These three lines of response (LORs) are parallel and at an angle β = (P + Q)/2. If the *P*s and *Q*s are contiguous detectors, these LORs are represented in the sinogram by contiguous horizontal samples on the line corresponding to the angle (P + Q)/2.

Each projection represents the counts acquired by a set of detector pairs that are all at the same angle, or whose LORs are parallel to one another. Figure 3.4 shows how a projection at the angle β = $(P_n + Q_n)/2$ has inputs from detectors that lie on contiguous parallel chords.

COMPONENTS OF A PET SYSTEM

A modern PET scanner is a highly sophisticated piece of equipment comprising a patient handling system, data-collection system, and image-reconstruction, display, and archival systems. Although the patient handling and image display components are the most conspicuous, the other systems play a vital role in image quality and patient throughput.

Collimators

Collimators in PET scanners are positioned to confine the radiation detected, which originates within the scanning field of view. Some early PET scanners (1,2) had one ring of detectors, and thick rings of lead were placed in front of and behind the plane of these detectors to reduce the probability of detecting annihilation photons from outside the slice being imaged. With the introduction of multislice scanners, the thick lead rings were maintained to define the external axial field of view, and thin lead or tungsten rings (1 to 5 mm thick), usually referred to as septa, were employed to define the individual imaging planes.

Most present-day commercial PET scanners now have these septa configured so they can be positioned to define the slices during two-dimensional (2D) PET studies, but they can be retracted during three-dimensional (3D) scans (see later discussion).

The collimators in PET are very different from those on a gamma camera. The common parallel-hole collimator on a gamma camera restricts the detection of gamma rays to those that are almost perpendicular to the crystal face. A high-resolution gamma camera collimator rejects almost all of the radiation emitted from a patient in the direction of the gamma camera, because most of it does not approach the crystal almost perpendicular to the surface.

Even in the 2D configuration, each element of a PET detector has a very wide field of view. The principle of coincidence detection provides an "electronic collimation" of the counts. One could think of the detector at one end of an LOR as identifying the point of detection and the other detector providing the angle of incidence.

The concept of electronic collimation is what makes PET imaging much more efficient (in terms of detected counts per injected dose) than other nuclear medicine procedures, because 99% of the radiation absorbed by the gamma camera's collimator goes undetected. The equivalent amount of single annihilation photons are detected by the PET system's detectors but are rejected by the coincidence circuit. Although the perforated lead gamma camera collimator is a passive system, each photon must be detected and paired with another to produce one count. In practice, the coincidence circuit rejects about 99% of the photons detected by the crystals. Because each detector can correctly identify only one photon at a time, a great deal of time is spent processing annihilation photons that will never correspond to a coincident count. This lost time is referred to as dead time and is a major limitation for image quality when doing PET studies with short-lived isotopes at high levels of injected activity levels. Modern cameras, scintillators, and electronics are designed to minimize dead-time problems.

Detectors

The detectors in a PET scanner perform much more efficiently than those in a gamma camera. As was mentioned in the previous section, they detect mostly single photons, which are later discarded, but are required to be ready to detect the annihilation photon pairs that are in coincidence. To do this successfully, the detectors in dedicated PET are much smaller than those of a gamma camera. Numerous small independent detectors result in lower dead-time losses.

Most radioisotopes used in nuclear medicine have relatively low energies (e.g., technetium-99m [^{99m}Tc] at 140 keV) and are detected with a very high efficiency by the relatively thin (6 to 10 mm) sodium iodide–thallium (NaI-Tl) crystal of a gamma camera. Thicker detectors are required to detect the 511-keV annihilation photons, and detectors with much higher stopping power are required.

To record a useful "count," both detectors must each detect its photon, so in PET, the probability of detecting a count depends on the square of the single detector's efficiency. For this reason, PET detectors are thicker than those in a gamma camera. The crystals in gamma cameras are made as thin as possible (while allowing for adequate efficiency) to improve their spatial resolution. Using very thick crystals to provide adequate efficiency for PET imaging, while providing good spatial resolution, appears to be a paradox.

To satisfy these seemingly contradictory requirements, early PET systems (1,2) used single crystals coupled to individual photomultipliers. This was mainly done to reduce the dead time. It also made them very expensive, particularly when the crystals were made very small to optimize the spatial resolution.

In the 1980s, a great variety of ideas to provide high detection efficiency and spatial resolution while keeping the cost reasonable were published. Most involved ways of putting many more than one crystal on one or more photomultiplier tubes (PMTs) and using some coding scheme to identify the crystal. The technique that survived was the "block detector," first described by Casey and Nutt (3).

Block detectors are made by cutting deep channels into a solid crystal and then filling these channels with non–light-conducting material to prevent the light from spreading from one section to the next.

PET scanners for human use today employ scintillation crystals coupled to photomultipliers as their detectors. The first PET scanners (1,2,4) used NaI crystals, the same material used in gamma cameras. However, most dedicated PET scanners use much denser crystals, and for more than 20 years, bismuth germanate (BGO) (5–7) has been the scintillator of choice due to its very high density and atomic number. Many other scintillators have been proposed and some of them have been used in PET scanners. The best-known ones are barium fluoride (8) and gadolinium oxyorthosilicate (9). The ideal scintillator would be very dense and rapidly convert most of the annihilation photon energy into light. The best one is cerium-doped lutetium oxyorthosilicate (LSO) (10). This is now used in the latest high-performance PET scanners (11).

The important properties of these crystals for PET are given in Table 3.2. The combination of high light output and a short time constant allow for very fast timing (i.e., a short coincidence window), which reduce the chance of random coincidences and reduce the dead time. They also enhance the crystal identification when these crystals are used in block detectors.

TABLE 3.2. *Properties of commonly used scintillators in PET*

Property	Detector thickness	Scintillator		
		NaI(Tl)	Bismuth germanate	Lutetium oxy-orthoscilicate
Relative light output	—	100	15	75
Decay constant (nsec)	—	230	300	40
Density (g/mL)	—	3.67	7.13	7.40
Effective atomic number	—	51	75	66
Singles efficiency at 511 keV	10 mm thick	29%	62%	58%
	25 mm thick	58%	91%	89%
Coincidence efficiency at 511 keV	10 mm thick	8.4%	38.4%	43.8%
	25 mm thick	33.6%	82.8%	79.2%
Singles efficiency at 133 keV	10 mm thick	93%	100%	100%

Circumferential ⟶

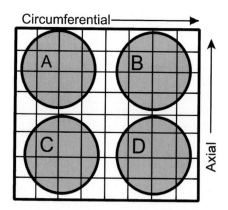

Axial ⟶

FIG. 3.5. Crystals (*squares*) and round photomultiplier tubes (*A through D*) in Siemens CTI ECAT Exact HR+ PET scanner detector block. (8 × 8 crystals; overall dimensions: 38 × 36 × 30 mm.)

Circumferential ⟶

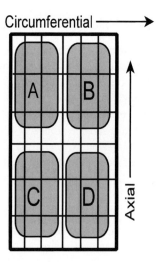

Axial ⟶

FIG. 3.6. Crystals and photomultiplier tubes (*A through D*) in the General Electric Advance PET scanner detector block. (6 × 6 crystals; overall dimensions: 26 × 51 × 30 mm.)

The efficiencies given in Table 3.2 provide an important insight into the effect of the scintillator material and its stopping power. The single-photon detection efficiency for 140-keV photons in a 10-mm thick NaI crystal is 93%, whereas the coincidence efficiency for the same crystal (i.e., the probability of detecting both 511-keV photons) is only 8.4%, making it a very poor choice for PET imaging even though it is excellent for single-photon emission computed tomography (SPECT) with ^{99m}Tc. On the other hand, 25 mm of BGO or LSO provides about 80% coincident detection for 511-keV photons, making these crystals superior for PET imaging. Thicker NaI crystals (25 mm) are used successfully in PET imaging, although their detection efficiency is about 40% of that for BGO crystals in the same physical geometry. The most common PET detector material is BGO.

In most dedicated PET scanners, each detector is a separate module, which can be replaced when required. The complete module contains either four PMTs or two dual PMTs, as well as the cut-block scintillation crystal, but no active electronic components, all housed in a light-tight thin metal enclosure. The enclosure provides electrical and magnetic shielding. The BGO crystal dimensions are about 40 × 40 × 30 mm and this is cut into between 6 × 8 and 8 × 8 individual crystals. Diagrams of the crystals and the PMTs for two commonly used PET scanners are shown in Figs. 3.5 and 3.6.

Signal Processing Electronics

Each PET block detector has signal cables for each PMT and requires one high-voltage (1,600 to 1,800 V) connection for the whole module. The signals from each PMT are amplified and filtered and then summed to provide a signal proportional to the energy from which the arrival time of the annihilation photons is determined. The time at which this signal triggers a constant fraction discriminator is measured with respect to a very fast systemwide clock that records the time to the nearest 1 or 2 ns. The PMT signals are combined in

a way similar to the signals from the PMTs on a gamma camera, which is commonly referred to "Anger-logic," in honor of Hal Anger, the inventor of the gamma camera. With the PMTs referred to as A, B, C, and D, the following equations allow an initial position estimate of the incoming photons:

$$X = \frac{[B - A] + [D - C]}{A + B + C + D}$$

$$Y = \frac{[C - A] + [D - B]}{A + B + C + D}$$

$$E = [A + B + C + D]$$

These three signals can be digitized with eight-bit analog-to-digital converters (ADCs). If the four signal outputs are properly balanced, a crystal identification pattern like the one shown in Fig. 3.7 is obtained. The signal processing module is able to adjust the gains of the individual signals and make it look like that shown in Fig. 3.7. The dots in this figure show the peak signal surrounded by the territory associated with each crystal element. The *X* and *Y* values, from the equations above, are used to address a small memory (on the signal processing module), which provides the crystal address. The sum, or energy, signal is scaled with a factor for that crystal and compared with lower and upper discriminator settings to determine if the photon has an acceptable energy. If it does, the crystal address and the arrival time of the photon are sent to the coincidence circuit. The crystal address includes the ring number and the crystal position in the ring. Other information, such as the energy window, may also be included in the identification.

Coincidence Circuit

Analog coincidence circuits were used in older scanners, but today there are so many crystals it would be very difficult

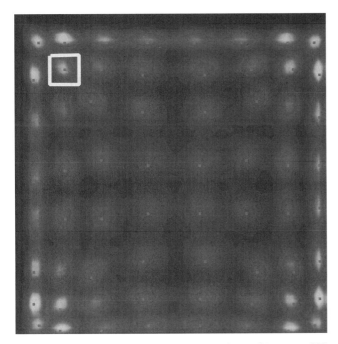

FIG. 3.7. Crystal identification pattern for a Siemens CTI HR+ 8- × 8-crystal block with the territory of one crystal element mapped out (*the white square*).

to do this. Instead the time stamps from the detector modules are compared and accepted as coincident when they are equal or nearly equal. The allowable time difference is called the coincidence resolving time and is given the symbol τ.

The time stamps from annihilation photon pairs, which differ by a small fixed time, are also compared. These are not in coincidence because the time difference is too large, but these events are representative of the random coincidences and are used to estimate how many random coincidences have occurred.

Data-acquisition Computer

Most modern PET scanners have a data-acquisition computer system (DACS) separate from the workstation used to set up, control, and display the scans. The DACS is comparatively simple as far as functions go, but it requires very large random access memory and disks. Some idea of the size requirements can be appreciated by considering that a PET scanner with a 15-cm field of view divided into D (24 for the General Electric [GE] Advance or 32 for the Siemens CTI ECAT HR+) crystals deep and 288 detectors in each ring requires $(32 \times 32 \times 288 \times 288)/4$ (more than 21 million) memory locations that may receive counts during the acquisition of one image. If this is a gated study, 16 times more memory is required. Twice as much memory is needed for dual-energy or simultaneous emission/transmission scans. Although a typical static PET scan may take about 10 minutes, some dynamic scans have frame times of only a few seconds and may be as long as 30 frames (more than 600 megabytes of memory is required).

Usually some form of compaction is done, such as combining two or four adjacent bins into one when short frame times are used. However, while acquiring any one frame of an image, all of this memory must be available. We can contrast this to a SPECT scanner with which one projection angle is acquired at a time, so typically only 128×128 (i.e., 16,384) memory locations are required to acquire the counts at any camera angle. Typically a PET scanner requires 1,000 times more memory during a scan than a SPECT scanner, even though the size of the final reconstructed image matrix (about $128 \times 128 \times 64$) is about the same.

Reconstruction, Display, and Image Analysis Systems

Most common PET scanners use separate systems for image reconstruction, image display, and image analysis. Reconstructing PET images, particularly 3D ones, is a very computation-intensive task, and this is usually handled by special purpose computers called array processors. These have many small processors, which work in parallel all doing the same task, but each working on different parts of the image to reconstruct it in a timely way. These require access to the raw data in the DACS memory. Image reconstruction is discussed in Chapter 4. During the process, the reconstructor must access not only the data acquired during the emission scan, but also data from a normalization scan to calibrate the detector-pair efficiencies, as well as a blank and transmission scan data to correct for attenuation and scattered radiation. Each of these data sets is very large.

An image display facility must be available to the scanner operator to verify that the images are technically satisfactory. Most other imaging modalities produce images much faster than PET scanners. (Ultrasound scanners produce real-time images, SPECT scanners can show each projection as it is being acquired, and x-ray computed tomography [CT] scanners can now reconstruct images in a few seconds.) Because PET deals with much more input data, PET scans are usually reconstructed asynchronously and are not normally displayed as they are reconstructed. One possible reason for this is that the 3D reconstructions process the whole volume at once, so it is only at the end of the process that all images become available at once. Another reason is perhaps that until recently PET was used more for research than for clinical reasons. The increased use of PET as a clinical tool is already creating a need for faster image reconstruction and more accessible images of recent scans. Off-line viewing facilities are almost as necessary as a quick display on the operator's console. PET scanning software now provides for the export of images to nearby workstations and centralized viewing facilities.

PET DETECTOR AND COLLIMATOR CONFIGURATIONS

Since the early 1970s when PET started, there have been three basic detector configurations: rings of discrete detec-

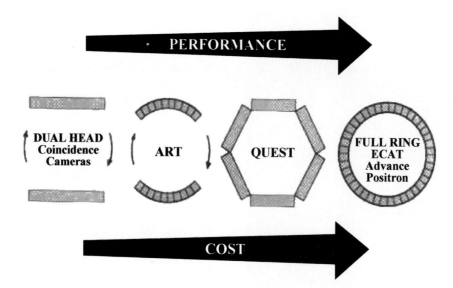

FIG. 3.8. Available geometries for PET detectors. The first two require rotation of the detectors to acquire all projections needed to form an image. (ART, partial-ring bismuth-4-germanium-3-oxygen-12 scanner; QUEST, full-ring sodium iodide scanner, similar to "C-PET." (From Phelps ME, Cherry SR. The changing design of positron imaging systems. *Clin Positron Imaging* 1998;1:31–45, with permission.)

tors (1,2), two planar area detectors (4), and polygons (12, 13) (hexagons and octagons). The vast majority of dedicated PET systems today are in the ring configuration. The discussion so far in this chapter has assumed this configuration. If a scanner is to be used for PET and SPECT, this is not the configuration of choice, even though it is probably the best for dedicated PET systems. An overview of the history of PET geometries and their relative sensitivities by Phelps and Cherry (14) gives some valuable insight into the sensitivity and cost of various systems; Fig. 3.8, showing a cost comparison, and Fig. 3.9, showing the comparative sensitivities, are reproduced from this article.

Ring of Scintillation Crystals with "Block" Detectors

The most common dedicated PET detector systems today consist of individual detector modules in which an array or

cut block of BGO scintillation crystals is coupled to four PMTs, as discussed previously. Two of these modules from the Siemens CTI ECAT Exact HR+, and the GE Advance are shown as Figs. 3.5 and 3.6. These have several advantages. (1) Each detector is a small independent system. The probability of two annihilation photons interacting with a small detector during the scintillator's decay time is obviously smaller than with a larger detector, so the dead time of the individual detectors is very small and the system dead time is small. (2) Each detector is a light-tight field replaceable module often with only one connector. This reduces the time to repair, compared with that of replacing a faulty module, which improves the availability of the scanner. (3) The symmetry that comes with a ring design provides uniform sampling at all angles.

A disadvantage of this design arises from the great depth

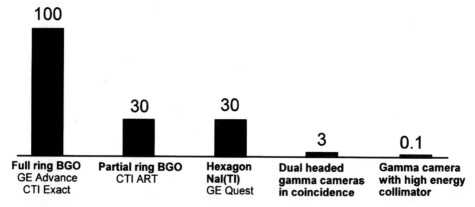

FIG. 3.9. Relative efficiencies of different PET detector configurations. (Based on Phelps ME, Cherry SR. The changing design of positron imaging systems. *Clin Positron Imaging* 1998;1:31–45, with permission.)

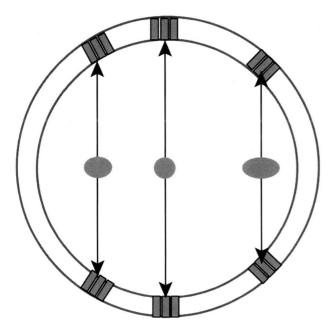

FIG. 3.10. Radial blurring is caused when the PET crystals are very deep compared with their width. Photons from objects near the edge of the field of view may penetrate one or more crystals before being detected. The uncertainty of the crystal in which they are detected causes the image to be blurred radially.

of the crystals required to detect 511-keV annihilation photons efficiently. When one attempts to improve the spatial resolution by making the crystals very thin, but retain efficiency by making them long, the photons near the edge of the imaging field may not be detected in the first crystal they enter, but pass through one or two crystals. This effect, referred to as radial blurring, is characteristic of ring systems. It results in a point source near the edge of the image field appearing in the image as an ellipse, which has its major axis along the radius of the scanner. The cause of this effect is illustrated in Fig. 3.10.

Planar Detectors

The very first PET scanners had planar (flat) detectors (4), but until quite recently, these went out of fashion. The loss of interest in this configuration was mainly due to its dead time. The most common configuration for planar detectors is the conventional gamma camera with a thicker than normal crystal. Using typical Anger-logic readout, a gamma camera can only handle one annihilation photon at a time. Because, as was shown in the section on electronic collimation, there are far more unpaired than paired photons detected, and both cause equal dead times, the coincidence count rates in these systems are very limited. Modern gamma cameras use individual ADCs for each PMT, and the computation of the point of incidence is done digitally. The advantage is that only PMTs in the region of the peak signal intensity are used to compute the position. If two annihilation

photons strike the crystal face at the same time, but at some distance apart, each is processed separately. This has the effect of reducing the effective area of the gamma as far as dead time is concerned to about one tenth of the total size.

Another detector configuration that was in vogue before ring systems became dominant was the hexagonal or octagonal configuration. The PETT IV and early ECAT systems are examples of this configuration. To provide adequate sampling, these systems had to rotate, and in some cases, the detectors also moved along their peripheral direction, making them mechanically quite complex. The recent "panel detectors" used in a high-resolution research tomograph represent a revival of this concept (12). This new system features a dual-layer scintillator to minimize radial blurring and interpolation in the dead zones where the panels join. This, in theory, allows the detectors to remain stationary.

PET Emission Imaging Modes

Many recent PET scanners have septa that are inserted for some studies and retracted for others. These allow the scanner to perform both 2D (Fig. 3.11) and 3D (Fig. 3.12) imaging. Although each has advantages and disadvantages, there is a trend toward 3D imaging.

2D PET Imaging

2D imaging is performed by positioning thin lead or tungsten annuli (called septa) between adjacent rings of crystals (Fig. 3.11). The outer diameter of the septa is just less than the inner diameter of the detector ring. The inner diameter is just wider than the patient scanning aperture. This divides the axial field into clearly defined planes. Annihilation photons approaching the detectors from beyond its plane must travel either through many septa (if they originate far from that slice) or very obliquely through one or two septa. In either case, the path length through the lead is long even though each septum is only 1 or 2 mm thick.

2D images are formed as direct or cross slices (Fig. 3.11). The thinnest slices are obtained when only annihilation photons that interact with crystals in the same ring are accepted. These are called direct slices, as opposed to cross slices, in which the annihilation photons interact with detectors in adjacent rings. The direct slices are slightly thinner than the cross slices, particularly near the edge of the field of view. The sensitivity of the scanner can be improved at the expense of axial resolution, by allowing the direct slices to be augmented from the addition of events whose photons come from crystals that are two rings apart and the cross slices made from crystals that are three rings apart.

2D images are quite well defined and contain very little contamination from events outside their axial extent. In this mode, the scanner is relatively insensitive to scattered radiation from within the plane because to reach a detector, a photon would probably have to scatter twice or be scattered through a very small angle to be detected in the same plane.

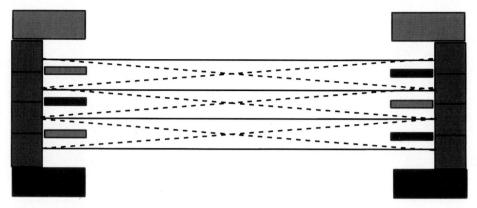

FIG. 3.11. Multislice PET scanner with septa configured for two-dimensional imaging with both direct slices (*solid*) and cross slices (*dashed*).

Until recently, 2D imaging was considered more quantitative than 3D imaging, but more accurate and faster 3D scatter correction algorithms are now available, so the trend is toward 3D imaging for all emission scans. However, 3D imaging with BGO detectors is limited in quality relative to 2D imaging, particularly in the abdomen.

3D PET Imaging

The septa in newer PET scanners can be retracted, exposing the detectors to oblique and transaxial annihilation photon pairs (Fig. 3.12). This increases the efficiency for unscattered rays by about five times depending on the range of oblique angles accepted. At the same time, the sensitivity to scattered rays goes up by about 20 times, so scatter fractions are much higher in 3D than 2D imaging. In most cases, the additional scattered rays have scattered only once in 3D imaging, so correction algorithms based on single, rather than multiple, scattering can be used and do very well in correcting the image for the loss of contrast due to the detection of scattered radiation. Scatter can severely degrade the quality of whole-body tumor images, particularly in large

patients, and it remains common for oncological imaging studies to be performed using only 2D PET.

PET scanners with planar detectors do not have septa, so they always work in the 3D mode.

ATTENUATION CORRECTION AND TRANSMISSION SCANS

PET is considered a quantitative imaging technique, so the images can be calibrated in units of activity concentration (kilobecquerel per milliliter, or nanocurie per milliliter). For this to be true, the images must be corrected for the effects of attenuation. The 511-keV annihilation photons in PET have less attenuation in body tissue than the 140-keV gamma rays from ^{99m}Tc, although both rays must emerge and be detected in PET, whereas only one is recorded in single-photon imaging. An important distinction between PET and SPECT is that in PET the measurement of attenuation can be made completely independent of the isotope distribution (Fig. 3.13). A positron annihilating at the point represented by the black dot produces two photons, one of which travels d_1 and the other d_2. The probability of each of them emerging

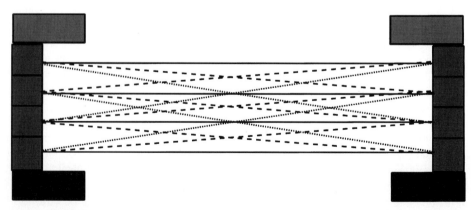

FIG. 3.12. A PET scanner without septa configured for three-dimensional imaging can accept direct slices (*solid*), cross slices (*dashed*), and oblique slices (*dotted*).

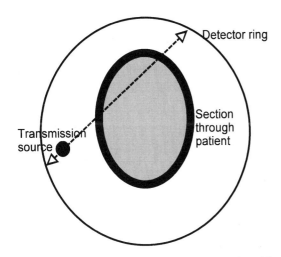

FIG. 3.13. The transmission source is outside the object to be scanned. Because the attenuation along any line is independent of the source position, the attenuation in the body can be measured using an external source.

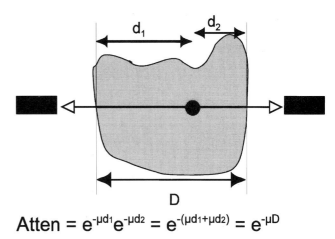

$$\text{Atten} = e^{-\mu d_1}e^{-\mu d_2} = e^{-(\mu d_1 + \mu d_2)} = e^{-\mu D}$$

FIG. 3.14. Attenuation is independent of the location of the annihilation along the line of response.

from the body is $e^{-\mu d_1}$ and $e^{-\mu d_2}$, but the probability of both of them emerging is the product of the probabilities, or as shown in the following equation, $e^{-\mu D}$.

$$A_1 = e^{-\mu d_1}$$

$$A_2 = e^{-\mu d_2}$$

$$A_1 \cdot A_2 = e^{-\mu(d_1 + d_2)}$$

$$A = e^{-\mu D}$$

The importance of this is that the attenuation along a particular LOR is independent of the point at which the positron annihilates. In fact, a simple extension of this equation to a case of nonuniform attenuation can be made, that is, where μ varies along the path and the photon encounters fat, lung, and bone on its path toward the detector.

$$A = e^{-\int_0^D \mu(l)\,dl}$$

Figure 3.14 shows an isolated point of activity that is outside the body. Even though it is outside the body, the preceding equation still applies, and this is used to make an independent measurement of the attenuation in the section being imaged. This type of image is called a transmission scan. The primary purpose of this procedure is for attenuation correction, but the data can also be used to make anatomic images if it is collected and processed correctly.

Transmission scans are acquired with one or more orbiting external sources, as shown previously. To form an image or provide data for attenuation correction, the number of events in each bin of the transmission scan's sinogram $T(r, \beta)$ are divided into the number of events obtained during the equivalent time during a blank scan $B(r, \beta)$ (i.e., with nothing in the scan field). A ''ratio'' sinogram is produced $R(r, \beta)$, and

this is used to correct the emission counts in each bin while reconstructing the emission scan. If the natural logarithm of this ratio is taken, and the resulting attenuation sinogram $A(r, \beta)$ reconstructed, an attenuation image is produced, as illustrated in the following equation:

$$R(r,\beta) = \frac{B(r,\beta)}{T(r,\beta)}$$

$$A(r,\beta) = \ln\left(\frac{B(r,\beta)}{T(r,\beta)}\right)$$

An image that resembles a low-contrast x-ray CT scan is obtained. The contrast is lower because the range of variation in tissue attenuation is lower at higher energies. These images can be useful in identifying anatomic regions, particularly if they are compared feature for feature with CT or magnetic resonance imaging (MRI), as they map the tissue density, not function.

Rod Sources

The fact that the attenuation for the pair of annihilation photons is independent of the location of the positron is used very effectively in the most common technique for measuring attenuation. One or three thin rods of germanium-68 are introduced as close as is practical to the inner surface of the septa and collimators. During a transmission scan, these sources orbit the scan field just outside the aperture through which the patient is imaged. During a transmission scan, only pairs of detectors that are colinear with the current location of the source are enabled to store counts. The fact that these scans are done with the septa in place, and that the source and detectors are colinear, prevents almost all scattered radiation from being detected, and this provides a very accurate measurement of the attenuation along all LORs.

The main advantage of this method is its potential accuracy. The main limitation is due to the very high count rate received by detectors that are near the current source. To obtain sufficient counts for a good quality transmission scan, one must count either at a high rate or for a long time. The former imposes an upper limit due to dead time and pulse pileup in the detectors near the source, and the latter makes for longer scanning times.

^{137}Cs Point Sources

To improve the counting statistics in transmission scans, some scanners now use one or more point sources of ^{137}Cs. This isotope has a 662-keV gamma ray (t½ = 30.1 years) and is available with very high specific activity so very concentrated small point sources can be made. The point source orbits the scan field in a spiral fashion, and the line joining the distant detector and the current point source is extrapolated to the point at which it intersects the near detector surface. This identifies a dummy detector with which the second photon would have interacted had the source been a positron rather than a single gamma emitter. This is accomplished using real-time electronics that use lookup tables to perform the calculations.

The main advantage of this method is the lack of dead time in the near detector, which allows for much stronger sources and faster scans. The disadvantage is that the lack of colinearity allows much more scattered radiation to be detected. Because this technique is commonly used with 3D scanning, the scatter fraction in these scans is very high, so the contrast is lower. The higher primary energy of the annihilation photons also reduces the contrast, so the final scan is often segmented by computer algorithms into zones corresponding to soft tissue, bones, and lung tissue, and the appropriate values for the attenuation at 511 keV are then associated with each region.

Use of Images from CT or MRI for Attenuation Correction

Another technique that can be used for attenuation correction is to import cross-sectional images of the same body sections from CT or MRI. For this to work, the tissue must be segmented based on the contrast mechanism in MRI or attenuation at much lower energies in the case of CT images, and each pixel assigned an appropriate attenuation coefficient at 511 keV. Image registration is a significant problem with this technique. The beds of both PET and CT scanners will probably be a different shape, and the patient will probably be positioned differently, making this a serious problem. Recently, PET-CT scanners have been introduced to overcome this problem.

Postinjection Attenuation Scans

The previous sections assume that there is no radioactivity in the patient. If there is, it will be detected along with that from the external source, and this will reduce the contrast

and by implication, the attenuation values obtained during the transmission scan. When several bed positions are required to investigate a large axial extent of the patient, it may be necessary to have the patient scanned twice, once for the attenuation measurement and again after a tracer injection, followed by an uptake period of about 40 minutes for the emission scan. This requires a very long scan time. It is unrealistically long for the patient and motion can occur, degrading the image quality. It also has a severe impact on the number of patients who can be scanned in a day.

Simultaneous Emission/Transmission Scans

Using the colinearity condition set up by the location of the rods, we have shown that an attenuation scan that is free from contamination can be obtained. But what about detector pairs that are nowhere near colinear with the rod position? These can still record counts from the radioactivity injected in the patient. This allows the possibility of simultaneous emission/transmission scans. Here, there are two sinograms for each patient section. High-speed electronics (using lookup tables) determine, on an event-by-event basis, if the line joining the two detectors is or is not colinear with the current position of the source. The yes/no result decides whether the event is considered an emission or transmission count, and the appropriate bin of the correct sinogram is incremented.

SOURCES OF NOISE IN PET IMAGES

All medical imaging techniques are limited by signal-to-noise considerations. In most cases, image quality improves with longer measurement times to provide more photons. PET is no exception to this, and there are more sources of noise in PET images than in conventional nuclear medicine single-photon imaging.

Poisson Counting Noise

All nuclear medicine techniques involve "counting photons." These photons are emitted from the body, unlike x-ray imaging, which measures (but rarely actually counts) the photons that are not absorbed by the body. To minimize the radiation dose, only enough tracer is injected to form a useful image because all organs are exposed to the injected radiation, whereas the external x-ray beam is collimated to match the detector area. After the tracer is injected, the patient is exposed to its radiation for a long time compared with the scanning time, whereas he or she is only exposed while the x-ray beam is on. For an equivalent radiation dose, far more x-ray photons will be absorbed by the detector than during the acquisition of a nuclear medicine image.

In the case of a digitally acquired planar gamma camera image, the number of counts in each pixel is directly proportional to the pixel area and the effective counting time (i.e., the decay-corrected counting time). Because radioactive decay is a random process, the number of counts acquired in two measurements will not be the same. In fact, the number of counts N acquired per unit time has an uncertainty such that the standard deviation is $\sqrt{N}$. Images acquired for short times have far more noise, which is expressed as a percentage of the mean counts (i.e., $100 \times \sqrt{N}/N$, or $100\sqrt{N}$). For the same reason, images divided into more smaller pixels show more noise.

The propagation of noise into a reconstructed image from projections is outside the scope of this chapter, but the noise does propagate, and the more noise in the projections, the more noise in the final image.

Scattered Counts

When annihilation photons are scattered before reaching the detector, the LOR joining the two detectors no longer passes through the point of annihilation, resulting in a loss of contrast. The contrast can be restored by making an estimate of the scattered counts in each LOR and subtracting it from the observed counts. The estimate is often made by convolving each projection (horizontal line in a sinogram) with a smoothing function, which is characteristic of the scattering probability in that projection. When this is done, the scatter profile is a smooth function that extends beyond the true-count profile. When this is subtracted, the resulting total-scatter projection will have the same total noise as previously, but because something is subtracted, the percentage of noise will increase, as $100 \times \sqrt{N}/(N - S) > 100 \times \sqrt{N}/(N)$.

Random Counts

Random counts are unique to PET imaging and represent an additional source of noise, which must be estimated and removed to prevent a loss of image contrast. Random counts arise when two photons from different annihilations strike two detectors nearly simultaneously. As discussed previously, each detector records many single counts for each coincident count. When there is a lot of activity, it is very likely that two of these single counts will occur within the time window τ, during which two detected annihilation photons are considered simultaneous. If two crystals have single count rates of S_1 and S_2, then the random count rate R for these detectors will be

$$R = 2\tau S_1 S_2$$

To correct for random counts, the count rate is first estimated and then subtracted from each point in the sinogram. The most common way of doing this is to use two timing windows, one for prompt counts and another that is delayed by a few tens of nanoseconds. In this window, a true coincidence (i.e., one arising from the same annihilation) is impossible, but a random coincidence is just as likely to occur as it would be in the normal timing window.

There is an uncertainty associated with making this measurement, so this is an additional source of noise. If R is the random coincidence rate, the percentage of noise in this measurement is $100 \times \sqrt{R}/R$. To obtain the true count rate associated with any LOR, we must use the measured count rate N, less the scattered S and random R count rates, so

$$T = N - S - R$$

Dead Time

As stated previously, the electronic collimation used in PET requires that all annihilation photons that interact with the detector be initially processed and then probably discarded when they are found not to be in coincidence. Each detector can record only one photon at a time. If another interacts with the detector while it is still scintillating after the last one, both the energy and the position of both photons will be wrong, and the timing signal from the second one will be lost. Because the PMT signals are filtered to measure their values more precisely, the minimum time to process each interaction is about 1,000 ns for BGO crystals and about 200 ns for LSO and NaI crystals, which are both faster and emit more light. Although this may not seem like a very long time, if the singles count rate in a crystal is a few hundred thousand counts per second (cps), it will be unable to respond much of the time. This time during which it is unavailable is called the dead time. It depends on the total count rate in each detector. Making the detectors smaller reduces their count rates and this is a major consideration in PET detector design. The area of a gamma camera crystal is many times that of a PET detector, although the newer gamma cameras can process more than one incident gamma ray at a time if they interact with the crystals sufficiently far apart.

The Concept of Noise-effective Counts

The noise due to counting photons is only part of the story in PET images. There are both true unscattered photon pairs detected, which are the only source of signal and are subject to normal poisson counting statistical noise, and there are also scattered and random counts, which contribute no signal, only noise, to the image. The noise in PET images is worse than it would be in a simple planar counting study for a given number of true counts recorded, but there would be many more true counts detected for a given activity concentration than there would be in a conventional gamma camera image.

One can think of the true PET counts being "devalued" due to the corrections for random and scattered counts. This concept is referred as a noise-effective count (NEC) rate. It is the equivalent rate for true counts had the other sources of noise not been present. If N is the coincidence count rate, T is the true count rate, S is the scattered count rate, and R is the random count rate, then

$$NEC = \frac{T}{1 + \dfrac{S}{T} + \dfrac{2fR}{T}}$$

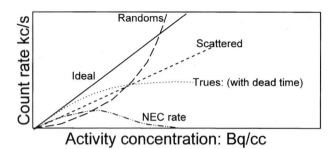

FIG. 3.15. An ideal PET scanner with no dead time would have a count rate directly proportional to the activity concentration. The scattered counts are a constant fraction of the true counts, whereas the random count rate increases with the square of the activity concentration. Dead time limits the efficiency as the activity concentration increases. The noise-effective count rate first rises then plateaus and eventually falls.

The terms S/T and R/T (which are always positive) serve to reduce the effective counting rate. The scatter fraction S/T is constant for a given imaging situation, but the random rate increases as the activity and count rate increases. The NEC is depicted in Fig. 3.15, along with the ideal performance of a scanner. Figure 3.15 also shows the true, random, and scattered count rates. High activity concentrations serve to limit the NEC and the NEC actually falls if the activity concentration is increased. An analogy can be made with the scatter fraction S/T by saying it is like the sales (or value-added) tax on an article in a shop, which is the same for everyone. The random fraction R/T, however, increases like income tax, so the more you earn, proportionally the more you pay!

Out-of-Field Counts

The scanner can only detect true counts from within its filed of view. However, activity outside the field can contribute large numbers of single photons, which will contribute to the random counts and scattered counts. The septa used in 2D imaging are quite effective at attenuating out-of-field counts, but 3D studies are much more prone to contamination due to out-of-field counts. This is particularly problematic with dual-headed coincidence cameras, which are poorly shielded against out-of-field events.

Noise From Attenuation Correction

To obtain quantitative PET images, one must correct for attenuation. Failure to do so results in an overestimation of the activity concentration at the edge of the body, and an artificially high activity concentration is observed in low-density tissue regions like the lungs. There has been a significant debate in recent PET literature on whether to do attenuation correction at all if all one needs is to "see" a hot spot.

Attenuation correction using transmission scans takes time and adds noise to the emission image.

Because the attenuation correction or an image from a transmission scan is the result of dividing the data in the blank scan's bins by the data in the transmission scan's bins, the noise in the attenuation correction map or image is substantial. LORs containing more activity have higher counts and thus lower noise in an emission scan. However, if a LOR passes through a region of high attenuation, it will have lower counts in the transmission scan. Because each bin is divided into a blank scan bin, the resulting bin will contain a bigger number. Thus, the noise in regions of higher attenuation is higher than in regions of lower attenuation. If the transmission scan is acquired for a short time on an obese patient, it is possible that some sinogram bins will contain no counts at all. This would result in dividing by zero.

Some preprocessing of the transmission scan data is always done, including interpolation of all zero and negative bins and smoothing the transmission sinogram before dividing it into the blank scan.

Some postprocessing in the form of image segmentation is often performed. The basis for this comes from the observation that there are really only four likely values of attenuation coefficient in PET imaging, those for air, lung tissue, water-equivalent tissue, and bone. Boundary finding and artifact detecting algorithms are applied to categorize each region in the attenuation image, and the most probable value assigned to each region. When properly applied, these can eliminate the noise from transmission scans and permit quantitative imaging in a timely fashion.

PET IMAGING MODES

Static Emission Scans

A static PET image is one made during a period when the activity distribution is fairly stable and the counting time is long enough to obtain a good quality image. Typical applications are in the measurement of the glucose metabolism of the brain or heart using the tracer fluorodeoxyglucose (FDG). The half-life is long, and the whole brain or heart can be imaged in one scan if the axial scan field is about 15 cm. Another example is in cerebral blood flow "activation" studies with $H_2{}^{15}O$. If the scan is started about 15 seconds after injection and lasts 1 minute, the scan captures a fairly constant count rate at the peak of the activity concentration in the brain. In both of these cases, a model exists to derive the functional parameter (glucose utilization or blood flow) from a single image.

Dynamic Emission Scans

Dynamic studies are used in cases in which it is necessary to follow the activity over a long period to apply a more complex model of the underlying physiology. This is done to extract several rate constants for the biologic process.

Measurement of oxygen consumption and neuroreceptor and neurotransmitter studies often require dynamic scans.

Dynamic scans are performed with the subject stationary, using a series of imaging frames, which normally get longer as the study progresses. Often they are accompanied by either arterial or venous blood sampling to provide an "input function" representing the activity concentration of the tracer in the blood during the scanning session. Each image is reconstructed as if it were acquired independently of the others.

The time series of images can be analyzed by placing regions of interest (ROIs) over important areas in one image and having a suitable image analysis program provide a time-activity curve (TAC) where the activity concentration in becquerels per milliliter is provided as a function of time. These data and the input function's TAC are input to the model to provide the biologic rate constants for each region chosen.

Studies to measure oxygen consumption are often done with 5- to 10-second frames over 2 to 3 minutes. Receptor studies usually take more than an hour with the frame time changing from 10 seconds at the start to 5 minutes near the end.

Only one attenuation scan is required and it is used to correct all frames. The subject must remain very still, to ensure that the ROIs chosen on one frame correspond to the same tissue throughout the study and that the attenuation map remains registered with the correct body section throughout the study.

Whole-body Scans

Whole-body scans are the fastest growing application of PET. These studies, which rarely cover the whole body (i.e., they often extend from the upper neck through the mid thighs), provide one of the most effective means of looking for tumor metastases. FDG is the tracer of choice in these studies because of its excellent accumulation in tumors, its long half-life, and its ease of availability. The studies are performed in several "bed positions" by acquiring an emission scan for 5 to 10 minutes and then moving the patient by a distance that is somewhat less than the scanner's axial field of view. Sometimes an emission scan series is done, followed by a transmission scan series in the same bed positions. Transmission and emission scans are often done in an interleaved fashion. The former is subject to misregistration of the data due to intervening patient movement, and the latter requires reconfiguring the scanner (acquisition mode, transmission sources, and possibly septa) and can waste a lot of time during the session.

These studies are reconstructed as a series of slices, which are saved as a "volume" of perhaps $128 \times 128 \times 2,048$ pixels. The volume is then resliced horizontally or vertically with respect to the prone patient and they provide slices through the body in the coronal or sagittal planes. Many examples of these scans are given elsewhere in this book.

QUALITY CONTROL OF PET IMAGING

A number of steps must be taken to ensure that the scanner produces consistently high-quality images.

Quantitative Imaging versus "Making Pictures"

When PET scanners are used to produce whole-body scans, it is the human interpretation of the images in the context of the suspected disease that is the end product of the PET scan. Nuclear medicine physicians are trained to evaluate "images," and with experience, they can often distinguish between an artifact and a region of an image that is suspicious for cancer or an infarct. The most common parameter extracted from these images is the standard uptake value (SUV). This is related to the injected dose per body mass and is usually higher in tumors than in healthy tissue. To make this measurement, one must perform an attenuation scan and use it to correct the emission scan. In the interpretation of these images, the suspicious region is identified visually and then appropriate software tools provide the SUV in that region.

Other applications of PET in cardiology or neurology require dynamic scanning. The estimation of parameters from these scan sequences is more complex and requires greater attention to issues related to scanner calibration.

Calibration of Individual Detectors

The calibration of individual detectors produces a pattern that looks like the one in Fig. 3.9. Here, the eight rows and columns of detectors in a CTI HR + block are easily distinguished, and a dot marks the peak of each crystal's territory in the map. If one PMT is weak, the pattern is "pulled away" from it and the result is a distorted picture. Examination of the individual detector patterns is not routinely performed as part of daily quality control but is an important assessment or a part of more extensive service. The detectors must all be working properly before other calibration procedures are performed.

Daily Blank Scans

As mentioned in the section on attenuation correction, a blank scan (one with nothing in the scan field) is required to estimate the attenuation coefficients for each LOR. This scan is used to correct many studies. To prevent noise in this scan being propagated to all other scans, it makes sense for this scan to be noise free. Many newer scanners are equipped to do this scan without an operator present. This allows the blank scan to be performed for about an hour during the night when the equipment would not be in use. This type of quality control is typically performed each day the scanner is used for imaging.

Examination of this scan will show up faults like a bad detector (which appears as a diagonal band on a sinogram).

An automated analysis tool can compare today's blank scan with recent ones and report changes that indicate that the system requires recalibration or repair.

During a blank scan, the transmission sources are exposed, so the scanner becomes a source of radiation without a patient present. Although this seems appropriate from the radiation exposure point of view, it is not a normal procedure with other radiation emitting devices (e.g., a radiation therapy machine or x-ray system that suddenly turned itself on during the night would not be considered safe). Those involved in radiation safety should be alerted to the fact that the PET scanner does this.

Normalization of Detector Systems

The normalization of the LORs is required to produce uniform images. Some systems require separate normalization for 2D and 3D imaging, so both a strong and a weak source are required. A 20-cm diameter source is usually placed in the center of the field of view and counted for a long time. From the size of the source, the length of the chords through it, and the number of counts obtained in each LOR, a calibration factor is obtained for all the LORs that pass through the source. The other LORs are normalized based on the coincidence efficiencies of each detector, as measured along the chords that intersect the source.

Calibration of Each Image Plane

It is possible to calibrate the individual slices of a PET scanner with an object of known size whose activity concentration is known. This calibration is not only essential for quantitative imaging, but also very important in the production of whole-body scans. The efficiency of each plane can be very different. Even in 2D imaging, the cross planes (odd-numbered ones) are more efficient than the direct planes (even-numbered ones), as illustrated in Fig. 3.16 (for the CTI HR +), because there are more detectors available for cross planes than direct planes. The sensitivity in 3D imaging is very much greater near the axial center of the field of view due to the contribution of the oblique planes to the central region. Figure 3.17 shows the sensitivity of the CTI HR + in the 3D mode. The vertical scales on Figs. 3.16 and 3.17 are different by almost a factor of seven. The plane sensitivity numbers, in counts per second divided by becquerels per milliliter, for each plane (Figs. 3.16 and 3.17) are used as calibration factors during image reconstruction.

Cross-calibration: Isotope Calibrator, PET Scanner, Well Counter

Patient doses are usually measured in an ionization chamber (radioisotope calibrator). This instrument is a shielded

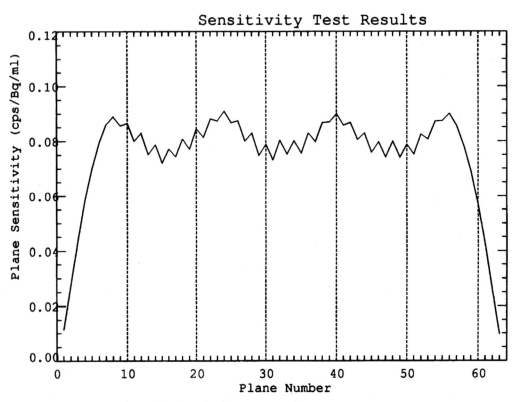

FIG. 3.16. Plane-by-plane sensitivity for 63 slices of a Siemens CTI ECAT HR + scanner in the two-dimension mode, tested with a 20-cm-diameter NEMA flood phantom filled with germanium-68 plastic resin. The saw-tooth pattern is due to the fact that more detectors contribute to the cross slices than to the direct slices. The four peaks are due to the fact that the crystals in the center of each block are more efficient than those at the edge.

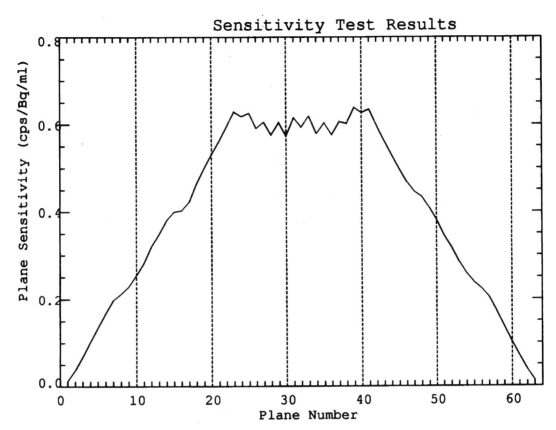

FIG. 3.17. Plane-by-plane sensitivity for 63 slices of a Siemens CTI ECAT HR+ scanner in the three-dimension mode, tested with a 20-cm-diameter NEMA flood phantom filled with germanium-68 plastic resin. The peak sensitivity is about nine times more than in the two-dimension mode. The sensitivity falls off rapidly outside the central one third of the axial field. For this reason, there is great value in positioning the organ of interest in the central region.

well-shaped ionization chamber, into which a small vial or the syringe containing the patient dose is placed. It is designed for measuring high activities and is unsuitable for measuring blood samples. The PET scanner is calibrated to provide quantitative images in becquerels per milliliter (or nanocuries per milliliter). A well counter, used for measuring blood samples, is a well-shaped NaI crystal connected to a counting system, which normally provides a reading in counts per second.

The suppliers of calibration sources include a small sample of the activity from the calibration source that can fit in the well counter. The activity in the sample and the date of the measurement are provided by the supplier, so it is possible to calibrate the well counter in becquerels per counts per second or in "how many atoms decay for each count recorded." An efficient well counter has an efficiency of about 0.4 Bq/cps, so it can detect 40% of the atoms that decay within the well.

PET scanner efficiencies are usually quoted as counts per second divided by becquerels per milliliter, as discussed in the previous section. However, these are measured from either the entire source volume, to obtain the total efficiency, or the slice volume, as noted above. The PET values must be corrected for the slice or total source volume to get these in the same units. If the slices are assumed to have the thickness of the crystals (e.g., 0.4 cm) and the calibration source has a radius of 10 cm, the slice volume is 25 cm². In this example, the plane sensitivity near the center of a 3D PET scanner is about 0.6 cps/(Bq/mL) divided by slice volume (0.024 cps/Bq). Thus, the central planes of a PET scanner will detect about 2.4% of the atoms that decay.

A very useful check on the cross-calibration of a PET scanner is to take a typical patient dose and add it to distilled water in a cylinder the same size as that used to calibrate the PET scanner. If the dose is first measured in the ionization chamber, and a known volume from the diluted solution is measured in the well counter, it is possible to cross-calibrate the isotope calibrator, scanner, and well counter if the times and dilution factor are recorded.

SUMMARY

Coincidence imaging is the key to the high sensitivity and excellent spatial resolution of PET. The highest photon detection efficiency is achieved with dedicated full-ring PET scanners. Cameras are evolving with newer detectors and CT sources for transmission correction, and these are important innovations.

REFERENCES

1. Robertson J, Marr R, Rosenbaum B. Thirty-two crystal positron transverse section detector. In: Freedman G, ed. *Tomographic imaging in nuclear medicine.* New York: New York Society of Nuclear Medicine, 1973:151–153.

2. Derenzo S, Budinger T, Cahoon J, et al. The Donner 280 crystal high resolution positron tomograph. *IEEE Trans Nucl Sci* 1979;26: 2790–2793.

3. Casey ME, Nutt R. A multicrystal two dimensional BGO detector system for positron emission tomography. *IEEE Trans Nucl Sci* 1986;33: 460–463.

4. Anger H. Multiple plane tomographic scanner. In: Freedman G, ed. *Tomographic imaging in nuclear medicine.* New York: New York Society of Nuclear Medicine, 1973:2–15.

5. Weber MJ, Monchamp RR. Luminescence of $Bi_4Ge_3O_{12}$: spectral and decay properties. *J Appl Phys* 1973;44:5495–5499.

6. Cho ZK, Farhuki MR. Bismuth germanate as a potential scintillator in positron cameras. *J Nucl Med* 1977;18:840–844.

7. Thompson CJ, Yamamoto YL, Meyer E. Positome II: a high efficiency positron imaging device for dynamic brain studies. *IEEE Trans Nucl Sci* 1979;26:585–589.

8. Wong WH, Mullani NA, Wardworth G, et al. Characteristics of small barium fluoride (BaF_2) scintillation for high intrinsic resolution time-of-flight positron emission tomography. *IEEE Trans Nucl Sci* 1984; 31:381–386.

9. Takagi K, Fukazawa T. Cerium-activated Gd_2SiO_5 single crystal scintillator. *Appl Phys Lett* 1983;42:43–45.

10. Melcher CL, Schweitzer JS. Cerium-doped lutetium oxyorthosilicate: a fast, efficient, new scintillator. *IEEE Trans Nucl Sci* 1992;39:502–505.

11. Wienhard K, Scmannd M, Casey ME, et al. The ECAT HRRT: performance evaluation of the new high resolution research tomograph. Paper presented at: *PET-2000 ECAT Users' Meeting*; August 2000; Barcelona, France.

12. Williams CW, Crabtree MC, Burgiss SG. Design and performance characteristics of a positron emission computed axial tomograph ECAT-II. *IEEE Trans Nucl Sci* 1979;26:619–627.

13. Hoffman EJ, Phelps ME, Huang SC. Performance evaluation of a positron tomograph designed for brain imaging. *J Nucl Med* 1983;24:245–257.

14. Phelps ME, Cherry SR. The changing design of positron imaging systems. *Clin Positron Imaging* 1998;1:31–45.

CHAPTER 4

Data Analysis and Image Processing

Robert A. Koeppe

The goal of positron emission tomography (PET) is to make use of tracers labeled with positron-emitting radionuclides for diagnostic imaging. PET, a nuclear medicine imaging procedure, differs from standard radiologic x-ray procedures in that the radiation detected by the imaging device originates and is emitted from the subject's body, rather than originating from an external source and being transmitted through the body. PET studies, like all nuclear medicine radioisotope emission procedures, yield images that represent the distribution of the radiotracer within the body. This distribution or pattern of uptake and incorporation depends on the physiologic, pharmacologic, and/or biochemical state of the individual's body. In contrast, images produced by conventional x-ray procedures reflect x-ray attenuation and are governed by the physical composition of the body. Thus, nuclear medicine procedures in general and PET procedures in particular are capable of providing information concerning how the body is functioning at a physiologic or biochemical level, whereas x-ray procedures such as computed tomography (CT) primarily depict human anatomy. Although PET does provide limited anatomic information, and some functional information can be derived from CT, each technique is useful in its own way. As we will see later in this and other chapters, recent advances in both hardware and software allow the combination of functional and anatomic information, improving both the ability to answer scientific questions and the overall diagnostic utility of tomographic imaging methods.

PET procedures have the additional potential of providing quantitative measures of radiotracer concentration in a living biologic system at spatial resolutions of a few millimeters and with subminute temporal resolution. Methods for obtaining quantitative images of radiotracer concentration from PET involve a technique called image reconstruction from projections. For many PET applications, these quantitative measures of radiotracer concentration can be extended to yield more pertinent measures of biologic function through the use of compartmental analysis and tracer kinetic modeling. Analysis of a *temporal sequence* of radiotracer images allows estimates of parameters representing specific physio-

logic processes such as blood flow, glucose metabolism, protein synthesis, neurotransmitter or enzyme levels, and receptor or binding site density.

This chapter discusses the basic principles involved in the production and processing of PET images and describes various methods used to analyze the quantitative data produced by PET. The goal of image reconstruction and its associated steps is to produce the most accurate images of radiotracer concentration possible, with the highest signal-to-noise ratio (SNR) and at the highest spatial resolution. The primary goal of compartmental modeling is to provide more valuable information related to the functional state of the subject than can be provided by images of radioactivity distribution alone. The overall goal of image display techniques is to provide both spatial and functional information in a visually optimal manner. The following sections describe the theoretical concepts of and methods for (a) image reconstruction from projections including the additional steps and corrections specific to PET data; (b) compartmental modeling including data-acquisition requirements, curve fitting, parameter estimation, and model validation; and (c) methods for combining and displaying both functional and anatomic information for multiple imaging studies.

IMAGE RECONSTRUCTION FROM PROJECTIONS

In conventional planar nuclear medicine gamma camera imaging or in simple x-ray imaging, information from the three dimensions of a human subject gets collapsed onto a two-dimensional (2D) image. There is ambiguity in such images, because all information from one dimension is represented by a single point or pixel of the 2D image. For gamma camera images, radioactivity from different locations within the body appears overlaid upon itself. Tomography, or slice imaging, is a method that allows a three-dimensional (3D) object to be depicted as a series or stack of thin 2D cross-sectional images. Each image of the series represents only two dimensions of an object, whereas information on the third dimension is contained in the different images of the series. Although this appears simple in concept, imaging devices have the inherent problem of recording information from three dimensions on 2D detector surfaces. Thus, each acquired data point recorded still represents information integrated along one dimension of the object. These integrals or weighted sums are referred to as projections or projection rays. Image reconstruction from projections is the mathematical technique or groups of techniques that allow the construction of the set of cross-sectional images, each representing only two dimensions of information.

Historical Background

The beginnings of image reconstruction from projections occurred with a 1917 paper published by the Austrian mathematician J. Radon (1). In this work, he proved that a 2D or 3D object can be reconstructed exactly from the full set of its projections, a projection again representing the object integrated along one dimension. It was not until the 1950s to 1970s—when this result was rediscovered by people in several different fields, including mathematics (2,3), radio astronomy (4), and electron microscopy (5), in addition to medical imaging (6–8)—that applications for image reconstruction from projections began to be found. Although the first suggestions of using positron-emitting radionuclides for medical imaging arose in the 1950s (9–12) and the first positron tomographic imaging devices appeared in the 1960s (13) and 1970s (14), the practical application of PET imaging followed that of single-photon emission computed tomography (SPECT) (15,16) and did not occur until the mid to late 1970s.

As the field exploded throughout the 1970s, hundreds of papers relating to image reconstruction from projections were published in prominent journals from the fields of mathematics, physics, engineering, and biomedicine. Several reviews of reconstruction algorithms were written (17–19), summarizing the few different general approaches and the many different specific implementations of image-reconstruction algorithms.

Reconstruction Algorithms

Although reconstruction algorithms can be categorized in several different ways, most algorithms for PET can be classified into two general approaches: reconstruction by filtered back-projection (FBP) and iterative reconstruction. Before discussing these approaches, we review some concepts common to both.

Projection Data

The data acquired directly by a PET scanner represents the sum or integral of radioactivity along the lines connecting any given pair of detectors, often referred to as lines of re-

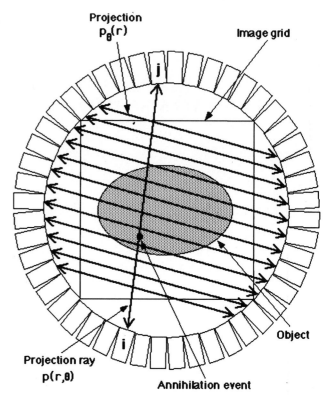

FIG. 4.1. Projection data for two-dimensional PET acquisition. The diagram represents a single detector ring containing 48 detectors. A coincidence line of response between a given pair of detectors i and j is called a projection ray, $p(r,\theta)$, and can be defined in terms of an angle θ and the distance r that the line passes from the center of the field of view. The projection ray data give the sum or integral of radioactivity along the line connecting the two detectors. A set of all projection rays having the same angle θ is referred to as a projection and is denoted by $p_\theta(r)$. Each projection p_θ represents one complete view of the object.

sponse (LORs). This is true for both 2D and 3D data acquisition. In the following paragraphs, we describe the basics of 2D image reconstruction, most of which applies to 3D reconstruction as well. 3D image reconstruction is discussed later in this chapter.

Assume the true 2D radiotracer distribution that we are imaging is given by the function $f(x,y)$, where x and y are standard Cartesian coordinates. The measured PET data, as depicted in Fig. 4.1, can be represented by

$$p\theta(x') \equiv p(x',\theta) = \int f(x,y)\, dy' \qquad [4.1]$$

where (x') and (y') are the coordinates in a Cartesian system rotated by the angle θ.

$$x' = \cos(\theta)x + \sin(\theta)y$$
$$y' = \cos(\theta)y - \sin(\theta)x \qquad [4.2]$$

Each (x',θ) pair of the projection data represents a single line integral that in turn corresponds to a specific pair of detectors (LOR). A given $p(x',\theta)$ often is called a projection ray. The collection of projection rays with the same angle θ is referred to as a projection. Thus, we also can define $p_\theta(x')$ as an equivalent representation of the projection data, but one used when referring to the collection of projection rays as a whole rather than the individual rays $p(x',\theta)$. All the rays of a given projection $p_\theta(x')$ are parallel, where x' is a simple linear measure of the position of each ray within the projection. It is important to note that each projection p_θ of the 2D object has only *one* dimension. Thus, the 2D projection data defined by $p(x',\theta)$ can also be thought of as a *set* of one-dimensional (1D) projections $p_\theta(x')$. Each individual member of this set of projections is defined by a single angle (θ) and represents one complete view of the object. By a complete view, we mean that each point of the object $f(x,y)$ is included in one and only one ray of each projection. Thus, in a perfect noise-free system, the sum over all rays of a given projection is the same for all projections and is proportional to the total radioactivity in the object.

$$\sum_{x'} p_\theta(x') = \int\int f(x,y)\, dx dy \qquad \text{for all } \theta \qquad [4.3]$$

The entire collection of projection data when plotted as θ versus x' is called a sinogram because a point source in the object traces a sinusoidal pattern (see Color Plate 1 following page 394). It is not mandatory to group the projection rays into parallel collections, as described here, but one can choose other groupings such as all rays that contain a common detector. For 2D data, this particular grouping of projection rays would create a fan-shaped projection and thus is referred to as fan-beam geometry (x-ray CT terminology). Note though that a single projection still consists of a complete view of the object. Specific groupings may be beneficial for specific applications; however, throughout this chapter, we retain the parallel-ray geometry.

Filtered Back-projection

One method of reconstructing images from their projections is called FBP. As the name implies, this involves two principal steps: filtering the projections and then back-projecting them to create the reconstructed image. The operation of back-projection in terms of the projection data, $p(x',\theta)$, from our 2D object, $f(x,y)$, is given by

$$b(x,y) = \int_0^{2\pi} p(x',\theta)\, d\theta \qquad [4.4]$$

Back-projection in one sense is the converse operation to the forward-projection that occurs naturally during PET data acquisition; that is, the act of PET data acquisition itself

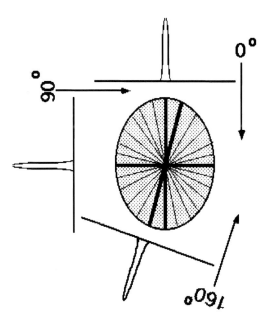

FIG. 4.2. Two-dimensional back-projection. Depicted is an object containing a single point of radioactivity located at the center of the field of view. Each projection contains a single peak representing the radioactivity from this point. Back-projection (without filtering) consists of taking the data from each projection and "smearing" them back along the rays of the projection. Note that the arrows are shown in the opposite direction, representing the operation of *back*-projection, than those of Color Plate 1 (following page 394) that represent the inherent *forward*-projection operation of data acquisition. The dark lines correspond to the back-projections along three angles 0, 90, and 160 degrees. The lighter lines correspond to back-projections along other projection angles. The resultant back-projected image, however, is not a single point, but a starlike pattern centered on the location of the point. This result demonstrates why "filtering" the projections is necessary before the back-projection step.

transforms a 2D array of values into sets of projections or line integrals, whereas back-projection converts the projection set back to a 2D array. Note, however, that forward-projection followed by simple back-projection does not yield the original object. As shown in Fig. 4.2, an object consisting of a single point source is represented by projection data having a single nonzero value at each projection angle. Because these data are back-projected, each angle θ creates a line in the reconstructed image. Thus, a point-source object yields an image with a starlike pattern. To arrive back at the true object, the projection data must be modified or filtered before back-projection.

Before describing the filtering step, the concept of the Fourier transform must be introduced. A one dimensional Fourier transformation of a one dimensional function $f(x)$ is a *frequency space* representation of $f(x)$. By this we mean that any function $f(x)$ can be described as the sum of *sin* or *cos* functions having varying frequencies and magnitudes,

$F(v)$. The value of $F(v)$ gives the magnitude of the sinusoidal function with frequency v. The Fourier transform is defined mathematically as

$$F(v) = \int_{-\infty}^{+\infty} f(x) \, e^{-i2\pi xv} \, dv \qquad [4.5]$$

The Fourier transform of $F(v)$ yields the original function $f(x)$. This transform from $F(v)$ back to $f(x)$ is called an inverse Fourier transformation, although the mathematical formulas for both transforms are identical.

From Radon's work, it can be shown that if the Fourier transformation of the projection data at angle θ

$$P\theta(v) = \int_{-\infty}^{+\infty} p(x',\theta) \, e^{-i2\pi x'v} \, dv \qquad [4.6]$$

is multiplied by v,

$$P_\theta^F(v) = |v| \, P_\theta(v) \qquad [4.7]$$

then the inverse Fourier transform of P_θ^F

$$p^F(x',\theta) = \int_{-\infty}^{+\infty} P_\theta^F(v) \, e^{-i2\pi vx'} \, dx' \qquad [4.8]$$

yields a filtered projection, $p^F(x',\theta)$, which under noise-free conditions yields the true object when back-projected.

$$f(x,y) = b^F(x,y) = \int_0^{2\pi} p^F(x',\theta) \, d\theta \qquad [4.9]$$

The frequency-space filter v is commonly known as a "ramp" filter. To summarize, image reconstruction by FPB consists of four steps applied to each projection θ from 0 to 2π: (a) Fourier transform the projection, (b) filter the transformed projection in frequency space, (c) inverse Fourier transform the filtered frequency-space projection, and (d) back-project the filtered projection.

A major limitation of PET image reconstruction using FBP is statistical noise. The distribution of spatial frequencies (the power spectrum) of the actual (i.e., noise-free) radiotracer distribution tends to decline at higher frequencies while statistical noise tends to have a fairly uniform frequency distribution, close to "white" noise. The multiplication in frequency space by a ramp filter amplifies the higher frequencies that tend to be dominated by noise, thus causing a decreased SNR in the reconstructed images. To control noise, a post-reconstruction smoothing filter can be applied, or more commonly, the ramp filter is modified to preferentially reduce higher frequencies in the projection data. Although many different filter functions have been employed (Butterworth, Hamming, Parzen), all have the same general property that they "roll off" at higher frequencies (Fig. 4.3). While filters that have a sharper roll-off suppress more noise, they also reduce high-frequency signal, thereby creating an inherent trade-off between noise and spatial resolution. In practice, projection data are not continuous but discrete. Shannon's sampling theorem states that the maximum frequency that can be represented by the data, called the Nyquist frequency (v_N), equals 1 divided by twice the sampling frequency, $v_N = 1/(2x')$. Trying to recover higher frequencies produces errors in the reconstruction images called aliasing artifacts. Thus, the frequency-space filter extends from zero to the Nyquist frequency.

Fourier transforms, although useful, are not essential for FBP. This is because of an equivalence between the convolu-

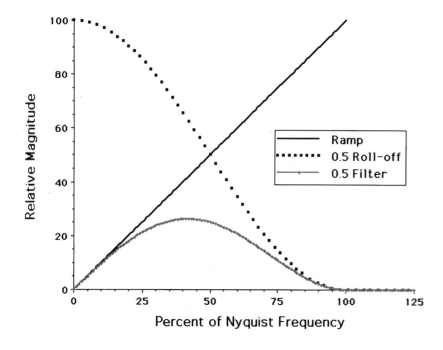

FIG. 4.3. Back-projection filters. For noise-free data, a linearly increasing "ramp" function in Fourier space gives the appropriate filter necessary for exact reconstruction of the object. The noise in PET data, however, has a fairly uniform frequency distribution; thus, a ramp filter amplifies the high-frequency noise and results in noisy-looking images. To limit noise propagation, the ramp filter is rolled off at higher frequencies. The roll-off function (shown for a Hamming 0.5 filter) is multiplied by the ramp filter to yield the final filter function.

tion of two functions and the product of their Fourier transforms.

$$g(x) \otimes h(x) = \int_{-\infty}^{+\infty} g(u)\, h(x-u)\, du = G(v) \times H(v) \quad [4.10]$$

By applying this principle to Eqs. 4.7 and 4.8, the filtered projection $p^F(x',\theta)$ can be obtained by taking the inverse Fourier transform of the frequency-space filter $W(v)$ and convolving it with the raw projection data $p(x',\theta)$.

$$F^{-1}\{P_\theta^F(v)\} = F^{-1}\{[W(v) \times P_\theta(v)]\} \quad [4.11]$$

and thus

$$p^F(x',\theta) = [F^{-1}\{W(v)\}] \otimes [p(x',\theta)] \quad [4.12]$$

where F^{-1} represents the inverse Fourier transform.

The noise properties of FBP for low-count studies, such as occur in many whole-body fluorine-18-fluorodeoxyglucose (^{18}F-FDG) scans, plus the additional noise and significant artifacts associated with transmission scanning and patient movement (see attenuation correction, below), have prompted much effort in the development of alternative algorithms for image reconstruction. Most of these techniques fall into the category of iterative reconstruction techniques.

Iterative Reconstruction

Iterative reconstruction techniques are not a recent development but have been available and used for PET as long as FBP. The main limitation in the past has been the greater computational requirements for iterative methods than for FBP. This section outlines the basic steps of iterative reconstruction. The following section describes advances that have made iterative techniques readily available for routine use.

Rather than using an analytic solution to produce an image from the projection data, iterative reconstruction makes a series of estimates of the image, compares forward-projections of these estimates to the measured data, and refines the estimates by optimizing an objective function until a satisfactory result is obtained. Iterative methods have several advantages over FBP. They allow more accurate modeling of the data-acquisition system than the line-integral model used by FBP and more accurate modeling of the statistical noise in emission and transmission images. An additional advantage is that iterative methods can incorporate *a priori* information about the object being scanned into the reconstruction process. For example, because we are imaging radiotracer concentration, we know all image values must be greater than or equal to zero. Thus, a nonnegativity constraint can be included in the optimization. Another use of *a priori* information is the incorporation of anatomic boundaries from co-registered CT or magnetic resonance (MR) scans with a constraint designed to allow differences across boundaries but penalize differences within boundaries.

The three key steps of an iterative algorithm are (a) determination of a model describing the data-acquisition system (including noise), (b) a calculation using the objective function quantifying how well the image estimate matches the measured data, and (c) an algorithm that determines the next estimate of the image. The model for the measured data takes the general form $\mathbf{p} = \mathbf{Af}$, where $\mathbf{p} = \{p_j,\ j = 1, \ldots, m\}$ is a vector containing all m values of the measured projection ray data (i.e., $p(x',\theta)$ for all (x',θ) pairs), $\mathbf{f} = \{f_i,\ i = 1, \ldots, n\}$ is a vector containing the values of all image voxels (i.e., $f(x,y)$ for all (x,y) pairs) and $\mathbf{A} = \{A_{ij}\}$ is a forward-projection matrix for mapping $\mathbf{f}$ into $\mathbf{p}$. Matrix $\mathbf{A}$ is often called the system, design, or transition matrix. The elements of the matrix A_{ij} contain the probabilities of a positron annihilation event occurring in voxel i being detected in projection ray j. Several additional unwanted processes, such as random and scattered coincidences, as will be discussed below, affect the measured projection data, thus complicating the general model. These can be incorporated into a system model of the form $\mathbf{p} = \mathbf{Af} + \mathbf{r} + \mathbf{s}$, where $\mathbf{r}$ and $\mathbf{s}$ are vectors representing the random and scattered events including the measured projection data $\mathbf{p}$. A discussion of more complex system models is beyond the scope of this chapter. The objective function includes any *a priori* constraints such as nonnegativity and smoothness. Typical objective functions include the Poisson likelihood and the chi-square error (the Gaussian likelihood). The iterative algorithm must ensure that successive estimates of the image converge toward a solution that maximizes (or minimizes) the objective function. The algorithm must also have an exiting criterion that defines when to terminate the iteration process.

The most extensively studied iterative algorithm is the maximum-likelihood expectation-maximization (ML-EM) (20), which seeks to maximize the logarithm of the Poisson likelihood.

$$L(\boldsymbol{p} \mid \boldsymbol{f}) = \sum_{j=1}^{n} \left[\ln\left(\sum_{i=1}^{n} A_{ij} f_i \right) - \sum_{i=1}^{n} A_{ij} f_i \right] \quad [4.13]$$

In practice, the logarithm of the likelihood function is maximized instead of the likelihood function itself for computation reasons, and because they both are maximized for the same image $\mathbf{f}$.

The EM algorithm updates the voxel values (f_i) by

$$f_i^{k+1} = \frac{f_i^k}{\sum\limits_{j=1}^{m} A_{ij}} \sum_{j=1}^{m} \left[A_{ij} \frac{p_j}{\sum\limits_{i'=1}^{n} A_{i'j} f_i^k} \right] \quad [4.14]$$

where f^k and f^{k+1} are the image estimates from iteration k and $k+1$, respectively. Note the double summations over i and j. These steps make the algorithm computationally demanding.

Reduction in Computational Load

As mentioned earlier, the main limitation of iterative reconstruction is its high computational load. For many algorithms, one iteration requires about twice the time of FBP. Thus, considerable effort has been directed not only toward maximizing algorithm performance with respect to image quality, but also toward the development of schemes that converge rapidly. If sufficient quality image estimates can be obtained in 5 instead of 50 iterations, the computation time of iterative routines might well be acceptable.

A significant breakthrough in iterative reconstruction speed occurred with the introduction of reconstruction using "ordered subsets" (OSs) of projection data (21). The concept of OSs can be applied to any iterative algorithm; however, the initial paper and most implementations have paired OS with the EM algorithm (OSEM). For OSEM, the projection data are grouped into subsets. A standard EM algorithm is then applied to one of the subsets using the appropriate rows of the system matrix. The resulting reconstruction becomes the starting value to be used with the next subset. A single iteration of OSEM is completed when each of the subsets has been used once. Assuming mutually exclusive and exhaustive subsets (i.e., each projection ray is a member of one and only one subset), a single OSEM iteration requires approximately the same computation time as one standard EM iteration. However, "convergence" is much faster. Further iterations can be performed by making additional passes through the same OSs. Results from Hudson and Larkin's paper show that one or two iterations with either 32 or 16 subsets yield images with lower chi-square and mean-square error than images with 20 to 30 iterations with standard EM. Reconstructed images appear visually similar as well. In general, to achieve a reconstruction with a given error level, the number of iterations required is inversely proportional to the number of subsets used.

For implementation with PET, each subset may include several projection angles (a projection being the complete set of parallel projection rays at one angle). The order in which the projections are processed is arbitrary from the standpoint of the algorithm, but particular orders improve image quality and accelerate convergence. For example, selecting projections that are widely and evenly spaced, and hence contain substantially different information, is better than selecting projections that are close in angle and hence do not vary considerably from one another. For the detector configuration of the ECAT Exact scanner, a single 2D sinogram consists of 192 projections, 168 rays per projection. A 32-subset implementation of OSEM uses only six projections per subset (192 projections per 32), with 30 degrees between each projection of the subset.

A problem with the OSEM algorithm is that, except for noise-free data, the solution does not converge to the maximum-likelihood solution. Other rapid statistical algorithms, including row-action maximum likelihood and space-alternating generalized maximum likelihood have been developed. These also make application of iterative techniques possible on a routine basis, but they do converge to the true maximum-likelihood solution. Another potential problem

with OSEM, as with the original EM and many other iterative algorithms, is that they produce images with high variance at large numbers of iterations. Such images have a grainy appearance and are visually unappealing. The process to control this is called regularization. Regularization can be accomplished by various means including stopping after a limited number of iterations, post-reconstruction smoothing, or incorporation of constraints, penalties, or other *a priori* information as described earlier.

With faster computers and with the improvements made in the implementation of the algorithms, as described in the proceeding paragraphs, iterative reconstruction for 2D projection sets became practical on a routine basis by the mid-1990s. With a clear advantage in SNR over FBP, iterative techniques have become the method of choice for 2D PET image reconstruction. This advantage is greater in lower count whole-body imaging than in higher count brain studies. However, at about the same time, 3D PET acquisition also became readily available, increasing the computation demands on reconstruction algorithms by more than an order of magnitude, and thus a new set of challenges was encountered.

Image Reconstruction for 3D PET

The introduction of 3D data acquisition marked a tremendous advance in PET imaging. Although not without its own unique set of problems, 3D acquisition with the interslice septa removed increases scanner sensitivity by a factor of 6 to 8 or more depending on the axial field of view (FOV) of the scanner, thereby increasing the noise-equivalent counts (NECs) typically by a factor of 3 to 5. With this large increase in SNR, particularly in high statistical quality brain studies, the advantages that iterative techniques have over FBP are not as pronounced. Furthermore, the computational load of 3D reconstruction is much greater than that of 2D reconstruction. Therefore, analytic techniques, which have a speed advantage over iterative ones, once again appear more attractive. However, with the recent dramatic increase in clinical PET using ^{18}F-FDG, particularly whole-body oncology imaging, minimizing scan time is essential both for patient comfort and cooperation and for efficient patient throughput. Thus, the statistical quality of clinical scans is limited even with 3D acquisition, so iterative algorithms will continue to provide a means of improving image SNR. In this section, alternatives for reconstruction of projection data from 3D PET are summarized. A more thorough discussion of 3D acquisition and image-reconstruction methods, as well as other topics, can be found in a recent book covering both theoretical and practical aspects of 3D PET (22).

3D Projection Data

Assuming the true 3D radiotracer distribution we are imaging is given by the function $f(x,y,z)$, then the measured 3D

PET data, considering a spherical geometry, can be represented by

$$p_{\theta,\phi}(x',y') \equiv p(x',y',\theta,\phi) = \int f(x,y,z) \, dz' \qquad [4.15]$$

where x', y', and z' are the coordinates within the rotated plane that is perpendicular to a line with in-plane angle θ and azimuthal (out-of-plane) angle ϕ. There is not a perfect correspondence to the 2D case in which the projection data $p(x',\theta)$ can be thought of as a set of one dimensional projections $p_\theta(x')$, where the different members of the set are defined by a *single* angle θ. Three-dimensional projection data needs to be thought of as a set of two dimensional projections $p_{\theta,\phi}(x',y')$, where the members of the set are defined by *two* angles θ and ϕ. This concept is easily visualized by thinking of a radiographic chest film as being a 2D projection of the 3D chest, with two angles needed to define its orientation (anteroposterior vs. lateral and superior vs. inferior).

Reconstruction of a 3D object from a complete set of its 2D projections can be performed analytically by 3D FBP in a manner analogous to the use of 2D FBP for reconstructing a 2D object from a complete set of its 1D projections. However, unlike the 2D case in which a full ring of PET detectors (which completely encircle a 2D object) can provide the complete set of projections, it is not practical to construct a PET scanner that has full solid-angle coverage of a 3D object, the human body. Thus, one cannot acquire the complete set of 2D projections necessary for 3D FBP. Many projections are either truncated or missing entirely. Applying 3D FBP to incomplete projection data can result in severe image artifacts.

3D FBP with Reprojection

To address this problem, an algorithm referred to as 3D back-projection with reprojection (23) was developed, which produces estimates of the missing or truncated projection data. With these estimates of projection data for the unmeasured angles, 3D FBP can then be applied to the completed set of 2D projections. The estimates of the missing projections are calculated as follows. First, the projections that would be acquired from 2D acquisition—that is, the complete set of 1D projections for each transverse slice—are extracted from the entire set of measured projection data. These 1D projection sets are reconstructed by standard 2D reconstruction to form a first-pass estimate of the 3D object. Next the line integrals for all missing or incomplete projections are calculated by forward-projection through the first-pass estimate of the 3D volume. These calculated projections are then merged with the measured projections to obtain the complete projection set, which are then used for reconstruction of a final 3D image using the standard 3D FBP algorithm. The computation time to reconstruct a 3D data set using 3D FBP with reprojection is more than an order of magnitude greater than the comparable 2D data sets. This

is due simply to the tremendous number of projection rays that need to be back-projected. Typical 3D data sets contain as many as 20 to 80 million projection rays. Therefore, considerable effort continues to be put into the development of methods to reduce computational loads and reconstruction time.

One simple means of reducing reconstruction time that is commonly provided by commercial vendors is data reduction by combining neighboring projections. For 3D acquisition, this has been accomplished by averaging projections across both the in-plane polar angles (θ) and the azimuthal angles (ϕ) now present due to removal of the septa. This reduction is sometimes called ''mashing.'' With current scanners, an in-plane mashing factor of 2 is typical, which reduces the number of polar angles by 2. The azimuthal angle data reduction is somewhat more complex but follows the same general principle of making the angular projection grid coarser. Reconstruction performance needs to be assessed to ensure that this combining of projections does not cause artifacts that result from undersampling projection space. Threefold to eightfold reductions in the number of LORs are usually possible without degrading imaging quality significantly. Three-dimensional data sets can thus be reduced to a much more manageable size of around 10 megabytes per scan on current systems.

Rebinning Algorithms

Other analytic approaches have been introduced for 3D reconstruction (24–27), and although they provide satisfactory performance, none have reduced reconstruction time relative to 3D FBP with reprojection by more than a factor of two. Thus, alternative approaches to the problem have received considerable attention. Because 2D reconstructions are more than an order of magnitude faster than 3D, methods that convert the projections from 3D data into approximations of projections from 2D data (one sinogram per transverse slice) are very attractive. A method for converting 3D to 2D data is commonly referred to as a rebinning algorithm.

It is easier to understand rebinning if we consider the 3D projection data as coming from a cylindrical geometry instead of the spherical geometry used for equation 4.15.

$$[p(x',y',\theta,\phi)]_{spherical} \Leftrightarrow [p(x',\theta,z,\delta)]_{cylindrical} \qquad [4.16]$$

where z is the distance along the axial extent of the scanner and δ is a measure of off-axis tilt. For a scanner with detectors in a cylindrical geometry, consider a plane perpendicular to the long axis of the scanner. All the projection rays within this plane are defined by x' and θ just as in the 2D case. Because all these rays are perpendicular to the scanner's axis, the off-axis tilt δ is zero, and if this plane goes through the center of the axial FOV, z also is zero. This projection set can be reconstructed by a 2D algorithm to yield an image of the transverse slice running through the middle of the axial FOV. Other projection sets that exist in different but parallel planes to this set still would have $\delta = 0$ but would have different values of z. Two-dimensional reconstruction of the additional sets yields images of other transverse slices. However, most of the projection rays in 3D PET acquisition are not perpendicular to the long axis of the scanner ($\delta \neq 0$), so the job of rebinning is to convert data for all projection rays with nonzero δ to rays with zero δ. These data can then be sorted into sets of projections, one for each transverse slice of the scanner, z.

$$p(x',\theta,z,\delta) \Rightarrow p(x',\theta,z) \equiv p_z(x',\theta) \quad [4.17]$$

which can then be reconstructed by a rapid 2D algorithm. In practice, the z value of a given projection ray is defined simply by the average z coordinate of the two detectors represented by this ray. The value of $\delta = \tan(\phi)$, the angle between the projection ray and the transaxial plane, can be calculated from the ring offset and the physical distance between the two detectors.

Rebinning methods must be fast and accurate, and must incorporate the entire 3D data set to maintain the advantage of increased sensitivity provided by 3D acquisition. Rebinning can be approximate or exact; however, approximate methods can be implemented more efficiently and thus offer a speed advantage. One very rapid and simple method of rebinning is single-slice rebinning (SSRB) (28), in which any projection ray at a given azimuthal (out-of-plane) angle is rebinned into the transverse slice that is located halfway axially between the two detectors, that is, merely setting δ to 0. Thus, using SSRB, the conversion of equation 4.17 becomes

$$p(x',\theta,z,\delta) \approx p(x',\theta,z,0) = p_z(x',\theta) \quad [4.18]$$

Although fast, this method is not very accurate for events that occur a large distance from the central axis. If the azimuthal angle of the accepted projection rays is not too large, this method can provide an improved SNR for regions located near the center of the FOV. It should be pointed out that this general technique is in fact used in all standard 2D acquisitions. Even in the very first multislice scanners, a cross-plane was produced by rebinning the projection rays that came from detectors that are one ring apart (a small but nonzero δ). Current-generation scanners typically operate under the SSRB principle by accepting rays from detectors that are offset from one another by 0, ± 2, and ± 4 rings for "true" planes and ± 1, ± 3, and ± 5 rings for cross-planes.

FORE Rebinning

A significant advance in 3D reconstruction came with the introduction of a new rebinning technique based on taking 2D Fourier transforms of the projection data called Fourier rebinning (FORE) (29). The 2D Fourier transform of each oblique projection with respect to x' and θ is given by

$$P(\nu_{x'},k,z,\delta) = \int_{-\infty}^{+\infty} dx' \int_{0}^{2\pi} d\theta\, (e^{-i2\pi x' \nu_{x'}})\, p(x',\theta,z,\delta) \quad [4.19]$$

The equation 4.17 conversion using FORE is accomplished in Fourier space instead of projection space.

$$P(\nu_{x'},k,z,\delta) \cong P\left(\nu_{x'},k,z - \frac{k\delta}{\nu_{x'}},0\right) = P(\nu_{x'},k,z',0) \quad [4.20]$$

Following the FORE approximation, the inverse 2D Fourier transform yields

$$p_{z'}(x',\theta) = p(x',\theta,z',0) = F^{-1}[P(\nu_{x'},k,z',0)] \quad [4.21]$$

Two-dimensional reconstructions are then performed on each set of projections (defined by z') to yield the stack of transverse images defining the 3D volume. The 2D reconstructions can be either FBP or iterative. Many groups have applied FORE and have shown that the method produces images comparable to 3D FBP with reprojection, but with computational savings of greater than an order of magnitude when following FORE with 2D FBP.

The introduction of FORE made the job of processing large numbers of 3D PET scans, such as are needed for repeated $H_2^{15}O$ scans or long multiframe dynamic studies, much easier. The next logical step was to combine the advantages of the increased sensitivity of 3D scanning with the noise-reduction properties of iterative reconstruction through the use of both rebinning methods, such as FORE, and computation reduction techniques, such as OSs. Several papers have been published recently using FORE + OSEM. Reconstruction performance of the combined FORE + OSEM technique has been compared with 3D FBP with reprojection (30), with FORE + 2D FBP (31) and FORE + PWLS (penalized weighted least squares (32), an alternative to ML-EM optimization, and to fully 3D OSEM (33). FORE + OSEM was found to outperform 3D FBP with reprojection in terms of contrast and SNR while requiring less time to perform. FORE + OSEM outperformed FORE + 2D FBP. FORE + PWLS was found to be superior to FORE + OSEM when attenuation correction was not incorporated into the system matrix. However, FORE + OSEM with attenuation correction incorporated into the system matrix performed very similarly to FORE + PWLS but is faster computationally. FORE + OSEM was found to perform nearly as well as 3D OSEM, but with time savings of greater than a factor of 10.

Fully 3D Iterative Approaches

We have seen that reconstruction techniques, including iterative approaches, are now available to handle heavy loads of 3D PET data. This does not mean that current-day reconstruction methodology should be considered fully mature. In one sense, the quest for better image reconstruction may never end. As new scanners are developed that have higher and higher intrinsic resolution, such as the many recently developed small-animal scanners, more detected events are needed per unit volume to approach this resolution in the reconstructed images. This in turn requires better models for describing data acquisition and for characterizing the noise properties of the PET data. To this end, work continues on the implementation of fully 3D iterative techniques that avoid even the relatively minor problems associated with techniques such as FORE and OSEM. Qi et al. have implemented fully 3D iterative techniques for human (34) and animal (35) imaging, attempting to obtain the highest quality images possible. This same group has recently published a review of the current state of the art in regard to statistical approaches to image reconstruction in PET (36).

Data Corrections

Accurate quantitative images of radiotracer concentration are not obtained by direct reconstruction of the raw projection data acquired from a PET scanner. To ensure optimal quantification, several corrections must be made to the projections before or during the reconstruction process. These corrections are important and require as much attention as is given to the reconstruction algorithms.

Normalization

With thousands of detectors in current PET scanning systems, it is unreasonable to assume that all detectors will respond uniformly to a given number of incident radiation events. Some detectors will have a lower response than average while others will have a higher response. Furthermore, the geometry between a pair of detectors in coincidence is not fixed but varies for several reasons, so there are inherent differences in detector response due to geometric considerations. Even if all the detectors did respond with the same efficiency to a fixed radiation source, the coincidence pair responses (the projection rays) would vary. Therefore, the entire set of projection data for each acquired PET scan must be normalized for differences in detector response throughout the scanner. As suggested above, the components of the normalization can be separated into two categories: those related to the relative efficiencies of the individual detectors and those related to the physical or geometric arrangement of the detectors. Thus, even though a major portion of the normalization correction accounts for variations in *individual* detector responses, the overall correction is applied on a ray-by-ray basis.

There are two general approaches for determining the correction factors used for normalization. The first is a direct measurement of the factors. In this approach, a low-radioactivity source (typically a rotating ^{68}Ge rod) is used to generate or measure a correction factor for each coincidence pair by acquiring a scan in the same manner as one acquires a

"blank" scan. For the 2D case, this correction takes the form

$$N(r,\theta) = \frac{\left[\sum_{r=1}^{j}\sum_{\theta=1}^{k} P_N(r,\theta)\right]\left[j \times k\right]}{P_N(r,\theta)} \quad [4.22]$$

where $N(r,\theta)$ is the normalization factor for projection ray sum r of angle θ, $P_N(r,\theta)$ is the uncorrected projection data from the normalization scan, and the summations are over all k projection angles and all j projection rays per angle. The normalized projection data are simply

$$P_{corr}(r,\theta) = N(r,\theta) \times P(r,\theta) \quad [4.23]$$

where $P(r,\theta)$ is the uncorrected projection ray measured from any arbitrary PET scan, $N(r,\theta)$ is the correction factor for this ray determined from the normalization scan as given by equation 4.22, and $P_{corr}(r,\theta)$ is the corrected projection raw value. This approach, in a single measurement, accounts for both the individual detector efficiencies and the differences in geometry between the various detector pairs.

A second correction technique separates the individual detector efficiencies from the geometric effects. In this approach a set of normalization factors for the individual detectors (instead of coincidence pairs) is generated, and then the product of any two detectors efficiencies yields an estimate of the coincidence pair sensitivity. This value is then corrected further for differing geometric effects based the physical locations of the two detectors. This method can be considered an indirect or calculated correction. The are at least two geometric effects that must be considered. One is the differential response depending on how closely the LOR for the two detectors passes to the center of the FOV. For 3D acquisition, this effect has both transverse and axial components. A second effect is based on the block detectors in use on current PET systems where many detector crystals are coupled to a few photomultiplier tubes. The location of a particular detector crystal within a block (center or edge) is important. The overall normalization factor for a detector pair using an indirect or calculated approach takes the form

$$N(i_m,j_n) = \frac{1}{E(i_m) \times E(j_n) \times G(r,\theta,m,n) \times B(k_{ij},r,\theta,m,n)} \quad [4.24]$$

where $N(i_m, j_n)$ is the normalization factor for the projection ray between detector i of ring m and detector j of ring n, $E(i_m)$ and $E(j_n)$ are the individual efficiencies for those two detectors, $G(r,\theta,m,n)$ is the geometric efficiency between two detectors and $B(k_{ij},r,\theta,m,n)$ is the block-related correction factors, with k_{ij} defining the relative positions within a block of detectors i and j.

Current PET scanners are more stable than early scanners, so normalization typically must be performed only weekly to monthly. A directly measured normalization determines the entire set of normalization factors every time. For an indirect or calculated normalization, however, the individual detector efficiencies $E(i_m)$ are measured weekly to monthly, whereas the geometric factors G and B can be measured once carefully and stored, then retrieved each time to calculate the normalization factors for a given PET scan.

The relative advantages and disadvantages of the two general approaches, the additional considerations for 3D versus 2D normalization, and the interaction between this correction and other corrections (particularly scatter) are beyond the scope of this chapter. Bailey et al. (37) present an excellent and more detailed discussion of normalization.

Detector Dead-time

During the time a detector is processing a detected event, it is unable to process any additional events. If an event occurs during this time, it goes unprocessed and is lost. Such losses are referred to as dead-time losses. As count rate increases, the probability of having a lost event increases and scanner "dead time" increases. These losses are not simply related to the singles and the coincidence count rates, but also are dependent on the analog and digital electronics of the system. Dead time is further complicated by the block detector design of current scanners. It is extremely difficult to calculate dead time for PET scanners entirely from first principles. In practice, one can assess dead time by plotting the measured count rate of a decaying source over time. Assuming the source is a single radionuclide, one can calculate the "true" count rate from the half-life of the nuclide and plot this versus the actual measured count rate. At low activity and hence low count rates, the plot will be linear. At higher count rates, a nonlinearity arises as the expected number of events exceeds the measured number. The ratio of the measured to the expected events yields an estimate of scanner dead time. For the majority of present-day scanners, an empirical relationship between count rate and dead time is provided by the manufacturer as part of the software package. Typically, corrections are fairly accurate up to at least 50% and as high as 75% to 80% dead time. For current scanners, dead-time corrections are accurate to better than $\pm 5\%$ for count rates up to at least 5 μCi/mL (in a 20-cm-diameter phantom) for 2D acquisitions and up to at least 1 μCi/mL for higher sensitivity 3D acquisition.

Random and Multiple Coincidences

As described in Chapter 3, the detection of the two nearly colinear 511-keV photons within a specified amount of time τ, called the coincidence window or coincidence resolving time, forms the basis for PET imaging. The near simultaneous ($\leq$10-ns) detection of two photons is called a coincidence event. Remembering that it is highly likely that only one of the two annihilation photons is detected, usually only a single event is recorded by the scanner during a given time interval τ. Therefore, as the detected count rate increases, the probability that one event is detected from each of two

separate positron annihilations within the coincidence window increases as well. This type of event is defined as random coincidence, sometimes also called an accidental coincidence. As shown in Color Plate 2 (following page 394), the coincidence line connecting the two detectors for a random coincidence gives erroneous information about the position of the positron decay, causing image-reconstruction artifacts if not accounted for. Because the scanner cannot distinguish "true" coincidences from "random" coincidences on an event-by-event basis, an alternative scheme is required.

Two distinct methods have been used for random coincidence correction. The first requires that the singles detection rates be recorded for each detector of the scanner. The random coincidence rate for a given projection ray of PET scan i, $C_R(i)$ is given by the product of twice the coincidence resolving time τ, multiplied by the singles rates of the two detectors $C_{S_1}(i)$ and $C_{S_2}(i)$.

$$C_R(i) = 2\tau\, C_{S_1}(i)\, C_{S_2}(i) \qquad [4.25]$$

Note that because the singles count rates increase linearly with the amount of radioactivity in the FOV, the randoms count rates increase as the square of the amount of radioactivity. Thus, at low count rates, randoms are insignificant while at high count rates, the randoms rates easily can exceed the true coincidence rates. This method of correction is applied to each projection ray separately, but only once per scan.

$$C_T(i) = C_M(i) - C_R(i) \qquad [4.26]$$

where $C_M(i)$ and $C_T(i)$ are the measured and corrected true coincidence count rates, respectively.

The second method involves setting up two distinct coincidence windows. The first window is the standard coincidence window of width τ. As before, both true and random coincidences are recorded in this window, which for this approach is called the "prompt" coincidence window. A second coincidence circuit is set up, but with one of the two inputs being delayed by a time considerably greater than the resolving time τ. Rather than searching for two events that occur within a single 10-ns window (as is done in the "prompt" circuit), this circuit searches for events that occur in two separate 10-ns windows offset by, for example, 100 ns. This offset window produces what are called "delayed" coincidence events. The probability that a true coincidence occurs in the "delayed" window is zero, whereas the probability that a "random" coincidence occurs is the same as in the "prompt" window. Thus, the "prompt" window records true plus random coincidences, whereas the "delayed" window records only randoms. Subtracting "delayed" from "prompt" coincidences yields an estimate of "true" coincidences. The advantage of this approach is that it can be implemented on-line and requires no postacquisition processing. During data acquisition, a memory location exists for each detector pair whose projection ray subtends the FOV. For every "prompt" coincidence event detected, the memory location representing the appropriate projection ray is incremented by one. For each "delayed" event detected, the memory location is decremented by one. This commonly used decrementing procedure ruins the Poisson statistical model that is the theoretical basis for equation 4.13 and the ML-EM (and OSEM) iterative reconstruction algorithms. Alternative reconstruction methods have been proposed for PET measurements that are precorrected for random coincidences (38,39).

Scattered Coincidence Events

At 511-keV energies, two types of photon interactions occur: Compton scattering and photoelectric absorption. Scintillation detectors are designed to maximize the number of photoelectric interactions while minimizing the probability of Compton scattering. This is accomplished by a material with high effective atomic number and high density. However, due to the lower effective atomic number in the body, most interactions in human tissue occur via Compton scattering, as depicted in Color Plate 2 (following page 394). As was the case for random coincidence events, detection of events in which one or both of the photons have undergone at least one Compton scatter causes the location of the annihilation to be misplaced. Inclusion of scattered events causes a relatively uniform background, decreasing image contrast and reducing the SNR. Naturally, we would like to record only unscattered photon events, but it is not possible to identify with complete certainty whether a particular event is scattered. Scintillation detectors with higher light output do, however, have better energy resolution and thus are better able to distinguish unscattered from scattered events.

Accurate correction for Compton-scattered photons is extremely complex, with hundreds of papers having been written on quantifying its effects as well as developing and testing methods for correction. For 2D acquisition, scatter was only moderately important, with 15% to 20% of the detected events being scattered. Image quality was not affected greatly, so scatter correction was often ignored without major impact. With 3D scanning, 35% to 50% of the detected events may be scattered and correction has become much more critical. Current scatter corrections fall into three basic groups: (a) those using multiple energy windows; (b) those based on direct calculation from analytic formulas for Compton scatter or on Monte Carlo calculations; and (c) methods involving a variety of techniques such as convolution, deconvolution, or the fitting of analytic functions to areas of the image void of radioactivity (thus, representing only scattered events).

Although each of these three general techniques has its own advantages and limitations, details of such methods are beyond the scope of this text. The reader is referred to Bailey et al. (40) for a more thorough discussion of scattered events and correction methods to account for their occurrence. Here, we describe briefly only the direct calculation approach. It is assumed that the true radioactivity distribution can be reconstructed accurately when the measured PET data, emission and transmission, contain only unscattered events. The measured PET data, however, include both true and scattered events. The correction is performed iteratively. The original measured data are reconstructed as an initial estimate of the true radioactivity distribution. From these images and the analytic formulas for Compton scatter, the scatter component to the raw projection data is estimated. This scatter component is subtracted from the measured PET data as the next approximation to the scatter-free projection data. This new projection set is reconstructed as the next approximation to the true radioactivity distribution. These steps are repeated until the images reconstructed from the current estimate of the scatter-free projection data yield predicted scatter that when added to the scatter-free data equal the measured projection data. In practice, successive approximations to the scatter-free distribution can be made during the normal iterations of the OSEM reconstruction algorithm.

Attenuation

A final but extremely important correction to the projection data is that which accounts for the effects of photon attenuation in the body. For a true coincidence event to be detected, both photons must exit the body. This is less likely for annihilations located deep within the body than for ones occurring near the body's surface. One convenient aspect of PET imaging is that the attenuation correction factor for any given projection ray is the same for a positron annihilation occurring anywhere along the ray. The net attenuation is simply the product of the probabilities that each photon escapes without interacting:

$$e^{-\mu x_1} e^{-\mu x_2} = e^{-\mu(x_1 + x_2)} \qquad [4.27]$$

where μ is the linear attenuation coefficient for 511-keV photons in tissue, and x_1 and x_2 are the distances the two photons must travel through tissue. Because the sum $x_1 + x_2$ always equals the total path length l through the body, the attenuation-correction factor is given by $e^{+\mu l}$. Independence of the position of the annihilation along the ray is true even if the attenuation coefficient varies across the path due to multiple tissue types (lung, soft tissue, and bone).

Again, there are two general approaches used to account for photon attenuation. First is a calculated or analytic method, where the path length for each projection ray is estimated in some fashion and the value for μ is assumed. The attenuation-correction factor, as indicated above, is simply $e^{+\mu l}$. The two main limitations of this approach are (a) it is not always easy to determine the path length of all projection rays and (b) variations in μ are not easily accounted for. A major advantage is that there is no statistical noise associated with the correction. This approach has been used for brain imaging where the shape of the head can be approximated by an ellipse and the attenuation is uniform except for a thin rim of skull.

Blank Scan   **Transmission Scan**

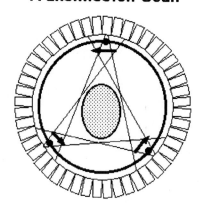

Corrected Emission = Raw Emission x (Blank/Trans)

FIG. 4.4. Schematic for measured attenuation correction. As described in the text, measured attenuation is performed by acquiring two scans: a "blank" scan and a "transmission" scan. Both scans are performed using radioactive sources that are rotated around the gantry in front of the detectors. The blank scan measures the coincidence rate from the sources when *nothing* is in the field of view. The transmission scan measures the coincidence rate when the *object* being imaged is in the field of view. The ratio between these two measures is used, ray by ray, to correct the emission projection data.

A second method is to measure the attenuation factors directly. This approach typically uses external rod sources that are rotated around the FOV. Most sources contain the positron emitter ^{68}Ge, which has a 0.75-year half-life. Two scans are acquired (Fig. 4.4), a "blank" scan that is acquired with nothing in the FOV (similar in nature to the normalization scan described above) and a "transmission" scan where the subject is in the FOV in the identical position as the emission scan. After appropriate corrections, the ratio of the measured projection data from the blank scan divided by the transmission scan yields a correction factor for the emission data. If a particular projection ray has 400 counts in the blank scan, but only 50 counts in the transmission scan, the correction factor for the emission data will be 8.

Although measured attenuation avoids the problems associated with the analytic approach, several other potential problems arise. Statistical uncertainty in the blank and particularly the transmission scan propagates into the reconstructed emission images. This problem is particularly bad in the abdomen, where attenuation is high and thus detected transmission events low. Subject motion between the times of the transmission and emission scans can cause significant errors in the correction factors for particular projection rays, resulting in severe artifacts when motion is substantial. Such artifacts are considerably worse for FBP than for iterative approaches. Transmission scans also take considerable time. If a subject can reasonably be expected to remain still for 1 to 2 hours, we would want to spend the entire time acquiring emission data. For body scans, however, nearly as much time is required for transmission as emission imaging. Fur-

thermore, for clinical FDG scans that have a 50-minute incorporation period, it becomes problematic to perform all transmission scanning before injection of the radiotracer. This is due to both subject motion and study duration issues. If transmission scans are performed after injection, then the contribution of the FDG events to transmission data must be taken into account.

Over the past decade, much work has been done to improve attenuation correction. The two most significant advances are described here. The first was to provide the capability of performing postinjection transmission scans. Before this advance, a typical clinical protocol might include 30 minutes of transmission scanning, injection of ^{18}F-FDG, and then a 50-minute uptake period, followed by 30 to 60 minutes or more of emission imaging. Thus, a subject would have to lie still for more than 2 hours. This is difficult on the patient and it occupies the scanner for long periods of time even when no data are being acquired. Furthermore, registration between transmission and emission scans may be jeopardized by the length of time between the acquisitions. Through the use of rotating rod sources instead of a continuous ring of radioactivity, postinjection transmission scanning is possible. For discrete rod sources, only a small fraction of the projection rays contain valid "transmission" coincidences at any given time. Only rays that pass through one of the rod sources can have coincidences that originate from the rod. All other events come from FDG decay. Thus, most of the emission coincidences that occur at any given time are rejected based on the known positions of the rods.

The second major advance was the development of a combination calculated/measured attenuation correction that makes use of the advantages of each approach. A transmission scan is acquired, but rather than performing the correction based on the ray-by-ray difference between blank and transmission data, this scan is reconstructed into a map of attenuation coefficients. Although individual rays are noisy, the reconstructed transmission image allows segmentation into different tissue types. Each pixel of the image is *assigned* an attenuation coefficient based on the segmentation. The segmented images, in practice, are smoothed and then used to calculate attenuation factors for the emission data. This process greatly reduces noise propagation from the transmission measurements into the reconstructed emission images. Color Plate 3 (following page 394) shows a 2D whole-body transaxial slice reconstructed with measured attenuation on the left side and with segmented attenuation correction on the right side. Clearly demonstrated is the noise propagation from the transmission data into the emission image when attenuation correction is performed without segmentation. In addition, reconstructions were performed with both FBP and with an iterative OSEM algorithm. The better noise properties of iterative reconstruction are demonstrated clearly. In particular, notice the reduction in streak artifacts with OSEM that plague back-projection techniques. Keeping in mind that both images are derived from the identical projection data, the improvement from the upper-left image to the lower-right image (which has both segmented attenuation correction and iterative reconstruction) truly is impressive.

A variety of additional issues arise when determining attenuation corrections for 3D PET. A major difficulty is that the radioactivity level of the rod sources required for adequate statistics in 2D studies causes excessive dead time and random coincidence rates in 3D studies. Currently, transmission scans are performed in 2D mode, reconstructed, and then forward-projected into the full set of 3D projection rays. Considerable work by Fessler et al. has been performed to maximize the quality of the reconstructed transmission data (41,42).

A recent advance worth mentioning is the use of CT for attenuation correction. With the advent of combined PET-CT, the need for rotating rod sources for such systems is alleviated altogether. Although the effective photon energy of CT is much lower than 511 keV, a calculation to convert attenuation coefficients from ''CT'' to ''511-keV'' attenuation coefficients is relatively straightforward. Therefore, combining PET and CT not only provides the capability to image functional and anatomic information in the same setting, but the CT can be used for attenuation correction. CT images are of much higher quality than rod source images, thus nearly no noise is introduced by the correction. In addition, because CT scans require much less time, the 30% to 40% of the scan time currently used for transmission imaging is unnecessary and can be used either to shorten the study or for additional emission imaging.

COMPARTMENTAL MODELING

Image reconstruction in conjunction with the appropriate corrections to the measured projection data yields quantitative measures of a PET tracer's spatial radioactivity distribution within the human body. However, this distribution is not static over the course of the study, but varies with time, depending on the different processes that govern its uptake and subsequent biologic fate in the body. By acquiring a dynamic sequence of PET measurements, we obtain information about the *in vivo* behavior of the particular radiotracer being imaged, which can be used to provide measurements of specific biologic functions. This is accomplished through the use of an analysis process commonly referred to as compartmental or tracer kinetic modeling.

Compartmental modeling techniques are mathematical constructs that involve the concept of different spaces or compartments in which the tracer can reside plus a set of model rate constants or parameters that describe how rapidly the tracer moves between compartments. With some knowledge of the radiotracer and the biologic properties that govern its *in vivo* behavior, these rate constants are then assumed to represent specific physiologic or biochemical processes such as blood flow, glucose metabolism, protein synthesis, neurotransmitter level, enzyme activity, and receptor or binding site density.

The following sections describe the fundamentals of compartmental modeling and tracer kinetic techniques. The steps required for selection, implementation, and validation of a compartmental model are discussed, including consideration of practical issues that affect the use of compartmental model strategies. Models for two specific applications, measurement of blow flow and glucose metabolism, are reviewed in more detail. We include examples of applications for neurologic, cardiac, and oncologic studies.

Fundamentals of Compartmental Modeling

Radiotracers allow for the investigation of physiologic and biochemical processes *without altering* the normal functions of the biologic system. The mathematical description of the movement of radioactive tracer material within the system is known as tracer kinetics. Biologic systems can be represented or modeled as a collection of compartments, sometimes referred to as pools or spaces, linked by kinetic processes that provide a mechanism for exchange of tracer between adjoining compartments. A compartmental model consists of a finite number of compartments, each of which is assumed to behave as a single homogeneous, well-mixed, distinct component of the overall biologic system.(43) Different compartments may represent either *distinct* physical spaces, such as blood plasma versus brain tissue, or different chemical forms (FDG vs. FDG 6-PO$_4$) or pharmacologic states (bound vs. unbound) of the radiotracer that occupy the *same* physical space.

The various compartments of a tracer kinetic model are linked by a set of parameters commonly called rate constants

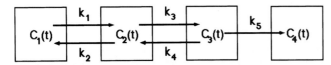

FIG. 4.5. Generalized compartmental model. The system described by this hypothetical model consists of four compartments that contain a given radiotracer at concentrations C_1, C_2, C_3, and C_4. The radiotracer is exchanged or transferred between compartments at rates proportional to the five rate constants k_1 through k_5. Exchange between compartments 1 and 2 and between compartments 2 and 3 is reversible, whereas exchange of radiotracer between compartments 3 and 4 is irreversible.

(Fig. 4.5). The values of these parameters represent the rates at which the radiotracer is exchanged between the various compartments. In the case in which two compartments represent different distinct physical spaces, the parameters that link them represent the rates of flow or transport across that particular physical boundary. In the case in which two compartments share the same physical space but represent different chemical forms or pharmacologic states, the parameters represent the rates of transformation from one chemical form or state of the substance to the other.

The amount or concentration of the radiotracer in the model compartments can be described as a function of time by a set of first-order differential equations in terms of the model parameters. The basis for the differential equations is derived from the law of conservation of mass, or mass balance. Mass balance, for tracer applications, means that the amount of radioactive tracer that enters a compartment per unit time (the influx) minus the amount of tracer that leaves the compartment per unit time (the efflux) is equal to the amount of tracer accumulated in the compartment per unit time. The amount of radiotracer typically is measured in either microcuries or megabecqurels (MBq). Under steady-state or equilibrium conditions, the influx of radiotracer is equal to the efflux, and the net change in the amount or concentration of radiotracer over time is zero.

Figure 4.5 depicts a hypothetical compartmental system consisting of four compartments and a total of five rate constants. In some fields of compartmental modeling, a rate constant is written with two subscripts depicting both the compartments that it links. For example, the rate constant describing transfer of material from compartment 1 to compartment 2 is written as k_{21} while the rate constant describing transfer of material from compartment 3 to compartment 1 is written as k_{13}. In the field of nuclear medicine, it has been more common to use a single subscript (Fig. 4.5), with transfer from compartment 1 to compartment 2 being referred to as k_1 and transfer from compartment 2 to compartment 1 being referred to as k_2. Rate constants representing transfer between subsequent model compartments are referred to as k_3, k_4, k_5, and so on. In this chapter, we adopt the nuclear medicine convention using only single sub-

scripts. The differential equations describing the concentration of material in each compartment are written in the same form as the mass balance equation and appear as follows:

$$dC_1(t)/dt = k_2C_2(t) - k_1C_1(t)$$
$$dC_2(t)/dt = [k_1C_1(t) + k_4C_3(t)] - [k_2C_2(t) + k_3C_2(t)]$$
$$dC_3(t)/dt = k_3C_2(t) - [k_4C_3(t) + k_5C_3(t)] \qquad [4.28]$$
$$dC_4(t)/dt = k_5C_3(t)$$

where dC_i/dt is the rate of change in concentration of radiotracer in compartment i; the positive terms describe influx, and the negative terms describe efflux. Note that the amount of radiotracer leaving a compartment by any route is proportional to the concentration in that compartment. The proportionality constants between the quantities of radiotracer leaving and the concentrations in the compartments are the model rate constants. These rate constants appear as the coefficients for the efflux and influx terms in equation 4.28. A rate constant generally has units of inverse time (min^{-1}) and describes the fraction of radiotracer leaving a compartment in a given amount of time. For example, a rate constant of 0.1 min^{-1} indicates that an amount of tracer equal to 10% of that in the compartment will be transported out of the compartment every minute. For this model because all the rate constants appear to the first power, all processes governing radiotracer exchange between the model compartments are first order and thus the system is said to obey first-order kinetics.

Steps Required for Design and Implementation of a Compartmental Model

Although there are many ways to group the steps required for using compartmental models, the general procedures common to all PET applications are summarized briefly here. Examples given in this section are specific to the application of $H_2{}^{15}O$ for the measurement of blood flow. Subsequent sections in the chapter go into more detail about some of these steps and give examples of how other compartmental models are applied for PET radiotracers designed to measure other biologic functions.

Define the Dynamic Process to be Measured

The first step is to be clear what specific biologic process or processes are to be measured. For "blood flow," we are measuring the mass specific rate of tissue perfusion—that is, the amount of blood supplied to a given volume of tissue per unit time, typically in units of milliliters (blood) and $min^{-1}mL^{-1}$ (tissue).

Select an Appropriate Radiotracer

This is obviously a crucial step in the overall process. The entire field of PET radiochemistry research is devoted to developing radiotracers for measuring a vast array of bio-logic processes. Many PET tracers have been developed for measuring blood flow, including $H_2^{15}O$, $C^{15}O_2$, $CH_3^{18}F$, ^{11}C-butanol, ^{15}O-butanol, $^{13}NH_3$, and ^{62}Cu-PTSM. Of these, $H_2^{15}O$ has been used most often.

Understand the Physiology and Biochemistry of the Radiotracer

Application of a compartmental model requires adequate knowledge of the *in vivo* behavior of the radiotracer and should include understanding of the following:

1. The mechanism of transport between blood and tissue (diffusion, carrier-mediated transport)
2. Possible trapping, metabolism, synthesis, or breakdown of the tracer
3. Possible reversal of any trapping or metabolic processes
4. Distribution in blood (e.g., binding to plasma proteins, red blood cells)
5. Possible creation and presence of radiolabeled metabolites in the blood
6. Possible creation and presence of radiolabeled metabolites in the tissue

The following is the pertinent information for $H_2^{15}O$. Oxygen-15 has a half-life of 122 seconds. This requires short scans and thus high counting rates but allows multiple scans to be performed easily. Water is transported across the plasma membrane into the body tissues by passive diffusion. Water is not trapped or metabolized. This means that a single tissue compartment representing free $H_2^{15}O$ should suffice for describing the *in vivo* distribution of water in the body. Blood vessels are highly permeable to water, so water can diffuse rapidly into and out of tissue and therefore is said to be "freely" diffusible. Plasma proteins do not bind water. Water does diffuse into red cells, but red cells equilibrate very rapidly with plasma; thus, radioactivity in the red cells can be considered to be available for transport in tissue. The body produces no labeled metabolites of water. Similar information needs to be obtained for any other tracer proposed for use with PET.

Develop a Workable Compartmental Model

With knowledge concerning the *in vivo* behavior of $H_2^{15}O$, we propose a single tissue compartment model, sometimes called a two-compartment model when arterial plasma is considered as a separate compartment. Figure 4.6 depicts this simple model containing the blood pool, a single tissue compartment, and two rate constants describing the exchange of $H_2^{15}O$ between the plasma and tissue. C_T represents the concentration of $H_2^{15}O$ in tissue ($\mu Ci\ mL^{-1}$ of tissue), C_P represents the concentration of $H_2^{15}O$ in arterial plasma ($\mu Ci\ mL^{-1}$ of blood), K_1 is the rate constant for transport of $H_2^{15}O$ from plasma across the blood–brain bar-

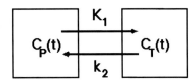

FIG. 4.6. Compartmental model for $H_2^{15}O$. The model consists of a compartment representing arterial plasma and a single tissue compartment representing $H_2^{15}O$ in tissue. Other tissue compartments are not required because water is neither trapped nor metabolized in tissue. C_P and C_T represent the concentration of radiotracer in arterial plasma and tissue, respectively. K_1 and k_2 are the rate parameters describing transport of the radiotracer across the capillary membrane.

rier (BBB) to brain (mL blood $min^{-1}mL^{-1}$ tissue), and k_2 is the rate constant for back-diffusion from tissue back to blood (min^{-1}). The rate constant K_1 is written in uppercase to denote the difference in units from those of k_2 or other rate constants. This is because the units of C_P are $\mu Ci\ mL^{-1}$ of blood and not mL^{-1} of brain like the concentration of the tissue compartment.

Understand Model Assumptions

Most compartmental model applications involve a certain number of assumptions that must be valid if the measures obtained about the biologic system are to be correct. These assumptions separate into two categories: (a) those that relate to the biologic system and to the radiotracer used and (b) those that relate to the specific experimental procedures employed to make the measurements. The first of these two categories is discussed here, while later sections of the chapter that describe particular applications contain examples of those in the second group.

All processes of the biologic system that influence the kinetic behavior of the radiotracer are assumed to be in steady state throughout the duration of the experiment. This does not mean that the radiotracer concentration has to be in the steady state. Before continuing, it is important to distinguish between the terms steady state and equilibrium. For radiotracer applications, the existence of steady state means that the concentration of radiotracer in each compartment remains constant over time. This does not necessitate the existence of an equilibrium condition, where there is zero net transfer of radiotracer between compartments, but only that the net rate at which a substance enters a compartment must equal the net rate at which it leaves.

Steady state refers to a change in concentration of radiotracer *within* a compartment that has one or more inputs and one or more outputs. Equilibrium refers to the exchange of radiotracer *across* the interface *between* compartments and exists only when the exchange is equal in both directions. Thus, a *single* compartment can (or cannot) be at steady state while *two* compartments can (or cannot) be in equilibrium with each another.

In practice, the requirement of steady state means that the concentration or amount of *parent* substance in any compartment must remain constant during the experiment, and consequently that the rates of transport or metabolism of the parent substance also must remain constant during the time frame of the study. It is important to note again that the steady-state requirement applies only to the biologic system and not to the radiotracer. For example, the concentration of systemic glucose in the capillaries and tissue, and the concentration of glucose 6-phosphate in tissue must remain constant throughout the PET study, thus keeping the net rates of the processes we are attempting to measure, glucose transport and phosphorylation, constant. Note that although a steady state is required for the systemic substance glucose, glucose is not in equilibrium because there is always a net flux of glucose from blood to tissue and from free glucose to glucose 6-phosphate. In contrast, the concentration of radiotracer (the glucose analogue ^{18}F-FDG) in the various model compartments varies freely over time.

In most applications, the concentration of radiotracer introduced into the system is assumed to be negligible such that it does not affect or perturb the system by its presence in any way. If this assumption is violated, then the measurement may provide information about effects induced by the presence of the radiotracer instead of the systemic process that we want to measure. Compliance with this assumption ensures that the processes that govern the kinetic behavior of the radiotracer remain first order and that the conservation laws of mass transport are valid.

Each compartment of the system must be *spatially* homogeneous with respect to the concentrations of both tracer and any systemic substances (in addition to the *temporal* homogeneity requirements described above). To accommodate this, one assumes complete and instantaneous mixing of all materials within a compartment. Although mixing obviously is not instantaneous, in practice it must be rapid compared with the exchange rates between compartments.

Write/Solve the Differential Equations Describing Tracer Exchange Between Model Compartments

From Fig. 4.6 while following the format of equation 4.28, the linear first-order differential equation for the single tissue compartment model is

$$dC_T(t)/dt = K_1 C_P(t) - k_2 C_T(t) \qquad [4.29]$$

where $dC_T(t)/dt$ is the first derivative of the $H_2^{15}O$ time course in tissue with respect to time and represents the rate of change in radiotracer concentration.

The solution to a first-order linear differential equation of this form is

$$C_T(t) = K_1 C_P(t) \otimes e^{-k_2 t} \qquad [4.30]$$

where $\otimes$ denotes the mathematical operation of convolution. Because a PET scanner cannot measure radiotracer instanta-

neously, equation 4.30 requires integration of the duration of the scan, yielding

$$PET_i = \int_{t-start_i}^{t-stop_i} C_T(t)\, dt = K_1 \int_{t-start_i}^{t-stop_i} C_P(t) \otimes e^{-k_2 t}\, dt$$

$$[4.31]$$

where PET_i represents the ith frame of the dynamic PET study and $t\text{-}start_i$ and $t\text{-}stop_i$ are the scan start and stop times for frame i. The sequence of i PET measurements for any given region describes the time course of the radioactivity in that tissue and is commonly referred to as a time-activity curve (TAC). Note that the tissue concentration is linearly scaled by the uptake rate constant K_1. This means that if the net uptake of a radiotracer is doubled, the entire PET TAC is doubled. Only the parameter k_2 affects the shape of the TAC. This is true for more complex PET models as well. The parameter K_1 always describes the overall *scale* of the measured PET data, whereas the remaining rate constants (k_2, k_3, k_4, etc) describe the *shape* of the measured data.

Define the Measured Quantities and Unknown Parameters

Equation 4.31 has two measured quantities, the tissue radioactivity concentration estimated from the dynamic data PET_i and the arterial plasma radioactivity concentration, usually estimated from discrete arterial blood samples, and two unknowns to be estimated, K_1 and the clearance exponential coefficient, k_2. More detailed discussion of the measurement of arterial plasma curves and the methods for estimating the model parameters from the measured data are described in later sections of this chapter.

Understand Biologic Significance of Model Parameters

Compartmental modeling applications become useful only when a relationship can be made between the mathematical parameters (model rate constants) and the physiologic or biochemical parameters associated with the particular function under investigation. For example, the essential information to be obtained from a $H_2^{15}O$ PET study is not actually the value of K_1 or k_2 but is the rate of tissue perfusion.

The physiologic definition and hence significance of K_1 can be derived as shown by Gjedde (44) and is the same for most compartmental model applications with PET.

$$K_1 = f(1 - e^{-PS/f}) = f\, E_0 \ \text{(mL blood min}^{-1}\text{mL}^{-1}\text{ brain)}$$

$$[4.32]$$

where f is blood flow (called mass- or volume-specific flow because it is given per unit mass or volume) with the same units as K_1, mL blood min^{-1}mL^{-1} tissue, PS is the capillary permeability surface area product with permeability in units of cm min^{-1} and surface area in cm^2 mL^{-1}. Because cubed centimeter is equivalent to milliliter, the *PS* product has the appropriate units of mL blood $min^{-1}mL^{-1}$ tissue. The term $(1 - e^{-PS/f})$ ranges from near zero if *PS* is much smaller than *f* to near unity if *PS* is much larger than *f*. This term is often referred to as the single-pass extraction fraction and is designated by E_0. E_0 gives the fraction of radiotracer in the arterial plasma that crosses the plasma membrane and enters the tissue during a single capillary transit.

The radiotracer does not have to remain in the tissue but may cross back into the blood during the same capillary transit or may even cross the plasma membrane several times during a single transit. K_1 therefore is equal to the mass specific blood flow multiplied by the fraction of radiotracer that is extracted during a capillary transit. Because the total rate of passage of radiotracer through a capillary is given by $f C_P$, and the rate of uptake by tissue is given by $K_1 C_P$, we see that the fraction of radiotracer that is carried into the tissue from the blood, E_0, is given by $K_1 C_P / f C_P$ (i.e., the uptake rate divided by the total rate of radiotracer passage through the capillary). This equals K_1/f and is consistent with the definition of E_0 given in equation 4.32.

Typically, the rate constant K_1 is referred to as the uptake rate constant and describes the unidirectional rate of transfer of the radiotracer from blood to tissue. The value of K_1 is dependent on both blood flow and capillary membrane permeability. For $H_2^{15}O$, which is considered to be freely diffusible, K_1 can be interpreted further by making the assumption that the permeability surface area product is large enough relative to blood flow that the extraction fraction term of K_1 is equal to one ($E_0 = 1$) Therefore, for $H_2^{15}O$, K_1 is equal to blood flow. Although mass-specific flow is commonly given in units of milliliters of blood per minute per 100 g of tissue (mL min^{-1} 100 g^{-1}), PET measurements yield tissue concentrations in microcuries per unit volume, not per unit mass, as the definitions given above reflect this fact. However, multiplying flow values given in milliliter blood $min^{-1}mL^{-1}$ tissue by the density of tissue (mL g^{-1}), which is only slightly greater than unity, then multiplying by 100 converts flow estimates into the familiar units of milliliter min^{-1} 100 g^{-1}.

The coefficient k_2 is a pure rate constant in that it has units of min^{-1} and describes the rate of clearance of radiotracer or parent substance from tissue back to blood. As discussed previously, a pure rate constant gives the fraction of radioactivity that is removed from tissue per unit time. Typically, the rate constant k_2 is referred to as the clearance rate constant and, like K_1, is also related to both blood flow and capillary membrane permeability. The mean transit time in tissue, τ_m, of water or other nontrapped or metabolized radiotracers is given by the inverse of the clearance rate constant k_2. Similarly, the *biologic* half-clearance time $\tau_{1/2}$ of a tracer in a compartment (not to be confused with the *physical* half-life of the radioisotope $t_{1/2} = \ln 2/\lambda$) is defined as the time it takes to clear out one half of the tracer from the compartment and is given by τ_m multiplied by the natural log of 2.

Not only do individual rate constants have physiologic

meaning, but often ratios of certain rate constants have significance. Consider equation 4.29 under steady-state conditions for water. By definition (no net change in concentration over time), the term $dC_P(t)/dt$ equals zero and thus

$$K_1[C_P(t)]_{ss} = k_2[C_T(t)]_{ss} \qquad [4.33]$$

or rearranging

$$K_1/k_2 = [C_T(t)/C_P(t)]_{ss} \qquad [4.34]$$

This steady-state ratio of the concentration in tissue to blood is defined as the volume of distribution, V_d, or the tracer's tissue-to-blood partition coefficient, *p*. Formally, the volume of distribution is given in units of milliliter blood mL^{-1} tissue, and the partition coefficient is given in mL blood g^{-1} tissue (45), the difference being only that of the density of tissue. We see from equation 4.34 that the ratio K_1/k_2 is equal to the steady-state distribution volume of water. Therefore, by using dynamic PET measurements and compartmental modeling, one can estimate the volume of distribution of a radiotracer by estimating the rate constants K_1 and k_2, while *never* achieving steady-state conditions for the radiotracer at any time during the PET study.

For the single tissue compartment model for $H_2^{15}O$, we can now rewrite equations 4.29 through 4.31 using the physiologic meanings for the rate constants. Because K_1 equals flow and K_1/k_2 equals the distribution volume of water, the clearance rate constant k_2 can be expressed as f/V_d, yielding

$$dC_T(t)/dt = fC_P(t) - (f/V_d) C_T(t) \qquad [4.35]$$

$$C_T(t) = fC_P(t) \otimes e^{-(f/V_d)t} \qquad [4.36]$$

and finally

$$PET_i = \int_{t-start_i}^{t-stop_i} C_T(t) \, dt = f \int_{t-start_i}^{t-stop_i} C_P(t) \otimes e^{-(f/V_d)t} \, dt$$

$$[4.37]$$

noting that the influx or uptake is determined entirely by blood flow while the efflux or clearance rate is determined both by blood flow and by the tissue distribution volume of the radiotracer. Translating equation 4.37 back into words, we see that the measured PET data are equal to the blood flow multiplied by the integral of the arterial plasma radioactivity input time course (commonly called an input function) convolved with the exponential clearance or "washout" of activity from tissue.

$$PET_i = CBF \int_i input \, function \otimes clearance \qquad [4.38]$$

Develop Mathematical Schemes for Estimating Model Parameters

Once all the data have been acquired, images reconstructed, and a compartmental model selected, a method to obtain estimates of the model parameters from the dynamic data must be employed to translate *kinetic* information into *physiologically* and/or *biochemically meaningful* information. This step and the following two (sensitivity analysis/model optimization and model validation) are linked. Together, they are used to ensure that estimates of a parameter assumed to reflect a particular biologic process is indeed a good measure or index of that process. As stated before, a compartmental model is a mathematical description of a biologic system. The job of the parameter estimation algorithm is to determine what *values* of the parameters of this mathematical description, when entered into the compartmental model, optimally describe the measured tissue TACs.

One aspect of parameter estimation is the assessment of the goodness of fit, which quantifies how well the model describes the measured data. Such measures help determine the appropriateness of a particular model configuration and to compare the performance of different configurations, thus aiding in the determination of the optimal implementation of a tracer kinetic model. The entire process of estimating model parameters to describe a measured data set is often referred to as curve fitting. A thorough discussion of parameter estimation techniques and curve fitting for PET applications by Carson (46) provides further information on this subject.

The criteria used for optimization and the methods employed for determining the parameter values are discussed in more detail in the "Parameter Estimation" section.

Sensitivity Analysis/Model Optimization

Analysis of model sensitivity is a crucial step in compartmental modeling applications for PET. The goal of this analysis is to quantify the effects that statistical noise and compartmental model assumptions have on the estimated parameters. Sensitivity analysis uses a combination of simulated data and when possible measured PET data. Typically, a comprehensive model more complex than the actual model that will be implemented is used to derive the mathematical relationships and equations that are best thought to describe the *in vivo* kinetic behavior of the radiotracer.

By using a range of values covering those typically expected for the model parameters, the equations of the *comprehensive* model are used to calculate "noise-free" radiotracer concentrations across the duration of the study. Statistical noise and/or biases from potential violations in model assumptions are then added to the noise-free data. Finally, the *practical* model that will be used with the measured PET data is applied to the simulated "noisy" and/or "biased" data and estimates of the model parameters are obtained.

When many sets of simulated data are generated for the same "true" conditions, the mean, standard deviation, bias, uncertainty, and overall accuracy for the estimates of each model parameter can be calculated. Sensitivity analysis not only can predict how well a particular PET radiotracer and proposed compartmental model will perform but also is helpful in optimizing the specific model implementation, the parameter estimation technique used, and the experimental design and acquisition protocols.

Model Validation

When a compartmental model is finally applied to human PET studies, one must validate that the model can accurately predict the measured concentration time course of the radiotracer. In addition, one also must validate that the parameter estimation technique can provide accurate quantitative values for the physiologic parameters that are of interest in the study. It may be the case that more than one model configuration can describe the measured data sufficiently well, yet different configurations will yield different estimates of the same parameter.

Care must be taken to ensure that the model is not only mathematically appropriate but also physiologically appropriate. One must ask whether the model is capable of providing *meaningful* estimates of the biologic process or processes being measured. More specifically, one needs to address the following two questions. When the biologic process of primary interest in the study changes, does the compartmental model yield changes in the parameter or combination of parameters that are interpreted as reflecting that process (i.e., is the model sensitive)? Conversely, when another biologic process changes, one that is not of interest, does the compartmental model yield unchanged estimates of the parameter of interest (i.e., is the model specific)?

Modeling results should be compared with more direct measures of the parameter under investigation whenever possible. Many of these more direct measures may come from studies in animals or an isolated human study in which more invasive procedures are performed. Measures that are widely accepted can serve as "gold standards" for comparison with newly proposed techniques. Examples of such validation studies include (a) measuring cerebral blood flow using a diffusible radiotracer simultaneously with a well accepted microsphere method and (b) comparing neurotransmitter or enzyme activity levels measured with PET with levels determined by direct chemical assay.

More detailed examples of validation studies for two particular radiotracers are given in the "Model Validation" section.

Practical Considerations

The best designed experiments with a perfect radiotracer, a state-of-the-art PET scanner and image reconstruction, a validated compartmental model, and a thorough sensitivity analysis still can yield meaningless data if certain practical issues are overlooked. The length of study that can be tolerated by some patients is one very important consideration. If 2 or more hours of data are required to obtain results with an acceptable degree of accuracy, patients who are very ill may not be able to complete the procedure. Only a certain degree of motion within a study can be accounted for before results are rendered useless. The probability of being able to obtain a useful data set should be considered.

Another consideration relates to the amount of data that

may need to be acquired, worked up, and stored. Consider a case in which a sensitivity analysis indicates that scans should be acquired every 10 seconds for the first few minutes of the study, and 40 frames are needed to provide optimal results. However, a model simplification is possible that requires only ten frames but decreases the accuracy of the estimated parameters by a few percentage points. This most likely is a good practical trade-off. Sometimes by simplifying a procedure and reducing the work and cost associated with acquiring and processing the data, additional subjects can be studied and with a greater probability of success per subject, thereby improving the power of the experiment by an increase in sample size.

Tracer Models with Multiple Tissue Compartments

The information derivable from radiotracers that can be modeled by a single tissue compartment is limited to the transport rate constants and to simple volumes of distribution. Although these may be sufficient for some applications, they may limit the study of more complex biologic systems. When models with multiple tissue compartments are employed, then the solution to the differential equations describing the model, the parameter estimation routine, and the interpretation of the physiologic significance of the rate parameters naturally become more complex. Here, we discuss the implementation and interpretation of data from multitissue compartment models, using ^{18}F-FDG as the primary example of a two-tissue compartment model.

The solution to the set of differential equations derived from more complex models such as that for FDG becomes increasing complicated as the number of compartments increases. This solution takes the general form

$$PET_i = \int_i input\ function \otimes tissue\ impulse\ response \quad [4.39]$$

where the measured tissue data (PET_i) equals the integral of the arterial plasma input curve convolved with a term called the tissue impulse response function. The tissue impulse response is what the measured PET concentration curve or *tissue response would be* if the arterial plasma input function were a perfect bolus or delta function *impulse*. This can be seen from equation 4.39 and the fact that a delta function is the identity function for mathematical convolution—that is, for any arbitrary function $g(t) \otimes \delta(t) = g(t)$. The physiologic parameters to be estimated are contained in the tissue impulse response. The actual arterial plasma input function is never a perfect bolus, so the measured PET data are never equivalent to the impulse response function. Because the radiotracer input to the tissue is spread over time, the measured PET data are a "spread-out" or "smeared" transformation of the impulse response. The more blunted the arterial input, the more smeared the measured PET data. The form of the impulse response is defined by the specific configuration of the compartmental model. For example from equation 4.30, we see that the general form of the impulse

response for a single-tissue model is $K_1 e^{-k_2 t}$. The parameters of the impulse response function are linked to the model rate constants and can be estimated from the input function and PET data by a general technique referred to as deconvolution. By deconvolution, we mean that if $A(t) = B(t) \otimes C(t)$, then $B(t)$ deconvolved from $A(t) = C(t)$. In other words, if we take the PET data and deconvolve the measured input function from it, we get an estimate of the tissue impulse response. Deconvolution methods are described in more detail in the "Parameter Estimation" section.

The complexity of the impulse response function is governed by the complexity of the compartmental model. For a two-tissue compartment model, such as that used for ^{18}F-FDG (Fig. 4.7), the general form of the impulse response I_r becomes

$$I_r(t) = A_1 e^{-\alpha_1 t} + A_2 e^{-\alpha_2 t} \quad [4.40]$$

Note that unlike the single-tissue model in which the I_r parameters corresponded directly to the compartmental model parameters, the four parameters of the two-tissue I_r (A_1, A_2, α_1, α_2) do not correspond exactly to the compartmental model parameters, but they can be converted easily.

$$\alpha_1 = \frac{\sqrt{(k_2 + k_3 + k_4) - [(k_2 + k_3 + k_4)^2 - 4k_2 k_4]}}{2}$$

$$\alpha_2 = \frac{\sqrt{(k_2 + k_3 + k_4) + [(k_2 + k_3 + k_4)^2 - 4k_2 k_4]}}{2} \quad [4.41]$$

$$A_1 = \frac{K_1(k_3 + k_4 - \alpha_1)}{(\alpha_2 - \alpha_1)}; \quad A_2 = \frac{K_1(\alpha_2 - k_3 - k_4)}{(\alpha_2 - \alpha_1)}$$

Volumes of Distribution for Multicompartment Models

Before examining the compartmental model for FDG, the physiologic meaning of various combinations of rate constants must be revisited. At this time, it is necessary to introduce the concepts of reversible and irreversible models. Consider a model with two tissue compartments and rate constants K_1 through k_4 (Fig. 4.7). Note that the exchange across all compartment boundaries is bidirectional. We refer to this model configuration as reversible. In this case, it is possible for radiotracer that exists in any compartment to reverse its steps and clear from the tissue. On the other hand, consider a radiotracer that undergoes a metabolic process represented by k_3 that is *ir*reversible. In this case, there would be no process represented by k_4 (i.e., $k_4 = 0$) and a radiotracer that enters the second tissue compartment becomes irreversibly trapped in the tissue. Thus, a model configuration in which exchange across at least one compartment boundary is unidirectional is said to be an irreversible model. The differential equations for the two tissue compartments of a reversible model become

$$dC_f(t)/dt = K_1 C_p(t) - k_2 C_f(t) - k_3 C_f(t) + k_4 C_m(t)$$

$$dC_m(t)/dt = k_3 C_f(t) - k_4 C_m(t) \quad [4.42]$$

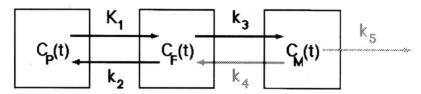

FIG. 4.7. A two-tissue compartmental model for fluorine-18-fluorodeoxyglucose (^{18}F-FDG). The model consists of a compartment representing arterial plasma and two tissue compartments, representing free (unmetabolized FDG) and trapped (FDG-6-PO$_4$; the chemical form of FDG after the first step of metabolism). C_P, C_F, and C_M represent the concentrations of radiotracer in the arterial plasma, the free pool, and the trapped pool, respectively; k_1 and k_2 are the rate parameters describing transport of the radiotracer across the blood–brain barrier, and k_3 and k_4 are the parameters describing rates of the processes of trapping and possible release (phosphorylation and dephosphorylation for FDG). For ^{18}F-FDG, the rate of dephosphorylation is very slow and is sometimes ignored (*the lighter gray arrow and rate constant* k$_4$). Also for ^{18}F-FDG, no further metabolism occurs past phosphorylation, so k_5 is zero. However, for the parent substance that FDG traces, namely glucose, further metabolism does occur and is irreversible (*striped light gray arrow and rate constant* k$_5$).

which simplify to the following equations for an irreversible two-tissue compartment model.

$$dC_f(t)/dt = K_1 C_p(t) - k_2 C_f(t) - k_3 C_f(t)$$

$$dC_m(t)/dt = k_3 C_f(t) \qquad [4.43]$$

For a single tissue compartment model, there is only one route of clearance from tissue, and thus when steady state occurs (i.e., when $dC_T(t)/dt = 0$), the net exchange between tissue and blood is also zero and thus conditions for equilibrium are satisfied. Therefore, for a single tissue compartment model, steady-state and equilibrium conditions are satisfied simultaneously, and thus, the equilibrium and steady-state distribution volumes are identical. Similarly for two-tissue compartment models that are reversible, steady-state and equilibrium conditions are satisfied simultaneously. However, for irreversible two-tissue compartment models, steady-state and equilibrium conditions may not occur simultaneously. The compartments representing free and metabolized radiotracer, C_f and C_m, can never reach equilibrium unless k_3 is zero. Although the metabolized compartment also cannot be in steady state unless k_3 is zero, the free compartment can reach *steady state* if $K_1 C_P$ equals $(k_2 + k_3)C_f$. Rearranging, we can see that this occurs when the ratio of radiotracer concentration in the free compartment relative to that in plasma equals $K_1/(k_2 + k_3)$. Note, however, that the free compartment is in *equilibrium* with the blood, when $K_1 C_P$ equals $k_2 C_f$. This occurs when free radiotracer concentration relative to that in plasma equals K_1/k_2. The steady-state and equilibrium distribution volumes of the free compartment are given by

$$[V_{d(f)}]_{ss} = K_1/(k_2 + k_3)$$

$$[V_{d(f)}]_{eq} = K_1/k_2 \qquad [4.44]$$

In practice, equilibrium is never achieved unless k_3 is zero and then $[V_d]_{ss}$ would equal $[V_d]_{eq}$. When k_3 is nonzero; however, the steady-state volume is always lower than the

equilibrium volume due to the continual removal of the radiotracer by the irreversible pathway.

Returning to the reversible model, by similar logic we see that the distribution volume for the free compartment (either equilibrium or steady state) is equal to K_1/k_2. If, in addition, the free and metabolic compartments are in equilibrium, then $dC_m(t)/dt = 0$, and $k_3 C_f(t)$ must equal $k_4 C_m(t)$, and therefore, the equilibrium ratio of the metabolized to free concentration equals k_3/k_4. Since the equilibrium ratio of the free to plasma concentration is K_1/k_2, then the distribution volume of the metabolized compartment relative to plasma is $(K_1/k_2) \times (k_3/k_4)$.

The total distribution volume would be the sum of the volumes of distribution; therefore, the distribution volumes for the individual compartments, as well as the total, are given by

$$V_{d(f)} = K_1/k_2$$

$$V_{d(m)} = (K_1/k_2) \times (k_3/k_4) \qquad [4.45]$$

$$V_{d(tot)} = V_{d(f)} + V_{d(m)} = (K_1/k_2) \times (1 + k_3/k_4)$$

As we will see later, distribution volume estimates can be used as an index for many biochemical and pharmacologic processes.

Compartmental Model For ^{18}F-FDG

The most commonly used and successful PET radiotracer to date has been the glucose analog ^{18}F-fluorodeoxyglucose. This tracer is used routinely to provide local measures of glucose utilization for metabolic studies of the brain and heart, and for localization of tumors that readily incorporate ^{18}F-FDG. The general model for ^{18}F-FDG is the two-tissue compartment model presented in Fig. 4.7. As defined in the original work using ^{14}C-deoxyglucose by Sokoloff et al. (47), and later using ^{18}F-FDG (48–50), the metabolic rate of glucose (MR_{glc}) is the net rate at which glucose is converted to glucose 6-phospate.

$$MR_{glc} = C_P[K_1k_3/(k_2 + k_3)] \text{ (mg min}^{-1} \text{ 100 g}^{-1}) \quad [4.46]$$

where C_P is the arterial plasma concentration of stable glucose (mg mL^{-1}) and K_1, k_2, and k_3 are the rate constants for *glucose*. Note that the net rate of utilization is dependent both on the transport rates (K_1 and k_2) and on the rate of phosphorylation (k_3).

In practice, we do not measure the rate constants for glucose, but instead, we can measure the steady-state arterial plasma glucose concentration and the rate constants for FDG; thus, equation 4.46 can be rewritten as:

$$MR_{glc} = (C_P/LC)[K_1^*k_3^*/(k_2^* + k_3^*)] \text{ (mg min}^{-1} \text{ 100 g}^{-1})$$
$$[4.47]$$

where K_1^* through k_3^* are the rate constants for ^{18}F-FDG and LC, referred to as the lumped constant, is a combination of terms representing the ratio of the metabolic rates of FDG and glucose. The lumped constant takes into account the relative rates of transport and phosphorylation for FDG and glucose, which in turn are dependent on the steady-state distribution volumes and on the Michaelis–Menton constants (V_{max}, K_m) of FDG and glucose.

From Equation 4.47, we see that a measurement of the cold glucose level in plasma, an assumed value for the lumped constant, and estimates of K_1^*, k_2^*, and k_3^* from a dynamic sequence of PET scans, provides a measure of the metabolic rate of glucose. However, one of the reasons that ^{18}F-FDG has been so widely used in PET is that a simplified approach can be used that provides reliable estimates of the rate of metabolism. As first described for animal autoradiography using ^{14}C-deoxyglucose by Sokoloff et al. (47) and as later adapted to PET, an approximation of MR_{glc} can be derived from a set of data acquired at a relatively late time postinjection. This was extremely important for autoradiographic studies, in which only one data point can be obtained (because the animal is sacrificed), but also allows for human PET studies to be accomplished more conveniently.

This approach works because of the kinetics of deoxyglucose and FDG. The rate of phosphorylation is reasonably high while the rate of dephosphorylation is very low; thus, the radiotracer essentially is trapped once phosphorylated. The fraction of radiotracer residing in the trapped pool increases throughout the study. Because the clearance from tissue is relatively rapid, by 40 to 50 minutes the majority of radiotracer in tissue has been phosphorylated and a single "late" static image closely reflects the relative metabolic rate of glucose (Fig. 4.8). By assuming "population" average values for the individual rate constants for ^{18}F-FDG

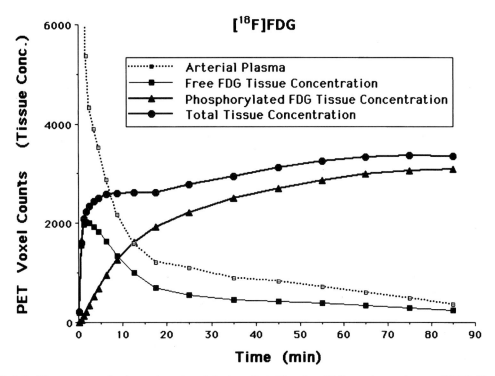

FIG. 4.8. Time courses for free, phosphorylated, and total fluorine-18-fluorodeoxyglucose (FDG). Shown is the arterial plasma input function measured from discrete samples (*dashed line*), the calculated time courses for the radioactivity concentration in the free (*squares*) and phosphorylated (*triangles*) compartments, and the total tissue concentration measured by PET (*circles*). Note that the fraction of total measured radioactivity that is in the phosphorylated tissue compartment increases as time progresses. Because the activity in this compartment is metabolized FDG, a "late" PET scan 40 to 60 minutes or more after the injection serves as a reliable index of glucose metabolism.

(dropping the asterisks) and given a value for the cold glucose concentration in plasma, we calculate a "*population*" average MR_{glc}.

$$[MR_{glc}]_{pop} = (C_P/LC)[(K_{1pop}k_{3pop})/(k_{2pop} + k_{3pop})] \quad [4.48]$$

MR_{glc} for an *individual* is then calculated by "correcting" the population average metabolic rate based on the static PET and arterial plasma input function measurements. The method assumes that the best correction factor for estimating an individual's regional metabolic rate is given by the ratio of the regional ^{18}F-FDG concentration in the phosphorylated compartment for the individual, $[C_m]_{ind}$, to the population average, $[C_m]_{pop}$. Because $[C_m]_{ind}$ cannot be determined directly, it is best estimated by subtracting a calculation of the expected free concentration, $[C_f]_{pop}$, from the measured PET value, $[C_{tot}]_{ind}$.

$$[MR_{glc}]_{ind} = [MR_{glc}]_{pop} \times [\{C_{tot}]_{ind} - [C_f]_{pop}\}/[C_m]_{pop}]$$
$$[4.49]$$

Note that $[C_{tot}]_{ind}$ is the measured PET data for the individual while $[C_f]_{pop}$ and $[C_m]_{pop}$ are the calculated values of the free and phosphorylated compartments based on *population* average rate constants, but the *individual's* arterial input function. $[C_f]_{pop}$ and $[C_m]_{pop}$ can be estimated from the solutions to their differential equations given in equation 4.42 and the relationships described in equation 4.41.

$$C_f(t) = [K_1/(\alpha_2 - \alpha_1)][k_4 - \alpha_1)e^{-\alpha_1 t}$$
$$+ (\alpha_2 - k_4)^{-\alpha_2 t}] \otimes C_P(t) \quad [4.50]$$
$$C_m(t) = [K_1 k_3/(\alpha_2 - \alpha_1)][e^{-\alpha_1 t} - e^{-\alpha_2 t}] \otimes C_P(t)$$

where $\alpha_{1,2}$ are defined in equation 4.41 and all ks are *population* average rate constants for ^{18}F-FDG.

Two alternative formulations (51,52) have been proposed for the correction factor in equation 4.49. Both the original and these alternative calculations are approximations of the true metabolic rate. Which approximation works best is dependent on how the individual's rate constants differ from the population average values. Propagation of errors for each of the methods differs and depends on several factors, as discussed these two articles. It should also be emphasized that although there are some errors in each of these approximations, each has been shown to be relatively small in magnitude under most conditions and the general FDG method has proved to be an excellent technique for the measurement glucose metabolism.

An example of how the concept of the steady-state volume of distribution is applied to PET is seen in the use of ^{18}F-FDG for measuring glucose metabolism. The rate at which glucose is transferred from the free to the 6-PO_4 tissue compartment is equal to the rate of phosphorylation of glucose and is given by $k_3 C_f$, as seen in equation 4.43. Thus, if we are interested in measuring the metabolic rate of glucose

using kinetic modeling, we need to estimate not only the rate constant for phosphorylation, k_3, but also the concentration of parent glucose in the free tissue compartment. However, C_f is not known or easily measured. Because glucose is assumed to be in the steady state during the study, the steady-state volume of distribution of glucose in the free tissue compartment is given by equation 4.44 and is equal to $K_1/(k_2 + k_3)$. Multiplying the arterial plasma concentration of glucose, C_P, by the steady-state volume of distribution yields an estimate of C_f for glucose. Therefore, $k_3 C_f$, the rate at which glucose is metabolized, is given by k_3 times the plasma glucose concentration multiplied by the volume of distribution volume for free glucose, or $k_3 C_P[K_1/(k_2 + k_3)]$ just as given in equation 4.46.

Model Complexity: Trade-off in Bias vs. Precision

The *in vivo* behavior of many PET radiotracers is complex. A comprehensive model describing the kinetics of a tracer may require a compartmental configuration with many compartments and many rate parameters. Because of the statistical limits of the data, and because PET measures only the *sum* of the radioactivity across all compartments, the actual models used for analysis must be simplified. Most PET radiotracers can support models with two to at most six parameters under the best of circumstances. When one attempts to estimate a large number of model parameters from a single dynamic PET study, parameter variance tends to be high. Variability in parameter estimates may be too high to permit reliable interpretation of the data, so the most accurate model descriptions become impractical to implement with PET. However, as less complex models are employed, parameter estimates may become biased and thus may yield useless information. A trade-off exists between bias and uncertainty in the model estimates that is controlled largely by the complexity of the model configuration. Methods of reducing model complexity include combining or lumping compartments (assuming that the compartments equilibrate rapidly) and assuming that values for certain model parameters are known. The optimal degree of model complexity must be considered carefully for each application.

The appropriate level of model complexity is dependent on which parameter is of greatest interest. The uncertainty in a model parameter that is of little physiologic interest can be high as long as the error in its estimate does not propagate into the parameter of interest. Validity of the simplifying assumptions is also important. If, for example, a parameter is held at a fixed value in the model and the value may be in error by $\pm 50\%$ but causes only a $\pm 5\%$ bias in the parameter of interest, then this reduction in complexity is acceptable. However, if failure of a simplifying assumption is found to cause a 50% bias in the parameter of interest, then the model simplification is inappropriate. One should also consider whether the biases introduced by a given assumption are of approximately the same magnitude (and direction) across both regions and subjects. If so, then this model reduction may well be acceptable; if not, the simplification should not be made. The ability to find the optimal level of model complexity is extremely important for successful interpretation of PET data. An analysis of model sensitivity can be used in conjunction with *a priori* knowledge of the expected parameter values and the particular hypotheses being investigated to determine the compartmental configuration with the optimal level of complexity. Other discussions on this topic are available for further reference (53–55).

Compartmental Models for Pharmacologic Studies

Figure 4.9A depicts the general compartmental model for pharmacologic studies consisting of the arterial plasma compartment C_P and three tissue compartments representing free ligand in tissue (C_F), nonspecifically bound ligand (C_{NS}), and specifically bound ligand (C_{SP}). Six rate parameters describe exchange between the model compartments. As discussed in the preceding section, the statistical quality of PET data usually is not sufficient for estimating this number of parameters, so the complexity of the model must be reduced. The first simplifying assumption made in most pharmacologic applications is that the free and nonspecific binding compartments equilibrate rapidly. This allows combining them into a single compartment (C_{F+NS}). This two-tissue compartment configuration (Fig. 4.9B) has rate parameters defined as

$$K_1 = f(1 - e^{-PS/f}) = f E_0$$

$$k_2' = K_1/V_{d(F+NS)} = (K_1/V_{d(F)})/(1 + V_{d(NS)}/V_{d(F)})$$

$$k_3' = (k_{on}B_{max})/(1 + V_{d(NS)}/V_{d(F)}) \quad [4.51]$$

$$k_4 = k_{off}$$

and thus,

$$k_3'/k_4 = (k_{on}B_{max}/k_{off})/(1 + V_{d(NS)}/V_{d(F)})$$

$$= (B_{max}/K_D)/(1 + V_{d(NS)}/V_{d(F)}) \quad [4.52]$$

where $V_{d(F)}$, $V_{d(NS)}$, and $V_{d(F+NS)}$ are the steady-state tissue distribution volumes of free ligand, nonspecifically bound ligand, and their sum respectively, k_{on} is the bimolecular association rate between ligand and receptor (g pmol^{-1}min^{-1}), B_{max} is the binding site density or concentration of unoccupied binding sites (pmol g^{-1}), k_{off} is the dissociation rate of ligand from the binding site complex (min^{-1}), and KD is the equilibrium dissociation constant for the specific binding site (pmol g^{-1} or nanomolar). The prime symbols on k_2' and k_3' are used to differentiate these rate constants from the true k_2 and k_3 that describe rates of exchange from the compartment containing only free ligand. The ratio B_{max}/K_D is commonly called the ''binding potential'' while the term $(1 + V_{d(NS)}/V_{d(F)})$ reflects the apparent increase in the volume of the binding precursor pool when combining free and nonspecific compartments. Thus, $1/(1 + V_{d(NS)}/V_{d(F)})$

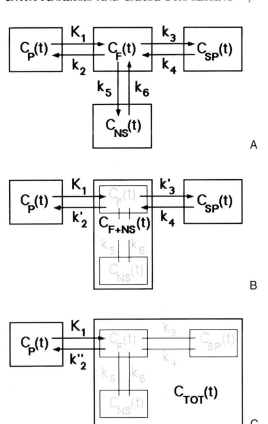

FIG. 4.9. Compartmental model configurations for pharmacologic PET studies. **A:** A generalized model configuration describing many of the radioligands designed as pharmacologic markers. The model consists of the arterial plasma compartment C_P and three tissue compartments representing free ligand in tissue (C_F), nonspecifically bound ligand (C_{NS}), and specifically bound ligand (C_{SP}). In most applications, the statistical quality of the data cannot support estimation of the six rate constants; thus, simpler configurations are required for practical implementation. **B:** The most common simplification of combining free and nonspecific compartments is by assuming they equilibrate rapidly with one another. The kinetics of four rate constants k_2, k_3, k_5, and k_6 are approximated by two new parameters k_2' and k_3', which are equivalent to $k_2/(1 + k_5/k_6)$ and $k_3/(1 + k_5/k_6)$, respectively. The prime notation is used to indicate the lumping of two compartments into one. Note that the ratio k_5/k_6 is equivalent to the ratio of distribution volumes of the nonspecific to the free compartment as described in equation 4.51. **C:** A model configuration that can be used when all tissue compartments equilibrate rapidly. In this scenario, a single tissue "clearance" constant k_2'' approximates five rate constants k_2 through k_6 by the relationship $k_2'' = k_2/(1 + k_3/k_4 + k_5/k_6)$. The ratio k_1/k_2'' yields the total tissue distribution volume $V_{d(TOT)}$. This approach may be useful when the ratio k_3/k_4 is the dominating component of the term $(1 + k_3/k_4 + k_5/k_6)$. This is equivalent to saying that the specific distribution is the dominating component of the total distribution volume ($V_{d(TOT)} = V_{d(F)} + V_{d(NS)} + V_{d(SP)}$).

$[= V_{d(F)}/(V_{d(F)} + V_{d(NS)})]$ describes the fraction of radiolabel available ("free") either for transport back to plasma or binding and is equivalent to the term f_2 often used to designate the free fraction in tissue. The distribution volumes of free plus nonspecific, specific, and total binding sites are defined in the same manner as those in equation 4.45.

$$V_{d(F+NS)} = K_1/k_2'$$

$$V_{d(SP)} = (K_1/k_2') \times (k_3'/k_4)$$

$$= (K_1/k_2) \times (k_3/k_4) = V_{d(F)}(B_{max}/K_D)$$

$$V_{d(tot)} = V_{d(F+NS)} + V_{d(SP)}$$

$$= (K_1/k_2') \times (1 + k_3'/k_4)$$

$$= V_{d(F+NS)} + V_{d(F)}(B_{max}/K_D)$$

[4.53]

An additional model simplification can be made if the rates of association and dissociation from the specific binding site are rapid compared with the transport parameters, K_1 and k_2, reducing the model to a single tissue compartment (Fig. 4.9C), described by K_1 and only an additional rate constant k_2'', giving the *net* clearance from tissue. The total volume of distribution $V_{d(tot)}$ ($= K_1/k_2''$) has the same definition as in the two-tissue compartment configuration given by equation 4.53. How closely the $V_{d(tot)}$ estimates from the two model configurations agree will depend on how rapidly free and bound compartments equilibrate (i.e., the validity of the simplifying assumption).

The primary goal of a pharmacologic study is to provide a reliable index of binding site density or whatever other pharmacologic parameter is being studied. In the ideal, this would be a direct quantitative measure of B_{max}, the density of available binding sites; however, for practical reasons, this may not be possible. As defined in Eqs. 4.51 through 4.53, other parameters or combinations of parameters relate to binding density, which might provide more reliable measures of binding density. These include k_3 ($= k_{on}B_{max}$), k_3/k_4 ($= B_{max}/K_D$), k_3'/k_4 ($= f_2B_{max}/K_D$), $V_{d(SP)}$ ($= V_{d(F)}[B_{max}/K_D]$), and $V_{d(tot)}$ ($= V_{d(F+NS)} + V_{d(F)}[B_{max}/K_D]$). The distribution volume estimates, particularly $V_{d(tot)}$, are functions of more than just binding site density and therefore contain additional intrinsic bias compared to either k_3 or k_3/k_4. However, the precision of distribution volume estimates typically is much better than that of individual rate constants.

For every radiotracer, one needs to determine which measure yields the optimal trade-off between bias and precision and the greatest sensitivity to changes in binding site density.

Data Acquisition Considerations for Compartmental Modeling

In general, compartmental modeling and tracer kinetic analysis require the acquisition of two sets of data, the radioactivity time courses in blood and tissue, to yield estimates of physiologic parameters. This section discusses the methodologic issues related to measuring these two sets of data.

It is very obvious that the quality of the PET data directly affects the reliability of the estimated model parameters. It should be stressed that for compartmental modeling applications that require arterial input functions, equal attention should be paid to obtaining accurate estimates of the arterial plasma concentration curves.

Measurement of the Radiotracer Concentration in Arterial Plasma

Interpretation of the kinetic behavior of a radiotracer, as indicated by equation 4.39, requires knowledge of the amount of radiotracer being supplied to the tissue. In other words, the level of radioactivity in a particular tissue at any given time is dependent both on the amount of radioactivity delivered to the tissue (the input function) and by what happens to the radiotracer once in the tissue (the tissue response function). Measurement of the amount of radioactivity delivered to the tissue typically is accomplished by acquiring discrete arterial plasma samples, usually from a radial artery, and measuring the radioactivity in a well counter. For cardiac applications, it is possible to derive the input function from PET imaging of the heart blood pool. Although this is relatively straightforward, several additional issues must be considered.

Red Blood Cell Radioactivity

For many PET radiopharmaceuticals, the radioactivity in arterial plasma is the portion of the total bloodborne radioactivity that is available for transport into the tissue. This is not the case for all radiotracers. If the radiotracer can diffuse rapidly between plasma and red cells, then radioactivity in red cells is available for transport into the tissue. However, if the equilibration time between red cells and plasma is much longer than a single capillary transit, then only radiotracer in the plasma is available for transport, and thus, the concentration time course in plasma alone should be used as the input function.

Binding to Plasma Proteins

Another consideration is whether the radiotracer binds to plasma proteins. If this is the case, as occurs with many highly lipophilic tracers, there will be a decreased amount of radiotracer available for transport, resulting in a decreased extraction fraction and hence an apparent decrease in BBB permeability. As with red cells, the possibility of tracer bound to plasma proteins being able to dissociate and cross the capillary membrane during a single capillary transit must be considered.

Radiolabeled Metabolites

Another consideration for determining the arterial input function is the possibility of the radiolabel being converted to a chemical form different from that of original radiotracer. This is an issue in many neuroreceptor studies in which radiolabeled metabolites of the authentic ligand are found in blood. Because radiolabeled metabolic byproducts are formed *in vivo,* the fraction of metabolites in the blood generally increases with time, necessitating a time-dependent correction. This correction is often possible by chromatographic analysis of each or selected blood samples to determine the fraction of plasma radioactivity that is in the form of the authentic ligand (56). There is, however, a requirement that the labeled metabolites are not transported from blood into tissue. Any labeled metabolites that can enter tissue would require inclusion in the compartmental model, necessitating a second input function for the radiolabeled metabolite and a second set of rate constants describing the kinetic behavior of the metabolite in tissue. The statistical quality of PET data generally does not support the estimation of these additional parameters, so PET ligands that produce metabolites that cross the capillary membrane are poor candidates for success.

Figure 4.10 shows a typical input function obtained from a radioligand study of the benzodiazepine receptor system using ^{11}C-flumazenil (FMZ). The top panel is a semilog plot showing both total radioactivity in the arterial plasma (*filled circles*) and the level of authentic ^{11}C-FMZ only (*open triangles*). The bottom panel shows the fraction of total activity in the plasma that arises from radiolabeled metabolites. Note that the metabolite fraction monotonically increases, with most rapid production of metabolites early after administration of ^{11}C-FMZ, followed by an apparent equilibration between metabolites and authentic ligand pools at a ratio of about 3 or 4 : 1. The corrected input function shown in the top panel equals the total plasma radioactivity, multiplied by one minus the metabolite fraction.

Measurement of the Tissue Time-activity Curves

The second set of data required for kinetic modeling is the tissue concentration time course measured by the PET scanner. For quantitative modeling studies, we assume that all appropriate corrections were made to the acquired PET data and that the image-reconstruction algorithms have provided the best possible estimate of the radiotracer's concentration in tissue. In addition, the sensitivity analysis can be used to help determine the scanning sequence required for kinetic analysis. Radiotracers having more rapid kinetics require shorter duration scan frames. Figure 4.11 shows typical PET TACs in the brain for four different radiotracers: $H_2^{15}O$ (*upper left*); ^{11}C-FMZ a benzodiazepine antagonist for measuring receptor density (*upper right*); ^{13}N-ammonia for measuring myocardial perfusion (*lower left*); and ^{11}C-acetate for measuring oxidative metabolism (*lower right*). Note that due to the different half-lives of the tracers, the range of scan times can vary dramatically. Some tracers such as $H_2^{15}O$ and ^{11}C-FMZ enter and leave the tissue rapidly, others such as ^{11}C-acetate enter and leave much more slowly, and others

such as ^{13}N-NH$_3$ are trapped in tissue for long periods of time.

Contribution of Bloodborne Radioactivity

An important issue not addressed to this point is that the measured PET data include detected events from any body component that happens to be in the FOV. Although we have stated that a PET scan measures the radiotracer concentration in *tissue,* every region imaged, whether it is heart, brain, tumor, or another organ, is composed of a mixture of *tissue* and *blood* because these cannot be separated completely at PET resolution. Unless the tissue and blood concentrations are identical, the tissue concentration cannot equal exactly the concentration measured by the tomograph. For example, shortly after a bolus administration, the blood concentration is much higher than the tissue concentration. Thus, even though only a small fraction of the space being imaged is blood, the detected events coming from bloodborne radioactivity may comprise a considerable portion of the total signal (57). This is a considerable problem for cardiac studies in which the VOIs are directly adjacent to large blood pools and it is hard to obtain data without vascular contamination, made even more difficult by heart motion due to both the cardiac and respiratory cycles.

The bloodborne component is more important for radiotracers with low extraction fractions since the tissue concentration rises more slowly. PET measurements, rather than being a direct estimate of the radiotracer concentration in tissue $C_T(t)$ are given by

$$PET_i = CBV \int_i C_{blood}(t) + (1 - CBV) \int_i C_T(t) \quad [4.54]$$

where $C_{blood}(t)$ is the mean concentration in the blood pool within the region and *CBV* is the cerebral blood volume given as a fraction of the total imaging volume (mL blood mL^{-1} imaging volume). It should be emphasized that the total blood concentration time course $C_{blood}(t)$ is not the same as the input function $C_P(t)$, because blood consists of red cell, plasma, and plasma protein components; arterial, capillary, and venous components; and may include radiolabeled metabolites. The appropriate model equations for the tissue concentration $C_T(t)$, such as those for single- or two-compartment models, are inserted into equation 4.51. *CBV* can be considered as an additional model parameter that can be either (a) estimated in the fitting procedures, (b) estimated by some additional measurement, or (c) assumed to be known and fixed at a constant value.

Parameter Estimation

Parameter estimation routines should provide optimal estimates of the model parameters. To be ''optimal,'' there must be a particular criterion that is used as a measure of goodness of fit. This criterion is often called the cost function or optimization function. Values for the parameters are ad-

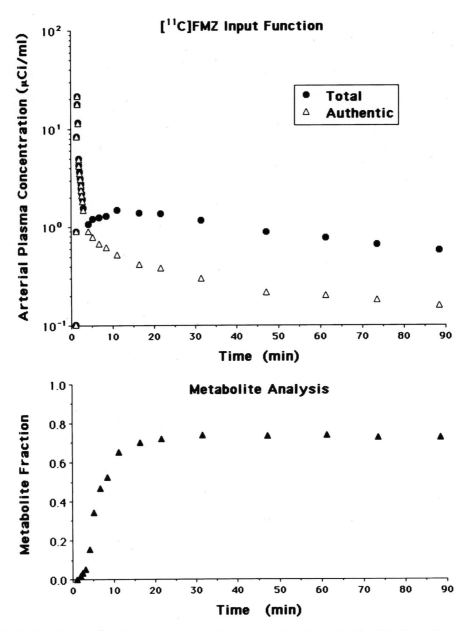

FIG. 4.10. Arterial input function measurement. A measured input function **(top)** for the radiotracer ^{11}C-flumazenil (FMZ), a benzodiazepine antagonist. Shown is the total radioactivity concentration (*filled circles*) measured by a sodium iodide well counter from discrete blood samples acquired from the radial artery and spun in a centrifuge separating plasma from red blood cells. As with many PET ligands, radiolabeled metabolites may form in the blood or peripheral tissues and must be accounted for. The relative amounts of authentic and metabolized radiotracer can be determined by chromatographic techniques. Shown are the results **(bottom)** of such a determination, plotting the fraction of total radioactivity in the plasma that is in the form of labeled metabolites over the duration of the study. ^{11}C-FMZ metabolites are seen to increase rapidly after administration and appear to equilibrate rather quickly at a fraction of about 75%. The metabolite component is then removed from the measure of total radioactivity, to yield just the concentration of authentic ^{11}C-FMZ (*open triangles in the top*). This curve is used as the input function for compartmental analysis.

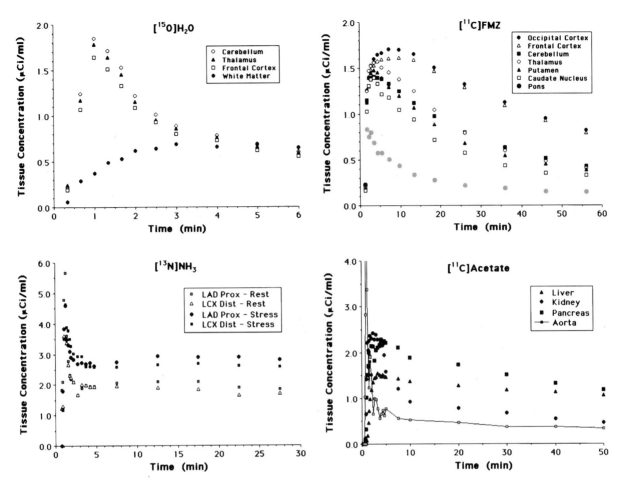

FIG. 4.11. PET time-activity curves (TACs). Shown are typical PET TACs for four different radiotracers: $H_2{}^{15}O$ used for measuring blood flow **(upper left)**; ^{11}C-flumazenil for measuring receptor density **(upper right)**; ^{13}N-NH_3 for measuring myocardial blood flow **(bottom left)**; and ^{11}C-acetate for measuring oxidative metabolism **(bottom right)**. The two sets of curves on the top are from brain studies. Cerebral blood flow is seen to be high in gray-matter structures and low in white matter. Benzodiazepine receptor density is high in cortical structures, moderate in cerebellum, deep gray nuclei, and very low in pons and other brainstem structures. The cardiac ammonia study shows curves for both rest and dipyridamole (a coronary vasodilator) stress studies in the regions of the proximal left anterior descending artery *(LAD prox)* and the distal left circumflex artery *(LCX dist)*. There is increased uptake of ^{13}N-NH_3 during the stress study, indicating increased flow. Very different tissue kinetics are observed between kidney, liver, and pancreas for the oxidative metabolism study using ^{11}C-acetate.

justed so that the cost function is either minimized or maximized depending on the function. The most commonly used optimization criterion in PET studies is least squares, where the cost function is defined as the squared discrepancy between the measured PET data and the values predicted by the compartmental model equations summed over the temporal sequence of scans. The optimal parameter values are defined to be those that yield the minimum sum of squared discrepancies, or as the name implies, the least squares fit to the data. Included in the calculation is appropriate weighting of the data based on the known or measured variances in the reconstructed image values. The weighted sum of squared discrepancies is termed the chi-square value (χ^2).

Another optimization criterion is maximum likelihood, as is commonly used in iterative reconstruction, in which parameter values are selected such that the measured data values are statistically the most probable to have occurred. The cost function for maximum likelihood estimation varies depending on the assumptions about the data. Least squares estimation provides the maximum likelihood estimation under the conditions that the errors in the measured data are independent, uncorrelated, follow a Gaussian distribution, and have uniform error variance across the measurements. In practice, however, some or all of these conditions are not met, and the least squares solution is only an approximation of the maximum likelihood solution.

Nonlinear Regression Techniques

The most common methods for obtaining least squares estimates from kinetic PET studies fall into the category of regression techniques. Both linear and nonlinear regression methods are used. Although most PET studies require nonlinear regression, simpler linear regression methods can be applied in some cases. A model is said to be linear, so linear techniques can be applied if the model equation consists only of terms that are linear with respect to each of the model parameters to be estimated. Linear regression has the advantage of being a very rapid means for estimating parameters because there is an analytic solution that provides the least squares solution to the regression equations.

Most PET radiotracers are not described by linear models and thus require nonlinear regression. In general, nonlinear regression cannot be performed analytically but must be approached in an iterative manner, which as we noted for image reconstruction is far more computationally intensive. The standard procedure is to provide initial estimates of each of the unknown model parameters. From this guess, an initial chi-square value is calculated. Consider an n-dimensional set of chi-squared values comprising all numerical combinations of the n parameters. The goal is now to search this n-dimensional space for the global minimum. This location specifies the optimal or best-fit set of model parameters (K_1, k_2, ... k_n).

There are several possible routines to "search" chi-squared space for the minimum. One common approach, referred to as a gradient search, as described by Marquardt (58) and Bevington (59), updates all parameters simultaneously. The local gradient in chi-square space is calculated at the point specified by the current set of parameter values. The direction in the n-dimensional parameter space along which the value of χ^2 changes most rapidly is determined. The magnitudes of the parameter values are adjusted so that the travel on the chi-squared surface is along the direction of steepest descent. An updated χ^2 value is calculated for the new point in parameter space and is compared with the previous value. This procedure is repeated until the difference between the current and previous χ^2 value is less than some prespecified limit.

The methods of linear and nonlinear regression analysis are designed to provide the least squares or optimal estimates for the parameters of a given model. However, this does not guarantee that the model applied was appropriate or even if appropriate that the optimal values provide stable and reproducible estimates of the model parameters. The χ^2 value also can be used to assess how well the predicted data values describe the actual measured results. The reduced chi square, χ^2_ν, is defined as chi squared divided by the number of degrees of freedom, which is given by the number of independent observations (data points) minus the number of parameters estimated from the data minus 1. It can be shown that χ^2_ν is equivalent to the ratio of the estimated variance of the fit to the estimated true variance in the data. The estimated variance of the fit is dependent on both the dispersion of the

data and the accuracy of the fit, whereas the true variance is dependent only on the dispersion of the data. Thus, the reduced chi square provides a useful measure of goodness of fit. If the fitting function for the compartmental model contributes no additional variance, then χ^2_ν will have a value of 1.0. Therefore, if the model describing the measured data is appropriate, the χ^2_ν value will be close to unity; however, if the model does not fit the data well, the estimated variance increases and χ^2_ν values will be significantly greater than 1.

An additional use of the reduced χ^2 value is to assess the relative performance of two different model configurations, as when testing whether a single tissue compartment model is sufficient to describe the kinetics of a radiotracer or whether two tissue compartments are required. The ratio of two χ^2_ν distributions can be shown to follow an F distribution. The F statistic is used to assess if inclusion of additional model parameters significantly improves the goodness of fit.

Another method of assessing the goodness of fit is to examine a plot of the difference between the measured and predicted data values, termed the residuals. If the model configuration accurately describes the measured data, then the residuals from the least squares fit will be distributed randomly about zero. The plots of the residuals versus time (Fig. 4.12) demonstrate the utility of visual examination. The upper panels show a data set and the least squares fit for a single tissue compartment model on the left and the plot of the residuals from this fit on the right. The lower panels show the same data set with the least squares fit for a model with two tissue compartments (*left*) and the plot of its residuals (*right*). Note that although the goodness of fit for the two models are visually similar, with the more complex model yielding only a modestly better fit (as can be seen from the points around the peak concentration), examination of the residuals clearly indicates the superiority of a model with two tissue compartments for describing the data.

Specialized Graphical Approaches

There are certain applications in which a simplified graphical or linear approach can be used to provide estimates of the quantity of interest. Although the compartmental model may not be linear with respect to all model parameters, it is sometimes possible to reformulate the model equations so a linear relationship exists between the data and the primary quantity being measured. Two such approaches deserve mention, because they have been used for analysis in hundreds of PET studies. One approach is used with irreversible radiotracers and is called a Patlak plot while the other is used with reversible radiotracers and is called a Logan plot. For both methods, the linear fitting procedure provides excellent stability against the noise from the dynamic PET measurements.

Patlak analysis (60) estimates the net rate of radiotracer accumulation in an irreversible compartment. This approach was applied initially for estimation of glucose metabolic rate

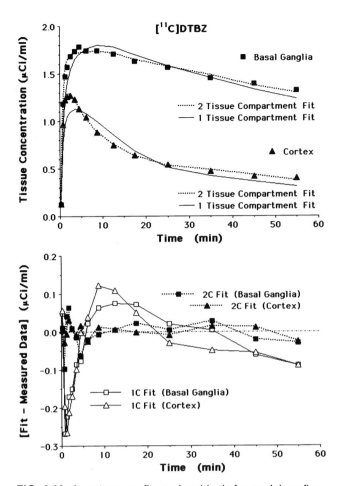

FIG. 4.12. Least square fits and residuals for model configurations with one- and two-tissue compartments. Shown are the time activity curves **(top plot)** for the vesicular monoamine transporter marker ^{11}C-dihydrotetrabenazine and best-fit model solutions using least squares optimization. Shown are fits to basal ganglia (*squares*) and cortex (*triangles*) using both a single-tissue compartment with two rate parameters (*solid lines*) and a two-tissue compartment with four rate parameters (*dashed lines*). Although the appearance of the fits for the two model configurations is similar, analysis of the residuals indicates that goodness of fit is superior for the more complex model, particularly at time points near the peak radioactivity concentration. These differences can be seen more clearly in the residuals shown in the **bottom plot.** The residuals give the difference between the best-fit model prediction and the measured data. There are large negative errors shortly after injection for the one-compartment fits. These fits then consistently overestimate the measured data between about 5 and 25 minutes after injection and finally again underestimate the later time points. This is compared with the relatively small and random errors resulting from fits using a model configuration with two tissue compartments (*dashed lines*).

from dynamic data, rather than from a static scan requiring assumptions about the population average rate constants. Patlak analysis yields an estimate of $K_1 k_3/(k_2 + k_3)$, which is the combination of parameters needed to calculate MR_{glc} as given in equation 4.47. This is accomplished by perform-

ing linear regression on the tissue concentration divided by the plasma concentration as a function of the integral of the plasma concentration divided by the plasma concentration.

$$\frac{C_T(T)}{C_P(T)} = [K_1 k_3/(k_2 + k_3)] \frac{\int_0^T C_P(t)\, dt}{C_P(T)} + [K_1 k_2/(k_2 + k_3)^2]$$

[4.55]

This plot, the Patlak plot, becomes linear over time with a slope of $K_1 k_3/(k_2 + k_3)$ (sometimes written as K) and an intercept of $K_1 k_2/(k_2 + k_3)^2$. Visual examination of a Patlak plot provides an indication of whether the irreversibility assumption is valid. Although this approach is excellent for measuring *net* incorporation—that is, $K_1 k_3/(k_2 + k_3)$—one should not assume that every radiotracer that yields a linear Patlak plot should be analyzed by this approach. In many applications such as receptor studies using irreversible ligands, binding site density is the biologic function of interest. The parameter k_3 and not the combination of parameters $K_1 k_3/(k_2 + k_3)$ yields an index of binding. The Patlak slope is dependent both on the binding or trapping rate and on the transport rate constants, K_1 and k_2. This is appropriate for estimating MR_{glc} but not receptor density. When the value of k_3 is high relative to the transport parameters, $k_3/(k_2 + k_3)$ approaches 1.0 and the slope reflects K_1, not binding. Under such conditions, uptake is said to be flow or delivery limited. It is interesting to note this is the exact principle on which radiolabeled microsphere flow measurements are based. One measures the *net* trapping of the microspheres, yet because trapping is instantaneous ($k_3 \to \infty$), the rate of trapping directly reflects flow.

Logan analysis (61) provides a related approach for analysis of reversible radiotracers. The Logan plot is based on the relationship

$$\frac{\int_0^T C_T(t)\, dt}{C_T(T)} = [V_{d(TOT)}] \frac{\int_0^T C_P(t)\, dt}{C_T(T)} + [INT] \quad [4.56]$$

where $V_{d(TOT)}$ is determined by linear regression of the integral of the tissue activity divided by the instantaneous activity versus the integral of the plasma activity divided by the tissue activity. What is particularly useful is that this approach is applicable for models with any number of serial compartments as long as each is reversible. The plot eventually becomes linear with a slope equal to the total radiotracer volume of distribution. For a tracer that can be described by a single tissue compartment, the plot is linear over all time. As additional compartments are required, the time to reach linearity increases. The intercept (*INT*) has physiologic meaning and for a single-compartment model is approximately equal to k_2^{-1}. Thus, the slope divided by the negative of the intercept yields an estimate of the transport parameter, K_1.

Parameter Estimation without Arterial Input Functions

Another group of specialized parameter estimation techniques are those that avoid the need for arterial plasma sampling. Because arterial sampling is somewhat invasive, is often labor intensive, and can increase errors in the parameter estimates if not performed properly, an approach that does not require blood samples appears very attractive. Although there have been several very different strategies for avoiding blood sampling, the most common has been the use of "reference regions" for the analysis of neuroreceptor binding studies. We focus on this particular strategy in this section, giving examples of three specific reference region approaches. A "reference region" is defined as a region within the image FOV that contains no specific binding sites. For each of these approaches, it is assumed that the reference region has the same free plus nonspecific volume of distribution as all other regions. Thus, the reference region can be used as a measure of the amount of free plus nonspecific uptake to subtract from the $V_{d(TOT)}$ to arrive at an estimate of the *specific* binding.

Logan et al. (62) developed a reference region method based on an extension of their work described in the preceding section. In the reference region Logan plot, the ratio of distribution volumes (*DVR*) between a given tissue region and the reference region is determined from the slope of the straight-line portion of a plot of the following relationship.

$$\frac{\int_0^T C_T(t)\,dt}{C_T(T)} = [DVR]\frac{\left[\int_0^T C_{RR}(t)\,dt + C_{RR}(T)/k_2\right]}{C_T(T)} + [INT]$$

[4.57]

where C_{RR} is the PET measure for the reference region and $DVR = V_{d(TOT)}/V_{d(RR)}$. The ratio of the slope over the negative of the intercept is related to the ratio of transport rate constants (K_1R) between target and reference volumes. The binding potential (*BP*) is then given by

$$BP = V_{d(SP)}/V_{d(RR)} = (V_{d(TOT)} - V_{d(RR)})/V_{d(RR)} = DVR - 1$$

and is equal to the estimate of the slope of the plot, *DVR*, minus 1.

The reference tissue model (RTM) of Lammertsma and Hume (63) has several similarities to the Logan approach. The RTM equation is derived from the differential equations describing the time rate of change in the tracer's concentration in both tissue and reference regions based on a common arterial plasma input. The simultaneous solution to those equations, eliminating the blood term yields

$$\int_0^T C_T(t)\,dt = [K_1R]\int_0^T C_{RR}(t)\,dt$$
$$+ [k_2 - K_1R/(1 + BP)]\int_0^T C_{RR}(t)\,dt$$

[4.59]

$$\otimes e^{-[k_2/(1+BP)]t}$$

This model has three parameters, K_1R, k_2, and *BP*. Standard nonlinear least squares analysis yields estimates of the three terms in square brackets, and hence, the three model parameters.

The final reference region approach is to use estimates of the equilibrium ratio of the radiotracer's tissue concentrations in the tissue and in the reference region. *BP* is given simply by

$$BP = (C_{T[eq]} - C_{RR[eq]})/C_{RR[eq]}$$

[4.60]

where the concentrations are measured directly by PET under equilibrium conditions, thus requiring a continuous infusion protocol, rather than a simple bolus injection of the radiotracer.

Model Validation

Once parameters have been estimated, one should quantify the overall performance of the kinetic model. One should establish not only how well the model configuration describes the kinetics of the radiotracer and how accurately the parameters can be estimated, but also that the final results make sense and are consistent with known information about the system being measured.

Besides comparison to other direct or accepted measures, as mentioned previously, another means of physiologic validation is to show that as biologic processes change, the compartmental analysis can detect these changes and also to show that these changes are specific to the appropriate parameters of the model. For example, if a compartmental model is used to measure the brain uptake and binding density of a particular ligand, then the compartmental model should be able to distinguish between changes in the delivery of ligand to the brain and the density of binding. Two experiments are performed to validate this specificity: (a) an intervention that changes delivery but not binding and (b) an intervention that changes binding density. An example of a pair of such experiments for ^{11}C-FMZ, a rapidly reversible benzodiazepine antagonist analyzed using a single tissue compartment model, is shown in Color Plates 4 and 5 following page 394. The first intervention was performed using an eyes closed/eyes open paradigm to change cerebral blood flow and hence tracer delivery (64). Color Plate 4 (following page 394) shows that K_1 increased 30% in the visual cortex during the stimulus scan, while $V_{d(TOT)}$ was unchanged. For the second intervention, scans were acquired before and after a partial blocking dose of 0.012 mg of cold FMZ per kilogram of body weight. This was administered 40% by bolus just before the second study and 60% by constant infusion over the duration of the scan. Color Plate 5 (following page 394) shows that specific binding estimates were decreased by about 40% throughout the brain.

A similar validation study was performed using the radiotracer N-^{11}C-methylpiperidinyl propionate (PMP), a substrate for hydrolysis by the enzyme acetylcholinesterase

(AChE). Carbon-11-PMP is irreversibly hydrolyzed by AChE, so a two-tissue compartment three parameter model (65) is used to analyze the data. Two PET studies were acquired, preadministration and postadministration of a dose of the AChE inhibitor physostigmine (66) designed to inhibit approximately 50% of the AChE activity. Compartmental estimates of the model parameter k_3, the index for AChE enzyme activity, are shown in Color Plate 6 (following page 394) and are seen to be 40% to 50% decreased after physostigmine administration.

CO-REGISTRATION OF 3D DATA SETS

Many scientific and clinical questions can be answered better through the use of *multiple* sets of 3D image data. For applications involving PET, this includes many scenarios: (a) a dynamic sequence of scans after the injection of a single radiotracer, as is acquired for most compartmental modeling studies; (b) a scan after each of several injections of the same radiotracer, as is acquired for functional activation studies using repeated injections of $H_2^{15}O$; (c) scans after the injection of different radiotracers, such as the use of both ^{11}C-raclopride and ^{11}C-dihydrotetrabenazine (DTBZ) to image multiple aspects of the dopamine system, or both ^{11}C-methionine and ^{18}F-FDG in a clinical study on a brain tumor patient; (d) scans from different modality imaging techniques in addition to PET, such as or SPECT, MR, or x-ray CT, the latter two providing the capability of matching function with structure; and (e) scans across different individuals.

To make the best use of these multiple 3D images sets, one needs to be certain that extraction (either visual or quantitative) of information from the different data sets is accomplished in a consistent manner. An important first step is to be able to co-register the various image sets to one another: both intramodality and intermodality and intrasubject and intersubject. Co-registration may involve only rigid-body transformation (translate, rotate) for intrasubject applications but may also involve nonlinear deformations to register images to a standardized coordinate system.

Intrasubject, Intramodality Registration

The simpler of the above scenarios are the ones involving multiple PET data sets acquired from a single subject. All scans from a single subject have the same underlying anatomy and all scans acquired using the same modality have many additional similarities, such as resolution. The early strategies to ensure co-registration of multiple scans from the same subject involved physical restraints. Even with such devices, the small amount of movement that occurs cannot be ignored (67). Another early strategy was to use external positron-emitting markers (68). This approach worked reasonably well for brain studies; however, application of external marker methods to whole-body imaging proved problematic. There is greater physiologic motion and variation in

patient positioning during imaging and it soon became evident that skin surface anatomy did not always accurately reflect the location of internal structures. Even for brain studies, the skin is not rigidly fixed to the skull, and therefore, registration accuracy is limited. Although external landmark methods were very fast, they were not sufficiently accurate.

The next step in registration involved user-defined landmarks within the image sets. This approach relies on the ability of an expert user identifying a series of points that represent identical locations in each image set. For rigid-body registration, only three points are needed in each image set, whereas for nonlinear deformation many more points are needed. The obvious limitation of such approaches, even for rigid-body registration, is that specification of such points cannot be accomplished with perfect accuracy. One way found to improve accuracy of rigid-body registration involves selecting more than three landmarks and using a fitting routine known as the ''Procrustes algorithm'' to minimize the sum of the squared discrepancies between homologous landmarks (69). It was demonstrated empirically that about 15 landmarks provided registration accuracy of about 0.5 mm (70). These methods, while providing reasonably accurate rigid-body registration, are not as practical for registration that requires nonlinear deformations. Furthermore, the time required for the user to accurately specify the landmarks is substantial.

The limitations encountered in the above approaches prompted work on registration algorithms that are fully or near fully automated. Various automated registration routines were proposed in the early 1990s, all based on image similarity but with several different criteria or cost functions used to optimize registration of the two image sets. These have included maximizing the cross-correlation between image sets (71), minimizing the variance in the ratio of image sets (72), minimizing either the absolute or the squared difference between images (73), and maximizing the number of voxels within a fixed difference between two image sets (74). All of these techniques are robust, work well with PET data, are easy to implement, and are rapid to perform. Registration of multiple $H_2^{15}O$ scans can be accomplished with an accuracy of better than 0.5 mm for translations and 0.5 degrees for rotations. The final criterion uses an adjustable threshold instead of just the random noise properties, and thus is less sensitive to the noise level in the images

For the image sets that differ greatly from one another, registration strategies not relying on image similarity become necessary. One such method is based on mutual information (MI) or relative entropy (75,76). Such routines are applicable for intramodality registration but are particularly useful for intermodality registration, and thus are discussed below.

Intrasubject, Intermodality Registration

Accurate registration of PET with other modalities is becoming increasingly valuable. For brain studies, registration of functional and anatomic images has been used to correct for atrophy and as a means to define volumes of interest for subsequent data analyses. Both in research and more recently in clinical practice, there has been great interest in registering whole-body ^{18}F-FDG-PET with CT images from oncology patients, then overlaying the image sets for accurate viewing of the correspondence between regions of high FDG uptake and the underlying anatomic structure. There has also been considerable interest in using co-registered PET-CT images to aid in radiation therapy planning for lung and other cancers. The push for the ability to display multimodal or ''fused'' images showing both functional and structural information is such that combined PET-CT systems have recently been introduced by major medical imaging companies. Although having both PET and CT devices within the same gantry will greatly aid this cause, it still is essential to ensure that registration between the image sets is extremely accurate. Small misregistration of PET and MR causes large errors in tissue atrophy measures. Similarly, accurate registration of PET and CT is essential if PET is to be useful in radiotherapy treatment planning for oncology patients. We review briefly the methods, both historical and current, for functional/structural image registration.

Early registration methods used external contrast markers (radioactive sources for PET, gadolinium for MR, iodine for CT). These methods provide a reasonable first-order registration, but for the same reasons as for intramodality registration, their usefulness is limited.

Another general approach for PET-MR/CT registration is based on surface matching. Segmentation defining the body surface is performed on the transmission (or sometimes emission) PET data sets and on the MR or CT images. The two image sets are aligned by minimizing the sum of the distances or squared distances between corresponding points on the two 3D surfaces (77,78). This method has been shown to work reasonably well but still yields only 1.0- to 3.0-mm accuracy. Another method has been a user-driven interactive approach (79). This technique uses superimposed PET and MR (or CT) data sets, displayed simultaneously as transverse, coronal, and sagittal cuts through the body at user-selected levels. The user has full control over the three translation and the three rotational degrees of freedom. This approach is reproducible and again fairly accurate, with errors typically less than 2.0 mm. However, it requires considerable user expertise and time to register a pair of image sets. The Procrustes approach also has been used for cross-modality registration but suffers from the same problem related to time and user expertise.

As with intramodality registration, fully (or near fully) automated routines have become the standard. These are user independent, reproducible, and more accurate. The two most commonly used approaches for registration of PET data sets with either CT or MR are (a) a method referred to as automated image registration (AIR) based on the matching of voxel intensities and (b) methods based on maximization of mutual information (MI) as mentioned previously (80–83).

AIR is included as part of the statistical parametric mapping packages widely used for functional neuroimaging applications and available over the internet (e.g., SPM99, Wellcome Department of Cognitive Neurology; www.fil.ion.ucl.ac.uk/spm). The voxel intensity approach used by AIR requires segmentation of the anatomic image set into tissue types and some degree of image preprocessing before registration. Accuracy is dependent on the quality of both functional and anatomic data, but with current systems, errors are on the order of 1.0 mm.

MI has proven to be a very useful approach to multimodality image registration. MI is a basic information theory concept that measures the statistical dependence between two random variables or for this application, two image sets. Thus, MI quantifies the amount of information that an image set from one modality contains about the image set from the other modality. Because no assumptions are made regarding the relationship between the voxel values of the two sets, the method is general and can be applied automatically. For these reasons, MI offers greater flexibility than AIR. The algorithm requires little or no preprocessing and minimal user interaction (user removal of external body tissues is not required).

The MI between two variables (or image sets) X and Y is defined as

$$I(X,Y) = \sum_x \sum_y p_{XY}(x,y) \log\left(\frac{p_{XY}(x,y)}{p_X(x)\, p_Y(y)}\right) \quad [4.61]$$

where p_X and p_Y are the probability density functions of X and Y, respectively, and $p_{X,Y}$ is their joint probability function. MI is also related to entropy by

$$I(X,Y) = H(X) + H(Y) - H(X,Y) \quad [4.62]$$

where $H(X)$ and $H(Y)$ give the entropy of X and Y, respectively, and $H(X, Y)$ gives their joint entropy.

$$H(X) = -\sum_x p_X(x) \log(p_X(x))$$

$$H(Y) = -\sum_y p_Y(y) \log(p_Y(y)) \quad [4.63]$$

$$H(X,Y) = -\sum_x \sum_y p_{XY}(x,y) \log(p_{XY}(x,y))$$

The implementation of MI at the University of Michigan by Meyer et al. (MiamiFuse) allows for either affine or nonlinear warping registration via thin-plate splines (TPS) (84). The basic routine consists of the following steps. Approximate control points are selected in each image set. From these points, the geometric mapping from one image set (homologous) to the other (reference) is computed. This transform is then applied to the entire homologous data set to obtain data set pairs for this current estimate of the co-registration. From these data pairs, the joint 2D histogram is created and the MI calculated. Next, an optimizing algorithm adjusts the coordinates of the control points from the homologous image set with the goal of maximizing the resultant

MI between the reference and the transformed homologous image set. From the adjusted control points for the homologous image set and the original control points of the reference set, a new mapping is computed. This process is repeated until the MI is maximized.

Color Plates 7 and 8 (following page 394) demonstrate two applications of intermodality registration. Color Plate 7 shows results from a research study using ^{11}C-DTBZ to measure VMAT2 binding site density. Two parametric image sets are obtained from the dynamic sequence of PET scans. One represents the transport rate (K_1) of radioligand into the brain *(upper left)* and the second represents its total tissue distribution volume ($V_{d(TOT)}$), an index of the vesicular transporter density *(upper right)*. These were estimated by kinetic analysis following intermodality co-registration of the dynamic PET data set. The center image shows the comparable slice from an MR study on the same subject after co-registration by MI maximization. Overlays of both functional PET parameters on the co-registered MR are shown in the bottom images.

Color Plate 8 (following page 394) shows images of a co-registered ^{18}F-FDG PET scan with x-ray CT for a cancer patient. Two different transaxial levels of the PET study are shown on the left, while the corresponding levels of the CT, after registration by MI, are shown on the right. The middle pair of images presents the fusion of functional and anatomic information.

Intersubject Registration

We conclude this section with a brief description of methods to register data sets across subjects. Intersubject registration is important when assessing the same PET measures across one or more groups of subjects. Standardized coordinate systems have been used for a variety of imaging applications for more than a decade, with the vast majority focused on the brain. The first PET study attempting to co-register different individuals into a standardized coordinate system (85) employed the stereotactic atlas of Talairach and Tournoux (86), thus the use of the term ''stereotactic coordinates.'' In this original approach, transformation of the PET data set into stereotactic coordinates was based on the use of both a PET scan and a lateral skull x-ray for determining the line connecting the anterior and posterior commissures (AC-PC line). Subsequently, routines have been developed that require only the PET data, first an interactive routine (87) and then a completely automated approach (88,89). Initial implementations used only linear scaling of the image sets and did not include nonlinear warping. It was soon understood that nonlinear warping was needed to improve registration across subjects. The first fully automated method for nonlinear warping of PET images used a 3D thin-plate spline (TPS) approach (90). Other ''standardized'' coordinate systems have been introduced, such as the brain atlas developed by The International Consortium on Human Brain Mapping (ICBM) (91). A current typical procedure for registering brain scans across subjects starts by intrasubject, intermodality affine registration of each subject's PET and MR (or CT) scans. This is followed by nonlinear warping of the subject's MR image set (because MR has better anatomic detail than PET) to the ICBM standard brain via TPS and MI. The same mapping is then applied to the subject's co-registered PET data to transform the functional images into ICBM coordinates.

The introduction of functional MRI has been responsible for a tremendous increase in the amount of work done in the area of registration and nonlinear warping. Currently, much of the work related to intersubject registration and nonlinear deformation of data occurs outside the field of PET. A more detailed discussion of these endeavors is outside the scope of this chapter.

SUMMARY

Optimal reconstruction of PET image sets is essential to obtain maximum information about the physiologic, pharmacologic, and biochemical status of the person being studied. The techniques and algorithms to reconstruct tomographic images have received extensive study and have incorporated data obtained from a variety of scientific disciplines. The two most common approaches are filtered back projection (FBP) and iterative reconstruction. FBP suffers from propagation of statistical noise while the iterative reconstruction algorithms have great computational requirements. The iterative methods are considered to be more accurate, particularly for lower count studies, and they are proving to be possible and useful in everyday clinical practice as advances are made in handling the vast amounts of data produced.

Achieving optimal sensitivity for PET requires 3D data sampling. Algorithms have been developed for reconstructing 3D PET data sets and progress is being made in reducing the time to process the tremendous amount of data necessary for image reconstruction. Further refinements to correct 3D images of the body for scatter and random events remain important areas for research.

To more fully measure functions in the human body with PET, it is necessary to obtain kinetic data and express it in quantitative units. Compartmental modeling is used to mathematically express and quantify the kinetic processes by which radioactive tracers move from one space or pharmacologic state—that is, one compartment—to another. The assumptions presupposed by each model must be validated and it is important to establish an appropriate model for the specific biologic function being investigated. The quantitative data obtained from compartmental modeling make it possible to accurately compare sequential studies in the same patient or data obtained from two or more groups of patients.

Co-registration of functional and anatomic imaging modalities is gaining in importance and the use of PET-CT in oncology and PET-MRI in neurologic applications has been the subject of intensive research in both academic and commercial arenas.

Advances in image reconstruction, kinetic modeling, and image registration are expected to continue and will further enhance the utility of PET.

REFERENCES

1. Radon J. Über die Bestimmung von Funktionen durch ihre integralwere längs gewisser Mannigfaltigkeiten (On the determination of functional from their integrals along certain manifolds). *Ber Saechs Akad Wiss Leipzig Math-Phys Kl* 1917;69:262–277.
2. Cormack A. Representation of a function by its line integrals, with some radiological applications. *J Appl Phys* 1963;34:2722–2727.
3. Cormack A. Representation of a function by its line integrals, with some radiological applications. *J Appl Phys* 1963;35:2908–2913.
4. Bracewell RN. Strip integration in radio astronomy. *Aust J Phys* 1956: 9;189–217.
5. DeRosier DJ, Klug A. Reconstruction of three-dimensional images from electron micrographs. *Nature* 1968;217:130–134.
6. Oldendorf WH. Isolated flying spot detection of radiodensity discontinuities—displaying the internal structural pattern of a complex object. *IRE Trans Biomed Electronics BME* 1961;8:68–72.
7. Kuhl DE, Edwards RQ. Image separation radioisotope scanning. *Radiology* 1963;80:653–661.
8. Hounsfield GN. Computerized transverse axial scanning (tomography): part 1, description of system. *Br J Radiol* 1973;46:1016–1022.
9. Wrenn FR, Good ML, Handler P. The use of positron-emitting radioisotopes for the localization of brain tumors. *Science* 1951;113:525–527.
10. Sweet WH. Uses of nuclear disintegrations in the diagnosis and treatment of brain tumors. *N Engl J Med* 1951;245:875.
11. Brownell GL, Sweet WH. Localization of brain tumors with positron emitters. *Nucleonics* 1953;11:52.
12. Anger HO, Rosenthal DJ. Scintillation camera and positron camera. In: *Medical radioisotope scanning.* Vienna: The International Atomic Energy Agency and the World Health Organization, 1959:59–82.
13. Rankowitz S, Robertson JS, Higinbotham. Positron scanner for locating brain tumors. *IRE Int Conv Rec* 1962;10:49–56.
14. Robertson JS, Marr RB, Rosenblum B, et al. 32-crystal positron transverse section detector. In: Freedman GS, ed. *Tomographic imaging in nuclear medicine.* New York: Society of Nuclear Medicine, 1973: 142–153.
15. Kuhl DE, Edwards RQ. The Mark 3 scanner: a compact device for multiple-view and section scanning of the brain. *Radiology* 1970;96: 563–770.
16. Kuhl DE, Edwards RQ, Ricci AR, et al. The Mark IV system for radionuclide computed tomography of the brain. *Radiology* 1976;121: 405–413.
17. Gordon R, Herman GT. Three-dimensional reconstruction from projections: a review of algorithms. *Int Rev Cytol* 1974;38:111–151.
18. Brooks RA, DiChiro G. Principles of computer assisted tomography (CAT) in radiographic and radioisotopic imaging. *Phys Med Biol* 1976; 21:689–732.
19. Budinger TF, Gullberg GT. Three dimensional reconstruction in nuclear medicine emission imaging. *IEEE Trans Nucl Sci* 1974;21:20.
20. Shepp LA, Vardi Y. Maximum likelihood reconstruction for emission tomography. *IEEE Trans Med Imaging* 1982;2:113–122.
21. Hudson HM, Larkin RS. Accelerated image reconstruction using ordered subsets of projection data. *IEEE Trans Med Imaging* 1994;13: 601–609.
22. Defrise M, Kinihan PE. Data acquisition and image reconstruction for 3D PET. In: Townsend DW, ed. *The theory and practice of 3D PET.* Dordrecht, The Netherlands: Kluwer Academic Publishers, 1998:1–53.
23. Kinihan PE, Rogers JB. Analytic 3D image reconstruction using all detected events. *IEEE Trans Nucl Sci* 1989;36:964–968.
24. Cho ZH, Ra JB, Kilal SK. True three-dimensional reconstruction—application of algorithm towards full utilization of oblique rays. *IEEE Trans Med Imaging* 1983;2:6–18.
25. Stearns CW, Chesler DA, Brownell GL. Accelerated image reconstruction for a cylindrical positron tomograph using Fourier domain methods. *IEEE Trans Nucl Sci* 1990;37:773–777.
26. Defrise M, Townsend DW, Clack R. *FAVOR: a fast reconstruction algorithm for volume imaging in PET; conference recording of the IEEE Nuclear Science Symposium; Santa Fe, NM; 1991.* 1992: 1919–1923.
27. Stazuk MW, Rogers JG, Harrop R. Full data utilization in PVI using the 3-D Radon transform. *Phys Med Biol* 1992;37:689–704.
28. Daube-Witherspoon ME, Muehllehner G. Treatment of axial data in three-dimensional PET. *J Nucl Med* 1987;28:1717–1724.
29. Defrise M, Kinihan PE, Townsend DW, et al. Exact and approximate rebinning algorithms for 3-D PET data. *IEEE Trans Med Imaging* 1997; 16:145–158.
30. Kinihan PE, Defrise M, Townsend DW, et al. *Fast iterative image reconstruction of 3D PET; conference recordings IEEE Nuclear Science Symposium, Santa Fe, NM; 1996.* 1997:1918–1922.
31. Comtat C, Kinihan PE, Defrise M, et al. Fast reconstruction of 3D data with accurate statistical modeling. *IEEE Trans Nucl Sci* 1998;45: 1083–1089.
32. Fessler JA. Penalized weighted least-squares image reconstruction for positron emission tomography. *IEEE Trans Med Imaging* 1994;13: 290–300.
33. Liu X, Comtat C, Michel C, et al. Comparison of 3-D reconstruction with 3D-OSEM and with FORE-OSEM for PET. *IEEE Trans Med Imaging* 2001;20:804–814.
34. Qi J, Leahy RM, Hsu C, et al. Fully 3D Bayesian image reconstruction for the ECAT EXACT HR +. *IEEE Trans Nucl Sci* 1998;45: 1096–1103.
35. Qi J, Leahy RM, Cherry SR, et al. High-resolution 3D Bayesian image construction using the microPET small-animal scanner. *Phys Med Biol* 1998;43:1001–1013.
36. Leahy RM, Qi J. Statistical approaches in quantitative positron emission tomography. *Stat Comput* 2000;10:147–163.
37. Bailey DL, Grootoonk S, Kinahan PE, et al. Quantitative procedure in 3D PET. In: Townsend EW, ed. *The theory and practice of 3D PET.* Dordrecht, The Netherlands: Kluwer Academic Publishers, 1998: 88–98.
38. Yavuz M, Fessler JA. Penalized-likelihood estimators and noise analysis for randoms-precorrected PET transmission scans. *IEEE Trans Med Imaging* 1999;18:665–674.
39. Yavuz M, Fessler JA. Maximum likelihood emission image reconstruction for randoms-precorrected PET scans. Conference recordings of the 2000 IEEE Nuclear Science Symposeum. *Med Imaging Conf* 2000.
40. Bailey DL, Grootoonk S, Kinahan PE, et al. Quantitative procedure in 3D PET. In: Townsend EW, ed. *The theory and practice of 3D PET.* Dordrecht, The Netherlands: Kluwer Academic Publishers, 1998: 57–87.
41. Erdogan H, Fessler JA. Monotonic algorithms for transmission tomography IEEE. *Trans Med Imaging* 1999;18:801–814.
42. Erdogan H, Fessler JA. Ordered subsets algorithms for transmission tomography. *Phys Med Biol* 1999;44:2835–2851.
43. Godfrey K. *Compartmental models and their application.* New York: Academic Press, 1983.
44. Gjedde A. Calculation of cerebral glucose phosphorylation from brain uptake of glucose analogs *in vivo*: a re-examination. *Brain Res Rev* 1982;4:237–274.
45. Lassen NA, Perl W. *Tracer kinetic methods in medical physiology.* New York: Raven Press, 1979.
46. Carson RE. Parameter estimation in positron emission tomography. In: Phelps ME, Mazziotta JC, Schelbert HR, eds. *Positron emission tomography and autoradiography, principles and applications for the brain and heart.* New York: Raven Press, 1986:347–390.
47. Sokoloff L, Reivich M, Kennedy C, et al. The (C-14) deoxyglucose method for the measurement of local cerebral glucose utilization: theory, procedure and normal values in the conscious and anesthetized albino rat. *J Neurochem* 1977;28:897–916.
48. Reivich M, Kuhl D, Wolf A, et al. The [18F]Fluorodeoxyglucose method for the measurement of local cerebral glucose utilization in man. *Circ Res* 1977;44:127–137.
49. Phelps ME, Huang SC, Hoffman EJ, et al. Tomographic measurement of local cerebral glucose metabolic rate in humans with (F-18)2-Fluoro-2-Deoxy-D-Glucose: validation of method. *Ann Neurol* 1979;6: 371–388.
50. Huang S-C, Phelps ME, Hoffman EJ, et al. Non-invasive determination of local cerebral metabolic rate of glucose in man. *Am J Physiol* 1980; 238:E69–E82.

51. Brooks RA. Alternative formula for glucose utilization using labeled deoxyglucose. *J Nucl Med* 1982;23:540–549.
52. Hutchins GD, Holden JE, Koeppe RA, et al. Alternative approach to single-scan estimation of cerebral glucose metabolic rate using glucose analogs, with particular application to ischemia. *J Cereb Blood Flow Metab* 1984;4:35–40.
53. Huang S-C, Phelps ME. Principles of tracer kinetic modeling in positron emission tomography and autoradiography. In: Phelps ME, Mazziotta JC, Schelbert HR, eds. *Positron emission tomography and autoradiography, principles and applications for the brain and heart.* New York: Raven Press, 1986:287–346.
54. Graham MM. Model simplification: complexity versus reduction. *Circulation* 1985;72[Suppl 4]:63–68.
55. Koeppe RA. Compartmental modeling alternatives for kinetic analysis of PET neurotransmitter/receptor studies. In: Kuhl DE, ed. *Frontiers in nuclear medicine:in vivo imaging of neurotransmitter functions in brain, heart, and tumors.* Washington, DC: American College of Nuclear Physicians, 1990:113–139.
56. Frey KA, Koeppe RA, Mulholland GK, et al. Parametric *in vivo* imaging of benzodiazepine receptor distribution in human brain. *Ann Neurol* 1991;30:663–672.
57. Koeppe RA, Hutchins GD, Rothley JM, et al. Examination of assumptions for local cerebral blood flow studies in PET. *J Nucl Med* 1987; 28:1695–1703.
58. Marquardt DW. An algorithm for least-squares estimation of nonlinear parameters. *J Soc Ind Appl Math* 1963;11(2):431–441.
59. Bevington PR. *Data reduction and error analysis for the physical sciences.* New York: McGraw-Hill, 1969:232–241.
60. Patlak C, Blasberg RG, Fenstermacher JD. Graphical evaluation of blood-to-brain transfer constants from multiple-time uptake data. *J Cereb Blood Flow Metab* 1983;3:1–7.
61. Logan J, Fowler JS, Volkow ND, et al. Graphical analysis of reversible radioligand binding from time-activity measurements applied to [*N*-11C-methyl]-(−)-cocaine PET studies in human subjects. *J Cereb Blood Flow Metab* 1990;10:740–747.
62. Logan J, Fowler JS, Volkow ND, et al. Distribution volume ratios without blood sampling from graphical analysis of PET data. *J Cereb Blood Flow Metab* 1996;16:834–840.
63. Lammertsma AA, Hume SP. Simplified reference tissue model for PET receptor studies. *Neuroimage* 1996;4:153–158.
64. Holthoff VA, Koeppe RA, Frey KA, et al. Differentiation of radioligand delivery and binding in the brain: validation of a two-compartment model for [C-11]flumazenil. *J Cereb Blood Flow Metab* 1991;11(5): 745–752.
65. Koeppe RA, Frey KA, Snyder SE, et al. Kinetic modeling of *N*-[11C]methylpiperidinyl propionate: alternatives for analysis of an irreversible PET tracer for measurement of acetylcholinesterase activity in human brain. *J Cereb Blood Flow Metab* 1999;19:1150–1163.
66. Kuhl DE, Koeppe RA, Minoshima S, et al. *In vivo* mapping of cerebral acetylcholinesterase activity in aging and Alzheimer's disease. *Neurology* 1999;52:691–699.
67. Phillips RL, London ED, Links JM, et al. Program for PET image alignment: effects on calculated differences in cerebral metabolic rates for glucose. *J Nucl Med* 1990;31:2052–2057.
68. Wilson MW, Mountz JM. A reference system for neuroanatomical localization on functional reconstructed cerebral images. *J Comput Assisted Tomogr* 1989;13:174–178.
69. Schonemann PH. A generalized solution to the orthogonal Procrustes problem. *Psychometrica* 1966;31:1–10.
70. Evans AC, Merritt S. Anatomical-functional correlation analysis of the human brain using three dimensional imaging systems. *SPIE Med Imag III: Image Proc* 1989;1092:264–274.
71. Junck L, Moen JG, Hutchins GD, et al. Correlation methods for the centering, rotation, and alignment of functional brain images. *J Nucl Med* 1990;31(7):1220–1226.
72. Woods RP, Cherry SR, Mazziotta JC. Rapid automated algorithm for aligning and reslicing PET images. *J Comput Assisted Tomogr* 1992; 16:620–633.
73. Eberl S, Kanno I, Fulton RR, et al. Automatic 3D spatial alignment for correcting interstudy patient motion in serial PET studies. In: Uemura K, Lassen NA, Jones T, et al, eds. *Quantification of brain function—tracer kinetics and image analysis in brain PET* [International Congress Series 1030]. Tokyo: Excerpta Medica, 1993:419–428.
74. Minoshima S, Koeppe RA, Fessler JA, et al. Integrated and automated data analysis method for neuronal activation studies using O-15 water PET. In: Uemura K, Lassen NA, Jones T, et al, eds. *Quantification of brain function—tracer kinetics and image analysis in brain PET* [International Congress Series 1030]. Tokyo: Excerpta Medica, 1993: 409–418.
75. Vajda I. *Theory of statistical inference and information.* Dordrecht, The Netherlands: Kluwer Academic Publishers, 1989.
76. Cover TM, Thomas JA. *Elements of information theory.* New York: Wiley, 1991.
77. Levin DN, Pelizzari CA, Chen GTY, et al. Retrospective geometric correlation of MR, CT, and PET images. *Radiology* 1988;169: 817–823.
78. Pelizzari CA, Chen GTY, Spelbring DR, et al. Accurate three-dimensional registration of CT, PET, and or MR images of the brain. *J Comput Assisted Tomogr* 1989;13:20–26.
79. Pietrzyk U, Herholz K, Heiss WD. Three-dimensional alignment of functional and morphological tomograms. *J Comput Assisted Tomogr* 1990;14:51–59.
80. Woods RP, Mazziotta JC, Cherry SR. MRI-PET registration with automated algorithm. *J Comput Assisted Tomogr* 1993;17:536–556.
81. Woods RP, Grafton ST, Holmes CJ, et al. Automated image registration, I: general methods and intrasubject, intramodality validation. *J Comput Assisted Tomogr* 1998;22:139–152.
82. Maes F, Collignon A, Vandermeulen D, et al. Multimodality image registration by maximization of mutual information. *IEEE Trans Med Imaging* 1997;16:187–198.
83. Meyer CR, Boes JL, Kim B, et al. Demonstration of accuracy and clinical versatility of mutual information for automatic multimodality image fusion using affine and thin plate spline warped geometric deformations. *Med Image Analysis* 1997;3:195–206.
84. Bookstein FL. *Morphometric tools for landmark data: geometry and biology.* Cambridge, UK: Cambridge University Press, 1991.
85. Fox PT, Perlmutter JS, Raichle ME. A stereotactic method of anatomical localization for positron emission tomography. *J Comput Assisted Tomogr* 1985;9:141–153.
86. Talairach J, Tournoux P. *Co-planar stereotaxic atlas of the human brain.* New York: Thieme Medical Publisher, 1988.
87. Friston KJ, Passingham RE, Nutt JG, et al. Localisation in PET images. Direct fitting of the intercommissural (AC-PC) line. *J Cereb Blood Flow Metab* 1989;9:690–695.
88. Minoshima S, Berger KL, Lee KS, et al. An automated method for rotational correction and centering of three-dimensional functional brain images. *J Nucl Med* 1992;33:1579–1585.
89. Minoshima S, Koeppe RA, Mintun MA, et al. Automated detection of the intercommissural line for stereotactic localization of functional brain images. *J Nucl Med* 1993;34:322–329.
90. Minoshima S, Koeppe RA, Frey KA, et al. Anatomic standardization: linear scaling and nonlinear warping of functional brain images. *J Nucl Med* 1994;35:1528–1537.
91. Mazziotta JC, Toga AW, Evans A, et al. A probabilistic atlas of the human brain: theory and rationale for its development. The International Consortium for Brain Mapping (ICBM). *Neuroimage* 1995;2: 89–101.

Principles of Cancer Imaging with Fluorodeoxyglucose

Richard L. Wahl

Anatomic imaging has been the fundamental approach to cancer imaging for more than 100 years. The robustness of anatomic methods is supported by their daily use in managing individual patients with cancer in the third millennium. A limitation of anatomic imaging is that it detects a phenotypic alteration that is sometimes, but not invariably, associated with cancer—a mass. Often with anatomic imaging, we do not know if masses are due to malignant or benign etiologies, such as can occur in solitary pulmonary nodules or border-line-sized lymph nodes. Small cancers are undetectable with traditional anatomic methods, as they have not yet formed a mass. After surgery or other treatment, it is even more difficult to assess for the presence or absence of recurrent tumor with anatomic methods. Posttreatment scans are complicated by dependence on comparisons with normal anatomy to detect altered morphologic findings due to cancer. Anatomic methods do not predict response to treatment and do not quickly reveal those tumors responding to therapy (1–3). Despite these challenges, anatomic images remain routine in cancer management. Positron emission tomography (PET), a functional imaging method, helps address many of the limitations of anatomic imaging, and when combined with anatomic images in fusion images, PET is emerging as a particularly valuable tool, providing both anatomic precision and functional information in a single image set (3) (Table 5.1.1).

MOLECULAR AND FUNCTIONAL ALTERATIONS IN CANCER

The molecular bases of neoplasia are increasingly well defined. Mutations in genomic DNA precede development of overt neoplasia (4). With sufficient alterations in genotype, phenotypic changes occur (Table 5.1.2). These genotypic and phenotypic changes in cancer antedate development of discrete mass lesions and represent potential targets for innovative imaging agents.

The concept of an altered "genome," "proteome," and resulting alterations in metabolism are consistent with an altered "metabolosome" and are concepts increasingly recognized as present in cancers. PET, due to its superb sensitivity to low signal levels, is able to detect signals from tracers targeting such alterations preferentially present in cancer.

PET has led the growing field of "molecular imaging" to the clinic not only because of the quantitative capabilities of PET and the sensitivity of electronic collimation, but also due to the choice of a proper radiotracer for cancer imaging. Although a wide variety of molecular, proteomic, and metabolic alterations occur in cancers and many of these can or may ultimately be imaged using PET, the most useful target in the clinical practice of PET to date has been the increased glucose metabolism present in most cancers. Other PET tracers, such as those targeting hypoxia, proliferation, amino acid transport, blood–brain barrier permeability, and protein synthesis, are discussed to a limited extent in several chapters of this book. This section focuses on the use of fluorodeoxyglucose (FDG) in cancer imaging.

GLUCOSE METABOLISM AS A TARGET

Accelerated glucose metabolism has been known to be present in cancers for nearly 70 years (5). Increased glucose metabolism is not specific for cancer, however. Indeed, the dominant tracer used in clinical PET imaging to date, 2-(fluorine-18)fluoro-2-deoxy-D-glucose (^{18}F-FDG) was developed as a tracer to study the initial steps of glucose metabolism in the brain (6). This tracer is transported into glucose-consuming cells, such as those in the brain or cancers, phosphorylated by hexokinase, typically type II, to FDG 6-phosphate, and then retained and can be imaged by PET (Fig. 5.1.1).

The development of FDG as a tumor imaging agent was not as rapid as its use in brain imaging. Although the Brookhaven group and others recognized and showed the promise of FDG for tumor targeting in animal models, this agent achieved only limited application to visceral imaging in this

TABLE 5.1.1. *Limitations of anatomic imaging methods for cancer assessment*

- Masses adjoining normal structures such as bowel are commonly undetected
- Commonly fail to detect small tumor foci
- Do not define the composition of the mass
- Lymph nodes are detected but not characterized as malignant or benign
- Often impossible to interpret after surgery due to altered anatomy
- Do not predict what therapy should be chosen
- Do not quickly determine whether tumor is responding to therapy
- Often do not provide prognostic information

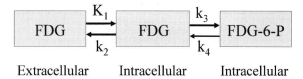

FIG. 5.1.1. Fluorodeoxyglucose kinetic modeling. K_1 is in part facilitated by Glut-1 glucose transporter molecules. k_3 is due to hexokinase activity. k_4 is due to glucose-6-phosphatase, which is typically at low levels in most cancers.

period (7,8). As early as 1982, the feasibility of imaging brain tumors and colorectal cancer with PET was shown in humans (9,10). Several other reports of successful tumor imaging with FDG and either planar imaging or PET appeared in small clinical studies in the late 1980s (11–13). Pioneering studies were being performed simultaneously by investigators in Japan using carbon-11 (^{11}C)-L-methionine (14).

The tumor targeting properties of FDG were further developed in a series of animal studies performed in the late 1980s (15–16). In these studies, the targeting of FDG to a wide variety of human tumor xenografts was evaluated in nude mice and compared with the targeting ability of monoclonal antibodies, which were the more typical agents of that time. My colleagues and I found that across a very wide range of human tumors, including breast, lung, renal, bladder, ovarian, testicular, head and neck, and lymphoma and melanoma, the uptake of FDG was very much higher (in terms of tumor-to-background uptake ratios) than that which was seen with the higher molecular weight, and in theory, more "specific" monoclonal antibody (MAb) tracers. Higher tumor/blood uptake ratios were commonly seen within a few hours of

intravenous tracer injection. Similarly, targeting to tumor metastases in lymph nodes was very high in comparison to targeting seen with comparable MAB agents. These preclinical data strongly suggested that tumor imaging of both primary and metastatic disease would be possible.

In brief, in nearly every circumstance in which animal models predicted that FDG would allow for successful imaging of tumors, the human studies showed the same: FDG targeted and imaged well breast cancer, renal cancer, bladder cancer, ovarian cancer, melanoma, lung cancer, and germ cell tumors (17–22). Many groups made similar observations in humans in a variety of cancers (23–26). It quickly became abundantly clear that FDG PET imaging would be a useful technique for cancer imaging.

UNDERSTANDING THE SIGNAL SEEN WITH FDG PET

Although superb images of many common kinds of cancer are feasible using FDG PET, it is important to understand the mechanisms of tracer uptake in cancers to fully understand the images and, most practically, the causes of false-positive and false-negative imaging results. In the past decade, improved understanding of some of the molecular alterations in glucose metabolism in cancer has been achieved. For example, overexpression of facilitative glucose transporters is common, and the Glut-1 transporter is often over-expressed in cancer (27). This is the molecular species that aids FDG transit from outside the cancer cell to inside the cell. Similarly, some of the hexokinase enzymes, such as hexokinase II, can be overexpressed in cancer. These are important proteins in the early phases of glucose metabolism, most notably the transport and phosphorylation of glucose to glucose 6-phosphate. Glucose 6-phosphate is metabolized further, but the tracer ^{18}F-FDG is not further metabolized after this step. FDG-6-phosphate has been shown to be the major species accumulated and imaged within cancers using FDG PET. By contrast, renal and genitourinary (GU) activity seen with PET, which can be vexing in image interpretation, are actually in the form of FDG.

In general, the extent of FDG uptake in tumors seems, at least in untreated tumors, quite directly related to the viable

TABLE 5.1.2. *Molecular and functional alterations in cancer*

Function	Increased	Decreased
Glucose metabolism	X	
Amino acid transport	X	
Protein synthedsis	X	
DNA Synthesis	X	
Blood flow	X	X
Receptors	X	
Oxygen tension		X
Apoptosis	X	X
Membrane turnover	X	
Signal transduction	X	
Vascular density	X	
Vascular permeability	X	
Oncogene products	X	
Many other genetic markers	X	X

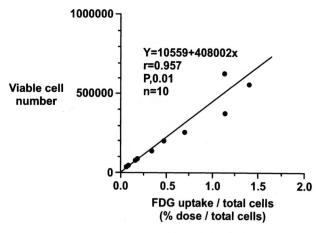

FIG. 5.1.2. Relationship between viable cell number and fluorodeoxyglucose (FDG) uptake. This is shown in an adenocarcinoma line, but the relationship holds across many cell lines of varying etiologies. Uptake of FDG is more related to living cancer cell numbers than to the cell cycle, thus differing from agents imaging proliferation.

cell number (Figs. 5.1.2 and 5.1.3), both *in vitro* and *in vivo* (27–31). In our hands, the number of viable cancer cells expressing Glut-1 appears best correlated with the extent of FDG uptake in a given type of cancer (see Color Plate 9 following page 394). Most cancer cells only modestly depend on insulin for FDG uptake, using little in the way of insulin-sensitive Glut-4 transporters. The heart, however, is very dependent on Glut-4. Thus, preparation of patients for cardiac FDG studies is completely different than for tumor

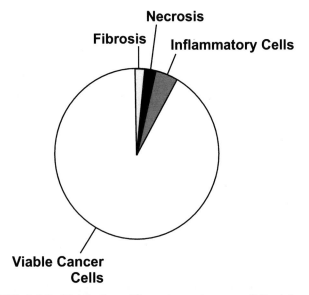

FIG. 5.1.3. Distribution of fluorodeoxyglucose activity determined with quantitative autoradiographic techniques in breast cancer after intravenous delivery. The bulk of uptake in the untreated tumor is in viable cancer cells, but some uptake occurs into nonmalignant elements.

TABLE 5.1.3. *Factors affecting fluorodeoxyglucose uptake in tumors*

Factor	Increased	Decreased
Viable cell number	X	
Tumor perfusion	X	
Hypoxia	X	
Inflammatory cells	X	
Necrosis		X
Hyperglycemia		X
Insulin		X
Adenosine triphosphate levels	X	
Glucose transporter expression	X	
Hexokinase activity	X	
Receptor agonists	X	
Receptor blockade		X
Chemotherapy acute	X	
Chemotherapy effective		X
Radiation acute	X	
Radiation chronic		X

imaging. Glucose loading and insulin treatment are not generally warranted to achieve optimal cancer imaging in the euglycemic patient. Preclinical and clinical studies also clearly showed that high glucose levels in the blood would impair tumor targeting with FDG. Thus, close attention to dietary preparation is needed with FDG when the goal is optimal tumor imaging (32–34). The relationships between cancer cell number, glucose transporters, flow, hexokinase levels, insulin levels, oxygen tension, cell-cycle status, adenosine triphosphate levels, receptor status, and the ^{18}F signal seen at PET are complex (Table 5.1.3). Of some note is that FDG uptake and Glut-1 expression rise markedly *in vitro* in cancer cells that are made hypoxic. Tumors with low flow and high FDG uptake might well be expected to by hypoxic. We also have seen high frequencies of Glut-1–positive cancer cells near necrotic regions, suggesting these border-zone cells are hypoxic (35,36).

Determining which process—delivery of tracer to the tumor, transport of FDG into the cancer cell, or phosphorylation of the tracer into the form of FDG—is rate limiting has been a topic of some discussion. In the brain, delivery of FDG is excellent, transport is high, and the phosphorylation rate k_3 is generally felt to represent the rate-limiting step in FDG accumulation into normal brain, with the accumulated ^{18}F activity in the form of FDG 6-phosphate (6). Tumors are somewhat different in that their perfusion rate is lower than normal brain, on average, and they have areas of very low perfusion, which are hypoxic in many cases. Thus, delivery of tracer and transport may be more critical than the phosphorylation rate in some of these tumors or at least in areas of the tumors. This area is quite complex and controversial (37,38).

It is clear that higher levels of transporter molecules alone, such as in transgenic animals with an overexpression of Glut-1, can result in lower serum glucose levels, greater total body glucose utilization, and lesser susceptibility to the development of diabetes. This supports the concept that glucose transport can have important influences on glucose consumption rates, seemingly separate from the influence of the hexokinase levels (38). Using kinetic modeling approaches, their studies have shown that tumors with higher standard uptake values (SUVs) actually had lower k_3 values than a group of tumors with high k_3 values (lung k_3 averaged lower than breast k_3, but lung SUVs were much higher than breast SUVs). This supports the importance of delivery and transport of the tracer to the net ^{18}F accumulation in tumors (39). Studies have also shown that when flow is measured by $H_2^{15}O$ and compared with FDG uptake, they correlate reasonably strongly, suggesting tumor ^{18}F uptake and flow are reasonably well linked. Thus, factors other than Glut-1–positive viable tumor cell number contribute to the net accumulation of FDG in the form of FDG 6-phosphate in tumors, but the signal is clearly correlated with the number of living, glycolytically active cancer cells in the tumor.

Knowing FDG to be a tracer of a general process altered in cancers and not a tumor-specific process helps us understand false-positive results. Inflammatory cells can accumulate FDG. This high FDG uptake can lead to confusion with cancer in some instances. However, the high tracer uptake in infections can also serve as a useful tool to detect infections and inflammation in some circumstances. Inflammation can cause false-positive results after therapy (40–42).

FDG uptake can rise in tumor cells for other reasons. For example, receptor stimulation by receptor binding of agonists can increase tracer uptake, as can an acute cellular response to irradiation or chemotherapy, with which the cell uses glucose at an increased level in response to the "shock" of treatment in the early phases posttreatment (43).

We are still learning about FDG uptake and its mechanisms and alterations relative to specific therapies (44,45). It seems quite clear that caution must be exercised if inflammation is believed to be present or if there is very recent therapy. Obviously, stability in measurements of glucose metabolism will depend on careful attention to detail in replicating study preparation conditions. With careful attention to detail, PET with FDG can serve as an excellent method to monitor response of cancers to therapy (45). Much like high FDG uptake, low FDG uptake in certain tumors can be understood mechanistically. For example, bronchioloalveolar carcinomas often have low tracer uptake, as do mucinous adenocarcinomas (46). These tumors have much lower cellularity than many other tumors. It is important that the mechanisms of uptake of FDG and other new molecular imaging tracers are well understood at the cellular level to best understand the scans we interpret.

FDG is currently the most commonly used and versatile tracer for cancer imaging. It has limitations, however, and although exceedingly useful in answering many common questions in cancer imaging, other tracers currently available or in development may provide additional valuable information. Various processes use glucose, which can be confusing. Examples include infection, inflammation, normal brain, the heart, and others. Further, FDG is excreted by the kidneys to a much greater extent than glucose due to lesser renal reabsorption of FDG than glucose. This intense FDG uptake in the GU system and brain can be confusing and make lesion detection difficult. FDG competes with glucose for uptake in tissues, so diabetics can have low FDG uptake in tumors if their serum glucose levels are high. FDG uptake does not vary markedly over the cell cycle, so if proliferation rate imaging is desired, FDG may not be the optimal tracer. Finally, some tumors have low enough FDG uptake that they are sometimes not detectable, such as some prostate cancer (47). Alternative tracers of a variety of types are under study. Choline-based compounds are showing promise in prostate and other cancers (48).

PRACTICAL ISSUES IN PET IMAGING OF THE CANCER PATIENT WITH FDG

To successfully detect cancer in patients with FDG PET, images of consistently high technical quality must be obtained and consistent interpretation criteria applied by skilled physician interpreters. Excellent interpreters cannot overcome the limitations of poor-quality images, but poor interpreters can cause excellent-quality images to be misinterpreted.

The determinants of lesion detectability in PET are several fold and are reviewed, in part, in later sections of this text. With FDG, as with other tracers, there must be a sufficient signal detected by the PET scanner versus background activity for lesion detection (49). The absolute intensity of the signal is dependent on the biology of the lesion and the injected dose of radiotracer. For example, untreated breast cancer and prostate cancers have lower FDG uptake, on average, than similarly sized untreated lung cancers or melanomas (39). The images obtained from obese patients have substantially fewer of the usable high-quality counts per millicurie injected than those from thin patients. Detectability will depend not only on the radioactivity levels in the tumor but also on the background levels in adjoining healthy tissues, the resolution and sensitivity of the scanning device, the reconstruction algorithm chosen, and the experience of the interpreting physician.

IMAGING DEVICE

PET imaging devices continue to evolve in terms of their performance capabilities. Dedicated PET devices are typically fairly expensive, in part because the thick detector materials required to stop the energetic 511-keV photons resulting from positron annihilation. Typically bismuth-germanate (BGO) or other materials such as lutetium oxy-orthosilicate (LSO) or germanium orthosiliate (GSO), and occasionally sodium iodide (NaI) are used. For high sensitivity from a PET scanner, there is presently no substitute for high-quality detector materials. Many high-quality "true" coincidence counts are needed to produce PET images of excellent quality.

Attempts to convert thin crystal, such as $\frac{3}{8}$- to $\frac{3}{4}$-inch-thick NaI gamma cameras, even dual- and triple-head devices, into collimated gamma cameras for detection of the high-energy 511-keV photons have been disappointing. This occurs because many counts are rejected by thick collimators and because such devices do not take advantage of coincidence detection. In general, such systems have difficulty detecting small tumors, and when these systems have been compared with dedicated PET imaging, up to half of small lesions, smaller than 3 cm, were not detected with the collimated gamma camera but were detected with dedicated PET (50). Although some cancers can be seen with this method, and results in lung nodules of adequate size have been somewhat promising in some studies, collimated FDG single-photon emission computed tomography (SPECT) imaging is not recommended for clinical use due to its insensitivity for small lesions (51). Medicare in the United States will not reimburse FDG imaging with such a device, practically making the technique unused for tumor imaging. Collimated FDG-SPECT systems are more useful for assessing myocardial viability.

There has been a much greater level of interest and substantial progress in modifying dual- or triple-headed gamma cameras with NaI crystals as devices for positron imaging. These devices use coincidence circuitry as in dedicated PET and have spatial resolution comparable to that of high-quality gamma cameras. The cameras have a lower efficiency for detecting true coincidences than dedicated full-ring PET cameras and detect many more scatter events due to their need to use three-dimensional (3D) imaging to have good sensitivity.

The lower efficiency of NaI crystals and the large crystal size result in more potential acceptance of scattered counts. Although these cameras can work reasonably well in thin patients and in the thorax and neck in many clinical studies, they produce significantly inferior lesion detection statistics for lesions smaller than 2 to 3 cm, particularly those in the abdomen (52). These cameras may have utility in some limited settings, such as evaluating a large mass for viability; however, if dedicated PET is available, it is the preferred method for imaging.

The technology of these cameras has improved rapidly, and more recent generation scanning devices with thicker crystals, attenuation correction, some septa present (to be two and a half dimension, not 3D), and sophisticated iterative reconstruction programs have led to improved quality of images. However, the limited amount of detector material and its composition in these devices has generally resulted in images that are inferior to those obtained with traditional two-dimensional (2D) dedicated PET devices (53). Recognition of the lower accuracy of the hybrid devices led U.S. Medicare to substantially limit the use of these devices in PET imaging. This limitation on reimbursement has slowed dissemination of this form of technology.

Clearly, camera technology continues to evolve, and it is possible that dedicated PET scanners will ultimately largely be transformed to combination PET/computed tomography (CT) scanners in a few years. The move from radionuclide to x-ray sources for transmission correction occurred in bone densitometry and this same scenario may occur for PET transmission imaging. The CT images, in addition to being of higher photon flux and possibly allowing more accurate or more robust transmission scans, also offer the possibility of diagnostic localization of tumors with greater accuracy. The author has had early access to PET-CT technology and it appears to be disseminating rapidly.

PATIENT SELECTION FOR PET

PET costs more than most other noninvasive imaging methods and exposes patients to radiation. Obviously, it is important to use the test wisely so clinically relevant questions can be answered. Specific indications for PET are discussed in multiple sections of this book, but a few general principles should apply in patient selection. Issues we face often are requests of a referring physician to evaluate a lesion smaller than 5 mm in size, either in the thorax or elsewhere in the body. This is asking a lot from PET, because many lesions of this size that are malignant are not detected on PET, due to resolution and count limitations (49). Although some can be seen, positive scan results are much more useful and reliable than negative scan results when the lesions are small. The issues faced with each patient should be thoroughly discussed with the referring physician and the pros and cons of doing or not doing the PET study should be understood by all—including the patient—before the study is done. If there are clear indications that the data from the PET study will not be helpful in the care of a certain patient, then it is the nuclear medicine physician's responsibility to discourage doing it.

Another frequently asked question is whether there is a tumor present after surgery. Trying to answer such a question a few days after surgery is difficult with PET, because there is normally uptake in surgical wounds and scars. If a wound is infected, and the question is whether a tumor is present or not, this is also quite difficult to resolve, because PET results are often positive in infections, whether a tumor is present or not (42). Again, discussion with the referring physician may result in a postponement of the PET study for several months or until the infection has resolved.

Similarly, claustrophobic patients, patients with severe movement disorders (who cannot lie still for the scan), patients who are morbidly obese, patients who cannot lie on their back or side, and poorly controlled diabetics are not optimal candidates for FDG PET. Access to all relevant history and correlative information is also quite important for optimal PET imaging. Education and discussion with the referring physician are essential to ensure that PET is used wisely and the risks and benefits of the test are known.

PATIENT PREPARATION

In contrast to cardiac PET imaging in which insulin levels must be increased to target FDG to the cardiac muscle, in cancer imaging, the goal is to have low insulin levels at the time of FDG injection and a low blood sugar level. This optimizes tumor uptake and minimizes FDG uptake into skeletal muscle. This is typically achieved by making the patient fast for 4 or more hours before the scan. Often, patients are encouraged to drink water to maintain a good hydration level for the scans. This can enhance urinary excretion. Patients are usually instructed to avoid extensive physical activity before the PET scan so there is not FDG uptake into skeletal muscle.

Patient Interview

It is recommended that patients be interviewed before they are scanned. Often, the history supplied by the referring physician is inadequate or limited. The timing of correlative imaging studies and their availability and results are important issues to securing the proper diagnosis. Particularly important is securing historical information related to whether there have been recent surgical procedures, biopsies, and therapies, as well as regarding the patients medications. For example, sites of recent biopsies can have increased tracer uptake. Similarly, patients who have just received effective chemotherapy are less likely to have their tumors visualized than patients who have not had recent therapy (e.g., chemotherapy can reduce tumor signal) (45). Bone metastases will be more difficult to detect in patients who have recently received colony-stimulating factors, because these increase the marrow signal (54). Obviously, exclusion of pregnancy in female patients is as important as securing information regarding claustrophobia or difficulty lying stationary for the scans. Thus, as in any nuclear medicine procedure, historical information can be very important.

INJECTION AND IMAGING

Various approaches to injected dose size and imaging duration have been studied. One important issue is the simple one of where to inject the dose. FDG is generally given intravenously, but the choice of vein is important. If FDG is extravasated in the arm, it will accumulate in draining lymph nodes with great avidity (15). Thus, if the goal is to evaluate the right axilla of the patient for possible tumor involvement, injection of the right arm would not be preferred. Either the left arm or a foot vein would be preferable to minimize the possibility of a small amount of tracer extravasating and localizing to the draining regional lymph nodes.

The choice of the injected millicurie dose of FDG will be partly dependent on the scanning device chosen. With 2D BGO PET scanners, injected doses in the 10- to 15-mCi range are common, with doses of 20 mCi not unusual. With 3D scanners, lower injected doses are typically given. With NaI detector full-ring scanners, an injected dose of 5 mCi or so may be completely adequate. The emitted photon flux differs between small and large patients due to attenuation effects. Larger patients may need a higher millicurie dose than small patients. Most oncologic PET with BGO scanners

is done in the 2D mode to minimize scattered and random event detection.

The duration of imaging is dependent to some extent on the injected dose. If more millicuries are given, a shorter acquisition will be feasible for comparable statistical quality. Typically 5 to 10 minutes of acquisition per imaging level is performed (emission), although the exact and optimal duration is not well established. The author currently acquires each scan level for 5 minutes based on an average 15-mCi injected dose per patient.

If the goal is to detect a very small lesion, a larger injected dose and longer duration may be required.

A decision must be made as to whether to perform attenuation correction of images or not. Attenuation correction adds time to the study and adds noise. There has been a trend toward reducing the duration of time used in acquiring the attenuation correction data and efforts to reduce noise (55). With perfect attenuation correction, PET is a precisely quantitative procedure, but perfect attenuation correction is not achieved due to statistical limitations, and in many instances, precise quantitation is not required diagnostically. For lesion detection, experienced readers can often detect nearly as many lesions with attenuation correction as without, and if there is a motion artifact or a low-quality attenuation scan, the nonattenuation-corrected images can be more diagnostically useful than the attenuation-corrected ones. Many institutions, including the author's, use attenuation correction with a segmented method to minimize noise and time requirements, and also reconstruct the nonattenuation-corrected data sets for examination. The availability of quick and accurate attenuation correction would make attenuation correction routine. CT-based attenuation maps may allow this to be achieved, and there is a trend toward CT tubes as the source for attenuation maps (56).

The extent of the body imaged depends on the clinical question. For most cancers, images of the body from the acoustic meatus through the mid thigh are viewed as adequate. Imaging of the full brain is not routine in most centers unless the patient has melanoma or known or strongly suspected brain metastases. This limitation to imaging the brain is due to the fact that a significant fraction of metastases do not have intense tracer uptake and may fail to be detected. The lower extremities are generally imaged if there is a specific question related to that portion of the body. For example, in patients with a history of melanoma of the foot, imaging the entire lower extremities is very appropriate. Imaging the entire body takes a long time and may necessitate shorter acquisition protocols per imaging level to be feasible. If a clinical question is focused only on the brain, then brain-only imaging is appropriate. If the clinical question is mainly regarding the head and neck, then more limited imaging for a longer duration may be most rational.

After patients are injected intravenously with FDG, they are asked to remain still and quiet and to not exert themselves, and at the appropriate time, they are asked to void and then imaging is begun. Voiding is done before PET emission imaging to minimize the FDG signal from the bladder and kidneys, where it is excreted. ^{18}F has a half-life of less than 2 hours, so the longer the uptake phase, the fewer the total counts available. Thus, even though it is known that FDG uptake in tumors generally rises as a fraction of the injected dose from the time of injection until the time of imaging, emission images are usually begun between 50 and 60 minutes after the tracer is injected. Longer delays can provide better target-to-background ratios, but it is not clear that this results in improved accuracy in most cases, and it clearly results in lower statistical image quality. It is important that the FDG imaging protocol be followed carefully to achieve reproducible results. Because FDG uptake after injection rises with time, the lesion uptake changes with time. Performing repeated FDG studies at precisely the same time after injection maximizes the chances of achieving reproducible results.

Image reconstruction algorithms and filters are discussed elsewhere, but their choice is important for optimal imaging. It must be realized that to avoid very noisy appearing images, some image smoothing, or filtering, must take place. This means that the resolution of the scanner in patient studies is not as good as the potential optimal resolution of the scanner using, for example, a ramp filter in phantoms (49). The choice of reconstruction algorithm varies, but in many centers, the venerable filtered back-projection method is still often used in high-count brain PET studies. Iterative algebraic methods such as the ordered subset expectation maximization (OSEM) are more commonly used for visceral imaging. These algebraic methods reduce streak artifacts but can produce other distortions such as ''hot spots,'' not ''hot lines.'' The interpreting physician and physicist for the facility must make a rational choice of filter type, filter cutoff and reconstruction algorithms for the camera, and injected dose and must use them consistently to maximize reproducibility of PET studies.

Interpretation of PET images requires considerable clinical experience. It is recommended that images be read in an interactive fashion on a computer monitor with the ability to display coronal, sagittal, transverse, and maximum-intensity projection or rotating views. The ability to vary the gray scale is very important. Although images can be read on film, most centers prefer to read soft-copy image sets. A familiarity with normal structures and their variants is important (see Chapter 5.2).

QUANTITATIVE MEASUREMENTS

Quantitative and semiquantitative methods can be used in PET image interpretation, although most centers use qualitative interpretation techniques. The only semiquantitative technique relatively routinely applied is the SUV (57). This value was originally defined as:

$$SUV = [mCi/mL \text{ (decay corrected) in tissue}]/[mCi \text{ of tracer injected into the patient/body weight in grams}]$$

The value becomes unitless if it is assumed that 1 g of body weight is equal to 1 mL. The SUV calculated in this manner is also known as SUV_{bw}.

The SUV would equal 1 if a tracer was completely and uniformly distributed throughout the body after injection and if there was no excretion. In fact, however, FDG does not distribute normally throughout the body. In the fasting state, little FDG goes to fat or muscle, so these tissues have low SUVs, under one in many instances. By contrast, liver and blood SUVs are often higher than 1.

The SUV can be helpful and in some studies has been able to separate malignant from benign tissues fairly well (e.g., in lung nodules with an SUV higher than 2.5, cancer is more probable than in low SUV lesions). Similarly, the SUV can be very helpful in a given patient in monitoring the response of a cancer to therapy. The SUV is quite reproducible from study to study, typically within 10% to 15%,

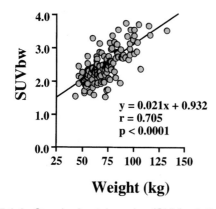
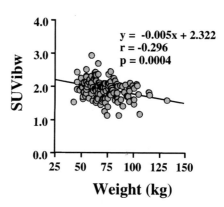

FIG. 5.1.4. Standard uptake value (SUV) relationship with weight. SUV **(left)** calculated based on total body mass (SUV_{bw}) is higher in normal blood in heavy patients. SUV **(right)** corrected to ideal body weight (SUV_{ibw}) is less dependent on weight but does show dependence and is an overcorrection. (From Sugawara Y, Zasadny KR, Neuhoff AW, et al. Reevaluation of the standardized uptake value for FDG: variations with body weight and methods for correction. *Radiology* Nov 1999;213(2):521–525, with permission.)

TABLE 5.1.4. *Formulas used in the calculation of standardized uptake values*

Parameter for denominator	Calculation
SUV_{bw} (using only body weight)	Weight the patient
SUV_{ibw} (using ideal body weight)	IBW = 45.5 + 0.91 (height − 152) or IBW + weight if IBW > weight
SUV_{lbm} (using lean body mass)	LBM = 1.07 height − 148 (weight/height)^2
SUV_{bsa} (using body surface area)	BSA = (weight)$^{0.425}$ × (height)$^{0.725}$ × 0.007184

BSA, body surface area; IBW, ideal body weight; LBM, lean body mass; SUV, standardized uptake value.

TABLE 5.1.5. *Technical factors affecting measurements of standardized uptake values with fluorodeoxyglucose*

Factor	Effect
Uptake period after tracer injection	Longer generally results in higher SUV than shorter
Size of ROI	Smaller ROI gives higher SUV
Pixel size of PET image	Higher pixel images give higher maximum SUV values
Reconstructed resolution of PET images	Higher resolution produces higher SUV for small ROIs
Body mass index	Obese patients have higher tumor and normal SUVs than thin patients
Serum glucose level	In fasting state, higher glucose levels reduce tumor FDG uptake
Quality of tracer injection	Partly extravasated doses reduce SUV

FDG, fluorodeoyglucose; ROI, region of interest; SUV, standardized uptake value.

and this is more precise than some of the parameters used in kinetic modeling, such as the k_3, which is far more variable when evaluated in a test–retest setting. The SUV is not independent of body size. The SUV rises in blood and healthy tissues with increasing body weight. Thus, obese patients have higher SUVs in normal blood and liver than thin patients. This is because FDG does not distribute into fat in the fasting state, and obese patients have a disproportionate fraction of their body mass in the form of fat. This means that SUVs for tumors and healthy tissue are higher in the obese patient and can be misleading (Fig. 5.1.4). A simple correction, using lean body mass (LBM) or body surface area (BSA) can avoid these problems quite effectively. Thus, we use the SUV_{lean} or SUV calculated by replacing the actual weight of the patient with the LBM in the denominator of the SUV calculation (Table 5.1.4). SUV_{lean} tends to be lower than SUV, in general. SUV_{bsa} is a valuable index, but the conversion factor leads to numbers far from the typical SUV (Fig. 5.1.5). Methods for calculating LBM and BSA are shown in Table 5.1.4, which includes the most recent method of LBM calculation (58).

The region of interest (ROI) size can have an impact on the SUV calculation. Large ROIs produce lower SUV than small regions placed over maximal tumor activity (45). The maximal pixel value in tumor is often used and is quite reproducible. In a given center, it is important to be consistent with the way the ROIs are drawn to achieve optimal reproducibility. Typically, we record the maximum SUV in a tumor and note the maximum uptake in a 1.2-cm square ROI. It has been argued that SUV multiplied by the volume of the lesion is a very critical value. This value may be of considerable relevance in treatment-response assessment. This parameter is quite reproducible in experienced hands. A summary of factors that can affect SUV is shown in Table 5.1.5.

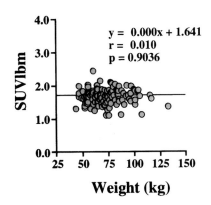
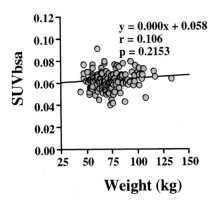

FIG. 5.1.5. Standard uptake values (SUVs) corrected for lean body mass (SUV$_{lbm}$) **(left)** or body surface area (SUV$_{bsa}$) **(right)** are independent of patient weight. These are the preferred parameters. Because of the small units for SUV$_{bsa}$, most use SUV$_{lbm}$ **(left)** if patients are obese. (From Sugawara Y, Zasadny KR, Neuhoff AW, et al. Reevaluation of the standardized uptake value for FDG: variations with body weight and methods for correction. *Radiology* Nov 1999;213(2):521–525, with permission.)

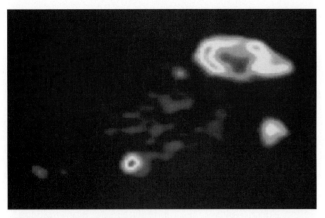

FIG. 5.1.6. Fluorodeoxyglucose PET scan of a patient with breast cancer, showing the difficulty in anatomically locating "hot spots" representing tumor. This transverse scan shows the large primary tumor on the patient's left, a left axillary node and posterior uptake in the spine or possibly the lung. (From Wahl RL, Cody RL, Hutchins GD, et al. PET imaging of breast cancer with ^{18}F-FDG. *Radiology* 1989;173:419P, with permission.)

FUSION OF FORM AND FUNCTION

FDG has a high level of targeting to many cancers, which is highly desirable on most counts. However, an early and obvious limitation seen in our earliest clinical studies of breast cancer in 1989 showed a disadvantage of being successful in targeting a radiopharmaceutical almost too well to cancer. The problem was that the tumors could be seen, but it was difficult to tell precisely where they were located anatomically. An early image we obtained of breast cancer shows this clearly; there are tumors present, but where exactly are they located anatomically (Fig. 5.1.6)? Anatomy is still needed. Working with my colleague Chuck Meyer at Michigan, we developed methods to fuse the anatomic information of CT with PET into "anatometabolic images" (1). These images show what the functional activity is and where. However, they are challenging to generate in some circumstances and are prone to misalignment unless great caution is taken in positioning patients identically between the PET and CT or magnetic resonance imaging studies (1). Thus, a need for better fusion was clearly needed.

Although FDG is a potent, but simple, molecular imaging tracer and has been the cornerstone of clinical PET imaging in cancer, PET methods while anatomically precise are limited in their accuracy for precisely localizing lesions. A major practical problem has been that PET can find the specific molecular alteration, but it can be very difficult to know what to do about it clinically if it cannot be localized or biopsied to add certainty to the diagnosis. Some years ago, the technique of "anatometabolic fusion imaging" was described by the author and his colleagues, detailing the fusion of PET and CT data sets via software. This ability to use software and more recently dedicated hardware solutions to present PET molecular imaging data in a clear and well-understood anatomic context is key to the progress of molec-

ular imaging. However, software approaches require extreme attention to detail to be successful and are very difficult to use reliably, other than in the brain.

Beyer et al. (56) fused the PET method and CT method using hardware and software, by combining a PET and a CT scanner in the same hybrid device so the patient has both types of scans performed during a single acquisition period (56). This technology was of obvious utility and the fusions were of high quality. Several manufacturers were able to see the obvious benefits of this type of approach. We were fortunate at Johns Hopkins Hospital to have installed the first commercially produced PET-CT scanner in the United States and have used it in diagnosing cancer in several hundred clinical cancer patients. The benefits of this technology were immediately apparent to those interpreting studies on a daily basis, but they are being rigorously studied to determine where this technology is clearly cost-effective versus alternative methods. An example of a combined PET-CT scan obtained with this equipment is shown in Color Plate 10 (following page 394). To date, fusions obtained from our dedicated PET-CT scanner have been of very high quality. The method appears useful not only for precisely localizing FDG avid tumors, but also for achieving increased certainty that healthy structures with FDG uptake are not confused with cancer.

Anatomolecular imaging using FDG and PET-CT is a clinical reality and PET-CT will increasingly be adopted as the new clinical standard for noninvasive imaging the cancer patient.

COST-EFFECTIVENESS

Excellent examples of cost-effectiveness studies and a review of cost-effectiveness with an emphasis on PET have recently appeared in the literature (59,60). Suffice it to say that in many instances, PET is the most accurate diagnostic test for cancer and it often costs less than or no more than performing CT scans of multiple levels of the body, with and without contrast. The major cost savings with PET occur, however, when PET provides diagnostic information that reduces the frequency of alternative expensive procedures—for example, avoiding thoracotomy in lung or esophageal cancer or eliminating the need for surgery in patients with colorectal cancer. In the United States, the cost/efficacy ratio of PET has recently improved, as Medicare has lowered reimbursement for PET. Lower PET costs make PET more cost-effective. Although PET has been considered an "expensive" imaging test by many, it is clear that the improved quality of decisions resulting from PET and lower costs for PET based on improved throughput have served to make the test one considered effective and necessary by referring physicians, not one in which a careful cost/benefit decision must be made in each case of intended use.

SUMMARY

Anatomic imaging of cancer using x-rays has proven very useful for more than 100 years but has clear limitations.

Anatomic methods reliably show whether a large mass is present or absent, but not what the mass is composed of. Imaging additional phenotypic alterations of the altered genotype of cancers with PET adds clinically valuable information for patient management. Although many molecular alterations are present in cancer, the one by far most exploited in clinical practice and research has been the accelerated glucose metabolism present in most cancers. This process is imaged well with the radiotracer ^{18}F-FDG. The ability to spatially localize the molecular alterations of cancer, either through qualitative cognitive methods by the imaging specialist, through computer fusion of image sets, or through fused "anatomolecular" image sets using dedicated PET-CT, is key to optimal use of the imaging methods, as is careful attention to consistency in scan acquisition.

REFERENCES

1. Anzai Y, Carroll WR, Quint DJ, et al. Recurrence of head and neck cancer after surgery or irradiation: prospective comparison of 2-deoxy-2-[F-18]fluoro-D-glucose PET and MR imaging diagnoses. *Radiology* 1996;200(1):135–141.
2. Sugawara Y, Zasadny KR, Grossman HB, et al. Germ cell tumor: differentiation of viable tumor, mature teratoma, and necrotic tissue with FDG-PET and kinetic modeling. *Radiology* 1999;211(1):249–256.
3. Wahl RL, Quint LE, Cieslak RD, et al. "Anatometabolic" tumor imaging: fusion of FDG-PET with CT or MRI to localize foci of increased activity. *J Nucl Med* 1993;34(7):1190–1197.
4. Zhang W, Laborde PM, Coombes KR, et al. Cancer genomics: promises and complexities. *Clin Cancer Res* 2001;7(8):2159–2167.
5. Warburg O. *The metabolism of tumors.* New York: Richard R. Smith, Inc, 1931:129–169.
6. Phelps ME, Huang SC, Hoffman EJ, et al. Tomographic measurement of local cerebral glucose metabolic rate in humans with (^{18}F)2-fluoro-2-deoxy-D-glucose: validation of method. *Ann Neurol* 1979;6(5):371–388.
7. Som P, Atkins HL, Bandoypadhyay D, et al. A fluorinated glucose analog, 2-fluoro-2-deoxy-D-glucose (^{18}F): nontoxic tracer for rapid tumor detection. *J Nucl Med* 1980;21(7):670.
8. Larson SM, Weiden PL, Grunbaum Z, et al. Positron imaging feasibility studies, II: characteristics of 2-deoxyglucose uptake in rodent and canine neoplasms: concise communication. *J Nucl Med* 1981;22(10):875–879.
9. Patronas NJ, Di-Chiro G, Brooks RA, et al. Work in progress: [^{18}F] fluorodeoxyglucose and positron emission tomography in the evaluation of radiation necrosis of the brain. *Radiology* 1982;144(4):885–889.
10. Yonekura Y, Benua RS, Brill AB, et al. Increased accumulation of 2-deoxy-2-[^{18}F]fluoro-D-glucose in liver metastases from colon carcinoma. *J Nucl Med* Dec 1982;23(12):1133–1137.
11. Kern KA, Brunetti A, Norton JA, et al. Metabolic imaging of human extremity musculoskeletal tumors by PET. *J Nucl Med* Feb 1988;29(2):181–186.
12. Paul R. Comparison of fluorine-18-2-fluorodeoxyglucose and gallium-67 citrate imaging for detection of lymphoma. *J Nucl Med* Mar 1987;28(3):288–292.
13. Strauss LG, Clorius JH, Schlag P, et al. Recurrence of colorectal tumors: PET evaluation. *Radiology* 1989;170(2):329–332.
14. Fujiwara T, Matsuzawa T, Kubota K, et al. Relationship between histologic type of primary lung cancer and carbon 11 L methionine uptake with positron emission tomography. *J Nucl Med* 1989;30(1):33–37.
15. Wahl RL, Kaminski MS, Ethier SP, et al. The potential of 2-deoxy-2[^{18}F]fluoro-D-glucose (FDG) for the detection of tumor involvement in lymph nodes. *J Nucl Med* 1990;31(11):1831–1835.
16. Wahl RL, Hutchins GD, Buchsbaum DJ, et al. ^{18}F-2-deoxy-2-fluoro-D-glucose uptake into human tumor xenografts. Feasibility studies for cancer imaging with positron-emission tomography. *Cancer* 1991;67:1544–1550.
17. Wahl RL, Cody RL, Hutchins GD, et al. PET imaging of breast cancer with ^{18}FFDG. *Radiology* 1989;173:419P.
18. Wahl RL, Cody R, Hutchins GD, et al. Primary and metastatic breast carcinoma: initial clinical evaluation with PET with the radiolabeled glucose analog 2-[^{18}F]-fluoro-deoxy-2-D-glucose (FDG). *Radiology* 1991;179:765–770.
19. Wahl RL, Harney J, Hutchins G, et al. Imaging of renal cancer using positron emission tomography with 2-deoxy-2-(^{18}F)-fluoro-D-glucose: pilot animal and human studies. *J Urol* Dec 1991;146(6):1470–1474.
20. Harney JV, Wahl RL, Liebert M, et al. Uptake of 2-deoxy, 2-(^{18}F) fluoro-D-glucose in bladder cancer: animal localization and initial patient positron emission tomography. *J Urol* 1991;145(2):279–283.
21. Wahl RL, Hutchins GD, Roberts J. FDG-PET imaging of ovarian cancer: initial evaluation in patients. *J Nucl Med* 1991;32(5):982.
22. Gritters LS, Francis IR, Zasadny KR, et al. Initial assessment of positron emission tomography using 2-fluorine-^{18}fluoro-2-deoxy-D-glucose in the imaging of malignant melanoma. *J Nucl Med* Sep 1993;34(9):1420–1427.
23. Kubota K, Matsuzawa T, Amemiya A, et al. Imaging of breast cancer with [^{18}F]fluorodeoxyglucose and positron emission tomography. *J Comput Assist Tomogr* 1989;13(6):1097–1098.
24. Dahlbom M, Hoffman EJ, Hoh CK, et al. Whole-body positron emission tomography: part I: methods and performance characteristics. *J Nucl Med* 1992;33:1191–1199.
25. Rosenfeld SS, Hoffman JM, Coleman RE, et al. Studies of primary central nervous system lymphoma with fluorine-18-fluorodeoxyglucose positron emission tomography. *J Nucl Med* Apr 1992;33(4):532–536.
26. Hoh CK, Hawkins RA, Glaspy JA, et al. Cancer detection with whole-body PET using 2-[^{18}F]fluoro-2-deoxy-D-glucose. *J Comput Assist Tomogr* Jul/Aug 1993;17(4):582–589.
27. Brown RS, Wahl RL. Over expression of Glut-1 glucose transporter in human breast cancer: an immunohistochemical study. *Cancer* 1993;72(10):2979–2985.
28. Brown R-S, Fisher S-J, Wahl R-L. Autoradiographic evaluation of the intra-tumoral distribution of 2-deoxy-D-glucose and monoclonal antibodies in xenografts of human ovarian adenocarcinoma. *J Nucl Med* Jan 1993;34(1):75–82.
29. Higashi K, Clavo AC, Wahl RL. Does FDG uptake measure proliferative activity of human cancer cells? *In vitro* comparison with DNA flow cytometry and tritiated thymidine uptake. *J Nucl Med* Mar 1993;34:414–419.
30. Brown RS, Leung JY, Fisher SJ, et al. Intratumoral distribution of tritiated-FDG in breast carcinoma: correlation between Glut-1 expression and FDG uptake. *J Nucl Med* Jun 1996;37(6):1042–1047.
31. Brown RS, Leung JY, Kison PV, et al. Glucose transporters and FDG uptake in untreated primary human non-small cell lung cancer. *J Nucl Med* Apr 1999;40(4):556–565.
32. Wahl RL, Henry CA, Ethier SP. Serum glucose: effects on tumor and normal tissue accumulation of 2-[^{18}F]-fluoro-2-deoxy-D-glucose in rodents with mammary carcinoma. *Radiology* Jun 1992;183(3):643–647.
33. Torizuka T, Fisher SJ, Brown RS, et al. Effect of insulin on uptake of FDG by experimental mammary carcinoma in diabetic rats. *Radiology* Aug 1998;208(2):499–504.
34. Torizuka T, Fisher SJ, Wahl RL. Insulin-induced hypoglycemia decreases uptake of 2-[F-18]fluoro-2-deoxy-D-glucose into experimental mammary carcinoma. *Radiology* Apr 1997;203(1):169–172.
35. Clavo AC, Brown RS, Wahl RL. Fluorodeoxyglucose uptake in human cancer cell lines is increased by hypoxia. *J Nucl Med* Sep 1995;36(9):1625–1632.
36. Clavo AC, Wahl RL. Effects of hypoxia on the uptake of tritiated thymidine, L-leucine, L-methionine and FDG in cultured cancer cells. *J Nucl Med* Mar 1996;37(3):502–506.
37. Aloj L, Caraco C, Jagoda E, et al. Glut-1 and hexokinase expression: relationship with 2-fluoro-2-deoxy-D-glucose uptake in A431 and T47D cells in culture. *Cancer Res* 15 Sep 1999;59(18):4709–4714.
38. Hansen PA, Marshall BA, Chen M, et al. Transgenic overexpression of hexokinase II in skeletal muscle does not increase glucose disposal in wild-type or Glut1-overexpressing mice. *Biol Chem* 21 Jul 2000;275(29):22381–22386.
39. Torizuka T, Zasadny KR, Recker B, et al. Untreated primary lung and breast cancers: correlation between F-18 FDG kinetic rate constants and findings of *in vitro* studies. *Radiology* Jun 1998;207(3):767–774.
40. Kubota R, Yamada S, Kubota K, et al. Intratumoral distribution of

fluorine-18-fluorodeoxyglucose *in vivo:* high accumulation in macrophages and granulation tissues studied by microautography. *J Nucl Med* 1992;33(11):1972–1980.

41. Brown RS, Leung JY, Fisher SJ, et al. Intratumoral distribution of tritiated fluorodeoxyglucose in breast carcinoma, I: are inflammatory cells important? *J Nucl Med* 1995;36(10):1854–1861.

42. Sugawara Y, Braun DK, Kison PV, et al. Rapid detection of human infections with fluorine-18 fluorodeoxyglucose and positron emission tomography: preliminary results. *Eur J Nucl Med* 1998;25(9):1238–1243.

43. Higashi K, Clavo AC, Wahl RL. *In vitro* assessment of 2-fluoro-2-deoxy-D-glucose, L-methionine and thymidine as agents to monitor the early response of a human adenocarcinoma cell line to radiotherapy. *J Nucl Med* 1993;34(5):773–779.

44. Minn HR, Zasadny KR, Quint LE, et al. Lung cancer: reproducibility of quantitative measurements for evaluating 2-[F-18]-fluoro-2-deoxy-D-glucose uptake at PET. *Radiology* 1995;196:167–173.

45. Wahl RL, Zasadny KR, Hutchins GD, et al. Metabolic monitoring of breast cancer chemohormonotherapy using positron emission tomography (PET): initial evaluation. *J Clin Oncol* 1993;11(11):2101–2111.

46. Higashi K, Ueda Y, Seki H, et al. Fluorine-18-FDG-PET imaging is negative in bronchioloalveolar lung carcinoma. *J Nucl Med* Jun 1998;39(6):1016–1020.

47. Shreve PD, Grossman HB, Gross MD, et al. Metastatic prostate cancer: initial findings of PET with 2-deoxy-2-[F-18]fluoro-D-glucose. *Radiology* Jun 1996;199(3):751–756.

48. Kobori O, Kirihara Y, Kosaka N, et al. Positron emission tomography of esophageal carcinoma using (11)C-choline and (18)F-fluorodeoxyglucose: a novel method of preoperative lymph node staging. *Cancer* 1999;86(9):1638–1648.

49. Raylman RR, Kison PV, Wahl RL. Capabilities of two- and three-dimensional FDG-PET for detecting small lesions and lymph nodes in the upper torso: a dynamic phantom study. *Eur J Nucl Med* Jan 1999;26(1):39–45.

50. Macfarlane DJ, Cotton L, Ackermann RJ, et al. Triple-head SPECT with 2-[fluorine-18]fluoro-2-deoxy-D-glucose (FDG): initial evaluation in oncology and comparison with FDG-PET. *Radiology* Feb 1995;194(2):425–429.

51. Mastin ST, Drane WE, Harman EM, et al. FDG SPECT in patients with lung masses. *Chest* Apr 1999;115(4):1012–1017.

52. Shreve PD, Steventon RS, Deters EC, et al. Oncologic diagnosis with 2-[fluorine-18]fluoro-2-deoxy-D-glucose imaging: dual-head coincidence gamma camera versus positron emission tomographic scanner. *Radiology* May 1998;207(2):431–437.

53. Delbeke D, Sandler MP. The role of hybrid cameras in oncology. *Semin Nucl Med* Oct 2000;30(4):268–280.

54. Sugawara Y, Fisher SJ, Zasadny KR, et al. Preclinical and clinical studies of bone marrow uptake of fluorine-1-fluorodeoxyglucose with or without granulocyte colony-stimulating factor during chemotherapy. *J Clin Oncol* Jan 1998;16(1):173–180.

55. Wahl RL. To AC or not to AC: that is the question. *J Nucl Med* Dec 1999;40(12):2025–2028.

56. Beyer T, Townsend DW, Brun T, et al. A combined PET/CT scanner for clinical oncology. *J Nucl Med* Aug 2000;41(8):1369–1379.

57. Zasadny KR, Wahl RL. Standardized uptake values of normal tissues at PET with 2-[fluorine-18]-fluoro-2-deoxy-D-glucose: variations with body weight and a method for correction. *Radiology* Dec 1993;189(3):847–850.

58. Sugawara Y, Zasadny KR, Neuhoff AW, et al. Reevaluation of the standardized uptake value for FDG: variations with body weight and methods for correction. *Radiology* Nov 1999;213(2):521–525.

59. Park KC, Schwimmer J, Shepherd JE, et al. Decision analysis for the cost-effective management of recurrent colorectal cancer. *Ann Surg* 2001;233(3):310–319.

60. Valk PE. Clinical trials of cost effectiveness in technology evaluation. *Q J Nucl Med* 2000;44(2):197–203.

Normal Variants in FDG PET Imaging

Paul D. Shreve and Chuong Dac Huy Bui

Advances in positron emission tomography (PET) capability and widespread recognition of the value of fluorodeoxyglucose-positron emission tomography (FDG PET) in oncology has led to the routine whole-body (torso or abdomen) imaging for most oncologic indications. The high FDG uptake by most malignancies relative to the level of FDG distributed throughout much of the body facilitates identification of malignant neoplasms. Compared with conventional anatomic approaches, whole-body FDG PET often permits much more rapid and accurate identification of the presence and extent of malignant disease. Focal FDG tracer accumulation due to cancer, however, must be distinguished from normal, normal variant, and benign pathologic sources of FDG uptake. This is a principal task in the interpretation of whole-body FDG PET scans applied to oncologic diagnoses.

FDG tracer uptake depicts tissue glucose metabolism. Hence, in addition to the abnormal glucose metabolism associated with malignant neoplasm, both normal variations in glucose metabolism and increased glucose metabolism due to various pathologies are revealed on FDG PET. Interpretation of whole-body FDG PET requires knowledge of normal and normal variant patterns of FDG uptake, as well as familiarity with the many benign pathologic causes of increased FDG uptake. Frequently, both anatomic and physiologic knowledge is needed to reliably identify sites of FDG uptake with normal, variant, or benign pathologic etiologies.

NORMAL WHOLE-BODY FDG DISTRIBUTION

On whole-body PET performed between 1 and 2 hours after intravenous administration of FDG, the brain, heart, and urinary tract are the most prominent sites of tracer accumulation (Fig. 5.2.1). The brain, an obligate user of glucose, is always prominent relative to the rest of the body. Both supratentorial and infratentorial gray matter are FDG avid, and the level of FDG uptake is in the range typical of FDG-avid malignancies. The myocardium has similar FDG avidity in the fed state, but with a sufficiently long fast (typically more than 12 hours), the myocardial metabolism shifts to fatty acids as a source of energy, and the myocardial uptake

becomes largely indistinguishable from blood pool tracer activity. FDG follows a urinary excretory route, and in the absence of aggressive hydration, diuretics, and urinary catheterization, FDG is present in the bladder and to varying degrees in the upper urinary tract.

Elsewhere, tracer activity is distributed at low levels in recognizable anatomic structures on attenuation-corrected images (Fig. 5.2.1). Cardiac and mediastinal great vessel blood pool is discernible against the very low tracer activity of the lungs (Fig. 5.2.2). The liver and spleen are associated with slightly higher FDG activity than blood pool levels and are reliably identified in the abdomen, as are the kidneys. The pancreas is normally not discretely identified. Bowel is seen to varying degrees, as is the stomach, due to widely variable levels of FDG uptake in the alimentary tract. Bone marrow normally is associated with FDG accumulation at levels higher than blood pool activity, and vertebral bodies are consistently identified, as well as other major marrow-containing skeletal structures such as the pelvis, hips, and sternum. Lymphoid tissue in the neck that is associated with the palatine tonsils is consistently FDG avid and typically clearly identified. FDG activity in the neck associated with laryngeal musculature or thyroid tissue is frequently seen. Glandular tissue of the breast is associated with low-level uptake, slightly greater than blood pool in younger women (Fig. 5.2.2).

NORMAL VARIANT FDG DISTRIBUTION

Myocardium

Uptake of FDG in myocardium in patients who fast for 4 to 18 hours is variable, ranging from uniform and intense to nearly absent. In the fed state, FDG uptake in intact myocardium is intense, on the order of brain gray matter. With a sufficient fast, the heart will shift energy metabolism from glucose to fatty acids (1) and demonstrate little FDG uptake. In practice, however, even with overnight fasting, FDG uptake in myocardium is not reliably absent. With contemporary PET images and image-reconstruction software, the presence of intense FDG uptake in the myocardium does not

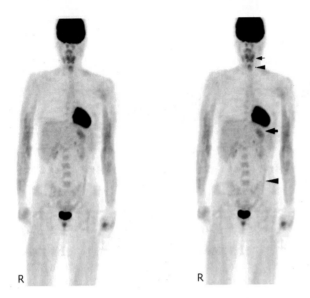

FIG. 5.2.1. Normal whole-body distribution of fluorodeoxyglucose. Attenuation-corrected anterior projection image. Intense tracer activity is present in the brain, heart, and bladder. In the neck, parapharyngeal tonsillar lymphoid activity (*small arrow*) and minimal thyroid/laryngeal muscle activity is seen (*small arrowhead*). Inferior to the heart is low-level gastric activity (*large arrow*) and the outlines of the liver, spleen, and kidneys are discernible. Normal bone marrow tracer activity defines the vertebral bodies and pelvis. Vertical linear activity in the left abdomen and pelvis is the left colon (*large arrowhead*). Some increased muscle uptake is present in the arms.

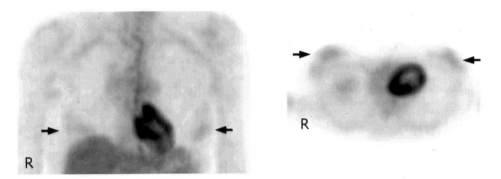

FIG. 5.2.2. Normal distribution of fluorodeoxyglucose in the chest. Attenuation-corrected anterior projection image and transaxial image. Normal breast glandular tissue is present (*arrows*). The blood pool in the mediastinum is seen due to the very low level of tracer activity in the lungs. Myocardial uptake is heterogeneous but intense. Normal liver and spleen activity is delineated in the upper abdomen.

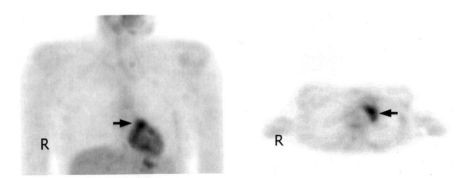

FIG. 5.2.3. Inhomogeneous myocardial fluorodeoxyglucose (FDG) uptake. Attenuation-corrected anterior projection image and transaxial image. Myocardial FDG uptake is inhomogeneous as heart muscle shifts from glycolytic to fatty acid metabolism in fasted patients. The base of the heart is often the last to lose FDG uptake, resulting in focal uptake in the mediastinum that should not be mistaken for mediastinal lymph nodes.

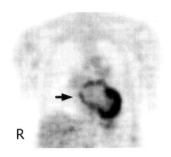
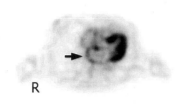

FIG. 5.2.4. Atrial muscle fluorodeoxyglucose uptake. Attenuation corrected coronal and transaxial images. Uptake in atrial myocardium is often detected, can be irregular and may be associated with somewhat focal activity. This pattern should not be mistaken for mediastinal lymph nodes.

generally present limitations in interpretation, except perhaps abnormalities associated with the pericardium or directly adjacent lung. The transition from the intense FDG uptake of dominant glycolytic myocardial metabolism to absent FDG uptake of dominant fatty acid metabolism is frequently nonuniform. The base of the left ventricular myocardium tends to be the last portion to lose glucose avidity. An irregular distribution of FDG in the left ventricular myocardium can be observed in patients who have fasted 4 to 18 hours. This may give the appearance of discrete foci at the base of the heart, which could be misinterpreted as FDG-avid mediastinal lymph nodes if anatomic relationships are not appreciated (Fig. 5.2.3). In addition, atrial tissue is sometimes discernible, and again irregular FDG distribution can occur and appear to be small focal abnormalities in the mediastinum (Fig. 5.2.4). In the fed state, right ventricular myocardium is typically seen at low levels but can become as prominent as left ventricular myocardium in the setting of right ventricular hypertrophy.

Skeletal Muscle

At rest, skeletal muscle relies on fatty acid oxidative metabolism for energy. With increased energy demand, glycolysis becomes the major source of energy for skeletal muscle and depends on relative oxygen delivery and tissue oxidative capacity. Fast-twitch muscle fibers, with sparse mitochondria and limited oxidative capacity, are associated with a consistently high glucose demand. Extraocular muscles routinely demonstrate elevated FDG accumulation (2). Skeletal muscle composed of slow-twitch fibers will demonstrate glucose uptake during active contraction or after glycogen depletion. Skeletal muscle undergoing active contraction during the FDG uptake phase (largely, the first 30 minutes after tracer administration) will demonstrate elevated FDG accumulation. Heavy use of skeletal muscle before injection of FDG may also result in FDG uptake, likely related to replenishment of glycogen stores (3). For this reason, patients are typically advised to refrain from heavy exercise the day before their FDG PET examination, and after FDG administration, they are asked to sit semirecumbent or lie quietly. Insulin increases muscle uptake of glucose and insu-

lin given before or immediately after FDG administration will result in diffusely increased muscle uptake (4).

Low-level uptake in the forearm muscles is relatively common (Fig. 5.2.1). Major truncal muscles can be prominent with patients who have been physically active even hours before FDG injection (Fig. 5.2.5). Heavy ventilatory efforts associated with physical exertion or pulmonary disease commonly result in identifiable intercostal muscles (Fig. 5.2.5) and diaphragmatic crura (Fig. 5.2.6). Symmetric uptake in the strap muscles of the neck and thoracic paravertebral musculature (Figs. 5.2.5 and 5.2.7) is frequently seen and has been attributed in some instances to patient anxiety

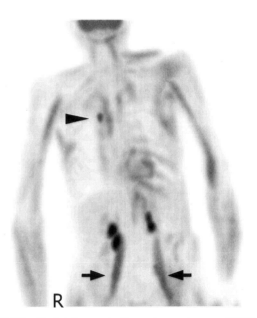

FIG. 5.2.5. Skeletal muscle fluorodeoxyglucose (FDG) uptake. Attenuation-corrected posterior projection image. Vigorous exercise even before FDG administration can manifest as prominent FDG uptake in major muscle groups. Uptake defining portions of musculature in the arms, shoulders, paraspinal, intercostal, and psoas muscles (*arrows*) is evident. Focal tracer activity bilaterally at the cephalad aspects of the psoas muscle activity is FDG in the intrarenal collecting systems. A small focus of tracer in the chest (*arrowhead*) is an FDG-avid lung nodule.

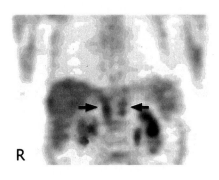
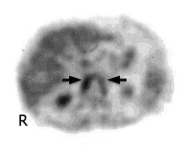
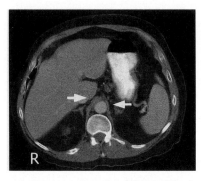

FIG. 5.2.6. Fluorodeoxyglucose (FDG) uptake in diaphragmatic crura muscle. Attenuation-corrected coronal and transaxial images, and corresponding transaxial computed tomography. Elevated ventilatory efforts during the FDG uptake phase, such as in patients with severe chronic obstructive pulmonary disease, may result in FDG uptake in intercostal and diaphragmatic muscles. Focal FDG uptake in the diaphragmatic crural muscles can occur, but typically it is seen as the somewhat elongated configuration of the crura and should not be mistaken for FDG-avid retroperitoneal lymph nodes.

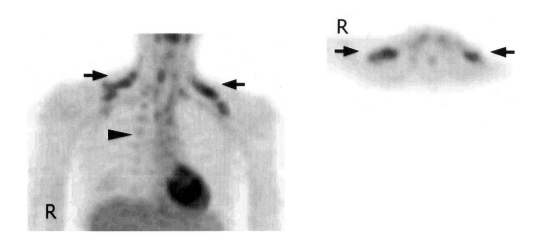

FIG. 5.2.7. Fluorodeoxyglucose (FDG) uptake in the strap muscles of the neck. Attenuation-corrected anterior projection and transaxial images. FDG uptake is present in portions of the supraspinatus and scalene muscles (*arrows*). Repeated isolated foci corresponding to the paraspinal muscles (*arrowhead*) are also present. Muscle insertions and origins associated with the base of the neck and the clavicles frequently demonstrate FDG uptake, which can be focal and mistaken for supraclavicular lymph nodes or nodal groups at the neck base.

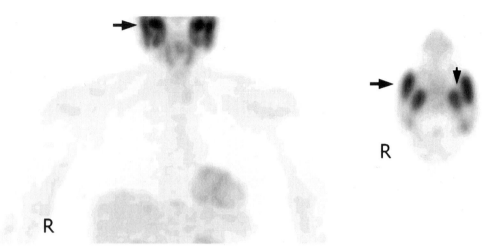

FIG. 5.2.8. Fluorodeoxyglucose (FDG) uptake in the muscles of mastication. Attenuation-corrected anterior projection and transaxial images. Intense FDG uptake in the masseter (*arrow*) and lateral pterygoid (*short-tailed arrow*) muscles. Activities such as gum chewing before or during the FDG uptake phase can result in intense FDG accumulation in these muscles. In patients who have undergone head and neck surgery, altered muscle balance can result in FDG uptake in an asymmetric or isolated pattern in muscles such as pterygoids, which should not be confused with infratemporal fossa tumor recurrence or a metastasis.

(5,6). Although the symmetry and configuration of muscle FDG uptake generally permit correct identification (Fig. 5.2.8), FDG uptake does not always appear in the entire muscle. Focal activity at the origin or insertion of muscle occurs frequently, particularly with the musculature associated with the head and neck, where supraclavicular foci of FDG uptake due to muscle uptake can be difficult to distinguish from nodal abnormalities, particularly when symmetry is absent. Likewise, imbalance in muscle groups due to disease or associated treatment such as surgery can result in focal asymmetric FDG uptake, which in certain locations such as the neck can lead to potential misdiagnosis (7). Recently, increased uptake into fat in the neck has been described as being a normal variant (RL Wahl, personal communication).

Speech during the uptake phase of FDG increases FDG activity in the laryngeal muscles and the tongue (8). In the absence of prior related surgery, laryngeal musculature uptake is nearly always symmetric (Fig. 5.2.9) and readily appreciated as normal. Tongue uptake varies from mild to intense, typically involves the entire tongue, and is easily recognizable on projection and sagittal images. Isolated focal uptake can be seen, however (Fig. 5.2.10). Prior surgery involving the larynx or tongue can yield focal asymmetric muscle uptake that may be indistinguishable from residual or recurrent malignancy. Asymmetric or isolated major muscle FDG uptake can be confounding in the shoulder girdle musculature. The teres minor muscle is commonly seen and should not be confused with a metastasis or other pathology in the shoulder region (Fig. 5.2.11).

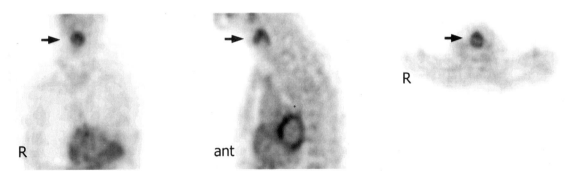

FIG. 5.2.9. Laryngeal musculature fluorodeoxyglucose (FDG) uptake. Attenuation-corrected projection, sagittal, and transaxial images. If the patient uses muscles associated with vocalization during the FDG uptake phase, he or she may show increased tracer accumulation. Symmetry and location usually allow identification, as in this example (*arrow*), where the cricothyroid and cricoarytenoid muscles form a symmetric ring of activity on the transaxial image. Surgery in this area can alter muscle symmetry and balance, as well as result in focal unilateral or asymmetric tracer activity that is very difficult to distinguish from recurrent or metastatic neoplasm.

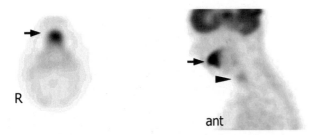

FIG. 5.2.10. Fluorodeoxyglucose (FDG) uptake in the tongue. Attenuation-corrected transaxial and sagittal images. The tongue is usually seen as low-level tracer activity, but vocalization during the FDG uptake phase can result in intense FDG uptake, typically comprising the entire tongue. Focal uptake (*arrow*), however, can occur, which is potentially indistinguishable from a tongue neoplasm. Low-level laryngeal musculature is also present (*arrowhead*). Surgery, including resection of neoplasm and reconstruction, can alter tongue musculature balance, which can also lead to focal muscle tracer activity that is very difficult to distinguish from recurrent or metastatic neoplasm.

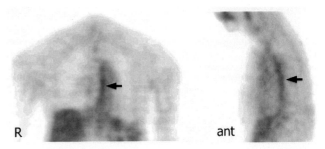

FIG. 5.2.12. Normal esophageal fluorodeoxyglucose (FDG) uptake. Attenuation-corrected coronal and sagittal images. FDG uptake slightly above blood pool is present throughout much of the esophagus (*arrow*).

Alimentary Tract

FDG uptake in the alimentary tact, from esophagus to rectosigmoid colon, is widely variable, in terms of both distribution and intensity. The etiology of FDG uptake in the alimentary tract is presently not understood and may reflect different normal and benign pathologic phenomena in different portions of the alimentary tract.

The esophagus occasionally is associated with low-level activity throughout its extent (Fig. 5.2.12). Relatively intense fusiform and extended FDG uptake occurs in the presence of esophagitis (Fig. 5.2.13), which is indistinguishable from the configuration of esophageal cancer. Esophagitis is common and often asymptomatic; hence, FDG uptake in the esophagus is not specific for esophageal malignancy. A small focus of FDG activity is frequently seen at the gastroesophageal junction (Fig. 5.2.14), possibly related to the lower esophageal splinter, and likewise should not be presumed to be related to malignancy.

The normal stomach commonly shows FDG uptake that is usually somewhat greater than FDG activity in the liver and readily identifiable based on location and configuration (Fig. 5.2.15). Gastric FDG uptake can be intense if the stomach is contracted and it may appear as an isolated FDG-avid mass that is potentially indistinguishable from a malignant tumor. Location and configuration of the stomach, as well as distribution of FDG uptake in the gastric wall, can be variable and in some instances may require careful anatomic correlation to confirm that the FDG uptake is of gastric origin (Fig. 5.2.16). Gastric lymphoma and gastric carcinoma are not reliably diagnosed on FDG PET alone. The propensity for gastric FDG uptake is maintained in hiatal hernias but those must be differentiated from esophageal concerns (Fig. 5.2.17).

Bowel, particularly the right colon (Fig. 5.2.16), commonly demonstrates FDG uptake. The bowel uptake appears to be in the wall and may reflect to varying degrees active smooth muscle, metabolically active mucosa, bowel wall lymphoid tissue, swallowed secretions, or colonic microbial activity. Uptake is typically segmental or contiguous in the colon, and the appearance of projection images can be reminiscent of radiographic contrast studies of the colon (Fig. 5.2.18). Small-bowel FDG activity is usually lower in intensity than FDG activity observed in the colon and is typically seen in the lower pelvis (Fig. 5.2.19). The continuous or

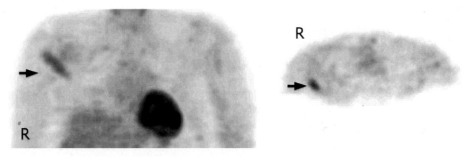

FIG. 5.2.11. Shoulder muscle fluorodeoxyglucose uptake. Attenuation-corrected anterior projection and transaxial images. For unclear reasons, the teres minor muscle frequently is seen, typically in a unilateral pattern.

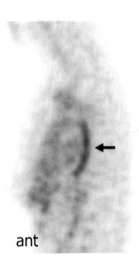
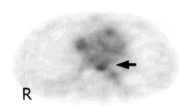

FIG. 5.2.13. Esophageal fluorodeoxyglucose (FDG) uptake associated with esophagitis. Attenuation-corrected sagittal and transaxial images. Long segmental FDG uptake (*arrow*) in the esophagus, corresponding to endoscopic findings of esophagitis. Esophageal cancer can yield a similar, but generally more intense and focal, pattern of tracer activity.

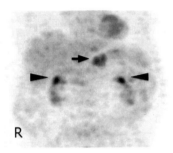
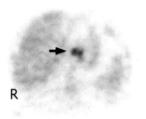
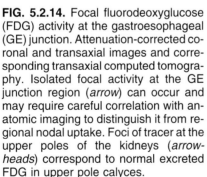
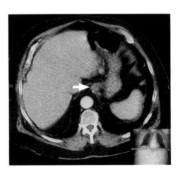

FIG. 5.2.14. Focal fluorodeoxyglucose (FDG) activity at the gastroesophageal (GE) junction. Attenuation-corrected coronal and transaxial images and corresponding transaxial computed tomography. Isolated focal activity at the GE junction region (*arrow*) can occur and may require careful correlation with anatomic imaging to distinguish it from regional nodal uptake. Foci of tracer at the upper poles of the kidneys (*arrowheads*) correspond to normal excreted FDG in upper pole calyces.

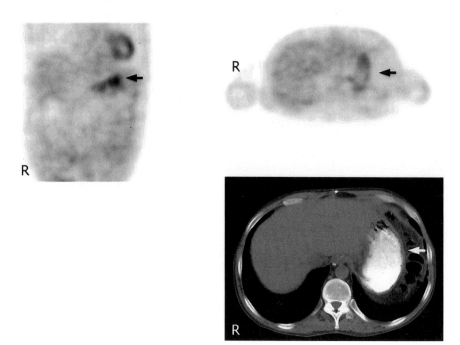

FIG. 5.2.15. Gastric fluorodeoxyglucose (FDG) uptake. Attenuation-corrected coronal and transaxial images and corresponding transaxial computed tomography. Location and configuration usually readily identify FDG uptake in the stomach wall (*arrow*).

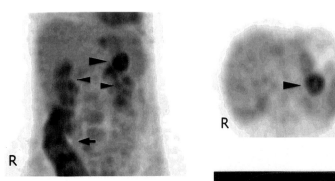

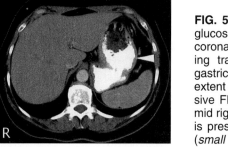

FIG. 5.2.16. Gastric and colonic fluorodeoxyglucose (FDG) uptake. Attenuation-corrected coronal and transaxial images and corresponding transaxial computed tomography. Focal gastric activity corresponding to the posterior extent of the stomach (*large arrowhead*). Extensive FDG uptake is seen in the proximal and mid right colon (*arrow*). Excreted urinary tracer is present in the intrarenal collecting systems (*small arrowheads*).

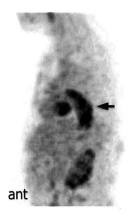

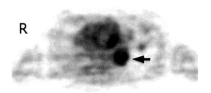

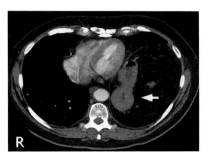

FIG. 5.2.17. Intrathoracic gastric fluorodeoxyglucose (FDG) uptake in a partially intrathoracic stomach. Attenuation-corrected sagittal and coronal images and corresponding transaxial computed tomography. When the stomach is in an unusual location gastric uptake requires anatomic correlation to confirm the physiologic origin.

segmental components of its appearance make proper identification possible.

Focality of FDG uptake in either the large or the small bowel can be confounding, because peritoneal metastatic implants or mesenteric lymph node pathology may be entirely indistinguishable. In some instances, careful anatomic correlation can be helpful in assigning isolated focal FDG uptake in the abdomen or pelvis to bowel origin (Fig. 5.2.20). The clinical significance of focal FDG uptake is not yet established, although preliminary reports have attributed such uptake to villous adenomas or carcinoma (9). Inflammatory bowel disease is known to cause diffuse or segmental FDG uptake (10). Some investigators have reported success in reducing bowel FDG uptake using smooth-muscle relax-

ants immediately before FDG administration (11) or isosmotic bowel preparations the evening before the examination (12). These are not well-established methods, however.

Genitourinary Tract

Unlike glucose, FDG is not well reabsorbed by the tubular cells of the kidney, and the excretory route of FDG in the

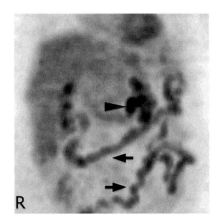

FIG. 5.2.18. Bowel fluorodeoxyglucose (FDG) uptake. Attenuation-corrected anterior projection image. Segments or the entire colon frequently are associated with increased FDG uptake (*arrows*). Excreted urinary tracer in the renal calyces and left renal pelvis is also present (*arrowhead*).

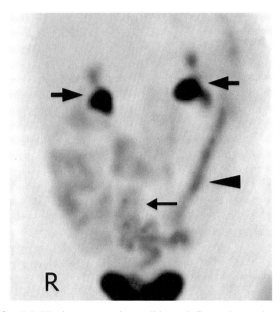

FIG. 5.2.19. Large- and small-bowel fluorodeoxyglucose (FDG) uptake. Attenuation-corrected anterior projection image. FDG uptake in the right colon, left colon (*arrowhead*) extending into the sigmoid colon. FDG uptake in the distal small bowel adjacent to the cecum is also present (*arrow*). Urinary FDG activity is present in the renal pelves (*short-tailed arrows*).

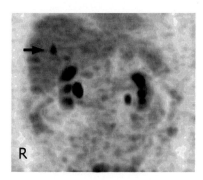

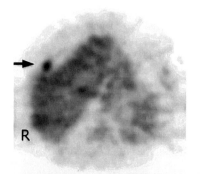

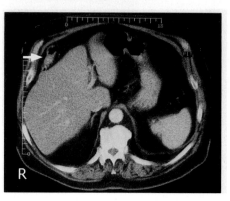

FIG. 5.2.20. Small focal colonic fluorodeoxyglucose (FDG) uptake. Attenuation-corrected anterior projection and transaxial images and corresponding computed tomography transaxial image. Focal, in contrast to segmental, bowel uptake can be difficult to assign to bowel, particularly when in an atypical location. Focal activity in the interposed hepatic flexure (*arrow*) would be nearly impossible to assign to bowel without anatomic correlation.

urine results in intense tracer activity in the intrarenal collecting systems, ureters, and bladder (Fig. 5.2.21). The presence of urinary tracer in the intrarenal collecting systems and ureters is dependent on the degree of hydration and renal function of the patient. Both hydration and use of furosemide

have been advocated to facilitate clearance of FDG from the intrarenal collecting systems and ureters (13). In most instances, however, the intensity and location of the urinary FDG permits correct identification of the calyces, renal pelves, and ureters.

The dependent location of the upper pole renal calyces in the supine patient frequently results in urinary tracer pooling (Fig. 5.2.22), which should not be confused with abnormal tracer uptake in adjacent structures such as the adrenal. Likewise, abnormalities in the upper urinary tract such as urinary diversions, redundant and dilated ureters, diverticula, or communicating cysts can result in focal tracer activity that could be confused with an FDG-avid mass (Fig. 5.2.23); correlation with anatomic imaging can be essential in such circumstances.

Occasionally, ureteral activity will be limited to a small isolated focus (Fig. 5.2.24), which can be very difficult to differentiate from a retroperitoneal lymph node. With contemporary image-reconstruction algorithms, intense urinary tracer activity in the bladder does not significantly compromise assessment of regional structures, and anatomic alterations such as diverticula or transurethral resection of the prostate (TURP) defects are discernible (Fig. 5.2.25). Tracer activity in the bladder can be reduced by use of urinary bladder catheterization and lavage (13).

Uterine endometrium can demonstrate elevated FDG uptake, which should not be confused with uterine or presacral neoplasm (14). Moderately intense FDG uptake occurs in the testes (Fig. 5.2.26), which is a consistently normal finding, and tends to decline with advancing age (15).

FIG. 5.2.21. Urinary tract. Attenuation-corrected anterior projection image. Excreted urinary fluorodeoxyglucose tracer is present in the intrarenal collecting systems (*short-tailed arrow*), ureters (*arrowheads*), and bladder (*arrow*).

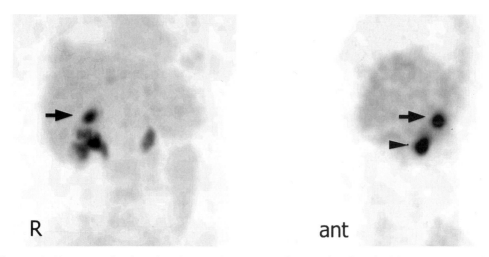

FIG. 5.2.22. Upper renal pole calyx. Attenuation-corrected coronal and sagittal images. Urinary fluoro-deoxyglucose tracer often pools in the dependent portion of the intrarenal collecting system. Upper pole calyceal tracer activity (*arrow*), and tracer in renal pelvis (*arrowhead*).

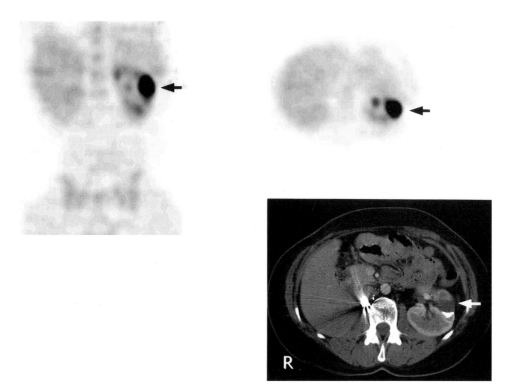

FIG. 5.2.23. Calyceal diverticulum. Attenuation-corrected coronal and axial images and corresponding transaxial computed tomography. Urinary tracer accumulation in a left renal calyceal diverticulum (*arrow*).

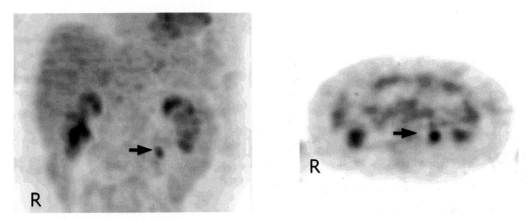

FIG. 5.2.24. Isolated ureteral fluorodeoxyglucose (FDG) urinary activity. Attenuation-corrected coronal and transaxial images. Focal tracer activity in a ureter (*arrow*) can be difficult to distinguish from an FDG-avid retroperitoneal lymph node.

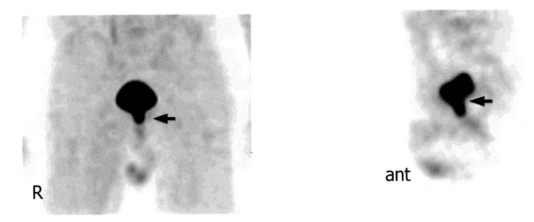

FIG. 5.2.25. Urinary bladder fluorodeoxyglucose activity. Attenuation-corrected anterior projection and sagittal images. Anatomic alterations of the bladder such as this transurethral resection of the prostate defect (*arrow*) are analogous to images obtained with contrast radiographs or computed tomography.

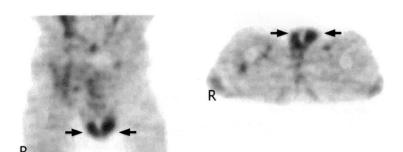

FIG. 5.2.26. Testicular fluorodeoxyglucose (FDG) uptake. Attenuation-corrected coronal and transaxial images. Testicular FDG uptake (*arrows*) is a normal finding.

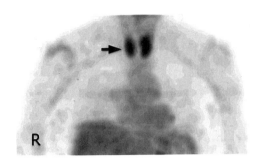
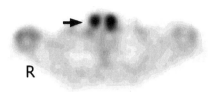
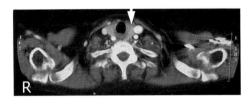

FIG. 5.2.27. Thyroid fluorodeoxyglucose (FDG) uptake. Attenuation-corrected anterior projection and transaxial images, and corresponding transaxial computed tomography. FDG uptake can be absent, mild, or present at relatively high levels in euthyroid patients.

Thyroid

Healthy thyroid tissue can demonstrate moderate to intense FDG uptake (Fig. 5.2.27). In one series, one third of clinically euthyroid patients demonstrated observable thyroid tissue FDG uptake in both lobes of the gland (16). The etiology and implications of this are not entirely understood, although thyroiditis is associated with a similar or more intense degree of FDG uptake (Fig. 5.2.28).

Bone Marrow

Bone marrow normally has mild to moderate FDG uptake, roughly equivalent to that of liver. Marrow is commonly identified in the vertebral bodies, pelvis, hips, proximal long bones, and the sternum. Any process disturbing marrow distribution will alter the marrow-related FDG distribution. For example, vertebral body marrow activity is diminished with loss of vertebral body height in patients with insufficiency

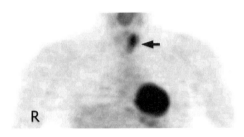
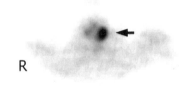
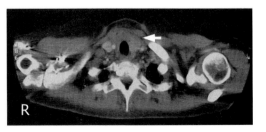

FIG. 5.2.28. Thyroiditis. Attenuation-corrected anterior projection and transaxial images, and corresponding transaxial computed tomography. Somewhat focal activity in the left lobe of the thyroid corresponding to surgically proven thyroiditis. The left thyroid lobe and isthmus were surgically removed.

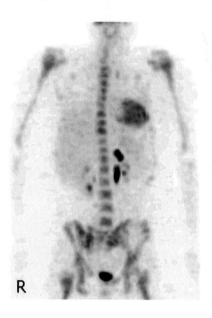
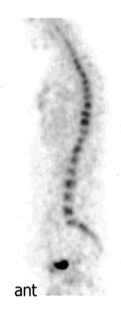

FIG. 5.2.29. Bone marrow under hematopoietic stimulation. Attenuation-corrected anterior projection and sagittal images. This patient with lymphoma had been treated with a chemotherapy regimen that included colony stimulating factor. Normal bone marrow fluorodeoxyglucose uptake is increased.

compression deformities or fractures, resulting in apparent relatively "hot" vertebral bodies that could be misinterpreted as metastatic foci in vertebral bone marrow. Patients undergoing treatment with hematopoietic stimulants such as granulocyte colony-stimulating factor will have increased bone-marrow FDG uptake (Fig. 5.2.29), which can be intense and extensive and should not be confused with disseminated tumor in the marrow (17).

Lymphoid Tissue

Lymphoid tissue in certain locations is associated with sufficient FDG uptake to be routinely identified. The palatine tonsils are almost always identified and can have fairly intense tracer uptake (Fig. 5.2.30), and usually this is where

the associated lymphoid tissue of Waldeyer ring is discernible (2). The thymus is well delineated in young patients with FDG uptake modestly above blood pool, and it is usually easily identified based on configuration, particularly on projection image reconstructions (Fig. 5.2.31).

FDG UPTAKE IN NONMALIGNANT TUMORS

The increased glycolysis and cellular glucose uptake associated with malignant transformation underlies the detection of cancer using FDG PET. Certain benign tumors have increased FDG uptake, and they can have an intensity that is entirely within the range of malignant neoplasms. Goitrous thyroid can be associated with increased FDG uptake, with

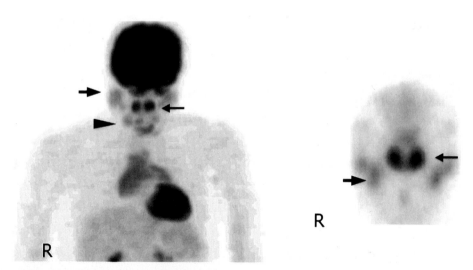

FIG. 5.2.30. Salivary gland and tonsillar fluorodeoxyglucose (FDG) uptake. Attenuation-corrected anterior projection and transaxial images. Salivary glands such as parotid (*arrow*) and submandibular glands (*arrowhead*) are typically identified by modest FDG uptake. Palatine tonsils are almost always identified and can exhibit relatively prominent FDG uptake (*small arrows*).

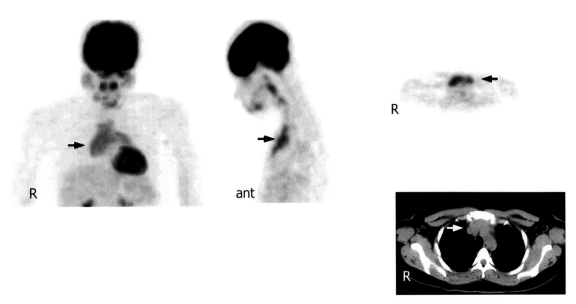

FIG. 5.2.31. Thymus. Attenuation-corrected anterior projection, sagittal, and transaxial images, as well as corresponding transaxial computed tomography. In young patients, the thymus is normally associated with moderate FDG uptake. Due to its bulk and configuration, it is readily seen on fluorodeoxyglucose PET, as in this 25-year-old woman who is 12 months after undergoing chemotherapy for lymphoma.

the size, configuration, and inhomogeneity entirely reminiscent of a radionuclide thyroid scan (Fig. 5.2.32). Benign thyroid nodules can also result in focal FDG uptake, which could be mistaken for malignancy (Fig. 5.2.33).

Although FDG PET has been reported to have a high level of accuracy in the diagnosis of adrenal nodules due to metastatic disease (18), benign hypertrophy of the adrenals can yield identifiable FDG uptake (Fig. 5.2.34). Anatomic correlation is essential when adrenal FDG uptake is present. Gynecomastia in men can result in unexpected somewhat focal areas of FDG uptake in the chest wall (Fig. 5.2.35). Again, anatomic correlation is essential in determining the benign etiology of such findings.

BENIGN PATHOLOGIC FDG UPTAKE DUE TO INFLAMMATION

Inflammation in myriad manifestations is the most significant cause of FDG uptake that can be mistaken for malignant disease. Glycolytic metabolism is elevated in the leukocyte infiltration associated with inflammatory processes (19), so sterile, pyogenic, and granulomatous inflammation are associated with increased FDG uptake. In some instances, the configuration and/or location of FDG uptake is easily identified as due to inflammation. In other instances, careful anatomic correlation is required to confirm the benign etiology, and finally in many cases such as with lymph nodes, it is not possible to distinguish benign inflammatory FDG uptake from malignancy.

Normal wound healing is associated with an inflammatory response and modest FDG uptake is associated with healing wounds (Fig. 5.2.36). Similarly, the inflammatory response associated with tissue resorption results in modest FDG uptake in a resolving hematoma or thrombus. FDG is quite sensitive to inflammation, with focal uptake readily seen at the entrance site of uncomplicated indwelling percutaneous tubes or lines (Fig. 5.2.37) or even small cutaneous carbuncles (Fig. 5.2.38). Ostomies will show modest FDG uptake.

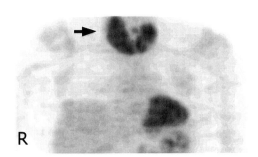

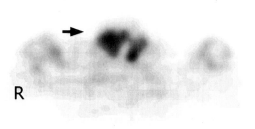

FIG. 5.2.32. Thyroid goiter. Attenuation-corrected anterior projection and transaxial images. Goitrous thyroid exhibits increased fluorodeoxyglucose uptake with discernible heterogeneity.

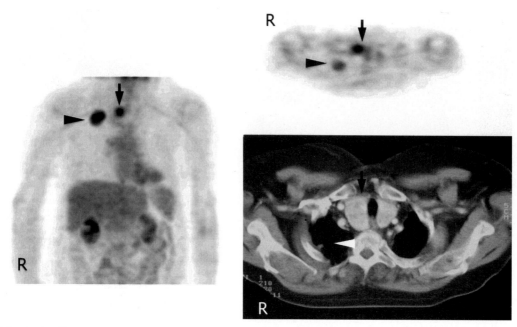

FIG. 5.2.33. Thyroid nodule. Attenuation-corrected anterior projection and transaxial images and corresponding transaxial computed tomography. Benign thyroid nodules can exhibit focal increased tracer uptake (*arrow*), as in this patient with an incidental benign thyroid nodule. Focal tracer in right lung apex (*arrowhead*) is a primary lung cancer.

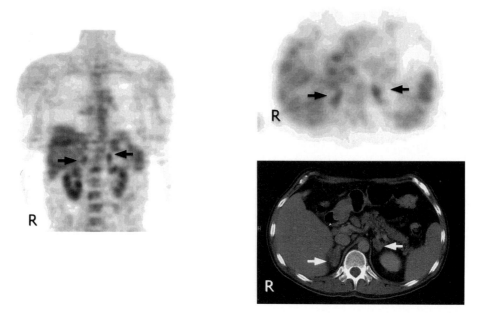

FIG. 5.2.34. Adrenal hypertrophy. Attenuation-corrected anterior projection and transaxial images and corresponding transaxial computed tomography. Adrenal hypertrophy is associated with modest fluorodeoxyglucose uptake (*arrows*).

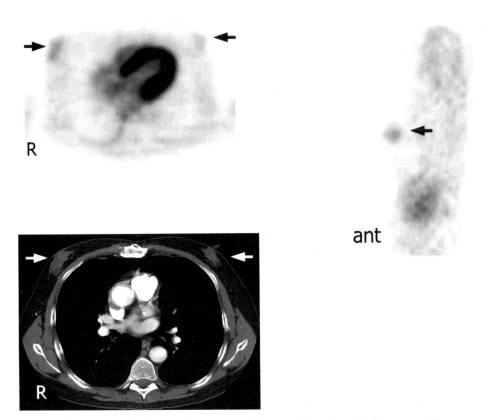

FIG. 5.2.35. Gynecomastia. Attenuation-corrected transaxial and sagittal images with corresponding transaxial computed tomography. Small foci of glandular tissue are associated with moderate fluorodeoxyglucose uptake (*arrows*).

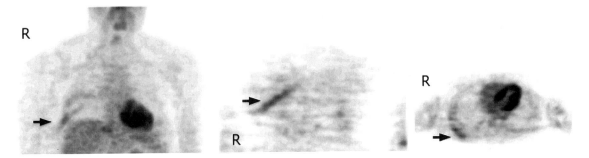

FIG. 5.2.36. Wound healing. Attenuation-corrected anterior projection, coronal, and transaxial images. Linear fluorodeoxyglucose uptake along a healing incision in the right posterior chest (*arrow*) in a patient 2 months after undergoing right thoracotomy.

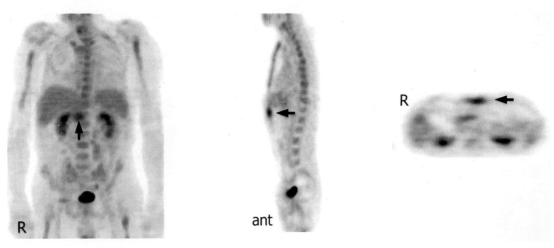

FIG. 5.2.37. Percutaneous tube insertion. Attenuation-corrected anterior projection and sagittal and transaxial images. Focal fluorodeoxyglucose accumulation (*arrow*) at the uncomplicated insertion site of an indwelling percutaneous gastric feeding tube.

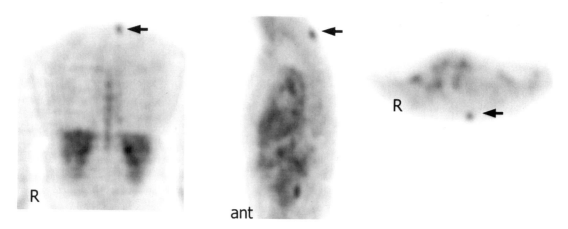

FIG. 5.2.38. Cutaneous carbuncle. Attenuation-corrected coronal, sagittal, and transaxial images. Small focus of fluorodeoxyglucose uptake (*arrow*) associated with a clinically insignificant cutaneous carbuncle.

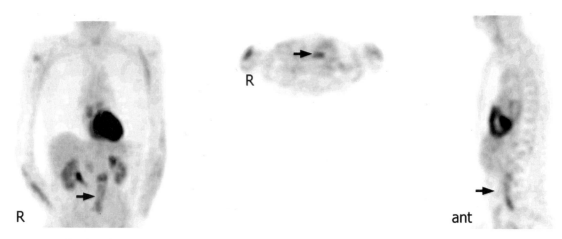

FIG. 5.2.39. Aortic graft. Attenuation-corrected anterior projection and transaxial and sagittal images. Tubular pattern of fluorodeoxyglucose accumulation (*arrow*) in the retroperitoneum corresponding to a normal established aortic graft. This was an incidental finding in a patient years after undergoing graft placement.

128

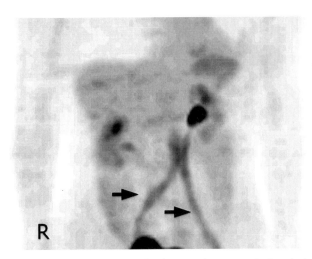

FIG. 5.2.40. Bifemoral graft. Attenuation-corrected anterior projection image. Fluorodeoxyglucose (FDG) accumulation (*arrow*) in bifemoral grafts. Normal colon and urinary FDG uptake is also seen.

Vascular grafts are associated with moderate FDG uptake and are frequently observed (Figs. 5.2.39 and 5.2.40). The presence of FDG uptake does not indicate infection, although infected grafts would be expected to be FDG avid. Major arterial vessels involved with advanced atheromatous disease such as the abdominal or thoracic aorta will often be unexpectedly conspicuous due to FDG uptake in the vessel wall (20) (Fig. 5.2.41).

Pyogenic infections, such as abscesses and pneumonia, can be associated with intense FDG uptake (21). Pneumonia typically causes diffuse relatively uniform FDG activity that is easily recognized. However, with cavitation the appearance can be indistinguishable from certain cavitating neoplasms such as squamous cell carcinomas. Likewise, abscesses, which typically are defined by a rim of intense FDG uptake, can have an appearance indistinguishable from a malignant mass with a necrotic center.

Focal FDG uptake occurs in both uncomplicated and complicated pancreatitis (22). Diffuse FDG uptake is typically seen in acute pancreatitis, although focality can occur. Complications such as an abscess or a phlegmonous mass can be associated with intense focal FDG uptake, even in relatively asymptomatic patients months after initial disease presentation (Fig. 5.2.42).

Healing fractures demonstrate increased FDG uptake weeks into the healing process (23). Healing sternotomy (Fig. 5.2.43) and rib fractures (Fig. 5.2.44) are a common source of FDG uptake in bone that could be misinterpreted as osseous metastatic disease. Degenerative or inflammatory joint disease can give rise to elevated FDG uptake (Fig. 5.2.45). Sternoclavicular joints, and to a lesser extent the acromioclavicular, which frequently demonstrate elevated tracer uptake on bone scans, are seen far less frequently on FDG scans. Anterior rib ends likewise occasionally demonstrate focal FDG uptake. Costovertebral joints occasionally show modest uptake, and this may be difficult to distinguish from paravertebral musculature.

The sequela of radiation therapy are associated with FDG uptake even months after therapy (24) and is usually equivalent to slightly greater than blood pool activity (Fig. 5.2.46). Radiation pneumonitis can, however, be intense (Fig. 5.2.47) and difficult to differentiate from active infection or neoplasm (25).

Although FDG PET is more specific than anatomic criteria in determining the presence or absence of malignancy, the specificity is limited by FDG uptake in lymph nodes secondary to inflammatory changes. Active granulomatous diseases such as tuberculosis (26) and sarcoidosis (27) frequently cause high FDG uptake that is well into the range of FDG uptake observed with FDG-avid malignancy such as lung cancer (Fig. 5.2.48). Similarly, chronic inflammation associated with occupational lung disease is associated with FDG-avid mediastinal lymph nodes, in addition to lung and pleural-based inflammation associated FDG uptake (Fig. 5.2.49). The generalized inflammatory response of regional

(*text continues on page 135*)

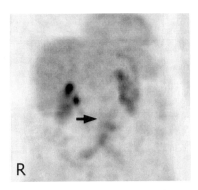
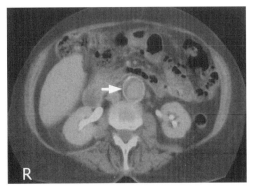

FIG. 5.2.41. Atherosclerosis. Attenuation-corrected anterior projection image and transaxial computed tomography. Moderate fluorodeoxyglucose accumulation associated with atherosclerosis and associated changes in the abdominal aorta (*arrow*). Similar findings are common in the aortic arch.

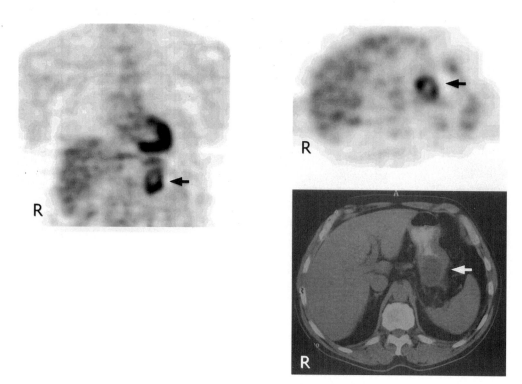

FIG. 5.2.42. Pancreatitis. Attenuation-corrected anterior projection and transaxial images and transaxial computed tomography. Phlegmonous changes in the tail of the pancreas extend to the gastric wall, resulting in high fluorodeoxyglucose uptake (*arrow*) months after the clinical symptoms of the pancreatitis had resolved.

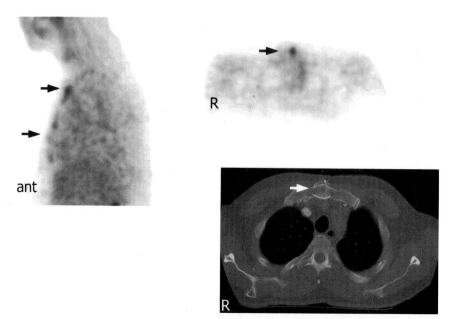

FIG. 5.2.43. Healing sternotomy. Attenuation-corrected sagittal and transaxial images and transaxial computed tomography. Moderate fluorodeoxyglucose uptake in a discontinuous pattern (*arrows*) in a patient 6 months after undergoing sternotomy.

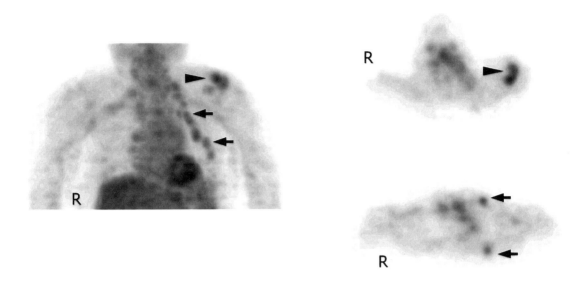

FIG. 5.2.44. Healing fractures. Attenuation-corrected anterior projection and selected transaxial images. Focal fluorodeoxyglucose uptake in multiple healing rib fractures (*arrows*) and an acromial fracture (*arrowhead*) in a patient 2 weeks after experiencing trauma.

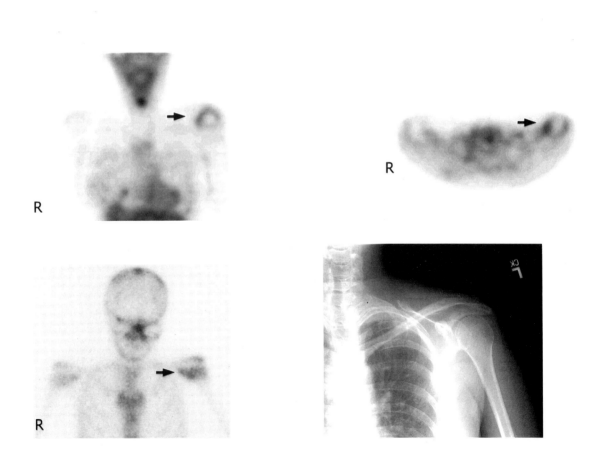

FIG. 5.2.45. Capsulitis. Attenuation-corrected anterior projection and transaxial images, and anterior view technetium-99m bone scan and radiograph. Longstanding left shoulder pain diagnosed as "frozen shoulder" demonstrates fluorodeoxyglucose (FDG) uptake in the joint capsule with associated inflammation on FDG PET(*arrow*).

131

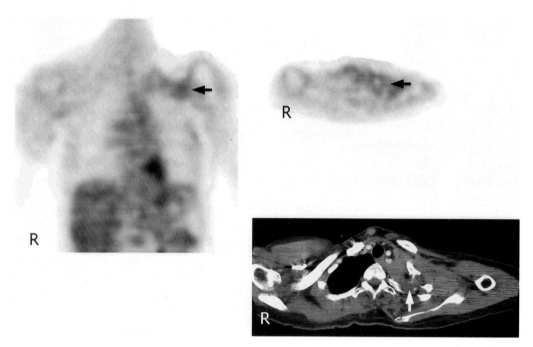

FIG. 5.2.46. Radiation therapy sequela. Attenuation-corrected anterior projection and transaxial images and corresponding transaxial computed tomography. Moderate fluorodeoxyglucose uptake (*arrow*) in soft tissue scarring, sequela of radiation therapy that was present several years after completion of therapy.

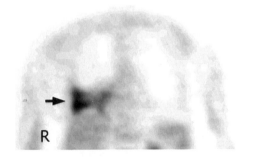

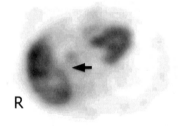

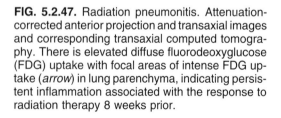

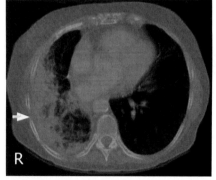

FIG. 5.2.47. Radiation pneumonitis. Attenuation-corrected anterior projection and transaxial images and corresponding transaxial computed tomography. There is elevated diffuse fluorodeoxyglucose (FDG) uptake with focal areas of intense FDG uptake (*arrow*) in lung parenchyma, indicating persistent inflammation associated with the response to radiation therapy 8 weeks prior.

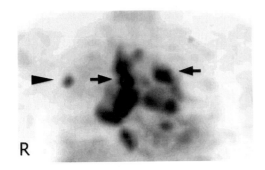
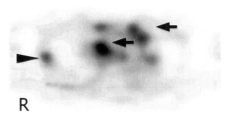

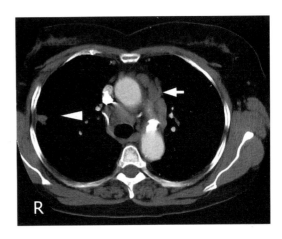

FIG. 5.2.48. Sarcoidosis. Attenuation-corrected anterior projection and transaxial images and corresponding transaxial computed tomography. Intense fluorodeoxy-glucose uptake is seen in mediastinal and hilar adenopathy (*arrows*) in an asymptomatic patient with sarcoidosis. The subpleural right lung nodule (*arrowhead*) was non–small cell lung cancer. Mediastinal lymph nodes were characterized by granulomatous changes only at thoracotomy.

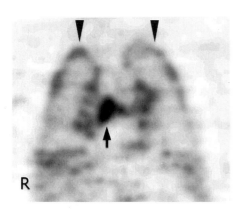
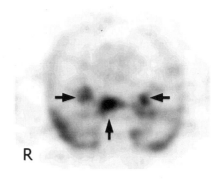

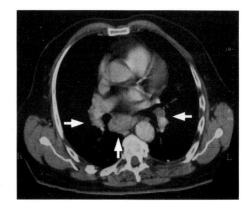

FIG. 5.2.49. Occupational lung disease. Attenuation-corrected anterior projection and transaxial images and corresponding transaxial computed tomography. Moderate fluorodeoxyglucose (FDG) uptake in the pleural/peripheral lung parenchyma (*arrowheads*) and intense FDG uptake in subcarinal and hilar lymphadenopathy (*arrows*) are seen in a retired quarry worker with known occupational lung disease.

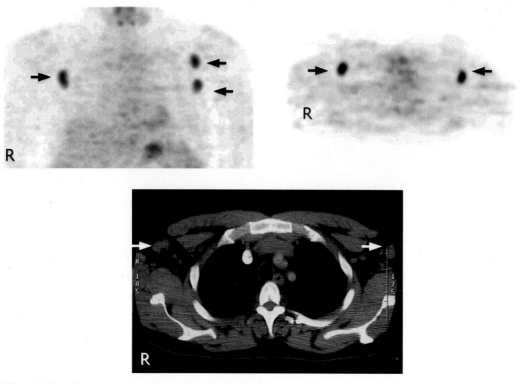

FIG. 5.2.50. Inflammatory lymph nodes. Attenuation-corrected anterior projection and transaxial images and corresponding transaxial computed tomography. There is intense fluorodeoxyglucose uptake in axillary lymph nodes (*arrows*) in this patient with rheumatoid arthritis. Excised nodes showed follicular hyperplasia.

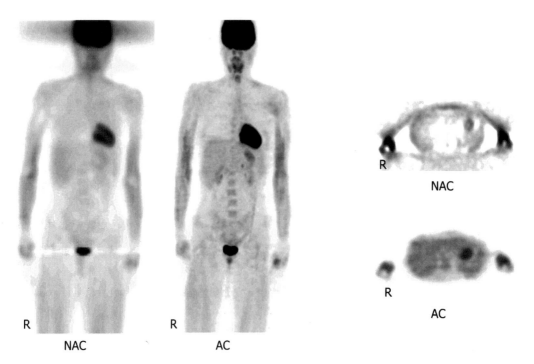

FIG. 5.2.51. Non–attenuation-corrected versus attenuation-corrected images. Whole-body anterior projection images and transaxial images using non–attenuation-corrected *(NAC)* filtered back-projection reconstruction and attenuation-corrected *(AC)* reconstruction using segmented transmission scan with statistical reconstruction methods. Attenuation artifact results in less apparent activity centrally, with much greater apparent activity on the skin surface. Details appear lost due to the nonuniformity and geometric distortion on the NAC images, although such are actually present.

134

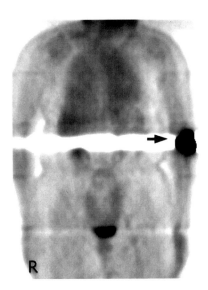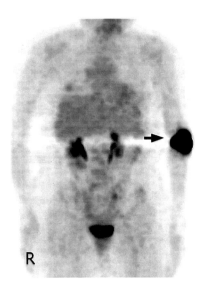

FIG. 5.2.52. Reconstruction artifact. Whole-body anterior projection images using non–attenuation-corrected filtered back-projection reconstruction **(left)** and attenuation-corrected reconstruction using segmented transmission scan with statistical reconstruction methods **(right).** Reconstruction artifacts due to intense tracer activity in the left arm injection site, and less so in the bladder. Such artifacts are reduced by statistical reconstruction methods.

lymph nodes to infection or recent instrumentation is a common source of elevated FDG uptake in noncancerous lymph nodes, and FDG-avid lymph nodes near sites of known infection or recent instrumentation must be interpreted with caution (27). The immunologic challenge to lymph nodes draining the aeroepithelium accounts for the generalized false-positive rate of up to 10% to 15% for lymph nodes in the neck and mediastinum (28,29). For somewhat similar reasons, false-positive lymph nodes occur, although less frequently, in the axilla and inguinal nodal basins (Fig. 5.2.50). Although not common, persistent inflammation associated with prior surgery can yield intense abnormal FDG uptake.

ARTIFACTS DUE TO IMAGE RECONSTRUCTION

Due to the current rapid development of PET technology and image-reconstruction algorithms, the interpretive pitfalls associated with image reconstruction vary among equipment and image-acquisition and image-reconstruction protocols. Before recent advances, whole-body FDG PET was performed without attenuation correction, yielding images with radial nonuniformity and distortion, which can make recognition of familiar anatomic landmarks and relationships difficult (Fig. 5.2.51). Presently whole-body studies are usually performed using attenuation correction, a trend further advanced by new combined PET/computed tomography images (30). Because current statistical image-reconstruction algorithms can yield apparent focal increased activity from movement artifacts or generalized noise, it is also advisable to have non–attenuation-corrected filtered back-projection images for confirmation of such suspect abnormalities. Re-construction artifacts due to large areas of high concentration of tracer such as the heart, bladder, or extravasation at an injection site are minimized by statistical reconstruction (Fig. 5.2.52).

SUMMARY

Tumors generally have high FDG uptake that allows detection by PET. Because glucose metabolism is a widespread process, there is normal uptake of FDG in many locations throughout the body. Infections and inflammation can have high glucose utilization. Knowledge of the variable normal distribution of FDG is essential to separate pathologic from physiologic uptake. This chapter reviews many normal variants that can mimic pathology.

REFERENCES

1. Schelbert HL. Myocardial metabolism. Assessment of blood flow and substrate metabolism in the myocardium of the normal human heart. In: Schwaiger M, ed. *Cardiac positron emission tomography.* Norwell: Kluwer Academic Publishers, 1996:207–216.
2. Jabour BA, Choi Y, Hoh CK, et. al. Extracranial head and neck: PET imaging with 2-[F-18]fluoro-2-deoxy-D-glucose and MR imaging correlation. *Radiology* 1993;186:27–35.
3. Pappas GP, Olcott EW, Drace JE. Imaging skeletal muscle function using (18)FDG-PET: force production, activation, and metabolism. *J Am Phys* 2001;90:329–337.
4. Kelley DE, Williams KV, Price JC. Insulin regulation of glucose transport and phosphorylation in skeletal muscle assessed by PET. *Am J Phys* 199;277:3610–3619.
5. Barrington SF, Maisey MN. Skeletal muscle uptake of fluorine-18-FDG: effect of oral diazepam. *J Nucl Med* 1996;37:1127–1129.
6. Cook GJR, Fogelman I, Maisey MN. Normal physiological and benign pathological variants of 18-fluoro-2-deoxyglucose positron-emission

tomography scanning: potential for error in interpretation. *Semin Nucl Med* 1996;26:308–314.

7. Shreve PD, Anzai Y, Wahl RL. Pitfalls in oncologic diagnosis with FDG-PET imaging: physiologic and benign variants. *RadioGraphics* 1999;19:61–77.

8. Kostakoglu L, Wong JCH, Barrington SF, et al. Speech-related visualization of laryngeal muscles with fluorine-18-FDG. *J Nucl Med* 1996; 37:1771–1773.

9. Seiei Y, Fujii H, Nakahara T, et al. 18-F-FDG-PET detection of colonic adenomas. *J Nucl Med* 2001;42:989–992.

10. Meyer MA. Diffusely increased colonic F-18 FDG uptake in acute enterocolitis. *Clin Nucl Med* 1995;20:434–435.

11. Stahl A, Weber W, Avril N, et al. The effect of *N*-butylscopolamine on intestinal uptake of F-18 fluorodeoxyglucose in PET imaging of the abdomen. *Eur J Nucl Med* 1999;26(P):1017.

12. Miraldi F, Vesselle H, Faulhaber PF, et al. Elimination of artifactual accumulation of FDG in PET imaging of colorectal cancer. *Clin Nucl Med* 1998;23:3–7.

13. Vesselle HJ, Miraldi FD. FDG-PET of the retroperitoneum: normal anatomy, variants, pathologic conditions, and strategies to avoid diagnostic pitfalls. *RadioGraphics* 1998;18:805–823.

14. Brigid GA, Flanagan FI, Dehdashti F. Whole-body positron emission tomography: normal variations, pitfalls, and technical considerations. *AJR Am J Roentgenol* 1997;169:1675–1680.

15. Kosuda S, Fisher S, Kison PV, et al. Uptake of 2-deoxy-2[^{18}F]fluoro-D-glucose in the normal testis: retrospective PET study and animal experiment. *Ann Nucl Med* 1997;11:195–199.

16. Conti PS, Durski JM, Singer PA, et al. Incidence of thyroid gland uptake of F-18 FDG in cancer patients. *Radiology* 1997;205(P):220.

17. Sugawara Y, Fisher SJ, Zasadny KR, et al. Pre-clinical and clinical studies of bone marrow uptake of fluorine-18-fluorodeoxyglucose with or without granulocyte colony-stimulating factor during chemotherapy. *J Clin Oncol* 1998;16:173–180.

18. Erasmus JJ, Patz EF Jr, McAdams HP, et al. Evaluation of adrenal masses in patients with bronchogenic carcinoma using 18F-fluorodeoxyglucose positron emission tomography. *AJR Am J Roentgenol* 1997; 168:1357–1360.

19. Weisdorf DJ, Craddock PR, Jacob HS. Glycogenolysis versus glucose transport in human granulocytes: differential activation in phagocytosis and chemotaxis. *Blood* 1982;60:888–893.

20. Yun M, Yeh D, Araujo LI, et al. F-18 FDG uptake in the large arteries: a new observation. *Clin Nucl Med* 2001;26:314–319.

21. Stumpe KDM, Dazzi H, Schaffner A, et al. Infection imaging using whole-body FDG-PET. *Eur J Nucl Med* 2000;27:822–832.

22. Shreve PD. Focal fluorine-18 fluorodeoxyglucose accumulation in inflammatory pancreatic disease. *Eur J Nucl Med* 1998;25:259–264.

23. Meyer M, Gast T, Raja S, et al. Increased F-18 FDG accumulation in acute fracture. *Clin Nucl Med* 1994;19:13–14.

24. Lowe VJ, Hebert ME, Anscher MS, et al. Serial evaluation of increased chest wall F-18 fluorodeoxyglucose (FDG) uptake following radiation therapy in patients with bronchogenic carcinoma. *Clin Positron Imaging* 1998;1:185–191.

25. Frank A, Lefkowitz D, Jaeger S, et al. Decision logic for retreatment of asymptomatic lung cancer recurrence based on positron emission tomography findings. *Int J Radiat Oncol Biol Phys* 1995;32: 1495–1512.

26. Goo JM, Im JG, Do KH, et al. Pulmonary tuberculoma evaluated by means of FDG-PET: findings in 10 cases. *Radiology* 2000;216: 117–121.

27. Yamada Y, Uchida Y, Tatsumi K, et al. Fluorine-18-fluorodeoxyglucose and carbon-11 methionine evaluation of lymphadenopathy in sarcoidosis. *J Nucl Med* 1998;39:1160–1166.

28. Stuckensen T, Kovacs AF, Adams S, et al. Staging of the neck in patients with oral cavity squamous cell carcinomas: a prospective comparison of PET, ultrasound, CT and MRI. *J Cranio-Maxillo-Facial Surg* 2000; 28:319–324.

29. Gupta NC, Tamim WJ, Graeber GG, et al. Mediastinal lymph node sampling following positron emission tomography with fluorodeoxyglucose imaging in lung cancer staging. *Chest* 2001;120:521–527.

30. Shreve PD. Adding structure to function. *J Nucl Med* 2000;41: 1380–1382.

Central Nervous System

Michael J. Fulham

The common presentations of patients with tumors of the central nervous system (CNS) include focal or generalized seizures, unaccustomed headache, personality and cognitive changes, and focal neurologic signs (1,2). Individual clinical features generally depend on the location of the tumor, its histologic type, and its rate of growth. CNS tumors include cerebral metastases and primary tumors. The main emphasis in this chapter is primary CNS tumors, but for completeness, the role of positron emission tomography (PET) in the assessment of cerebral metastases is also discussed.

Loeffler et al. (3) suggest that cerebral metastases are up to 10 times more common than primary brain tumors. Although cerebral metastases may be detected before or at the same time the primary malignancy is found, in more than 80% of cases, they are found after a diagnosis of systemic cancer is made and they occur in 20% to 40% of these patients. Primary CNS tumors, affecting the brain and spinal cord, have an incidence of 2 to 19 cases per 100,000 persons per year in the United States (4). There are two main peaks: one in childhood, where CNS tumors are the second leading cause of cancer-related death; and a second in later life, between ages 65 and 79 years. The tumor types and the locations at which they occur in these two age groups are distinctly different.

Primary CNS tumors are separated by their cell of origin, which is the basis of the new World Health Organization (WHO) classification (5). The primary CNS tumors may have a neuroepithelial, meningeal, hematopoietic, nerve sheath, or germ-cell origin, with a miscellaneous group including cysts and tumor-like lesions such as epidermoids, dermoids, colloid cysts, Rathke cleft cysts, and others. In children, the most common form of tumor is the primitive neuroectodermal tumor (including medulloblastomas), followed by diffuse infiltrating neuroepithelial tumors; these tumors are much more common in the posterior fossa, diencephalon, and brainstem. Neuroepithelial tumors in adults comprise more than 90% of the primary brain tumors, and collectively, they are called gliomas. They include astrocytomas, oligodendrogliomas, and ependymomas. Unfortunately, no single pathologic classification for gliomas is accepted by all and used universally. Various classifications have been introduced since the middle of last century and some continue to be used routinely today, which remains a continuing source of confusion for clinicians (6–9). For the purposes of this chapter, the WHO classification will be used, with increasing grade indicating increasing degree of malignancy: grade I pilocytic astrocytoma (PA), grade II astrocytoma (low grade), grade III anaplastic astrocytoma, and grade IV glioblastoma multiforme (GBM). Oligodendrogliomas and ependymomas are classified as WHO grade II, with the anaplastic-equivalent tumors as grade III.

The initial step in the evaluation of a patient with a suspected primary CNS tumor, after a history and neurologic examination, is to perform some form of neuroimaging. This is usually anatomic imaging with computed tomography (CT) or magnetic resonance imaging (MRI). Both techniques can depict anatomy exquisitely and assess the integrity of the blood–brain barrier through the application of contrast media. When an assessment of the degree of tumor vascularity is needed, conventional cerebral angiography and sometimes magnetic resonance angiography are done. Initial management decisions are then made on the basis of the grade of the suspected tumor, its size and location, and the patient's age, clinical symptoms, and performance status (2,10,11). Whenever possible in high-grade tumors (grades III and IV), some form of neurosurgical resection is performed to obtain a tissue sample and improve symptoms.

Although pathologic examination of the excised tissue is regarded as the gold standard for determination of tumor biology, it is problematic because the pathologic interpretation is heavily dependent on the experience of the pathologist, and sampling error may mean that the specimen obtained does not accurately reflect tumor aggressivity. Heterogeneity is a consistent characteristic of gliomas (12). The tumor margin often shows atypical but not definitively neoplastic cells. Deeper within the macroscopic abnormality seen on imaging, there may be regions of low-grade tumor admixed with areas of increased cellularity, pleomorphism, and vascular proliferation. Still other regions within the tumor may show foci of hemorrhage or necrosis but without neoplastic cells.

After the initial surgical procedure and the pathologic assessment of the tumor type and grade, the patient may be merely observed, treated with adjuvant external beam radiotherapy, sometimes radiosurgery or brachytherapy, and chemotherapy. In most circumstances, some type of sequential anatomic imaging is then done in the follow-up period. Tumor relapse may be treated with further surgery, chemotherapy, or radiotherapy provided the tolerance of the CNS to radiation has not been reached and the patient has a good performance status. Anatomic imaging is also the tool used most frequently for stereotactic biopsy and volumetric resection (13–16). Further, treatment decisions after surgery and the assessment of tumor response are often predicated on the degree of contrast enhancement seen in the tumor on anatomic imaging (17). However, the shortcomings of anatomic imaging modalities in evaluating tumor biology and response to therapy are recognized by experienced clinicians (10,18–22).

Functional imaging can refine the noninvasive evaluation of brain tumors and improve management and patient outcomes through the measurement of tumor metabolism and metabolites. Although magnetic resonance spectroscopy (MRS) is used in some centers to provide functional imaging data, it has a number of limitations and PET is the premier functional imaging modality for this patient group (20,23). Although PET has been used extensively in research with a variety of ligands to provide insight into many aspects of CNS tumor biology, the bulk of the work in the last decade that has had an impact on patient management and outcome has been carried out with fluorine-18-fluorodeoxyglucose (^{18}F-FDG PET).

TECHNICAL ISSUES RELATED TO BRAIN TUMOR IMAGING

Imaging Protocol

For FDG PET scans, adult patients are studied after a 6-hour fast. Because PET is a functional imaging modality and can be affected by a variety of environmental factors, including medications (see later discussion), it is important to standardize the performance of the scan as much as possible. An uptake period of 30 to 40 minutes is allowed before the patient is positioned on the scanning bed, and in our center, the patient's eyes are patched and ears are plugged from just before the injection of isotope to the end of data acquisition on the scanner. Data acquisition depends on the tomograph used but can vary from 15 to 45 minutes. Many centers perform neurologic FDG PET studies without measurement of glucose utilization; however, we routinely perform quantitative studies with blood sampling using a simplified "arterialized venous" method, because we believe that it aids in interpretation (24,25). We also measure the attenuation of photons with a postinjection algorithm, rather than use a calculated method. This approach, coupled with an uptake period that is performed "off camera," allows for accurate attenuation correction and increased patient throughput (26).

"Noisy" Images

Hyperglycemia results in decreased cerebral FDG uptake, with resultant "noisy" and poor-quality images, because the tracer dose of FDG competes with glucose for uptake. Head motion during the acquisition period also degrades image quality, and although a number of centers have developed algorithms to correct for motion (27–29), it is still better to limit motion rather than to correct for it later. Thus, some form (e.g., thermoplastic mask) of head restraint is used, together with careful patient positioning in the scanner gantry.

Video Electroencephalogram Monitoring

It is important to remember that seizures are a common accompaniment of CNS tumors, and furthermore, clinically inapparent seizures may occur more commonly than is recognized. Seizures produce glucose hypermetabolism that occurs in the cell body and at the efferent terminals of the epileptic site. Epileptic foci responsible for seizures in patients with brain tumors are often located in the cortex at the edge of the imaging abnormality. If a subclinical seizure occurs during the uptake or acquisition period of an FDG PET scan, there can be focal glucose hypermetabolism. This is important to recognize because it may be interpreted, erroneously, as evidence of a high-grade tumor. MRI is also similarly affected and we have seen changes on T2-weighted images and disruption of the blood–brain barrier with gadolinium–diethylenetriamine pentaacetic acid (Gd-DTPA) enhancement. This issue is discussed in detail later in this chapter. In our center, we routinely perform video electroencephalogram (EEG) monitoring on all patients with suspected or proven brain tumors to help identify those patients with subclinical seizure activity.

Image Co-registration/Alignment

Image co-registration of anatomic and functional imaging data sets is increasingly being employed to aid diagnosis and lesion localization. A variety of algorithms have been developed both to register functional data sets to one another (30,31) and to CT and MR data (32). In our center, we use an alignment program to register sequential studies to the initial scan, and it is particularly valuable in following low-grade gliomas or in assessing response to treatment (30). Before frameless stereotaxy, the FDG PET data are registered to the CT and MR data (32). The recent development, by the main PET scanner vendors, of a high-end PET scanner coupled to a helical CT scanner is a major advance not just for whole-body PET studies, but also for neurologic studies.

Image Interpretation

There is avid FDG uptake into the CNS, because glucose is the only fuel that the brain uses for energy metabolism, and the main requirements for energy in mammalian nervous tissue occur at the synaptic terminals, rather than cell soma. Thus, FDG PET images reflect synaptic activity that may be excitatory or inhibitory because both types of synaptic transmission require energy utilization. However, there are two exceptions: (a) high-grade CNS tumors (Fig. 5.3.1) and (b) seizure foci during the ictus, where somal glucose use predominates. An underlying principle of FDG PET in the assessment of CNS tumors is that the higher the grade of malignancy, the greater the glucose metabolism, which is due in part to greater "anaerobic glycolysis" with increasing grade of malignancy and expression of specific glucose transporters (GLUTs) (34–36).

Hypermetabolism and Hypometabolism

Because normal cortex and the deep nuclei are characterized by relatively avid glucose uptake when compared with white matter, one approach to determine if a tumor is "benign" or malignant is to compare the peak glucose metabolism in the lesion to glucose metabolism in a reference region. Our practice is to use the white matter of the centrum semiovale of the contralateral cerebral hemisphere (37,38). The reasoning behind this approach is as follows: (a) White matter contains glial cells and axons of neurons, (b) axons have minimal glucose utilization (33); thus, (c) white matter best reflects normal glial glucose metabolism and (d) malignant brain tumors have higher rates of glucose utilization than normal glia.

Di Chiro et al. (39) showed in 1982 that glucose hypermetabolism relative to white matter is seen in high-grade tumors (anaplastic astrocytoma, GBM), whereas in low-grade tumors, glucose metabolism is less than, equal to, or only slightly greater than it is in white matter. These findings have been duplicated by many other centers (40–42), with one exception (43). Tyler et al. (43) found no correlation between glucose metabolism and grade in 16 (2 low-grade astrocytomas) patients. However, they compared average, rather than maximal, tumoral glucose metabolism with contralateral brain with an early generation PET scanner. The surprisingly low metabolic values seen in their high-grade tumors could be explained by partial volume error and region-of-interest placement that included areas of necrosis (37,43). In a large number of patients, we reported that the average value for the ratio of tumor to white matter glucose metabolism is 1.3 for low-grade tumors, 4.2 for anaplastic astrocytomas, and 6.5 for GBM (38). Delbeke et al. (44) suggested a "cutoff" ratio of 1.5 to separate low-grade from high-grade gliomas.

It is self-evident, but nevertheless important, to appreciate the characteristics (and limitations) of the PET device when interpreting PET scans. It is not surprising that a PET device with a 5- to 7-mm in-plane and z-axis resolution will have difficulty detecting a 1- to 2-mm-thin rim of tumor because of partial volume effects, and similarly, 5-mm-thick transaxial MR sections coupled with a 5-mm interspace gap may miss similarly sized lesions.

Cerebellar Diaschisis

Asymmetric glucose metabolism is often seen in the cerebellar hemispheres in patients with primary supratentorial brain tumors. "Crossed" cerebellar diaschisis (CCD) was the term used by Baron et al. (45) in 1980 when it was first noted on some of the early PET scans carried out in patients with cerebral ischemia. Although the original patients had strokes and a PET blood-flow tracer was used, the observation was confirmed by others and extended to patients with cerebral gliomas (46). CCD refers to an obvious reduction in glucose metabolism in the cerebellar hemisphere contralateral, hence "crossed," to the supratentorial lesion. The term diaschisis was first introduced by Von Monakow in 1910 to describe a " . . . state of reduced or abolished function . . . after a brain injury and acting on a neural region remote from the lesion" (47). The mechanism for this phenomenon is an interruption to the corticopontocerebellar (CPC) pathway from the cerebral hemispheres to the opposite cerebellar cortex. The CPC pathway arises from all lobes of the cerebral hemispheres, but the major inputs are from prefrontal, sensorimotor cortex, and the occipital lobes (45, 48). The first synapse in the CPC pathway is in the ipsilateral pons and second-order neurons cross to the contralateral cerebellar hemisphere via the middle cerebellar peduncle to terminate in the cerebellar cortex (49). Fulham et al. (48) showed with FDG PET in patients with brain tumors that there is ipsilateral pontine glucose hypometabolism consistent with this hypothesis and that there is relative preservation of glucose metabolism in the dentate nucleus of the hypometabolic cerebellar hemisphere. Cerebellar diaschisis does not appear to have a clinical accompaniment, at least to standard bedside tests of cerebellar function, and can be seen with any supratentorial injury be it tumor, stroke, gliosis, trauma, or other. It has a variable time course (50) and reversibility is seen in stroke, but in patients with brain tumors, the cerebellar diaschisis is often persistent.

Effects of Corticosteroids and Other Medication

Corticosteroids are commonly administered, often for prolonged periods, to patients with brain tumors for the symptomatic relief of cerebral edema. Common consequences of long-term steroid therapy include centripetal obesity with cushingoid facies, abdominal striae, disordered sleep patterns, and neuropsychiatric disturbances, which range from a mild behavioral change to psychosis (51). Adrenal glucocorticoids are known to affect cell glucose utilization throughout the body, and experimental studies have shown there is an effect on brain glucose utilization, but the mechanism for the neuropsychiatric abnormalities in patients with long-term corticosteroid therapy is unclear (52,53). Investigators at the National Institutes of Health reported a marked reduction in cerebral glucose metabolism in patients with brain tumors who were cushingoid after prolonged exogenous corticosteroid therapy, which may provide insights into the neuropsychiatric effects of corticosteroids (54). They measured cerebral glucose metabolism with FDG PET in 45 patients (56 studies) with unilateral gliomas. The main findings were that in the cushingoid patients, there was a significant reduction in cerebral glucose metabolism when compared with healthy volunteers and two other patient groups (no dexamethasone plus or minus prior radiotherapy). In addition, serial FDG PET scans were done in eight patients, and there was a progressive reduction in glucose metabolism over time. In one patient, steroids were stopped and there was a concomitant increase in cerebral glucose metabolism. This reduction in glucose metabolism was not a reflection of tumor infiltration or cerebral atrophy and was independent of radiotherapy, concurrent anticonvulsant medication, transhemispheric functional disconnection (transhemispheric diaschisis), and blood sugar level. In a practical sense, high-dose steroids produce a marked reduction in cortical glucose utilization and the end result is that image quality is degraded and the usual topographic landmarks on the PET scan are poorly defined. Sedatives, including barbiturates and major tranquilizers, and to a lesser extent anticonvulsant medications, also reduce cerebral glucose metabolism (55–58). From a practical sense, it is important to appreciate that when the usual pattern of metabolism in the cortex relative to white matter and the tumor is disturbed, it may be due to the effects of medication.

THE IMPORTANT CLINICAL QUESTIONS

There are a number of critical issues in the clinical management of patients with proven or suspected primary brain tumors. PET can help with most but not all. The major questions for clinicians who look after patients with brain tumors are as follows: (a) Is the lesion a high-grade or low-grade tumor? A related question is what is the best tool for the initial staging of a suspected primary tumor? (b) What is the cell type? (c) If the tumor cannot be resected, what is the best site in the lesion to biopsy so the patient does not suffer a deficit and yet the tissue that is obtained reflects the biologic behavior of the tumor? (d) Has this presumed or proven low-grade glioma undergone malignant degeneration? (e) Has the tumor responded to treatment? (f) What is responsible for the patient's clinical deterioration after primary treatment? Other pertinent issues are as follows: (g) How far does the tumor extend into the surrounding tissue and (h) what is the role of PET in the assessment of cerebral metastases?

The Suspected High-grade Glioma—Does PET Help?

As stated earlier for a patient with a suspected brain tumor, the histologic grade and tumor type determines the outcome.

Ever since the first report from Di Chiro et al. (39), FDG PET has proven superior to anatomic imaging in grading gliomas. However, the first investigation that is carried out in most institutions is a brain CT or MR scan because of their ready availability when compared with PET. It is an accepted general principle that in this clinical context, a mass lesion that enhances after intravenous contrast (iodinated or paramagnetic) agents is considered to be a high-grade tumor. Similarly, a lesion with minimal or no enhancement is regarded as a low-grade tumor (7,59–63). There are a few exceptions (see "Special Tumors" section below) (38, 64–66).

The following is a typical clinical scenario. A 67-year-old man has a short history of severe unaccustomed headache and aphasia. There is no other relevant past medical history, in particular, no history of a malignancy, and on examination, there is a mild expressive aphasia. Anatomic imaging shows an irregularly enhancing lesion in the white matter and cortex of the left anterior temporal lobe (Fig. 5.3.1). The radiologic interpretation indicates an enhancing mass with probable necrosis that is likely to be a primary brain tumor. Does PET have a role in the preoperative assessment of the degree of malignancy in this patient? The answer is probably no. The patient is symptomatic and tissue is required for a diagnosis and further imaging is not needed. The neurosurgeon will use frameless stereotaxis to resect some or all of the macroscopic abnormality that is found at surgery while being ever careful to avoid an injury to the patient.

Prospective comparisons of FDG PET to MRI with Gd-DTPA have been done (67,68). Davis et al. (67) reported findings in 22 gliomas while Melisi et al. (68) analyzed 160 FDG PET studies from 113 patients with gliomas. Both studies reported similar findings that, in general, FDG PET and enhanced MRI were complementary, but Melisi et al. (68) noted that in 20% of cases, there was a lack of correspondence between FDG PET and MRI. Although it has been argued that such a correspondence diminishes the value of PET in this setting, this argument does not reflect the practical difficulties in the daily management (69). The 20% of instances in which there was a disparity between the MR scan and the FDG PET scans, reported by Melisi et al. (68), includes patients with primary high-grade tumors that did not enhance. Figure 5.3.2 illustrates such a case in which the lack of enhancement on MRI and a stereotactic biopsy that revealed findings consistent with a low-grade glioma led the neurosurgeon to adopt a conservative approach despite the marked increase in glucose metabolism detected with FDG PET. The subsequent clinical deterioration and death within 6 months of the PET scan was unfortunate. Figures 5.3.1 and 5.3.2 also show that FDG PET scans in patients with high-grade gliomas are notable for the heterogeneity within the tumor proper and the tumoral rim that often surrounds a necrotic center. This heterogeneity is appreciated less well on anatomic imaging, in which although the tumoral wall may vary in thickness, it shows homogene-

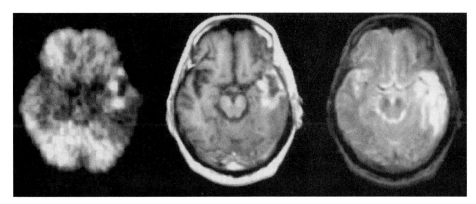

FIG. 5.3.1. Co-registered transaxial ^{18}F-fluorodeoxyglucose positron emission tomography (FDG PET), T1-weighted with gadolinium–diethylenetriamine pentaacetic acid, and T2-weighted magnetic resonance (MR) images **(from left to right)** in a 67-year-old man with a recent history of severe unaccustomed headache, aphasia, and a glioblastoma multiforme. FDG PET shows a heterogeneous rim of increased glucose metabolism that surrounds an ametabolic center in the dominant anterior left *(L)* anterior temporal lobe; there is glucose hypometabolism in the posterior L temporal lobe due to edema. MR scans show a ragged region of enhancement and marked edema in the L temporal lobe. There is a lack of complete correspondence between enhanced MR and hypermetabolism on FDG PET; the regions of hypermetabolism best reflect tumor biology. (Note: For this and all subsequent FDG PET scans in this chapter regions of high glucose utilization [hypermetabolism] are seen as white; and regions of reduced glucose utilization [hypometabolism] are gray.)

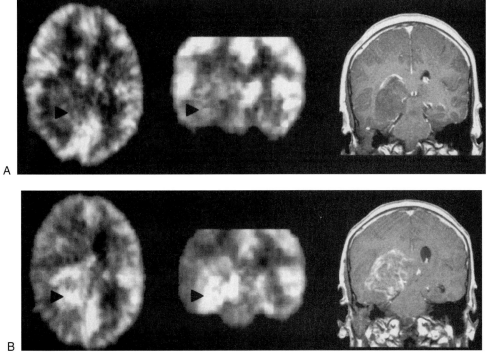

FIG. 5.3.2. Serial transaxial and coronal ^{18}F-fluorodeoxyglucose positron emission tomography (FDG PET) and coronal enhanced magnetic resonance imaging (MRI) images in a 46-year-old man who presented with a generalized tonic-clonic seizure. Stereotactic biopsy done before FDG PET revealed a low-grade astrocytoma. **A:** Initial FDG PET showed a heterogeneous pattern of increased glucose metabolism in the mass *(arrowhead)* in the right temporal white matter, consistent with a high-grade tumor. The mass did not enhance on MRI. **B:** Four months later, the patient deteriorated and radiotherapy was carried out. A second FDG PET done 2 months after the clinical deterioration showed markedly increased metabolism in the large right mesial temporal mass with avid enhancement after gadolinium-diethylenetriamine pentaacetic acid. The patient rapidly deteriorated and coned 2 days after the FDG PET scan. A glioblastoma multiforme was found at surgery.

ous enhancement. The neurosurgeon is generally reluctant to attempt to biopsy or resect a thick rim of enhancement that abuts the central sulcus. Further, a different approach is needed for an enhancing mass that is located in eloquent cortex or deep in a hemisphere or the brainstem. Thus, although it is accepted that FDG PET may not be required in the primary assessment of all suspected high-grade gliomas, it adds value where identification of tumoral heterogeneity can be used to guide stereotactic biopsy and resection.

How to Select the Best Site in the Lesion to Biopsy and Resect

A number of investigators have shown that FDG PET improves the diagnostic yield of stereotactic biopsy. When focal hypermetabolism seen with FDG PET is targeted, it is more likely that tissue that reflects the tumor biology will be obtained than when only anatomic imaging is used (70–72). Levivier et al. (71) reported improved yields when FDG PET was used to guide stereotactic biopsy, compared with CT, in 38 patients with supratentorial brain tumors (Fig. 5.3.3). Massager et al. (72) applied a similar technique, but with FDG PET compared with MRI, to brainstem lesions and showed that a combined PET-MR approach improved the accuracy of targeting. Importantly, this combined approach reduced the number of trajectories needed to obtain representative tissue, thereby limiting the risk for neurologic damage at this critical site (72).

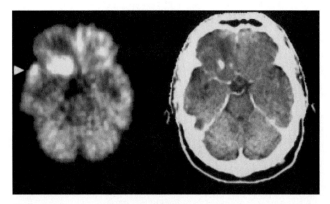

FIG. 5.3.3. Co-registered (^{18}F-fluorodeoxyglucose positron emission tomography [FDG PET] and computed tomography [CT]) transaxial images in a 49-year-old man who presented after a generalized tonic-clonic seizure. A right inferior frontal lesion seen on anatomic imaging was thought to be a low-grade glioma and a biopsy showed a low-grade astrocytoma. The patient was referred to the author's institution 9 months later and FDG PET showed a focal region of markedly increased glucose metabolism in the posterior aspect of the right gyrus rectus, together with another focus in the anterior right temporal lobe (*arrowhead*). These foci did not enhance with CT or magnetic resonance imaging (not shown); a small focus of calcification is seen anterior to the main region of glucose hypermetabolism. FDG PET was used to guide resection, and pathology revealed an anaplastic oligodendroglioma.

The Suspected Low-grade Glioma—Does PET Help?

Patients with low-grade gliomas are generally thought to have mass lesions with indistinct margins that are hyperintense on T2-weighted and flair MR images and that do not enhance after contrast. The lesion may have been detected asymptomatically or the patient may have presented with headache or a seizure, but focal neurologic signs are usually absent (Fig. 5.3.4). However, a number of reports demonstrate the unreliability of contrast enhancement in determining tumor grade and tumor extent. Chamberlain et al. (72a) showed that 31% of highly anaplastic and 54% of moderately anaplastic astrocytomas did not enhance on CT. In smaller series, Kondziolka et al. (22) and Kelly et al. (73) noted a similar lack of enhancement with MRI (between 47% and 90%) in anaplastic astrocytomas. In our center, an FDG PET scan is done to (a) confirm that the mass lesion is hypometabolic and consistent with a low-grade glioma and (b) determine if there are any regions of increased glucose metabolism, which implies focal anaplasia (Figs. 5.3.2 and 5.3.3). The management of patients with proven or suspected low-grade gliomas is controversial. Some clinicians use surgery, followed by radiation therapy; others perform a biopsy, followed by radiotherapy. Still others perform a biopsy, and if the pathologic findings are consistent with a low-grade glioma, they may then manage the patient conservatively with serial anatomic imaging. Finally, some clinicians do not perform a biopsy in a well patient with anatomic imaging findings that are consistent with a low-grade glioma and instead await clinical deterioration before intervention (1,2,74–77). However, there is less controversy regarding the management algorithm for an anaplastic tumor identified on biopsy or resection. The treatment of an anaplastic tumor typically includes radiotherapy and in some centers, chemotherapy.

In this author's opinion, for a patient with a hypometabolic lesion on FDG PET, there is a very strong argument to adopt a conservative approach and follow the patient with serial PET scans, given that (a) the natural history of low-grade gliomas is uncertain, (b) patients have been followed with proven low-grade gliomas upwards of 15 years, (c) cerebral irradiation has long-term deleterious cognitive effects, (d) sampling error can occur with stereotactic biopsy without PET, and (e) the desire to obtain a tissue for "diagnostic certainty" is usually quelled when the lesion is located in eloquent cortex (75,78–81).

What is the Cell Type?

The realization that low-grade gliomas, in particular oligodendrogliomas, tend to have a protracted clinical course and some are chemosensitive when they transform to aggressive tumors has emphasized the importance of an accurate histologic diagnosis (78,79). Unfortunately, there is no current imaging technique that can reliably predict histologic cell type. The ragged pattern of enhancement seen on MRI in an untreated patient is likely to indicate a high-grade

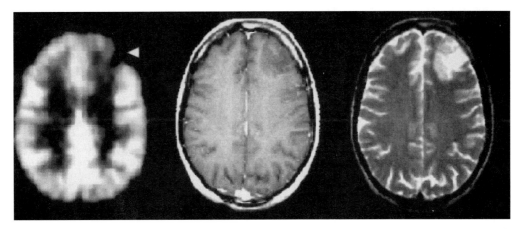

FIG. 5.3.4. Co-registered transaxial images of a 34-year-old man who presented with a generalized tonic-clonic seizure. Focal glucose hypometabolism in the left frontal lobe is seen on ^{18}F-fluorodeoxyglucose positron emission tomography (*arrowhead*). This region does not enhance on the T1-weighted image, but hyperintensity is seen on the T2-weighted magnetic resonance scan.

tumor, but the underlying tumor may be a cystic anaplastic astrocytoma, a necrotic GBM, or a cystic/necrotic oligodendroglioma. The pattern is nonspecific and a similar picture is seen in demyelination, in abscess formation, and in brain tumors after treatment. Calcification on CT and MR can be found in oligodendrogliomas, but again this finding does not have the specificity to be clinically valuable because calcification is found in other types of tumors including ganglioglioma and craniopharyngiomas. FDG PET can provide valuable clues to the underlying histology, but as with CT and MR, not the certainty required to be diagnostically valuable. For instance, FDG PET can detect markedly hypometabolic regions within an irregular hypermetabolic mass lesion that can indicate necrosis in GBMs, but cystic areas are also ametabolic. Cerebral lymphomas have markedly increased glucose metabolism, and a focal hypermetabolic lesion adjacent to the lateral ventricle is very suggestive of a primary cerebral lymphoma, although very high values for glucose metabolism can be seen in solid GBMs, anaplastic astrocytomas, and anaplastic oligodendrogliomas.

Has This Presumed/Proven Low-grade Glioma Undergone Malignant Degeneration?

A large percentage of presumed and proven low-grade gliomas—some investigators argue all—will undergo malignant degeneration. Thus, the recognition that low-grade gliomas are considered to be only relatively "benign." The important question is, when does this malignant transformation occur? In our center, FDG PET scans are performed yearly on patients with proven or presumed low-grade gliomas. The scan is done earlier if there are changes in the clinical features, for example, an increase in seizure or headache frequency without a clearly identifiable cause, particularly in patients older than 50 years. This decision is arbitrary, and unfortunately there are no data to predict the average time to malignant change. When increased metabolism is seen in the lesion on FDG PET, regardless of the MRI findings, that is the time to reevaluate the options for treatment and tissue sampling (82,83). An example is shown in Fig. 5.3.5, a 51-year-old man who presented with a generalized tonic-clonic seizure 5 years before the FDG PET scan was performed. At the time of the FDG PET scan, the patient was seizure-free and asymptomatic. The tumor involved eloquent cortex and the focus of glucose hypermetabolism was seen deep in white matter. Despite the FDG PET findings, it was decided that the patient be observed. Ten months later, he developed right arm weakness, and on the second FDG PET scan, the focus of glucose hypermetabolism was much larger and biopsy revealed a GBM. This patient illustrates an important issue: When a hypermetabolic focus is detected on FDG PET, when is the best time to intervene? The results for high-grade tumors treated with aggressive local therapies such as brachytherapy or radiosurgery are better if the tumor volume is small (84). But is intervention justified when the patient is asymptomatic? Most neurosurgeons are reluctant to operate on patients who are asymptomatic, but FDG PET data, first reported by Patronas et al. (85) and later by others (41,86,87), demonstrate that patients with brain tumors with glucose hypermetabolism have shortened survival. FDG PET is essential in the longitudinal follow-up of patients with low-grade tumors and its ability to detect malignant change is undisputed. Trials to provide data for the optimal management for these patients are now required.

Has the Tumor Responded to Treatment?

In addition to clinical findings and performance status, the degree of enhancement on MRI is currently used as the gold standard to measure tumor response in clinical trials (17). However, this approach has limitations. Cairncross et al. (88) showed that contrast enhancement on anatomic im-

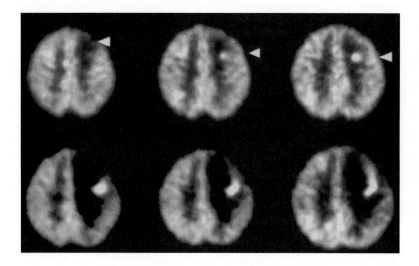

FIG. 5.3.5. Transaxial ^{18}F-fluorodeoxyglucose positron emission tomography (FDG PET) images obtained in a 51-year-old man with malignant degeneration of a low-grade astrocytoma. Diagnosis of a low-grade glioma was made 5 years earlier after presentation with a seizure. The lesion was located in eloquent cortex. At the time of the first FDG PET scan **(top row)**, the patient was asymptomatic. FDG PET showed a region of glucose hypometabolism in the left frontal lobe (*arrowhead in left image top row*) with a small focus of glucose hypermetabolism (*arrowhead*) in the deep component of the lesion **(middle and far right images).** At time of the second scan 10 months later **(bottom row)**, the patient had a right hemiparesis and seizure frequency had increased; FDG PET showed extensive hypometabolism affecting the left frontal lobe and the region of hypermetabolism is much larger. The lesion was partially resected and a glioblastoma multiforme that had arisen in a low-grade glioma was found at pathology.

aging performed 4 days after operation could be due to postsurgical changes, rather than residual tumor. In addition, corticosteroids have a profound effect on the degree of contrast enhancement, peritumoral edema, and to a lesser extent, the apparent volume of enhancing tumor by partial restoration of the blood–brain barrier (89–92). Up to a 50% reduction in the enhancing volume of anaplastic tumors has been reported to occur after corticosteroid administration (89).

Is it not more sensible to use functional imaging to assess response? Data that support the utility of PET in the assessment of tumor response continue to mature (93). FDG PET has been used to assess response to therapy longitudinally in patients with brain tumors (Fig. 5.3.6). The exact timing

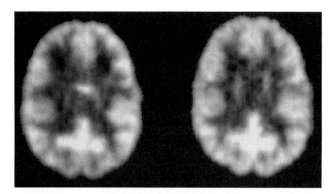

FIG. 5.3.6. Aligned transaxial ^{18}F-fluorodeoxyglucose positron emission tomography (FDG PET) scans performed before **(left)** external beam radiotherapy (59 Gy) and 6 months after **(right)** completion of therapy in a 37-year-old woman with an anaplastic astrocytoma. On FDG PET before therapy, focal glucose hypermetabolism was seen in the midline in the corpus callosum; biopsy showed an anaplasia glioma. Six months later, the hypermetabolic focus had completely resolved and normal metabolism in the bodies of the caudate nuclei was seen on either side of midline. The patient remained well and asymptomatic for another 4 years.

for the assessment of response is uncertain. Ideally, it would be valuable to know early in the course of treatment if the modality is having the desired effect. In this context, we have recently performed early time point FDG PET studies in a group (n = 6) of patients with high-grade gliomas who were given an orally active chemotherapeutic agent (Fig. 5.3.7A and B). A reduction of glucose metabolism was seen after 1 week of therapy in this patient group and predicted response. Although the number of patients is small, these data suggest that a reduction in glucose metabolism may identify the patients who may respond to therapy. Recent data from other tumor types have shown similar trends (94, 95). Further, although not applied to brain tumors, carbon-11 (^{11}C)-thymidine (see below) has been used to assess response in four patients with non–small cell lung cancer and two patients with sarcomas, prior to and 1 week after commencing therapy. Shields et al. (96) reported that the decrease in ^{11}C-thymidine uptake predated a reduction in glucose metabolism. Carbon-11-thymidine has also been used in the experimental setting to assess response to thymidylate synthetase inhibitors (97).

What is Responsible for the Patient's Clinical Deterioration After Primary Treatment for a Brain Tumor?

Clinical deterioration in a patient with glioma months or years after treatment is generally thought to be due to tumor recurrence and sometimes radiation or chemonecrosis. Anatomic imaging reveals a mass, often with surrounding edema and marked contrast enhancement. Unfortunately, these radiologic imaging findings are nonspecific and merely reflect disruption of the blood–brain barrier, which can be due to previous surgery, radiotherapy, and chemotherapy. Unsuspected seizure activity should be added to the differential diagnosis. It is important that discussions about the presence

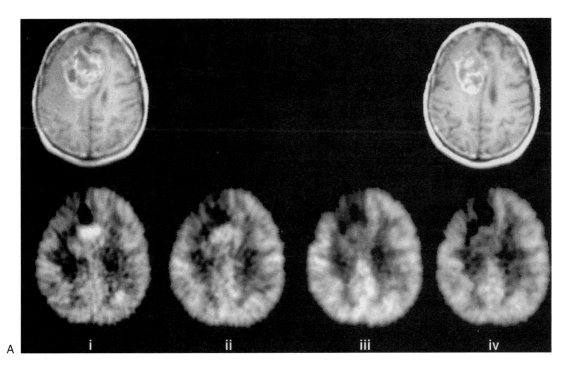

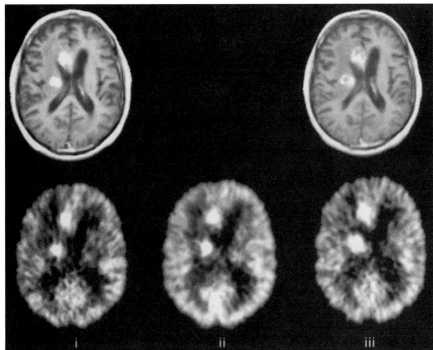

FIG. 5.3.7. Transaxial early time point ¹⁸F-fluorodeoxyglucose positron emission tomography (FDG PET) scans in two patients with high-grade gliomas performed before and after treatment. **A:** A 41-year-old man with an anaplastic astrocytoma who relapsed 14 months after radiotherapy. Co-registered magnetic resonance (MR) scans with gadolinium–diethylenetriamine penta-acetic acid (Gd-DTPA) were performed before **(upper left)** and at the completion of two cycles of chemotherapy 2 months later **(upper right)**. Co-registered FDG PET scans were done before *(i)*, at day 7 *(ii)*, day 21 *(iii)*, and at same time as the second MR scan *(iv)*. A marked reduction in tumoral glucose metabolism was seen at the end of 1 week, minimal glucose metabolism was seen after 3 weeks, and at 2 months there was almost a complete response. The large enhancing mass lesion was still seen with MR in the right frontal lobe and corpus callosum, and the lesion still enhanced markedly at 2 months and only fulfilled anatomic criteria of a partial response. The patient remained well with a good performance status for a further 8 months. **B:** A 59-year-old man with a glioblastoma multiforme who relapsed 5 months after primary therapy. Co-registered MR scans with Gd-DTPA were performed before **(upper left)** and 3 weeks later **(upper right)** when the patient continued to deteriorate clinically. Co-registered FDG PET scans were done before *(i)* and at days 7 *(ii)* and 21 *(iii)* after the commencement of therapy. On MR imaging, there were two enhancing lesions: one in the right frontal lobe and a second in the white matter of the right centrum semiovale; at day 21, the lesions were slightly larger and partly necrotic, but they did not meet the criteria for progressive disease. On FDG PET, the lesions did not change significantly at day 7 and at day 21 were larger and more metabolically active, consistent with progressive disease. Chemotherapy was stopped and the patient died 6 weeks later.

or absence of recurrence versus treatment-related necrosis on imaging studies should not be done in isolation. It is essential to relate the findings to the patient's clinical history and the management options that are available. In some instances, surgical resection may be appropriate for both tumor recurrence and radiation necrosis.

Patronas et al. (98) and Di Chiro et al. (99) first reported that FDG PET was able to differentiate hypometabolic radiation necrosis and chemonecrosis from recurrent hypermetabolic tumor. Doyle et al. (100) and Valk et al. (101) reported similar findings in patients with malignant gliomas who had been treated with interstitial brachytherapy. Valk et al. (101) also compared the PET results with clinical outcomes and found an overall accuracy of 84%. Recently, these findings have been challenged (102). Although the limitations of the study by Ricci et al. (102) could be discussed at length, it is more relevant to identify the relevant factors that should be considered in this clinical setting.

Radiation necrosis generally appears a year or more after irradiation with doses greater than 50 Gy, and it is rare less than 3 months after completion of therapy. The development of radiation necrosis is proportional to the dose and is inversely proportional to the number of fractions or time during which the radiation is administered (103,104). Some investigators regard it as an idiosyncratic phenomenon that cannot always be predicted or explained on the basis of dose, distribution, and fractionation of the radiotherapy. However, in our experience, when conventional radiotherapy doses are given (50 to 55 Gy), it is more common in the elderly and in patients with underlying vascular disease, hypertension, and diabetes (Fig. 5.3.8). With aggressive treatment protocols that deliver high doses of radiation locally (e.g., gamma knife and/or brachytherapy), necrosis is an expected therapeutic effect (84). The pathologic injury of radiation necrosis is mainly confined to white matter, whereas with chemonecrosis the gray matter is also affected. It is mainly a vascular injury and vessels undergo fibrinoid necrosis (105).

The pathologic diagnosis of radiation necrosis is not an easy task. Generally, tissue specimens that are removed from radionecrotic areas contain large irregular distorted tumor cells that are regarded as ''viable,'' as well as necrotic cells. But the pathologist is often unable to determine if these ''viable'' cells are capable of replicating. Unequivocal evidence for tumor recurrence depends on the presence of pseudopalisading surrounding necrotic areas, but this is generally not the rule (105). Often, there is evidence for both tumor recurrence and radiation necrosis on the pathologic specimen and the clinical dilemma is what to do next. The simple answer is that it depends on the clinical situation. For the patient in Fig. 5.3.8, treatment with small doses of corticosteroids was able to maintain a good performance status. If glucose hypermetabolism is seen on the PET scan, chemotherapy could be considered, but it was not used in this patient because of the deep location of the abnormality in the dominant hemisphere.

Finally, for PET practitioners, nonconvulsive status epilepsy (NCSE) should be considered in this setting. Focal glucose hypermetabolism, due to seizure activity rather than recurrent tumor, in the cortex adjacent to the site of the original tumor can be responsible for focal and global neurologic impairment in a patient with a brain tumor. NCSE is underemphasized in the literature and underrecognized clinically but is an eminently treatable cause of clinical deterioration in a patient with a brain tumor. In our experience, there is hardly ever the typical motor or sensory accompaniment; patients may be merely obtunded or have focal deficits. EEG is not always helpful, but FDG PET provides the

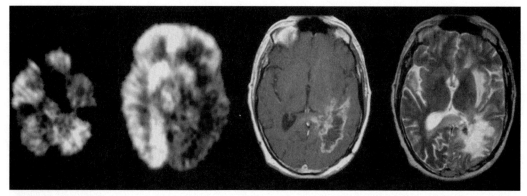

FIG. 5.3.8. Transaxial ^{18}F-fluorodeoxyglucose positron emission tomography (FDG PET) and enhanced magnetic resonance imaging (MRI) scans of a 48-year-old man with insulin-dependent diabetes and hypertension performed 18 months after completion of radiotherapy for an anaplastic astrocytoma. FDG PET scans showed right crossed cerebellar diaschisis and extensive glucose hypometabolism in the left temporooccipital lobes. On MRI, there was a ragged region of enhancement in the deep left temporooccipital lobes with edema that extends into the left insula. The deep enhancing mass was biopsied and revealed radiation necrosis. The patient developed new tumor foci in the left frontal lobe and died from progressive disease 8 months later.

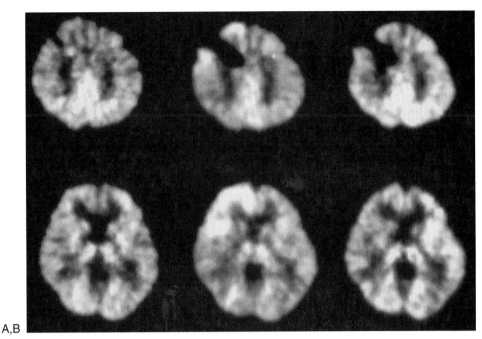

A,B   C

FIG. 5.3.9. Serial aligned transaxial ^{18}F-fluorodeoxyglucose positron emission tomography (FDG PET) scans in a 32-year-old woman treated with surgery and radiotherapy 12 years previously for a right frontal anaplastic astrocytoma. She was readmitted after increasing headache and focal seizures. Imaging showed an enhancing mass in the right frontal lobe that was removed at surgery and found to be consistent with recurrent tumor. **A:** Preoperative FDG PET showed a focus of glucose hypermetabolism in white matter of the right frontal lobe; the lower slice shows normal metabolism in the midfrontal cortex. Postoperatively, she was obtunded with a dense left hemiparesis, dysphagia, and dysarthria. **B:** A second FDG PET performed 7 days after surgery showed the ametabolic surgical defect and glucose hypermetabolism in the surrounding cortex in the right superior and midfrontal lobe. **C:** On a third FDG PET study 1 week later, there was a marked reduction in cortical hypermetabolism after effective anticonvulsant therapy accompanied by resolution of clinical signs and a return to a normal mental state.

clue and there is a dramatic improvement in performance status with anticonvulsant medication alone (Fig. 5.3.9).

How Far Does the Tumor Extend Into the Surrounding Tissue?

Delineating the "true" extension of a glioma into the adjacent brain, be it low grade or high grade, has been a difficult task with the available technologies. The problem is that of microscopic invasion beyond the macroscopic abnormality seen at operation and on anatomic imaging studies (73,106,107). Although it remains to be proven, there is a theoretical argument that removing all neoplastic cells that extend beyond the macroscopic margin of the tumor would offer better local control and perhaps a real possibility of cure. Early work with ^{11}C-methionine PET suggested that this tracer was better at delineating the tumor margin, particularly for low-grade gliomas, when compared with anatomic imaging (108). Subsequent work suggests that this probably only applies to low-grade oligodendrogliomas (109). Nevertheless, there are significant practical difficulties in translating these findings to the operating room. Accurate co-registration is difficult with the poor anatomic definition seen

with the "noisy" ^{11}C-methionine images. Once resection begins in the operating room, anatomic landmarks are further affected. In addition, neurosurgeons have an inherent reluctance to resect "normal-looking brain" at operation. Unfortunately, this is the usual case when the advancing margin of a diffusely infiltrating low-grade tumor is seen under the operating microscope.

What is the Role of PET in the Assessment of Cerebral Metastases?

In this clinical setting, a number scenarios may be encountered. First, a patient with a known malignant tumor, for example, melanoma, presents with neurologic symptoms suggestive of a CNS tumor, for example, headache or a generalized convulsion. Should a cerebral PET scan be done to determine if the patient has a cerebral metastasis? In most experienced PET centers, the answer is generally, no. PET does not currently have the spatial resolution to detect small cerebral metastases and the best imaging tool is a contrast-enhanced MR scan. FDG PET is compromised because most metastases occur at the gray-white junction and it is often impossible to separate a small hypermetabolic focus of metastatic tumor with little surrounding edema from the normal cortical glucose utilization. Although other ligands, ^{11}C-methionine and ^{11}C-thymidine, are not taken up by normal brain to a marked degree, the poorer signal-to-noise ratio of these ligands makes them unlikely diagnostic tools in this situation. Griffeth et al. (110) reported findings in 19 patients who had 31 metastases and FDG PET detected these in only 68%. Although many of the patients had already been treated with radiotherapy and/or chemotherapy and an early generation PET scanner was used, not only was there difficulty detecting small lesions, but four lesions 1.2 cm in diameter were missed. We believe that the explanation relates to the nature of CNS metastases. In our experience, although many

cerebral metastases appear to have homogeneous enhancement on MRI on FDG PET, they have a central ametabolic core, due to necrosis or cystic change, with a very thin rim (1 to 2 mm) of increased glucose metabolism (Fig. 5.3.10A). Current PET scanner technology is often unable to resolve this thin rim of active tumor, so PET does not offer any advantage over anatomic imaging.

In the setting of a single large enhancing lesion in a patient with known cancer, where the differential diagnosis includes a primary brain tumor, we may perform a PET scan to aid the neurosurgeon in planning surgery and/or biopsy. In a similar context, PET has an additional role in the evaluation of a patient who presents with a cerebral metastasis as the

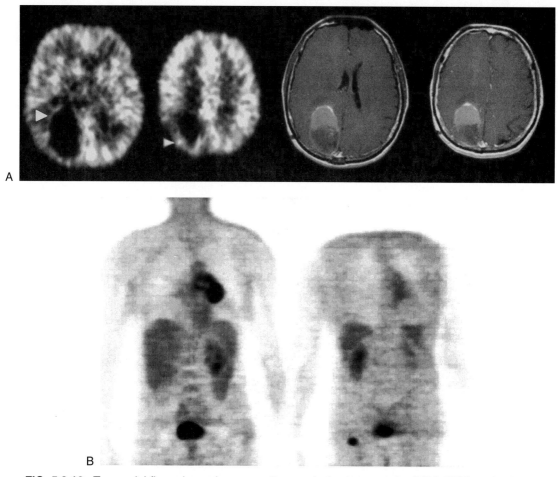

FIG. 5.3.10. Transaxial fluorodeoxyglucose positron emission tomography (FDG PET) and enhanced magnetic resonance imaging (MRI) scans in a 59-year-old man with a short history of unaccustomed headache and visual disturbance. He was a heavy smoker and a preoperative chest radiograph revealed a left hilar mass. **A:** The signal-to-noise ratio in the FDG PET scan was poor due to high-dose dexamethasone (16 mg/d); it showed an ametabolic mass in the right occipital lobe with a thin rim of increased glucose metabolism (*arrowheads*). On enhanced MRI, the lesion was partly hemorrhagic and also had a thin rim of enhancement. At surgery, a necrotic and hemorrhagic adenocarcinoma was removed. Thoracic surgery was planned to remove the primary tumor because there was no evidence of other metastatic disease. **B:** Coronal whole-body FDG PET images were performed to stage the patient's non–small cell lung cancer. A glucose-avid left hilar tumor extended directly into the mediastinum with nodal involvement and there was a glucose-avid focus in the right buttock, which was a subcutaneous metastasis. Surgery was not considered with evidence of mediastinal and another site of extrathoracic disease.

initial manifestation of a systemic malignancy. The underlying tumor is often only apparent after the solitary cerebral metastasis has been removed at surgery. In our center, we then perform a whole-body FDG PET scan, both to detect and to stage the underlying primary tumor because there are direct management implications; for example, a primary non–small cell lung cancer may be resected if there is no evidence of regional or other systemic spread (Fig. 5.3.10B).

SPECIAL TUMOR TYPES

A number of rarer primary CNS tumors are included in the classification of brain tumors (5), but their functional and anatomic imaging characteristics have only recently been described. Some of these tumors may be encountered in a clinical PET program and their features on FDG PET are important to recognize.

Pilocytic Astrocytoma

The pilocytic astrocytoma (PA) is regarded as a low-grade astrocytoma with a good prognosis (12). It occurs in a younger age group than astrocytomas and is most commonly seen in the midline cerebellum and hypothalamus, less frequently in the optic nerves and brainstem, and when found in the cerebral hemispheres, it usually occurs in the temporal lobes (12). Fulham et al. (38) reported functional and anatomic imaging results in five patients with PAs and noted that glucose metabolism in these tumors was similar to that found in anaplastic astrocytomas and much higher than that seen in low-grade gliomas. All tumors enhanced avidly on anatomic imaging and there was little surrounding edema. Given the accepted interpretation of tumoral glucose hypermetabolism, these data provoked the following questions: (a) Was the prognosis for pilocytic tumors poor, (b) was there a subset of pilocytic tumors with aggressive behavior, (c) do these findings invalidate the FDG PET assessment of brain tumors and violate the general principle that low-grade tumors have reduced glucose metabolism and high-grade tumors are hypermetabolic, or (d) do these data reveal an important exception to these principles and reflect a biologic peculiarity in pilocytic tumors? The patients noted in the report of Fulham et al. (38) were all stable and showed no evidence of disease progression after a long follow-up despite the PET and MR findings and the tumors seemed to behave in a benign fashion. However, it is apparent that pilocytic tumors have a number of atypical features. Although they are regarded as benign, they may undergo malignant degeneration and metastasize many years after the original diagnosis (111,112). They can have high proliferative indices, using Ki-67 labeling, and chromosomal abnormalities, both of which are usually seen in high-grade tumors (113–116). If the Daumas-Duport grading system, which is claimed to correlate well with clinical outcome, were used to grade these tumors, they would be incorrectly classified as aggressive tumors (7). Their vascular endothelium has

poorly developed tight junctions, which explains the intense enhancement on structural imaging, and vessels of this type are also usually found in malignant tumors (117,118). Although the mechanism for the paradoxical increase in glucose utilization in these tumors remains unexplained, the authors speculated that it was related to expression of the GLUT proteins.

Thus, it is important to remember that a PA should be considered in the differential diagnosis when there is a hypermetabolic tumor seen (a) in combination with intense enhancement on MRI, (b) where there is little surrounding edema, (c) in a young patient, and (d) the lesion is located in the optic chiasm, cerebellum, hypothalamus, or temporal lobes.

Ganglioglioma

These tumors are composed of well-differentiated but atypical neuronal elements and neoplastic glia. They are slow growing and rarely undergo anaplastic change (12). They occur at any age, and although commonly found in the temporal lobes where they can produce refractory epilepsy, they may be found anywhere in the neuraxis. The tumors may be solid or cystic and have areas of calcification; temporal lobe tumors are more likely to be solid (64). In a large series reported by Zentner et al. (65), enhancement on MRI was found in 16 of 36 patients. In our experience, these tumors are hypometabolic on FDG PET (Fig. 5.3.11), consistent with the findings of Kincaid et al. (119), who reported hypometabolism in 11 patients. There is one report of increased glucose metabolism in a temporal lobe tumor in a 13-year-old boy with refractory complex partial seizures (120). Unfortunately, details of the scanning protocol and whether or not EEG monitoring was done were not provided. The tumor was resected and proven to be low grade. Although the authors suggest caution when judging the malignant potential of a tumor with FDG PET ''in children or young adults with uncharacteristic findings,'' in this author's opinion, an alternative explanation is that the glucose hypermetabolism was due to unsuspected seizure activity in the uptake or scan period.

Dysembryoplastic Neuroepithelial Tumor

Dysembryoplastic neuroepithelial tumors (DNETs) were first identified in tissue resected from patients with refractory epilepsy by Daumas-Duport et al. (121). The pathologic, clinical, and radiologic findings of the ''simple'' and ''complex'' forms of these tumors can be found in a recent review (122). They have only been described in the supratentorial compartment and can be found in the mesial temporal lobes, the perirolandic region, and the parietal and occipital lobes. The main pathologic features are (a) a cortical location, (b) nodular architecture with the nodule having features of astrocytomas, oligodendrogliomas, or oligoastrocytomas, (c) foci of dysplastic cortex, and (d) presence of a ''glioneuronal'' element arranged in columns perpendicular to the cortex.

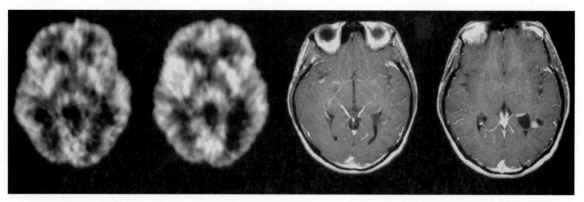

FIG. 5.3.11. Transaxial ^{18}F-fluorodeoxyglucose positron emission tomography (FDG PET) and magnetic resonance scans in a 23-year-old man after his first tonic-clonic convulsion. Anatomic imaging revealed a cystic lesion adjacent to the posterior horn of the left ventricle with a solid enhancing component. On FDG PET, the lesion was hypometabolic, consistent with a low-grade tumor. A ganglioglioma was found at surgery.

Patients typically have long-standing epilepsy, and on MRI, the involved cortex is expanded and hyperintense on T2-weighted images. In the complex forms, the large cortical nodules may appear to be located in white matter. None of the original tumors described by Daumas-Duport showed contrast enhancement. There are limited data with FDG PET, but at our center, DNETs have all shown glucose hypometabolism in the regions of abnormal signal intensity on MRI (Fig. 5.3.12). There are no regions of markedly increased glucose metabolism.

Pleomorphic Xanthoastrocytoma

In 1979, Kepes et al. (123) described the histologic and clinical features of pleomorphic xanthoastrocytomas (PXAs). These tumors are characterized by a superficial location, often involving the meninges, and pleomorphic lipid-laden glial fibrillary acid protein–positive neoplastic cells,

which are associated with an abundant reticulin network. The tumors tend to occur in young adults but have been described at any age. They are usually found in the temporal lobes and less commonly in the frontal and parietal lobes (12). Until recently, all reported tumors were located in the supratentorial compartment, but cerebellar tumors were described in two patients (124,125). Interestingly, in both cases, the cerebellar tumors appeared more than a decade after an initial PXA had been removed. All of these tumors enhance avidly on CT and MRI (126–128).

There is a single report of FDG PET findings in a 19-year-old man with a recurrent PXA (126). The tumor recurred 10 and 15 months after the original subtotal resection, and on each occasion, recurrence was associated with clinical and radiologic deterioration. The tumor was hypermetabolic relative to white matter and peak glucose utilization in the lesion was similar to that seen in anaplastic astrocytomas (38,126), which was consistent with the clinical behavior,

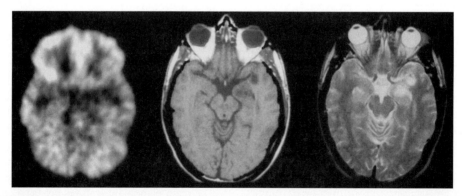

FIG. 5.3.12. Transaxial ^{18}F-fluorodeoxyglucose positron emission tomography (FDG PET) and magnetic resonance imaging (MRI) scans in a 21-year-old man with refractory epilepsy. On FDG PET, the left anteromesial temporal lobe was hypometabolic and corresponded to the complex hypointense lesion on T1-weighted images and the extensive region of hyperintensity on T2-weighted MRI. The lesion did not enhance with contrast. A dysembryoplastic neuroepithelial tumor was found at surgery.

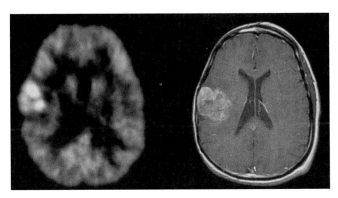

FIG. 5.3.13. Transaxial ¹⁸F-fluorodeoxyglucose positron emission tomography (FDG PET) and enhanced magnetic resonance images in a 25-year-old man with a recurrent pleomorphic xanthoastrocytoma. The original tumor in the right parietal lobe had been resected at age 7 and the patient received postoperative radiotherapy. On FDG PET, the tumor is markedly hypermetabolic and the hypermetabolism closely matches the regions of gadolinium-diethylenetriamine pentaacetic acid enhancement.

although necrosis and mitoses were not seen in the original specimen. Although additional FDG PET studies are required to determine if all PXAs demonstrate increased glucose utilization, we have studied another two patients with PXAs. In one patient, the tumor (Fig. 5.3.13) recurred in the parietal lobe 18 years after the original resection, and the other was studied on presentation and had a left temporal lobe lesion. In both cases, the tumors were hypermetabolic.

Gliomatosis Cerebri

Nevin (129) first used the term gliomatosis cerebri to describe a diffuse overgrowth of the nervous system with neoplastic glia in 1938. However, Russell and Rubinstein (12) regard it as an example of a diffuse astrocytoma. It is reported in all age groups and has a peak incidence in the fifth decade. It is notoriously difficult to diagnose because the initial symptoms are vague or nonspecific. Seizures, headache, and focal neurologic signs typically appear late in the course of the disease. The white matter is usually extensively infiltrated with bland neoplastic astrocytes, but occasionally it can be confined to gray matter. The neoplastic cells have a proliferative potential similar to that of low-grade gliomas (130). CT and MRI underestimate the extent of the disease (131,132). There are two PET reports in patients with gliomatosis cerebri. Mineura et al. (133) used ¹¹C-methionine PET in a 32-year-old patient with bilateral gray and white matter involvement of the temporooccipital lobes. Extensive areas of abnormal ¹¹C-methionine uptake corresponded to signal-intensity changes on MRI (133). Dexter et al. (134) reported FDG PET and MRI findings in a 16-year-old girl who presented with an isolated third-nerve palsy as the initial manifestation of gliomatosis cerebri, which was largely confined to gray matter. The tumoral involvement was hypometabolic on FDG PET, consistent with a low-grade tumor.

Spinal Cord Tumors

There is a paucity of data on the role of PET in the evaluation of patients with proven or suspected spinal cord tumors. There were two early reports but the patient numbers were small (135,136). Di Chiro et al. (136) studied seven patients, two with an early generation device (ECAT II) and five with the NeuroPET, which was a head-only tomograph. There was only one true spinal tumor and it was studied with the ECAT II, which had an in-plane resolution of 17 mm; the remaining tumors were brainstem tumors. Alavi et al. (135) reported a single case of a patient with a cervical cord GBM who was assessed after treatment for recurrent tumor versus radiation necrosis; the PET was hypermetabolic. They used the PENN PET system with sodium iodide detectors.

The availability of whole-body PET systems now allows functional imaging of the spinal cord. In a recent study, Wilmshurst et al. (137) reported their findings in 14 patients with intramedullary tumors (n = 13) and one schwannoma. They compared the PET findings with MRI findings and found a close correlation in the patients scanned on presentation (n = 8). Further, they commented that the PET uptake was in keeping with the low-grade histology, but PET did not provide additional useful information. In our center, we have had a different approach and have now scanned a cohort of patients (n = 33) with a diagnosis of proven spinal cord tumor or suspected spinal cord tumor. The diagnosis was based on neurologic findings compatible with a cord lesion and MRI findings that suggested that the likely diagnosis was an intramedullary spinal cord tumor. Our findings differ from those of Wilmshurst et al. in that (a) all the low-grade intramedullary spinal cord tumors showed increased glucose metabolism relative to the spinal cord (Fig. 5.3.14) and to values for glucose metabolism obtained in healthy subjects. This finding is in direct contrast to low-grade gliomas in the brain and posterior fossa. (b) However, FDG PET is able to differentiate spinal cord infarction, ischemia, and inflammation (demyelination) because these processes are hypometabolic on FDG PET. The absence of glucose hypermetabolism clearly identified the nontumorous lesions and was valuable in management.

OTHER PET LIGANDS

Various PET ligands other than FDG have been used to provide insights into tumor biology, and they range from tumoral glucose and oxygen metabolism, to blood flow, pH, status of the blood–brain barrier, amino acid uptake, and receptor binding. They can also assess the pharmacokinetics of chemotherapy delivery and the distribution of labeled drugs. These ligands have been mostly used in a research setting and few have made the translation into the clinical setting. The largest experience, outside of FDG, has been

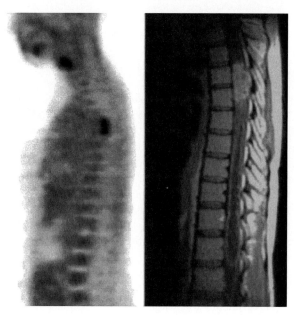

FIG. 5.3.14. Sagittal whole-body ^{18}F-fluorodeoxyglucose positron emission tomography (FDG PET) and enhanced magnetic resonance images in a 25-year-old woman with a proven ependymoma. On FDG PET, the tumor, despite its benign pathology, was relatively glucose avid when compared with normal spinal cord and it enhanced avidly after contrast enhancement.

directed at obtaining data about tumoral protein synthesis with a variety of tracers, but particularly with ^{11}C-methionine.

^{11}C-methionine and Amino Acid Transport

The initial hope was that PET ligands such as ^{11}C-methionine would be incorporated into tumoral proteins and provide insights into tumor activity and proliferative capacity. Although its exact mechanism of uptake is still not completely understood, it is apparent that ^{11}C-methionine uptake is related mainly to a saturable process—carrier-mediated amino acid transport—rather than incorporation into tumor proteins. In early work with small patient numbers, ^{11}C-methionine PET was compared with CT and MRI without Gd-DTPA and was found to be better at delineating the tumor margin, particularly for low-grade gliomas (60,108, 138).

A number of larger series can be found in the literature, but the actual role of ^{11}C-methionine in the important management questions for brain tumor patients (discussed above) is still uncertain (109,139–141). These later studies differ in the numbers of tumors in the different pathologic grades, the scanning methodologies employed, and the time points for data analysis, which may explain some of the disparities in the findings. Ogawa et al. (141) reported data from a series of 50 patients (32 high- and 18 low-grade gliomas). These investigators found that although there was

a significant difference in tracer uptake between high-grade and low-grade tumors, in an individual case it was difficult to evaluate the degree of malignancy from ^{11}C-methionine accumulation alone. Herholz et al. (139) reported data that included 83 untreated gliomas of varying grades and found that ^{11}C-methionine could distinguish between different grades of glioma, but high tracer uptake was seen in pituitary adenomas, meningiomas, and ependymomas. Kaschten et al. (140) found that although ^{11}C-methionine uptake was increased in GBMs, it could not separate low-grade from anaplastic astrocytomas. Further, tracer uptake was increased in oligodendrogliomas but was decreased in anaplastic oligodendrogliomas. The more marked ^{11}C-methionine uptake into oligodendrogliomas when compared with astrocytomas has been noted by Derlon et al. (109) in 22 patients, 10 of whom had low-grade oligodendrogliomas. Interestingly, in the low-grade astrocytomas in this study ^{11}C-methionine uptake was normal (compared with the contralateral normal brain) or low. This suggests that investigators in the earlier (60,108,138) and more recent reports (141) may have studied oligodendrogliomas. Finally, it is unclear if ^{11}C-methionine can detect malignant degeneration or separate recurrent tumor from radiation necrosis (142).

Various other PET tracers that all use amino acid transport mechanisms have been synthesized and used in similar clinical settings. These include ^{18}F-fluorotyrosine, ^{18}F-fluoroethyltyrosine, ^{18}F-fluorophenylalanine, ^{11}C-aminocyclopentane carboxylic acid, ^{11}C-α-aminoisobutyric acid, and ^{11}C-methyl-α-aminoisobutyric acid; however, none has made a notable impact on clinical practice.

FMISO and Tumor Hypoxia

There has been renewed interest in the evaluation of tumor hypoxia with the recent greater understanding of tumor angiogenesis and the introduction of improved radiation sensitizers such as tirapazamine (143). It is a general principle in radiation oncology that tumor cells, which are irradiated under normal oxygen tensions, are more sensitive to radiation than hypoxic tumor cells (144–146). It has been hypothesized that intratumoral hypoxia explains some of the radioresistance seen in high-grade gliomas in humans and animals (147,148). Research effort has been directed at altering the tumor milieu with chemical radiosensitizers and bioreductive agents with the hope of improving cell kill with radiotherapy, and tirapazamine is a product of this research.

Unfortunately, the identification of tumor hypoxia *in vivo* in humans is not a trivial task and requires the invasive placement of oxygen electrodes into the tumor. However, Rasey et al. (149) developed ^{18}F-fluoromisonidazole (^{18}F-FMISO) as a hypoxic imaging agent. Misonidazole and fluoromisonidazole have high electron affinity and are selectively reduced and incorporated into viable hypoxic cells.

Later, Valk et al. (150) used ^{18}F-FMISO to depict tissue hypoxia in three patients with high-grade gliomas. In two patients (anaplastic astrocytoma, GBM), there was marked uptake, and in the third patient, also with a GBM, there was no tracer uptake. Although these data were preliminary, they suggest that the detection of tumor hypoxia might be useful in the selection of patients for treatment with radiosensitizers and perhaps to measure response to radiation and chemotherapy.

[11]C-thymidine

Thymidine is easily taken up by cells and is incorporated into DNA. Labeled with carbon-14 and hydrogen-3, it has been used to assess cell growth and proliferation in the laboratory (151). Kubota et al. (152) demonstrated many years ago that DNA and protein synthesis decline more sharply after therapy than with FDG. Preliminary data with ^{11}C-thymidine PET were published by Vander Borght et al. (153). They noted ^{11}C-thymidine uptake in gliomas, regardless of grade, and benign meningiomas. Eary et al. (154) studied 13 patients with brain tumors and found that the qualitative results of ^{11}C-thymidine PET differed from those with FDG PET and MRI in 50% of cases, but the significance of this is, as yet, uncertain. Regardless, this ligand shows great promise for the future evaluation of tumor response, as indicated in the previous section.

The Others

In the 1980s glioma oxygen metabolism was studied by Rhodes et al. (155), who showed that gliomas extract a lower fraction of oxygen than normal brain, suggesting that gliomas are adequately oxygenated. Rottenberg et al. (156) demonstrated, surprisingly, that brain tumors had an alkaline pH level relative to normal brain. They used ^{11}C-dimethyl-2,4-oxazolidinedione PET (156), and this was later confirmed with phosphorus-31 MRS (157). Carbon-11-putrescine was proposed as a tracer for tumoral DNA synthesis in the late 1980s because putrescine serves as a precursor to the polyamines and increased polyamine metabolism is associated with malignancy (158). However, subsequent PET studies showed that ^{11}C-putrescine was merely a good tracer to depict blood–brain barrier disruption (159,160).

Experimental data suggested that benzodiazepines may regulate glial cell proliferation via the peripheral benzodiazepine receptors (PBRs) (161) and binding studies done on postmortem human tissue showed a high density of PBR binding sites in brain tumors. It was hoped that ligands directed at these receptors might be used as a marker of cell density in human gliomas (162,163). Two PBR ligands, Ro-5-4864 and PK-11195, were labeled with ^{11}C and were used in human PET studies. For ^{11}C-Ro-5-4864, there was no specific binding to astrocytomas (164,165). However, ^{11}C-PK-11195 uptake was found in human gliomas, but definitive evidence of the specificity of it binding to tumoral PBRs was not provided (165), although it was later reported by Pappata et al. (166) in a single patient. In the small series of Junck et al. (167) (9 patients) no meaningful data on tumor grading were obtained and additional work found that PBR binding occurs in ischemic and inflammatory lesions, which also suggested that PBR ligands may not be useful in separating recurrent tumor from radiation necrosis.

Is There a "Best" PET Ligand?

It is this author's opinion that although FDG has limitations, it is still the most versatile PET ligand to answer many of the critical questions that should be addressed for the effective management of patients with brain tumor, as suggested by Di Chiro (168) a decade ago. With the advances in radiochemistry and PET instrumentation, it is likely that a multiligand approach to management will be achieved in the near future. Such algorithms may use a combination of ligands to measure proliferative capacity, tumor angiogenesis, glucose metabolism, and receptor binding in the diagnostic, prognostic, and treatment settings.

REFERENCES

1. Jaeckle KA. Clinical presentation and therapy of nervous system tumors. In: Bradley WG, Daroff RB, Fenichel GM, et al, eds. *Neurology in clinical practice,* 1st ed. Massachusetts: Butterworth-Heinemann, 1991:1008–1030.
2. Wen PY, Black PM. Clinical presentation, evaluation and preoperative preparation of the patient. In: Berger MS, Wilson CB, eds. *The gliomas.* Philadelphia: WB Saunders, 1999:328–336.
3. Loeffler JS, Patchell RA, Sawaya R. Treatment of metastatic cancer. In: DeVita VT, Hellman S, Rosenberg SA, eds. *Cancer: principles & practice of oncology,* 5th ed. Philadelphia: Lippincott–Raven Publishers, 1997:2523–2536.
4. Levin VA, Leibel SA, Gutin PH. Neoplasms of the central nervous system. In: DeVita VT, Hellman S, Rosenberg SA, eds. *Cancer: principles & practice of oncology,* 5th ed. Philadelphia: Lippincott–Raven Publishers, 1997:2022–2082.
5. Kleihues P, Burger PC, Scheithauer BW. The new WHO classification of brain tumors. *Brain Pathol* 1993;3:255–268.
6. Burger PC, Vogel FS, Green SB. Glioblastoma and anaplastic astrocytoma: pathologic criteria and prognostic considerations. *Cancer* 1985; 56:1106–1111.
7. Daumas-Duport C, Scheithauer B, O'Fallon J, et al. Grading of astrocytomas: a simple and reproducible method. *Cancer* 1988;62: 2152–2165.
8. Kernohan JW, Mabon RF, Svien HJ, et al. A simplified classification of the gliomas. *Proc Staff Mtg Mayo Clin* 1949;24:71–75.
9. Ringertz N. Grading of gliomas. *Acta Pathol Microbiol* 1950;27: 51–64.
10. Jaeckle KA. Neuroimaging for central nervous system tumors. *Semin Oncol* 1991;18(2):150–157.
11. Shapiro WR, Shapiro JR. Primary brain tumors. In: Asbury AK, McKhann GM, McDonald WI, eds. *Diseases of the nervous system: clinical neurobiology,* 2nd ed. Philadelphia: WB Saunders, 1992: 1074–1092.
12. Russell DS, Rubinstein LJ. Tumors of central neuroepithelial origin. In: *Pathology of tumors of the nervous system,* 5th ed. Baltimore: Williams & Wilkins, 1989:83–350.
13. Barker FG, Gutin PH. Surgical approaches to gliomas. In: Berger MS, Wilson CB, eds. *The gliomas.* Philadelphia: WB Saunders, 1999: 349–360.
14. Kelly PJ. Computer assisted volumetric stereotactic resection of superficial and deep seated intra-axial brain mass lesions. *Acta Neurochir* 1991;52:26–29.
15. Kelly PJ. Stereotactic resection and its limitations in glial neoplasms. *Stereotact Funct Neurosurg* 1992;59(1-4):84–91.
16. Macuinas R. Interactive image-guided surgical technology for glial tumor resection. In: Berger MS, Wilson CB, eds. *The gliomas.* Philadelphia: WB Saunders, 1999:409–420.

17. Macdonald DR, Cascino TL, Schold SC, et al. Response criteria for phase II studies of supratentorial malignant glioma. *J Clin Oncol* 1990; 8:1277–1280.

18. Byrne TN. Imaging of gliomas. *Semin Oncol* 1994;21(2):162–171.

19. Di Chiro G. Positron emission tomography using [¹⁸F]fluorodeoxyglucose in brain tumors: a powerful diagnostic and prognostic tool. *Invest Radiol* 1987; 22:360–371.

20. Fulham MJ, Di Chiro G. Positron emission tomography and ¹H-spectroscoic imaging. In: Berger MS, Wilson CB, eds. *The gliomas*. Philadelphia: WB Saunders, 1999:295–317.

21. Gruber ML, Hochberg FH. Editorial: systematic evaluation of primary brain tumors. *J Nucl Med* 1990;31:969–971.

22. Kondziolka D, Lunsford LD, Martinez AJ. Unreliability of contemporary neurodiagnostic imaging in evaluating suspected adult supratentorial (low-grade) astrocytoma. *J Neurosurg* 1993;79:533–536.

23. Fulham MJ, Bizzi A, Deitz MJ, et al. Metabolite mapping of brain tumors with proton MR spectroscopic imaging: clinical relevance. *Radiology* 1992;185:675–686.

24. Eberl S, Anayat AR, Fulton RR, et al. Evaluation of two population-based input functions for quantitative FDG PET studies. *Eur J Nucl Med* 1997;24(3):299–304.

25. Phelps ME, Huang SC, Hoffman EJ, et al. Tomographic measurement of local cerebral glucose metabolic rate in humans with [¹⁸F]2-fluoro-2-deoxy-D-glucose: validation of method. *Ann Neurol* 1979;6: 371–388.

26. Hooper PK, Meikle SR, Eberl S, et al. Validation of post injection transmission measurements for attenuation correction in neurologic FDG PET studies. *J Nucl Med* 1996:128–136.

27. Fulton RR, Eberl S, Meikle SR, et al. A practical 3D tomographic method for correcting patient head motion in clinical SPECT. *IEEE Trans Nucl Sci* 1999;46(3):667–672.

28. Fulton RR, Meikle SR, Eberl S, et al. Use of an optical motion tracking system to measure patient head movements in positron emission tomography (PET). *IEEE Trans Nucl Sci* 2002 *(in press)*.

29. Green MV, Seidel J, Stein SD, et al. Head movement in normal subjects during simulated PET brain imaging with and without head movement. *J Nucl Med* 1994;35(9):1538–1546.

30. Eberl S, Kanno I, Fulton RR, et al. A general automated inter-study image registration technique for SPECT and PET studies. *J Nucl Med* 1996:137–145.

31. Woods RP, Cherry SR, Mazziotta JC. Rapid automated algorithm for aligning and reslicing PET images. *J Comput Assisted Tomogr* 1992; 16:620–633.

32. Ardekani BA, Braun M, Hutton BF, et al. A fully automatic multimodality image registration algorithm. *J Comput Assisted Tomogr* 1995; 19(4):615–623.

33. Kadekaro M, Vance WM, Terrell ML, et al. Effects of antidromic stimulation of the ventral root on glucose utilization in the ventral horn of the spinal cord in the rat. *Proc Natl Acad Sci* 1987;84:5492–5495.

34. Guerin C, Laterra J, Drewes LR, et al. Vascular expression of glucose transporter in experimental brain neoplasms. *Am J Pathol* 1992;140: 417–425.

35. Pessin JE, Bell GI. Mammalian facilitative glucose transporter family: structure and molecular regulation. *Annu Rev Physiol* 1992;54: 911–930.

36. Warburg O. *Metabolism of tumors*. London: Arnold & Constable, 1930.

37. Di Chiro G, Brooks RA. PET-FDG of untreated and treated cerebral gliomas. *J Nucl Med* 1988;29:421–422.

38. Fulham MJ, Melisi JW, Nishimiya J, et al. Neuroimaging of juvenile pilocytic astrocytomas: an enigma. *Radiology* 1993;189:221–225.

39. Di Chiro G, DeLaPaz R, Brooks RA, et al. Glucose utilization of cerebral gliomas measured by [¹⁸F]Fluorodeoxyglucose and positron emission tomography. *Neurology* 1982;32:1323–1329.

40. Kim CK, Alavi JB, Alavi A, et al. New grading system of cerebral gliomas using positron emission tomography with F-18 fluorodeoxyglucose. *J Neurooncol* 1991;10:85–91.

41. Alavi JB, Alavi A, Chawluk J, et al. Positron emission tomography in patients with glioma: a predictor of prognosis. *Cancer* 1988;62: 1074–1078.

42. Coleman RE, Hoffman JM, Hanson MW, et al. Clinical application of PET for the evaluation of brain tumors. *J Nucl Med* 1991;32:616–622.

43. Tyler JL, Diksic M, Villemure J-G, et al. Metabolic and hemodynamic evaluation of gliomas using positron emission tomography. *J Nucl Med* 1987;28:1123–1133.

44. Delbeke D, Meyerowitz C, Lapidus RL, et al. Optimal cutoff levels of F-18 fluorodeoxyglucose uptake in the differentiation of low grade from high-grade brain tumors with PET. *Radiology* 1995;195:47–52.

45. Baron JC, Bousser MG, Comar D, et al. Crossed cerebellar diaschisis in human supratentorial infarction [Abstract]. *Ann Neurol* 1980;8:128.

46. Patronas NJ, Di Chiro G, Smith BH, et al. Depressed cerebellar glucose metabolism in supratentorial tumors. *Brain Res* 1984;291: 93–101.

47. West JR. The concept of diaschisis: a reply to Markowitsch and Pritzel. *Behav Biol* 1978;22:413–416.

48. Fulham MJ, Brooks RA, Hallett M, et al. Cerebellar diaschisis revisited: pontine hypometabolism and dentate sparing. *Neurology* 1992; 42:2267–2273.

49. Brodal A. The cerebellum. In: *Neurological anatomy in relation to clinical medicine*. New York: Oxford University Press, 1981: 294–391.

50. Feeney DM, Baron JC. Diaschisis. *Stroke* 1986;17:817–830.

51. Carlstedt-Duke J, Gustafsson J-A. The molecular mechanism of glucocorticoid action. In: Ludecke DK, Chrousos GP, Tolis G, eds. *ACTH, Cushing's syndrome and other hypercortisolemic states*. New York: Raven Press, 1990:7–14.

52. Muncke A. Glucocorticoid inhibition of glucose uptake by peripheral tissues: old and new evidence, molecular mechanism and action. *Perspect Biol Med* 1971;14:265–289.

53. Kadekaro M, Ito M, Gross PM. Local cerebral glucose utilization is increased in acutely adrenalectomized rats. *Neuroendocrinology* 1988;47:329–334.

54. Fulham MJ, Brunetti A, Aloj L, et al. Decreased cerebral glucose metabolism in patients with brain tumors: an effect of corticosteroids. *J Neurosurg* 1995:657–664.

55. Blacklock JB, Oldfield EH, Di Chiro G, et al. Effect of barbiturate coma on glucose utilization in normal brain versus gliomas. Positron emission tomography studies. *J Neurosurg* 1987;67:71–75.

56. Gaillard WD, Zeffiro T, Fazilat S, et al. Effect of valproate on cerebral metabolism and blood flow: an ¹⁸F-2-deoxyglucose and ¹⁵O water positron emission tomography study. *Epilepsia* 1996;37:515–521.

57. Leiderman DB, Balish M, Bromfield EB, et al. Effect of valproate on human cerebral glucose metabolism. *Epilepsia* 1991;32:417–422.

58. Pahl JJ, Mazziotta JC, Bartzokis G, et al. Positron-emission tomography in tardive dyskinesia. *J Neuropsychiatry Clin Neurosci* 1995;7: 457–465.

59. McCormack BM, Miller DC, Budzilovich GN, et al. Treatment and survival of low-grade astrocytoma in adults—1977–1988. *Neurosurgery* 1992;31:636–642.

60. Lilja A, Bergstrom K, Spannare B, et al. Reliability of computed tomography in assessing histopathological features of malignant supratentorial gliomas. *J Comput Assisted Tomogr* 1981;5:625–636.

61. Joyce P, Bentson J, Takahashi M, et al. The accuracy of predicting histologic grades of supratentorial astrocytomas on the basis of computerized tomography and cerebral angiography. *Neuroradiology* 1978;16:346–348.

62. Butler AR, Horii SC, Kricheff II, et al. Computed tomography in astrocytomas. *Radiology* 1978;129:433–439.

63. Leeds NE, Elkin CM, Zimmerman RD. Gliomas of the brain. *Semin Roentgenol* 1984;19:27–43.

64. Castillo M, Davis PC, Takei Y, et al. Intracranial ganglioglioma: MR, CT, and clinical findings in 18 patients. *AJNR* 1990;11(1):109–114.

65. Zentner J, Wolf HK, Ostertun B, et al. Gangliogliomas: clinical, radiological, and histopathological findings in 51 patients. *J Neurol Neurosurg Psychiatry* 1994;57(12):1497–1502.

66. Lee Y-Y, van Tassel P, Bruner JM, et al. Juvenile pilocytic astrocytomas: CT and MR characteristics. *AJR Am J Roengenol* 1989;152: 1263–1270.

67. Davis WK, Boyko OB, Hoffman JM, et al. [¹⁸F]2-fluoro-2-deoxyglucose-positron emission tomography correlation of gadolinium-enhanced MR imaging of central nervous system neoplasia. *AJNR* 1993; 14(3):515–523.

68. Melisi JW, Fulham MJ, Patronas N, et al. *Comparison of Gd-DTPA enhanced MRI with PET-FDG in assessment of gliomas: proceedings of the Congress of Neurological Surgeons, Orlando, FL, 1991*. 1991: 264–266.

69. Olivero WC, Dulebohn SC, Lister JR. The use of PET in evaluating

patients with primary brain tumors: is it useful? *J Neurol Neurosurg Psychiatry* 1995;58:250–252.

70. Hanson MW, Glantz MJ, Hoffman JM, et al. FDG-PET in the selection of brain lesions for biopsy. *J Comput Assisted Tomogr* 1991;15: 796–801.

71. Levivier M, Goldman S, Pirotte B, et al. Diagnostic yield of stereotactic brain biopsy guided by positron emission tomography with [18F]fluorodeoxyglucose. *J Neurosurg* 1995;82:445–452.

72. Massager N, David P, Goldman S, et al. Combined magnetic resonance imaging– and positron emission tomography–guided stereotactic biopsy in brainstem mass lesions: diagnostic yield in a series of 30 patients. *J Neurosurg* 2000;93:951–957.

72a. Chamberlain MC, Murovic JA, Levin VA. Absence of contrast enlargement on CT brain scans of patients with supratentorial malignant gliomas. *Neurology* 1998;38:1371–1374.

73. Kelly PJ, Daumas-Duport C, Scheithauer B, et al. Stereotactic histological correlations of computerized tomography– and magnetic resonance imaging–defined abnormalities in patients with glial neoplasms. *Mayo Clin Proc* 1987;62:450–459.

74. Cairncross JG. The biology of astrocytomas: lessons learned from chronic myelogenous leukemia—hypothesis. *J Neurooncol* 1987;5: 11–27.

75. Cairncross JG. Low-grade glioma: to treat or not to treat? *Arch Neurol* 1989;46:1238–1239.

76. Laws ERJ, Taylor WF, Clifton MB, et al. Neurosurgical management of low-grade astrocytoma of the cerebral hemisphere. *J Neurosurg* 1984;61:665–673.

77. Peipmeier JM. Observations on the current treatment of low-grade astrocytic tumors of the cerebral hemispheres. *J Neurosurg* 1987;67: 177–181.

78. Cairncross JG, MacDonald DR. Successful chemotherapy for recurrent malignant oligodendroglioma. *Ann Neurol* 1988;23:360–364.

79. Bauman GS, Cairncross JG. Multidisciplinary management of adult anaplastic oligodendrogliomas and anaplastic mixed oligo-astrocytomas. *Semin Radiat Oncol* 2001;11:170–180.

80. Peterson K, DeAngelis LM. Weighing the benefits and risks of radiation therapy for low-grade glioma. *Neurology* 2001;56:1255–1256.

81. Surma-aho O, Niemela M, Vilkki J, et al. Adverse long-term effects of brain radiotherapy in adult low-grade glioma patients. *Neurology* 2001;56:1285–1290.

82. Francavilla TL, Miletich RS, Di Chiro G, et al. Positron emission tomography in the detection of malignant degeneration of low-grade gliomas. *Neurosurgery* 1989;24:1–5.

83. Fulham MJ. PET with [18F]fluorodeoxyglucose (PET-FDG): an indispensable tool in the proper management of brain tumors. In: Hubner KF, Collmann J, Buonocore E, et al, eds. *Clinical positron emission tomography.* St. Louis: Mosby–Year Book, 1992:50–60.

84. Gutin PH, Leibel SA, Wara WW, et al. Recurrent malignant gliomas: survival following interstitial brachytherapy with high-activity iodine-125 sources. *J Neurosurg* 1987;67:864–873.

85. Patronas NJ, Di Chiro G, Kufta C, et al. Prediction of survival in glioma patients by means of positron emission tomography. *J Neurosurg* 1985;62:816–822.

86. Holzer T, Herholz K, Jeske J, et al. FDG PET as a prognostic indicator in radiochemotherapy of glioblastoma. *J Comput Assisted Tomogr* 1993;17(5):681–687.

87. Schifter T, Hoffman JM, Hanson MW, et al. Serial FDG PET studies in the prediction of survival in patients with primary brain tumors. *J Comput Assisted Tomogr* 1993;17(4):509–516.

88. Cairncross JG, Pexman JHW, Rathbone MP, et al. Postoperative contrast enhancement in patients with brain tumor. *Ann Neurol* 1985;17: 570–572.

89. Cairncross JG, Macdonald DR, Pexman JH, et al. Steroid-induced CT changes in patients with recurrent malignant glioma. *Neurology* 1988; 38:724–726.

90. Hatam A, Bergstrom M, Yu Z-Y, et al. Effect of dexamethasone treatment on volume and contrast enhancement of intracranial neoplasms. *J Comput Assisted Tomogr* 1983;7:295–300.

91. Muller W, Kretzschmar K, Schicketanz K-H. CT-analyses of cerebral tumors under steroid therapy. *Neuroradiology* 1984;26:293–298.

92. Crocker EF, Zimmerman RA, Phelps ME, et al. The effect of steroid on the extravascular distribution of radiographic contrast material and technetium pertechnetate in brain tumors as determined by computed tomography. *Radiology* 1976;119:471–474.

93. Eary JF, Krohn KA. Positron emission tomography: imaging tumor response. *Eur J Nucl Med* 2000;27:1737–1739.

94. Hoekstra O, Ossenkoppele G, Golding R. Early treatment response in malignant lymphoma, as determined by planar fluorine-18-fluorodeoxyglucose scintigraphy. *J Nucl Med* 1993;34:1706–1710.

95. Schelling M, Avril N, Nahrig J, et al. Positron emission tomography using [(18)F]fluorodeoxyglucose for monitoring primary chemotherapy in breast cancer. *J Clin Oncol* 2000;18:1689–1695.

96. Shields AF, Mankoff DA, Link JM, et al. Carbon-11-thymidine and FDG to measure therapy response. *J Nucl Med* 1998;39:1757–1762.

97. Young H, Brock C, Wells P, et al. Monitoring response to treatment in the development of anti-cancer drugs using positron emission tomography. *Drug Information J* 1999;33:237–244.

98. Patronas NJ, Di Chiro G, Brooks RA, et al. Work in progress: [18F]Fluorodeoxyglucose and positron emission tomography in the evaluation of radiation necrosis of the brain. *Radiology* 1982;144:885–889.

99. Di Chiro G, Oldfield E, Wright DC, et al. Cerebral necrosis after irradiation and/or intraarterial chemotherapy for brain tumors: PET and neuropathologic studies. *AJNR* 1987;8:1083–1089.

100. Doyle W, Budinger TF, Valk PE, et al. Differentiation of cerebral radiation necrosis from tumor recurrence by [18F]FDG and 82Rb positron emission tomography. *J Comput Assisted Tomogr* 1987;11: 563–570.

101. Valk PE, Budinger TF, Levin VA, et al. PET of malignant cerebral tumors after interstitial brachytherapy: demonstration of metabolic activity and clinical outcome. *J Neurosurg* 1988;69:830–838.

102. Ricci PE, Karis JP, Heiserman JE, et al. Differentiating recurrent tumor from radiation necrosis: time for re-evaluation of positron emission tomography? *AJNR* 1998;19:407–413.

103. Sheline GE, Wara WM, Smithe V. Therapeutic irradiation and brain injury. *Int J Radiat Oncol Biol Phys* 1980;6:1215–1228.

104. Marks JE, Wong J. The risk of cerebral radionecrosis in relation to dose, time and fractionation. *Prog Exp Tumor Res* 1985;29:210–218.

105. Burger PC, Boyko OB. The pathology of central nervous system radiation injury. In: Gutin PH, Leibel SA, Sheline GE, eds. *Radiation injury to the nervous system.* New York: Raven Press, 1991:191–210.

106. Burger PC, Dubois PJ, Schold SC. Computerized tomographic and pathologic studies of untreated, quiescent, and recurrent glioblastoma multiforme. *J Neurosurg* 1983;58:159–169.

107. Earnest F, Kelly PJ, Scheithauer BW, et al. Cerebral astrocytomas: histopathologic correlation of MR and CT contrast enhancement with stereotaxic biopsy. *Radiology* 1988;166:823–827.

108. Mosskin M, Ericson T, Hindmarsh T, et al. Positron emission tomography compared with magnetic resonance imaging and computed tomography in supratentorial gliomas using multiple stereotactic biopsies as reference. *Acta Radiol* 1989;30:225–232.

109. Derlon J-M, Petit-Taboue M-C, Chapon F, et al. The *in vivo* metabolic pattern of low-grade brain gliomas: a positron emission tomographic study using 18F-fluorodeoxyglucose and 11C-L-methylmethionine. *Neurosurgery* 1997;40:276–288.

110. Griffeth LK, Rich KM, Dehdashti F, et al. Brain metastases from non-central nervous system tumors: evaluation with PET. *Radiology* 1993; 186(1):37–44.

111. Obana WG, Cogen PH, Davis RL, et al. Metastatic juvenile pilocytic astrocytoma: a case report. *J Neurosurg* 1991;75:972–975.

112. Mishima K, Nakamura M, Nakamura H, et al. Leptomeningeal dissemination of cerebellar pilocytic astrocytoma. *J Neurosurg* 1992;77: 788–791.

113. Murovic JA, Nagashima T, Hoshino T, et al. Pediatric central nervous system tumors: a cell kinetic study with bromodeoxyuridine. *Neurosurgery* 1986;19:900–904.

114. Tsanaclis AM, Robert F, Michaud J, et al. The cycling pool of cells within human brain tumors: in situ cytokinetics using the monoclonal antibody Ki-67. *Can J Neurol Sci* 1991;18:12–17.

115. Germano IM, Ito M, Cho KG, et al. Correlation of histopathological features and proliferative potential of gliomas. *J Neurosurg* 1989;70: 701–706.

116. Jenkins RB, Kimmel DW, Moertel CA, et al. A cytogenetic study of 53 gliomas. *Cancer Genet Cytogenet* 1989;39:253–279.

117. Long DM. Capillary ultrastructure and the blood brain barrier in human malignant brain tumors. *J Neurosurg* 1970;32:127–144.

118. Sato K, Rorke LB. Vascular bundles and wickerworks in childhood brain tumors. *Pediatr Neurosci* 1989;15:105–110.

119. Kincaid PK, El-Saden SM, Park SH, et al. Cerebral gangliogliomas: preoperative grading using FDG-PET and 201Tl-SPECT. *AJNR* 1998; 19:801–805.

120. Meyer PT, Spetzger U, Mueller HD, et al. High F-18 FDG uptake in

a low-grade supratentorial ganglioglioma: a positron emission tomography case report. *Clin Nucl Med* 2000;25(9):694–697.

121. Daumas-Duport C, Scheithauer BW, Chodkiewicz JP, et al. Dysembryoplastic neuroepithelial tumor: a surgically curable tumor of young patients with intractable partial seizures. *Neurosurgery* 1988;23: 545–556.

122. Daumas-Duport C. Dysembryoplastic neuroepithelial tumors. *Brain Pathol* 1993;3:283–295.

123. Kepes JJ, Rubinstein LJ, Eng LF. Pleomorphic xanthoastrocytoma: a distinctive meningocerebral glioma of young subjects with a relatively favorable prognosis: a study of 12 cases. *Cancer* 1979;44:1839–1852.

124. Lindboe CF, Cappelen J, Kepes JJ. Pleomorphic xanthoastrocytoma as a component of a cerebellar ganglioglioma: a case report. *Neurosurgery* 1992;31:353–355.

125. Glasser RS, Rojiani AM, Mickle JP, et al. Delayed occurrence of cerebellar pleomorphic xanthoastrocytoma after supratentorial pleomorphic xanthoastrocytoma removal. *J Neurosurg* 1995;82:116–118.

126. Bicik I, Raman R, Knightly JJ, et al. PET-FDG of pleomorphic xanthoastrocytoma. *J Nucl Med* 1995;36:97–99.

127. Blom RJ. Pleomorphic xanthoastrocytoma. CT appearance. *J Comput Assisted Tomogr* 1988;12:351–354.

128. Rippe DJ, Boyko OB, Radu M, et al. MRI of temporal lobe pleomorphic xanthoastrocytoma. *J Comput Assisted Tomogr* 1992;16(6): 856–859.

129. Nevin S. Gliomatosis cerebri. *Brain* 1938;61:170–191.

130. Hara A, Sakai N, Yamada H, et al. Assessment of proliferative potential of gliomatosis cerebri. *J Neurol* 1991;238:80–82.

131. Koslow SA, Classen D, Hirsch WL, et al. Gliomatosis cerebri: a case report with autopsy correlation. *Neuroradiology* 1992;34:331–333.

132. Artigas J, Cervos-Navarro J, Iglesias JR, et al. Gliomatosis cerebri: clinical and histological findings. *Clin Neuropathol* 1985;4:135–148.

133. Mineura K, Sasajima T, Kowada M, et al. Innovative approach in the diagnosis of gliomatosis using carbon-11-L-methionine positron emission tomography. *J Nucl Med* 1991;32:726–728.

134. Dexter MA, Parker GD, Besser M, et al. MR and positron emission tomography with fludeoxyglucose F18 in gliomatosis cerebri. *AJNR* 1995;16:1507–1510.

135. Alavi A, Kramer E, Wegener W, et al. Magnetic resonance and fluorine-18 deoxyglucose imaging in the investigation of a spinal cord tumor. *J Nucl Med* 1990;31:360–364.

136. Di Chiro G, Oldfield E, Bairamian D, et al. Metabolic imaging of the brain stem and spinal cord: studies with positron emission tomography using ^{18}F-2-deoxyglucose in normal and pathological cases. *J Comput Assisted Tomogr* 1983;7(6):937–945.

137. Wilmshurst JM, Barrington SF, Pritchard D, et al. Positron emission tomography in imaging spinal cord tumors. *J Child Neurol* 2000; 15(7):465–472.

138. Ericson K, Lilja A, Bergstrom M, et al. Positron emission tomography with ([^{11}C]methyl)-L-methionine, [^{11}C]D-glucose, and [^{68}Ga]EDTA in supratentorial tumors. *J Comput Assisted Tomogr* 1985;9:683–689.

139. Herholz K, Holzer T, Bauer B, et al. ^{11}C-methionine PET for differential diagnosis of low grade-gliomas. *Neurology* 1998;50:1316–1322.

140. Kaschten B, Stevenaert A, Sadzot B, et al. Preoperative evaluation of 54 gliomas by PET with fluorine-18-fluorodeoxyglucose and/or carbon-11-methionine. *J Nucl Med* 1998;39:778–785.

141. Ogawa T, Shishido F, Kanno I, et al. Cerebral glioma: evaluation with methionine PET. *Radiology* 1993;186:45–53.

142. Lilja A, Lundqvist H, Olsson Y, et al. Positron emission tomography and computed tomography in differential diagnosis between recurrent or residual glioma and treatment-induced brain lesions. *Acta Radiol* 1989;30:121–128.

143. von Pawel J, von Roemeling R, Gatzemeier U, et al. Tirapazamine plus cisplatin versus cisplatin in advanced non–small-cell lung cancer: a report of the international CATAPULT I study group. Cisplatin and Tirapazamine in Subjects with Advanced Previously Untreated Non–Small-Cell Lung Tumor. *JCO* 2000;18(6):1351–1359.

144. Bush RS, Jenkins RDT, Allt WC, et al. Definitive evidence for hypoxic cells influencing cure in cancer therapy. *Br J Cancer* 1978; 37[Suppl III]:302–306.

145. Mottram JC. Factors of importance in the radiosensitivity of tumors. *Br J Radiol* 1936;9:606–614.

146. Powers WE, Tolmach LJ. A multi-component x-ray survival curve for mouse lymphosarcoma cells irradiated *in vivo*. *Nature* 1963;197: 710–711.

147. Kayama T, Yoshimoto T, Fujimoto S, et al. Intratumoral oxygen pressure in malignant brain tumors. *J Neurosurg* 1991;74:55–59.

148. Moulder JE, Rockwell S. Hypoxic fractions of solid tumors: experimental techniques, methods of analysis and a survey of existing data. *Int J Radiat Oncol Biol Phys* 1984;10:695–712.

149. Rasey JS, Koh WJ, Grierson JR, et al. Radiolabelled fluoromisonidazole as an imaging agent for tumor hypoxia. *Int J Radiat Oncol Biol Phys* 1989;17(5):985–991.

150. Valk PE, Mathis CA, Prados MD, et al. Hypoxia in human gliomas: demonstration by PET with fluorine-18-fluoromisonidazole. *J Nucl Med* 1992;33:2133–2137.

151. Cleaver JE. Thymidine metabolism and cell kinetics. In: *Frontiers of biology*. Amsterdam: North-Holland Publishing, 1967.

152. Kubota K, Ishiwata K, Kubota R, et al. Tracer feasibility for monitoring tumor radiotherapy: a quadruple tracer study with fluorine-18-fluorodeoxyglucose or fluorine-18-fluorodeoxyuridine, L-[methyl-^{14}C]methionine, [6-3H]thymidine and gallium-67. *J Nucl Med* 1991; 32:2118–2123.

153. Vander Borght T, Pauwels S, Lambotte L, et al. Brain tumor imaging with PET and 2-[carbon-11]thymidine. *J Nucl Med* 1994;35:974–982.

154. Eary JF, Mankoff DA, Spence AM, et al. 2-[C-11]thymidine imaging of malignant brain tumors. *Cancer Res* 1999;59(3):615–621.

155. Rhodes CG, Wise RJ, Gibbs JM, et al. *In vivo* disturbance of the oxidative metabolism of glucose in human cerebral gliomas. *Ann Neurol* 1983;14:614–624.

156. Rottenberg DA, Ginos JZ, Kearfott KJ, et al. *In vivo* measurement of brain tumor pH using [^{11}C]DMO and positron emission tomography. *Ann Neurol* 1985;17:70–79.

157. Radda G. The use of NMR spectroscopy for the understanding of disease. *Science* 1986;233:640–645.

158. Hiesiger E, Fowler JS, Wolf AP, et al. Serial PET studies of human cerebral malignancy with [1-^{11}C]putrescine and [1-^{11}C]2-deoxy-D-glucose. *J Nucl Med* 1987;28:1251–1261.

159. Hiesiger EM, Fowler JS, Logan J, et al. Is [1-^{11}C]putrescine useful as a brain tumor marker. *J Nucl Med* 1992;33:192–199.

160. Rottenberg DA. Carbon-11-putrescine: back to the drawing board [Editorial]. *J Nucl Med* 1992;33:200–201.

161. Pawlikowski M, Kunert-Radek J, Radek A, et al. Inhibition of cell proliferation of human gliomas by benzodiazepines *in vitro*. *Acta Neurol Scand* 1988;77:231–233.

162. Starosta-Rubinstein S, Ciliax BJ, Penney JB, et al. Imaging of a glioma using peripheral benzodiazepine receptor ligands. *Proc Natl Acad Sci U S A* 1987;84:891–895.

163. Black KL, Ikezaki K, Santori E, et al. Specific high affinity binding of peripheral benzodiazepine receptor ligands to brain tumors in rat and man. *Cancer* 1990;65:93–97.

164. Bergstrom M, Mosskin M, Ericson K, et al. Peripheral benzodiazepine binding sites in human gliomas evaluated with positron emission tomography. *Acta Radiol* 1986;369:409–411.

165. Junck L, Olson JMM, Ciliax BJ, et al. PET imaging of human gliomas with ligands for the peripheral benzodiazepine binding site. *Ann Neurol* 1989;26:752–758.

166. Pappata S, Cornu P, Samson Y, et al. PET study of carbon-11-PK 1195 binding to peripheral type benzodiazepine sites in glioblastoma: a case report. *J Nucl Med* 1991;32:1608–1610.

167. Benavides J, Cornu P, Dennis T, et al. Imaging of human brain lesions with an omega 3 site radioligand. *Ann Neurol* 1988;24:708–712.

168. Di Chiro G. Which PET radiopharmaceutical for brain tumors [Editorial]. *J Nucl Med* 1991;32:1346–1348.

CHAPTER 5.4

Head, Neck, and Thyroid

Homer A. Macapinlac

Head and neck cancers are found with increasing frequency and account for up to 5% of all malignancies. There is a clear association of head and neck cancer with the use of tobacco and/or excess alcohol ingestion (1). The most important adverse prognostic factor is increasing T and N stages. This is assessed by proper physical inspection and palpation when possible, with indirect mirror examination and direct endoscopy when necessary. Computed tomography (CT) and magnetic resonance imaging (MRI) supplement the ability to stage the extent of disease, particularly the appropriate nodal drainage areas of the neck. The treatment options depend on the extent of disease and have evolved to become multimodal—for example, combining surgery and radiotherapy in early stage disease, with chemotherapy being added for advanced disease.

This chapter is a guide to clinicians seeking to apply fluorodeoxyglucose positron emission tomography (FDG PET) imaging in head and neck cancers for more accurate staging of tumor extent, discrimination of posttreatment changes from recurrent disease, and evaluation of response to multimodality therapy. PET is unique in this disease group, because it is more demanding in terms of interpretation, because smaller structures are imaged and the mobility of the neck makes it more difficult for anatomic correlation with CT or MRI to localize any abnormalities identified.

PATIENT PREPARATION

Nondiabetic patients are fasted for at least 4 to 6 hours before FDG injection. This is done because FDG is a glucose analogue that competes with native glucose for its accumulation, and its targeting is also dependent on insulin levels. Fasting results in low serum glucose and insulin levels, which allow good tumor uptake with minimal skeletal muscle activity. To further minimize activity in the myocardium, which facilitates detection of secondary tumors in the aerodigestive tract, patients are encouraged to consume a high-protein low-carbohydrate diet before fasting (Fig. 5.4.1). If the patient is nervous or is known to have posttherapeutic neuromuscular deficiencies or muscle spasm, a diazepam

tablet (5 to 10 g orally) can be prescribed to be taken 1 hour before injection of FDG. This may reduce normal skeletal muscle uptake that can mimic or obscure nodal disease (Fig. 5.4.2). The patients are encouraged to drink water before the injection of FDG because this enhances clearance of the tracer in the urinary collecting system, which is the main route of excretion. Diabetic patients are also asked to titrate their glucose levels to the reference range at the scheduled time of injection. Typically, they are advised to eat an early 5 a.m. breakfast and take their insulin injection or oral medication and are scheduled for FDG injection at about noon (2). Another approach is to have patients fast overnight and have the scan early in the morning, to minimize insulin effects.

Our current protocol at MD Anderson Cancer Center (MDACC) involves intravenous catheter placement in the

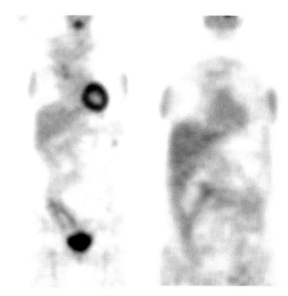

FIG. 5.4.1. Coronal ^{18}F-fluorodeoxyglucose positron emission tomography scans of the same patient on two occasions. One scan **(left)** was acquired after a 6-hour fast and showed intense myocardial activity. A second scan **(right)** was acquired after a 6-hour fast with carbohydrate restriction.

157

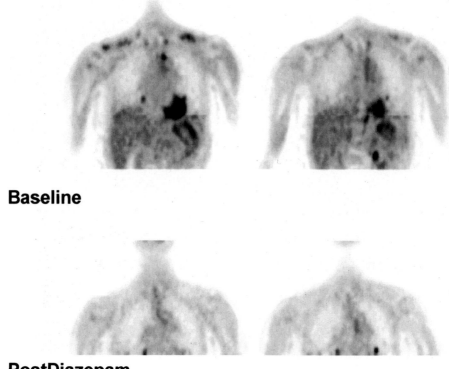

Baseline

PostDiazepam

FIG. 5.4.2. Coronal ^{18}F-fluorodeoxyglucose (FDG) positron emission tomography scans of a patient with thyroid cancer and lung metastases. The **upper row** demonstrates intense muscle uptake in the trapezius and neck muscles, making it difficult to distinguish possible tumor in the neck from tracer uptake in tense muscles. The patient returned a few days later and was given diazepam (10 mg orally) 1 hour before injection of FDG. The **lower row** demonstrates resolution of muscle uptake, with retention of uptake in the lung metastases.

antecubital fossa using an aseptic technique. A blood glucose sample is obtained and then 10 to 20 mCi of FDG is injected (bolus), followed by a 10-mL saline flush. The residual activity is then measured in a dose calibrator to determine the net injected dose, which is used for calculating standard uptake values (SUVs). The patient is then kept in a sitting or recumbent position and is asked not to talk, to keep vocalis muscle activity to a minimum, which is important in patients with laryngeal cancer. They are asked not to drink, to minimize activity in the muscles of deglutition, particularly FDG uptake in the muscles of the tongue, which becomes important when imaging patients with cancer at this site. Immediately before scanning, they are asked to drink water to rinse retained saliva in the mouth and esophagus and then to empty their bladder.

IMAGE ACQUISITION

At MDACC, we acquire two-dimensional (2D) emission scans at 5 minutes per field of view (FOV) and 3-minute transmission scans are acquired sequentially for attenuation correction. This acquisition format is using a Siemens/CTI

HR+ scanner, and the author has used similar parameters with a General Electric Advance Scanner. Scans should encompass the skull base by starting at the top of the ear as an external landmark and covering the thorax and upper abdomen. This is accomplished with three to four FOVs and the intent is to detect metastases and secondary tumors in the lungs or esophagus, which have an increased incidence in head and neck cancers (Fig. 5.4.3). The imaged field is extended to cover the pelvis in the evaluation of patients with an unknown primary. Images are reconstructed with vendor-supplied software (ordered subsets–expectation maximization and IRSAC) and standard SUV formulas are used. We have adopted a cutoff value, maximum SUV equals 2.5, as being suggestive of malignancy. This is done with caveats discussed elsewhere about size criteria, volume averaging, limits of resolution, body mass index, and normal variant activity. We are currently performing pilot studies using three-dimensional imaging by acquiring 3-minute emission and 2-minute transmission scans. This may allow faster scanning that is more efficient and better tolerated by patients. This has practical importance in patients with head and neck cancer, as they may have tracheostomies *in situ* or difficulty with airway maintenance. It should be noted that

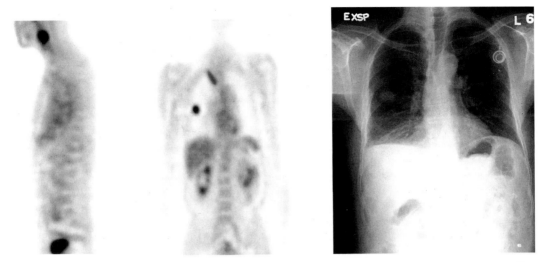

FIG. 5.4.3. A 44-year-old patient with a history of epiglottic cancer treated with radiotherapy. The ¹⁸F-fluorodeoxyglucose positron emission tomography scan reveals recurrence in the neck in the sagittal scan **(left)**, with two secondary sites in the right lung **(middle)**. Chest x-ray **(right)** demonstrates the right mid lung lesion. The less active right apical lesion demonstrated chronic infection and the right mid lung lesion was malignant on biopsy.

most of the results reported in the world literature in head and neck cancer have been acquired using 2D acquisition techniques.

NORMAL PATTERNS AND VARIANTS

Familiarity with the normal structures in the head and neck region is crucial to interpretation and awareness of the distribution of lymphoid tissue and thymic tissue, which is more prominent in younger patients, is very important (Fig. 5.4.4). It is important to have the CT or MRI for anatomic correlation with FDG PET, because both modalities complement each other in localization of both normal and abnormal tissue. A complete treatment history is vital to the interpretation; for example, recent chemotherapy may cause increased uptake in marrow in the spine and prior radiotherapy may demonstrate the opposite finding of hypometabolism in marrow. Postradiation changes with diminution of activity in the normal lymphoid tissues in the neck, which in turn are age dependent, should be anticipated. The extent of radiotherapy should be known, because this may cause protracted posttreatment changes manifested as increased uptake in lungs (Fig. 5.4.5), thyroid, and myocardium. Intense activity in muscle flaps should be noted (Fig. 5.4.6) and normal gastroesophageal junction activity may sometimes be pronounced in reflux esophagitis.

STAGING

Most head and neck cancers are squamous cell carcinomas of the larynx, pharynx, hypopharynx, and oral cavity with nodal metastases. FDG PET complements the CT and MRI

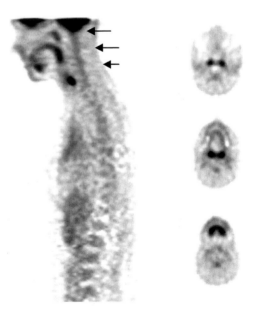

FIG. 5.4.4. ¹⁸F-Fluorodeoxyglucose positron emission tomography scan of a 29-year-old woman with a history of thyroid cancer after total thyroidectomy. The sagittal view **(left)** demonstrates normal thymic activity; the corresponding transaxial scan levels are also demonstrated (*the three arrows*). Also shown are normal lymphoid tissue **(top)** in the palatine tonsils, the level of the lingual tonsils **(middle)**, and the muscles (mylohyoid) of the floor of the mouth **(bottom)**.

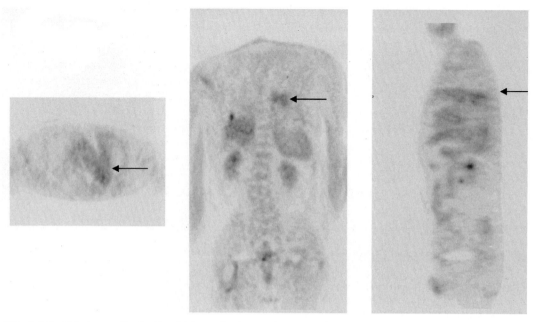

FIG. 5.4.5. This is a patient with a history of colorectal cancer with suspected recurrence due to a rising carcinoembryonic antigen (CEA) levels. The patient had previously been treated with radiotherapy to the left lung. Indicated are the (*arrows*) linear discrete and relatively faint postradiotherapy changes in the left mid lung. The focal area in the right lung base is the lung metastasis that is probably causing the elevated CEA levels.

in more accurately detecting the presence of tumor and nodal metastases. FDG PET improves the sensitivity and specificity of detecting malignancy in borderline or normal-sized nodes, plus the inherent value of the body survey for detecting occult distant metastases. However, limitations include acute inflammatory processes that may manifest as false-positive results and small lesions (less than 5 mm) that may be below the sensitivity of dedicated full-ring PET cameras. A prospective study by Wong et al. (3) of 54 patients, 31 patients with primary disease and 23 patients with suspected recurrence, showed that PET detected all the 31 primary

tumors. To determine the ability of PET to detect cervical nodal disease in 16 patients who underwent neck dissections, the sensitivity and specificity of FDG PET for nodal disease were 67% and 100%, respectively. This is better than the comparison with clinical assessment, which demonstrated sensitivities and specificities of 58% and 75%, whereas those for CT/MRI scans were 67% and 25%, respectively. FDG PET had an accuracy of 100% in 13 patients with previously treated neck disease, whereas CT/MRI was accurate only in 7 of the 13 patients. This study concluded that FDG PET was more accurate than CT and MRI for identifying both

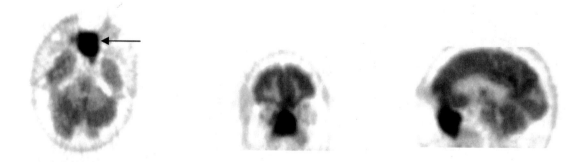

FIG. 5.4.6. This is a scan of a 58-year-old patient with a history of nasal cavity squamous cell cancer, which was resected, and a flap overlies the middle of the face. This hypermetabolic (*arrow*) area corresponds to the muscle in the reconstructive flap, as seen on the transaxial **(left)**, coronal **(middle)**, and sagittal **(right)** ^{18}F-fluorodeoxyglucose positron emission tomography scans. Only with complete clinical history and anatomic correlation could a tumor be excluded in this patient.

primary and recurrent tumors, as well as metastatic lesions in the neck (3). A larger prospective study of 106 patients with oral cavity cancers who underwent subsequent neck dissection (a total of 2,196 nodes examined) were evaluated with FDG PET, ultrasound, and CT scans. The results of the study were as follows: PET had a sensitivity of 70%, specificity 82%, accuracy 75%; ultrasound 84%, 68%, and 76%; CT 66%, 74%, and 70%; and MRI 64%, 69%, 66%, respectively. This study showed that PET had the highest specificity, but ultrasound had the highest sensitivity. PET alone detected 10 secondary cancers in these patients. However, multiple small nodes in the neck involved by cancer were identified (at pathology) and missed by imaging, so neck dissection is still recommended (4).

The incremental advantage of PET over conventional imaging appears to be even more promising in the posttreatment setting when previous surgery, radiation, or chemotherapy results in an alteration of the anatomy, which diminishes the specificity and sensitivity of CT or MRI. This was essentially the conclusion of a review of several prospective series by McGuirt et al. (5), in which FDG PET scanning was comparable to conventional imaging of head and neck cancers in detecting primary and metastatic disease, with its greatest role being in the evaluation of patients postradiotherapy. Anzai et al. (6) compared FDG PET with MRI or CT in a small series of 12 patients with suspected recurrence and found that FDG PET yielded a sensitivity and specificity of 88% and 100%, respectively, whereas those for MRI and/or CT were 25% and 75%, respectively. Lapela et al. (7) saw similar findings in 15 patients with suspected recurrence of head and neck cancers. Their results showed a sensitivity of 88% and a specificity of 86% (7). Detection of early primary or recurrent laryngeal cancer also appears to be an important application, because the CT results may be negative or normal appearing in this clinical situation. FDG PET was shown to provide excellent ability to detect lesions in the T1-2 region of the larynx (8).

It is difficult to distinguish residual or recurrent tumor from postradiation edema or soft-tissue and/or cartilage necrosis in patients treated for laryngeal carcinoma (Fig. 5.4.6). Recurrent tumor in this setting is often submucosal, requiring multiple deep biopsies before a diagnosis can be established (9,10). The superior accuracy of FDG PET to distinguish postradiation necrosis from recurrent laryngeal cancer was demonstrated to be 79% versus 61% for conventional imaging (i.e., CT), and (41%) for clinical examination (11). This is of practical clinical utility, because biopsy or intervention could be temporized if the PET scan is negative and spares the patient an unnecessary procedure. Furthermore, if the PET study is positive, more accurate staging could be performed to assist in treatment planning or to serve as a baseline before initiating chemotherapy.

An increasing application of FDG PET is the determination of metabolic response to therapy. The European Organization for Research and Treatment of Cancer has proposed a set of guidelines in determining complete, partial, stable,

or progressive disease by comparing baseline and posttreatment SUVs based on body surface area (12). Guidelines in assessing response should include consistency in patient preparation, post-FDG injection uptake time and/or conditions, time since the last dose of chemotherapy or radiotherapy, and identical scan acquisition. All of these are to minimize the already known variations in SUVs by using consistent clinical protocols for scanning all patients.

A study by Lowe et al. (13) demonstrated promising results in the accuracy of FDG PET in classifying response to chemotherapy in 26 patients with advanced head and neck cancer. They used tissue biopsies to document complete response or residual disease (Fig. 5.4.7). The sensitivity and specificity of PET for residual cancer after therapy were 90% and 83%, respectively. Two patients had initially negative biopsy results, but PET showed persistent disease. Pathology review and a second biopsy led to confirmation of the PET results in these cases, giving a sensitivity of 90% for initial tissue biopsy (13).

The timing of PET scanning after therapy becomes an important factor in distinguishing acute posttherapy changes from residual disease. In a prospective study of 44 patients who manifested symptoms of recurrence after therapy, the accuracy of FDG PET was the highest (94%) in patients who were imaged more than 12 weeks after the end of therapy. The use of SUV based on lean body mass appeared to be helpful in evaluating patients scanned less than 12 weeks posttreatment (14).

Patients with cervical nodal disease from an unknown primary constitutes only 1% to 5% of cases, but FDG PET has demonstrated a role in the proper management of these patients by finding the primary in 10% to 60% of cases. Although variable in terms of different studies, each successful case is essentially a "home run," because it spares the patient from undergoing unnecessary extensive treatment. Plus, most cases referred for these studies have already undergone extensive conventional imaging to find the tumor. A practical clinical clue is to pay attention to the histologic type of tumor in the lymph node; for example, if it is squamous, look hard at the head and neck, and if it is an adenocarcinoma look in the lung and gastrointestinal tract.

An early series by Braams et al. (15) showed that FDG PET identified the primary tumor in 30% of 13 patients who had undergone conventional imaging. A subsequent larger series by Kole et al. (16) consisting of 28 patients identified the primary tumor in 24% of patients: 2 in the nasopharynx, 1 in the tongue, 2 in the breast, and 1 each of lung and colon. In the series by Jungehulsing et al. (17), FDG PET revealed an unknown primary carcinoma in 7 (26%) of 27 patients: 2 lung, 2 nasopharynx, 1 parotid gland, 1 hypopharynx, and 1 tonsil. In the series by Bohuslavizki et al. (18), 20 (37.8%) of 53 patients had FDG PET results that were true-positive for a primary in the lungs (n = 10), the head and neck region (n = 8), the breast (n = 1), and the ileocolonic area (n = 1). Assar et al. (19) showed 9 (52%) of 17 patients had primary lesions identified as directed by PET. None of the five patients with negative FDG PET studies manifested evi-

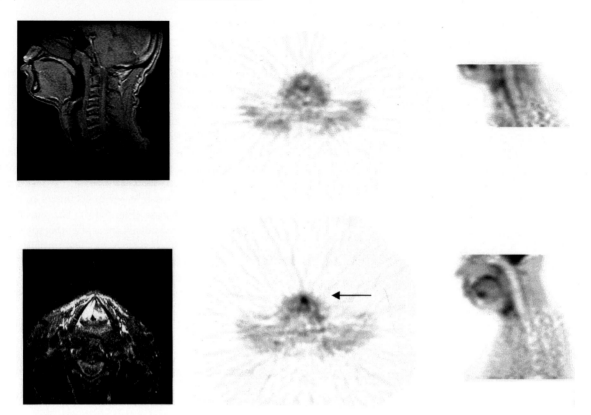

FIG. 5.4.7. Top: Sagittal magnetic resonance imaging **(left)**, transaxial **(middle)**, and sagittal **(right)** PET scans that demonstrate no uptake in the laryngeal cancer treated with radiotherapy. **Bottom:** This scan demonstrates recurrence in the focal area of hypermetabolism (*arrow*).

dence of a primary site of disease during follow-up of 8 to 42 months (mean, 29 months).

However, one has to reemphasize the value of PET in terms of specificity and the ability to detect distant metastases or secondary tumors. Because FDG suffers from the inability to differentiate benign inflammatory nodes, the use of other tracers such as carbon-11 (^{11}C)-methionine and ^{11}C-tyrosine has been studied in an effort to improve PET specificity. The difficulty with these tracers is related to normal salivary gland activity, which makes it difficult to localize nodes or tumors within or close to them (20). Chao et al. (21) demonstrated the feasibility of using copper-62 (^{62}Cu)-ATSM (diacetyl-bis(N(4)-methylthiosemicarbazone) as a tracer for measuring head and neck tumor hypoxia and using PET images and CT co-registration for intensity-modulated radiotherapy planning. The fraction of hypoxic cells is of great interest, because the evidence indicates that they are the more radioresistant clones of cells in tumor. The theory behind this effort is to deliver a more precise and higher dose of radiotherapy to these "resistant" regions while sparing healthy tissues.

THYROID CANCER

There is usually no FDG uptake in the thyroid gland in FDG PET scanning. Early FDG PET studies showed variable avidity in both benign (autonomous nodules) and malig-nant tumors. FDG PET studies have also demonstrated the potential of identifying occult thyroid tumors (22).

The standard therapy for well-differentiated thyroid cancer is surgical resection, followed by radioiodine (iodine-131 [^{131}I]) ablation. Despite this effective treatment, the overall recurrence rate of thyroid cancer is about 20% (23). Conventional imaging modalities used for surveillance are CT for detecting lung metastases, MRI for brain lesions, and ultrasonography for detecting cervical nodal metastases. The most commonly used combination for detecting recurrent or residual disease from thyroid cancer is ^{131}I imaging and serum thyroglobulin (Tg) levels. It is known that the FDG avidity of well-differentiated thyroid cancer is low while there is increased FDG uptake in the more poorly differentiated subtypes such as Hürthle cell cancer and Tall cell variants. Conversely, these poorly differentiated FDG-avid lesions lose their iodine avidity, which is sometimes called the "flip-flop" phenomenon (Fig. 5.4.8).

The clear indication for the use of FDG PET in thyroid cancer is in those patients who have negative ^{131}I scans with elevated serum Tg levels (23). FDG PET imaging localizes these non–iodine-avid metastases and allows either surgical or radiotherapeutic approaches if disease is localized, or systemic therapy for disseminated disease. In an early series by Grunwald et al. (24) of 33 patients (26 papillary and 7 follicular) with thyroid cancer, discrepancies between ^{131}I scanning and FDG PET were described. In highly differen-

was reduced in those older than 45 years, those with distant metastases, PET positivity, high rates of FDG uptake, and a high volume of the FDG-avid disease (more than 125 mL). Survival did not correlate with more traditional prognostic indicators such as gender, initial histology, or grade. The single strongest predictor of survival by multivariate analysis was the volume of FDG-avid disease. The 3-year survival probability of patients with FDG volumes of 125 mL or less was 0.96 (95% confidence interval [CI], 0.91–1.0), compared with 0.18 survival probability (95% CI, 0.04–0.85) in patients with FDG volume greater than 125 mL. Only one death (of leukemia) occurred in the PET-negative group (n = 66). Of the 10 patients with distant metastases and negative PET scans, all were alive and well. Patients older than 45 years with distant metastases that concentrate FDG are at the highest risk. FDG PET can identify high- and low-risk subsets in patients with distant metastases from thyroid cancer.

Early studies demonstrated that the lower sensitivity of bone scanning for detecting osseous metastases was because osteolytic lesions were missed. A prospective study comparing bone scanning with single-photon emission computed tomography (SPECT) and fluorine-18 (^{18}F) PET was done on 44 patients with known prostate, lung, or thyroid carcinoma (27). PET showed 96 metastases (67 of prostate carcinoma and 29 of lung or thyroid cancer), whereas bone scans revealed 46 metastases (33 of prostate carcinoma and 13 of lung or thyroid cancer). All lesions found with bone scans were detected with ^{18}F PET. The area under the receiver operating characteristic curve was 0.99 for ^{18}F PET and 0.64 for bone scans.

In a study by Pineda et al. (28) of 17 patients with negative ^{131}I scans and elevated Tg levels, all treated with 150 to 300 mCi of ^{131}I, therapy effectiveness was demonstrated with interval diminution of serum Tg levels and posttherapy ^{131}I scans that became negative. The current availability of FDG PET scans could allow them to be used as a method for response evaluation after empiric treatment of patients with ^{131}I instead of relying on Tg levels alone. Retinoic acids have been used as redifferentiating agents to attempt to induce iodine uptake as an alternative method of therapy in these patients who really have very few options. Somatostatin analogues have also been used as tumoristatic agents. The use of FDG PET after treatment with both redifferentiating (29) and tumoristatic agents (30) has been demonstrated to be helpful in monitoring the response.

Future directions of PET imaging for thyroid cancer would include the use of iodine-124 (^{124}I)-sodium iodide PET imaging, which has a 4.2-day half-life, has been demonstrated to be useful for imaging, and has improved dosimetry. Because ^{124}I is a positron emitter, the superior image resolution and inherent quantitative ability of PET imaging allow more precise determination of tracer kinetics by tumors. The fairly long half-life may be advantageous to tracers with prolonged biologic half-lives such as monoclonal antibodies

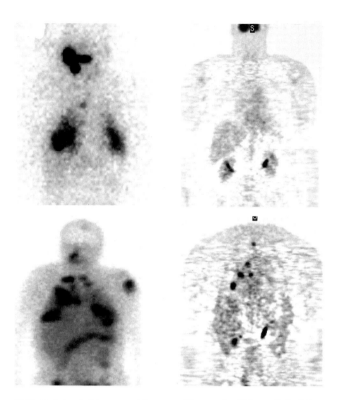

FIG. 5.4.8. A 61-year-old man with poorly differentiated thyroid cancer with bilateral lung uptake **(upper left)** on a post–iodine-131 (^{131}I) therapy scan. The ^{18}F-fluorodeoxyglucose positron emission tomography (FDG PET) scan was negative **(upper right)** and this patient is still clinically stable. A 66-year old man with follicular thyroid cancer with lung and bone metastases seen on the post–^{131}I therapy scan **(lower left)**, with an FDG PET scan **(lower right)** demonstrating bilateral lung uptake. This man died after 3 years despite multimodality therapy.

tiated tumors, ^{131}I scintigraphy had a high sensitivity, whereas in poorly differentiated carcinomas, FDG PET was superior (Fig. 5.4.9). Wang et al. (25) performed FDG PET on 37 patients with differentiated thyroid cancer after surgery and radioiodine ablation who had negative diagnostic ^{131}I whole-body scans. FDG PET localized occult disease in 71% of patients with elevated Tg levels, with one false-positive, and it was false-negative in five patients, most of whom had small cervical nodes. FDG PET changed the clinical management in 19 of the 37 patients. FDG PET had a positive predictive value of 92% in patients with elevated Tg levels and had a negative predictive value of 93% in patients with low Tg levels. This study also showed that hypothyroidism (high thyroid-stimulating hormone level) did not increase the ability to detect lesions with FDG PET.

Wang et al. (26) also set out to evaluate the prognostic implications of FDG uptake by poorly differentiated thyroid cancer in 125 patients who had previous thyroidectomies and were studied with diagnostic ^{131}I whole-body scans, serum Tg measurements, and additional imaging studies as clinically indicated (26). During a 41-month follow-up, 14 patients died. Univariate analysis demonstrated that survival

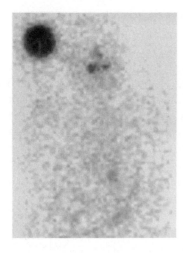
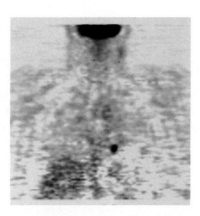
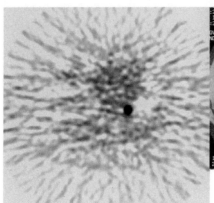
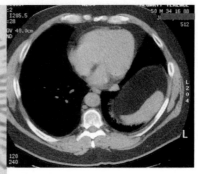

FIG. 5.4.9. A 50-year-old man with papillary thyroid cancer had a negative whole-body iodine-131 scan **(upper left).** The ^{18}F-fluorodeoxyglucose positron emission tomography study demonstrates a solitary lesion in the left lower lobe of the lung on the coronal **(upper right)** and transaxial scans **(lower left).** This was subsequently demonstrated on the computed tomography scan of the chest **(lower right).** This nodule was surgically removed and showed poorly differentiated thyroid cancer.

(31). Iodine-124-NaI has been demonstrated to be useful in PET imaging of patients with poorly differentiated thyroid cancer, with the potential advantage of more precise dosimetry to predict ^{131}I dose delivery and improved image quality (32). Issues of availability involve the need for medium-energy cyclotrons and adequate target preparation. Nevertheless, it is an interesting tracer because we have a wealth of experience with various iodinated diagnostic and therapeutic agents such as monoclonal antibodies, peptides, oligonucleotides, tyrosine kinase agents, and antiangiogenesis agents to use this isotope (Fig. 5.4.10).

SUMMARY

FDG PET has proven to be valuable in head and neck cancer imaging. Although it is somewhat better than CT or MRI for staging newly diagnosed head and neck cancer, its greatest utility is in assessing efficacy of therapy and detecting recurrence in patients who have been treated.

In thyroid cancer, PET with FDG has a growing role in assessing patients with rising Tg levels after treatment. PET often detects non–iodine-avid lesions and can lead to changes in the therapeutic plans. Iodine-124 is a promising radionuclide under study for thyroid disease.

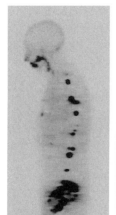
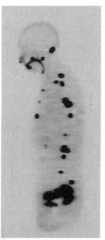
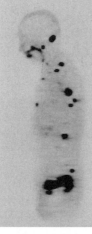

FIG. 5.4.10. These are sagittal iodine-124-sodium iodide PET images of a patient with follicular thyroid cancer with known extensive osseous metastases in the calvarium, spine, and pelvis.

REFERENCES

1. Spitz MR. Epidemiology and risk factors for head and neck cancer. *Semin Oncol* 1994;21(3):281–288.
2. Macapinlac HA, Yeung HWD, Larson SM. Defining the role of FDG PET in head and neck cancer. *Clin Positron Imaging* 1999;6:311–316.
3. Wong WL, Chevretton EB, McGurk M, et al. A prospective study of PET-FDG imaging for the assessment of head and neck squamous cell carcinoma. *Clin Otolaryngol* 1997;22(3):209–214.
4. Stuckensen T, Kovacs AF, Adams S, et al. Staging of the neck in patients with oral cavity squamous cell carcinomas: a prospective comparison of PET, ultrasound, CT and MRI. *J Craniomaxillofac Surg* Dec 2000;28(6):319–324.
5. McGuirt WF, Greven K, Williams D III, et al.. PET scanning in head and neck oncology: a review. *Head Neck* 1998;20(3):208–215.
6. Anzai Y, Carroll WR, Quint DJ, et al. Recurrence of head and neck cancer after surgery or irradiation: prospective comparison of 2-deoxy-2-[F-18]fluoro-D-glucose PET and MR imaging diagnoses. *Radiology* 1996;200(1):135–141.
7. Lapela M, Grenman R, Kurki T, et al. Head and neck cancer: detection of recurrence with PET and 2-[F-18]fluoro-2-deoxy-D-glucose. *Radiology* 1995;197(1):205–211.
8. Lowe VJ, Kim H, Boyd JH, et al. Primary and recurrent early stage laryngeal cancer: preliminary results of 2-[fluorine 18]fluoro-2-deoxy-D-glucose PET imaging. *Radiology* 1999;212(3):799–802.
9. Greven KM, Williams DW, Keyes JW, et al. Can positron emission tomography distinguish tumor recurrence from irradiation sequelae in patients treated for larynx cancer? *Cancer J Sci Am* 1997;3(6):353–357.
10. Macapinlac HA, Larson SM. Positron emission tomography (PET)—measured biochemical response to radiotherapy of laryngeal tumors. *Cancer J Sci Am* 1997;3(6):333–335.
11. Young H, Baum R, Cremerius U, et al. Measurement of clinical and subclinical tumour response using [^{18}F]-fluorodeoxyglucose and positron emission tomography: review and 1999 EORTC recommendations. European Organization for Research and Treatment of Cancer (EORTC) PET Study Group. *Eur J Cancer* Dec 1999;35(13):1773–1782.
12. McGuirt WF, Greven KM, Keyes JW, et al. Laryngeal radionecrosis versus recurrent cancer: a clinical approach. *Ann Otol Rhinol Laryngol* 1998;107(4):293–296.
13. Lowe VJ, Dunphy FR, Varvares M, et al. Evaluation of chemotherapy response in patients with advanced head and neck cancer using [F-18] fluorodeoxyglucose positron emission tomography. *Head Neck* 1997; 19(8):666–674.
14. Lonneux M, Lawson G, Ide C, et al. Positron emission tomography with fluorodeoxyglucose for suspected head and neck tumor recurrence in the symptomatic patient. *Laryngoscope* 2000;110(9):1493–1497.
15. Braams JW, Pruim J, Kole AC, et al. Detection of unknown primary head and neck tumors by positron emission tomography. *Int J Oral Maxillofac Surg* 1997;26(2):112–115.
16. Kole AC, Nieweg OE, Pruim J, et al. Detection of unknown occult primary tumors using positron emission tomography. *Cancer* 15 Mar 1998;82(6):1160–1166.
17. Jungehulsing M, Scheidhauer K, Damm M, et al. 2[F]-Fluoro-2-deoxy-D-glucose positron emission tomography is a sensitive tool for the detection of occult primary cancer (carcinoma of unknown primary syndrome) with head and neck lymph node manifestation. *Otolaryngol Head Neck Surg* Sep 2000;123(3):294–301.
18. Bohuslavizki KH, Klutmann S, Kroger S, et al. FDG PET detection of unknown primary tumors. *J Nucl Med* May 2000;41(5):816–822.
19. AAssar OS, Fischbein NJ, Caputo GR, et al. Metastatic head and neck cancer: role and usefulness of FDG PET in locating occult primary tumors. *Radiology* Jan 1999;210(1):177–181.
20. Chisin R, Macapinlac HA. The indications of FDG-PET in neck oncology. *Radiol Clin North Am* 2000;38(5):999–1012.
21. Chao KS, Bosch WR, Mutic S, et al. A novel approach to overcome hypoxic tumor resistance: Cu-ATSM-guided intensity-modulated radiation therapy. *Int J Radiat Oncol Biol Phys* 15 Mar 2001;49(4):1171–1182.
22. Ramos CD, Chisin R, Yeung HW, et al. Incidental focal thyroid uptake on FDG positron emission tomographic scans may represent a second primary tumor. *Clin Nucl Med* 2001;26(3):193–197.
23. Macapinlac HA. Clinical usefulness of FDG PET in differentiated thyroid cancer. *J Nucl Med* Jan 2001;42(1):77–78.
24. Grunwald F, Schomburg A, Bender H, et al. Fluorine-18 fluorodeoxyglucose positron emission tomography in the follow-up of differentiated thyroid cancer. *Eur J Nucl Med* Mar 1996;23(3):312–319.
25. Wang W, Macapinlac H, Larson SM, et al. [^{18}F]-2-fluoro-2-deoxy-D-glucose positron emission tomography localizes residual thyroid cancer in patients with negative diagnostic (^{131})I whole body scans and elevated serum thyroglobulin levels. *J Clin Endocrinol Metab* 1999;84(7):2291–2302.
26. Wang W, Larson SM, Fazzari M, et al. Prognostic value of [^{18}F]fluorodeoxyglucose positron emission tomographic scanning in patients with thyroid cancer. *J Clin Endocrinol Metab* 2000;85(3):1107–1113.
27. Schirrmeister H, Guhlmann A, Elsner K, et al. Sensitivity in detecting osseous lesions depends on anatomic localization: planar bone scintigraphy versus ^{18}F PET. *J Nucl Med* 1999;40(10):1623–1629.
28. Pineda JD, Lee T, Ain K, et al. Iodine-131 therapy for thyroid cancer patients with elevated thyroglobulin and negative diagnostic scan. *J Clin Endocrinol Metab* May 1995;80(5):1488–1492.
29. Grunwald F, Menzel C, Bender H, et al. Redifferentiation therapy-induced radioiodine uptake in thyroid cancer. *J Nucl Med* Nov 1998;39(11):1903–1906.
30. Robbins RJ, Hill RH, Wang W, et al. Inhibition of metabolic activity in papillary thyroid carcinoma by a somatostatin analogue. *Thyroid* 2000;10(2):177–183.
31. Pentlow KS, Graham MC, Lambrecht RM, et al. Quantitative imaging of I-124 using positron emission tomography with applications to radioimmunodiagnosis and radioimmunotherapy. *Med Phys* May-Jun 1991;18(3):357–366.
32. Erdi YE, Macapinlac HA, Larson SM, et al. Radiation dose assessment for I-131 therapy of thyroid cancer using I-124 PET imaging. *Clin Positron Imaging* 1999;1(2):41–46.

CHAPTER 5.5

Lung

Val J. Lowe

Cancer is running a close second to ischemic heart disease as a leading cause of mortality in the United States (1). As much as cancer therapy has been advanced in the past years, it has largely been disappointing in reducing the death rate from cancer (2). Lung cancer death rates have fluctuated in recent years, and not surprisingly, the changes parallel the regional trends in cigarette smoking (3). Mortality rates from lung cancer for women older than 55 years have increased more than fourfold in the last 20 years, likely reflecting changes in smoking habits that occurred decades ago (2). Today lung cancer is responsible for 32% of all cancer deaths in men and 25% in women in the United States (4).

These facts emphasize the importance of prevention in the fight against lung cancer. They have, along with award spending from cigarette company lawsuits, led to a new war of words in lung cancer prevention. Advertisements, which used to sing the praises of smoking and offer to all who inhale the hope of a glamorous life, are now replaced by descriptions of early aging or even prolonged ventilator dependency as an award for "lighting up." Prevention efforts had led to a decline in smoking. The decline, however, reached a plateau in the past few years, and rates of teenage smoking have begun to increase. In 1997, smoking rates among high school students in the United States were 32% higher compared with those for 1991 (5). Smoking prevention, it appears, will be a battle not soon won. Sadly, cancer caused by smoking will continue to be the reality for years to come, because smoking is common the world over.

In the medical setting, advances in lung cancer detection and treatment must therefore continue. New low-dose computed tomography (CT) may provide a way of more accurately screening populations at risk for lung cancer. Positron emission tomography (PET) imaging is another imaging method that is making its way into standard clinical practice. Although technologic developments in PET were nearly suffocated by government bureaucracy and regulatory blunders, PET is now rapidly growing in its applications.

LUNG NODULES

With the advent of better CT, it is becoming more and more obvious that the solitary nodule may be somewhat of a misnomer. Quite commonly multiple nodules are being detected on high-resolution CT scans when only a single nodule was seen on chest radiograph. These multiple nodules may be very tiny and their appropriate clinical assessment, if any, is yet to be determined. The dilemma in evaluation now becomes increasingly more difficult as small size and multiplicity make biopsy decisions challenging. In the coming years, large trials for nodule evaluation are being contemplated and will hopefully help answer some of these clinical questions.

Several invasive modalities are available to assist in the diagnosis of lung nodules that are large enough. However, negative results from either transbronchial or transthoracic biopsies cannot be accepted as reliable negatives. For example, the sensitivity of transthoracic needle aspiration (TTNA) for malignancy is reported to be only 42% for nodules of nonbronchogenic origin (6). This is a significantly higher false-negative rate than what has been reported in primary bronchogenic nodules. Certainly in patients with malignancy, the nodule could be of either etiology. In addition, up to 40% of nondiagnostic TTNA results have been shown to be malignant (6).

Most studies report a sensitivity of 75% to 86% for malignancy in TTNA-biopsied lung nodules (7,8). One study compared the use of TTNA and PET in the investigation of indeterminate nodules. The sensitivity and specificities were 100% and 78%, respectively, for PET, and 81% and 100%, respectively, for TTNA (9). These data suggest that more malignancies may in fact be missed using a traditional TTNA approach than with PET when triaging patients for thoracotomy. There are also risks to these more aggressive and invasive diagnostic maneuvers. Of note is that 9 (26%) of the 33 patients in this series required chest tube placement for pneumothoraces secondary to the TTNA.

In addressing these issues of accuracy and morbidity, some have suggested that patients who are well enough to undergo surgery should not have TTNA for assessment of lung nodules but go directly to surgical resection for diagnosis (7). This may not be the common view held in most of medical practice today, but reasoning along these lines is justifiable. It is easy to see that the evaluation of lung nodules has many potential variations and a "one size fits all" clinical pathway is not appropriate. Patient risk for malignancy, respiratory status, and interest in having the nodule removed will also certainly play a role in deciding what the appropriate course of action will be.

An accurate, noninvasive test for evaluating indeterminate pulmonary lesions would avoid considerable patient morbidity and potentially reduce the cost from invasive procedures. In many cases, patients would probably opt for such a procedure if the accuracy and risks of all available procedures were thoroughly explained to them.

Published data have demonstrated the ability of PET to accurately characterize lung abnormalities as malignant or benign and have been particularly encouraging. After the identification of a pulmonary abnormality by an anatomic study such as a chest radiograph, fluorodeoxyglucose positron emission tomography (FDG PET) imaging can be performed to evaluate the metabolic activity of the lesion in an attempt to distinguish a benign from a malignant process. In general, nodule uptake of FDG greater than blood pool activity at 50 to 70 minutes after injection is considered "positive." Semiquantitative analysis is also used and standard uptake values (SUVs) of more than 2.5 (or sometimes lower) are considered very worrisome for cancer.

Table 5.5.1 includes a short list of published papers discussing FDG PET studies in patients with solitary pulmonary nodules (10–16). Many more articles have been published, but some include duplicate patient groups. Articles selected for Table 5.5.1 are the last articles published by single institutions (in the case of single-institution studies) using similar patient groups to avoid double sampling of the patients included. Some investigators have included only solitary pulmonary nodules (SPNs) while others included any suspicious opacity (this is detailed in Table 5.5.1). The data show that dedicated PET scanners using FDG perform well in the group, with an average sensitivity and specificity of 95% and 81%, respectively, for the detection of malignancy in lung nodules. Figure 5.5.1 shows examples.

The sensitivity of PET is high enough that a negative PET examination could be reasonably considered to rule out malignancy in a population at low to moderate risk for malignancy. Depending on the population studied, some false-positive study results will be encountered. It would not, for example, be unexpected to find many false-positive PET study results in a community in which a high likelihood for pulmonary infection (e.g., tuberculosis) is being encountered. The clinical setting the test is used in, as is true for all diagnostic tests, will determine its clinical value. A recent metaanalysis also concluded that this is true (17). In this metaanalysis, the authors conclude that the sensitivity of PET is such that in a low-risk population (20% risk), the posttest probability of malignancy after having a negative PET scan result is about 1%.

It should be pointed out that most studies of PET in SPNs have been in lesions 7 mm or larger. False-negative results are probable in smaller lesions than this. Furthermore, false-negative results are more common in some types of lung cancer, particularly bronchioloalveolar cancer and carcinoid tumors of the lung.

The other question relating to solitary nodule evaluation is whether hybrid gamma cameras with coincidence capability are accurate enough to be used in the evaluation of lung nodules. In the metaanalysis by Gould et al. (17), the authors looked at the accuracy of dedicated scanners compared with coincidence gamma cameras and determined that the accuracy reported in the literature is not significantly different. They also stated that the confidence intervals for the coincidence scanner accuracy are wide, because their data come from only a few small studies, and that more study is therefore needed before making a definitive conclusion (17). It is likely that a direct comparison between the two technologies in the same patients will also be needed to determine if hybrid systems can perform at the level of dedicated scanners. In general, coincidence gamma cameras have lower sensitivity for small lesions (less than 1.5 cm) than dedicated PET.

The costs and benefits of different approaches are being evaluated. One report has suggested that a noninvasive approach using FDG PET can be more cost-effective without compromising patient survival (18). These investigators looked at immediate surgery and various combinations of noninvasive testing of SPNs using decision tree analysis. They suggested that given a low prevalence of malignant SPNs (less than 50%), either using PET with radiologic fol-

TABLE 5.5.1. *Studies of pulmonary opacities or solitary pulmonary nodules*

Author, yr (reference no.)	Patients: no. malignant/benign	PET criteria: standard uptake value or visual	Sensitivity	Specificity
Kubota et al., 1990 (10)	12/10	>2.0	83%	90%
Duhaylongsod et al., 1995 (11)	59/28	≥2.5	97%	82%
Bury et al., 1996 (12)	33/17	Visual	100%	88%
Knight et al.,1996 (13)	32/16	>2.5	100%	63%
Gupta et al.,1996 (14)	45/16	Visual	93%	88%
Lowe et at., 1997 (15)	120/77	≥2.5	96%	77%
Lowe et al., 1998 (16)	60/29	≥2.5	92%	90%
Totals	361/194	Averages	95%	81%

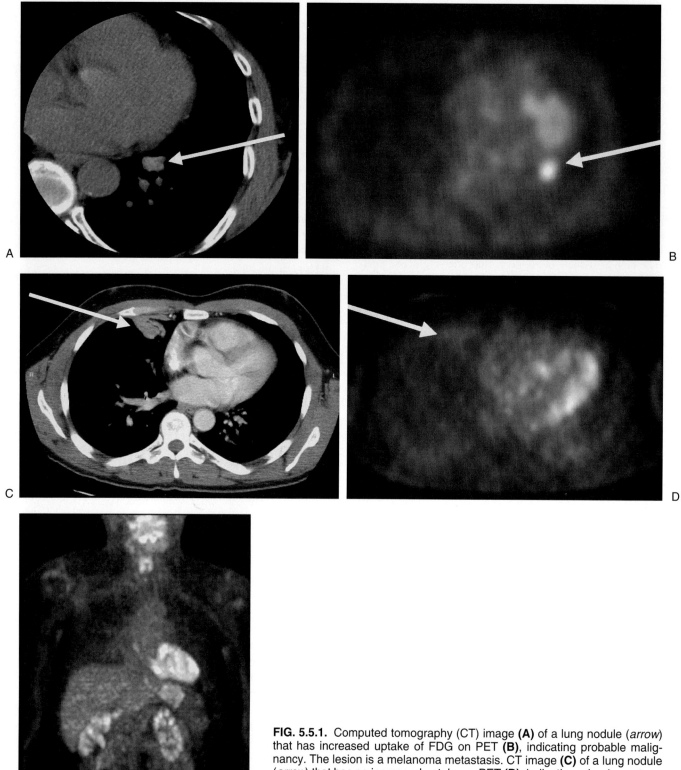

FIG. 5.5.1. Computed tomography (CT) image **(A)** of a lung nodule (*arrow*) that has increased uptake of FDG on PET **(B)**, indicating probable malignancy. The lesion is a melanoma metastasis. CT image **(C)** of a lung nodule (*arrow*) that has no increased uptake on PET **(D)**, indicating a benign nature. The coronal PET view confirming low tracer uptake in the lesion is also shown **(E)**. The lesion is rounded atelectasis.

low-up for 2 years or using PET and CT with follow-up resulted in a net cost reduction over using CT alone with follow-up. The majority of the savings would be from reducing the numbers of invasive procedures.

LUNG CANCER STAGING

Tumor

The majority of PET imaging work has been done in non–small cell lung cancer due to the need for regional and distant staging information in guiding therapy. Lung cancer staging is based on the TNM system and requires accurate characterization of the primary tumor (T), regional lymph nodes (N), and distant metastases (M). The appropriate categorization of stage presently relies on the information that can be obtained clinically. Traditionally this information has been obtained by CT and depends on anatomic abnormalities detectable by CT. This can be most helpful when determining the direct extension and involvement of the tumor into structures that can change disease stage. Tumors are described as T1 when they are 3 cm or less in greatest dimension arising distal to a main bronchus. A T2 tumor is one that is larger than 3 cm, invades the visceral pleura, or has local atelectasis or obstruction associated with it and is located greater than 2 cm from the carina. A T3 tumor invades the chest wall, diaphragm, mediastinal pleura, or pericardium or is associated with diffuse atelectasis or obstruction, and it can be 0 to 2 cm from the carina without involving the carina. A T4 tumor is one that invades vital mediastinal structures such as heart, great vessels, trachea, carina, or vertebral bodies or has a malignant effusion or separate tumor nodules in the same lobe. These stages are largely intended to distinguish what is and is not resectable—all but T4 being resectable. These tumor stages are components of the TNM staging classification.

PET has limited anatomic resolution and thus cannot be expected to accurately assess these levels of tumor involvement. Certainly, when a lesion is surrounded by lung and no other disease is detected, PET can rule out higher stage disease. However, when a tumor is directly adjacent to vital mediastinal structures, PET cannot clearly determine the extent of invasion. In some situations, this can be better detected by CT. Likewise, CT may be limited in sensitivity in detecting thoracic invasion, although it can be very specific if clear invasion is seen. Therefore, invasion of the tumor directly into thoracic structures is often evaluated best at surgery.

When anatomic abnormalities preclude the identification of a primary lung malignancy, PET may be of help. The accuracy of PET in this situation will depend on the inflammatory nature of any coexisting disease that may be hampering CT evaluation. Nodules causing bronchial obstruction are commonly difficult to evaluate, as the exact margin of the tumor versus the consolidation may not be clear. Like-wise, when effusions make tumor detection difficult, PET may be of help (Fig. 5.5.2).

Lymph Nodes

The presence of metastatic disease in lymph nodes correlates closely with worsening survival. N0 status indicates no nodal metastases. An N1 status implies a metastasis to ipsilateral peribronchial, lobar, or interlobar nodes. N2 implies a metastasis to ipsilateral mediastinal or subcarinal nodes. N3 indicates involvement of contralateral lymph nodes, scalene, or supraclavicular nodes. N0 status correlates with a 60% 5-year survival rate and N1 disease correlates with a 30% 5-year survival rate. Only a 10% to 20% survival rate or less is seen once N2-level nodes are involved. Generally, those with N3 lymph node disease do not survive 5 years.

The noninvasive assessment of mediastinal nodes for tumor involvement is relatively difficult with CT. Because of the possibility of nodal enlargement from reactive or inflammatory lung diseases or even congestive heart disease, there is ample probability that enlarged nodes may not be involved with tumor. The nodal size limit of normality used in CT imaging is about 1 cm for the short area of the lymph node. Therefore, any lymph node containing tumor that is less than 1 cm inside will not be called abnormal. Any lymph nodes that are larger than 1 cm will be called abnormal and suggestive of a metastasis in a patient with a lung cancer history. Many such enlarged nodes do not contain malignant cells but are enlarged due to other causes.

Alternatively, invasive sampling with mediastinoscopy can be performed to assess lymph node status. This procedure is unable to assess all lymph nodes with a single point of access. Specifically the aortopulmonary lymph nodes cannot be assessed without a different approach to the lymph nodes. The result is that the selection of lymph nodes for biopsy by the mediastinoscopy technique is based on accessibility. This results in a high, albeit imperfect, sensitivity for mediastinal disease of about 90% (19,20). It is unlikely that this will improve due to the limitations of the technique. Transbronchial needle biopsy of lymph nodes is also useful but is limited in sensitivity in part due to its "blind" nature and due to areas that cannot be sampled.

PET imaging relies on the metabolic activity level of the cells in the lymph node, so it measures information not "seen" by the CT scan. It also provides complete image sampling of the mediastinum, which is superior to what can routinely be obtained with mediastinoscopy. The use of PET imaging has produced an improvement in the accuracy of detecting lymph node disease or other metastases. Examples are shown in Figs. 5.5.3 and 5.5.4. Table 5.5.2 lists papers that have compared the accuracy of PET and CT in staging lung cancer in mediastinal lymph nodes (21–29). Most of the selected studies were blinded, prospective studies with histologic gold standards and were performed in single institutions. Some of the reports only list the nodal status of

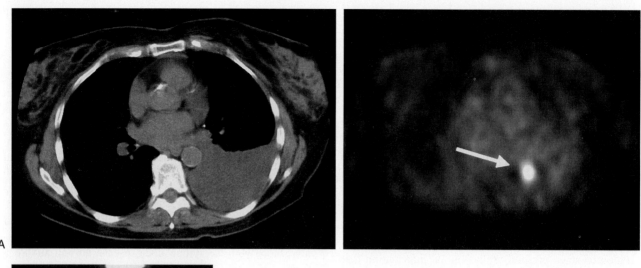

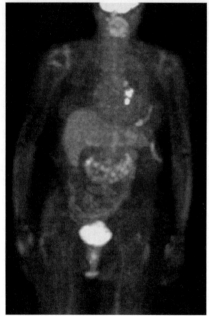

FIG. 5.5.2. Computed tomography (CT) image **(A)** of a left pleural effusion from which biopsy demonstrated adenocarcinoma. The primary malignancy was not identified on chest CT, mammography, abdominal CT, pelvic CT, or colonoscopy. Axial PET **(B)** indicated probable malignancy in the left lower lobe that was obscured on CT. The coronal whole body PET **(C)** showed the lung primary and mediastinal nodal disease and no other malignancy.

TABLE 5.5.2. *Studies comparing PET and CT in mediastinal staging of lung cancer*

Author, yr reference no.	Patient no.	Nodal status: no. malignant/benign (numbers indicative of)	Sensitivity PET	Specificity PET	Sensitivity CT (size criteria)	Specificity CT	Statistical significance PET vs. CT
Wahl et al., 1994 (21)	23	11/16 (sides)	82%	81%	64% (1.0 cm)	44%	$p < 0.05$
Patz et al., 1995 (22)	42	23/39 (stations)	83%	82%	43% (1.0 cm)	85%	$p < 0.01$
Scott et al., 1994 (23)	62	10/65 (stations)	100%	98%	60% (1.0 cm)	93%	$p = 0.031$
Sasaki et al., 1996 (24)	29	17/54 (stations)	76%	98%	65% (1.0 cm)	87%	$p < 0.05$
Steinert et al., 1997 (25)	47	58/133 (stations)	89%	99%	57% (0.7–1.1 cm)	94%	$p = 0.013$
Sazon et al., 1996 (26)	32	16/16 (patients)	100%	100%	81% (1.0 cm)	56%	$p < 0.01$
Valk et al., 1995 (27)	76	24/52 (sides)	83%	94%	63% (1.0 cm)	73%	$p < 0.01$
Vansteenkiste and Mortelmans 1995 (28)	105	47/643 (stations)	89%	99%	79% (1.5 cm)	54%	$p < 0.0003$
Pieterman et al., 2000 (29)	102	32/70 (patients)	91%	86%	75% (1.0 cm)	66%	$p < 0.001$
Totals	518	Weighted averages	88%	91%	63%	76%	

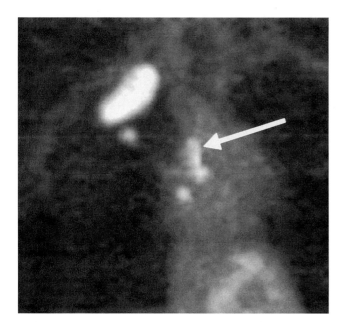

FIG. 5.5.3. PET obtained in a patient with a right lung tumor and mediastinal disease (*arrow*). No enlarged mediastinal lymph nodes were seen on computed tomography. Positive nodes were found at mediastinoscopy.

individual patients while others detail the number of positive nodes. The average sensitivity and specificity of the studies for nodal disease were 88% and 91%, respectively, for PET and 63% and 76%, respectively, for CT. This average sensitivity of PET for nodal disease is the same as that reported for mediastinoscopy and is clearly superior to CT in these data. All of the studies published to date, including those not referenced here, conclude that there is an advantage of PET over CT in mediastinal staging.

The less than 100% specificity of PET for mediastinal staging is often due to tracer uptake into inflammatory reactive lymph nodes. White cells have increased metabolism in these nodes, which results in more avid tracer uptake.

The study by Vansteenkiste et al. (30) probably demonstrates the most comprehensive nodal sampling of all of the studies and this was a particular goal of the investigators. Of note is the lower sensitivity reported by Sasaki et al. (24) for nodal disease. They used a PET scanner with lower spacial resolution (14 mm) and may therefore have had difficulty identifying smaller tumor volumes and obtaining results comparable to those obtained by the other investigators. This emphasizes the need to use high-resolution PET scans when attempting to stage the mediastinum. Because the sensitivity for small amounts of disease in small nodes should be optimized, the highest resolution dedicated PET scans would be the best choice for these evaluations. Coincidence gamma cameras can detect mediastinal nodal metastases but have difficulty detecting small lesions.

Staging the mediastinum using other PET tracers has been evaluated. Carbon-11-methionine and carbon-11 (^{11}C)-choline have been used as PET tracers to find mediastinal disease, and in small lesions, both appear to have done as well as FDG (31,32). It is difficult to consider using these tracers without demonstrating a clear advantage over FDG, particularly in light of the regulatory issues that would need to be overcome to lead to approval and reimbursement for these agents. If a clear advantage can be established at some point, certainly they could make their way into clinical practice. To be more practical for clinical use, fluoride labeling may be needed to be used, given the 20-minute half-life of ^{11}C.

Given the improved detection of mediastinal disease with PET, it is logical that radiation therapy planning would benefit from using PET information in planning radiation ports.

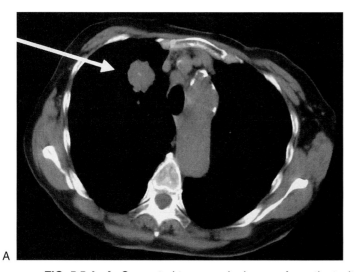

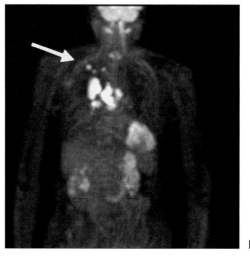

A B

FIG. 5.5.4. A: Computed tomography image of a patient with a history of right lung cancer (*arrow*), on which no adenopathy was described. **B:** The PET image shows hypermetabolism in the right lung tumor and multiple mediastinal and supraclavicular lymph nodes (*arrow*). Nodal disease was confirmed.

It has been shown that in patients with non–small cell lung cancer considered for curative radiation treatment, assessment of locoregional lymph node tumor extension by PET will improve tumor coverage and in selected patients will reduce the volume of normal tissues irradiated, and thus toxicity (33). It is not yet certain if this improved coverage will result in improved survival, but using PET should maximize the chances of survival as best as we can presently.

Staging the mediastinum with PET also appears to be cost-effective as a routine procedure. Gambhir et al. (18) evaluated the cost-effectiveness of FDG PET staging of lung cancer. These authors show that one can reduce management costs by $1,154 per patient by including PET.

Distant Metastases

When performing a PET scan, a whole-body image can be obtained to assess distant metastatic disease. Imaging from the head to the toes can be performed in the same imaging session. It is generally low yield to image the lower limbs, and this can add significantly to the time required for the scan. This is certainly an issue that should be discussed with the referring physician because some may expect the lower limbs to be imaged.

PET has not been shown to be effective in evaluating patients with lung cancer for the presence of brain metastases, particularly when they are asymptomatic (34). There is in fact some controversy over whether asymptomatic patients with lung cancer should be scanned for brain metastases at all. Generally, clinical guidelines suggest that it is not useful. In patients with other evidence of metastatic disease, it may be more prudent. Again consultation with the ordering physician should be left to guide this decision and may differ according to the clinical scenario presented. Many centers would perform an MRI or CT examination of the brain instead of FDG PET if brain metastases were suspected.

Images spanning from the middle of the neck to the pelvis should be considered as a minimum standard approach when imaging for distant metastases from lung cancer. Imaging beginning at the middle of the neck (to include all supraclavicular nodes) is extremely important, because PET can add information about supraclavicular node status that is frequently overlooked on CT. Supraclavicular disease has the added advantage of being easily accessible to needle biopsy. Imaging of the pelvis may be somewhat less important, as the likelihood of a metastasis solely to the pelvis is believed to be low. Consideration of the patient's ability to tolerate the PET scan or the referring physician's wishes is important when considering pelvic imaging.

Many authors have reported that PET has the ability to detect distant disease that may be otherwise undetectable (27,35,36). These studies have shown that at a minimum, 11% of the patients who undergo PET are shown to have a distant metastasis that was not detected by CT or other imaging methods. Unsuspected disease identified on PET thus resulted in upstaging. The results imply that adding PET

TABLE 5.5.3. *FDG PET studies of lung cancer metastatic disease*

Author, yr (reference no.)	Patient no.	Study type	PET detected unsuspected metastasis in
Bury et al., 1997 (35)	109	Prospective	14%
Lewis et al., 1994 (36)	34	Retrospective	29%
Valk et al., 1995 (37)	99	Prospective	11%

data will often change the plans regarding advisability of tumor resection. In the study by Lewis et al. (36), the PET findings resulted in patient management changes in 41% of the cases (Table 5.5.3).

Additionally, and just as important to clinical decisions, many false-positive findings on CT (including findings outside of the chest such as adrenal enlargement) were correctly interpreted as negative by PET. PET imaging has been shown to have the ability to distinguish benign adrenal enlargement from metastatic disease. Boland et al. (37) showed that PET imaging was able to show a statistically significant difference in lesion metabolism between benign enlarged adrenal glands and those with malignancy. A study by Erasmus et al. (38) showed that in 27 patients (33 enlarged adrenal glands) with bronchogenic carcinoma, PET correctly identified all adrenal glands that had tumor (Fig. 5.5.5).

Bone scans are commonly ordered in patients with lung cancer to rule out bone metastases. The sensitivity of bone scanning is high, but the specificity can be problematic because chronic bone or joint disease or trauma can cause false-positive study results. PET has been compared with bone scintigraphy, and although the tests are very similar with high sensitivity for metastases, PET has a much higher specificity for malignant disease than bone scintigraphy (39). Imaging the lower limbs with PET would need to be performed to get the same skeletal information provided by the bone scan. It is reasonable to consider PET a substitute for bone scans if completed with this protocol. Imaging the skeleton with PET is discussed in more detail elsewhere in the book. An example of a patient with lung cancer and extensive bone metastases is shown in Fig. 5.5.6.

EVALUATION OF LUNG CANCER TREATMENT: RESPONSE OR RECURRENCE

Most patients diagnosed with bronchogenic carcinoma present with the disease in an advanced state, a fact that helps explain the poor prognosis and 5-year survival of only 13% for all comers (40). An accurate assessment of the efficacy of chemotherapy and radiation therapy might prove to be of enormous benefit in directing therapy for patients with advanced stages of lung cancer. Historically, clinicians have used tumor shrinkage to assess treatment efficacy, but this

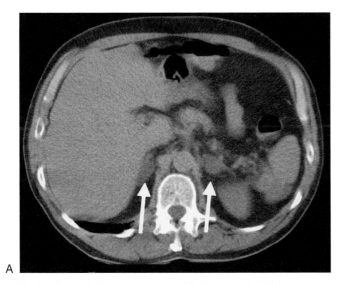
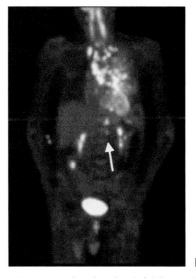

FIG. 5.5.5. A: Left lung cancer with chest and abdomen computed tomography showing left hilar and left mediastinal lymphadenopathy and bilaterally enlarged adrenal glands (*arrows*). **B:** PET showing bilateral mediastinal nodes, supraclavicular nodes, left adrenal hypermetabolism (*arrow*), and abdominal nodes all with increased FDG uptake.

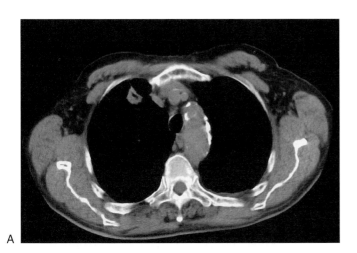

FIG. 5.5.6. Images of a patient who had chest pain while shoveling. He was evaluated in the emergency room for a heart attack and an indeterminate right lung mass was discovered **(A)**, as well as a left rib fracture. An indeterminate left lung mass was also seen **(B).** No adenopathy was seen. A few vertebral body fractures were noted. **C:** PET showed widespread metastases in bone and the thorax, as well as liver metastases that had not been seen previously.

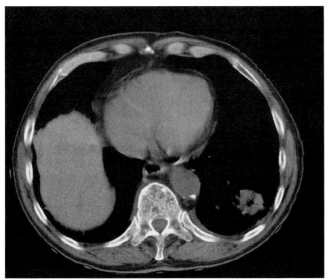
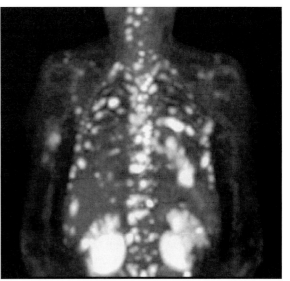

may not be the best indicator of response to therapy. FDG PET can identify changes in glucose uptake after treatment and may prove to be a better indicator of a favorable response to therapy. However, it may be important to differentiate between a decrease in FDG uptake and the complete absence of FDG uptake. Some investigators have concluded that a simple decrease in FDG uptake does not necessarily indicate a good prognosis (41). Rather, it has been suggested that a decrease in FDG uptake may only indicate a partial response due to death of cells sensitive to the therapy while other resistant cells continue to be metabolically active. In many tumors, it has been essential to quantify the decline in FDG uptake by measuring the SUV. In most tumors, the larger the decline in SUV, the more likely the tumor is to respond to therapy.

Much work remains to be done in the area of predicting prognosis with FDG PET. The design of studies in this area will need to involve long-term patient follow-up to determine the meaning of different degrees of metabolic change that may occur during or after therapy.

Posttreatment normalization of FDG uptake, on the other hand, appears to be a good prognostic sign. One study by Hebert et al. (41a) has demonstrated that negative PET findings after radiation therapy, even in the presence of nonspecific radiographic changes, are an indicator of a good response. Hebert et al. noted that all of their patients with negative PET findings were alive at 2 years after treatment, whereas 50% of patients with residual hypermetabolism, albeit reduced, had died within that same 2-year period. Other investigators have used this logic to justify further treatment of asymptomatic individuals whose PET scans demonstrate residual hypermetabolism after an initial course of therapy. Frank et al. (42) treated five such asymptomatic patients in their study, based solely on residual hypermetabolism and all were alive at 3 years.

Early diagnosis of recurrent lung cancer is another potential use of FDG PET. Radiologic changes such as scarring and necrosis that occur after therapy may obscure the identification of recurrent tumor unless significant tumor growth appears over time. The interpretation of recurrence is often not made until the disease progresses to the point of marked enlargement of questionable abnormalities. Unfortunately, a tissue biopsy that is negative for tumor in such situations is suspect, due to the inherent difficulty in identifying and accurately sampling the areas of viable tumor in the midst of scar. A PET evaluation of tumor recurrence can potentially assist in this determination. Patients who have chest radiographic findings that are suggestive of tumor recurrence can be accurately characterized by FDG PET imaging. Benign nonspecific pleural thickening is another example of a posttreatment change that may be difficult to differentiate from recurrent tumor. Pleural biopsy itself may be relatively unreliable when performed percutaneously. PET imaging can differentiate recurrent tumor from radiation-induced benign pleural thickening (43). The accuracy of differentiating treatment changes from recurrent disease with PET is high

and is better than CT performance in the same group of patients (11,44–46).

There are potential pitfalls for FDG PET when used for this purpose. Occasionally treatment can induce hypermetabolic inflammatory changes that may make it difficult to differentiate persistent tumor from treatment effect. This commonly occurs when radiation therapy has been used. Chemotherapy does not commonly induce the tissue damage that leads to inflammatory hypermetabolism. The likelihood of seeing moderate levels of hypermetabolism after radiation therapy diminishes as time passes (47). Scans are likely to be most reliable when a year or more has passed from the last radiation treatment. The most common finding indicative of posttherapy inflammatory hypermetabolism is diffuse, mildly elevated FDG accumulation in the soft tissues of radiation port regions. A cutoff SUV of 2.5 still appears to be accurate in differentiating tumor from benign changes in focal abnormalities identified in the posttreatment setting.

SMALL CELL LUNG CANCER

Very little has been written about the use of PET in small cell lung cancer. Primarily this is because small cell lung cancer is primarily treated by chemotherapy and information on PET about disease in the mediastinum would not add to the clinical decision process. There is some argument for using PET if therapy would be altered in the case of distant disease such as abdominal metastases. For limited stage disease (disease confined to a thoracic radiation port), therapy

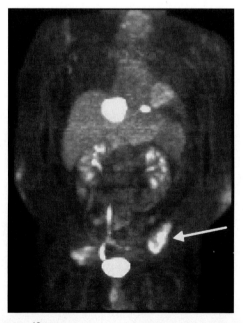

FIG. 5.5.7. ^{18}F-Fluorodeoxyglucose positron emission tomography image of a patient with small cell lung cancer in the left lower lobe who has a large liver metastasis and a left iliac bone metastasis (arrow), indicating extensive stage disease.

normally consists of chemotherapy and local radiation therapy with or without cranial irradiation. If extensive disease (disease outside a thoracic radiation port) is found, the therapy is felt to be palliative and different chemotherapy regimens are used. Radiation therapy in advanced disease would be performed to local areas for palliation only. In this setting, PET may be helpful to detect extensive disease. Small cell lung cancer is very metabolically active (Fig. 5.5.7), and there is good reason to believe that PET will perform with equivalent accuracy to non–small cell lung cancer. More study is needed in this tumor, however.

SUMMARY

Continuing advances in imaging technology have resulted in an improved ability to evaluate thoracic malignancies with PET. Published reports demonstrate that PET provides accurate, noninvasive detection of malignancy, which is useful in the characterization of nonspecific radiographic lung lesions, staging of known lung cancer, and identification of recurrent disease after treatment. Preliminary studies suggest that PET may also be able to accurately assess therapeutic response. The incorporation of PET into routine clinical practice has advanced rapidly and undoubtedly will continue to be an even more important and fully routine part of the clinical assessment of patients with lung malignancy.

REFERENCES

1. Beckett WS. Epidemiology and etiology of lung cancer. *Clin Chest Med* 1993;14:1–15.
2. Bailar JC III, Gornik HL. Cancer undefeated. *N Engl J Med* 1997;336:1569–1574.
3. Devesa SS, Grauman DJ, Blot WJ, et al. Cancer surveillance series: changing geographic patterns of lung cancer mortality in the United States, 1950 through 1994. *J Natl Cancer Inst* 1999;91:1040–1050.
4. Prager D, Cameron R, Ford J, et al. Bronchogenic carcinoma. In: Murray JF, Nadel JA, eds. *Textbook of respiratory medicine*. Philadelphia: WB Saunders, 2000:1415–1448.
5. Smith RA, Glynn TJ. Epidemiology of lung cancer. *Radiol Clin North Am* 2000;38:453–470.
6. Winning AJ, McIvor J, Seed WA, et al. Interpretation of negative results in fine needle aspiration of discrete pulmonary lesions. *Thorax* 1986;41:875–879.
7. Odell MJ, Reid KR. Does percutaneous fine-needle aspiration biopsy aid in the diagnosis and surgical management of lung masses [see Comments]? *Can J Surg* 1999;42:297–301.
8. Tsukada H, Satou T, Iwashima A, et al. Diagnostic accuracy of CT-guided automated needle biopsy of lung nodules. *AJR Am J Roentgenol* 2000;175:239–243.
9. Dewan NA, Reeb SD, Gupta NC, et al. PET-FDG imaging and transthoracic needle lung aspiration biopsy in evaluation of pulmonary lesions. A comparative risk-benefit analysis. *Chest* 1995;108:441–446.
10. Kubota K, Matsuzawa T, Fujiwara T, et al. Differential diagnosis of lung tumor with positron emission tomography: a prospective study. *J Nucl Med* 1990;31:1927–1932.
11. Duhaylongsod FG, Lowe VJ, Patz EJ, et al. Detection of primary and recurrent lung cancer by means of F-18 fluorodeoxyglucose positron emission tomography (FDG PET). *J Thorac Cardiovasc Surg* 1995;110:130–139.
12. Bury T, Dowlati A, Paulus P, et al. Evaluation of the solitary pulmonary nodule by positron emission tomography imaging. *Eur Respir J* 1996;9:410–414.
13. Knight SB, Delbeke D, Stewart JR, et al. Evaluation of pulmonary lesions with FDG-PET. Comparison of findings in patients with and without a history of prior malignancy. *Chest* 1996;109:982–988.
14. Gupta NC, Maloof J, Gunel E. Probability of malignancy in solitary pulmonary nodules using fluorine-18-FDG and PET [see Comments]. *J Nucl Med* 1996;37:943–948.
15. Lowe VJ, Duhaylongsod FG, Patz EF, et al. Pulmonary abnormalities and PET data analysis: a retrospective study [see Comments]. *Radiology* 1997;202:435–439.
16. Lowe VJ, Fletcher JW, Gobar L, et al. Prospective investigation of positron emission tomography in lung nodules. *J Clin Oncol* 1998;16:1075–1084.
17. Gould MK, Maclean CC, Kuschner WG, et al. Accuracy of positron emission tomography in the diagnosis of pulmonary nodules and mass lesions: a meta-analysis. *JAMA* 2001;285:914–924.
18. Gambhir SS, Shepherd JE, Shah BD, et al. Analytical decision model for the cost-effective management of solitary pulmonary nodules. *J Clin Oncol* 1998;16:2113–2125.
19. Van Schil PE, Van HRH, Schoofs EL. The value of mediastinoscopy in preoperative staging of bronchogenic carcinoma. *J Thorac Cardiovasc Surg* 1989;97:240–244.
20. Patterson GA, Ginsberg RJ, Poon PY, et al. A prospective evaluation of magnetic resonance imaging, computed tomography, and mediastinoscopy in the preoperative assessment of mediastinal node status in bronchogenic carcinoma. *J Thorac Cardiovasc Surg* 1987;94:679–684.
21. Wahl RL, Quint LE, Greenough RL, et al. Staging of mediastinal non–small cell lung cancer with FDG PET, CT, and fusion images: preliminary prospective evaluation. *Radiology* 1994;191:371–377.
22. Patz EJ, Lowe VJ, Goodman PC, et al. Thoracic nodal staging with PET imaging with ^{18}FDG in patients with bronchogenic carcinoma. *Chest* 1995;108:1617–1621.
23. Scott WJ, Schwabe JL, Gupta NC, et al. Positron emission tomography of lung tumors and mediastinal lymph nodes using [^{18}F]fluorodeoxyglucose; the members of the PET-Lung Tumor Study Group [Review]. *Ann Thorac Surg* 1994;58:698–703.
24. Sasaki M, Ichiya Y, Kuwabara Y, et al. The usefulness of FDG positron emission tomography for the detection of mediastinal lymph node metastases in patients with non–small cell lung cancer: a comparative study with x-ray computed tomography. *Eur J Nucl Med* 1996;23:741–747.
25. Steinert HC, Hauser M, Allemann F, et al. Non–small cell lung cancer: nodal staging with FDG PET versus CT with correlative lymph node mapping and sampling. *Radiology* 1997;202:441–446.
26. Sazon DA, Santiago SM, Soo HG, et al. Fluorodeoxyglucose-positron emission tomography in the detection and staging of lung cancer. *Am J Respir Crit Care Med* 1996;153:417–421.
27. Valk PE, Pounds TR, Hopkins DM, et al. Staging non–small cell lung cancer by whole-body positron emission tomographic imaging. *Ann Thorac Surg* 1995;60:1573–1581.
28. Vansteenkiste JF, Mortelmans LA. FDG-PET in the locoregional lymph node staging of non–small cell lung cancer: a comprehensive review of the Leuven Lung Cancer Group experience. *Clin Positron Imaging* 1999;2:223–231.
29. Pieterman RM, van Putten JW, Meuzelaar JJ, et al. Preoperative staging of non–small-cell lung cancer with positron-emission tomography [Comment]. *N Engl J Med* 2000;343:254–261.
30. Vansteenkiste JF, Stroobants SG, De LP, et al. Mediastinal lymph node staging with FDG-PET scan in patients with potentially operable non–small cell lung cancer: a prospective analysis of 50 cases. Leuven Lung Cancer Group. *Chest* 1997;112:1480–1486.
31. Yasukawa T, Yoshikawa K, Aoyagi H, et al. Usefulness of PET with ^{11}C-methionine for the detection of hilar and mediastinal lymph node metastasis in lung cancer. *J Nucl Med* 2000;41:283–290.
32. Hara T, Inagaki K, Kosaka N, et al. Sensitive detection of mediastinal lymph node metastasis of lung cancer with ^{11}C-choline PET. *J Nucl Med* 2000;41:1507–1513.
33. Vanuytsel LJ, Vansteenkiste JF, Stroobants SG, et al. The impact of (^{18})F-fluoro-2-deoxy-D-glucose positron emission tomography (FDG-PET) lymph node staging on the radiation treatment volumes in patients with non–small cell lung cancer. *Radiother Oncol* 2000;55:317–324.
34. Palm I, Hellwig D, Leutz M, et al. Brain metastases of lung cancer: diagnostic accuracy of positron emission tomography with fluorodeoxyglucose (FDG-PET). *Medizinische Klinik* 1999;94:224–227.
35. Bury T, Dowlati A, Paulus P, et al. Whole-body ^{18}FDG positron emis-

sion tomography in the staging of non–small cell lung cancer. *Eur Respir J* 1997;10:2529–2534.

36. Lewis P, Griffin S, Marsden P, et al. Whole-body ¹⁸F-fluorodeoxyglucose positron emission tomography in preoperative evaluation of lung cancer. *Lancet* 1994;344:1265–1266.

37. Boland GW, Goldberg MA, Lee MJ, et al. Indeterminate adrenal mass in patients with cancer: evaluation at PET with 2-[F-18]-fluoro-2-deoxy-D-glucose. *Radiology* 1995;194:131–134.

38. Erasmus JJ, Patz EJ, McAdams HP, et al. Evaluation of adrenal masses in patients with bronchogenic carcinoma using ¹⁸F-fluorodeoxyglucose positron emission tomography [see Comments]. *AJR Am J Roentgenol* 1997;168:1357–1360.

39. Bury T, Barreto A, Daenen F, et al. Fluorine-18 deoxyglucose positron emission tomography for the detection of bone metastases in patients with non–small cell lung cancer. *Eur J Nucl Med* 1998;25:1244–1247.

40. Recine D, Rowland K, Reddy S, et al. Combined modality therapy for locally advanced non–small cell lung carcinoma. *Cancer* 1990;66:2270–2278.

41. Ichiya Y, Kuwabara Y, Sasaki M, et al. A clinical evaluation of FDG-PET to assess the response in radiation therapy for bronchogenic carcinoma. *Ann Nucl Med* 1996;10:193–200.

41a.Herbert ME, Lowe VJ, Hoffman JM, et al. Positron emission tomography in the pretreatment evaluation and follow-up of non-small cell lung cancer patients treated with radiotherapy: preliminary findings. *Am J Clin Oncol* 1996;19:416–421.

42. Frank A, Lefkowitz D, Jaeger S, et al. Decision logic for retreatment of asymptomatic lung cancer recurrence based on positron emission tomography findings. *Int J Radiat Oncol Biol Phys* 1995;32:1495–1512.

43. Lowe VJ, Patz EF, Harris L, et al. FDG-PET evaluation of pleural abnormalities. *J Nucl Med* 1994;35:229P.

44. Patz EJ, Lowe VJ, Hoffman JM, et al. Persistent or recurrent bronchogenic carcinoma: detection with PET and 2-[F-18]-2-deoxy-D-glucose. *Radiology* 1994;191:379–382.

45. Inoue T, Kim EE, Komaki R, et al. Detecting recurrent or residual lung cancer with FDG-PET. *J Nucl Med* 1995;36:788–793.

46. Bury T, Corhay JL, Duysinx B, et al. Value of FDG-PET in detecting residual or recurrent nonsmall cell lung cancer. *Eur Respir J* 1999;14:1376–1380.

47. Lowe VJ, Hebert ME, Hawk TC, et al. Chest wall FDG accumulation in serial FDG-PET images in patients being treated for bronchogenic carcinoma with radiation. *J Nucl Med* 1994;35:76P.

CHAPTER 5.6

Lymphoma

Sven N. Reske and Inga Buchmann

Hodgkin's disease (HD) is a malignant disease of lymphoid cells and accounts for about 1% of all malignancies. In the United States, about 7,500 new patients are diagnosed with HD per year with a male-to-female ratio of 1.3 : 1. HD has a striking bimodal age distribution. In industrialized countries, the first peak occurs at approximately 20 to 30 years of age, and the second peak occurs during late adulthood. The incidence is 2.8 per 100,000. HD usually spreads in an orderly fashion from one lymph node group to a contiguous lymph node group. Extranodal disease is less common than in non-Hodgkin's lymphoma (NHL). Treatment strategies are based almost entirely on stage. The goal of treatment is cure. The main modalities of treatment are chemotherapy and/or radiation and combined treatment modalities in disease with unfavorable characteristics. Overall survival in stage less than II is 80% to 85% at 10 years and disease-free survival is 70% to 75% at 10 years. In stage III, overall survival is 65% to 70% and disease-free survival is 30% to 34% at 10 years. In stage IV, overall survival is about 42% and disease-free survival is about 18% at 10 years. The history of HD is also somewhat predictive of patient outcome.

NHL constitutes an extremely heterogeneous group of neoplasms of the immune system, each of which is characterized by its own particular histology, immunophenotype, and in some cases genotype. NHL is the sixth most common malignancy in the United States, with an annual incidence of 55,000 to 60,000 cases and 24,000 deaths per year. The peak incidence of NHL occurs after age 50. The incidence is about 16 per 100,000 and is rising for unknown reasons, increasing at a rate of approximately 3% to 4% per year for the past three decades. Unlike in HD, treatment planning for NHL takes into consideration not only stage but also the untreated natural history of the various entities that are broadly grouped into low-, intermediate-, and high-grade disease (1). The main modality of treatment is chemotherapy; novel approaches include immunotherapy and radioimmunotherapy (2,3), and stem-cell transplantation in relapsing disease. The goal of treatment is cure in aggressive and rapidly progressive NHL and prolongation of survival in low-grade NHL. The median survival time is 6 to 7 years in low-grade NHL and 3 to 4 years in aggressive NHL. The 5-year survival rate is 60% in rapidly progressive NHL.

The diagnosis of malignant lymphoma rests primarily on histopathologic examination of involved tissues. Conventionally, extent of disease is estimated by assessment of clinical findings; serologic tests; ultrasonography; computed tomography (CT) of the thorax, abdomen, and pelvis; bone marrow biopsy; magnetic resonance imaging; and skeletal scintigraphy in selected cases. In contrast to NHL, which is often disseminated at the time of diagnosis, HD spread usually follows sequential involvement of contiguous lymph nodes. Extranodal involvement as the first manifestation of HD is rare. According to the Ann Arbor classification (Table 5.6.1), patients with HD can be stratified into a limited stage (clinical stage II or less, absence of risk factors), intermediary stage (clinical stage II or less, presence of risk factors), or disseminated disease (4). The risk factors are defined as mediastinal bulk, extranodal involvement, more than three involved nodal areas, and an erythrocyte sedimentation rate

TABLE 5.6.1. *Ann Arbor classification; lymphoid structures: spleen, thymus, and Waldeyer's ring*

Stage I	Involvement of a single lymph node region or lymphoid structure or involvement of a single extralymphatic site (I_E).
Stage II	Involvement of two or more lymph node regions on the same side of the diaphragm (II), which may be accompanied by localized contiguous involvement of an extralymphatic organ or site (II_E).
Stage III	Involvement of lymph node regions on both sides of the diaphragm (III), which may also be accompanied by involvement of the spleen (III_S) or by localized contiguous involvement of an extralymphatic organ or site (III_E).
Stage IV	Diffuse or disseminated involvement of one or more extralymphatic organs or tissues, with or without associated lymph node involvement.

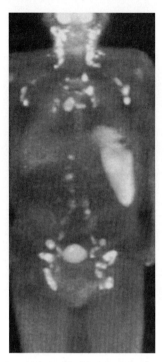

FIG. 5.6.1. PET scan (coronal view) of a patient with non-Hodgkin's lymphoma. There are extensive supradiaphragmatic and infradiaphragmatic, nodal lymphoma manifestations involving the cervical, supraclavicular/infraclavicular, bronchohilar, paraaortic, iliac, and inguinal areas. Diffuse spleen involvement with a lateral splenic infarct is also seen.

(ESR) of more than 50 mm per hour (associated with A-type symptoms) or an ESR of more than 30 mm per hour (associated with B-type symptoms).

The first report of increased ^{18}F-fluorodeoxyglucose (FDG) uptake in malignant lymphoma was published by Paul (5) in 1987. An example of whole-body fluorodeoxyglucose positron emission tomography (FDG PET) imaging of NHL with modern equipment is shown in Fig. 5.6.1. Paul (5) and others (6–9) found FDG imaging to be more sensitive than gallium-67 (^{67}Ga) imaging to detect malignant lymphomas. Later studies described a loose correlation of FDG uptake in untreated malignant lymphomas with the proliferative activity, grade of malignancy, and prognosis (6–8). Several authors found low FDG uptake and a decreased detection rate in low-grade lymphomas (6,7). This observation was not confirmed by others (Fig. 5.6.2) (10,11). FDG uptake is commonly seen in patients with low-grade lymphoma, but there are insufficient data to precisely define the overall sensitivity of FDG imaging in this group of patients. Uptake and transport rates of carbon-11 (^{11}C)-methionine have been found to be significantly increased in malignant lymphoma (12). The short half-life of ^{11}C and limited availability may preclude widespread use of this tracer for the detection and staging of patients with malignant lymphomas.

With the availability of whole-body PET scanners, the properties of FDG PET for staging and therapy monitoring have been systematically studied. Although FDG uptake rates are similar in lymphomas after overnight fasting and during euglycemic hyperinsulinemic clamp (which is used experimentally to keep serum glucose levels constant), increased muscle and other soft-tissue FDG uptake results in decreased lymphoma to soft-tissue contrast (13). Thus, a 4- to 12-hour fasting period is recommended for examining patients with malignant lymphomas with FDG PET. High-quality whole-body scans are necessary for exact staging. This is achieved by state-of-the-art ordered subsets–expectation maximization image reconstruction techniques (14). Attenuation correction can be used but is not necessary for staging as long as the reader is familiar with the image artifacts that are seen in non–attenuation-corrected images (15). In contrast, therapy control studies will require some quantitative approach such as determining the standard uptake value and thus attenuation correction is needed. One study reports encouraging results using a coincidence gamma camera and whole-body FDG imaging (16). These data have to be confirmed in larger patient series before general use of gamma camera coincidence PET can be recommended for staging malignant lymphoma. There are also some restrictions on the reimbursement for coincidence imaging in the United States and elsewhere.

Criteria for pathologic findings with FDG PET are unifocally or multifocally increased uptake in the location of node regions. Focal soft-tissue or bone marrow FDG uptake beyond areas of normal FDG accumulation such as brain, heart muscle, collecting system of the urinary tract and bladder, and to a variable degree large intestines is probably abnormal. Splenic uptake may be either diffuse or unifocal or multifocal in splenic lymphomatous involvement. During or immediately after radiotherapy or chemotherapy, nonspe-

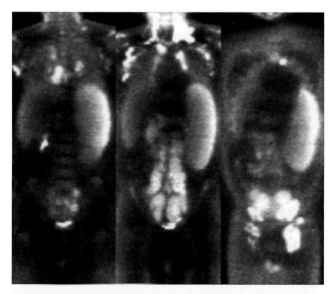

FIG. 5.6.2. Coronal PET scans of a patient with low-grade non-Hodgkin's lymphoma. There is disseminated, supradiaphragmatic, and infradiaphragmatic lymph node involvement and diffuse infiltration and enlargement of the spleen.

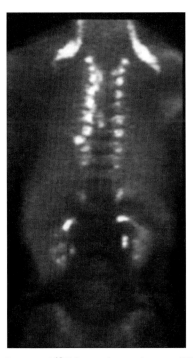

FIG. 5.6.3. A coronal ^{18}F-fluorodeoxyglucose (FDG) positron emission tomographic study demonstrates FDG uptake in the cervical, supraclavicular, and infraclavicular regions. It is likely in muscle, costovertebral muscle, and the region of the costovertebral joints. This pattern should not be confused with tumor uptake of FDG.

cific, usually symmetric, FDG uptake in cervical and supraclavicular and/or infraclavicular lymph nodes and costovertebral joints may be seen (Fig. 5.6.3). The underlying cause of this nonspecific FDG uptake is unknown. These findings usually resolve within 4 to 8 weeks after completion of radiotherapy or chemotherapy. In adolescents and younger adults, increased FDG uptake may temporarily be found in the thymus after chemotherapy (17). Also, nonspecific thymus FDG uptake generally resolves within several weeks after termination of chemotherapy. Further reasons for false-positive study results are radiation pneumonitis after radiotherapy and active tuberculosis or sarcoidosis (18).

STAGING

A pilot study evaluating FDG PET for staging in 16 patients was published by Newman et al. (19) in 1994. These authors reported excellent accuracy of FDG PET for thoracoabdominal lymphoma. All grades of NHL were successfully imaged. These results have been confirmed and extended by our group and by others. In 60 untreated patients (27 patients with HD, 33 patients with NHL), FDG PET was more accurate for detecting nodal involvement compared with CT and resulted in changing the stage, with an impact in management for 10% to 15% of patients (10,11). Extranodal staging with FDG PET was significantly superior to that

with CT and resulted in changes of tumor stage in 13 (16%) of 81 patients (11).

Spleen involvement is either demonstrated by diffuse increased FDG uptake or a nodular uptake pattern. FDG PET has great potential for demonstrating bone marrow involvement (20,21). Besides confirming lesions found at bone marrow biopsy, FDG PET provided additional information in 8 (10.3%) of 78 patients, which led to an upgrade of tumor stage. Bone marrow biopsy revealed marrow involvement not detected by FDG PET in 5.1% of patients. In these patients, diffuse marrow infiltration with less than 10% content of malignant cells was present and precluded detection by PET due to the low cellular density of tumor (20). FDG PET can completely replace bone scanning for assessing bone or bone marrow involvement (21). Excellent accuracy for both nodal and extranodal staging of malignant lymphoma has been confirmed in three recent studies (22–24), as well as in a prospective bicenter study (I. Buchmann et al., *unpublished data*).

In a prospective study of 18 patients, Hoh et al. (25) found an FDG PET–based staging algorithm more accurate and cost-effective than the conventional multimodality imaging approach. High predictive value of FDG PET for staging both HD and intermediate- and high-grade lymphoma has been confirmed in several recently published studies (16,18, 26).

In summary, nodal staging was roughly 10% more sensitive than conventional staging including CT and low-dose ^{67}Ga scanning (16), with a specificity of 85% to 90%, and led to a therapeutically relevant change of stage in about 10% of patients. For extranodal staging, a sensitivity of 95% to 100% and a specificity of 97% have been reported (11). For comparison, CT was 93% sensitive but only 63% specific for extranodal staging.

Performance of FDG PET in mucosa-associated lymphoid tissue has only been examined in a few patients by one group (7), and they reported a high diagnostic accuracy. Data on initial staging are shown in Table 5.6.2.

PREDICTING TREATMENT RESPONSE

Early evaluation of treatment response and persisting residual masses after the completion of therapy are well-recognized problems with morphologically based imaging techniques in the management of lymphoma. Using a planar detection technique, Hoekstra et al. (27) found a sharp reduction of FDG uptake within days after effective treatment before volume changes occurred, whereas FDG uptake persisted in nonresponders. These data were recently confirmed by Römer et al. (28), who described a 60% to 67% reduction of FDG uptake and metabolic rate as early as 7 days after initiation of therapy in patients with NHL responding to chemotherapy. Patients who subsequently relapsed displayed a significantly smaller reduction of FDG uptake assessed at 42 days after the start of therapy (28) (Table 5.6.2).

TABLE 5.6.2. *Literature of PET findings in lymphoma diagnosis*

Author, yr (reference no.)	Purpose	Total no. patients	Total no. studies	Total lesions	Sensitivity of PET %	Sensitivity of CT %	Specificity of PET %	Specificity of CT %	PPV PET %	PPV CT %	NPV PET %	NPV CT %	Accuracy of PET %	Accuracy of CT %
Initial staging														
Carr et al., 1998 (21)	M	50	50		81		76		62		90		78	
Moog et al., 1997 (10)	N	60		740	99									
Moog et al., 1998 (11)	M	81	56	58	97	63	100	93						
Moog et al., 1999 (33)	M bone	56					100					100		
Moog et al., 1998 (20)	T	78			81		100							
Rodriguez et al., 1997 (34)		8												
Buchmann et al., 2001 (26)	T	52	52	1297	99	83	100	99					99	96
Stumpe et al., 1998 HD/NHL (22)	T	35/15	10/7		88/83	88/75	100/100	100/33					90/86	89/57
Therapy monitoring/ residual mass														
Bangerter et al., 1998 (35)	TH	44	44		86									
Bangerter et al., 1999 (31)														
Cremerius et al., 1999 (30)	TH	72			88	84	83	31	50–90[b]				85	54
Römer et al., 1998 (28)	TH	11												
Zinzani et al., 1999 (36)	TH	44	44											
Cremerius 1998	TH	27	27		100	100	92	17	94	60	100	100	96	63
deWit et al., 1997 (29)	TH	34	34		100	86	73	3,7	557	19	100	50		
Lang et al., 2001 (37)	TH	51	63										91	62[a]
Hueltenschmidt et al., 2001 (18)	T/TH										96		96/91	56/62[a]
Stumpe et al., 1998 HD/NHL (22)	TH	35/15	43/11		85/100	75/100	96/100	38/83					96/100	50/89

[a] Conventional staging methods (MRI, ultrasound, CT).
[b] Independent of risk factor.

180

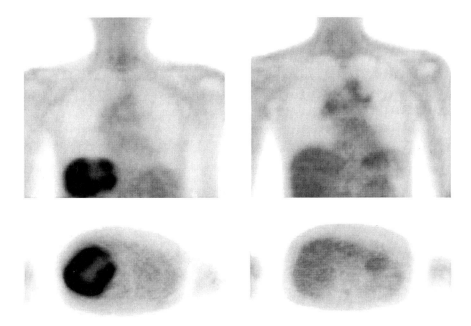

FIG. 5.6.4. Coronal and transverse PET scans of a patient with non-Hodgkin's lymphoma of the liver—**(left)** pretreatment and **(right)** 8 weeks posttreatment. Intense ^{18}F-fluorodeoxyglucose (FDG) uptake is seen in a hepatic lesion pretreatment. There is a good response, with no abnormal hepatic FDG uptake after chemotherapy.

A PET scan of a patient with a good treatment response is shown in Fig. 5.6.4.

EVALUATION OF RESIDUAL TUMOR VIABILITY

Assessment of the viability of residual lymphomatous masses after completion of therapy has been studied by several groups (29–31) (Table 5.6.2). The negative predictive value (NPV) of FDG PET was very high and predicted a complete response (Figs. 5.6.4 and 5.6.5A). Jerusalem et al. (32) have recently shown that persistent FDG uptake in residual masses or in progressive lymphoma (Fig. 5.6.5B) also has a very high predictive value for the presence of active disease and for prognosis.

The efficacy of FDG PET for detecting viable lymphoma after chemotherapy, mostly in CT-positive "residual masses," was examined in three papers with 162 patients. PET was 71% to 88% sensitive and 83% to 86% specific, compared with 88% sensitivity and 31% specificity for CT (30). Jerusalem et al. (32) reported a positive predictive value (PPV) of FDG PET of 100% and an NPV of 88%, compared with a 42% PPV and an 87% NPV for CT.

These authors reported a higher diagnostic and prognostic value for FDG PET than CT. Fifty-four patients with HD or NHL were evaluated after completion of chemotherapy. The progression-free survival rate at 1 year was 62% for patients with residual masses on CT versus 88% for patients without residual masses on CT. When FDG PET tumor activity was seen posttreatment, all patients had evidence of progression of disease at 1 year, whereas 86% of the patients with negative study results had a progression-free course for 1 year.

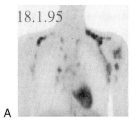
18.1.95

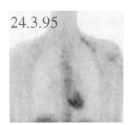
24.3.95

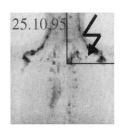
25.10.95

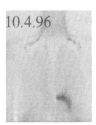
10.4.96

A

FIG. 5.6.5. Sequential ^{18}F-fluorodeoxyglucose (FDG) positron emission tomography scans of patients with non-Hodgkin's lymphoma with residual masses after chemotherapy. **A:** A nonmetabolically active residual mass indicates a high likelihood that there is no viable lymphoma present. *Figure continues*

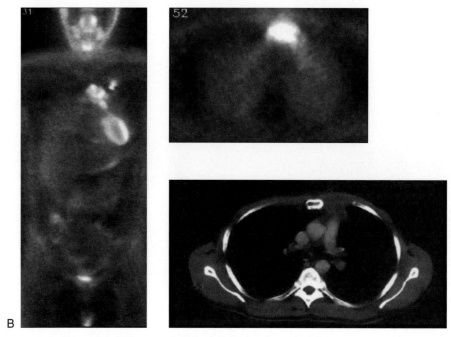

FIG. 5.6.5. *Continued.* **B:** A viable residual mass in the anterior mediastinum on computed tomography with coronal and transverse PET images shows increased FDG uptake, indicating active lymphoma after therapy.

SUMMARY

FDG PET is an efficient, noninvasive method for the primary staging of untreated HD and NHL. Compared with the standard imaging techniques, PET is significantly superior in detecting nodal and extranodal involvement, as well as lymphomatous bone marrow involvement. FDG PET is highly accurate in posttherapeutic differentiation of active residual disease and nonviable tumor masses.

Clinical use of FDG PET is indicated for staging of HD and NHL. In this latter patient group, it can be used most profitably in patients with intermediate-grade disease, because in this patient group, the highest impact of accurate staging on therapeutic strategy can be expected. In low-grade NHL, a watch-and-wait strategy is usually followed, whereas in high-grade NHL, an intense chemotherapeutic regimen is recommended irrespective of stage (1). Determination of viability of a residual mass after radiotherapy or chemotherapy is a firm indication for FDG PET both in HD and NHL.

REFERENCES

1. Segall GM. FDG PET imaging in patients with lymphoma: a clinical perspective. *J Nucl Med* 2001;42(4):609–610.
2. Bunjes D, Buchmann I, Duncker C, et al. Re-188-labeled anti-CD 66 (a,b,c,e) monoclonal antibody to intensify the conditioning regimen prior to stem cell transplantation for patients with high-risk acute myeloid leukemia or myelodysplastic syndrome: results of a phase I-II study. *Blood* 2001;98(3):565–572.
3. Reske SN, Bunjes D, Buchmann I, et al. Targeted bone marrow irradiation in the conditioning of high risk leukemia prior to stem cell transplantation. *Eur J Nucl Med* 2001 *(in press)*.
4. Diehl V, Engert A. An overview of the Second International Symposium on Hodgkin's disease. *Ann Oncol* 1992;3[Suppl 4]:1–3.
5. Paul R. Comparison of fluorine-18-2-fluorodeoxyglucose and gallium-67 citrate imaging for detection of lymphoma. *J Nucl Med* 1987;28:288–292.
6. Okada J, Yoshikawa K, Imazeki K, et al. The use of FDG-PET in the detection and management of malignant lymphoma: correlation of uptake with prognosis. *J Nucl Med* 1992;33:686–691.
7. Rodriguez M, Rehn S, Ahlström H, et al. Predicting malignancy grade with PET in non-Hodgkin's lymphoma. *J Nucl Med* 1995;36:1790–1796.
8. Okada J, Yoshikawa K, Itami M, et al. Positron emission tomography using fluorine-18-fluorodeoxyglucose in malignant lymphoma: a comparison with proliferative activity. *J Nucl Med* 1992;33:325–329.
9. Lapela M, Leskinen S, Minn HRI, et al. Increased glucose metabolism in untreated non-Hodgkin's lymphoma: a study with positron emission tomography and fluorine-18-fluorodeoxyglucose. *Blood* 1995;86:3522–3527.
10. Moog F, Bangerter M, Diederichs CG, et al. Lymphoma: role of whole-body 2-deoxy-2-[F-18]fluoro-D-glucose (FDG) PET in nodal staging. *Radiology* 1997;203:795–800.
11. Moog F, Bangerter M, Diederichs CG, et al. Extranodal malignant lymphoma: detection with FDG PET versus CT. *Radiology* 1998;206:475–481.
12. Leskinen-Kallio S, Ruotsalainen U, Nägren K, et al. Uptake of carbon-11-methionine and fluorodeoxyglucose in non-Hodgkin's lymphoma: a PET study. *J Nucl Med* 1991;32:1211–1218.
13. Minn H, Nuutila P, Lindholm P, et al. *In vivo* effects of insulin on tumor and skeletal muscle glucose metabolism in patients with lymphoma. *Cancer* 1994;73:1490–1498.
14. Hudson HM, Larkin RS. Accelerated image reconstruction using ordered subsets of projection data. *IEEE Trans Med Imaging* 1994;13(4):601–609.
15. Kotzerke J, Guhlmann A, Moog F, et al. Role of attenuation correction for fluorine-18 fluorodeoxyglucose positron emission tomography in the primary staging of malignant lymphoma. *Eur J Nucl Med* 1999;26:31–38.
16. Tatsumi M, Kitayama H, Sugahara H, et al. Whole-body hybrid PET with ¹⁸F-FDG in the staging of non-Hodgkin's lymphoma. *J Nucl Med* 2001;42:601–608.

17. Glatz S, Kotzerke J, Moog F, et al. Simulation of a mediastinal non-Hodgkin's lymphoma recurrence by a diffuse thymus hyperplasia in ^{18}F-FDG PET scan. *Rofo Fortschr Geb Rontgenstr Neuen Bildgeb Verfahr* 1996;165(3):309–310.

18. Hueltenschmidt B, Sautter-Bihl ML, Lang O, et al. Whole body positron emission tomography in the treatment of Hodgkin's disease. *Cancer* 2001;91:302–310.

19. Newman JS, Francis IR, Kaminski MS, et al. Imaging of lymphoma with PET with 2-[F-18]-fluoro-2-deoxy-D-glucose: correlation with CT. *Radiology* 1994;190:111–116.

20. Moog R, Bangerter M, Kotzerke J, et al. 18-F-fluorodeoxyglucose-positron emission tomography as a new approach to detect lymphomatous bone marrow. *J Clin Oncol* 1998;16:603–609.

21. Carr R, Barrington SF, Madan B, et al. Detection of lymphoma in bone marrow by whole-body positron emission tomography. *Blood* 1998;91:3340–3346.

22. Stumpe KDM, Urbinelli M, Steinert HC, et al. Whole-body positron emission tomography using fluorodeoxyglucose for staging of lymphoma: effectiveness and comparison with computed tomography. *Eur J Nucl Med* 1998;25:721–728.

23. Thill R, Neuerburg J, Fabry U, et al. Vergleich der befunde von 18-FDG-PET und CT beim prätherapeutischen staging maligner lymphome. *Nuklearmedizin* 1997;36:234–239.

24. Bumann D, deWit M, Beyer W, et al. Computertomographie und F-18-FDG-positronen-emissions-tomographie im staging maligner lymphome: ein vergleich. *Fortschr Röntgenstr* 1998;168:457–465.

25. Hoh CK, Glaspy J, Rosen P, et al. Whole-body FDG-PET imaging for staging of Hodgkin's disease and lymphoma. *J Nucl Med* 1997;38:343–348.

26. Buchmann I, Reinhardt M, Elsner K, et al. 2-(fluorine-18)fluoro-2-deoxy-D-glucose positron emission tomography in the detection and staging of malignant lymphoma. *Cancer* 2001;91:889–899.

27. Hoekstra OS, Ossenkoppele GJ, Golding R, et al. Early treatment response in malignant lymphoma, as determined by planar fluorine-18-fluorodeoxyglucose scintigraphy. *J Nucl Med* 1993;34:1706–1710.

28. Römer WR, Hanauske AR, Ziegler S, et al. Positron emission tomography in non-Hodgkin's lymphoma: assessment of chemotherapy with fluorodeoxyglucose. *Blood* 1998;91:4464–4471.

29. deWit M, Bumann D, Beyer W, et al. Whole-body positron emission tomography (PET) for diagnosis of residual mass in patients with lymphoma. *Ann Oncol* 1997;8:57–60.

30. Cremerius U, Fabry U, Kröll U, et al. Klinische wertigkeit der FDG-PET zur therapiekontrolle bei malignen lymphomen—ergebnisse einer retrospektiven studie an 72 patienten. *Nuklearmedizin* 1999;38:24–30.

31. Bangerter M, Kotzerke J, Griesshammer M, et al. Positron emission tomography with 18-fluorodeoxyglucose in the staging and follow-up of lymphoma in the chest. *Acta Oncol* 1999;38:799–804.

32. Jerusalem G, Beguin Y, Fassotte MF, et al. Whole-body positron emission tomography using ^{18}F-Fluorodeoxyglucose for posttreatment evaluation in Hodgkin's disease and non-Hodgkin's lymphoma has higher diagnostic and prognostic value than classical computed tomography scan imaging. *Blood* 1999;94:429–433.

33. Moog F, Kotzerke J, Reske SN. FDG PET can replace bone scintigraphy in primary staging of malignant lymphoma. J Nucl Med 1999;40:1407–1413.

34. Rodriguez M, Ahlstrom H, Sundin A, et al. [18F] FDG PET in gastric non-Hodgkin's lymphoma. *Acta Oncol* 1997;36:577–584.

35. Bangerter M, Moog F, Buchmann I, et al. Whole-body 2-[18F]-fluoro-2-deoxy-D-glucose positron emission tomography (FDG-PET) for accurate staging of Hodgkin's disease. *Ann Oncol* 1998;9:1117-1122.

36. Zinzani PL, Magagnoli M, Chierichetti F, et al. The role of positron emission tomography (PET) in the management of lymphoma patients. *Ann Oncol* 1999;10:1181–1184.

37. Lang O, Bihl H, Hultenschmidt B, et al. Clinical relevance of positron emission tomography (PET) in treatment control and relapse of Hodgkin's disease. *Strahlenther Onkol* 2001;177:138–144.

CHAPTER 5.7

Melanoma

Hans C. Steinert

Malignant melanoma is the most aggressive cancer of the skin. The incidence of cutaneous malignant melanoma is increasing dramatically in persons with light-colored skin throughout the world (1,2). No other tumor is increasing faster in number of new cases diagnosed. The death rate for melanoma has doubled in the last 35 years, with increases of approximately 5% per year in the older white population. As with most cancers, the causes of malignant melanoma are multifactorial. Numerous studies have demonstrated that the development and progression of melanoma are based on increasing levels of cutaneous solar exposure, particularly ultraviolet B radiation, in combination with the genotype, phenotype, and immunocompetence of the patient. The risk for a second melanoma is estimated to be about 5% in patients with a previous diagnosis of melanoma.

About 70% of melanomas are of the superficial spreading type. Nodular melanoma is the second most common type and comprises 20% to 30% of melanomas. Lentigo maligna melanoma comprises 5% to 10%, and acral lentiginous melanoma 2% to 8% of melanomas (3).

Melanomas can be located anywhere on the body but most commonly occur on the lower extremities in women and on the back in men. Malignant melanomas appear typically according to the "ABCD" rule with A being asymmetry of the lesion, B border irregularity, C color variation, and D diameter of more than 6 mm. Any pigmented lesion with a change in size, configuration, or color should be considered a potential melanoma, and an excision biopsy should be performed. Fortunately, in most developed countries, most patients are diagnosed early, so melanoma can generally be cured by surgical removal of the lesion. Nevertheless, late diagnosis is fairly common. The widely varying mortality reports in the literature depend more on stage at diagnosis than variations in surgical and treatment technique.

Histologic verification and accurate microstaging of tumor thickness are essential for treatment decisions and to predict the risk of metastases. For microstaging, two methods are used. The Clark method categorizes different levels of invasion that reflect increasing depth of penetration into the dermal layers and the subcutaneous fat (levels I, II, III,

IV, or V). The Breslow method measures the microscopic vertical height of melanomas using an optical micrometer. The American Joint Committee on Cancer (AJCC) has developed a four-stage system that allows subclassification of primary localized melanomas according to their malignant potential (Table 5.7.1).

For cutaneous melanomas, the proportion of patients presenting with AJCC stages I, II, III, and IV were 91.2%, 5.2%, 1.3%, and 2.2%, respectively. The 5-year survival rates for localized melanomas representing stages I and II were 92.5% and 74.8%, respectively. Lymph node–positive stage III patients had a 5-year survival rate of 49%, whereas stage IV patients with metastatic disease had a 5-year survival rate of only 17.9% (3).

It has been demonstrated that the total vertical height of a melanoma (Breslow thickness) is the single most important prognostic factor in stage I and II melanoma (5). Lesions with a Breslow thickness of less than 0.76 mm have an excellent prognosis, not differing significantly from that of a general population, whereas those with more than 4 mm in thickness have a 10-year survival rate of less than 40%. Once patients develop metastases, other prognostic factors must be considered. The dominant prognostic factors for patients with stage IV melanoma are as follows: the number of metastatic sites, the remission duration (less than 12 months vs. more than 12 months), and the site of metastases (visceral vs. nonvisceral) (6).

Surgical excision is the major therapeutic modality for primary malignant melanoma, applied in 95% of patients alone or with other modalities. Regional nodal metastases are the most common sites of metastatic melanoma. The number of involved lymph nodes has a significant impact on survival. The early diagnosis and immediate treatment are important. Surgical excision of metastatic nodes is the only effective treatment for cure or locoregional disease control. In some institutions, only clinically demonstrable metastatic nodes are excised. This type of excision has been termed therapeutic lymph node dissection (TLND). In other institutions, elective lymph node dissection (ELND) is performed. Even nodes that appear normal are excised because

TABLE 5.7.1. *Staging system for malignant melanoma adopted by the American Joint Committee on Cancer*

Stage	Description
IA	Localized melanoma ≤0.75 mm or level II[a] (T1 N0 M0)
IB	Localized melanoma 0.76–1.50 mm or level III[a] (T2 N0 M0)
IIA	Localized melanoma 1.51–4.00 mm or level IV[a] (T3 N0 M0)
IIB	Localized melanoma >4 mm or level V[a] (T4 N0 M0)
III	Regional lymph metastases and/or in-transit metastases (any T, N1 and N2, M0)
IV	Systemic metastases (any T, any N, M1)

[a] The American Joint Committee on Cancer Melanoma Committee recommended that when the thickness and level of invasion criteria are different, the measured tumor thickness should take precedence.

From Ketcham AS, Balch CM, Classification and staging systems. In: Balch CM, Milton GW, eds. *Cutaneous melanoma: clinical management and treatment results worldwide,* 2nd ed. Philadelphia: JB Lippincott Co, 1992: 213–220, with permission.

of the risk of occult or microscopic metastases. The issue of ELND is still in discussion. The melanoma thickness is an important factor for selecting patients who might benefit from ELND. Patients with thin melanomas (less than 1 mm) are usually cured by excision of the primary lesion. ELND would not provide a benefit in such patients. Patients with an intermediate melanoma thickness of 1 to 4 mm have an increased risk of occult regional nodal metastases but have a relatively low risk (less than 20%) of distant metastases. Patients with these lesions might benefit from ELND the most. Patients with melanomas more than 4 mm have a high risk (greater than 70%) of distant metastases. In these patients, ELND has only a palliative character. The major problem with ELND is that most patients suffer the morbidity associated with the operation of no potential benefit. In many locales, particularly in the United States, sentinel lymph node (SLN) localization and sampling have eliminated many full lymph node dissections. Indeed, if a SLN dissection is performed, it is only in a few cases that require a full lymph node dissection to be performed.

Recently, it has been shown that interferon-α-2b is an effective adjuvant treatment of high-risk resected melanoma (7–10). Additional adjuvant chemoimmunotherapy is variably used in node-positive disease.

The high mortality rate of patients with melanoma is due to its early hematogenous spread. The mechanism of hematogenous spread and implantation of melanoma cells is poorly understood, and the location of metastases is unpredictable. The skin, subcutaneous tissue, and distant lymph nodes are the most common sites of distant metastases, but melanoma can metastasize to all organs. Because of the poor response to chemotherapy and immunotherapy, early detection and surgical excision are important in improving the prognosis. As soon as distant metastases are diagnosed, the prognosis is poor, with a median survival time of 4 to 6 months (11). Vaccine therapies are in development for the management of patients with metastatic melanoma. The results of clinical trials of peptide vaccines for melanoma suggest that immune and clinical responses can be seen in patients with metastatic and resected disease (12–14).

For unknown primary melanomas, the distribution of metastases localized to a region or multiple sites at presentation is 43% and 57%, respectively. One must assume that the predominant origins of these unknown primary melanomas arise from a cutaneous melanoma that spontaneously regressed. Spontaneous regression is observed in up to 0.4% of melanomas (15) and is likely mediated by an immune mechanism. The 5-year survival rate in these patients (46.3%) is similar to the rate of survival of stage III cutaneous melanoma (49.0%). Several reports have shown that the surgical management of patients with lymph node disease from unknown primary melanomas fared as well as patients with known cutaneous primary sites (3).

The clinical course of melanoma can be characterized by the risk of recurrent disease and death well beyond 10 years after the initial diagnosis. Twenty-five percent of the patients who survive more than 10 years will experience recurrence. Among patients with stage III disease, about 70% relapse, and two thirds are at distant locations. Therefore, lifetime annual follow-up has been recommended and imaging studies are key to this follow-up.

STAGING OF MALIGNANT MELANOMA

Proper tumor staging is a key prerequisite for choosing the appropriate treatment strategy in melanoma. In the pretreatment evaluation, radiographic and PET imaging play an important role. After resection of the primary melanoma, the Breslow analysis gives an immediate estimate of the statistical likelihood of regional lymph node metastases and distant metastases. In patients with thin melanomas (Breslow thickness of less than 0.75 mm), the likelihood of metastases is so small that staging with imaging modalities is not cost-effective (16).

For staging of patients with increased risk for metastases of malignant melanoma (Breslow thickness of 1.5 mm or more), a variable combination of conventional imaging modalities have historically been used, such as chest x-ray, ultrasound of the abdomen and/or lymph nodes of the axilla, cervical region and groin, computed tomography (CT), and magnetic resonance imaging (MRI) of the body. The primary value of CT and MRI are the clear delineation of anatomic detail. However, these methods have generally been used to evaluate a specific region, rather than the entire body. Furthermore, specific identification of tumor tissue is difficult with these methods. Diagnosis of a lymph node metastasis with cross-sectional imaging modalities is mainly based on size, choosing 1.0 to 1.5 cm in short-axis nodal diameter as a cutoff value between benign and pathologic lymph nodes. However, using these criteria, metastases in small nodes can be missed and reactively enlarged nodes can cause false-positive results, limiting the value of the methods. CT often misses small metastases, particularly those in bowel and bone. These findings contribute to both the false-positive and the false-negative rates reported for CT scans. On ultrasound, in addition to size, criteria such as echogenicity can be used, increasing the results to a sensitivity of 76% (17). Melanoma metastases to bone are unusual as a single site of systemic disease, and investigation is only warranted when symptoms occur. Bone scintigraphy has proved to be an excellent screening modality for bone metastases, despite the better sensitivity reported in some studies using MRI (18).

Due to the limitations of morphologic imaging modalities, several radiopharmaceuticals have been used in nuclear medicine to visualize metastases of melanoma. These include gallium-67-citrate (19), immunoscintigraphy applying monoclonal antibodies against melanoma-associated antigens (20), indium-111-pentetreotide (21), technetium-99m methoxyisobutyl isonitrile (22), iodine-123 (^{123}I)-methyltyrosine (23), fluorine-18 (^{18}F)-fluoroethyl-tyrosine (24), ^{123}I-iodobenzofuran (25), ^{18}F-fluoro-DOPA (26,27), bromine-76-bromodeoxyuridine (28), and ^{18}F-fluorodeoxyuridine (29). However, these radiotracers did not offer any significant advantage in diagnostic sensitivity in screening for metastases of malignant melanoma. False-negative scan results were common because of the poor sensitivity. These radiotracers were suitable for imaging malignant melanoma only in exceptional cases. Several carbon-11 (^{11}C)–labeled radiopharmaceuticals have been used for experimental studies in malignant melanoma. Due to the short half-life of ^{11}C, the clinical use of these tracers is limited.

THE ROLE OF WHOLE-BODY FDG PET

Today, 2-[^{18}F]fluoro-2-deoxy-D-glucose (FDG) is the most widely used radiopharmaceutical for staging of malignant melanoma. *In vitro* and *in vivo* experiments with tumor cells demonstrated higher FDG uptake in melanoma than in other tumor types (30). FDG is a glucose analogue that is taken up by rapidly dividing cells. It is trapped in the first step of glucose utilization and accumulates in the cell. Whole-body positron emission tomography (PET) using FDG has been proven to be a highly effective and cost-saving modality to screen for metastases of malignant melanoma throughout the body. With the exception of the brain, whole-body FDG PET can largely replace the standard battery of imaging tests currently performed on high-risk patients (Fig. 5.7.1).

In 1993, Gritters et al. (31) compared the accuracy of regional FDG PET with that of CT in 12 patients with known metastatic melanoma. The sensitivity of PET was 100% for intraabdominal visceral and lymph node metastases. PET identified three lesions that were missed originally by CT.

Retrospectively, these lesions were also confirmed with CT. In this study, PET had a decreased sensitivity in detecting small pulmonary nodules identified by CT.

Our own group (32) analyzed the use of whole-body FDG PET in 33 patients with either known metastatic or newly diagnosed melanoma. Patients with suspected metastases also underwent CT, MRI, or both. Diagnoses were confirmed with histologic examination and/or with at least one imaging modality in addition to PET. Forty of 53 lesions evaluated proved to be melanoma metastases. Whole-body PET correctly depicted 37 sites of metastases. Three cutaneous metastases (smaller than 3 mm) were missed. The sensitivity of whole-body PET for the detection of malignant lesions was 92%. When no clinical information was provided (e.g., location of biopsy sites, surgery, and subcutaneous application of interferon), the specificity of PET was 77%, and with clinical information it increased to 100%. In 21% of patients, whole-body PET depicted previously unknown and unexpected new metastases. In four of six patients, the metastases could be surgically removed.

The excellent results in staging patients who have high-risk melanoma with whole-body FDG PET have been confirmed in larger patient studies in different PET centers worldwide (33–39). PET demonstrated high FDG uptake by nearly all untreated melanoma metastases in the lymph nodes and viscera (Fig. 5.7.2 through 5.7.4). Due to the results, whole-body FDG PET is reimbursed for patients with high-risk melanoma in many countries (Table 5.7.2).

Recently, this author has performed a metaanalysis of the literature for staging of high-risk melanoma with FDG PET (40). The study was conducted in collaboration with the Study Group of the German Society of Nuclear Medicine of PET in melanoma. In this study, a quality assessment of all articles was applied. PET studies for the microscopic tumor involvement of the SLN were excluded. Only PET studies with the definite confirmation of lesions were included. These pooled data were used for the metaanalysis. A total of 323 lesions could be included for the metaanalysis. An overall sensitivity of 90% (95% confidence level [CI], 86–94%) and an overall specificity of 87% (95% CI, 79–95%) were determined (Table 5.7.3). Other reviews of the FDG PET literature with different results have been published (41,42). Because studies for the detection of microscopic tumor involvement of lymph nodes were included in these analyses, the accuracy of FDG PET was lower.

FDG PET is clearly superior to CT in detecting most melanoma metastases. In 1995, Buzaid et al. (43) analyzed the value of CT in the staging of patients with locoregional metastases of melanoma. The records of 99 patients were reviewed. True-positive findings were observed in 7% and false-positive findings in 22% of patients. These results indicated a relatively low yield of CT in patients with locoregional disease. Because false-positive results were more common than true-positive findings, histologic verification was recommended. Holder et al. (35) compared FDG PET with CT in 76 patients with metastatic melanoma. PET scanning

(text continues on page 191)

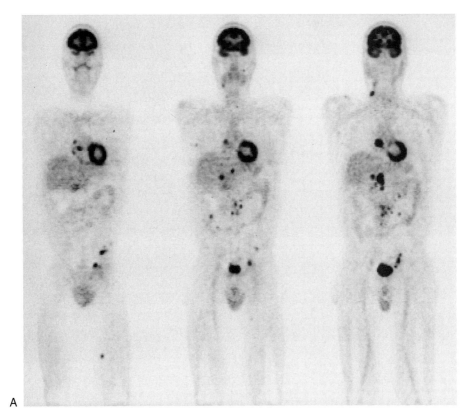

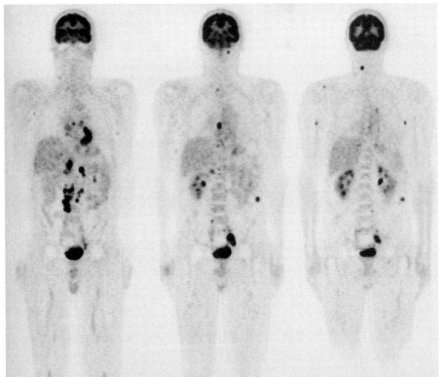

FIG. 5.7.1. A 48-year-old man had a history of metastatic melanoma. Whole-body ^{18}F-fluorodeoxyglucose positron emission tomography (FDG PET) detected several unknown metastases. **A, B:** Multiple coronal PET images showed high focal FDG accumulation in the right neck, posterior neck on the left side, in the right shoulder, and right arm, in the left axilla, supraclavicular region on the right side, in the right myocardium, in the porta hepatis, in both adrenal glands, and in paraaortic, interaortocaval, mesenteric, parailiac, and inguinal nodes on the left side, in the soft tissues of the left leg, and in multiple subcutaneous nodules. *Figure continues*

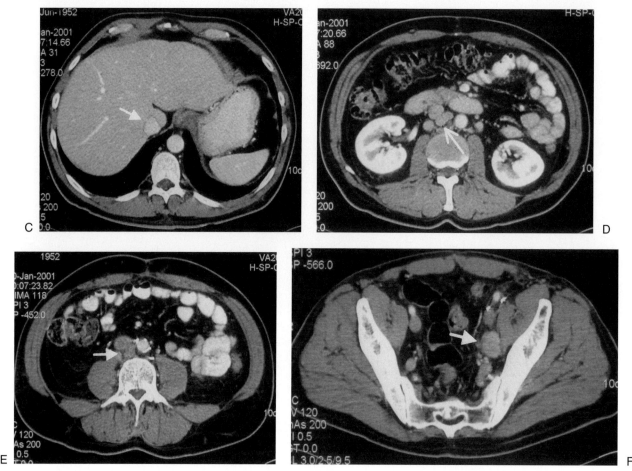

FIG. 5.7.1. *Continued.* Corresponding contrast-enhanced axial computed tomography (CT) scan of the **(C)** porta hepatis, of the **(D)** paraaortic and **(E)** interaortocaval regions, and of the **(F)** iliac nodal region. The other metastases depicted with PET were not described on CT.

TABLE 5.7.2. *Reimbursement status of FDG PET in malignant melanoma*

	Swiss reimbursement status	U.S. reimbursement status Medicare/BC-BS
Diagnosis of primary tumor	No	No
Diagnosis of sentinel lymph node	No	No
Staging in high-risk melanoman (Breslow ≥1.5 mm or known metastatic disease)	Yes	Yes
Restaging at relapse	Yes	Yes

TABLE 5.7.3. *Sensitivity and specificity of, FDG PET in malignant melanoma: results of literature search*

Literature	Method	Total lesions	Sensitivity	Specificity
(40)	Quality control of data,[a] metaanalysis of pooled data	323	90% (86–94%)[b]	87% (79–95%)[b]

[a] Only, PET studies with definite confirmation of lesions were included. PET studies for diagnosis of sentinel lymph nodes and microscopic tumor involvement were excluded.
[b] 95% confidence level.

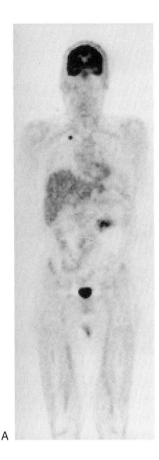

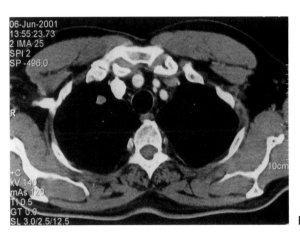

FIG. 5.7.2. A 53-year-old man had a surgically proven lung metastasis of a malignant melanoma. **A:** A coronal PET scan demonstrated a lesion with markedly increased ^{18}F-fluorodeoxyglucose uptake in the right anterior upper lung. **B:** The corresponding contrast-enhanced thoracic computed tomography (CT) scan showed a 1.5-cm nodule in the same location.

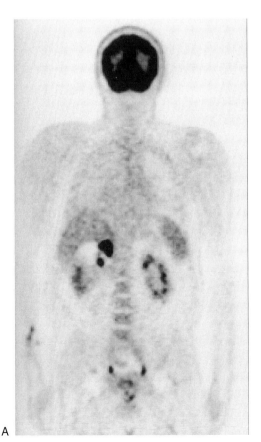

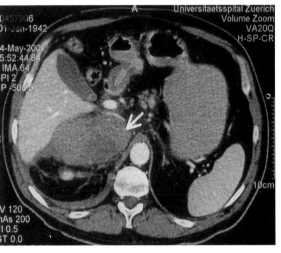

FIG. 5.7.3. **A:** A coronal PET image of a 53-year-old man with a primary melanoma in the left axilla demonstrated a photopenic structure in combination with a focal area of high ^{18}F-fluorodeoxyglucose accumulation above the right kidney. This finding was suggestive of a metastasis. **B:** A corresponding contrast-enhanced axial computed tomography (CT) scan showed a huge mass in the region of the right adrenal gland with heterogeneous densities. A metastasis to the right adrenal gland with adrenal hemorrhage was diagnosed.

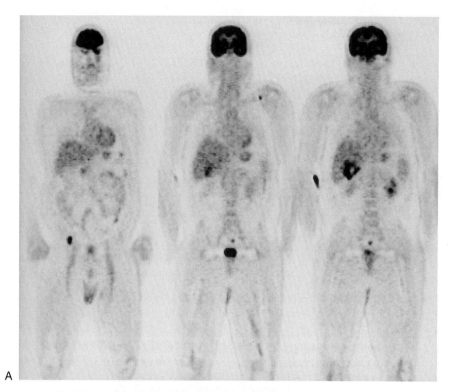

A

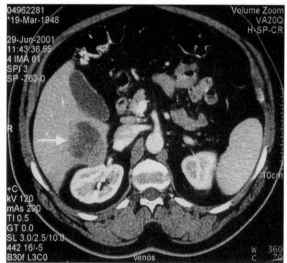

B

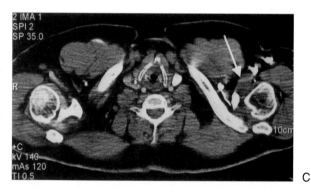

C

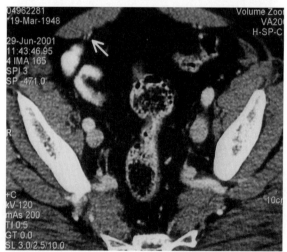

D

FIG. 5.7.4. Coronal PET scans of a 52-year-old man with a known liver metastasis of a malignant melanoma. **A:** In addition to the metastasis to the liver with central necrosis, the PET scans demonstrated previously unsuspected metastases to the right lower abdomen and in the left shoulder. **B:** A corresponding contrast-enhanced axial computed tomography (CT) scan showed the liver metastasis. **C, D:** The other metastases were found retrospectively after the PET scan had been performed.

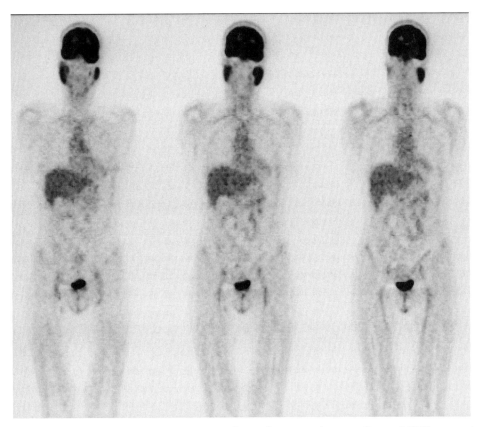

FIG. 5.7.5. A 54-year-old woman had a history of a malignant melanoma. Coronal PET scans demonstrated symmetric high ^{18}F-fluorodeoxyglucose uptake in both parotid glands due to proven sarcoidosis.

for the detection of melanoma metastases had a sensitivity of 94.2% compared with 55.3% for CT scanning. The four false-negative FDG PET scan results were thought to be due to smaller (less than 0.3 cm) lesions and diffuse areas of melanoma without significant mass effect.

A number of factors may interfere with the accuracy of PET scanning for metastases. It is well known that FDG is not a tumor-specific substance. False-positive results may be caused by an increased FDG uptake in inflammatory lesions or postoperative changes (44,45) (Fig. 5.7.5). Therefore, the clinical correlation of lesions with increased FDG uptake is obligatory to exclude tracer uptake in recent sites of surgery or infected or inflamed lesions, or at injection sites, for example. In most cases, these benign causes of FDG uptake can be specifically recognized and properly categorized. However, some nonmalignant solitary nodules with highly increased FDG accumulation can mimic metastases of melanoma in whole-body PET. Recently, our group analyzed whole-body FDG PET scans of more than 500 patients. Diagnoses were confirmed histopathologically. Ten patients (2%) showed hot spots with FDG PET that proved to be benign. Lesions were located in parotid glands, periarticular regions, and the colon, and they proved to be Warthin tumors (papillary cystadenoma lymphomatosum), villonodular synovitis, and colonic adenomas (46).

False-negative results may occur in patients with slow-growing tumors with a large necrotic component. Radiotherapy or chemotherapy may also influence the uptake of FDG due to cytolytic effects. Melanoma and small cell lung cancer are the most common tumors to metastasize to the brain. The brain is the site of recurrence in up to 20% of patients and usually occurs with widespread metastatic disease. Due to the physiologic high FDG uptake in the cortex, CT and MRI are generally superior to FDG PET in the detection of brain metastases. Brain scanning with CT or MRI should always be used in symptomatic patients to confirm the diagnosis. Patients with a single brain metastasis may benefit from surgical excision. PET may be useful to follow-up treatment response in known brain metastases undergoing therapy.

Micrometastatic disease cannot be detected with any imaging modality. The smallest metastases detected with dedicated PET scanners were 4 to 5 mm (Fig. 5.7.6). FDG PET accurately predicted regional node status in 88% of patients with melanoma (47). Crippa et al. (48) investigated the smallest detectable volume of melanoma metastases that could be determined. Analyzing 56 nodal basins, FDG PET detected 100% of metastases 10 mm or larger, 83% of metastases 6 to 10 mm, and 23% of metastases 5 mm or smaller. Our group examined the detectability of melanoma metasta-

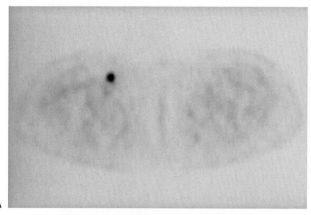 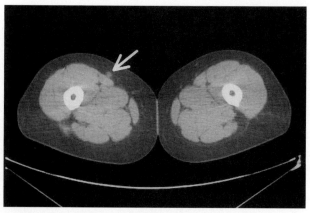

FIG. 5.7.6. A 54-year-old woman had a history of a malignant melanoma. The PET scan revealed a previously unknown and unsuspected single soft-tissue metastasis in the leg. **A:** An axial PET scan demonstrated a focal lesion with a markedly increased ¹⁸F-fluorodeoxyglucose uptake in the upper leg. **B:** The corresponding axial computed tomography (CT) scan showed a 5-mm lesion.

ses using coincidence emission scintigraphy and FDG (49). Detection of lesions smaller than 22 mm in diameter showed a reduced sensitivity versus detection in larger lesions. For whole-body staging of malignant melanoma, only dedicated PET scanners are recommended.

Lymphatic mapping of the SLN with radiolabeled colloid is a promising technique to investigate the draining nodal basins of cutaneous malignant melanomas. The lymphatic mapping of the SLN is followed by SLN biopsy. If there is microscopic lymph node involvement, the patient may benefit from a TLND (50), but distant metastases have to be excluded. In our institution, patients with a malignant melanoma with a Breslow thickness of more than 1.5 mm will generally first have a whole-body FDG PET. If metastatic disease is ruled out, SLN scintigraphy and biopsy are performed for the detection of microscopic metastases in the SLN. In other centers, SLN mapping is performed first, and if the SLN shows metastases, whole-body PET may be performed.

EFFECTIVENESS OF WHOLE-BODY FDG PET IN STAGING OF MELANOMA

In patients with thin melanomas (Breslow thickness of less than 0.75 mm), the likelihood of metastases is so small that staging with radiographic or PET imaging is not cost-effective. The inability of PET to identify microscopic disease suggests that it is of limited use in evaluating patients with stage I or II disease (38,51).

In recent studies, the cost-effectiveness of whole-body FDG PET in patients with melanoma has been studied. Our group (52) reviewed treatment records of 100 patients with newly diagnosed malignant melanoma and a Breslow thickness of more than 1.5 mm or known metastatic melanoma. In patients with known metastatic disease, all metastases had been removed. Two staging procedures were defined: (a) Conventional staging consisted of physical examination,

chest x-ray, and ultrasound of lymph nodes and abdomen. If suspicious lesions were found after conventional staging, then additional CT scans and histopathologic correlation were performed. (b) Staging with whole-body PET included inspection of the skin. Suspicious lesions were confirmed by biopsy or another imaging modality. The review evaluated many staging protocols for cost comparison. The total cost of conventional staging was 257,224 Swiss francs, compared with 261,650 Swiss francs for PET; thus, only 1.7% more. Among the 72 patients with metastatic disease, conventional staging costs were 227,445 Swiss francs while PET staging costs were 201,414 Swiss francs. In this subset, the PET protocol cost was 11.4% less than conventional staging. This author and his coworkers concluded that a Breslow tumor thickness of 1.5 mm or more is a cost-effective cutoff for deciding whether to use PET, because these patients have a higher risk of metastases (Fig. 5.7.7).

Gambhir et al. (53) compared the cost-effectiveness of the imaging strategies using conventional staging alone, including body CT and brain MRI, versus conventional staging with whole-body FDG PET. Sixty patients with suspected recurrence of malignant melanoma were included in the study. The study also evaluated predicted survival, using measures of life expectancy based on the literature, as well as savings due to changes in patient management resulting from the use of PET. The incremental cost-effectiveness ratio of the FDG PET strategy, compared with the conventional staging strategy, was $3,000 to $8,000 per year of life saved, a figure far below the standard of $50,000 per year of life saved used by U.S. health economists to characterize a cost-effective intervention.

In the author's experience, PET changes the treatment in 20% of patients with high-risk melanoma (32). Other groups reported an even higher influence of FDG PET on the diagnostic and therapeutic management of patients. In one study, PET resulted in a change in surgical management in 16 (36%) of 45 patients. The addition of FDG PET to the diag-

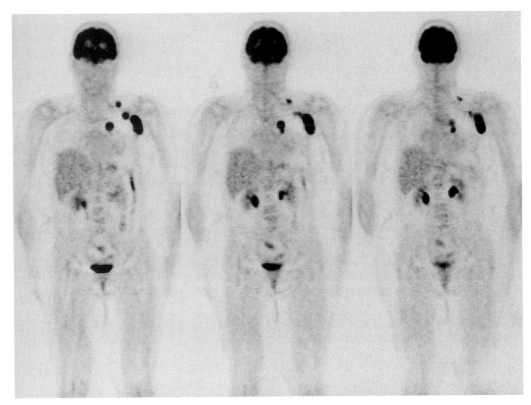

FIG. 5.7.7. A 60-year-old woman had known metastases in the left axilla and left supraclavicular region from malignant melanoma. The primary tumor was located in the right elbow (Breslow thickness of 1.5 mm) and had been resected 8 years before this presentation. In addition to the palpable axillary and supraclavicular metastases, coronal PET scans demonstrated metastases in the left lung that were not known to be present before PET.

nostic algorithm resulted in a savings-to-cost ratio of 2 : 1 because of the avoidance of unnecessary procedures (54).

SUMMARY

Whole-body FDG PET is a very effective imaging modality to screen for metastases in patients with malignant melanoma and at high risk for metastases (Breslow thickness of more than 1.5 mm or already known metastases). The advantage of PET, particularly in melanoma with its unpredictable spread of metastases, is that the whole body can be easily examined. Whole-body FDG PET has a major impact in the management of patients with melanoma. Surgical resection is the treatment of choice for regional lymph node metastases or for a single distant metastasis. Whole-body FDG PET should be used to exclude unknown metastases in patients in whom surgery is planned. If multiple metastases are present, patients are referred to chemoimmunotherapy. In extended metastatic disease, only palliative symptomatic therapy is indicated. Whole-body FDG PET plays an important role in the evaluation of patients when immunotherapy is being considered. Adjuvant treatment with recombinant interferon-α is only indicated in disease-free patients after resection of a high-risk cutaneous melanoma. PET can

also be useful in following response to various treatments and is becoming a standard diagnostic tool for patients with melanoma.

REFERENCES

1. Elwood JB, Koh HK. Etiology, epidemiology, risk factors, and public health issues of melanoma. *Curr Opin Oncol* 1994;6:179.
2. Armstrong BK, Kricker A. Cutaneous melanoma. *Cancer Surv* 1994; 19:219.
3. Chang AE, Karnell LH, Menck HR. The National Cancer Date Base report on cutaneous and noncutaneous melanoma. A summary of 84,836 cases from the past decade. *Cancer* 1998;83:1664–1678.
4. Ketcham AS, Balch CM. Classification and staging systems. In: Balch CM, Milton GW, eds. *Cutaneous melanoma: clinical management and treatment results worldwide,* 2nd ed. Philadelphia: JB Lippincott Co, 1992:213–220.
5. Balch CM, Murad TM, Soong S-J, et al. A multifactorial analysis of melanoma: prognostic histopathological features comparing Clark's and Breslow's staging methods. *Ann Surg* 1978;188:732–742.
6. Balch CM, Soong S-J, Murad TM, et al. A multifactorial analysis of melanoma, IV: prognostic factors in 200 melanoma patients with distant metastases (stage III). *J Clin Oncol* 1983;1:126–134.
7. Kirgwood JM, Strawderman MH, Ernsthoff MS, et al. Interferon alpha-2b adjuvant therapy of high-risk resected cutaneous melanoma: the Eastern Cooperative Oncology Group Trial EST 1684. *J Clin Oncol* 1996;14:7–17.
8. Cole BF, Gelber RD, Kirkwood JM, et al. Quality-of-life-adjusted survival analysis of interferon alfa-2b adjuvant treatment of high-risk re-

sected cutaneous melanoma: an Eastern Cooperative Oncology Group Study. *J Clin Oncol* 1996;14:2666–2673.

9. Hillner BE, Kirkwood JM, Atkins MB, et al. Economic analysis of adjuvant interferon alfa-2b in high-risk melanoma based on projections from Eastern Cooperative Oncology Group 1684. *J Clin Oncol* 1997; 15:2351–2358.

10. Grob JJ, Dreno B, de la Salmoniere P, et al. Randomised trial of interferon-alpha-2b as adjuvant therapy in resected primary melanoma thicker than 1.5 mm without clinically detectable node metastases. French Cooperative Group on melanoma. *Lancet* 1998;351: 1905–1910.

11. Silverberg E, Boring CC, Squires TS. Cancer statistics 1990. *CA Cancer J Clin* 1990;40:9–26.

12. Marchand M, van Baren N, Weynants P, et al. Tumor regressions observed in patients with metastatic melanoma treated with an antigenic peptide encoded by gene MAGE-3 and presented by HLA-A1. *Int J Cancer* 1999;80:219–230.

13. Nestle FO, Alijagic S, Gilliet M, et al. Vaccination of melanoma patients with peptide- or tumor lysate-pulsed dendritic cells. *Nat Med* 1998;4:328–332.

14. Thurner B, Haendle I, Roder C, et al. Vaccination with MAGE-3A1 peptide-pulsed mature, monocyte-derived dendritic cells expands specific cytotoxic T cells and induces regression of some metastases in advanced stage IV melanoma. *J Exp Med* 1999;190:1669–1678.

15. Baldo M, Schiavon M, Cicogna P, et al. Spontaneous regression of subcutaneous metastasis of cutaneous melanoma. *Plast Reconstr Surg* 1992;90:1073–1076.

16. Khansur T, Sanders J, Das SK. Evaluation of staging work-up in malignant melanoma. *Arch Surg* 1989;124:847–849.

17. Blessing C, Feine U, Geiger L, et al. Positron emission tomography and ultrasonography: a comparative retrospective study assessing the diagnostic validity in lymph node metastases of malignant melanoma. *Arch Dermatol* 1995;131:1394–1398.

18. Haubold-Reuter BG, Duewell S, Schicher BR, et al. The value of bone scintigraphy and fast spin-echo magnetic resonance imaging in staging of patients with malignant solid tumors: a prospective study. *Eur J Nucl Med* 1993;20:1063–106.

19. Kagan R, Witt T, Bines S, et al. Gallium-67 scanning for malignant melanoma. *Cancer* 1988;20:417–429.

20. Böni R, Huch-Böni R, Steinert HC, et al. Antimelanoma monoclonal antibody 225.28S immunoscintigraphy in metastatic melanoma. *Dermatology* 1995;191:119–123.

21. Hoefnagel CA, Rankin EM, Valdes Olmos RA, et al. Sensitivity versus specificity in melanoma using iodine-123 iodobenzamide and indium-111 pentetreotide. *Eur J Nucl Med* 1994;21:587–588.

22. Alonso O, Martinez M, Mut F, et al. Detection of recurrent malignant melanoma with ^{99m}Tc-MIBI scintigraphy. *Melanoma Res* 1998;8:355.

23. Steinert HC, Böni R, Huch-Böni R, et al. Jod-123-methyltyrosin-szintigraphie beim malignen *Melanom Nuklearmed* 1997;36:36–41.

24. Schreckenberger M, Kadalie C, Enk A, et al. First results of ^{18}F-fluoroethyl-tyrosine PET for imaging of metastatic malignant melanoma. *J Nucl Med* 2001;42[Suppl]:30P.

25. Steinert HC, Huch-Böni R, Böni R, et al. Dopamin-D$_2$-rezeptor szintigraphie mit jod-123-jodbenzofuran beim malignen. *Melanom Nuklearmed* 1995;34:146–150.

26. Ishiwata K, Kubota K, Kubota R, et al. Selective 2-fluorine-18-fluorodopa uptake for melanogenesis in murine metastatic melanomas. *J Nucl Med* 1991;32:95–101.

27. Mishima Y, Imahori Y, Honda C, et al. *In vivo* diagnosis of human malignant melanoma with PET using specific melanoma seeking fluorine-18-DOPA analogue. *J Neurooncol* 1997;33:163–169.

28. Böni R, Bläuenstein P, Dummer R, et al. Non-invasive assessment of tumour cell proliferation with positron emission tomography and ^{76}Br-bromodeoxyuridine. *Melanoma Res* 1999;9:569–573.

29. Vogg AT, Glatting G, Möller P, et al. ^{18}F5-fluoro-2′-desoxyuridine as PET-tracer for imaging of solid malignomas. *J Nucl Med* 2001; 42[Suppl]:30P.

30. Wahl RL, Hutchins GD, Buchsbaum DJ, et al. ^{18}F-2-deoxy-2-fluoro-D-glucose uptake into human tumour xenografts. *Cancer* 1991;67: 1544–1550.

31. Gritters LS, Francis IR, Zasadny KR, et al. Initial assessment of positron

emission tomography using 2-fluorine-18-fluoro-2-deoxy-D-glucose in the imaging of malignant melanoma. *J Nucl Med* 1993;34:623–648.

32. Steinert HC, Huch-Böni RA, Buck A, et al. Malignant melanoma: staging with whole-body positron emission tomography and 2-[F-18]-fluoro-2-deoxy-D-glucose. *Radiology* 1995;195:705–709.

33. Damian DL, Fulham MJ, Thompson E, et al. Positron emission tomography in the detection and management of metastatic melanoma. *Melanoma Res* 1996;6:325–329.

34. Rinne D, Baum RP, Hör G, et al. Primary staging and follow-up of high risk melanoma patients with whole-body ^{18}F-fluorodeoxyglucose positron emission tomography. *Cancer* 1998;82:1664–1671.

35. Holder WD Jr, White RL Jr, Zuger JH, et al. Effectiveness of positron emission tomography for the detection of melanoma metastases. *Ann Surg* 1998;227:764–769.

36. Hsueh EC, Gupta RK, Glass EC, et al. Positron emission tomography plus serum TA90 immune complex assay for detection of occult metastatic melanoma. *J Am Coll Surg* 1998;187:191–197.

37. Paquet P, Henry F, BelhocineT, et al. An appraisal of 18-fluorodeoxyglucose positron emission tomography for melanoma staging. *Dermatology* 2000;200:167–169.

38. Tyler DS, Onaitis M, Kherani A, et al. Positron emission tomography scanning in malignant melanoma. Clinical utility in patients with stage III disease. *Cancer* 2000;89:1019–1025.

39. Eigtved A, Andersson AP, Dahlstrom K, et al. Use of fluorine-18 fluorodeoxyglucose positron emission tomography in the detection of silent metastases from malignant melanoma. *Eur J Nucl Med* 2000;27:70–75.

40. Steinert HC, von Schulthess GK, Reuland P, et al. A meta-analysis of the literature for staging of malignant melanoma with whole-body FDG PET. *J Nucl Med* 2001;42[Suppl]:307P.

41. Gambhir SS, Czernin J, Schwimmer J, et al. A tabulated summary of the FDG PET literature. Oncologic applications: melanoma. *J Nucl Med* 2001;42[Suppl 1]:13S–15S.

42. Mijnhout GS, Hoekstra OS, van Tulder MW, et al. Systematic review of the diagnostic accuracy of 18F-fluorodeoxyglucose positron emission tomography in melanoma patients. *Cancer* 2001;91:1530–1542.

43. Buzaid AC, Sandler AB, Mani E, et al. Role of computed tomography in the staging of malignant melanoma. *J Clin Oncol* 1993;11:638–643.

44. Strauss LG. Fluorine-18 deoxyglucose and false-positive results: a major problem in the diagnostics of oncological patients. *Eur J Nucl Med* 1996;23:1409–1415.

45. Shreve PD, Anzai Y, Wahl RL. Pitfalls in oncologic diagnosis with FDG PET imaging: physiologic and benign variants. *Radiographics* 1999;19:61–77.

46. Steinert HC, Bode B, Boeni R, et al. Malignant melanoma: Non-malignant "hot spots" in whole-body FDG PET with radiologic pathologic correlation. *Radiology* 2000;217[Suppl]:359.

47. Macfarlane DJ, Sondak V, Johnson T, et al. Prospective evaluation of 2-[F-18]-fluoro-2-deoxy-D-glucose positron emission tomography in staging of regional lymph nodes in patients with cutaneous malignant melanoma. *J Clin Oncol* 1998;16:1770–1776.

48. Crippa F, Leutner M, Belli F, et al. Which kinds of lymph node metastases can FDG PET detect? A clinical study in melanoma. *J Nucl Med* 2000;41:1491–1499.

49. Steinert HC, Voellmy DR, Trachsel C, et al. Planar coincidence scintigraphy and PET in staging malignant melanoma. *J Nucl Med* 1998;39: 1892–1897.

50. Morton DL, Wen DR, Cochran AJ. Management of early-stage melanoma by intraoperative lymphatic mapping and selective lymphadenectomy or "watch and wait." *Surg Oncol Clin North Am* 1992;127: 247–259.

51. Acland KM, O'Doherty MJ, Russell-Jones R. The value of positron emission tomography scanning in the detection of subclinical metastatic melanoma. *J Am Acad Dermatol* 2000;42:606–611.

52. Von Schulthess GK, Steinert HC, Dummer R, et al. Cost effectiveness of whole-body PET imaging in non–small cell lung cancer and malignant melanoma. *Acad Radiol* 1998;5[Suppl 2]:S300–S302.

53. Gambhir SS, Hoh CK, Essner R, et al. A decision analysis model for the role of whole body FDG PET in the management of patients with recurrent melanoma. *J Nucl Med* 1998;39:94P.

54. Valk PE, Pounds TR, Tesar RD, et al. Cost-effectiveness of PET imaging in clinical oncology. *Nucl Med Biol* 1996;23:737–743.

CHAPTER 5.8

Breast

Farrokh Dehdashti

Breast cancer is the most common malignancy of women, accounting for approximately 30% of all cancers in women. It is estimated that in the year 2001, there will be nearly 193,700 new cases of breast cancer, and that there will be approximately 40,600 breast cancer–related deaths in the United States (1). Despite much progress in refining conventional imaging techniques and defining optimal multimodality treatment regimens, approximately one third of women who develop breast cancer will die of disseminated disease annually. This is in part attributable to persistent shortcomings in the methods currently used for the detection and evaluation of breast cancer.

The past decade has witnessed the emergence of functionally based methods such as positron emission tomography (PET) that have added new dimensions to the radiologic evaluation of breast cancer. Currently, the role of imaging is not limited to early detection of breast cancer but now involves staging and restaging, assessment of tumor behavior and prognosis, and monitoring response to therapy.

This chapter focuses on the current and potential clinical applications of PET, as well as its limitations, and discusses how this functional imaging modality can help resolve some of the shortcomings of conventional imaging modalities in the management of patients with breast cancer.

Although various biologic and functional characteristics of breast cancer, such as blood flow and receptor status, can be studied with PET, the clinical applications are mainly focused on the assessment of glucose metabolism using 2-(fluorine-18)fluoro-2-deoxy-D-glucose (FDG). This focus is related to tracer availability and the fact that PET assessment of some of the biologic features of breast cancer, such as tumor blood flow, does not appear to be clinically relevant. In addition, clinical and preclinical studies have shown increased FDG accumulation in breast cancer. In human breast cancer, marked overexpression of the glucose transporter GLUT-1 has been reported, and this is certainly an important factor contributing to the increased glucose accumulation within this cancer (2). *In vitro* studies of rat mammary tumors and human breast cancer cells (MCF-7 and HTB771P3) demonstrated an inverse relationship between extracellular glucose levels and tumor FDG uptake (3,4). In addition, it has been shown that tumor FDG uptake is closely related to the number of viable tumor cells (5).

FDG PET IMAGING PROTOCOL AND IMAGE ANALYSIS

[18]F-Fluorodeoxyglucose positron emission tomography (FDG PET) imaging protocols differ from institution to institution; however, several important issues should be considered for successful clinical FDG PET imaging of patients with breast cancer. In this group of patients, FDG should be administered intravenously via a vein in the arm opposite a suspected breast lesion or via a foot vein, to avoid increased FDG uptake in normal axillary lymph nodes as a result of extravasation of FDG at the injection site.

Patients should be fasted for at least 4 hours. *In vitro* studies of rodent and human mammary carcinoma cells in culture and *in vivo* studies in rodent tumor have demonstrated that acute hyperglycemia markedly impairs tumor FDG uptake (4). In addition, a significant decrease in tumor FDG uptake has been reported in the insulin-induced hypoglycemic state. Therefore, determination of blood glucose levels before FDG injection is recommended to identify patients with possible fasting hyperglycemia (4). Although patients are typically studied in the supine position, significantly greater FDG uptake in primary breast cancer has been reported with the patient in the prone position using scintimammography positioning techniques. Fewer motion-related artifacts and better separation of deep breast structures from the myocardium and liver, which may decrease scatter from FDG uptake in these organs, are seen in the prone position when compared with the supine position (6).

It has been reported that the tumor-to-nontumor uptake ratio is improved by obtaining delayed PET images 3 hours after administration of FDG (7). However, it is yet to be proven whether prone imaging or delayed imaging improves lesion characterization or detection sensitivity. Recently, to improve evaluation of the breasts, efforts have been focused on the development of high-resolution PET scanners dedicated to breast imaging (8), with the capability to co-register PET images and x-ray mammographic images (9).

FDG PET imaging is performed with or without attenuation correction. No significant difference has been demonstrated in lesion detectability of attenuation-corrected versus noncorrected images (10). However, attenuation correction is required for quantitative and semiquantitative assessment of tracer uptake.

Although clinical oncologic FDG PET images are most often interpreted qualitatively, semiquantitative measurements offer more objective criteria for differentiating benign from malignant lesions and monitoring response to therapy. The most commonly used semiquantitative methods include the standard uptake value (SUV), also known as the differential uptake ratio or the differential absorption ratio (DAR). SUV is an index of glucose metabolism based on tissue uptake of FDG normalized to body weight (or lean body mass or body surface area) and injected dose (11,12). Because in the fasting state, body fat has a much lower uptake of FDG, the SUVs of many tissues show a strong positive correlation with weight, and tissue SUVs may be overestimated in obese patients. This is very important in the assessment of response to therapy when FDG PET studies before and after cancer treatment are compared, because SUVs may not be comparable if the patient loses a significant amount of weight between the two PET studies. It has been shown that SUV normalized to lean body mass or body surface area instead of total body weight is a more accurate estimate that will not be affected by changes in body weight (11,12).

The Patlak graphical approach also has been used in a limited fashion for quantitative evaluation of the FDG metabolic rate in breast lesions. This graphical approach provides an estimate of the net FDG phosphorylation rate constant (in milliliters per minute per gram); this value is proportional to the glucose-utilization rate based on the assumptions that the flow of tracer is unidirectional into the cellular compartment and follows first-order kinetics, and that it occurs only in an irreversible manner if the tracer is metabolized, so the metabolites are also irreversibly trapped (13). Although this type of analysis may provide a more reliable estimate of regional glucose metabolism, it is time consuming and technically demanding, so it is not recommended for routine clinical studies of patients with cancer who are often too ill to tolerate the lengthy imaging required.

A recent study demonstrated similar diagnostic accuracy for visual and semiquantitative (SUV and Patlak) analysis in differentiating benign from malignant breast lesions (14). However, the average SUV normalized to body weight and blood glucose and corrected for partial volume averaging had the highest diagnostic accuracy, exceeding that achieved with either the Patlak method or both average and maximum SUV uncorrected for blood glucose level and partial volume averaging (14). In practice, Patlak analysis is rarely performed.

Physiologic accumulation of FDG in healthy breast tissue is variable, reflecting the amount of proliferative glandular breast tissue present. FDG uptake in normal breast is typically mild and diffuse, with focally increased uptake in the areolar complexes. However, FDG uptake is more prominent in premenopausal women with abundant proliferative glandular breast tissue and in postmenopausal women undergoing hormone-replacement therapy. The effect of the menstrual cycle on FDG accumulation in normal breast tissue is unknown. Intense FDG uptake has been reported in lactating breasts, but not in postpartum breasts of women who are not breast-feeding. FDG is detected in minimal amounts of breast milk despite intense uptake in the breast itself. Therefore, radiation exposure to an infant is mainly due to close contact with the mother's breast, rather than to ingestion of radioactive milk. Interruption of breast-feeding for approximately 8 hours should be sufficient to keep the infant's exposure to less than 500 mrem.

DETECTION OF BREAST CANCER

In randomized clinical trials, screening mammography has resulted in a reduction of the breast cancer mortality rate by about 25% to 45% in women older than 40 years (15). Recent significant progress in mammographic technique, as well as the appropriate use of supplementary imaging techniques, such as ultrasonography, has had a very important role in the early detection of breast cancer.

Currently, the diagnosis of breast cancer is based on breast self-examination, physical examination by trained personnel, mammography supplemented as necessary by ultrasonography, and histologic examination of identified breast lesions. Breast examination has low specificity and is not very sensitive for detection of small lesions, but it is useful for the detection of palpable breast masses.

Mammography has a relatively high sensitivity, ranging from 54% to 81% depending on age, breast density, and menopausal status (16). Although mammography has higher sensitivity for detecting breast cancer in fatty breasts, it is of limited value in several situations, such as in the detection of malignancy in dense breasts or postsurgical breasts (e.g., after breast augmentation, lumpectomy, or breast-conserving therapy for breast cancer), early detection of tumor recurrence after surgery, and monitoring response to therapy (17, 18). Mammography has a low positive predictive value (PPV) (10% to 35%) for nonpalpable cancers, and the frequency of positive biopsy findings after abnormal mammography results ranges from 10% to 50% (19–21). Due to the low specificity of mammography, most breast lesions are subjected to biopsy. Although the commonly employed fine-needle aspiration and stereotactic core biopsy are less invasive than excision biopsies, they suffer from sampling errors.

Recently, magnetic resonance imaging (MRI) of the breast has attracted significant attention, and although the initial results in assessing mammographically difficult-to-examine breasts are very promising, its clinical role in the evaluation of breast lesions has not yet been established.

PET imaging of the breast offers physiologic information

TABLE 5.8.1. *FDG PET results for differentiating benign from malignant breast masses*

Study, yr (reference no.)	No. of patients	Method of analysis	Sensitivity(%)	Specificity(%)
Tse et al., 1992 (22)[a]	14	Qualitative	80	100
Adler et al., 1993 (25)[b]	35	Semiquantitative	96	100
Hoh et al., 1993 (42)[a]	20	Qualitative	88	33
Nieweg et al., 1993 (23)[b]	20	Semiquantitative	91	100
Dehdashti et al., 1995 (36)[b]	32	Semiquantitative	88	100
Avril et al., 1996 (43)[b]	72	Semiqualitative	92	97
Scheidhauer et al., 1996 (24)[b]	30	Qualitative	91	86
Palmedo et al., 1997 (27)[b]	19	Qualitative	92	83
Kole et al., 1997 (26)[b]	13	Qualitative	100	67
Noh et al., 1998 (34)[b]	26	Semiquantitative	96	100
Rostom et al., 1999 (48)[a,b]	109	Qualitative	91	83
Avril et al., 2000 (28)[b]	144	Qualitative (CIR)	64	94
		(SIR)	80	75

[a] Whole-body imaging technique without attenuation correction.
[b] Attenuation-corrected images.
CIR, conventional image reading; SIR, sensitive image reading.

complementary to that achieved from conventional imaging techniques, and therefore, PET can be used to better characterize disease. However, PET has important limitations, such as limited availability, high cost, and limited resolution, suggesting that the clinical use of PET should be reserved for a selected subset of women with breast cancer.

FDG uptake is considerably higher in malignant tumors than in normal tissues. Several studies have demonstrated that FDG PET has a moderately high sensitivity (64% to 96%) and specificity (80% to 100%) for detection of primary breast cancer and for differentiating breast cancer from benign lesions (Table 5.8.1) (22–28,34,36,43,44,49). In a recent study of 144 patients with breast masses, visual qualitative analysis of parametric (SUV-normalized) FDG PET images was assessed. FDG PET images were evaluated using conventional image reading (CIR), in which only focal areas of markedly increased FDG accumulation were considered to represent malignancy, and sensitive image reading (SIR), in which those with diffuse or focal areas of moderately increased FDG accumulation were also considered to represent malignancy. Breast cancer was identified with a sensitivity of 64% and 80% using CIR and SIR, respectively. However, the increased sensitivity using SIR resulted in a significant decrease in specificity (94% to 75%) (28).

Avril et al. (28) also demonstrated that the diagnostic accuracy of FDG PET is dependent on tumor size. None of four stage pT1a tumors (0.5 cm or smaller) and only one of eight stage pT1b tumors (larger than 0.5 to 1.0 cm) were classified as malignant lesions by FDG PET. However, FDG PET had a high sensitivity (81% and 92% using CIR and SIR, respectively) for the detection of pT2 breast cancers (larger than 2.0 to 5.0 cm). Therefore, the limited sensitivity of FDG PET for the detection of small lesions makes this modality unsuitable for breast cancer screening, at least with whole-body PET scanners. False-positive results have been reported in infectious and inflammatory lesions, including

hemorrhagic inflammation after biopsy or surgery, due to accumulation of FDG in inflammatory cells (29,30). However, these conditions often can be easily recognized clinically. False-negative results are not limited to small lesions (typically those with less than a 1-cm diameter) but also are reported in slowly growing or well-differentiated tumors (such as tubular carcinomas, ductal carcinoma in situ, and lobular carcinomas) (23,28).

The sensitivity of FDG PET for the detection of breast cancer also is dependent on the degree of uptake within the lesion in comparison to uptake in the surrounding tissue (31). Therefore, it may be difficult to identify lesions of mild to moderate intensity against a background of diffusely increased activity, as can be seen in women with an abundance of proliferative glandular breast tissue (particularly young women).

Role of PET in Mammographically Difficult to Examine Breasts

One of the technical limitations of mammography is its reduced sensitivity for the detection of tumors in women with radiodense breasts and in those who have had breast surgery, including breast augmentation, lumpectomy, and breast-conservation therapy for breast cancer. The potential role of FDG PET in detecting breast cancer in mammographically difficult to examine breasts has been addressed in limited fashion as feasibility studies or as a component of other studies evaluating the role of PET in breast cancer (3,22,24, 32–34). These studies suggest that FDG PET has the potential to detect breast cancer before it becomes apparent clinically and may alleviate the need for biopsy or assist in obtaining histopathologic proof by directing the biopsy.

Other potential applications of FDG PET in breast imaging are in detecting an occult primary breast cancer in patients with known metastatic disease to an axillary node and in assessing the extent of breast cancer (detecting multicen-

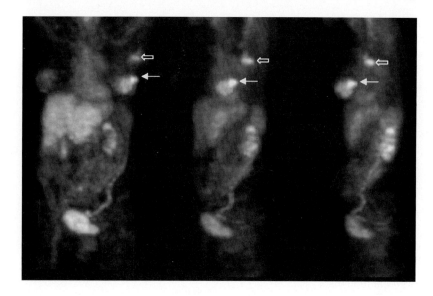

FIG. 5.8.1. PET detection of occult primary breast cancer. Anterior **(left)**, left anterior oblique **(middle)**, and left lateral **(right)** ¹⁸F-fluorodeoxyglucose (FDG) PET reprojection images demonstrate focal accumulation of FDG in the known axillary metastasis (*open arrows*) and in the retroareolar region (*solid arrows*) of the left breast.

tric or multifocal cancer) (Figs. 5.8.1 and 5.8.2) (24). Because breast conservation therapy has become the standard of care in early breast cancer and is preferred by many patients, determining the true extent of local disease has become extremely important in selecting the type of therapy. The finding of multicentric disease may significantly alter therapy (from breast-conservation therapy to mastectomy). Although routine use of FDG PET for the detection of multicentric or multifocal breast cancer is not recommended, it may be beneficial in patients with clinical suggestion of multiple lesions or those with extensive ductal carcinoma in situ, in whom multiple biopsies are not feasible.

Prognostic Value of PET

In untreated primary breast cancer, FDG uptake has been correlated with known prognostic factors by several investigators. In 86 patients with newly diagnosed breast cancer, Crippa et al. (35) compared tumor FDG uptake (SUV) with tumor histology, histopathologic grading, steroid-receptor levels (quantitative estrogen-receptor [ER] and progesterone-receptor [PR] concentrations), thymidine labeling index (LI), and expression of p53 (35). They reported a significant positive correlation between FDG uptake and tumor grade ($p < .004$) and p53 level ($p < .006$), but no significant correlation between FDG uptake and steroid-receptor status or LI. Similarly, we were unable to demonstrate any correlation between FDG uptake (SUV) and steroid-receptor status (ER or PR) in 43 untreated advanced breast cancers (36). Adler et al. (25) demonstrated a significant correlation between the nuclear grade of the tumor and normalized FDG uptake in a small number of patients.

In a study of 70 patients with primary breast cancer, patients with tumor FDG uptake (DAR) of 3.0 or more had a significantly worse prognosis for both overall survival ($p < .0005$) and disease-free survival ($p < .0001$) than the patients with a tumor DAR of less than 3.0 (37). In a multivariate analysis of the known prognostic factors such as histo-

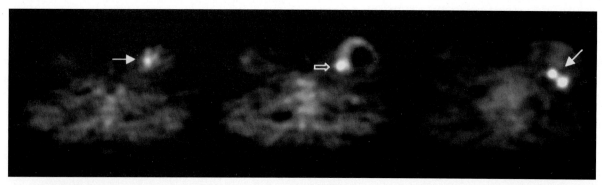

FIG. 5.8.2. PET detection of multicentric breast cancer. Transverse ¹⁸F-fluorodeoxyglucose (FDG) positron emission tomography images illustrate increased FDG accumulation in the known primary breast cancer in the inner quadrant of the left breast (*open arrow*). In addition, three foci of increased FDG accumulation are seen superior, as well as inferior and lateral, to the known cancer (*solid arrows*).

logic grade, tumor size, number of positive lymph nodes, microvessel density of the tumor, and tumor FDG uptake assessed by DAR, FDG uptake was an independent predictor of disease-free survival ($p = .0377$). Avril et al. (38) demonstrated a positive correlation between FDG uptake (SUV corrected for partial volume effect and normalized to blood glucose level) and histologic tumor type (ductal vs. lobular; $p = .003$), microscopic tumor growth pattern (nodular vs. diffuse; $p = .007$), and tumor cell proliferation ($p = .009$). No correlation was found between FDG uptake and tumor size, axillary lymph node status, presence of inflammatory cells, steroid-receptor status, expression of GLUT-1, or percentage of necrotic, fibrotic, and cystic components.

These studies demonstrate that tumor FDG uptake provides relevant and unique information about tumor biology, which predicts tumor behavior and prognosis preoperatively before histopathologic examination of breast cancer. These data may assist in the selection of the most appropriate therapy for an individual patient.

LYMPH NODE STAGING

The most common site of regional metastasis of breast cancer is the axillary lymph nodes. The status of axillary lymph nodes is the single most important prognostic variable in the staging of breast cancer; it has therapeutic importance and influences the selection of treatment for each patient. Patients with histologically negative axillary nodes have significantly better survival rates than patients with positive nodes. The relationship between prognosis and the number of involved axillary nodes has been well established; patients with one to three positive axillary nodes do better than patients with four or more involved nodes (39). The 10-year survival rate is significantly higher in patients with histologically negative axillary nodes (range, 65% to 80%) than in those with involvement of one to three nodes (range, 38% to 63%) or in those with more than three involved axillary nodes (range, 13% to 27%) (39). It has been shown that the likelihood of axillary nodal involvement is directly related to the size of the primary tumor at diagnosis (39). Approximately 50% of patients with breast cancer that is evident on physical examination have histologic evidence of axillary nodal involvement (39).

Clinical evaluation for predicting axillary nodal disease is inadequate, so lymph node dissection (either conventional or limited with the use of sentinel node localization) is routinely performed to assess axillary nodal status. Whether axillary nodal dissection has therapeutic benefit for regional control of breast cancer or is only of prognostic value in identifying patients who are at high risk for recurrence and need more aggressive therapy (chemotherapy and/or radiation therapy) remains controversial. Currently, conventional or limited axillary nodal dissection represents the standard of care in patients with invasive breast cancer (except those with less than a 5% risk of axillary nodal involvement; microinvasive breast cancer or grade 1 tumors less than 5 mm

when lymphatic invasion is not present). However, this procedure carries with it a relatively high cost and substantial morbidity. Therefore, a noninvasive test that could reliably evaluate the status and extent of nodal involvement would be of great interest in the management of patients with breast cancer. Accurate preoperative staging becomes even more important when one considers the increasing number of patients who are placed on neoadjuvant therapy before surgical removal of the primary tumor or lymph nodes. Thus, if ongoing clinical trials demonstrate significant survival benefits of systemic neoadjuvant therapy and such therapy becomes routine, the histopathologic information about the number of involved axillary lymph nodes and the size of the primary tumor will no longer be available, and other methods will have to be identified to provide similar prognostic information.

In preclinical studies of several types of tumors, Wahl et al. (40) demonstrated that FDG uptake in lymph nodes involved by metastatic tumor is greater than that in the normal lymph nodes. Since then, several studies have shown that FDG PET has the potential to be useful in noninvasive evaluation of locoregional nodal groups in patients with breast cancer and may reduce the number of patients requiring nodal dissection (Fig. 5.8.3) (Table 5.8.2) (22–25,35, 41–49). The reported sensitivities have ranged from 57% to 100% and specificities have ranged from 66% to 100% for detection of axillary nodal metastasis. False-negative results of PET occurred in patients with small deposits of tumors (typically smaller than 1 cm) (Table 5.8.2). Therefore, based

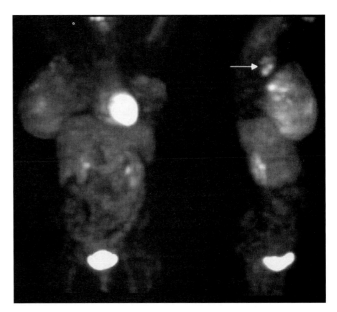

FIG. 5.8.3. PET detection of axillary nodal metastases. Anterior **(left)** and right lateral **(right)** reprojection ^{18}F-fluorodeoxyglucose (FDG) positron emission tomographic PET images demonstrate diffusely increased FDG accumulation in the enlarged right breast, consistent with inflammatory breast cancer. In addition, focal accumulation of FDG in several axillary lymph nodes (*solid arrow*) is seen.

TABLE 5.8.2. *FDG PET results for detection of axillary lymph node metastases*

Study, yr (reference no.)	No. of patients	Analysis	Sensitivity (%)	Specificity (%)
Wahl et al., 1991 (41)[a]	8	Qualitative	83	100
Tse et al., 1992 (22)[b]	10	Qualitative	57	100
Adler et al., 1993 (25)[a]	20	Qualitative	90	100
Hoh et al., 1993 (42)[b]	14	Qualitative	67	100
Nieweg et al., 1993 (23)[a]	5	Semiquantitative	100	N/A
Avril et al., 1996 (43)[a]	51	Qualitative	79	96
Scheidhauer et al., 1996 (24)[a]	18	Qualitative	100	89
Utech et al., 1996 (44)[a]	124	Qualitative	100	75
Crippa et al., 1998 (35)[a]	66	Qualitative	84	85
Adler et al., 1997 (46)[a]	20	Qualitative	95	66
Smith et al., 1998 (47)[a]	50	Qualitative	90	97
Rostom et al., 1999 (48)[a]	74	Qualitative	86	100
Schirrmeister et al., 2001 (49)[b]	85	Qualitative	79	92

[a] Attenuation-corrected images.
[b] Without attenuation correction.

on the current data, a positive FDG PET result may alleviate the need for axillary nodal dissection due to its high specificity; however, a negative FDG PET result does not preclude the need for axillary dissection considering its high false-negative rate (Table 5.8.2).

Avril et al. (43) demonstrated a positive correlation between PET detection of axillary nodal metastasis and the size of the primary tumor. In 51 patients using qualitative FDG PET, they reported a sensitivity and specificity of 94% and 100%, respectively, in patients with primary tumors larger than 2 cm in diameter and 33% and 100%, respectively, in patients with tumors smaller than 2 cm. They also demonstrated a positive correlation between the number of axillary nodes involved and PET detection of metastatic disease in the axilla; PET identified 1 of 4 patients with a single lymph node metastasis, 4 of 6 with two to five lymph node metastases, and all 10 patients with more than five lymph node metastases.

Recently, Schirrmeister et al. (49) demonstrated that FDG PET is superior to clinical evaluation for predicting axillary nodal involvement; the sensitivity and specificity were 79% and 92%, respectively, for FDG PET, and 41% and 96%, respectively, for clinical evaluation. Because of the limited resolution of PET, it is unlikely that this technique can detect small tumor deposits or determine accurately the number of involved axillary nodes. Thus, until more is known about the accuracy and the prognostic significance of a negative or a positive FDG PET scan in the axilla, treatment decisions should not be solely based on FDG PET results.

In addition to detection of axillary nodal involvement, FDG PET has the potential to detect involvement of other nodal groups, including the internal mammary and supraclavicular nodes. Involvement of the internal mammary nodes in the absence of axillary nodal involvement is uncommon (approximately 10%) (39). Prognosis in patients with internal mammary nodal metastases is comparable to that of patients with metastasis only to the axillary nodes (50). A worse prognosis has been reported when both nodal groups are involved (50).

Because detection of internal mammary nodal metastases is difficult with currently used staging methods and sampling is not routinely performed at surgery, the status of these lymph nodes has been largely ignored. However, with the use of the sentinel node technique (which can demonstrate that the primary route of drainage of the tumor is to the internal mammary nodes) and the increasing use of postsurgical adjuvant radiation therapy, the status of this nodal group has become important.

Knowledge of the status of supraclavicular lymph nodes also is very important because involvement of this nodal group is categorized as M1 disease and indicates a grave prognosis. The role of PET in noninvasive staging of these nodal groups is not known, and prospective trials are needed.

DISTANT METASTATIC DISEASE

Whole-body PET imaging has a major role in documenting the systemic extent of malignant disease in a single study because it can detect not only the primary tumor and nodal metastases, but also skeletal and visceral metastases. Several clinical studies have shown that FDG PET is more sensitive than currently used noninvasive techniques for demonstrating the true extent of metastatic disease (3,42,43) and will quite often reveal unsuspected metastatic disease (Fig. 5.8.4) (2,23,43). Avril et al. (43) studied 41 patients with breast cancer and reported that FDG PET demonstrated unsuspected distant metastatic disease in 12 of these patients (29%), with a resultant alteration in their management.

Breast cancer commonly metastasizes to bone. Overall, 8% of patients with breast cancer will develop osseous metastasis; however, the frequency is nearly 70% among patients with advanced disease (51). The median survival of patients with metastatic disease confined to the skeleton is 24 months and the 5-year survival rate is 20% (51). The

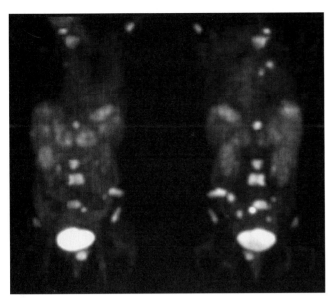

FIG. 5.8.4. PET detection of widespread metastatic breast cancer. Anterior and posterior ^{18}F-fluorodeoxyglucose positron emission tomography reprojection images demonstrate widespread osseous (spine, ribs, pelvis, proximal humerus) and hepatic (right and left lobes) metastases in a patient with treated left-sided breast cancer.

presence of osseous metastatic disease increases the morbidity and the cost of treatment.

Bone scintigraphy is currently the modality most widely used for evaluation of osseous metastatic disease from breast cancer, because it is highly sensitive and readily available. However, bone scintigraphy is not very specific and is somewhat limited in the evaluation of osteolytic metastatic foci. Cook et al. (52) compared technetium-99m (^{99m}Tc) methylene diphosphonate (MDP) bone scintigraphy with semiquantitative FDG PET in 23 patients with documented osseous metastatic breast cancer. They demonstrated that overall, FDG PET detected more osseous lesions than bone scintigraphy (mean, 14.1 vs. 7.8 lesions). This was most notable among the patients with osteolytic metastases (which were associated with a poor prognosis). Conversely, in patients with osteoblastic lesions, FDG PET detected significantly fewer lesions than bone scintigraphy ($p < .05$). Therefore, patients with a more aggressive breast cancer who tend to develop osteolytic metastatic lesions may benefit from earlier detection of osseous metastatic disease by FDG PET. Kao et al. (53) studied 24 patients with suspected or proven osseous metastatic breast cancer. A total of 89 lesions were found by bone scintigraphy and/or FDG PET; there were concordant results in 59 lesions and discordant results in 39 lesions (bone scintigraphy-positive/FDG-negative in 31 lesions and bone scintigraphy-negative/FDG-positive in 8 lesions). All 8 discordant lesions with bone scintigraphy-negative/FDG-positive and 11 of 31 discordant lesions with scintigraphy-positive/FDG-negative were confirmed to be metastatic sites; the remaining 20 discordant lesions were

benign. The difference between bone scintigraphy and FDG PET for detection of osseous metastases in breast cancer is likely related to the difference in the mechanism by which disease is detected by these modalities. Bone scintigraphy detects osteoblastic response to bone destruction by tumor cells and FDG PET mainly detects metabolic activity of the tumor cells. Both of these processes are important, so these techniques are complementary.

Recently, PET with ^{18}F-fluoride has been used to assess osseous metastatic disease in breast cancer. The bone uptake of ^{18}F is approximately twofold higher than that of ^{99m}Tc-MDP, and its blood clearance is faster, resulting in a higher bone-to-background ratio (54–57). Schirrmeister et al. (58) compared ^{18}F PET with conventional bone scintigraphy in 34 patients with breast cancer. In 17 patients, ^{18}F PET detected 64 lesions, whereas bone scintigraphy detected 29 lesions in 11 of these patients. The results of ^{18}F PET altered clinical management in four patients (12%). On a lesion-by-lesion basis, the area under the receiver operating characteristic (ROC) curve was 0.99 for ^{18}F PET and 0.74 for bone scintigraphy ($p < .05$). On a patient-by-patient basis, the area under the ROC curve was 1.00 for ^{18}F PET and 0.82 for bone scintigraphy ($p < .05$). Not surprisingly, because of the greater sensitivity of ^{18}F PET, the number of benign lesions detected by ^{18}F PET was higher than that detected by conventional bone scintigraphy, leading to a higher number of false-positive studies. With the improved image contrast and greater spatial resolution of PET, ^{18}F PET should allow for earlier detection of osseous metastases and more accurate definition of the extent of metastatic disease than is possible with conventional bone scintigraphy.

MONITORING RESPONSE TO THERAPY

A potentially important role of FDG PET in breast cancer is predicting the response of the tumor to therapy, as well as assessing the effectiveness of therapy. PET has the ability to quantify tracer distribution *in vivo*. This, coupled with the observation that changes in tumor metabolism occur shortly after initiation of therapy before any change in tumor size, makes this technique well suited for predicting and monitoring response to therapy. Conventional imaging modalities are limited in assessing response to therapy, and often a delay of several weeks after completion of therapy is required before the effectiveness of the treatment can be assessed. It would be very desirable to have the ability to predict response to therapy before therapy has begun or shortly after institution of therapy so nonresponders could be identified reliably so an alternative treatment could be substituted in these patients. In addition, the morbidity and costs associated with ineffective treatment could be avoided.

FDG PET has been used effectively to monitor therapy of several types of cancers, including breast cancer. Minn et al. (59) studied 10 patients with breast cancer before and after therapy (chemotherapy alone in 7 patients and in combination with radiotherapy in 3 patients) using qualitative planar FDG imaging. They demonstrated that an increase in FDG uptake in breast cancer over time was associated with tumor progression. In a prospective study, Wahl et al. (60) demonstrated an early and significant decrease in tumor glucose metabolism (both semiquantitatively and quantitatively) 8 days after institution of effective chemohormonotherapy in eight patients with locally advanced breast carcinoma; the reduction in tumor metabolism antedated changes in tumor size. No significant decline in tumor FDG uptake was noted in three nonresponders. Others have reported similar results in patients with advanced breast cancer (61,62).

In a recent study to assess the value of FDG PET in predicting response to therapy, Schelling et al. (63) studied 22 patients undergoing chemotherapy for locally advanced breast cancer. They compared semiquantitative tumor FDG uptake after the first (16 patients) and second (all 22 patients) courses of neoadjuvant chemotherapy with the histopathologic response after completion of therapy. After the first course of therapy, all responders (defined as pathologic complete response or minimal residual disease) were identified using a decline in tumor SUV to a level below 55% of baseline (100% [3 of 3 patients] sensitivity and 85% [11 of 13 patients] specificity). After the second course of therapy using the same threshold, all but one of the responders were identified (91% [5 of 6 patients] sensitivity and 94% [15 of 16 patients] specificity). In another study of 30 patients with advanced breast cancer, Smith et al. (64) compared semi-

quantitative and quantitative tumor FDG uptake before and after institution of chemotherapy (after the first, second, and fifth doses of therapy), as well as after the last dose of chemotherapy with histopathologic response. After the first pulse of chemotherapy, FDG PET predicted complete pathologic response with a sensitivity of 90% and a specificity of 74% using a decline in tumor SUV to a level below 20% of baseline.

With the increasing use of chemotherapy in conjunction with hematopoietic cytokines such as granulocyte colony-stimulating factor (G-CSF) and granulocyte-macrophage colony-stimulating factor (GM-CSF) in patients with breast cancer, it is important to be familiar with the effect of such therapy on FDG uptake of the bone marrow (Fig. 5.8.5). In a recent study, Sugawara et al. (65) studied the effects of G-CSF and GM-CSF in the biodistribution of FDG in rats and 11 patients with breast cancer. In rats, bone marrow activity was significantly higher in the group pretreated with G-CSF and GM-CSF compared with the control group not treated with cytokines ($p < .05$); however, the biodistribution in other normal tissues was comparable in both groups.

In patients with breast cancer, chemotherapy alone did not result in increased FDG uptake in bone marrow; however, bone marrow uptake increased after treatment with G-CSF. The SUV corrected for lean body mass (SUV_{lean}) of the bone marrow was 1.56 ± 0.23 at baseline, 3.13 ± 1.40 after one cycle ($p < .01$), 2.22 ± 0.85 after two cycles ($p < .05$), and 2.14 ± 0.79 after three cycles of therapy

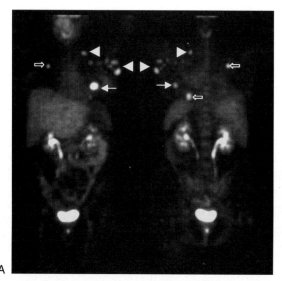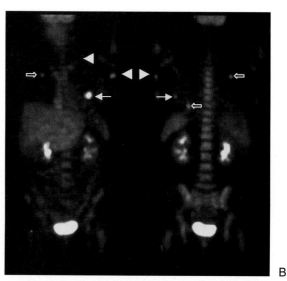

FIG. 5.8.5. PET assessment of response to therapy. **A:** Pretherapy anterior **(left)** and posterior **(right)** ^{18}F-fluorodeoxyglucose positron emission tomography (FDG PET) reprojection images demonstrate focal accumulation of FDG in the left primary breast (*solid arrow*), two pulmonary metastases (*open arrows*), a left supraclavicular, and multiple left axillary lymph nodes (*arrowheads*). **B:** Posttherapy anterior **(left)** and posterior **(right)** FDG PET reprojection images demonstrate partial response to therapy with significant residual disease at the site of primary tumor (*solid arrow*) and metastatic lesions (*open arrows* and *arrowheads*). In addition, there is diffusely increased FDG accumulation in the bone marrow, secondary to recent treatment with granulocyte colony-stimulating factor (G-CSF). Splenic uptake of FDG is slightly higher posttreatment as well. This is best seen on the posterior projection image, likely due to G-CSF treatment.

$(p < .5)$ (65). The dose of G-CSF and the duration of treatment were correlated with the extent of increase in FDG uptake in the bone marrow. After completion of treatment with G-CSF, FDG uptake in the bone marrow declined but was higher than the baseline level for up to 4 weeks after completion of therapy. In addition, markedly increased FDG uptake in the spleen was often noted after treatment with G-CSF, likely due to extramedullary hematopoiesis in the spleen (66). Therefore, a uniform increase in bone marrow or splenic activity should be interpreted with caution; a history of recent therapy with G-CSF agents would be helpful in making the distinction between diffuse metastatic disease and the drug effect. If possible, FDG PET should be delayed for a few weeks after completion of treatment with G-CSF or other hematopoietic cytokines because marked activity in bone marrow may interfere with accurate assessment of response to therapy.

RECURRENT DISEASE

Early detection and accurate restaging of recurrent breast cancer is important in the selection of the most appropriate mode of therapy and in identifying patients with limited disease amenable to curative therapy (Fig. 5.8.6). Conventional imaging modalities are limited in differentiating posttherapy changes from recurrent tumor, particularly in the region of prior surgery and/or radiation therapy. Moon et al. (67) studied 57 patients with a clinical suggestion of recurrent breast cancer after initial therapy (surgery with or without adjuvant chemotherapy or radiotherapy). They reported that non–attenuation-corrected whole-body FDG PET has sensitivity, specificity, PPV, and negative predictive values (NPVs) of 93%, 79%, 82%, and 92%, respectively, for the detection of recurrent breast cancer.

Lonneux et al. (68) studied 39 patients who were treated (surgery with or without adjuvant chemotherapy or radiotherapy) for breast cancer; 34 of these patients had an asymptomatic increase in tumor markers and 5 had clinical findings

suggestive of recurrent tumor. Thirty-three patients had recurrent disease at 39 sites and the remaining six patients had no evidence of tumor recurrence after a mean follow-up of 18 months (range, 12 to 24 months). FDG PET detected disease in 31 of 33 patients with disease recurrence (37 of 39 sites); however, conventional imaging results were positive in only 6 of these patients. Therefore, FDG PET had 94% (31 of 33 patients) sensitivity and 50% (3 of 6) specificity. Bender et al. (69) studied 75 patients with suspected recurrent breast cancer and demonstrated that FDG PET is a useful adjunct to MRI and/or CT in the detection of recurrent disease involving lymph nodes and visceral organs. For lymph node involvement, the sensitivity and specificity were 97% and 91%, respectively, for FDG PET and 74% and 95%, respectively, for CT and/or MRI. For the detection of recurrent disease in visceral organs, the sensitivity was 96% for FDG PET and 57% for CT and/or MRI.

Locoregional recurrence occurs in 7% to 30% of patients with breast cancer. Clinical detection of locoregional recurrence is limited because the signs and symptoms of locoregional recurrence often cannot be reliably distinguished from side effects of therapy. Conventional imaging techniques also are limited in differentiating posttherapeutic changes from tumor recurrence.

Hathaway et al. (70) compared FDG PET with MRI in evaluating the axillary and brachial plexus in 10 patients with suspected locoregional recurrence. MRI correctly detected disease in five patients and was indeterminate in four of nine patients with disease recurrence, whereas FDG PET detected locoregional recurrence in all nine patients as well as additional unsuspected disease in six of these patients (distant metastatic disease in five and local breast recurrence in one). Both FDG PET and MRI results were negative in the single patient without disease.

Bender et al. (69) demonstrated that MRI and/or CT were superior to FDG PET in the detection of local recurrence. FDG PET results were negative in four patients with 7- to 10-mm lesions; therefore, the sensitivity and specificity of

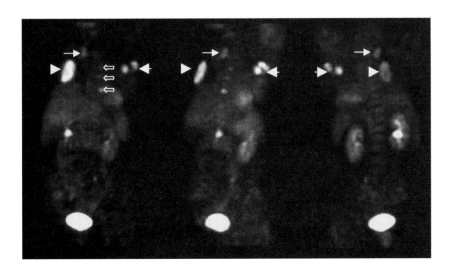

FIG. 5.8.6. PET detection of recurrent breast cancer. Anterior **(left)**, left anterior oblique **(middle)**, and posterior **(right)** ^{18}F-fluorodeoxyglucose positron emission tomographic reprojection images demonstrate several nodal (left internal mammary [*open arrows*], left axillary [*short solid arrows*], and right paratracheal [*long solid arrows*]) metastases and the right chest wall recurrence (*arrowheads*) in a patient with treated right breast cancer.

FDG PET were 80% and 96%, respectively, versus 93% and 98%, respectively, for CT and/or MRI (69). Ahmad et al. (71) studied 19 patients with signs and symptoms suggestive of recurrence in the region of brachial plexus; all but two of these patients had received local radiation therapy in the past. Fourteen patients had disease recurrence in the axilla and brachial plexus, one had disease in the sternum (which accounted for her symptoms), and four did not have recurrence. FDG PET results were positive in all 14 patients with locoregional recurrence; CT results were positive in three and negative in six of these patients who underwent CT. FDG PET results were normal in four patients without disease recurrence; two of these patients underwent CT and MRI, whose results were also negative for disease recurrence. The remaining patient did not have locoregional disease but had positive FDG PET findings for distant metastases in the sternum.

These studies indicate that FDG PET can quite reliably assess disease recurrence at distant and local sites and is a very useful adjunct to conventional imaging modalities.

RECEPTOR IMAGING

Most breast cancers are dependent on estrogen, progesterone, or both for their growth. The stimulatory effect is mediated through nuclear estrogen receptors (ERs) and progesterone receptors (PRs). Therefore, these receptors have been targeted by hormonal agents in an effort to control tumor growth. Both drugs are based on hormone antagonists and agonists and have been successfully used in the treatment of breast cancer. It has long been known that the ER (and PR) status of the tumor is an important prognostic factor in breast cancer (72,73); hormone-dependent tumors, as indicated by increases in the ER and PR content of the tumor, are less aggressive than ER-negative (or PR-negative) tumors. Because of the importance of these receptors, *in vitro* assays of tissue obtained at biopsy or surgery are routinely used to estimate the ER and PR content of breast cancer. The most commonly used methods included ligand binding assays, immunohistochemical analysis, and enzyme immunoassay. These assays have a number of shortcomings, most notably that they provide limited information about the functional status of the receptors and the responsiveness of tumor to hormone therapy; only 55% to 60% of patients with ER-positive disease respond to hormone therapy (vs. less than 10% of patients with ER-negative disease) (72,74).

ER status not only is important in predicting the likelihood of response to first-line hormone therapy but also predicts responsiveness to second-line and subsequent hormone therapy. However, in recurrent or metastatic breast cancer, the ER status of the lesions may not always be the same as that of the original primary tumor; approximately 20% of ER-positive primary breast cancers have ER-negative metastases (72). Indeed, the receptor status of recurrent or metastatic disease may be more predictive of response to hormone ther-

apy. Because some of these metastatic lesions are not amenable to biopsy, their receptor status cannot be easily determined. Therefore, a method that can reliably determine both the quantity and the functional status of tumor ERs in individual lesions would be of critical importance in identifying patients who have less aggressive disease and would benefit from hormone therapy.

Estrogen-receptor Imaging

Several decades ago, it was recognized that the presence of tumor receptors provides a mechanism for selective uptake of radiolabeled hormones as tumor imaging agents. The unique feature of PET, namely its ability to precisely quantify tracer distribution *in vivo*, has rendered it a very desirable method for evaluating receptors. The steroid-receptor systems in breast cancer, and particularly the ER, have attracted the interest of numerous investigators. Efforts to identify a radioligand with high affinity and selectivity for the ER and with properties suitable for imaging have been ongoing for more than two decades. Several steroidal and nonsteroidal estrogens labeled with bromine-77, bromine-75, iodine-123, and ^{18}F have been synthesized (75). One of the most promising positron-emitting radiolabeled estrogen analogues identified is 16α-(^{18}F)fluoro-17β-estradiol (FES). This radioligand has high specific activity, high selective ER binding *in vitro*, and high affinity for ER-positive target tissues (e.g., uterus and mammary tumors) in animal models (76–79). Because of its favorable characteristics, FES has been most extensively studied in patients with breast cancer. FES PET has been successfully used to image ER-positive breast cancers and to accurately determine the ER status of these tumors. An excellent correlation has been demonstrated between tumor FES uptake measured on PET images (expressed as the percentage of injected dose per milliliter) and the ER concentration of the tumor determined by conventional quantitative ligand binding assays of the primary breast cancer ($r = 0.96$; $p < .001$) (80).

In patients with known metastatic breast cancer, FES PET also has been shown to be highly sensitive (93%) for the detection of ER-positive metastatic foci (81). FES accumulation within metastatic lesions decreased after institution of tamoxifen therapy, presumably related to the nonavailability of ERs to interact with FES because the receptors were occupied by tamoxifen and its bioactive metabolites. This confirmed that the tumor uptake of FES is a receptor-mediated process and suggests that FES may be useful for evaluating the availability of functional ERs in breast cancer and predicting the likelihood of response to hormone therapy.

In patients (n = 43) with untreated advanced breast cancer, tumor uptake of FES was compared with *in vitro* ER levels and tumor uptake of FDG (36), to determine the relationship between FDG uptake and ER status of breast cancer. Although ER-negative tumors are expected to be more aggressive than ER-positive tumors, no significant relationship between FDG uptake and either the ER status or the FES uptake was seen (36). This study demonstrated a good correlation between the results of FES PET and *in vitro* ER assays and revealed that *in vitro* ER assays and/or FES PET provide unique information about tumor ER status that cannot be obtained indirectly from FDG PET. The overall rate of agreement between the results of *in vitro* ER assays and the results of FES PET was 88% (36). This level of agreement is similar to that observed between replicate *in vitro* assays (with disagreements explained by such factors as interlaboratory variability, interassay variability, and specimen variability). It is known that independent of the stage of disease, survival of women with ER-positive disease is superior to that of women with ER-negative disease. Similar results were found in this study; the median survival of patients with FES-negative disease was relatively short, at 21.6 months, whereas the median survival of FES-positive patients had not yet been achieved at a median follow-up interval of 22 months (82). In the same study, tumor heterogeneity and ER concordance between primary and metastatic lesions in individual patients also has been addressed with FES PET. Fifty individual metastatic lesions in 17 patients were evaluated with FES PET; concordance among multiple lesions within a patient was observed in 76% of patients (81). This level of concordance is comparable to that identified by *in vitro* ER determinations, when multiple sites have been biopsied.

Hormone-receptor status of breast cancer directs systemic therapy; patients with hormone-sensitive (ER-positive and/or PR-positive) advanced breast cancer are candidates for hormone therapy. Within 7 to 10 days after institution of hormonal treatment, 5% to 20% of patients experience a phenomenon known as the hormonal ''flare'' reaction, characterized by increased pain at sites of osseous metastatic disease, pain and erythema in soft-tissue lesions, hypercalcemia, and apparent disease progression on bone scintigraphy (83). Clinically, it is sometimes difficult to distinguish a flare reaction from disease progression. The clinical flare reaction has been shown to be predictive of response to such therapy in 80% of individuals (83–85) and is presumed to represent an initial agonist effect of the drug on the tumor before its antagonist effect supervenes (84).

Preclinical studies in immature female rats have shown that both tamoxifen and estrogen cause prompt increases in FDG accumulation in estrogen-responsive normal tissue (uterus) (86); presumably, both estrogen and tamoxifen initially stimulate cell proliferation and glucose metabolism and thus cause increased FDG uptake. These observations suggested that augmentation of tumor FDG uptake (''metabolic flare'') early during a course of tamoxifen treatment would be indicative of an agonist effect of the drug on functional ERs and predictive of a good response to therapy.

If ''metabolic flare'' can be detected early during the course of tamoxifen treatment, responders can be distinguished from nonresponders. In a recent prospective study of 11 patients with ER-positive advanced breast cancer, this hypothesis was tested. The presence of metabolic flare, indi-cated by an increase in quantitative (SUV) tumor FDG uptake 7 to 10 days after tamoxifen therapy over pretherapy values, discriminated patients who subsequently responded to tamoxifen therapy from those who did not respond (Fig. 5.8.7) (87). Additionally, the pretherapy FES uptake in the tumor and the magnitude of ER blockade by tamoxifen, as measured by a decrease in quantitative tumor FES uptake after tamoxifen therapy, were superior to *in vitro* ER and PR assays in predicting response to tamoxifen therapy (87).

These results recently have been confirmed in a larger series of patients (n = 40) with ER-positive advanced breast cancer (88). A multivariate logistic regression analysis of the results demonstrated that the baseline FES uptake and the percentage change in FDG uptake were the best predictors of response to tamoxifen therapy. We demonstrated that the PPV for response to tamoxifen of metabolic flare (if an increase in tumor FDG uptake of $\geq 10\%$ was arbitrarily selected as the cutoff criterion) was 91% and the NPV was 94%. The corresponding PPV and NPV for the baseline FES uptake (with a cutoff SUV of 2.0) were 79% and 88%, respectively (88). This study demonstrated that PET provides unique information about tumor response at the biochemical level early during therapy that could be used to guide therapy.

Progesterone-receptor Imaging

Although PR status is considered a weaker prognostic factor than ER status (72), the combination of ER and PR expression is a stronger predictor of response to hormone therapy than either alone (72,73,89,90). The presence of PR in a tumor is presumed to indicate a functionally intact estrogen-response mechanism, because it is produced by estrogen stimulation. Efforts at developing radiolabeled ligands for PRs have been less successful than those for ER imaging. Several radiolabeled progesterone analogues have been developed (91,92). 21-(^{18}F)fluoro-16α-ethyl-19-norprogesterone (FENP) is one such compound that has been developed for imaging by PET. Although FENP had favorable *in vitro* and *in vivo* characteristics in preclinical testing, imaging results with this compound in patients with breast cancer were disappointing due to the low target-to-background uptake ratio, poor correlation of tumor uptake with PR content of the tumor, and high nonspecific uptake (91,93–95). The search for a more suitable progesterone-based imaging compound continues and currently several new ^{18}F radioligands are being developed.

Imaging with Radiolabeled Antiestrogens

Fluorine-18-fluorotamoxifen, an analogue of tamoxifen, has been developed as a tracer to assess tumor ER status and to predict responsiveness to tamoxifen therapy (96,97). Limited clinical studies of ^{18}F-fluorotamoxifen in patients with breast cancer have demonstrated that this compound

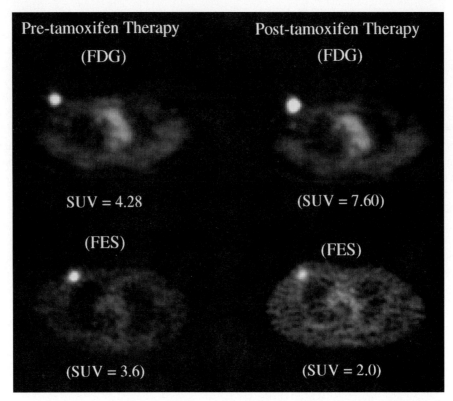

FIG. 5.8.7. "Metabolic flare." Anterior ^{18}F-fluorodeoxyglucose (FDG) positron emission tomographic **(top)** and ^{18}F-fluoroestradiol (FES) PET **(bottom)** images before **(left)** and after **(right)** tamoxifen therapy. On the pretreatment images, there is intense FDG and FES uptake in the right primary breast cancer. After 1 week of tamoxifen therapy, there is an increase in the tumor FDG uptake (reflected by an increase in the maximum standard uptake value of the tumor) and a concomitant decrease in FES uptake.

has low specific binding to ERs and high nonspecific binding in other tissues (97).

OTHER RADIOPHARMACEUTICALS

Protein Metabolism

In a pilot study, L-(methyl-^{11}C)methionine (Met) has been used to evaluate protein metabolism in breast cancer (98). Although tumor uptake of Met correlated with the S-phase fraction of the tumor measured by flow cytometry and response to systemic or radiotherapy, only lesions larger than 3 cm were reliably identified. This has significantly limited the use of Met PET in clinical or research settings. In a preliminary study, PET with L-(1-^{11}C)tyrosine (Tyr) has been studied in patients with primary breast cancer. Tyrosine has the potential to be useful in differentiating benign from malignant lesions, because high Tyr uptake was noted in malignant tumors while benign lesions had no uptake (26).

SUMMARY

The last decade has witnessed a striking increase in interest in clinical and investigational use of PET in breast cancer. The unique functional information provided by PET has

been shown to be of significant value for the evaluation of patients with breast cancer. PET is being increasingly used to resolve clinical questions that are not satisfactorily addressed by conventional imaging methods. The current literature suggests that PET not only can improve breast cancer detection, staging, and management, but also can provide prognostic information.

The functional information provided by PET can resolve some of the shortcomings of the conventional imaging methods in the evaluation of patients with breast cancer (e.g., patients with difficult-to-examine breasts). Although encouraging results have been shown in staging of regional lymph nodes with FDG PET, the role of PET in nodal staging has not been clearly defined. It is anticipated that the results of a recently completed prospective multicenter clinical trial will determine the utility of FDG PET in staging locoregional lymph nodes in early breast cancer.

There is increasing evidence that FDG PET is the preferred study to assess the extent of distant metastatic disease and is particularly useful in patients with high clinical suggestion of disease who have normal conventional imaging study results.

FDG PET has shown promise in assessing early response to chemotherapy and/or hormone therapy. In addition, significant progress in the development and testing of receptor imaging ligands, particularly ER-based ligands, has provided unique information about the biology and behavior of breast cancer, leading to more effective treatment of this cancer.

REFERENCES

1. Greenlee RT, Murray T, Hill-Harmon MB, et al. Cancer statistics, 2001. *CA Cancer J Clin* 2001;51:15–36.
2. Brown RS, Wahl RL. Over expression of Glut-1 glucose transporter in human breast cancer: an immunohistochemical study. *Cancer* 1993; 72:2979–2985.
3. Wahl RL, Cody RL, Hutchins GD, et al. Primary and metastatic breast carcinoma: initial clinical evaluation with PET with the radiolabeled glucose analogue 2-[F-18]-fluoro-2-deoxy-D-glucose. *Radiology* 1991; 179:765–770.
4. Wahl RL, Henry CA, Ethier SP. Serum glucose: effects on tumor and normal tissue accumulation of 2-[F-18]-fluoro-2-deoxy-D-glucose in rodents with mammary carcinoma. *Radiology* 1992;183:643–647.
5. Brown RS, Leung JY, Fisher SJ, et al. Intratumoral distribution of tritiated fluorodeoxyglucose in breast carcinoma, I: are inflammatory cells important? *J Nucl Med* 1995;36:1854–1861.
6. Yutani K, Tatsumi M, Uehara T, et al. Effect of patients being prone during FDG PET for the diagnosis of breast cancer. *AJR Am J Roentgenol* 1999;173:1337–1339.
7. Boerner AR, Weckesser M, Herzog H, et al. Optimal scan time for fluorine-18 fluorodeoxyglucose positron emission tomography in breast cancer. *Eur J Nucl Med* 1999;26:226–230.
8. Murthy K, Aznar M, Bergman AM, et al. Positron emission mammographic instrument: initial results. *Radiology* 2000;215:280–285.
9. Bergman AM, Thompson CJ, Murthy K, et al. Technique to obtain positron emission mammography images in registration with x-ray mammograms. *Med Phys* 1998;25(11):2119–2129.
10. Bleckmann C, Dose J, Bohuslavizki KH, et al. Effect of attenuation correction on lesion detectability in FDG PET in breast cancer. *J Nucl Med* 1999;40:2021–2024.
11. Zasadny K, Wahl RL. Standardized uptake values of normal tissues at FDG-PET: variations with body weight and a method for correction: "SUV-lean." *Radiology* 1993;189:847–850.
12. Sugawara Y, Zasadny KR, Neuhoff AW, et al. Reevaluation of the standardized uptake value for FDG: variations with body weight and methods for correction. *Radiology* 1999;213:521–525.
13. Patlak CS, Blasberg RG. Graphical evaluation of blood-to-brain transfer constant from multiple-time uptake data. Generalization. *J Cereb Blood Flow Metab* 1985;5:584–590.
14. Avril N, Bense S, Ziegler SI, et al. Breast imaging with fluorine-18-FDG PET: quantitative image analysis. *J Nucl Med* 1997;38:1186–1191.
15. Feig SA. Role and evaluation of mammography and other imaging methods for breast cancer detection, diagnosis, and staging. *Semin Nucl Med* 1999;29:3–15.
16. Whitman GJ. The role of mammography in breast cancer prevention. *Curr Opin Oncol* 1999;11(5):414.
17. Sickles EA. Mammographic features of early breast cancer. *AJR Am J Roentgenol* 1984;143:461–464.
18. Moskowitz M. The predictive value of certain mammographic signs in screening for breast cancer. *Cancer* 1983;51:1007–1011.
19. Kopans DB. Positive predictive value of mammography. *AJR Am J Roentgenol* 1992;158:521–526.
20. Franceschi D, Crowe J, Zollinger R, et al. Biopsy of the breast for mammographically detected lesions. *Surg Gynecol Obstet* 1990;171: 449–455.
21. Skinner M, Swain M, Simmons R. Nonpalpable breast lesions at biopsy: a detailed analysis of radiographic features. *Ann Surg* 1988;208: 203–208.
22. Tse NY, Hoh K, Hawkins RA, et al. The application of positron emission tomography with fluorodeoxyglucose to the evaluation of breast disease. *Ann Surg* 1992;216:27–34.
23. Nieweg OE, Kim EE, Wong WH, et al. Positron emission tomography with fluorine-18-deoxyglucose in the detection and staging of breast cancer. *Cancer* 1993;71:3920–3925.
24. Scheidhauer K, Scharl A, Pietrzyk, et al. Quantitative [18F]FDG positron emission tomography in primary breast cancer: clinical relevance and practicability. *Eur J Nucl Med* 1996;23:618–623.
25. Adler LP, Crowe JP, Al-Kaisi NK, et al. Evaluation of breast masses and axillary lymph nodes with [F-18] 2-deoxy-2-fluoro-D-glucose PET. *Radiology* 1993;187:743–750.
26. Kole AC, Nieweg OE, Pruim J, et al. Standardized uptake value and quantification of metabolism for breast cancer imaging with FDG and L-[1-11C]tyrosine PET. *J Nucl Med* 1997;38:692–696.
27. Palmedo H, Bender H, Grunwald F, et al. Comparison of fluorine-18 fluorodeoxyglucose positron emission tomography and technetium methoxyisobutyl isonitrile scintimammography in the detection of breast tumors. *Eur J Nucl Med* 1997;24:1138–1145.
28. Avril N, Rosé CA, Schelling M, et al. Breast imaging with positron emission tomography and fluorine-18 fluorodeoxyglucose: use and limitations. *J Clin Oncol* 2000;18(20):3495–3502.
29. Avril N, Dose J, Janicke F, et al. Metabolic characterization of breast tumors with positron emission tomography using F-18 fluorodeoxyglucose. *J Clin Oncol* 1996;14:1848–1857.
30. Bakheet SMB, Powe J, Kandil A, et al. F-18 FDG uptake in breast infection and inflammation. *Clin Nucl Med* 2000;25(2):100–103.
31. Torizuka T, Zasadny KR, Recker B, et al. Untreated primary lung and breast cancers: correlation between F-18 FDG kinetic rate constants and findings of *in vitro* studies. *Radiology* 1998;207:767–774(abst).
32. Wahl RL, Helvie MA, Chang AE, et al. Detection of breast mass after augmentation mammoplasty using 18-fluorodeoxyglucose-PET. *J Nucl Med* 1994;35:872–875.
33. Noh D-Y, Yun I-J, Kang H-S, et al. Detection of cancer in augmented breasts by positron emission tomography. *Eur J Surg* 1999;165: 847–851.
34. Noh D-Y, Yun I-J, Kim J-S, et al. Diagnostic value of positron emission tomography for detecting breast cancer. *World J Surg* 1998;22: 223–228.
35. Crippa F, Seregni E, Agresti R, et al. Association between [18F]fluorodeoxyglucose uptake and postoperative histopathology, hormone receptor status, thymidine labeling index and p53 in primary breast cancer: a preliminary observation. *Eur J Nucl Med* 1998;25:1429–1434.
36. Dehdashti F, Mortimer JE, Siegel BA, et al. Positron tomographic assessment of estrogen receptors in breast cancer. Comparison with FDG-PET and *in vitro* receptor assays. *J Nucl Med* 1995;36:1766–1774.
37. Oshida M, Uno K, Suzuki M, et al. Predicting the prognoses of breast carcinoma patients with positron emission tomography using 2-deoxy-2-fluoro[18F]-D-glucose. *Cancer* 1998;82:2227–2234.
38. Avril N, Menzel M, Dose J, et al. Glucose metabolism of breast cancer assessed by 18F-PET: histologic and immunohistochemical tissue analysis. *J Nucl Med* 2001;42:9–16.
39. Hellman S, Harris JR. Natural history of breast cancer. In: Harris JR, Lippman ME, Marrow M, et. al, eds. *Diseases of the breast,* 2nd ed. Philadelphia: Lippincott Williams & Wilkins, 2000:407–423.
40. Wahl RL, Kaminski MS, Either SP, et al. The potential of 2-deoxy-2-fluoro-D-glucose (FDG) for detection of tumor involvement in lymph nodes. *J Nucl Med* 1990;31:1831–1835.
41. Wahl RL, Cody RL, August D. Initial evaluation of FDG-PET for staging of the axilla in newly diagnosed breast cancer patients. *J Nucl Med* 1991;32:981.
42. Hoh K, Hawkins RA, Glaspy JA, et al. Cancer detection with whole-body PET using [18F]fluoro-2-deoxy-D-glucose. *J Comput Assisted Tomogr* 1993;17:582–589.
43. Avril N, Dose J, Jäniicke F, et al. Assessment of axillary lymph node involvement in breast patients with positron emission tomography using radiolabeled 2-(fluorine-18)-fluoro-2-deoxy-D-glucose. *J Natl Cancer Inst* 1996;88:1204–1209.
44. Utech CI, Young CS, Winter PF. Prospective evaluation of fluorine-18 fluorodeoxyglucose positron emission tomography in breast cancer for staging of the axilla related to surgery and immunocytochemistry. *Eur J Nucl Med* 1996;23:1588–1593.
45. Crippa F, Agresti R, Donne VD, et al. The contribution of positron emission tomography (PET) with 18F-fluorodeoxyglucose (FDG) in the preoperative detection of axillary metastases of breast cancer: the experience of the national cancer institute of Milan. *Tumori* 1997;83: 542–543.
46. Adler LP, Faulhaber PF, Schnur KC, et al. Axillary lymph node metastases: screening with [F-18]2-deoxy-2-fluoro-D-glucose (FDG) PET. *Radiology* 1997;203:323–327.
47. Smith I, Ogston KN, Whitford P, et al. Staging of the axilla in breast

cancer: accurate *in vivo* assessment using positron emission tomography with 2-(fluorine-18)-fluoro-2-deoxy-D-glucose. *Ann Surg* 1998; 228(2):220–227.

48. Rostom AY, Powe J, Kandil A, et al. Positron emission tomography in breast cancer: a clinicopathological correlation of results. *Br J Radiol* 1999;72:1064–1068.

49. Schirrmeister H, Kühn T, Guhlmann A, et al. Fluorine-18 2-deoxy-2-fluoro-D-glucose PET in the preoperative staging of breast cancer: comparison with the standard staging procedures. *Eur J Nucl Med* 2001; 28:351–358.

50. Morrow M, Harris JR. Local management of invasive breast cancer. In: Harris JR, Lippman ME, Marrow M, et al, eds. *Diseases of the breast*, 2nd ed. Philadelphia: Lippincott Williams & Wilkins, 2000: 515–560.

51. Coleman RE, Rubens RD. The clinical course of bone metastases from breast cancer. *Br J Cancer* 1987;55:61–66.

52. Cook GJ, Houston S, Rubens R, et al. Detection of bone metastases in breast cancer by [18]FDG PET: differing metabolic activity in osteoblastic and osteolytic lesions. *J Clin Oncol* 1998;16:3375–3379.

53. Kao C-H, Hsieh J-F, Tsai S-C, et al. Comparison and discrepancy of ^{18}F-2-deoxyglucose positron emission tomography and Tc-99m MDP bone scan to detect bone metastases. *Anticancer Res* 2000;20: 2189–2192.

54. Krishnamurthy GT, Thomas PB, Tubis M, et al. Comparison of ^{99m}Tc polyphosphate and F-18, I: kinetics. *J Nucl Med* 1974;15:832–836.

55. Hawkins RA, Choi Y, Huang SC, et al. Evaluation of skeletal kinetics of fluorine 18-fluoride ion with PET. *J Nucl Med* 1992;33:633–642.

56. Hoh CK, Hawkins RA, Dalbom M, et al. Whole body skeletal imaging with [F-18] fluoride ion with PET. *J Comput Assisted Tomogr* 1992; 17:34–41.

57. Schieper C, Nuyts J, Bormans G, et al. Fluoride kinetics of the axial skeleton measured *in vivo* with fluorine-18-fluoride PET. *J Nucl Med* 1997;38:1970–1976.

58. Schirrmeister H, Guhlmann A, Kotzerke J, et al. Early detection and accurate description of extent of metastatic bone disease in breast cancer with fluoride ion and positron emission tomography. *J Clin Oncol* 1999;17:2381–2389.

59. Minn H, Soini I. [18F]Fluorodeoxyglucose scintigraphy in diagnosis and follow up of treatment in advanced breast cancer. *Eur J Nucl Med* 1989;15:61–66.

60. Wahl RL, Zasadny K, Helvie M, et al. Metabolic monitoring of breast cancer chemohormonotherapy using positron emission tomography: initial evaluation. *J Clin Oncol* 1993;11:2101–2111.

61. Flanagan FL, Dehdashti F, Siegel BA. PET in breast cancer. *Semin Nucl Med* 1998;28:290–302.

62. Bassa P, Kim EE, Inoue T, et al. Evaluation of preoperative chemotherapy using PET with fluorine-18-fluorodeoxyglucose in breast cancer. *J Nucl Med* 1996;37:931–938.

63. Schelling M, Avril N, Nährig J, et al. Positron emission tomography using [18F]fluorodeoxyglucose for monitoring primary chemotherapy in breast cancer. *J Clin Oncol* 2000;18:1689–1695.

64. Smith IC, Welch AE, Hutcheon AW, et al. Positron emission tomography using [18F]-fluorodeoxy-D-glucose to predict the pathologic response of breast cancer to primary chemotherapy. *J Clin Oncol* 2000; 18:1676–1688.

65. Sugawara Y, Fisher SJ, Zasadny KR, et al. Preclinical and clinical studies of bone marrow uptake of fluorine-18-fluorodeoxyglucose with or without granulocyte colony-stimulating factor during chemotherapy. *J Clin Oncol* 1998;16:173–180.

66. Abdel-Dayem HM, Rosen G, El-Zeftawy H, et al. Fluorine-18 fluorodeoxyglucose splenic uptake from extramedullary hematopoiesis after granulocyte colony-stimulating factor stimulation. *Clin Nucl Med* 1999; 24:319–322.

67. Moon DH, Maddahi J, Silverman DHS, et al. Accuracy of whole-body fluorine-18-FDG PET for the detection of recurrent or metastatic breast carcinoma. *J Nucl Med* 1998;39:431–435.

68. Lonneux M, Borbath I, Berlière M, et al. The place of whole-body PET FDG for the diagnosis of distant recurrence of breast cancer. *Clin Positron Imaging* 2000;3(2):45–49.

69. Bender H, Kirst J, Palmedo H, et al. Value of ^{18}F-fluorodeoxygulcose positron emission tomography in the staging of recurrent breast carcinoma. *Anticancer Res* 1997;17:1687–1692.

70. Hathaway PB, Mankoff DA, Maravilla KR, et al. Value of combined FDG PET and MR imaging in the evaluation of suspected recurrent local-regional breast cancer: preliminary experience. *Radiology* 1999; 210:807–814.

71. Ahmad A, Barrington S, Maisey M, et al. Use of positron emission tomography in evaluation of brachial plexopathy in breast cancer patients. *Br J Cancer* 1999;79:478–482.

72. Elledge RM, Fuqua SAW. Estrogen and progesterone receptors. In: Harris JR, Lippman ME, Marrow M, et al., eds. *Diseases of the breast,* 2nd ed. Philadelphia: Lippincott Williams & Wilkins, 2000:471–488.

73. Vollenweider-Zerargui L, Barrelet L, Wong Y, et al. The predictive value of estrogen and progesterone receptors' concentrations on the clinical behavior of breast cancer in women: clinical correlation on 547 patients. *Cancer* 1986;57:1171–1180.

74. Ravdin PM, Green S, Dorr TM, et al. Prognostic significance of progesterone receptor levels in estrogen receptor-positive patients with metastatic breast cancer treated with tamoxifen: results of a prospective Southwest Oncology Group study. *J Clin Oncol* 1992;10:1284–1291.

75. Katzenellenbogen JA. Designing steroid receptor-based radiotracers to image breast and prostate tumors. *J Nucl Med* 1995;36[Suppl]:8–13.

76. Kiesewetter DO, Kilbourn MR, Landvatter SW, et al. Radiochemistry and radiopharmaceuticals. *J Nucl Med* 1984;25:1212–1221.

77. Mathias CJ, Welch MJ, Katzenellenbogen JA, et al. Characterization of the uptake of 16α-[18F] fluoro-17β-estradiol in DMBA-induced mammary tumors. *Int J Radiat Appl Instrum B* 1987;14:15–25.

78. Brodack JW, Kilbourn MR, Welch MJ, et al. Application of robotics to radiopharmaceutical preparation: controlled synthesis of fluorine-18 16α-fluoroestradiol-17β. *J Nucl Med* 1986;27:714–721.

79. Brodack JW, Kilbourn MR, Welch MJ, et al. NCA 16α-[18F]fluoroestradiol-17β: the effect of reaction vessel on fluorine-18 resolubilization, product yield and effective specific activity. *Int J Radiat Appl Instrum A* 1986;37:217–221.

80. Mintun MA, Welch MJ, Siegel BA, et al. Breast cancer: PET imaging of estrogen receptors. *Radiology* 1988;169:45–48.

81. McGuire AH, Dehdashti F, Siegel BA, et al. Positron tomographic assessment of 16α-[18F]fluoro-17β-estradiol uptake in metastatic breast carcinoma. *J Nucl Med* 1991;32:1526–1531.

82. Mortimer JE, Dehdashti F, Siegel BA, et al. Clinical correlation of FDG and FES-PET imaging with estrogen receptor and response to systemic therapy. *Clin Cancer Res* 1996;2:933–939.

83. Plotkin D, Lechner J, Jung W, et al. Tamoxifen flare in advanced breast cancer. *JAMA* 1978;240:2644–2646.

84. Legha S. Tamoxifen in the treatment of breast cancer. *Ann Intern Med* 1988;109:219–228.

85. Vogel C, Schoenfelder J, Shemano I, et al. Worsening bone scan in the evaluation of antitumor response during hormonal therapy of breast cancer. *J Clin Oncol* 1995;13:1123–1128.

86. Welch M, Bonasera T, Sherman E, et al. [F-18]fluorodeoxyglucose (FDG) and 16α [F-18]fluoroestradiol-17β (FES) uptake in estrogen-receptor (ER)–rich tissues following tamoxifen treatment: a preclinical study. *J Nucl Med* 1995;36:39.

87. Dehdashti F, Flanagan FL, Mortimer JE, et al. PET assessment of "metabolic flare" to predict response of metastatic breast cancer to antiestrogen therapy. *Eur J Nucl Med* 1999;26:51–56.

88. Mortimer JE, Dehdashti F, Siegel BA, et al. Metabolic flare: an indicator of hormone responsiveness in advanced breast cancer. *J Clin Oncol* 2001;19(11):2797–2803.

89. Sledge GJ, McGuire W. Steroid hormones receptors in human breast cancer. *Adv Cancer Res* 1983;38:61–75.

90. Hellman S, Harris JR. Prognostic and predictive factors. In: Harris JR, Lippman ME, Marrow M, et al, eds. *Diseases of the breast,* 2nd ed. Philadelphia: Lippincott Williams & Wilkins, 2000:489–514.

91. Pomper MG, Katzenellenbogen JA, Welch MJ, et al. 21-[18F]fluoro-16α-ethyl-19-norprogesterone: syntheses and target tissue selective uptake of a progestin receptor for positron emission tomography. *J Med Chem* 1988;31:1360–1363.

92. Pomper M, Pinney K, Carlson K, et al. Target tissue uptake selectivity of three fluorine-substituted progestins: potential imaging agents for receptor-positive breast tumors. *Nucl Med Biol* 1990;17:309–319.

93. Katzenellenbogen JA, Welch MJ, Dehdashti F. The development of estrogen and progestin radiopharmaceuticals for imaging breast cancer. *Anticancer Res* 1997;17:1573–1576.

94. Verhagen A, Studeny M, Luurtsema G, et al. Metabolism of a [18F]fluorine labeled progestin (21-[18F]fluoro-16-alpha-ethyl-19-norprogester-

one) in humans: a clue for future investigations. *Nucl Med Biol* 1994; 21:941–952.

95. Dehdashti F, McGuire AH, Brocklin HFV, et al. Assessment of 21-[18F]fluoro-16-alpha-ethyl-19-norprogesterone as a positron-emitting radiopharmaceutical for the detection of progestin receptors in human breast carcinomas. *J Nucl Med* 1991;32:1532–1537.

96. Yang D, Kuang LR, Cherif A, et al. Synthesis of [18F]fluoroalanine and [18F]fluorotamoxifen for imaging breast tumors. *J Drug Target* 1993;1:259–267.

97. Yang DJ, Li C, Kuang LR, et al. Imaging, biodistribution and therapy potential of halogenated tamoxifen analogues. *Life Sci* 1994;55:53–67.

98. Leskinen-Kallio S, Nagren K, Lehikoinen P, et al. Uptake of 11C-methionine in breast cancer studied by PET. An association with the size of S-phase fraction. *Br J Cancer* 1991;64:1121–1124.

CHAPTER 5.9

Esophagus

Richard L. Wahl

Esophageal carcinoma is a relatively uncommon cancer, with an estimated 13,200 new cases (9,900 men and 3,300 women) expected in the United States in 2001 (1). The cancer is extremely lethal and has an estimated death rate of 12,500 patients per year, with 9,600 men and 3,000 women dying. This very high mortality rate is consistent with a very low 5-year survival after diagnosis, which is only about 12% for all stages of the disease. Although the 5-year survival is still poor, it has improved slightly, but significantly ($p < .05$) from 5% to 7% in 1974 to 1976 to 12% in 1989 to 1996, presumably due to improved diagnosis and treatment (1,2).

Most esophageal cancers diagnosed worldwide are of squamous cell histology. However, in the Western world, there has been a substantial increase in the incidence and prevalence of adenocarcinoma of the esophagus, particularly those arising at the esophagogastric junction (2–5). Most, if not all, adenocarcinomas of the distal esophagus arise from areas with specialized intestinal metaplasia, which develop as a consequence of chronic gastroesophageal (GE) reflux. In some patients, it can be difficult to determine if tumors at the GE junction arose from the esophagus or the stomach itself. A substantial focus on the prevention of GE reflux disease (GERD), including prevention and treatment of Barrett esophagus, is an ongoing attempt to reduce the increase of adenocarcinoma of the esophagus in the Western world. Risk factors for esophageal carcinoma include achalasia, in addition to GE reflux. When gastric carcinomas occur in the fundus, they can be difficult to distinguish from esophageal carcinomas. These tumors occur in an additional 21,700 patients per year in the United States (1).

The most common sites of metastatic disease are the locoregional lymph nodes immediately adjoining the esophagus and the upper abdominal lymph nodes. Tumors in the lower esophagus and GE junction may metastasize to mesenteric nodes and tumors of the upper esophagus to the cervical nodes, as well as the liver, lungs, and other organs including bone.

Decisions concerning primary therapy of esophageal cancer are based on knowledge of the extent of the primary tumor. If surgery is planned, it is obviously best to remove all known cancer. Surgery for esophageal carcinoma is a major procedure and carries risks with it. Determining if aggressive "curative intent" surgery or palliation is appropriate is a key decision. The stage at presentation is important to prognosis and to rational management. Staging for esophageal carcinoma is commonly tabulated using the American Joint Committee on Cancers TNM system (2) (Table 5.9.1). Survival is dependent on stage and although poor in all stages, is much better for localized than locoregional or disseminated esophageal cancers (25%, 12%, and 2% 5-year survivals, respectively). Various methods have been used to stage esophageal cancer, including endoscopic ultrasound (EUS), computed tomography (CT), and more recently positron emission tomography (PET) imaging, particularly using ^{18}F-fluorodeoxyglucose (FDG). Imaging is key to defining stage and to planning management (2–7).

The management of esophageal cancer has been in evolution. Traditionally, surgery was the first choice for curative treatment, but the very low survival rates of esophageal cancer after surgery alone (5% or less for 5 years in many instances) showed that additional effective therapy was needed. Esophageal cancers are quite responsive to chemotherapy and external beam radiation therapy. Thus, combined treatment methods are increasingly common, although the results have been somewhat mixed. These treatment modalities have recently been reviewed (4,5). In many centers, aggressive chemotherapy, often neoadjuvant (to reduce tumor burden), has been performed before surgery, and assessing response to such therapy is of key importance. In at least some series, 5-year survival rates in excess of 50% have been reported in patients in whom a complete pathologic response is seen to neoadjuvant therapy (4,5).

PRIMARY TUMOR DETECTION

Nearly all localized primary esophageal carcinomas are detected first by clinical symptoms of dysphagia or in the context of endoscopy performed as part of an evaluation of the upper gastrointestinal (GI) tract for GE reflux. PET has not been used as a primary screening method for esophageal

TABLE 5.9.1. *Staging esophageal cancer*

TNM definitions

Primary tumor (T)

TX	Primary tumor cannot be assessed (cytologically positive tumor not evident endoscopically or radiographically)
TO	No evidence of primary tumor (e.g. after treatment with radiation and chemotherapy)
Tis	Carcinoma *in situ*
T1	Tumor invades lamina propria or submucosa, but not beyond it
T2	Tumor invades muscularis propria
T3	Tumor invades adventitia
T4	Tumor invades adjacent structures (e.g., aorta, tracheobronchial tree, vertebral bodies, pericardium)

Regional lymph node involvement (N)

NX	Regional nodes cannot be assessed
N0	No regional node metastasis
N1	Regional node metastasis

Distant metastasis (M)

MX	Presence of distant metastasis cannot be assessed
M0	No distant metastasis
M1	Distant metastasis
	Tumors of the lower thoracic esophagus
	M1a Metastasis in celiac lymph nodes
	M1b Other distant metastasis
	Tumors of the midthoracic esophagus
	M1a Not applicable
	M1b Nonregional lymph nodes and/or other distant metastasis
	Tumors of the upper thoracic esophagus
	M1a Metastasis in cervical nodes
	M1b Other distant metastasis

Stage grouping

Stage 0	Tis N0 M0
Stage I	T1 N0 M0
Stage IIA	T2 N0 M0
	T3 N0 M0
Stage IIB	T1 NI M0
	T2 NI M0
Stage III	T3 NI M0
	T4 any N M0
Stage IV	Any T any N M1
Stage IVA	Any T any N M1a
Stage IVB	Any T any N M1b

Adapted from Fleming ID, Cooper JS, Henson DE, et al., eds. *American Joint Commission on Cancer staging handbook. From the AICC staging manual,* 5th ed. Philadelphia: Lippincott–Raven Publishers, 1998:65–69.

carcinoma. The precursor lesion to many cases of adenocarcinoma of the esophagus is Barrett esophagus. It usually has a low total volume that would not be expected to be detected using whole-body PET imaging devices, although on rare occasions it can be (8). Similarly, some inflammations of the distal esophagus can have mild increased FDG uptake (8). Several studies have shown that the vast majority of primary esophageal cancers that are first diagnosed by other methods are detectable by ^{18}F-fluorodeoxyglucose positron emission tomography (FDG PET), with sensitivities in the 90% to 100% range (9–14) (Table 5.9.2). An example of PET visualization of a primary esophageal carcinoma lesion is shown in Fig. 5.9.1.

When PET results have been reported to be falsely negative in esophageal cancers, it has usually been because the tumor volume of the lesions was small, such as stage T1 primary lesions. Diagnostic challenges in esophageal cancer can include determining whether there is abnormal or physiologic uptake at the GE junction. There may be some uptake in this location normally, so detecting small esophageal cancers can be problematic. For these reasons, it is probable that early low-volume esophageal cancer can be much more easily detected by direct visualization using an endoscope than by PET.

LOCOREGIONAL NODAL DETECTION

The detection of nodal metastases with PET is dependent on the volume of tumor in the metastasis, the intensity of tracer uptake in the lesion, and the background tracer activity (as well as the injected dose of radiotracer and the performance and resolution of the scanner), as well as the interpretation criteria. CT detects nodal metastases based on their size, and what constitutes a ''positive or negative'' node by CT differs with different observers. The larger the node, the more likely it is to represent a node involved by cancer, although the optimal cutoff size for ''positive or negative'' nodes is not clear in esophageal cancer.

Both PET and CT can fail to detect small metastases of esophageal cancer to locoregional lymph nodes. Lesions smaller than 5 mm are not usually detected on PET with FDG, which is consistent with other detection challenges encountered with current FDG PET technology. To achieve high sensitivity with CT, small lymph nodes must be called ''positive.'' For example, 5-mm and larger nodes may be called abnormal in some CT studies, whereas others may choose a 10-mm-size cutoff. The smaller the cutoff for node size, the more likely cancer will be detected, but at the price of a lower specificity. This results in a considerable range in the sensitivity and specificity of PET for assessing tumor involvement in regional lymph nodes and an even greater range in accuracy of CT (Table 5.9.3).

In general, PET is not exceptionally sensitive, but it has a high specificity for the detection of locoregional lymph node metastases (typical sensitivities of 22% to 76%, but with specificities of about 90%). By contrast, reported CT

TABLE 5.9.2. *Accuracy of PET for detection of primary esophageal carcinoma in patients in whom esophageal cancer was first diagnosed by other methods*

Author (reference no.)	N	Sensitivity of PET	Specificity of PET	Accuracy of PET
Fukunaga et al. (9)	42	41/42 98%	11/11 100%	52/53 99%
Flanagan et at. (10)	29	29/29 100%	N/A	N/A
Kole et al. (11)	26	25/26 100%	N/A	N/A
Couper et al. (12)	14	13/14 93%	N/A	N/A
Flamen et al. (13)	74	70/74 95%	N/A	N/A
Weber et al. (14)	40	40/40 100%	N/A	N/A
Overall	225	218/225 97%		

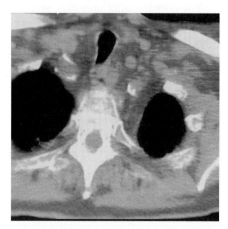
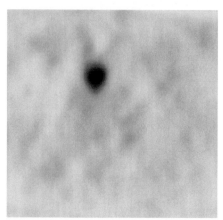
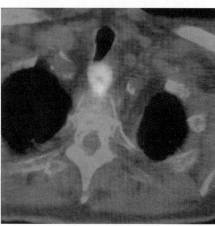

FIG. 5.9.1. Localized esophageal carcinoma in the upper esophagus. Images show a computed tomographic (CT), a PET, and a fused PET/CT image **(lower left)** obtained with a PET/CT scanning device.

TABLE 5.9.3. *Accuracy of PET versus CT for staging regional nodal metastases*

Author (reference no)	N	PET sensitivity	CT/EUS sensitivity	PET specificity	CT/EUS specificity	PET accuracy	CT/EUS accuracy
Lerut et al. (15)	39	22%	83%	—	—	48%	69%
Meltzer et al. (16)	47	41%	87%	90%	14%	—	—
Flamen et al. (13)	74	33%	81%	89%	67%	—	—
Choi et al. (17)	48	57%	18%	97%	99%	86%	78%
Rankin et al. (18)	19	24%	53%	—	—	—	—
Kole et al. (25)	26	—	—	—	—	62%	90%
Block et al. (19)	41	52%	29%	—	—	—	—
Luketich et al. (20)	35	45%	—	100%	—	—	—
Flanagan et al. (10)	29	76%	45%	—	—	—	—

EUS, endoscopic ultrasound.

TABLE 5.9.4. *Accuracy of PET in evaluating metastatic esophageal cancer*

Author (reference no.)	N	Sensitivity of PET	Sensitivity of CT	Specificity of PET	Specificity of CT	Accuracy of PET	Accuracy of CT
Lerut et al. (15)	42	86%	—	—	—	86%	62%
Luketich et al. (21)	100	69%	46%	93%	74%	84%	63%
Flamen et al. (25)	34	—	—	—	—	82%	64%
Block et al. (16)	58	100%	29%	—	—	—	—
Yeung et al. (22)	109	80%	68%	95%	81%	86%	73%

sensitivity/specificity pairs range from (18%/78% to 87%/14%), meaning CT can be either very insensitive and reasonably specific (though not as specific as PET) or very sensitive and extremely nonspecific. When directly compared, in several studies, PET was an equivalent or more accurate method for nodal staging than CT, but both are somewhat limited in accuracy (11,13,15–17).

EUS has been reported to be more sensitive than either PET or CT for staging regional nodes immediately contiguous with the esophagus, and it is reasonably specific. EUS is good at assessing tumor size and depth of invasion. There are no data showing that PET is accurate in evaluating the primary tumor stage of esophageal cancers. EUS has a significant learning curve and may not be routinely available. Further, EUS may be technically impossible if there is an esophageal stricture due to cancer, because it may be impossible to pass the endoscope beyond a tumor-induced stricture (3,7). There is some interest in using minimally invasive surgical techniques for staging esophageal cancer, and these are likely to be more sensitive than imaging but are clearly more invasive.

SYSTEMIC METASTASES

In virtually all studies to date, PET has been more accurate than other conventional diagnostic methods in detecting systemic metastases (Table 5.9.4). Reported sensitivities of PET in larger peer-reviewed manuscripts have been between 70% and 100%, whereas those of CT have been lower at 29% to 68% (10–23). The specificity of PET is high, typically in the mid 90% range, whereas that of CT is in the 74% to 81% range. A review of the literature, including abstracts with limited data and more heterogeneous patient groups, showed comparable results in 452 patients (24). It is quite clear that PET with FDG is the most accurate single noninvasive method for detecting systemic metastatic esophageal carcinoma. An example of a primary esophageal carcinoma with disseminated systemic metastases is shown in Fig. 5.9.2.

Although PET is the most effective single imaging method for detecting distant metastases from esophageal carcinoma, specific comparisons between other imaging methods and PET have been limited in some organ systems. For example,

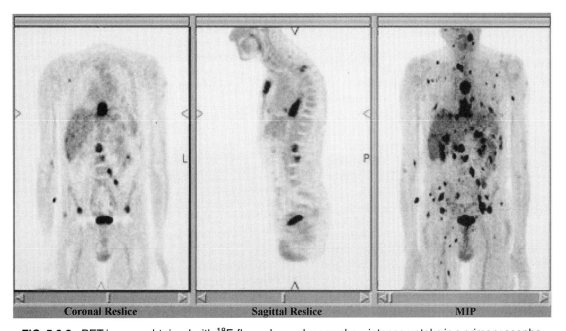

FIG. 5.9.2. PET images obtained with ^{18}F-fluorodeoxyglucose show intense uptake in a primary esophageal carcinoma in the thorax. There are also multiple metastatic foci to soft tissue, bone, liver, and other organs that are consistent with stage IV disease. MIP, maximum-intensity projection; L, left; P, posterior.

the accuracy of PET versus CT in detecting liver metastases is likely a situation in which PET is superior to CT. However, it is not clear that PET is superior to CT or MRI in the detection of metastases to the brain, and indeed it is probable that brain metastases are less well seen with FDG PET than with MRI, as is the case in lung cancer imaging. For this reason, the author would still recommend the use of anatomic imaging to assess the brain if there is a concern regarding the presence of brain metastases.

It is also likely that very small (a few millimeters) lung metastases will be detected better by CT than by PET. This would seem probable based on the known physical performance characteristics of PET for small lesions using current PET devices. The relative performance of PET versus bone scans in the detection of bone metastases is only reported to a limited extent. Given the relatively high uptake of FDG into esophageal cancers, it is likely that esophageal cancer will be detected well if metastatic, even if in bone.

INSTRUMENTATION AND REIMBURSEMENT

PET is currently approved by Medicare in the United States for a number of applications in esophageal cancer, including staging, restaging, and assessing response of cancers after therapy. Most of the literature is based on use of dedicated two-dimensional (2D) image acquisition using bismuth germanate (BGO) detector PET cameras. Some early experience in PET imaging of esophageal cancer was based on use of three-dimensional partial-ring detector PET systems. Such devices are somewhat more prone to detecting scattered events, which can lower target-to-background ratios unless accurate computer corrections are put in place. It is of interest that the only paper in which PET fared worse than CT in sensitivity was obtained using such a device (16).

No data exist to demonstrate that coincidence imaging with dual-head gamma cameras is an effective method for detecting small metastases of esophageal carcinoma. Medicare (CMS) rules specifically exclude hybrid gamma cameras from the list of devices approved for reimbursement for PET imaging of esophageal carcinomas, and these devices are used only infrequently in the United States for detection of esophageal cancer with FDG. Our initial data using 2D acquisitions with BGO PET with CT fusion (PET/CT device) has been encouraging and a representative image is included from our system (Fig. 5.9.1).

DETECTION OF RECURRENT DISEASE

Esophageal cancer commonly recurs, so detection of recurrence by imaging is an important clinical question. This has been addressed by Flamen et al (25) who evaluated 33 patients with 40 recurrent sites. PET was not as reliable in characterizing anastomotic recurrences as conventional diagnostic methods (CDMs), which included EUS. PET tended to have false-positive results in patients with benign strictures after dilation, although PET was very sensitive (sensitivity, specificity, and accuracy of 100%, 57%, and

74% for PET, respectively, vs. 100%, 93%, and 96%, respectively, for CDM). PET was very reliable for detecting systemic metastases, with sensitivity, specificity, and accuracy for PET of 94%, 82%, and 87%, respectively, compared with 81% sensitivity, 82% specificity, and 81% accuracy for CDM ($p = $ NS). Although the accuracy rates in these patients were comparable, PET provided additional information in about 27% of patients (25). PET appears to add incremental value to CDM but in this setting is not clearly proven superior to CDM. Based on available data, it seems the combination of CDMs and PET would be the most rational approach to detect recurrent disease.

ASSESSING RESPONSE TO THERAPY

Esophageal carcinomas, traditionally treated with surgery, are increasingly being treated with neoadjuvant chemotherapy, and often radiation therapy is included (5). In some studies, if complete pathologic remission is achieved after combined chemoradiation therapy, 5-year survival rates of more than 50% have been reported (4,5).

It has been suggested that it might be feasible to eliminate the need for surgery if it were possible to determine with imaging that there was no residual tumor present. Establishing whether treatment is effective early after it is started and thus likely to lead to a complete pathologic response, or after treatment is completed if it has or has not achieved a pathologic response, can help determine the next step in treatment and may reflect prognosis. Several reports have showed that FDG PET can measure the response of a variety of cancers to therapy. In breast cancer, early declines in FDG uptake in cancers antedate changes in tumor size and can predict response and outcome (26).

Pretreatment and posttreatment PET scans in 13 patients with esophageal carcinoma showed a change in FDG uptake paralleling the change in tumor size on CT. The largest reductions in FDG uptake were seen in patients who achieved a complete response, whereas a mild increase in FDG uptake was seen during therapy in two patients with progressive disease (12). In a similar study, 27 patients with histopathologically proven squamous cell carcinoma of the esophagus located at or above the tracheal bifurcation underwent neoadjuvant therapy consisting of external beam radiotherapy and 5-fluorouracil as a continuous infusion (27). FDG PET was performed before and 3 weeks after the end of radiotherapy and chemotherapy (before surgery). Quantitative measurements of tumor FDG uptake were correlated with histopathologic response and patient survival. After neoadjuvant therapy, 24 patients underwent surgery. Histopathologic evaluation revealed fewer than 10% viable tumor cells in 13 patients (responders) and more than 10% viable tumor cells in 11 patients (nonresponders). In responders, FDG uptake decreased by 72% ± 11%; in nonresponders, it decreased by only 42% ± 22%. Using a retrospectively determined threshold of a 52% decrease of FDG uptake compared with baseline, the sensitivity to detect response was 100%, with a corresponding specificity of 55%. The positive predictive value (PPV) and negative predictive value were 72% and 100%, respectively. The patients who failed to show a decrease in FDG uptake of more than 52% had a significantly worse survival after resection than those who had a larger decrease (26). These data are promising, but the relatively low PPV of a large decrease in FDG uptake for predicting patients' response is consistent with the limitation of PET in detecting small amounts of residual cancer noninvasively. Difficulties in detecting small tumor volumes are compounded by decreases in FDG uptake that follow treatment, which further reduce the detectable signal. Nonetheless, PET performed quite well in this setting.

Ideally, PET should be performed soon after treatment is started in an effort to determine longer-term response. PET scans before and at 14 days after the start of a platinum-based chemotherapy regime for treatment of esophageal carcinoma were performed in 40 patients. Response was assessed after 3 months of therapy by EUS and histology (14). Responding tumors had a decrease in tracer uptake of 54% ± 17%, whereas nonresponding tumors showed only a minimal decline in tracer uptake of 15% ± 21%. A cutoff value of a 35% decline was about 95% effective in separating tumors that ultimately responded from those that did not. Patients with greater declines in tumor FDG uptake were more likely to achieve a histologic complete response as well. The patients with a larger decline in FDG uptake also had significantly longer times to tumor progression and/or recurrence than those patients with only minimal drops in tracer uptake with treatment.

MANAGEMENT CHANGES AND COST-EFFECTIVENESS

A comprehensive review of the PET literature in esophageal cancer, including abstracts, suggested that PET changed management in 14% to 20% of patients (24). This often involved finding disseminated metastatic disease not detected by other methods but can also include clarifying that a ''positive'' abnormality on CT is in fact not ''positive'' on PET and thus not likely to represent a metastasis. The cost-effectiveness of PET in esophageal cancer has not been extensively studied, but when major surgery is avoided in 10% to 20% (or more) of patients after a PET study, the test is most likely cost-effective. This projection is based on a conservatively estimated 10-fold difference between the cost of PET versus the cost of surgery.

OTHER TRACERS FOR PET IN ESOPHAGEAL CANCER

PET has been used most extensively with FDG as a tracer in patients with esophageal cancer and the results have been very good. Only modest work has been performed with other PET tracers. Carbon-11 (^{11}C)-choline and FDG PET were compared for accuracy in 33 patients with biopsy-proven

esophageal carcinoma (16 patients with tumors classified as T1 and 17 patients with tumors classified as T2 through T4. Carbon-11-choline PET was more effective than FDG PET and CT in detecting very small metastases localized in the mediastinum. It was ineffective, however, in detecting metastases localized in the upper abdomen because of the normal uptake of ^{11}C-choline in the liver. These data were based on a small number of patients, but the authors believed PET with both tracers might be the most accurate approach for diagnosing esophageal carcinoma (28).

A follow-up paper evaluated 18 patients with esophageal carcinoma with both tracers. PET results were compared with surgical and histopathologic findings. FDG PET was able to detect all (100%) of the 16 malignant primary lesions, whereas ^{11}C-choline PET detected 73%. On a lesion basis, FDG PET detected 10 of 12 nonregional metastases (83% sensitivity), whereas ^{11}C-choline PET detected 5 of 12 (42% sensitivity). Standard uptake values were significantly higher for FDG (6.6 ± 3.5 vs. 5.5 ± 2.5 for ^{11}C-choline; $p = .04$). The authors concluded ^{11}C-choline PET was able to visualize esophageal carcinoma and its metastases but appeared to be inferior to FDG PET. The authors believed choline uptake in the liver, stomach wall, and upper abdomen made FDG the superior agent (29). Thus, FDG is the preferred agent for imaging esophageal carcinoma.

SUMMARY

PET with FDG is an accurate method for noninvasive detection of primary esophageal cancers, but endoscopy and EUS are more reliable methods for characterizing the size and local invasiveness of the untreated primary lesions. FDG PET is generally more specific than CT and is somewhat superior to CT in accuracy, but it can fail to detect small nodal metastases in many instances. EUS in skilled hands may be superior to PET for assessing locoregional periesophageal metastases to lymph nodes. FDG PET is clearly superior to other imaging methods for detecting systemic metastatic disease. Data to date on assessment of response to treatment suggest PET provides an early and quite accurate readout of the efficacy of therapy. PET is incapable of detecting residual microscopic disease at the conclusion of treatment due to resolution limitations. Tracers other than FDG, although of interest, have not demonstrated clear superiority to FDG in imaging this tumor.

REFERENCES

1. American Cancer Society. ACS cancer statistics, 2001. Available at: www.cancer.org.
2. Orringer MS. Esophageal surgery. In: Wells S, ed. *Scientific principles of surgery,* 1st ed. Philadelphia: Lippincott Williams & Wilkins.
3. Rice TW. Clinical staging of esophageal carcinoma. CT, EUS, and PET. *Chest Surg Clin N Am* Aug 2000;10(3):471–485.
4. Geh JI, Crellin AM, Glynne-Jones R. Preoperative (neoadjuvant) chemoradiotherapy in esophageal cancer. *Br J Surg* Mar 2001;88(3): 338–356.

5. Law S, Wong J. What is appropriate treatment for carcinoma of the thoracic esophagus? *World J Surg* Feb 2001;25(2):189–195.

6. Fleming ID, Cooper JS, Henson DE, eds. *AJCC staging manual,* 5th ed. Philadelphia: Lippincott–Raven Publishers, 1998:65–69.

7. Messman J, Schjlottmann K. Role of endoscopy in the staging of esophageal and gastric cancer. *Semin Surg Oncol* Mar 2001;20(2):78–81.

8. Bakheet SM, Amin T, Alia AG, et al. F-18 FDG uptake in benign esophageal disease. *Clin Nucl Med* Dec 1999;24(12):995–997.

9. Fukunaga T, Enomoto K, Okazumi S, et al. Analysis of glucose metabolism in patients with esophageal cancer by PET: estimation of hexokinase activity in the tumor and usefulness for clinical assessment using ^{18}F-fluorodeoxyglucose. *Nippon Geka Gakkai Zasshi* May 1994;95(5):317–325.

10. Flanagan FL, Dehdashti F, Siegel BA, et al. Staging of esophageal cancer with ^{18}F-fluorodeoxyglucose positron emission tomography. *AJR Am J Roentgenol* Feb 1997;168(2):417–424.

11. Kole AC, Plukker JT, Nieweg OE, et al. Positron emission tomography for staging of esophageal and gastroesophageal malignancy. *Br J Cancer* Aug 1998;78(4):521–527.

12. Couper GW, McAteer D, Wallis F, et al. Detection of response to chemotherapy using positron emission tomography in patients with esophageal and gastric cancer. *Br J Surg* Oct 1998;85(10):1403–1406.

13. Flamen P, Lerut A, Van Cutsem E, et al. Utility of positron emission tomography for the staging of patients with potentially operable esophageal carcinoma. *J Clin Oncol* 15 Sep 2000;18(18):3202–3210.

14. Weber WA, Ott K, Becker K, et al. Prediction of response to preoperative chemotherapy in adenocarcinomas of the esophagogastric junction by metabolic imaging. *J Clin Oncol* 15 Jun 2001;19(12):3058–3065.

15. Lerut T, Flamen P, Ectors N, et al. Histopathologic validation of lymph node staging with FDG-PET scan in cancer of the esophagus and gastroesophageal junction: a prospective study based on primary surgery with extensive lymphadenectomy. *Ann Surg* Dec 2000;232(6):743–752.

16. Meltzer CC, Luketich JD, Friedman D, et al. Whole-body FDG positron emission tomographic imaging for staging esophageal cancer comparison with computed tomography. *Clin Nucl Med* Nov 2000;25(11):882–887.

17. Choi JY, Lee KH, Shim YM, et al. Improved detection of individual nodal involvement in squamous cell carcinoma of the esophagus by FDG PET. *J Nucl Med* May 2000;41(5):808–815.

18. Rankin SC, Taylor H, Cook GJ, et al. Computed tomography and positron emission tomography in the pre-operative staging of esophageal carcinoma. *Clin Radiol* Sep 1998;53(9):659–665.

19. Block MI, Patterson GA, Sundaresan RS, et al. Improvement in staging of esophageal cancer with the addition of positron emission tomography. *Ann Thorac Surg* Sep 1997;64(3):770–776.

20. Luketich JD, Schauer PR, Meltzer CC, et al. Role of positron emission tomography in staging esophageal cancer. *Ann Thorac Surg* Sep 1997;64(3):765–769.

21. Luketich JD, Friedman DM, Weigel TL, et al. Evaluation of distant metastases in esophageal cancer: 100 consecutive positron emission tomography scans. *Ann Thorac Surg* Oct 1999;68(4):1133–1136.

22. Yeung H, Macapinlac H, Mazumdar M, et al. FDG PET in esophageal cancer: incremental value over computed tomography. *Clin Positron Imaging* 1999:255–260.

23. Skehan SJ, Brown AL, Thompson M, et al. Imaging features of primary and recurrent esophageal cancer at FDG PET. *Radiographics* May 2000;20(3):713–723.

24. Gambhir S, Czernin J, Schwimmer J, et al. A tabulated summary of the FDG PET literature. *J Nucl Med* 2001;42:1S–93S.

25. Flamen P, Lerut A, Van Cutsem E, et al. The utility of positron emission tomography for the diagnosis and staging of recurrent esophageal cancer. *J Thorac Cardiovasc Surg* Dec 2000;120(6):1085–1092.

26. Wahl RL, Zasadny KR, Helvie M, et al. Metabolic monitoring of breast cancer chemohormonotherapy using positron emission tomography (PET): initial evaluation. *J Clin Oncol* 1993;11(11):2101–2111.

27. Brucher BL, Weber W, Bauer M, et al. Neoadjuvant therapy of esophageal squamous cell carcinoma: response evaluation by positron emission tomography. *Ann Surg* Mar 2001;233(3):300–309.

28. Kobori O, Kirihara Y, Kosaka N, et al. Positron emission tomography of esophageal carcinoma using (^{11})C-choline and (^{18})F-fluorodeoxyglucose: a novel method of preoperative lymph node staging. *Cancer* 1 Nov 1999;86(9):1638–1648.

29. Jager PL, Que TH, Vaalburg WH, et al. Carbon-11 choline or FDG-PET for staging of esophageal cancer? *Eur J Nucl Med* Dec 2001;28(12):1845–1849.

CHAPTER 5.10

Colorectal, Pancreatic, and Hepatobiliary

Dominique Delbeke, William H. Martin, and Martin P. Sandler

COLORECTAL CARCINOMA

Colorectal carcinoma is the third most common noncutaneous malignancy in the United States, representing 13% of all malignancies. More than 133,000 new cases are detected annually, with almost 55,000 annual deaths.

FDG PET in the Preoperative Diagnosis of Colorectal Carcinoma

Only a small number of studies have been performed with ^{18}F-fluorodeoxyglucose positron emission tomography (FDG PET) in the preoperative diagnosis of colorectal carcinoma (1,2). In 48 patients with known or suspected primary colorectal carcinoma, FDG PET imaging identified all primary carcinomas (2). Neither FDG nor computed tomography (CT) was sensitive for detecting local lymph node involvement, with both methods missing about 70% of nodal metastases. FDG PET was, however, superior to CT for detecting liver metastases, with a sensitivity and specificity of 88% and 100%, respectively, compared with 38% and 97%, respectively, for CT. False-positive findings include abscesses, fistulas, diverticulitis, and occasionally adenomas. Although the sensitivity of FDG PET for the detection of a primary colon carcinoma is high, it presently plays no established role in the preoperative diagnosis or initial staging, except on occasion to define or identify hepatic or distant extrahepatic metastases.

Detection and Staging of Recurrent Colorectal Carcinoma

Although approximately 70% of patients are believed to be cured of their primary cancer with surgery, cancer will recur in one third of these patients within 2 years. In 25% of these patients, the recurrence will be isolated to a single site and be potentially curable by another surgical resection (3). For example, approximately 14,000 patients per year present with isolated liver metastases as their first recur-

rence, and 20% of these die with metastases exclusive to the liver. Hepatic resection may result in a cure in up to 25% of these patients, but the size and number of hepatic metastases and the presence of extrahepatic metastases all adversely affect prognosis. The presence of extrahepatic metastases is thought to represent a contraindication to hepatic resection. Accurate noninvasive detection of inoperable disease with imaging modalities plays a pivotal role in selecting patients who would benefit from partial hepatectomy.

Limitations of Conventional Modalities

Elevated circulating levels of carcinoembryonic antigen (CEA) occur in approximately two thirds of patients with colorectal carcinoma. Serial serum CEA determinations are used to monitor these patients for recurrence, and the sensitivity is 59% and the specificity is 84%. Imaging is necessary to localize the site of recurrence. Barium contrast studies can detect local recurrence with an accuracy in the range of 80% but are only 49% sensitive for overall recurrence (4). CT has been the conventional imaging modality used to localize recurrence. However, CT fails to demonstrate hepatic metastases in up to 7% of patients and underestimates the number of lobes involved in up to 33% of cases (5). Extrahepatic abdominal metastases are commonly missed on CT, and the differentiation of postsurgical changes from tumor recurrence is problematic. Among the patients with negative findings on CT, 50% are found to have nonresectable disease at the time of exploratory laparotomy. Superior mesenteric arterial CT portography is more sensitive (80% to 90%) than CT (70% to 80%) for the detection of hepatic metastases (6, 7,8) but has a high rate of false-positive findings, lowering the specificity and the positive predictive value (PPV) (9).

Although functional imaging does not replace anatomic imaging because of limitations related to resolution and lack of landmarks, functional imaging can be important in identifying and/or characterizing malignant lesions not seen or equivocal on anatomic imaging. Anatomic and functional images give complementary information, and in many circumstances, registration of both sets of images is necessary for correct interpretation. Registration is typically performed by visual comparison, but various computerized methods are being developed.

Functional imaging with single-photon emitters for the detection and staging of malignancies has well-known limitations. Radioimmunoscintigraphy is limited by difficulties with antigenic heterogeneity, modulation, and variable depiction of tumor and nontumor cells, as well as by physiologic hepatic and bowel activity. Moreover, due to slow blood pool clearance, images are not acquired for several days after injection, a major disadvantage. Two radiolabeled monoclonal antibodies are commercially available for imaging colorectal carcinoma. The B72.3 antibody (OncoScint) targets the tumor-associated glycoprotein TAG-72 and is labeled with indium-111 (^{111}In). CEA-Scan is a technetium-99m (^{99m}Tc)–labeled Fab' antibody fragment, targeting tumor cells that express CEA. Clinical trials have demonstrated that both antibodies are superior to CT for the detection of extrahepatic metastases, with a sensitivity of 55% to 74% compared with 32% to 57% for CT. However, due to high uptake of ^{111}In in normal liver parenchyma, radioimmunoscintigraphy is less sensitive than CT for the detection of liver metastases (41% to 63% for monoclonal antibodies vs. 64% to 84% for CT) (10).

FDG PET for Detection and Staging Recurrent Colorectal Carcinoma

Numerous studies have demonstrated an important role for FDG PET in identifying recurrences of colorectal carcinoma (11–27). A metaanalysis of 11 reports encompassing 281 patients determined that the overall sensitivity and specificity of FDG PET were 97% and 76%, respectively (28).

Valk et al. (19) compared the sensitivity and specificity of FDG PET with those of CT for specific anatomic locations and found that FDG PET was more sensitive than CT in all locations except the lung, where the two modalities were equivalent. The largest difference between FDG PET and CT was found in the abdomen, pelvis, and retroperitoneum, where more than one third of FDG PET–positive lesions were negative by CT. FDG PET was also more specific than CT at all sites except the retroperitoneum. Whole-body FDG PET is particularly useful for detecting distant metastatic disease, including abdominal nodal disease and pulmonary metastases (indeterminate lung nodules), as well as for differentiating postsurgical scarring from recurrent disease, all of which are problematic for CT (18,29).

Several studies have compared FDG PET with CT to differentiate scar from local recurrence (12,13,15,16,30,31) and others to identify hepatic metastases (16–19,30). For differentiation of posttherapy scar from local recurrence, FDG PET is clearly more accurate (90% to 100%) than CT (48% to 65%), and CT is often equivocal.

For hepatic metastases, overall, FDG PET is more accurate than CT. However, most of these studies suffered from a major limitation: FDG PET was performed prospectively while CT was reviewed retrospectively and performed at various institutions, resulting in variable quality. Vitola et al. (17) and Delbeke et al. (18) reported comparison of FDG PET with CT and CT portography for detecting both hepatic and extrahepatic metastases. CT portography, which is more invasive and more costly than PET or CT alone, has been regarded by many as the most reliable imaging modality for determining resectability of hepatic metastases. FDG PET has a higher accuracy (92%) than CT (78%) and CT portography (80%), despite the slightly higher sensitivity of CT portography (Fig. 5.10.1) (17).

In two small studies of patients with unexplained CEA elevation and no abnormal findings on conventional evaluation, including CT, FDG PET correctly demonstrated recurrent tumor in two thirds of the patients (19,32).

Impact of FDG PET on the Management of Patients with Colorectal Carcinoma

The greater sensitivity of FDG PET compared with CT in diagnosis and staging of recurrent tumor results from two factors. One is that early detection of abnormal tumor metabolism can detect changes before they become apparent by anatomic imaging. Another is that the global nature of whole-body FDG PET imaging permits diagnosis of tumor when it occurs in unusual and unexpected sites. Detection of metastases at unexpected sites usually leads to a change in management.

FDG PET makes it possible to avoid unnecessary surgery by demonstrating nonresectable tumor that is negative by CT in patients with known recurrence, and it allows earlier evaluation for treatment by diagnosing recurrence before it is detectable by CT. In a cumulative population of 532 patients, FDG PET imaging led to a change in management in 36% of the patients (16,18,19,26,27,29,31). In the study of Delbeke et al. (18), surgical management was altered by PET in 28% of patients, in one third by initiating surgery, and in two thirds by avoiding surgery (Figs. 5.10.2 and 5.10.3). The metaanalysis of the literature determined that FDG PET changed the management in 102 (29%) of 349 patients (28).

In a survey-based study of 60 referring oncologists, surgeons, and generalists, FDG PET had a major impact on the management of patients with colorectal cancer and contributed to a change in clinical stage in 42% (80% upstaged and 20% downstaged) and a change in the clinical management in more than 60%. As a result of the PET findings, physicians avoided major surgery in 41% of patients for whom surgery was the intended treatment (33).

Cost-effectiveness of FDG PET

Including FDG PET in the evaluation of patients with recurrent colorectal carcinoma has been shown to be cost-

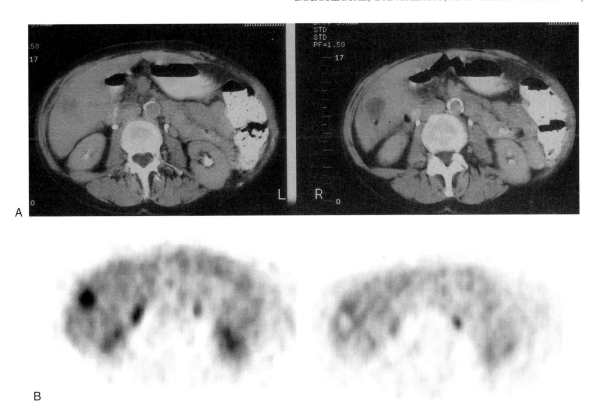

FIG. 5.10.1. A 69-year-old woman, with a history of colectomy for colon carcinoma and wedge resection of a hepatic metastasis 2 years prior, presented with a rising carcinoembryonic antigen level. **A:** The computed tomographic (CT) scan of the abdomen and pelvis was interpreted as no significant change in the postsurgical findings in the pelvis and the liver. **B:** Corresponding transaxial PET images with ^{18}F-fluorodeoxyglucose through the upper abdomen demonstrated a focus of increased uptake at the margin of resection (cold area) of the previous hepatic metastasis. Hepatic recurrence was confirmed at surgery and reexcised.

effective in studies using both a retrospective review of costs (19) and a decision-tree sensitivity analysis (34). In both studies, all cost calculations were based on Medicare reimbursement rates and a $1,800 cost for a PET scan. In a management algorithm in which recurrence at more than one site was treated as nonresectable, Valk et al. (19) evaluated cost savings in 78 patients undergoing preoperative staging of recurrent colorectal carcinoma. This study was limited to preoperative patients and demonstrated potential savings of $3,003 per patient resulting from diagnosis of nonresectable tumor by PET.

Gambhir et al. (34) used a quantitative decision-tree model, combined with sensitivity analysis, to evaluate cost effects in all patients with recurrent colorectal cancer. The conventional strategy, CEA levels and CT, for the detection of recurrence and determination of resectability was compared with combining this strategy with FDG PET for all patients presenting with suspected recurrence. The assumptions included a prevalence of resectable disease of 3%, a sensitivity and specificity of 65% and 45%, respectively, for CT, and 90% and 85%, respectively, for PET. The conventional strategy plus PET showed an incremental saving of $220 per patient.

Based on these data, patients referred for evaluation of potentially resectable recurrent colorectal carcinoma should undergo FDG PET imaging preoperatively. If limited hepatic metastases are seen, CT portography should be performed to evaluate their resectability and the possible presence of additional small metastases that are below PET resolution. If extrahepatic foci of uptake are present on the PET images (with or without liver metastases), a CT of the corresponding region of the body should be performed for anatomic correlation. This approach allows more accurate selection of the patients who will benefit from surgery and more importantly, patients who will not benefit from laparotomy and liver resection because of unsuspected or unrecognized extrahepatic disease.

Limitations of FDG PET Imaging

Tumor detectability depends on both the size of the lesion and the degree of uptake. False-negative lesions can be due to partial volume averaging, leading to an underestimation of the uptake in small lesions (smaller than 1 cm) or in necrotic lesions with a thin viable rim, classifying these lesions as benign instead of malignant. In the experience of

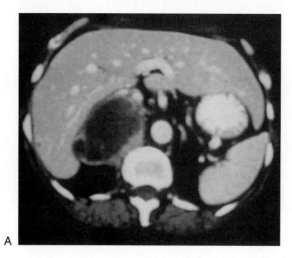

A

FIG. 5.10.2. A 57-year-old woman with a history of colectomy for colon carcinoma presented with rising carcinoembryonic levels. **A:** A computed tomographic (CT) scan demonstrated a large cystic lesion arising from the region of the right adrenal gland, and the patient was referred for surgical evaluation. **B:** Transaxial ¹⁸F-fluorodeoxyglucose positron emission tomography images through the chest and abdomen demonstrated a large area of uptake with a hypermetabolic necrotic center in the region of the right adrenal corresponding to the lesion seen on the CT scan. Four additional foci of uptake are seen: one at the base of the neck on the left, a second in the mediastinum, a third in the right lung field posteriorly, and a fourth adjacent to the right adrenal metastasis **(C, D)**.

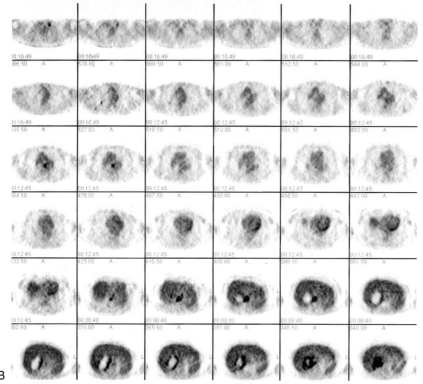

B

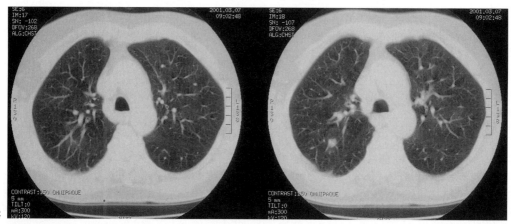

C

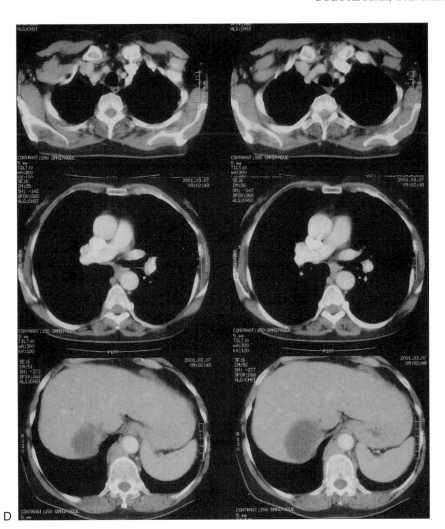

FIG. 5.10.2. *Continued.* A follow-up chest CT demonstrated a 1-cm lung nodule in the mid right lung field posteriorly **(C, bottom right)**, an 8-mm lymph node at the base of the left neck **(D, top left)**, a 1-cm lymph node anterior to the esophagus in the mediastinum **(D, middle row)**, and a large retrocrural lymph node **(D, bottom row)**. The surgery was canceled.

Vitola et al. (17), for example, approximately half of the hepatic lesions that were smaller than 1 cm had FDG uptake that could be easily identified visually.

The sensitivity of FDG PET for the detection of mucinous adenocarcinoma is lower than that for nonmucinous adenocarcinoma (41% to 58% vs. 92%), probably because of the relative hypocellularity of the mucinous tumors (35,36).

In view of the known high uptake of FDG by activated macrophages, it is not surprising that inflamed tissue demonstrates elevated FDG activity. Mild to moderate FDG activity seen along recent incisions, infected incisions, biopsy sites, drainage tubing, and catheters, as well as colostomy sites can lead to errors in interpretation if the history is not known. Some inflammatory lesions, particularly granulomatous ones, can accumulate significant amounts of FDG and can be mistaken for malignancies. This includes inflammatory bowel disease.

FDG activity is usually present in the gastrointestinal tract and can sometimes be difficult to distinguish from a malignant lesion, but the linear pattern of uptake, characteristic of bowel, is usually easy to recognize and is best seen on coronal views.

Monitoring Therapy of Colorectal Carcinoma

Two studies have shown that FDG PET can differentiate local recurrence from scarring after radiation therapy (12, 13). However, increased FDG uptake immediately after radiation may be due to inflammatory changes and is not always associated with residual tumor. The time course of postirradiation FDG activity has not been studied systematically; it is, however, generally accepted that FDG activity present 6 months after completion of radiation therapy most likely represents tumor recurrence.

Preliminary reports suggest that the response to chemotherapy in patients with hepatic metastases can be predicted with PET. It may be possible to separate responders from nonresponders after 4 to 5 weeks of chemotherapy with fluorouracil by measuring FDG uptake before and during therapy (37). Regional therapy to the liver by chemoembolization can also be monitored with FDG PET imaging. FDG uptake decreases in responding lesions. The presence of residual uptake in some lesions can help in guiding further regional therapy (38). A pilot study of 15 patients with unresected primary rectal carcinoma demonstrated that FDG PET imag-

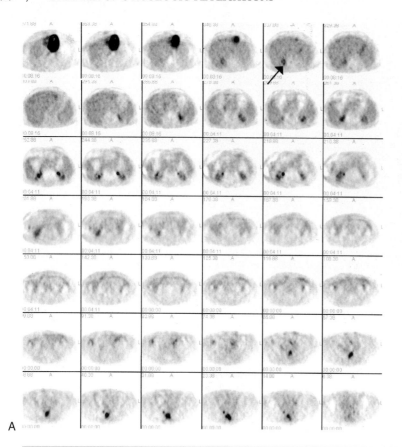

A

FIG. 5.10.3. A 57-year-old man was found to have a liver metastasis during surgical exploration at the time of colectomy for colon carcinoma. He was referred 3 months later for surgical evaluation of his liver metastasis. The ^{18}F-fluorodeoxyglucose positron emission tomography images **(A and B)** demonstrated a focus of uptake in the **(A)** right lobe of the liver posteriorly (*arrow*) corresponding to the known metastasis. Intense normal uptake is seen in the heart and gastrointestinal tract. A second focus of uptake was seen in the sacrum (best localized on the sagittal image) **(B)** (*arrow*), indicating a skeletal metastasis that was confirmed by magnetic resonance imaging. The hepatectomy was canceled.

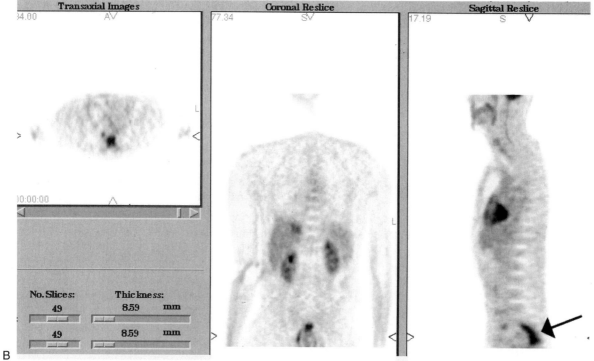

B

ing adds incremental information for assessing the response to preoperative radiation and 5-fluorouracil–based chemotherapy (39).

Summary: Colorectal Cancer

Evaluation of patients with known or suspected recurrent colorectal carcinoma is now an accepted indication for FDG PET imaging. FDG PET does not replace imaging modalities such as CT for preoperative anatomic evaluation but is indicated as the initial test for diagnosis and staging of recurrence and for preoperative staging of known recurrence that is considered to be resectable. PET imaging is valuable for (a) differentiation of posttreatment changes from recurrent tumor, (b) differentiation of benign from malignant lymph nodes, (c) evaluating a rising serum CEA level in the absence of a known source, (d) increasing the specificity of structural imaging when an equivocal lesion is detected, and (e) monitoring therapy. Addition of FDG PET to the evaluation of these patients reduces overall treatment cost by accurately identifying patients who will and will not benefit from surgical procedures.

PANCREATIC CARCINOMA

Pancreatic ductal adenocarcinoma is the fourth leading cause of death in the United States and is increasing in incidence. The preoperative diagnosis, staging, and treatment of pancreatic cancer remain challenging.

Limitations of Conventional Imaging Modalities

The suspicion for pancreatic cancer is often raised by sonographic or CT findings, including the presence of a low-attenuation pancreatic mass and dilatation of the pancreatic duct and/or biliary tree. CT is the most common diagnostic imaging modality used in the preoperative diagnosis of pancreatic cancer. CT is also important to assess vascular involvement and invasion of adjacent organs. In a multicenter trial (40), the diagnostic accuracy of CT for staging and resectability was 73%, with a PPV for nonresectability of 90%, but more recent studies have reported accuracy rates of 85% to 95%, likely related to improvements in CT technology (41,42).

Unfortunately, interpretation of the CT scan is sometimes difficult in the setting of mass-forming pancreatitis or questionable findings such as enlargement of the pancreatic head without definite signs of malignancy or a discrete mass (43, 44). The diagnosis of locoregional lymph node metastases is also difficult with CT, because they often are small. In addition, small hepatic metastases (smaller than 1 cm) cannot reliably be differentiated from cysts (45). Therefore, the reported negative predictive value for nonresectability is less than 30%. Despite recent technical improvements in magnetic resonance imaging (MRI), including magnetic reso-

nance cholangiopancreatography (MRCP), the diagnostic performance of MRI remains similar to that of CT (46–49).

Endoscopic ultrasound offers the possibility of tissue diagnosis with fine-needle aspiration (FNA) biopsy, but the field of view is limited (50–52). The accuracy of endoscopic retrograde cholangiopancreatography (ERCP) is 80% to 90% in differentiating benign from malignant pancreatic masses, including the differentiation of tumor from chronic pancreatitis because of the high degree of resolution of ductal structures. The limitations include false-negative findings when the tumor does not originate from the main duct, a 10% rate of technical failure, and up to 8% morbidity due to iatrogenic pancreatitis. The main advantages are the possibilities of FNA biopsy and interventional procedures. Although FNA biopsy may provide a tissue diagnosis with a high degree of accuracy, this technique suffers from significant sampling error (53,54), with a false-negative incidence of 8% to 17%.

The difficulty in making a preoperative diagnosis is associated with two types of adverse outcomes. First, less aggressive surgeons may abort attempted resection due to a lack of tissue diagnosis. This is borne out by the significant rate of "reoperative" pancreaticoduodenectomy performed at major referral centers (55–57). A second type of adverse outcome, generated by failure to obtain a preoperative diagnosis, occurs when more aggressive surgeons inadvertently resect benign disease. This is particularly notable in those patients who present with suspected malignancy without an associated mass on CT scan. This has been reported to occur in up to 55% of patients in some series (58).

FDG PET in the Preoperative Diagnosis of Pancreatic Carcinoma

To avoid these adverse outcomes, metabolic imaging with FDG PET can be used to improve the accuracy of the preoperative diagnosis of pancreatic carcinoma. Most malignancies, including pancreatic carcinoma, demonstrate increased glucose utilization due to an increased number of glucose transporter (GLUT) proteins and increased hexokinase and phosphofructokinase activity (59,60). There is recent evidence that the overexpression of GLUTs by malignant pancreatic cells contributes to the increased uptake of FDG by these neoplasms (61,62). In 11 studies (63–73), the performance of FDG PET to differentiate benign from malignant lesions ranged from 85% to 100% for sensitivity, 67% to 99% for specificity, and 85% to 93% for accuracy. In most of these studies, the accuracy of FDG PET imaging was superior to that of CT. For example, in the study of Delbeke et al. (73), the sensitivity and specificity of FDG PET imaging was 92% and 85%, respectively, compared with 65% and 62%, respectively, for CT.

The sensitivity of CT imaging improves with the size of the lesion, but the sensitivity of FDG PET is not as dependent on lesion size (74). However, these studies suffer from biases; the acquisition of the CT data is often not performed prospectively, and the quality of the CT images may be variable among different institutions. Together, these series support the conclusion that FDG PET imaging may represent a useful adjunctive study in the evaluation of patients with suspected pancreatic cancer.

Limitations of FDG PET Imaging

As with any imaging modality, FDG PET has limitations in the evaluation of pancreatic cancer. The high incidence of glucose intolerance and diabetes exhibited by patients with pancreatic pathology represents a potential limitation of this modality in the diagnosis of pancreatic cancer. Elevated serum glucose levels result in decreased FDG uptake in tumors due to competitive inhibition; low standard uptake values (SUVs) with false-negative FDG PET scans have been noted in hyperglycemic patients. Several studies have reported a lower sensitivity in hyperglycemic compared with euglycemic patients (66,70,73). For example, in a study of 106 patients with a disease prevalence of 70% (70), FDG PET had a sensitivity of 98% in a subgroup of euglycemic patients versus 63% in hyperglycemic patients. This has led some investigators to suggest that the SUV be corrected according to serum glucose level (75–78).

In the studies of Delbeke et al. (73) and Diederichs et al. (78), the presence of elevated serum glucose levels and/or diabetes mellitus may have contributed to false-negative interpretations; but correction of the SUV for serum glucose level has not significantly improved the sensitivity of FDG PET in the diagnosis of pancreatic carcinoma. The true impact of serum glucose levels on the accuracy of FDG PET in pancreatic cancer and other neoplasms remains somewhat controversial, although it is clear that elevated serum glucose levels can reduce tumor FDG uptake significantly.

False-negative study results may also occur when the tumor diameter is less than 1 cm (i.e., small ampullary carcinoma). Ampullary carcinomas arise from the ampulla of Vater and have a better prognosis than pancreatic carcinoma because they cause biliary obstruction and are diagnosed earlier in the course of the disease. The detection rate with FDG imaging is only 70% to 80%, probably because of their smaller size at the time of clinical presentation.

Both glucose and FDG are substrates for cellular mediators of inflammation. Some benign inflammatory lesions, including chronic and acute pancreatitis with or without abscess formation, can accumulate FDG and result in false-positive interpretations on PET images (66,69,79,80). Poststenotic pancreatitis can also obscure FDG uptake in the tumor itself. False-positive study results are more frequent in patients with elevated C-reactive protein (CRP) and/or acute pancreatitis, with a specificity as low as 50% (80,81). Therefore, screening for acute inflammatory disease with serum CRP has been recommended.

Preliminary reports suggest that the degree of FDG uptake has prognostic value. Nakata et al. (82) noted a correlation between SUV and survival in 14 patients with pancreatic

adenocarcinoma. Patients with an SUV higher than 3.0 had a mean survival of 5 months, compared with 14 months in those with an SUV lower than 3.0. In a multivariate analysis of 52 patients with pancreatic carcinoma (83), the median survival of patients with an SUV higher than 6.1 was 5 months, compared with 9 months for patients with an SUV lower than 6.1.

FDG PET imaging is complementary to CT in the evaluation of patients with pancreatic masses or in whom the diagnosis of pancreatic carcinoma is suspected. In view of the probable decreased sensitivity seen in patients with hyperglycemia, the acquisition of PET images should be performed under controlled metabolic conditions and in the absence of acute inflammatory abdominal disease.

FDG PET for Staging Pancreatic Carcinoma

Stage II disease is characterized by extrapancreatic extension (T stage), stage III by lymph node involvement (N stage), and stage IV by distant metastases (M stage). T staging can only be evaluated with anatomic imaging modalities, which demonstrate the relationship between the tumor, adjacent organs, and vascular structures. Functional imaging modalities cannot replace anatomic imaging in the assessment of local tumor resectability.

FDG imaging is not superior to helical CT for N staging but is more accurate than CT for M staging. In the study of Delbeke et al. (73), metastases were diagnosed both on CT and on PET in 10 of 21 patients with stage IV disease, but PET demonstrated hepatic metastases not identified or equivocal on CT and/or distant metastases unsuspected clinically in seven additional patients (33%). In four patients (19%), neither CT nor PET imaging showed evidence of metastases, but surgical exploration revealed carcinomatosis in three and a small liver metastasis in one patient. FDG PET is sensitive for detection of hepatic metastases, but false-positive findings have been reported in the liver of patients with dilated bile ducts and inflammatory granulomas (84).

Impact of FDG PET on the Management of Patients with Pancreatic Carcinoma

The rate at which FDG PET may lead to alterations in clinical management clearly depends on the specific therapeutic philosophy employed by the evaluating surgeon. In the study of Delbeke et al. (73), the surgeons advocated pancreaticoduodenectomy only for those patients with potentially curable pancreatic cancer. They also took an aggressive approach to resection, including en bloc retroperitoneal lymphadenectomy and selective resection of the superior mesenteric-portal vein confluence when necessary. Most patients with nonmalignant biliary strictures were managed without resection. In that series of 65 patients, the application of FDG PET imaging, in addition to CT, altered the surgical management in 41% of the patients, 27% by detecting CT-occult pancreatic carcinoma, and 14% by identifying unsuspected distant metastases, or by clarifying the benign nature of lesions equivocal on CT (73).

FDG PET for Monitoring Therapy and Detection of Recurrent Pancreatic Carcinoma

Preliminary studies suggest that neoadjuvant chemoradiation improves the resectability rate and survival of patients with pancreatic carcinoma (85,86). A pilot study determined that FDG PET imaging might be useful for the assessment of tumor response to neoadjuvant therapy and the evaluation of suspected recurrent disease after resection (74). Nine patients underwent FDG PET imaging before and after neoadjuvant chemoradiation therapy. FDG PET successfully predicted histologic evidence of chemoradiation-induced tumor necrosis in the four patients who demonstrated at least a 50% reduction in tumor SUV after chemoradiation. Among these patients, none showed a measurable reduction in tumor diameter, as assessed by CT. This is consistent with past data that showed a more rapid drop in tumor glucose metabolism levels than the changes in tumor size. The four patients who had FDG PET evidence of tumor response went on to successful resection, all showing 20% to 80% tumor necrosis in the resected specimen. Three patients showed stable FDG uptake and two showed increasing FDG uptake indicative of tumor progression. Among the two patients with progressive disease demonstrated by FDG PET, one showed tumor progression on CT, and the other demonstrated stable disease. Among the five patients who showed no response by FDG PET, the disease could be subsequently resected in only two, and only one patient who underwent resection showed evidence of chemoradiation-induced necrosis in the resected specimen.

Another pilot study suggests that the absence of FDG uptake at 1 month after chemotherapy is an indicator of improved survival versus patients in whom persistent uptake is present (87). Definitive conclusions regarding the role of FDG PET in assessing treatment response will obviously require evaluation in much larger populations of patients. However, given the poor track record of CT in assessing histologic response to neoadjuvant chemoradiation, the potential utility of FDG PET in this capacity deserves further investigation.

Most reports concerning the clinical utilization of FDG PET imaging for pancreatic malignancy have emphasized the identification of recurrent nodal or distant metastatic disease. In a preliminary study (74), eight patients were evaluated for possible recurrence because of either indeterminate CT findings or a rise in serum tumor marker levels (Fig. 5.10.4). All were noted to have significant new regions of FDG uptake: four in the surgical bed and four in new hepatic metastases. In all patients, metastases or local recurrence was confirmed pathologically or clinically. Another study of 19 patients concluded that FDG PET added important incremental information in 50% of the patients, resulting in a

change of therapeutic procedure (88). This included patients with elevated serum tumor marker levels but no findings on anatomic imaging. Therefore, FDG PET may be particularly useful when (a) CT identifies an indistinct region of change in the bed of the resected pancreas that is difficult to differentiate from postoperative or postradiation fibrosis, (b) for the evaluation of new hepatic lesions that may be too small to biopsy, and (c) in patients with rising serum tumor marker levels and a negative conventional workup. Given the poor prognosis of pancreatic cancer, it is not expected that large differences in patient outcome will result from such studies. However, it is probable that patients will benefit by giving the most appropriate treatment while eliminating treatments viewed as unlikely to be effective.

Summary: Pancreatic Cancer

FDG PET imaging appears to be a sensitive and specific adjunct to CT when applied to the preoperative diagnosis of pancreatic carcinoma, particularly in patients with suspected pancreatic cancer in whom CT fails to identify a discrete tumor mass. By providing preoperative documentation of pancreatic malignancy in these patients, laparotomy may be undertaken with a curative intent, and the risk of aborting resection due to diagnostic uncertainty is minimized. FDG PET imaging is also useful in the clarification of CT-occult metastatic disease, allowing nontherapeutic resection to be avoided altogether in this group of patients. As is true with other neoplasms, FDG PET holds promise in the restaging of patients posttherapy.

HEPATOBILIARY TUMORS

In the United States, metastases to the liver from various primary neoplasms occur 20 times more often than primary hepatic carcinoma and are often multifocal. Although many tumors may metastasize to the liver, the most common primaries producing liver metastases are colorectal, gastric, pancreatic, lung, and breast carcinoma. Ninety percent of malignant primary liver tumors are epithelial in origin: hepatocellular carcinoma and cholangiocarcinoma. Mesenchymal tumors such as angiosarcomas, epithelioid angioendothelioma, and primary lymphoma are relatively rare malignant tumors that can affect the liver.

Hepatocellular carcinoma arises from the malignant transformation of hepatocytes and is common in the setting of chronic liver disease such as viral hepatitis, cirrhosis, or in patients exposed to carcinogens. Hepatocellular carcinoma most frequently metastasizes to regional lymph nodes, lung, and the skeleton.

Cholangiocarcinomas arise from biliary cells and represent only 10% of the epithelial tumors. About 20% of patients who develop cholangiocarcinomas have predisposing conditions, including sclerosing cholangitis, ulcerative colitis, Caroli disease, choledochal cyst, infestation by the fluke

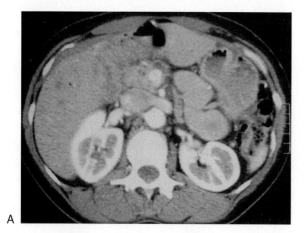

FIG. 5.10.4. A 50-year-old woman with a history of Whipple procedure for pancreatic carcinoma 2 years prior presented with back pain and epigastric pain. A computed tomography (CT) scan of the abdomen **(A)** was interpreted as postsurgical changes in the region of the pancreatic head. The coronal **(B)** and transaxial **(C)** ^{18}F-fluorodeoxyglucose (FDG) positron emission tomography images demonstrated a focus of uptake in the region of the head of the pancreas, indicating local recurrence and a focus of uptake in the left lung field consistent with a pulmonary metastasis. The focus at the base of the neck on the midline is due FDG uptake in the laryngeal muscles related to vocalization during FDG uptake phase.

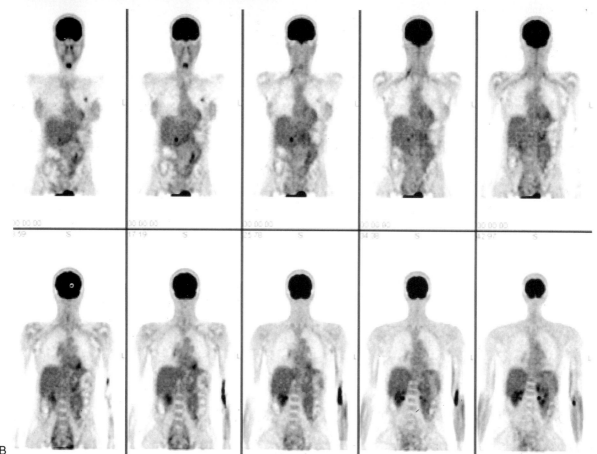

Clonorchis sinensis, cholelithiasis, or exposure to Thorotrast among others.

Approximately 50% of cholangiocarcinomas occur in the liver and the other 50% are extrahepatic. These tumors are often unresectable at the time of diagnosis and have a poor prognosis. Intrahepatic cholangiocarcinomas can be further subdivided in two categories: the peripheral type arising from the interlobular biliary duct and the hilar type (Klatskin tumor) arising from the main hepatic duct or its bifurcation. In addition, they can develop in three different morphologic types: infiltrating sclerosing lesions (most common), exo-phytic lesions, and polypoid intraluminal masses. Malignant tumors arising along the extrahepatic bile ducts are usually diagnosed early, because they cause biliary obstruction. Tumors arising near the hilum of the liver have a worse prognosis because of their direct extension into the liver. Distant metastases occur late in the disease and most often affect the lungs.

Gallbladder carcinoma is uncommon and is associated with cholelithiasis in 75% of the cases. These tumors are insidious, unsuspected clinically, and usually discovered at surgery or incidentally in the surgical specimen. They fre-

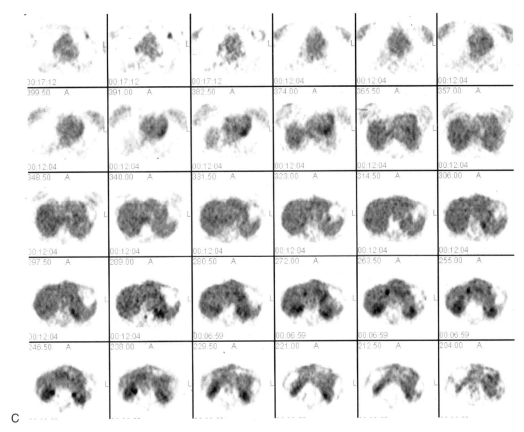

FIG. 5.10.4. *Continued.*

quently spread to the liver and can perforate the wall of the gallbladder metastasizing to the abdomen. Distant metastases may occur in the lungs, pleura, and diaphragm.

Conventional Imaging Modalities for Evaluation of Hepatic Lesions

The diagnostic issues addressed by conventional imaging include early detection of these tumors, differentiation from cirrhosis and other benign liver lesions, and evaluation of the response to therapy. Screening for hepatic lesions is commonly performed with transabdominal ultrasound. Ultrasound can detect lesions as small as 1 cm in diameter but is operator-dependent and inherently two-dimensional, and it suffers from poor specificity. Hepatic metastases can be hypoechoic, hyperechoic, or cystic or can have mixed echogenicity; isoechoic metastases are undetected. CT is the conventional method used for assessing the liver at many institutions and intravenous contrast is useful for the detection of liver metastases. Metastases may be better seen during the arterial or portal venous phase after contrast injection depending of the vascularity of the tumor. The development of the helical technique has resulted in a sensitivity comparable to that of MRI, although CT portography remains the most sensitive technique for the detection of small lesions.

Because hepatocellular carcinoma is often associated with elevated serum levels of α-fetoprotein (AFP), serum AFP measurements and ultrasound are the conventional methods for screening patients at risk for hepatocellular carcinoma. Differentiation of low-grade hepatocellular carcinomas from hepatic adenoma can be difficult even on core biopsy. Although a capsule is often present in small hepatocellular carcinomas, it is seldom seen in large ones. Invasion of the portal vein is often present, particularly with large hepatocellular carcinomas. Hepatocellular carcinoma can undergo hemorrhage and necrosis or demonstrate fatty metamorphosis. The presence of these characteristics on imaging studies is suggestive of hepatocellular carcinoma but requires high-resolution techniques for successful detection.

Dynamic multiphase gadolinium-enhanced MRI may be superior to dual-phase spiral CT for characterizing hepatocellular carcinoma (89). Although large lesions (more than 3 cm) may be visualized by CT and ultrasound, with a sensitivity from 80% to 90%, smaller lesions may be difficult to distinguish from the surrounding hepatic parenchyma, particularly in patients with cirrhosis and regenerating nodules. The sensitivity for small hepatocellular carcinomas is about 50%. CT portography is the most sensitive technique for detection of lesions smaller than 1 cm. Gallium-67 (^{67}Ga) or thallium-201 (^{201}Tl) scintigraphy may be helpful to identify hepatocellular carcinoma if the findings on other imaging modalities are equivocal. Seventy percent to 90% of hepatocellular carcinomas have ^{67}Ga or ^{201}Tl uptake greater than the liver, and ^{67}Ga scintigraphy has been used in conjunction with a sulfur colloid scan to differentiate hepatocellular carcinoma from regenerating nodules in cirrhotic patients (90).

Fibrolamellar carcinoma, a low-grade malignant tumor representing 6% to 25% of hepatocellular carcinomas, occurs in a younger population of patients without underlying cirrhosis. An avascular scar that may contain calcifications is characteristic. In contrast, avascular scar without calcifications characterizes focal nodular hyperplasia. MRI and single-photon emission computed tomography (SPECT) scintigraphy with radiolabeled red blood cells, ^{99m}Tc-sulfur colloid, or ^{99m}Tc-dimethyl iminodiacetic acid agents can help to further characterize some lesions (hemangioma, focal nodular hyperplasia, and adenoma).

Cholangiocarcinomas are often not seen on CT because they are small and isodense. When this is the case (most hilar tumors and 25% of peripheral tumors), the level of biliary ductal dilatation helps determine the location of the tumor. When the tumor is visible on CT, it most often appears as a nonspecific hypodense mass. Delayed retention of contrast material is characteristic and must be differentiated from cavernous hemangioma. A central scar or calcification is seen in 25% to 30% of the cases. On MRI, these tumors are usually hypointense on T1-weighted and hyperintense on T2-weighted images. The central scar is best seen as a hypointense structure on the T2-weighted images. After gadolinium administration, there is early peripheral enhancement with progressive concentric enhancement, as with CT. MRI may demonstrate tumors not seen on CT and should be used as a problem-solving tool (89).

MRCP used as an adjunct to conventional MRI may provide additional information regarding the extension of hilar cholangiocarcinoma for example. If MRCP can establish the resectability of the tumor, the patient may undergo immediate surgery and be spared a percutaneous cholangiogram (PTC) and biliary drainage procedure. PTC or ERCP is usually not indicated for peripheral tumors but can demonstrate hilar cholangiocarcinoma in most cases and is better than CT for evaluating the intraductal extent of the tumor.

PTC and ERCP are the procedures of choice for demonstrating the infiltrating and/or sclerosing type of cholangiocarcinoma. Typically, a malignant stricture tapers irregularly and is associated with proximal ductal dilatation, although it is difficult to differentiate from sclerosing cholangitis, one of the preexisting conditions. Some tumors are seen as intraluminal defects, but mucin, blood clots, calculi, an air bubble, or biliary sludge may have a similar appearance. ERCP/PTC is often performed at the same time as a biliary drainage procedure.

FDG PET in the Diagnosis of Malignant Hepatic Lesions

Differentiated hepatocytes normally have a relatively high glucose-6-phosphatase activity, which allows dephosphory-lation of intracellular FDG and its egress from the liver. Although experimental studies have shown that glycogenesis decreases and glycolysis increases during carcinogenesis, the accumulation of FDG in hepatocellular carcinoma is variable due to varying degrees of activity of the enzyme glucose-6-phosphatase in these tumors (91,92). It has been postulated that FDG PET evaluation of liver tumors, particularly hepatocellular carcinomas, will require dynamic imaging with blood sampling and kinetic analysis. Kinetic analysis is cumbersome to perform clinically and cannot be performed over the entire body, thus preventing staging. Studies using kinetic analysis have shown that the phosphorylation kinetic constant (k_3) is elevated in virtually all malignant tumors including hepatocellular carcinoma. The dephosphorylation kinetic constant (k_4) is low in metastatic lesions and in cholangiocarcinomas, resulting in intratumoral accumulation of FDG. But k_4 is similar to k_3 for hepatocellular carcinomas that do not accumulate FDG (93–95). Therefore, hepatocellular carcinomas are hypermetabolic, but many do not accumulate FDG due to their inability to retain FDG intracellularly.

There are three patterns of uptake for hepatocellular carcinoma: FDG uptake higher than, equal to, or lower than liver background (55%, 30%, and 15%, respectively). FDG PET detects only 50% to 70% of hepatocellular carcinomas (Fig. 5.10.5) but has a sensitivity of more than 90% for all other primaries (cholangiocarcinoma and sarcoma) and all metastatic tumors to the liver (96,97). All benign tumors, including focal nodular hyperplasia, adenoma, regenerating nodules, cysts, and hemangiomas demonstrate FDG uptake at the same level as normal liver, except for rare abscesses with granulomatous inflammation. In addition, a correlation has been found between the degree of FDG uptake, including both the SUV and k_3, and the grade of malignancy (95,96).

FDG imaging may have prognostic significance in the evaluation of patients with hepatocellular carcinoma. Hepatocellular carcinomas that accumulate FDG tend to be moderately to poorly differentiated and are associated with markedly elevated AFP levels (98,99). However, FDG PET has limited value for the differential diagnosis of focal liver lesions in patients with chronic hepatitis C virus infection, because of the low sensitivity for the detection of hepatocellular carcinoma and the high prevalence of this tumor in that population of patients (100).

There is preliminary evidence that FDG PET imaging may be useful in the diagnosis and management of small cholangiocarcinomas in patients with sclerosing cholangitis (101). It is more helpful in patients with nodular cholangiocarcinomas than in those with the infiltrating variety. False-positive findings can be seen in patients with biliary stents, probably related to inflammatory changes, as well as in patients with acute cholangitis.

FDG PET for Staging Hepatobiliary Tumors

In patients with hepatocellular carcinoma that accumulate FDG, PET imaging is able to detect unsuspected regional

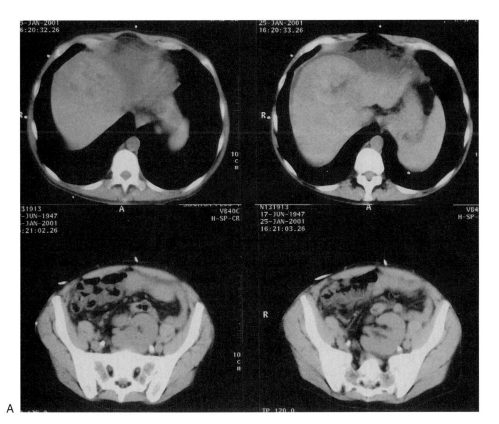

A

FIG. 5.10.5. A 53-year-old man with hepatic cirrhosis presented with right upper quadrant pain. The abdominal computed tomography (CT) scan **(A)** showed a 7-cm mass in the left lobe of the liver. Biopsy of the lesion demonstrated hepatocellular carcinoma, and the patient was referred for staging. The coronal ^{18}F-fluorodeoxyglucose positron emission tomography (FDG PET) images **(B)** demonstrated FDG uptake in the hepatic mass with central photopenia, indicating central necrosis. No focal extrahepatic uptake was seen to indicate metastases. The patient was treated with regional chemoembolization, and the therapeutic results were to be monitored with FDG PET imaging. In addition, the FDG PET images demonstrated the right kidney in the normal anatomic position and an incidental finding of a left pelvic kidney, which was seen on a follow-up pelvic CT **(A, bottom row)**.

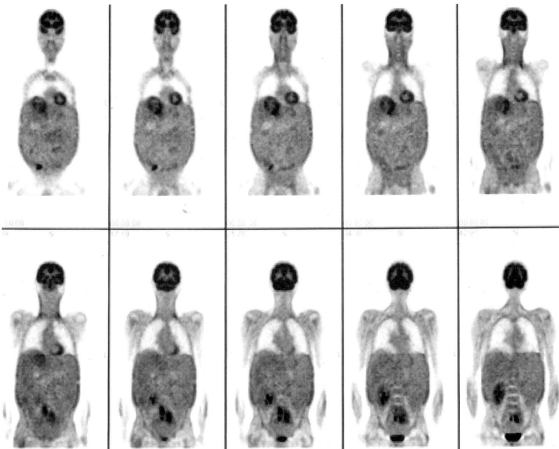

B

and distant metastases, as with other tumors. In some cases, FDG PET is the only imaging modality that can demonstrate the tumor and its metastases. In a series of 23 patients with hepatocellular carcinoma who underwent FDG PET imaging in an attempt to identify extrahepatic metastases, 13 (57%) of the 23 patients had increased uptake in the primary tumor and 4 (31%) of those 13 had extrahepatic metastases demonstrated by FDG PET images (102).

FDG PET for Monitoring Therapy and Detection of Recurrent Hepatobiliary Tumors

Because most patients with hepatocellular carcinoma have advanced-stage tumors and/or underlying cirrhosis with impaired hepatic reserve, surgical resection is often not possible. Therefore, other treatment strategies have been developed, including hepatic arterial chemoembolization, systemic chemotherapy, surgical cryoablation, ethanol ablation, radiofrequency ablation, and in selected cases, liver transplantation. In patients treated with hepatic arterial chemoembolization, FDG PET is more accurate than lipiodol retention on CT in predicting the presence of residual viable tumor. Due to the associated inflammatory response, it is recommended that FDG imaging be delayed for at least several weeks after ablative therapy. The presence of residual uptake in some lesions can help in guiding further regional therapy (103–105). It is expected but not yet demonstrated that FDG PET may surpass CT in determining the success of other ablative procedures in these patients.

Unsuspected gallbladder carcinoma is discovered incidentally in 1% of routine cholecystectomies. At present, most cholecystectomies are performed laparoscopically, and occult gallbladder carcinoma found after laparoscopic cholecystectomy has been associated with reports of gallbladder carcinoma seeding of laparoscopic trocar sites (106,107). Increased FDG uptake has been demonstrated in gallbladder carcinoma (108) and has been helpful in identifying recurrence in the area of the incision when CT could not differentiate scar tissue from malignant recurrence (109).

Summary: Hepatobiliary Cancers

Most malignant hepatic tumors, primary or secondary, are FDG avid, and most benign processes accumulate FDG to the same level as normal hepatic parenchyma and they are not detected with PET. Approximately one third of hepatocellular carcinomas do not accumulate FDG and are false-negatives. Therefore FDG imaging is not recommended for evaluation of focal hepatic lesions in patients with chronic hepatitis C or for screening for hepatocellular carcinoma in a population at increased risk. Small ampullary carcinoma and cholangiocarcinoma of the infiltrating type can be false-negative as well. Metastases from mucinous colorectal carcinomas and from neuroendocrine tumors such as carcinoid may also be false-negative. Foci of inflammation along biliary stents and granulomatous abscesses, including foci of acute cholangitis, accumulate FDG and can be misinterpreted as malignant. FDG imaging can detect unsuspected metastases and aid in monitoring therapy in patients with malignant tumors accumulating FDG, including hepatocellular carcinomas and cholangiocarcinomas.

COST AND REIMBURSEMENT ISSUES

Until recently, implementation of clinical PET was hindered by the high cost of PET systems, the need for access to a cyclotron and a support laboratory for FDG production. The high maintenance and operating expenses of scanners and cyclotrons, as well as the lack of reimbursement for clinical procedures by third-party payers, are other factors involved.

The recent increase in installation of cyclotrons and development of commercial FDG distribution centers has increased FDG availability, thereby greatly reducing radiopharmaceutical expense. The largest number of cyclotrons for medical radionuclide production exists in the United States (n = 66), followed by Europe (n = 48) and Japan (n = 33), although these numbers are rapidly rising. Approximately 20 of the U.S. cyclotron sites distribute FDG to hospitals that have imaging equipment without radiopharmaceutical production facilities, thereby greatly increasing the number of patients who can benefit from FDG imaging.

The third-party reimbursement situation for oncologic PET has also improved in recent years. In 1997, the Blue Cross/Blue Shield Technology Evaluation group concluded that published data supported the use of FDG PET imaging in the evaluation of solitary pulmonary nodules and the staging of non–small cell lung cancer, and other private insurers soon followed. In January 1998, the Health Care Financing Administration (HCFA) approved Medicare reimbursement for solitary pulmonary nodules that are smaller than 4 cm in diameter and indeterminate on CT scan, as well as for the initial staging of pathologically diagnosed non–small cell lung cancer. The HCFA also reviewed data supporting reimbursement for evaluation of other tumors and in July 1999 commenced reimbursement for recurrent colorectal carcinoma with serum CEA elevation, primary or recurrent lymphoma, and metastatic melanoma. In December 2000, the HCFA approved reimbursement of FDG PET for the evaluation of six body tumors: non–small cell lung carcinoma, colorectal carcinoma, lymphoma, melanoma, head and neck, and esophageal carcinoma, excluding monitoring therapy. The reimbursement is limited to studies performed on high-resolution PET scanners and was implemented in July 2001. This area is changing rapidly, however with coverage continuing to expand.

REFERENCES

1. Gupta NC, Falk PM, Frank AL, et al. Pre-operative staging of colorectal carcinoma using positron emission tomography. *Nebr Med J* 1993;78(2):30–35.
2. Abdel-Nabi H, Doerr RJ, Lamonica DM, et al. Staging of primary colorectal carcinomas with fluorine-18 fluorodeoxyglucose whole-

body PET: correlation with histopathologic and CT findings. *Radiology* 1998;206(3):755–760.

3. August DA, Ottow RT, Sugarbaker PH. Clinical perspectives on human colorectal cancer metastases. *Cancer Metastases Rev* 1984;3: 303–324.

4. Hughes KS, Simon R, Songhorabodi S, et al. Resection of liver for colorectal carcinoma metastases: a multi-institutional study of indications for resection. *Surgery* 1988;103:278–288.

5. Steele G Jr, Bleday R, Mayer R, et al. A prospective evaluation of hepatic resection for colorectal carcinoma metastases to the liver: Gastrointestinal Tumor Study Group protocol 6584. *J Clin Oncol* 1991;9:1105–1112.

6. Soyer P, Levesque M, Elias D, et al. Detection of liver metastases from colorectal cancer: comparison of intraoperative US and CT during arterial portography. *Radiology* 1992;183:541–544.

7. Nelson RC, Chezmar JL, Sugarbaker PH, et al. Hepatic tumors: comparison of CT during arterial portography, delayed CT and MR imaging for preoperative evaluation. *Radiology* 1989;172:27–34.

8. Small WC, Mehard WB, Langmo LS, et al. Preoperative determination of the resectability of hepatic tumors: efficacy of CT during arterial portography. *AJR Am J Roentgenol* 1993;161:319–322.

9. Peterson MS, Baron RL, Dodd GD III, et al. Hepatic parenchymal perfusion detected with CTPA: imaging-pathologic correlation. *Radiology* 1992;183:149–155.

10. Suckler LS, DeNardo GL. Trials and tribulations: oncological antibody imaging comes to the fore. *Semin Nucl Med* 1997;27:10–29.

11. Yonekura Y, Benua RS, Brill AB, et al. Increased accumulation of 2-deoxy-2-[18F]fluoro-D-glucose in liver metastases from colon carcinoma. *J Nucl Med* 1982;23:1133–1137.

12. Strauss LG, Clorius JH, Schlag P, et al. Recurrence of colorectal tumors: PET evaluation. *Radiology* 1989;170:329–332.

13. Ito K, Kato T, Tadokoro M, et al. Recurrent rectal cancer and scar: differentiation with PET and MR imaging. *Radiology* 1992;182: 549–552.

14. Gupta NC, Falk PM, Frank AL, et al. Pre-operative staging of colorectal carcinoma using positron emission tomography. *Nebr Med J* 1993;78:30–35.

15. Falk PM, Gupta NC, Thorson AG, et al. Positron emission tomography for preoperative staging of colorectal carcinoma. *Dis Colon Rectum* 1994;37:153–156.

16. Schiepers C, Penninckx F, De Vadder N, et al. Contribution of PET in the diagnosis of recurrent colorectal cancer: comparison with conventional imaging. *Eur J Surg Oncol* 1995;21:517–522.

17. Vitola JV, Delbeke D, Sandler MP, et al. Positron emission tomography to stage metastatic colorectal carcinoma to the liver. *Am J Surg* 1996;171:21–26.

18. Delbeke D, Vitola J, Sandler MP, et al. Staging recurrent metastatic colorectal carcinoma with PET. *J Nucl Med* 1997;38:1196–1201.

19. Valk PE, Abella-Columna E, Haseman MK, et al. Whole-body PET imaging with F-18-fluorodeoxyglucose in management of recurrent colorectal cancer. *Arch Surg* 1999;134:503–511.

20. Ruhlmann J, Schomburg A, Bender H, et al. Fluorodeoxyglucose whole-body positron emission tomography in colorectal cancer patients studied in routine daily practice. *Dis Colon Rectum* 1997;40: 1195–1204.

21. Flamen P, Stroobants S, Van Cutsem E, et al. Additional value of whole-body positron emission tomography with fluorine-18-2-fluoro-2-deoxy-D-glucose in recurrent colorectal cancer. *J Clin Oncol* Mar 1999;17(3):894–901.

22. Akhurst T, Larson SM. Positron emission tomography imaging of colorectal cancer. *Semin Oncol* 1999;26(5):577–583.

23. Kim EE, Chung SK, Haynie TP, et al. Differentiation of residual or recurrent tumors from post-treatment changes with F-18 FDG PET. *Radiographics* 1992;12:269–279.

24. Vogel SB, Drane WE, Ros PR, et al. Prediction of surgical resectability in patients with hepatic colorectal metastases. *Ann Surg* 1994;219: 508–516.

25. Imbriaco M, Akhurst T, Hilton S, et al. Whole-body FDG-PET in patients with recurrent colorectal carcinoma. A comparative study with CT. *Clin Positron Imaging* 2000;3(3):107–114.

26. Imdahl A, Reinhardt MJ, Nitzsche EU, et al. Impact of 18F-FDG-positron emission tomography for decision making in colorectal cancer recurrences. *Arch Surg* 2000;385(2):129–134.

27. Staib L, Schirrmeister H, Reske SN, et al. Is (18)F-fluorodeoxyglucose positron emission tomography in recurrent colorectal cancer a contribution to surgical decision making? *Am J Surg* 2000;180(1):1–5.

28. Huebner RH, Park KC, Shepherd JE, et al. A meta-analysis of the literature for whole-body FDG PET detection of colorectal cancer. *J Nucl Med* 2000;41:1177–1189.

29. Lai DT, Fulham M, Stephen MS, et al. The role of whole-body positron emission tomography with [18F]fluorodeoxyglucose in identifying operable colorectal cancer. *Arch Surg* 1996;131:703–707.

30. Ogunbiyi OA, Flanagan FL, Dehdashti F, et al. Detection of recurrent and metastatic colorectal cancer: comparison of positron emission tomography and computed tomography. *Ann Surg Oncol* 1997;4: 613–620.

31. Beets G, Penninckx F, Schiepers C, et al. Clinical value of whole-body positron emission tomography with [18F]fluorodeoxyglucose in recurrent colorectal cancer. *Br J Surg* 1994;81:1666–1670.

32. Flanagan FL, Dehdashti F, Ogunbiyi OA, et al. Utility of FDG PET for investigating unexplained plasma CEA elevation in patients with colorectal cancer. *Annals of surgery* 1998;227(3):319–323.

33. Meta J, Seltzer M, Schiepers C, et al. Impact of 18F-FDG PET on managing patients with colorectal cancer: The referring physician's perspective. *J Nucl Med* 2001;42:586–590.

34. Gambhir SS, Valk P, Shepherd J, et al. Cost effective analysis modeling of the role of FDG PET in the management of patients with recurrent colorectal cancer. *J Nucl Med* 1997;38:90P.

35. Whiteford MH, Whiteford HM, Yee LF, et al. Usefulness of FDG-PET scan in the assessment of suspected metastatic or recurrent adenocarcinoma of the colon and rectum. *Dis Colon Rectum* 2000;43(6): 759–770.

36. Berger KL, Nicholson SA, Dehadashti F, et al. FDG PET evaluation of mucinous neoplasms: correlation of FDG uptake with histopathologic features. *AJR Am J Roentgenol* 2000;174(4):1005–1008.

37. Findlay M, Young H, Cunningham D, et al. Noninvasive monitoring of tumor metabolism using fluorodeoxyglucose and positron emission tomography in colorectal cancer liver metastases: correlation with tumor response to fluorouracil. *J Clin Oncol* 1996;14:700–708.

38. Vitola JV, Delbeke D, Meranze SG, et al. Positron emission tomography with F-18-fluorodeoxyglucose to evaluate the results of hepatic chemoembolization. *Cancer* 1996;78:2216–2222.

39. Guillem J, Calle J, Akhurst T, et al. Prospective assessment of primary rectal cancer response to preoperative radiation and chemotherapy using 18-fluorodeoxyglucose positron emission tomography. *Dis Colon Rectum* 2000;43:18–24.

40. Megibow AJ, Zhou XH, Rotterdam H, et al. Pancreatic adenocarcinoma: CT versus MR imaging in the evaluation of resectability—report of the Radiology Diagnostic Oncology Group. *Radiology* 1995; 195(2):327–332.

41. Diehl SJ, Lehman KJ, Sadick M, et al. Pancreatic cancer: value of dual-phase helical CT in assessing resectability. *Radiology* 1998;206: 373–378.

42. Lu DSK, Reber HA, Krasny RM, et al. Local staging of pancreatic cancer: criteria for unresectability of major vessels as revealed by pancreatic-phase, thin section helical CT. *Am J Radiol* 1997;168: 1439–1444.

43. Johnson PT, Outwater EK. Pancreatic carcinoma versus chronic pancreatitis: dynamic MR imaging. *Radiology* 1999;212(1):213–218.

44. Lammer J, Herlinger H, Zalaudek G, et al. Pseudotumorous pancreatitis. *Gastrointest Radiol* 1995;10:59–67.

45. Bluemke DA, Cameron IL, Hurban RH, et al. Potentially resectable pancreatic adenocarcinoma: spiral CT assessment with surgical and pathologic correlation. *Radiology* 1995;197:381–385.

46. Bluemke DA, Fishman EK. CT and MR evaluation of pancreatic cancer. *Surg Oncol Clin North Am* 1998;7:103–124.

47. Catalano C, Pavone P, Laghi A, et al. Pancreatic adenocarcinoma: combination of MR angiography and MR cholangiopancreatography for the diagnosis and assessment of resectability. *Eur Radiol* 1998;8: 428–434.

48. Irie H, Honda H, Kaneko K, et al. Comparison of helical CT and MR imaging in detecting and staging small pancreatic adenocarcinoma. *Abdom Imaging* 1997;22:429–433.

49. Trede M, Rumstadt B, Wendl, et al. Ultrafast magnetic resonance imaging improves the staging of pancreatic tumors. *Ann Surg* 1997; 226:393–405.

50. Hawes RH, Zaidi S. Endoscopic ultrasonography of the pancreas. *Gastrointest Endosc Clin North Am* 1995;5:61–80.

51. Legmann P, Vignaux O, Dousset B, et al. Pancreatic tumors: comparison of dual-phase helical CT and endoscopic sonography. *AJR Am J Roentgenol* 1998;170:1315–1322.

52. Mertz HR, Sechopoulos P, Delbeke D, et al. EUS, PET, and CT scanning for evaluation of pancreatic adenocarcinoma. *Gastrointest Endosc* 2000;52(3):367–371.

53. Brandt KR, Charboneau JW, Stephens DH, et al. CT- and US-guided biopsy of the pancreas. *Radiology* 1993;187:99–104.

54. Chang KJ, Nguyen P, Erickson RA, et al. The clinical utility of endoscopic ultrasound-guided fine-needle aspiration in the diagnosis and staging of pancreatic carcinoma. *Gastrointest Endosc* 1997;45:387–393.

55. McGuire GE, Pitt HA, Lillemoe KD, et al. Reoperative surgery for periampullary adenocarcinoma. *Arch Surg* 1991;126:1205–1212.

56. Tyler DS, Evans DB. Reoperative pancreaticoduodenectomy. *Ann Surg* 1994;219:211–221.

57. Robinson EK, Lee JE, Lowy AM, et al. Reoperative pancreaticoduodenectomy for periampullary carcinoma. *Am J Surg* 1996;172:432–438.

58. Thompson JS, Murayama KM, Edney JA, et al. Pancreaticoduodenectomy for suspected but unproven malignancy. *Am J Surg* 1994;169:571–575.

59. Flier JS, Mueckler MM, Usher P, et al. Elevated levels of glucose transport and transporter messenger RNA are induced by ras or src oncogenes. *Science* 1987;235:1492–1495.

60. Monakhov NK, Neistadt EL, Shavlovskii MM, et al. Physiochemical properties and isoenzyme composition of hexokinase from normal and malignant human tissues. *J Natl Cancer Inst* 1978;61:27–34.

61. Higashi T, Tamaki N, Honda T, et al. Expression of glucose transporters in human pancreatic tumors compared with increased F-18 FDG accumulation in PET study. *J Nucl Med* 1997; 38:1337–1344.

62. Reske S, Grillenberger KG, Glatting G, et al. Overexpression of glucose transporter 1 and increased F-18 FDG uptake in pancreatic carcinoma. *J Nucl Med* 1997;38:1344–1348.

63. Bares R, Klever P, Hellwig D, et al. Pancreatic cancer detected by positron emission tomography with ^{18}F-labeled deoxyglucose: method and first results. *Nucl Med Commun* 1993;14:596–601.

64. Bares R, Klever P, Hauptmann S, et al. F-18-fluorodeoxyglucose PET *in vivo* evaluation of pancreatic glucose metabolism for detection of pancreatic cancer. *Radiology* 1994;192:79–86.

65. Stollfuss JC, Glatting G, Friess H, et al. 2-(Fluorine-18)-fluoro-2-deoxy-D-glucose PET in detection of pancreatic cancer: value of quantitative image interpretation. *Radiology* 1995;195:339–344.

66. Inokuma T, Tamaki N, Torizuka T, et al. Evaluation of pancreatic tumors with positron emission tomography and F-18 fluorodeoxyglucose: comparison with CT and US. *Radiology* 1995;195:345–352.

67. Kato T, Fukatsu H, Ito K, et al. Fluorodeoxyglucose positron emission tomography in pancreatic cancer: an unsolved problem. *Eur J Nucl Med* 1995;22:32–39.

68. Friess H, Langhans J, Ebert M, et al. Diagnosis of pancreatic cancer by 2[F-18]-fluoro-2-deoxy-D-glucose positron emission tomography. *Gut* 1995;36:771–777.

69. Ho CL, Dehdashti F, Griffeth LK, et al. FDG PET evaluation of indeterminate pancreatic masses. *Comput Assisted Tomogr* 1996;20:363–369.

70. Zimny M, Bares R, Fass J, et al. Fluorine-18 fluorodeoxyglucose positron emission tomography in the differential diagnosis of pancreatic carcinoma: a report of 106 cases. *Eur J Nucl Med* 1997;24:678–682.

71. Keogan MT, Tyler D, Clark L, et al. Diagnosis of pancreatic carcinoma: role of FDG PET. *AJR Am J Roentgenol* 1998;171:1565–1570.

72. Imdahl SA, Nitzsche E, Krautmann F, et al. Evaluation of positron emission tomography with 2-[^{18}F]fluoro-2-deoxy-D-glucose for the differentiation of chronic pancreatitis and pancreatic cancer. *Br J Surg* 1999;86(2):194–199.

73. Delbeke D, Chapman WC, Pinson CW, et al. F-18 fluorodeoxyglucose imaging with positron emission tomography (FDG PET) has a significant impact on diagnosis and management of pancreatic ductal adenocarcinoma. *J Nucl Med* 1999;40:1784–1792.

74. Rose DM, Delbeke D, Beauchamp RD, et al. 18-Fluorodeoxyglucose-positron emission tomography ([18]FDG-PET) in the management of patients with suspected pancreatic cancer. *Ann Surg* 1998;229:729–738.

75. Wahl RL, Henry CA, Ethier SP. Serum glucose: effects on tumor and normal tissue accumulation of 2-[F-18]-fluoro-2-deoxy-D-glucose in rodents with mammary carcinoma. *Radiology* 1992;183:643–647.

76. Lindholm P, Minn H, Leskinen-Kallio S, et al. Influence of the blood glucose concentration on FDG uptake in cancer—a PET study. *J Nucl Med* 1993;34:1–6.

77. Diederichs CG, Staib L, Glatting G, et al. FDG PET: elevated plasma glucose reduces both uptake and detection rate of pancreatic malignancies. *J Nucl Med* 1998;39:1030–1033.

78. Diederichs CG, Staib L, Vogel J, et al. Values and limitations of FDG PET with preoperative evaluations of patients with pancreatic masses. *Pancreas* 2000;20:109–116.

79. Zimny M, Buell U, Diederichs CG, et al. False positive FDG PET in patients with pancreatic masses: an issue of proper patient selection? *Eur J Nucl Med* 1998;25:1352.

80. Shreve PD. Focal fluorine-18-fluorodeoxyglucose accumulation in inflammatory pancreatic disease. *Eur J Nucl Med* 1998;25:259–264.

81. Diederichs CG, Staib L, Glasbrenner B, et al. F-18 fluorodeoxyglucose (FDG) and C-reactive protein (CRP). *Clin Positron Imaging* 1999;2(3):131–136.

82. Nakata B, Chung YS, Nishimura S, et al. ^{18}F-fluorodeoxyglucose positron emission tomography and the prognosis of patients with pancreatic carcinoma. *Cancer* 1997;79:695–699.

83. Zimny M, Fass J, Bares R, et al. Fluorodeoxyglucose positron emission tomography and the prognosis of pancreatic carcinoma. *Scand J Gastroenterol* 2000;35:883–888.

84. Frolich A, Diederichs CG, Staib L, et al. Detection of liver metastases from pancreatic cancer using FDG PET. *J Nucl Med* 1999;40:250–255.

85. Yeung RS, Weese JL, Hoffman JP, et al. Neoadjuvant chemoradiation in pancreatic and duodenal carcinoma. A Phase II Study. *Cancer* 1 Oct 1993;72(7):2124–2133.

86. Jessup JM, Steele G Jr, Mayer RJ, et al. Neoadjuvant therapy for unresectable pancreatic adenocarcinoma. *Arch Surg* May 1993;128(5):559–564.

87. Maisey NR, Webb A, Flux GD, et al. FDG PET in the prediction of survival of patients with cancer of the pancreas: a pilot study. *Br J Cancer* 2000;83:287–293.

88. Franke C, Klapdor R, Meyerhoff K, et al. [18]-F positron emission tomography of the pancreas: diagnostic benefit in the follow-up of pancreatic carcinoma. *Anticancer Res* 1999;19:2437–2442.

89. del Pilar Fernandez M, Redvanly RD. Primary hepatic malignant neoplasms. *Radiol Clin North Am* 1998;36(2):333–348.

90. Oppenheim BE. Liver imaging. In: Sandler MP, Coleman RE, Wackers FTJ, et al, eds. *Diagnostic nuclear medicine*. Baltimore, MD: Williams & Wilkins, 1996:749–758.

91. Weber G, Cantero A. Glucose-6-phosphatase activity in normal, precancerous, and neoplastic tissues. *Cancer Res* 1955;15:105–108.

92. Weber G, Morris HP. Comparative biochemistry of hepatomas, III: carbohydrate enzymes in liver tumors of different growth rates. *Cancer Res* 1963;23:987–994.

93. Messa C, Choi Y, Hoh CK, et al. Quantification of glucose utilization in liver metastases: parametric imaging of FDG uptake with PET. *J Comput Assisted Tomogr* 1992;16:684–689.

94. Okazumi S, Isono K, Enomoto D, et al. Evaluation of liver tumors using fluorine-18-fluorodeoxyglucose PET: characterization of tumor and assessment of effect of treatment. *J Nucl Med* 1992;33:333–339.

95. Torizuka T, Tamaki N, Inokuma T, et al. *In vivo* assessment of glucose metabolism in hepatocellular carcinoma with FDG PET. *J Nucl Med* 1995;36:1811–1817.

96. Khan MA, Combs CS, Brunt EM, et al. Positron emission tomography scanning in the evaluation of hepatocellular carcinoma. *J Hepatol* 2000;32:792–797.

97. Delbeke D, Martin WH, Sandler MP, et al. Evaluation of benign vs. malignant hepatic lesions with positron emission tomography. *Arch Surg* 1998;133:510–515.

98. Iwata Y, Shiomi S, Sasaki N, et al. Clinical usefulness of positron emission tomography with fluorine-18-fluorodeoxyglucose in the diagnosis of liver tumors. *Ann Nucl Med* 2000;14:121–126.

99. Trojan J, Schroeder O, Raedle J, et al. Fluorine-18 FDG positron emission tomography for imaging of hepatocellular carcinoma. *Am J Gastroenterol* 1999;94:3314–3319.

100. Schroder O, Trojan J, Zeuzem S, et al. Limited value of fluorine-18-fluorodeoxyglucose PET for the differential diagnosis of focal liver

Standard Tests and Imaging Procedures for Follow-up of Ovarian Cancer

Like the challenge of early diagnosis of ovarian cancer based on clinical presentation, physical examination and imaging procedures, observation, and frequent medical follow-up of patients with ovarian cancer to detect recurrent disease is an equally difficult task. Clinical findings and deterioration of performance status usually prompt laboratory tests and anatomic imaging procedures. The CA-125 tumor marker, CT, MRI, ultrasound, and monoclonal antibody (MoAb) scintigraphy are alternatives to surgical exploration. Laparotomy and laparoscopy are invasive and not always accurate in confirming the presence or absence of tumor. The overall false-negative rate is from 30% to 35% because some regions of the mesentery, the peritoneum, and areas obscured by adhesions cannot be explored by laparoscopy; this results in incomplete examinations of those patients.

CT and MRI techniques continue to improve with advances in technology and provide excellent localization and structural delineation with good sensitivity for staging advanced ovarian cancer. The Radiological Diagnostic Oncology Group sponsored by the National Cancer Institute reported the sensitivity and specificity of CT, MRI, and ultrasound specifically for detecting metastatic spread to the three common anatomic areas: the peritoneum, the lymph nodes, and the hepatic parenchyma (7). For peritoneal implants, the sensitivity and specificity were 92% and 82% for CT, 95% and 80% for MRI, and 69% and 93% for ultrasound. For lymph nodes, the sensitivity and specificity were 43% and 89% for CT, 38% and 84% for MRI, and 32% and 93% for ultrasound. For liver lesions, the sensitivity and specificity were 40% and 96% for CT, 40% and 96% for MRI, and 57% and 98% for ultrasound. It is noteworthy that the specificity for small lesions (2 cm or smaller) was 0% (zero of three patients) for CT, 33% (two of six) for MRI, and 63% (five of eight) for ultrasound.

The tumor marker CA-125 is elevated (more than 35 U/mL) in about 80% of cases with epithelial ovarian cancer and usually indicates persistent or recurrent disease. However, 35% of patients with normal CA-125 levels still can have persistent disease (13). When the CA-125 level continues to rise, further diagnostic tests must be considered.

Radioimmunoscintigraphy with radiolabeled MoAbs is an alternative and, in theory, is a potentially more tumor-specific diagnostic approach to recurrent ovarian cancer (14–17). Although initial expectations for this method were high, performance in practice has not met the promise of these very high expectations. A diagnostic accuracy of as high as 84% has been reported for this scintigraphic method in the setting of detection of recurrent ovarian cancer (16). However, the specificity of immunoscintigraphy can be rather low (37%), as reported by Lieberman et al. (17). Scintigraphy with MoAbs is quite effective in localizing peritoneal metastases and carcinomatosis (14,18), but quite insensitive in detecting liver metastases, in part due to high indium-111 uptake in the normal liver. There is also some concern about human antimouse antibody and the inconvenience of the several days delay between injection and imaging (19). With further development, MoAbs may play a larger role in the diagnosis and, more importantly, a probably greater role in the treatment of ovarian cancer. However, radioantibody imaging is quite limited in its clinical applications.

FDG PET Imaging in Ovarian Cancer

Considering the shortcomings of the conventional imaging techniques, particularly for detecting recurrent ovarian cancer, other diagnostic methods are being sought. Whole-body FDG PET metabolic imaging can detect viable proliferating tumor tissues including ovarian cancer. Wahl et al. (20) in a preliminary report and Hubner et al. (21) and Casey et al. (22) reported that ^{18}F-FDG PET is effective in detecting ovarian cancer. Other investigators have used FDG PET in clinical investigations for detecting, staging, and monitoring ovarian cancer, as indicated later in this chapter. Many of these reports focused on the detection of recurrent ovarian cancer.

PET Imaging Method

FDG PET examinations for ovarian cancer are now routinely performed with commercially available dedicated positron imaging devices or—at some institutions—much less frequently, with gamma cameras operated in coincidence mode. The most commonly used radiotracer in PET oncology is ^{18}F-FDG, administered in doses ranging between approximately 5 and 20 mCi (185 to 740 MBq).

Patients scheduled for PET scans generally should have nothing by mouth for at least 4 hours (preferably 6 to 12 hours) before injection of ^{18}F-FDG; furthermore, patients should be well hydrated and avoid strenuous work or exercise for 24 hours before the scan. Because elevated blood glucose levels diminish FDG uptake by tumor cells, pre-PET scan blood sugar determination is good practice. In oncology patients, blood sugar levels are usually not adjusted with dextrose or insulin, unlike in cardiac FDG viability studies, particularly in diabetics, in whom the quality of the PET examination is closely related to the blood sugar level.

Another important technical and logistic aspect of FDG PET examinations is the normal presence of intense FDG activity in the bladder, due to normal ^{18}F-FDG renal clearance, which may interfere with optimal interpretation of the images. Various methods of reducing or eliminating renal and bladder activity have been suggested. Instructions to the patient might include drinking up to eight glasses of water during the 24 hours before the PET scan. Some investigators suggest starting intravenous infusion of 500 mL of Ringer solution simultaneously with 20 mg of intravenous furosemide at the time of the FDG administration and have the patient void after the uptake period (45 to 60 minutes) before positioning the patient on the scanning table and starting scanning with the first bed position in the pelvis. This method is applicable to typical "static" body scans in multiple bed positions. However, if a dynamic PET study of the pelvis is desired, this cannot be done because data acquisition for dynamic studies starts at the time of injection. In that situation, irrigation of the bladder with 2 to 3 liters of USP sterile water will help to reduce interference from bladder activity. In practice, dynamic FDG studies are done mainly in the research setting and not in routine clinical practice.

For attenuation correction (required for quantifying uptake and for calculating standard uptake values [SUVs]), it is necessary to obtain transmission scans for each bed position. With current state-of-the-art whole-body PET scanners, transmission and emission scanning can be performed sequentially for each bed position. With future PET/CT hybrid scanners, a brief CT scan done just before or after the emission PET data are acquired to accomplish transmission and emission scanning more rapidly.

After an uptake period of 45 to 60 minutes, data acquisition for a body scan of a patient with ovarian cancer is typically started below the pelvis and finished at the shoulder level. Image reconstruction takes into account attenuation correction, correction for radioactive decay, and count losses due to "dead time." Filtered backprojection and/or iterative reconstruction (using the ordered subsets–expectation maximization algorithm) produce transaxial tomographic images, which are also the basis for coronal, sagittal, and projection images. If dynamic data acquisition is performed, the emitted counts are collected in specified time frames, such as six frames for 20 seconds each, three frames for 60 seconds each, seven frames for 300 seconds each, and one frame for 1,200 seconds (17 frames total). In routine practice, dynamic images are only infrequently obtained—most commonly in a research setting.

PET Image Data Analysis

Most PET studies in oncology are whole-body scans and are evaluated by visual interpretation. Various rating scales can be applied—for example, 0 for normal, 1 for probably normal, 2 for equivocal, 3 for probably abnormal, and 4 for definitely abnormal. Other rating schemes are based on activity concentration ratios taking uptake in presumably normal tissues such as the liver as point of reference.

PET images that are attenuation corrected can also be assessed using a calibration factor and correcting for body weight and injected dose. The resulting parametric images then display the standardized activity concentration for each image point (pixel). The SUV based on these assumptions is reflected in the following equation:

$$SUV_{BW} = \frac{ROI(camera\ cts/px) \times CF(\mu Ci/mL/camera\ cps/px)}{Dose\ (\mu Ci)/BW\ (mL)} = 0$$

where *ROI* is the region of interest, *cts* is counts per second,

px is pixels, *CF* is calibration factor, and *BW* is body weight.

Dynamic image data sets can also be analyzed quantitatively by plotting time-activity curves (TACs) or performing a graphical analysis, as introduced by Patlak and Blasberg (23). To avoid sampling of arterial blood, the input function for the plasma concentration of the radiotracer can be taken from the PET images by analyzing blood activity in large vessels identified in the images. In this way, the accumulation rate of FDG can be approximated for the regions of interest under study. In general, the higher the FDG uptake in a tissue, the more likely it is to be of malignant origin.

FDG Uptake Patterns in Ovarian (Particularly Recurrent) Cancer

FDG PET appears to be extremely sensitive in identifying primary and recurrent ovarian cancers, although it is much less studied in primary cancers. Ovarian cancer tends to invade local structures directly in its early stage and later spreads by intraperitoneal seeding, lymphatic invasion, and hematogenous routes. It is helpful to consider the typical patterns of tumor extension for the various subcategories of epithelial ovarian cancer (2–4) when interpreting FDG PET images. One should look for peritoneal implants on the omental and peritoneal surfaces, the right paracolic gutter, the right subdiaphragmatic and liver surface, and the mesentery. Involvement of spleen and bowel should also be considered. Extraabdominal metastases are less common and liver metastases occur late in the disease, although metastases to the peritoneal surface of the liver are quite common.

On CT, lymph nodes larger than 1.0 cm in short-axis dimension—typically in the paraaortic, external iliac, obturator, and hypogastric lymph node chains—are considered highly suggestive of metastatic invasion. Hydronephrosis, a fairly common complication of lymph node metastases in ovarian cancer due to ureteral obstruction, is easily recognized on whole-body FDG PET scans. Lymphatic spread into the anterior mediastinum and right thoracic duct via retrosternal lymphatic channels is less likely, but it does occur.

Metastases secondary to hematogenous spread can occur in liver, lung, spleen, pancreas, and kidney and are generally readily identifiable on PET images. However, renal metastases may present a problem because of the existing renal activity. This can be remedied, to some extent, by intravenous hydration, furosemide, and bladder irrigation. Another limitation regarding lesion detectability by PET is the spatial resolution. An axial resolution of 5.0 mm FWHM and a transaxial resolution of 8.0 mm FWHM or slightly better are possible with current state-of-the-art PET scanners. Thus, very small lesions (3.0 mm or smaller) are unlikely to be detected.

Results of FDG PET in Ovarian Cancer

Only a relatively few investigators have studied the clinical utility of FDG PET for patients with ovarian cancer. One of the reasons for this paucity of information is probably related to the fact that ovarian is not among the most common cancers and there has been no large cohort of patients with ovarian cancer studied near any PET center during the last 10 years. Although the number of patients reported in the literature is well below 1,000, the results are sufficiently good to justify use of FDG PET as a diagnostic tool for ovarian cancer, particularly in conjunction with other imaging modalities that facilitate anatomic correlation.

Results of FDG PET in primary untreated ovarian cancer and in cases of suspected recurrence reported in the early 1990s have consistently demonstrated a rather high sensitivity. In the early publications between 1991 and 1995, Wahl et al. (20), Hubner et al. (21), Casey et al. (22), Karlan et al. (24), Gupta et al. (25), Avril et al. (26), and Boland et al. (27) indicated that ovarian cancer can be recognized by PET based on the increased glucose utilization. The sensitivities ranged from 83% to 100%.

In contrast to the high sensitivity of FDG PET for ovarian cancer, the specificity of PET was not consistent and actually quite discordant not only in the earlier reports but also in publications after 1995. PET results presented in publications by Zimny et al. (29), Römer et al. (30), Garcia et al. (31), Fenchel et al. (32), Kubik-Huch et al. (33), and Grab et al. (34) suggested a considerable spread of specificity values ranging between 50% (33) and 54% (30) and up to 78% (32) and 86% (29).

The discrepancy in the specificity of FDG PET in detecting metabolically active ovarian cancer gives cause for some concern regarding the negative predictive value (NPV) of PET in ovarian cancer. This concern is clearly expressed by the results of the prospective study on characterizing ovarian cancer with FDG PET by Römer et al. (30), who found a specificity of only 54% for the presence of ovarian cancer. Although the total study population was only 24 patients, the low specificity obtained in this prospective study indicates that some degree of caution is in order regarding the use of FDG PET for assessing residual or recurrent ovarian cancer.

The discordant results, particularly in regard to the specificity of FDG PET for primary or recurrent ovarian cancer, may be due to a variety of factors such as patient selection criteria, tumor size, effectiveness and timing of surgery or chemotherapy, and the level of confidence based on the gold standard of surgical and histopathologic findings or based on specified survival times as an indicator of positive or negative PET results.

An extended, probably multiinstitutional, prospective study is needed to assess the impact of FDG PET on the management of ovarian cancer. In the meantime, currently available information regarding typical findings in FDG PET scans in ovarian cancer will have to suffice for this to be a useful tool for managing these patients. Special attention must be given to the natural behavior of this disease, a better understanding of the reasons for false-negative and false-positive results, and consideration of the nonspecific FDG uptake in normal tissues and pitfalls in interpreting FDG PET oncology studies. High technical quality of FDG PET studies is essential.

Knowing the metastatic spread pattern of ovarian cancer and the various underlying "benign" conditions leading to false-positive results helps to improve the accuracy of FDG PET in ovarian cancer. Recognizing nonspecific gastrointestinal (GI) and GU tract activity, postoperative changes, stoma sites, activity patterns secondary to urinary tract diversion, fibrotic changes, and bone marrow activity also help to avoid false-positive interpretations (35). In some cases, the SUVs and if available the slope of the TAC help distinguish "benign" and malignant processes. Image co-registration using conventional methods and hybrid PET/CT fusion technology can add a new level of sophistication to PET imaging and correlate metabolic information with the anatomy.

Benign conditions potentially leading to false-positive results include benign mucinous cystadenomas, endometrial and follicular cysts, corpus luteum cysts, fibromas, cystadenofibromas, misinterpreted GI tract activity, salpingo-oophoritis, and coexisting peritonitis, teratomas, dermoid cysts, tuboovarian abscesses, benign thecoma, and schwannoma. False-negative results include well-differentiated serous/mucinous cystadenocarcinoma, borderline tumors, disseminated carcinomatosis, and pT1a adenocarcinomas. It is of interest that carcinomatosis can be missed by FDG PET, likely because it is of low volume (30).

Early work by Hubner et al. (21) suggested that an SUV cutoff of 3.25 might be helpful to distinguish between benign and malignant ovarian lesions. By contrast, Römer et al. (30) could not find a statistically significant difference between SUVs of ovarian cancer and the SUVs of inflammatory or infectious processes. Based on the small numbers of PET studies in ovarian cancer that have evaluated the utility of SUVs, it is probably safe to say that SUVs are not routinely needed for interpretation of ovarian cancer PET studies, but they may be useful in some situations.

Römer et al. (30) achieved a sensitivity and specificity of 83% and 54%, respectively, when using an SUV of 3.25 as threshold, identical those of 83% and 54%, respectively, from using visual interpretation criteria. However, when infectious processes were excluded from the analysis, consideration of SUV helped to distinguish malignant from benign processes.

In general, there is good agreement on the SUVs for ovarian cancer, as reported by a small number of investigators with an average SUV of 5.32 with a range of 4.3 to 6.8. In our early work (21), we found the SUV for malignant lesions to be 6.12 ± 3.53, and for benign processes 3.08 ± 1.68. Based on cumulative distribution and receiver operating characteristic data analysis, an SUV of 3.25 was found to be an acceptable cutoff between benign and malignant lesions. Interestingly, the highest SUV (56.7) ever reported was observed by Zimny et al. (29) in a leiomyosarcoma.

Some examples of FDG PET are shown in Figs. 5.11.1

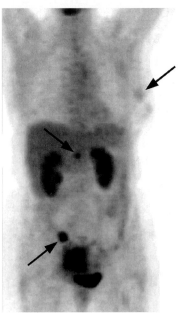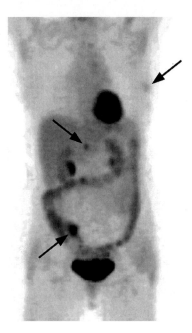

A,B

FIG. 5.11.1. Two ^{18}F-fluorodeoxyglucose (FDG) body scans of a 77-year-old woman with recurrent ovarian cancer. **A:** There is an approximately 6.5-cm area of increased FDG uptake in the lower mid-pelvis extending into the right pelvic wall. Adjacent to it in the region of the cecum is a focus suggesting a bowel implant of tumor (*lower arrow*). In addition, there is uptake in a right paraaortic lymph node (*middle arrow*). The standard uptake values in these areas range between 2.6 and 6.8. Faint focal FDG uptake in the left breast is noted on both studies (*upper arrows*). A follow-up mammogram was negative. The follow-up PET scan **(B)**, performed 9 months after additional chemotherapy, shows apparent resolution of the neoplastic process in the pelvis. Uptake in the right paraaortic lymph node is less intense and the focus in the region of the cecum is unchanged and presumed to be nonspecific. Renal and cardiac uptake show the not unexpected variability between the studies. The patient was well 9 months after the second PET scan **(B)**.

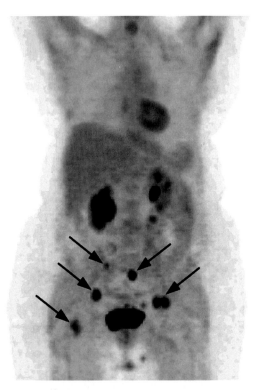

FIG. 5.11.2. ^{18}F-Fluorodeoxyglucose (FDG) whole-body scan of a 59-year-old woman status postsurgery and after chemotherapy for ovarian carcinoma. Rising cancer antigen 125 prompted this PET examination, showing multiple foci of intense FDG uptake in pelvic, inguinal, and femoral lymph nodes (*arrows*). There is prominent activity in the collecting system of both kidneys. Surgical exploration confirmed recurrence. After additional chemotherapy, the patient was alive 6 months later, presumably still with active disease.

through 5.11.4 to demonstrate the utility of PET, particularly in detecting recurrent ovarian cancer.

Discussion of FDG PET in Ovarian Cancer

PET using ^{18}F-FDG can detect not only primary but also recurrent or metastatic ovarian cancer with a high degree of accuracy, cost-effectiveness, and a significant impact on patient management. Whole-body FDG PET in our experience provides new information in approximately 30% to 40% of the patients with pelvic masses. Additional findings on dynamic or body PET studies may reveal evidence of metastatic disease or other primary cancers as coincidental findings in some patients.

FDG PET and CT have the highest accuracy both for diagnosing and for excluding ovarian cancer. PET can modify surgical approach in many cases and helps to identify patients who should receive chemotherapy and patients who would not benefit from surgery or should have further surgical debulking. A negative PET scan result together with a negative CT or MRI result may obviate other diagnostic procedures.

In some settings when suspected recurrence is based on CT scans, smaller "lesions" than 2.0 cm but still FDG-positive do not have to be debulked and can be treated with chemotherapy. A positive PET scan result in the presence of smaller than 1.5-cm suspicious lesions on CT can probably support the decision to forgo a laparotomy and to proceed directly to chemotherapy or intraperitoneal radionuclide treatment. One of the limitations of PET is its spatial resolution. However, lesions as small as 5.0 and 7.0 mm have been identified by FDG PET. In spite of possible pitfalls and limitations of the resolution of the various PET imaging devices, the sensitivity, specificity, and positive predictive

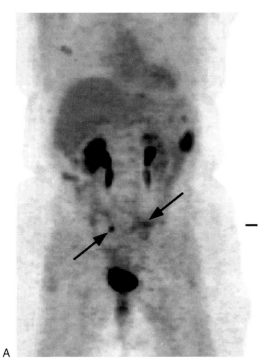

A

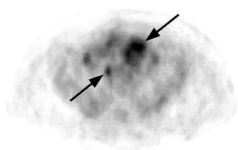

B

FIG. 5.11.3. ^{18}F-Fluorodeoxyglucose (FDG) body projection image of a 40-year-old woman with a history of ovarian cancer 3.5 years after completion of chemotherapy, clinical follow-up, and a cancer antigen 125 level of 90 IU. The scan shows an intense focus of FDG accumulation in the region of the splenic flexure, with a standard uptake value (SUV) of 5.9, and a less intense focus more superiorly. **A, B:** There is hazy FDG activity in the anterior abdomen (*right arrows*), with more intense uptake in the right lower abdomen with an SUV of 3.8 (*left arrows*). The diffuse uptake in the anterior abdomen is worrisome for omental implants. This was confirmed as malignant ascites, and with additional chemotherapy, the patient was doing well 9 months later.

value (PPV) of PET overall—particularly when combined with another imaging technique—are excellent.

In general, the essential diagnostic information from FDG PET can be derived from qualitative body images and no additional quantitative analysis of PET data is needed. In some cases, information from SUVs, which can be obtained from attenuation-corrected images, is helpful, and in some other situations, co-registration of PET images and concurrent CT images is useful in localizing abnormalities in question.

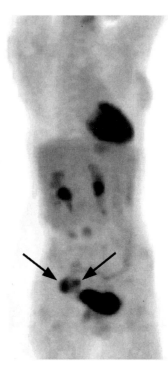

FIG. 5.11.4. ^{18}F-Fluorodeoxyglucose (FDG) positron emission tomography body scan of a 44-year-old woman with ovarian cancer, status after six cycles of chemotherapy and rising cancer antigen 125 level (105 IU). The projection image above is rotated to the patient's left to better show two foci of increased FDG accumulation in the region of the sigmoid colon (*arrows*). Laparoscopic biopsy revealed recurrent disease. Further chemotherapy was started.

Impact of PET on the Management of Patients with Ovarian Cancer

Based on the—albeit sparse—published data, it appears that FDG PET can be used to confirm disease or to monitor progression or regression of disease in more than 80% of patients with ovarian cancer. In 15% of patients examined for suspected recurrent ovarian cancer at the University of Tennessee Medical Center, the information obtained from FDG PET had a direct impact on the course of patient treatment, that is, whether to continue/change chemotherapy or recommend or negate second-look operations. The potential cost savings of using FDG PET to select the appropriate treatment for 57 patients and avoid second-look surgeries were approximated (36). The results of that study that related the PET results to surgical and histologic findings indicate potential significant cost savings when using FDG PET (37). The results indicated a range of $1,941 to $11,766 in cost savings if follow-up of patients with ovarian cancer involved the same diagnostic test for all of the patients in that study.

CERVICAL AND ENDOMETRIAL CANCER

Uterine cancer, including endometrial and cervical cancer, are the most common gynecologic cancers and tend to be diagnosed and treated at earlier stages than ovarian cancer. As a result, the 5-year survival rates are 94% for localized endometrial and 90% for early cervical cancer.

The overall experience with PET in these types cancer is limited. Nevertheless, it appears that endometrial cancers and cervical cancers are FDG avid (38) and accumulate L-methyl-^{11}C-methionine with mean SUVs higher than 8.0, as reported by Lapela et al. (39). As with other pelvic cancers, urinary tract activity may interfere with complete evaluation. Rose et al. (40) reported high FDG uptake in 91% of cervical cancers (N = 32). FDG PET imaging is a sensitive predictor of pelvic and paraaortic lymph node metastases. Sugawara et al. (41) found high FDG uptake in recurrent cervical cancer and lymph node metastases.

PET Applications for Cancer of the Genitourinary Tract and the Prostate

Renal Cancer

Reports on the utility of FDG PET in renal cancer are sparse, but there appears to be a place for FDG PET for clarifying equivocal diagnostic information from CT, MRI, angiography, or cyst aspiration. Wahl et al. (42) demonstrated the feasibility of PET imaging for renal cell carcinoma (RCC) in 1991; Goldberg et al. (43) applied FDG PET for the initial diagnosis of renal masses in 1997, and Hoh et al. (44) suggested using FDG PET for detecting metastases from RCC and for restaging. With renal cancers, as with neoplasms near the urinary bladder, interpretation may be difficult. Zhuang et al. (45) found FDG uptake values to be an unreliable indicator for malignant renal tumors. Gamma camera–based coincidence imaging has also been suggested to be effective for staging and restaging renal tumors (46). The normal FDG background uptake in the kidneys and collecting system can make detecting renal cancers more challenging than in other locations in the body.

Bladder Cancer

FDG PET has been used with some success in the diagnosis of bladder cancer and the detection of pelvic lymph node metastases and distant metastases (47–49). The main problem with FDG PET in primary bladder cancer is the presence of FDG activity in the urinary bladder. Nevertheless, sensitivity and specificity rates of 78% for both, with a $p = .30$ with pretest likelihood of spread has been reported. Kosuda et al. (49) had four false-negative results in 12 patients in spite of using retrograde bladder irrigation. Kosuda et al. (49) also measured the SUVs in primary bladder tumors and lymph node metastases and obtained values ranging between 2.19 to 6.17 and 1.72 to 4.79, respectively. In bladder cancer, the question of radiation-induced fibrotic changes and scarring versus residual/recurrent tumor cannot be answered by conventional imaging methods. This may be a situation in which FDG PET may be a useful adjunct to the other imaging procedures.

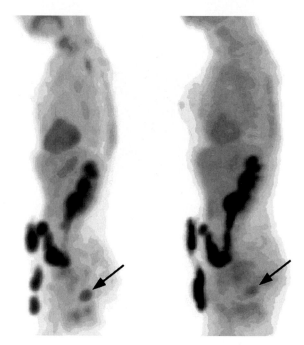

FIG. 5.11.5. ^{18}F-Fluorodeoxyglucose positron emission tomography body scans of a 62-year-old woman with bladder cancer diagnosed and treated in 1997. The initial PET scan (**left**) indicated residual tumor in the left lower pelvis with a standard uptake value (SUV) of 3.4 (*arrows*). A follow-up PET examination 4 months later (**right**) showed no change in the uptake pattern or in intensity (SUVs of 2.7 to 3.1). Chemotherapy was continued. (The projection images showing the lateral views of both examinations also demonstrate extensive normal urine activity that is present in an ileal conduit and external collection system.)

Some examples of PET images in bladder cancer (Figs. 5.11.5 through 5.11.7) demonstrate how metabolic imaging can help in guiding treatment of this type of cancer. The example in Fig. 5.11.7 also shows the aggressive nature of metastatic bladder cancer.

Testicular Cancer

FDG PET has been used effectively in germ-cell and non–germ-cell cancer of the testicle (50,51). Because many patients with testicular cancer can be cured, particularly with the currently available aggressive forms of treatment, accurate initial staging and close follow-up to detect metastatic disease early is extremely important. With evidence from FDG PET, initial staging is likely to be changed in one out of five patients; and in cases of suspected recurrence, PET is likely to change management in 50% of the patients. Hain et al. (52,53) found PPVs of 96% and NPVs of 90% when evaluating patients with suspected relapse of germ-cell tumors and obtained similar results when using PET for initial staging of germ-cell tumors. In another study by Cremerius et al. (54), 50 patients with testicular cancer were staged with FDG PET. In this cohort, PET detected metastases in

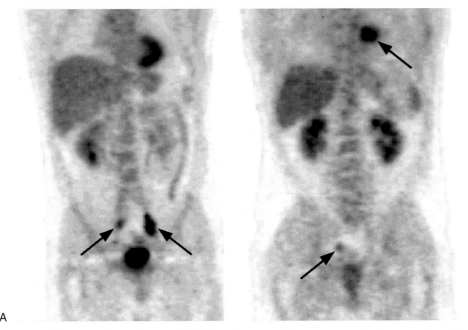

FIG. 5.11.6. ^{18}F-Fluorodeoxyglucose (FDG) positron emission tomography images of a 54-year-old man with bladder cancer. **A:** Focal uptake in iliac and paraaortic lymph nodes consistent with metastases (coronal image) (*arrows*). **B:** A follow-up scan 5 months later shows minimal residual activity in the right iliac lymph node chain (coronal image) (*lower arrow*); in addition, there is a new focus with intense FDG uptake in the left mid lung field, a new metastasis (*upper arrow*). The patient died 4 months later.

13 (87%) of 15 patients and excluded metastases in 33 (94%) of 35 patients. False-negative results were obtained in two patients with small (10.0 mm or smaller) retroperitoneal lymph nodes, and false-positive findings were the result of nonspecific muscular uptake and in one case by active sarcoidosis.

The shortcoming presented by the limited resolution of PET were pointed out by Albers et al. (55), who could not demonstrate viable tumors smaller than 5.0 mm in an FDG PET staging study of patients with germ-cell tumors. FDG PET for evaluating posttherapy changes in patients with testicular cancer is another potential application (56,57). Su-

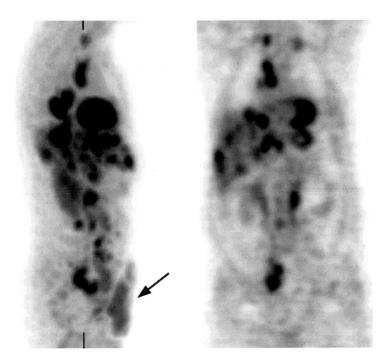

FIG. 5.11.7. ^{18}F-Fluorodeoxyglucose positron emission tomography body images (**left**, sagittal; **right**, coronal) of a 69-year-old man with a history of progressive metastatic spread from a bladder carcinoma. The scan shows multifocal abnormal uptake throughout the liver and abdomen. There is also urinary activity from urinary tract diversion (*arrow*). The patient died 7 days after the PET study with disseminated metastases.

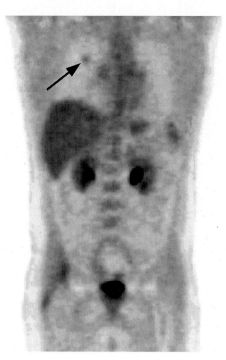

FIG. 5.11.8. ^{18}F-Fluorodeoxyglucose positron emission tomography body volume image of a 33-year-old man with a nonseminomatous germ-cell tumor of the left testis, stage III, which was treated with orchiectomy, chemotherapy, and autologous stem-cell transplantation. The PET scan taken 2 years later showed questionable worrisome (*arrow*) focal abnormalities in the upper lobe of the right lung and in the liver, suggesting metastatic disease. Additional chemotherapy and stem-cell transplantation were completed 4 months later. The patient remained clinically free of disease after the last PET scan.

gawara et al. (58) also showed that high FDG uptake was typical of viable germ-cell tumors. They also showed very low FDG uptake in scaring and viable benign teratoma after treatment. Kinetic modeling of dynamic data appeared capable of separating scar, which had low k_1 (flow), values from viable teratoma, which had high k_1 values. Two examples of testicular cancer (Figs. 5.11.8 and 5.11.9) also demonstrate the utility of FDG PET for monitoring response to treatment of testicular cancer.

Prostate Cancer

The incidence rates of prostate cancer have been rising during the last three decades. This type of cancer represents almost 30% of new cancers in American men. Prostate cancer has a tendency to spread into the pelvic/abdominal lymph nodes, to distant sites, and to bone. A more sensitive and specific diagnostic tool would be helpful for preoperative evaluation for metastatic disease in soft tissue and to differentiate benign bone "pathology" from bone metastases. One might have expected that FDG PET could provide this needed sensitivity and specificity. However, so far FDG PET

results in prostate cancer have been quite disappointing with low sensitivities (59–61). It is difficult to demonstrate FDG uptake in the primary prostate cancer versus uptake in normal prostate, because prostate cancer is not particularly FDG avid. Primary tumors and lymph node metastases have commonly been missed (62). Furthermore, metastatic bone le-

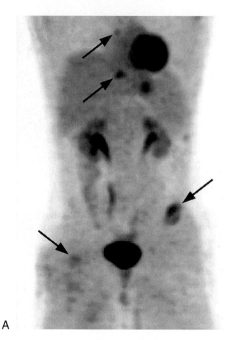

A

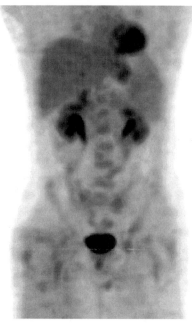

B

FIG. 5.11.9. Two fluorodeoxyglucose positron emission tomographic body scans of a 32-year-old man with testicular carcinoma showing evidence for bone metastases **(A)** in the sternum, spine, the left iliac crest, and the right femur (*arrows in order*). Right hydronephrosis and evidence for a right femoral prosthesis are also seen on the scan. There is **(B)** complete resolution of the abnormalities 4 months later. Moderate normal gastric activity was noted in both studies.

sions generally do not avidly concentrate FDG (60,61). FDG PET has been somewhat effective in documenting lymph node involvement, with lymph node metastases usually showing more intense uptake than the primary tumor in the prostate gland but FDG is not proved to be robust in this setting.

Several other radiotracers have been suggested for PET imaging of prostate cancer such as putrescine labeled with ^{18}F (63,64) or ^{11}C-labeled hydroxytryptophan (65). These approaches have not yet reached the level of clinical application. In addition, preliminary results have shown promise for ^{11}C-acetate for prostate cancer imaging (66).

Choline labeled with ^{11}C promises to be a useful radiotracer for detecting primary and metastatic prostate cancer (67). Kotzerke et al. (68) reported promising results with ^{11}C-choline, including detecting bone metastases from prostatic cancer. Unfortunately, the 20-minute half-life of ^{11}C does not permit facile commercialization or distribution of the agent and its use will be limited to scanners located near a cyclotron, in contrast to ^{18}F-labeled PET imaging agents. Therefore, the initial results obtained with ^{18}F-labeled choline in prostate cancer reported by the PET group at Duke University are exciting and may lead to a useful PET application for patients with prostate cancer (69). This agent is early in the evaluation phase, however.

SUMMARY

FDG PET appears to be the most accurate and cost-effective imaging procedure for detecting residual or recurrent ovarian cancer. This noninvasive test has a greater PPV and NPV than CT or MRI and in some respects may detect active tumor better than laparotomy or laparoscopy in areas of the abdomen that are not easily assessed at surgery. A combination of FDG PET and CT/MRI probably gives the highest accuracy for both diagnosis and exclusion of recurrent ovarian cancer. Of course, because of its limited spatial resolution, PET will fail to detect true microscopic tumor foci (5). PET rarely fails to detect large bulky tumors, and a negative PET scan result can obviate the need for an exploratory laparotomy. FDG PET helps to decide whether to operate and when to use chemotherapy. The impact of such information on patient management is obvious. FDG PET when used judiciously should reduce morbidity from unnecessary surgical procedures and/or chemotherapy and save money. It will also help in the selection of appropriate treatment and the initiation or change of treatment, and it should help gain valuable time when PET indicates ineffective treatment. In the context of the latter situation, FDG PET is probably a good choice for monitoring response to therapy in patients with ovarian cancer.

Although experience with FDG PET in renal, bladder, and cervical cancer is limited, the reported sensitivity and specificity rate for staging is close to 80%. If this level of accuracy holds up, FDG PET certainly has the potential to make a significant impact on the management of patients with these cancers.

In regard to testicular cancer, FDG PET has established itself in small studies as an effective method for staging and for detecting recurrent/metastatic disease. For prostate cancer, the utility of FDG PET has yet to be proven. The new tracer ^{18}F-choline holds promise to expand PET to this fairly common cancer of the male population. Carbon-11-acetate and ^{11}C-choline are also of interest, although they are logistically more challenging to use due to their short half-lives.

With all GU neoplasms when FDG is the tracer, considerable attention must be given to normal ^{18}F activity in the kidneys, ureters, bladder, and the bowel. Careful attention to detail to avoid false-positive interpretations due to normal structures is essential.

ACKNOWLEDGMENT

The author acknowledges the special effort of Mr. Shannon K. Campbell in preparing the illustrative figures presented in this chapter.

REFERENCES

1. Greenlee RT, Murray T, Bolden S, et al. Cancer statistics, 2000. *CA Cancer J Clin* 2000;50:7–33.
2. DiSaia PJ, Creasman WT. Epithelial ovarian cancer. In: DiSaia PJ, Creasman WT, eds. *Clinical gynecologic oncology,* 5th ed. St. Louis: Mosby, 1997:282–285.
3. Seewald VL, Goff BA, Greer BE, et al. Post-therapy surveillance in patients with epithelial ovarian cancer. In: Gershenson DM, McGuire WP, eds. *Ovarian cancer: controversies in management.* New York: Churchill Livingstone, 1998:310–311.
4. Fleischer AC, Rodgers WH, Rao BK, et al. Assessment of ovarian tumor vascularity with transvaginal color Doppler sonography. *J Ultrasound Med* 1991;10:563–568.
5. Weiner Z, Thaler I, Beck D, et al. Differentiating malignant from benign ovarian tumors with transvaginal color flow image. *Obstet Gynecol* 1992;79:159–162.
6. Schweitzer SF, Majid AS, Paredes VM. Imaging of ovarian malignancies. *Appl Radiol* 2000;29:9–13.
7. Tempany CM, Zou KH, Silverman SG, et al. Staging of advanced ovarian cancer: comparison of imaging modalities—report from the Radiological Diagnostic Oncology Group. *Radiology* 2000;215:761–767.
8. Friedman JB, Weiss NS. Second thoughts about second-look laparotomy in advanced ovarian cancer. *N Engl J Med* 1990;22:1079–1082.
9. Kawamoto S, Urban BA, Fishman EK. CT of epithelial ovarian tumors. *Radiographics* 1999;19:[Suppl]S85–S102.
10. Forstner R, Hricak H, White S. CT and MRI of ovarian cancer. *Abdom Imaging* 1995;20:2–8.
11. Luesley D, Lawton F, Blackledge G, et al. Failure of second-look laparotomy to influence survival in epithelial ovarian cancer. *Lancet* 1988;2:599–603.
12. Nicklin JL, Copeland LJ, Luesley DM, et al. Second look surgery. In: Gershenson DM, McGuire WP, eds. *Ovarian cancer: controversies in management.* New York: Churchill Livingstone, 1998:87.
13. Berchuck A, Boente MP, Bast RC Jr. The use of tumor markers in the management of patients with gynecologic carcinomas. *Clin Obstet Gynecol* 1992;35:45–54.
14. Sakahara H, Hosono M, Kobayashi H, et al. Immunoscintigraphy of ovarian cancer using a monoclonal antibody to CA-125. *J Nucl Med* 1994:210P(abst).
15. Abdel-Nabi H, Marchetti D, Erb D, et al. Imaging ovarian carcinoma patients with Tc-99M-88BV59, a totally human monoclonal antibody. *J Nucl Med* 1996;37[Suppl 5]:9P(abst).
16. Grana C, Fazio F, Magnani P, et al. Immunoscintigraphy before second

look: an alternative to surgery in ovarian cancer patients? *J Nucl Med* 1998;39[Suppl 5]:243P.

17. Lieberman G, Buscombe JR, Thakrar DS, et al. Radioimmunoscintigraphy with pan-adenocarcinoma antibody may have a low specificity in patients with suspected ovarian cancer. *J Nucl Med* 1998;39[Suppl 5]:150P.

18. Bohdiewicz PJ, Scott GC, Juni JE, et al. Indium-111 OncoScint CR/OV and F-18 FDG in colorectal and ovarian carcinoma recurrences. Early observations. *Clin Nucl Med* 1995;20:230–236.

19. Neal CE, Swenson LC, Fanning J, et al. Monoclonal antibodies in ovarian and prostate cancer. *Semin Nucl Med* 1993;23:114–126.

20. Wahl RL, Hutchins GD, Roberts J. FDG-PET imaging of ovarian cancer: initial evaluation in patients. *J Nucl Med* 1991;32:982(abst).

21. Hubner KF, McDonald TW, Niethammer JG, et al. Assessment of primary and metastatic ovarian cancer by positron emission tomography (PET) using 2-[18F]deoxyglucose (2-[18F]FDG). *Gynecol Oncol* 1993;51:197–204.

22. Casey MJ, Gupta NC, Muths CK. Experience with positron emission tomography (PET) scans in patients with ovarian cancer. *Gynecol Oncol* 1994;53:331–338.

23. Patlak CS, Blasberg RG. Graphical evaluation of blood-to-brain transfer constants from multiple uptake data. *J Cereb Blood Flow Metab* 1983;3:1–7.

24. Karlan BY, Hawkins R, Hoh C, et al. Whole-body positron emission tomography with 2-(18F)-fluoro-2-deoxy-D-glucose can detect recurrent ovarian carcinoma. *Gynecol Oncol* 1993;51:175–181.

25. Gupta N, Muths C, Casey M, et al. Detection of residual/recurrent ovarian cancer using PET-FDG imaging. *J Nucl Med* 1993;34[Suppl]:7P(abst).

26. Avril N, Janicke F, Dose J, et al. FDG-PET evaluation of pelvic masses suspicious for primary or recurrent ovarian cancer. *J Nucl Med* 1994;35[Suppl]:231P(abst).

27. Boland GW, Goldberg MA, Goff B, et al. PET for peritoneal carcinomatosis: correlation with surgery and CT. *Radiology* 1993;189[Suppl]:147(abst).

28. Hubner KF, Smith GT, Stephens TS, et al. Detecting recurrent ovarian cancer using F-18-FDG PET. *J Nucl Med* 1995;36[Suppl]:106P(abst).

29. Zimny M, Schroder W, Wolters S, et al. 18F-fluorodeoxyglucose PET in ovarian carcinoma: methodology and preliminary results [in German]. *Nuklearmedizin* 1997;36:228–233.

30. Römer W, Avril N, Dose J, et al. Metabolic characterization of ovarian tumors with positron-emission tomography and F-18 fluorodeoxyglucose [in German]. *Rofo Fortschr Geb Rontgenstr Neuen Bildgeb Verfahr* 1997;166:62–68.

31. Garcia AA, Crespo-Jara JM, Marti M, et al. Impact of whole body PET-FDG in the early detection of recurrent ovarian cancer. *J Nucl Med* 1999;40[Suppl]:105P(abst).

32. Fenchel S, Kotzerke J, Stohr I, et al. Preoperative assessment of asymptomatic adnexal tumors by positron emission tomography and F18 fluorodeoxyglucose [in German]. *Nuklearmedizin* 1999;38:101–107.

33. Kubik-Huch RA, Dorffler W, von Schulthess GK, et al. Value of (18F)-FDG positron emission tomography, computed tomography, and magnetic resonance imaging in diagnosing primary and recurrent ovarian carcinoma. *Eur Radiol* 2000;10:761–767.

34. Grab D, Flock F, Stohr I, et al. Classification of asymptomatic adnexal masses by ultrasound, magnetic resonance imaging, and positron emission tomography. *Gynecol Oncol* 2000;77:454–459.

35. Vesselle HJ, Miraldi FD. FDG PET of the retroperitoneum: normal anatomy, variants, pathologic conditions, and strategies to avoid diagnostic pitfalls. *Radiographics* 1998;18:805–824.

36. Smith GT, Hubner KF, McDonald T, et al. Avoiding second-look surgery and reducing costs in managing patients with ovarian cancer by applying F-18-FDG PET. *Clin Positron Imaging* 1998;1:263.

37. Smith GT, Hubner KF, McDonald T, et al. Cost analysis of FDG PET for managing patients with ovarian cancer. *Clin Positron Imaging* 1999;2:63–70.

38. Umesaki N, Tanaka T, Miyama M, et al. Early diagnosis and evaluation of therapy in postoperative recurrent cervical cancers by positron emission tomography. *Oncol Rep* 2000;7:53–56.

39. Lapela M, Leskinen-Kallio S, Varpula M, et al. Metabolic imaging of ovarian tumors with carbon-11-methionine: a PET study. *J Nucl Med* 1995;36:2196–2200.

40. Rose PG, Adler LP, Rodriguez M, et al. Positron emission tomography for evaluating para-aortic nodal metastasis in locally advanced cervical cancer before surgical staging: a surgicopathologic study. *J Clin Oncol* 1999;17:41–45.

41. Sugawara Y, Eisbruch A, Kosuda S, et al. Evaluation of FDG PET in patients with cervical cancer. *J Nucl Med* 1999;40:1125–1131.

42. Wahl RL, Harney J, Hutchins G, et al. Imaging of renal cancer using positron emission tomography with 2-deoxy-2-(18F)-fluoro-d-glucose. Pilot animal and human studies. *J Urol* 1991;146:1470–1474.

43. Goldberg MA, Mayo-Smith WW, Papanicolaou N, et al. FDG PET characterization of renal masses: preliminary experience. *Clin Radiol* 1997;52:510–515.

44. Hoh CK, Figlin RA, Belldegrun A, et al. Evaluation of renal cell carcinoma with whole body FDG PET. *J Nucl Med* 1996;37[Suppl]:141P(abst).

45. Zhuang H, Duarte PS, Pourdehnad M, et al. Standardized uptake value as an unreliable index of renal disease on fluorodeoxyglucose PET imaging. *Clin Nucl Med* 2000;25:358–360.

46. Montravers F, Grahek D, Kerrou K, et al. Evaluation of FDG uptake by renal malignancies (primary tumor or metastases) using a coincidence detection gamma camera. *J Nucl Med* 2000;41:78–84.

47. Harney JV, Wahl RL, Liebert M, et al. Uptake of 2-deoxy-2-(18F)-fluoro-D-glucose in bladder cancer: animal localization and initial patient positron emission tomography. *J Urol* 1991;145:279–283.

48. Kocher F, Grommel S, Hautmann R, et al. Preoperative lymph node staging in patients with kidney and urinary bladder neoplasm. *J Nucl Med* 1994;35[Suppl]:223P(abst).

49. Kosuda S, Kison PV, Greenough R, et al. Preliminary assessment of fluorine-18 fluorodeoxyglucose positron emission topography in patients with bladder cancer. *Eur J Nucl Med* 1997;24:615–620.

50. Hutchins GD, Schauwecker D, Fain R, et al. Evaluation of FDG uptake with PET in post-chemotherapy residual germ cell tumor radiographic abnormalities. *J Nucl Med* 1994;35[Suppl]:117P(abst).

51. Laubenbacher C, Block T, Avril N, et al. Lymph node status in patients with testicular cancer: assessment by FDG PET. *Eur J Nucl Med* 1995;22:888.

52. Hain SF, O'Doherty MJ, Timothy AR, et al. Fluorodeoxyglucose positron emission tomography in the evaluation of germ cell tumors at relapse. *Br J Cancer* 2000;83:863–869.

53. Hain SF, O'Doherty MJ, Timothy AR, et al. Fluorodeoxyglucose PET in the initial staging of germ cell tumors. *Eur J Nucl Med* 2000;27:590–594.

54. Cremerius U, Wildberger JE, Borchers H, et al. Does positron emission tomography using 18-fluoro-2-deoxyglucose improve clinical staging of testicular cancer? Results of a study in 50 patients. *Urology* 1999;54:900–904.

55. Albers P, Bender H, Yilmaz H, et al. Positron emission tomography in the clinical staging of patients with stage I and II testicular germ cell tumors. *Urology* 1999;53:808–811.

56. Hoh CK, Seltzer MA, Franklin J, et al. Positron emission tomography in urological oncology. *J Urol* 1998;159:347–356.

57. Cremerius U, Effert PJ, Adam G, et al. FDG PET for detection and therapy control of metastatic germ cell tumor. *J Nucl Med* 1998;39:815–822.

58. Sugawara Y, Zasadny KR, Grossman HB, et al. Germ cell tumor: differentiation of viable tumor, mature teratoma, and necrotic tissue with F-18-fluorodeoxyglucose positron emission tomography and kinetic modeling. *Radiology* 1999;211:249–256.

59. Wahl RL. *Emerging applications of PET in oncology: melanoma, lymphoma, and prostate cancer: proceedings of the Sixth Annual International PET Conference.* Fairfax, VA: Institute for Clinical PET, 1994.

60. Kanamaru H, Oyama N, Akino H, et al. Evaluation of prostate cancer using FDG-PET. *Hinoyokika Kiyo* 2000;46:851–853.

61. Kao CH, Hsieh JF, Tsai SC, et al. Comparison and discrepancy of 18F-2-deoxyglucose positron emission tomography and Tc-99m MDP bone scan to detect bone metastases. *Anticancer Res* 2000;20:2189–2192.

62. Liu IJ, Zafar MB, Lai YH, et al. Fluorodeoxyglucose positron emission tomography in diagnosis and staging of clinically organ-confined prostate cancer. *Urology* 2001;57:108–111.

63. Hwang D, Mathias CJ, Welch MJ, et al. Imaging prostate derived tumors with PET and N-(3-[F-18]fluoropropyl)putrescine (FPP). *Nucl Med Biol* 1990;17:525–532.

64. Hwang D, Lang L, Mathias CJ, et al. N-3-[F-18]fluoropropylputrescine

as potential PET imaging agent for prostate derived tumors. *J Nucl Med* 1989;30:1205–1210.

65. Kalkner KM, Ginman C, Nilsson S, et al. PET with C-11-5 hydroxy-tryptophan (5-HTP) in patients with metastatic hormone refractory prostatic adenocarcinoma. *Nucl Med Biol* 1997;24:319–325.

66. Oyama N, Jones LA, Sharp TL, et al. Androgenic control of glucose and acetate metabolism in rat prostate and prostate cancer tumor model. *J Nucl Med* 2001;42:26P(abst).

67. Kishi H, Kosaka N, Hara T, et al. Remarkable effect of hormonal therapy on advanced prostate cancer demonstrated by C-11 choline PET. *J Nucl Med* 1999;40[Suppl]:60P(abst).

68. Kotzerke J, Prang J, Neumaier B, et al. Experience with carbon-11 choline positron emission tomography in prostate carcinoma. *Eur J Nucl Med* 2000;27:1415–1419.

69. DeGrado TR, Coleman RE, Wang S, et al. Synthesis and evaluation of [18]-F-labeled choline as an oncologic tracer for positron emission tomography: initial findings in prostate cancer. *Cancer Res* 2000;61:110–117.

CHAPTER 5.12

Skeletal and Soft Tissue

Gary J.R. Cook

There is an increasing interest in the use of positron emission tomography (PET) tracers for the investigation of various aspects of skeletal disease, and this is particularly true for the diagnosis of bone metastases. Both fluorine-18-fluoro-deoxyglucose (^{18}F-FDG), as a tumor-specific tracer, and ^{18}F-fluoride ion, as a nonspecific bone tracer, have been assessed and early results suggest that both agents have roles to play in the clinical management of patients. There is also a body of work in primary bone and soft-tissue sarcomas using ^{18}F-FDG. The main areas where FDG PET is likely to be particularly helpful are in grading of tumors, recognizing metastatic disease at diagnosis, and assessing response to primary treatment.

BONE METASTASES

[18]F-fluoride

Fluorine-18-fluoride was first described as a bone-imaging agent in the 1960s (1) but was subsequently replaced by technetium-99m (^{99m}Tc)–labeled diphosphonate compounds that were more suitable for gamma camera imaging. The increased use of PET for clinical applications in recent years has renewed interest in the potential of using this agent for diagnostic purposes.

Uptake of ^{18}F-fluoride, as with other nuclear medicine bone tracers, depends on local blood flow and more importantly osteoblastic activity. It preferentially accumulates at sites of high bone turnover and remodeling by chemisorption onto bone surfaces, exchanging with hydroxyl groups in hydroxyapatite crystals to form fluoroapatite (2). Uptake of ^{18}F-fluoride occurs in both sclerotic and lytic metastases (3), with the majority of the latter being accompanied by an osteoblastic reaction and hence uptake of bone tracers.

The high resolution of modern PET systems, the routine acquisition of tomographic images, and the high contrast that is achievable between normal and abnormal bone as early as 1 hour after injection of ^{18}F-fluoride are factors that have led to the evaluation of ^{18}F-fluoride PET in patients with bone metastases (3–8).

Compared with conventional nuclear medicine imaging,

PET has the advantage of superior quantitative accuracy and the ability to measure regional skeletal metabolic parameters in absolute numbers (3). Using such methods, the regional plasma clearance of ^{18}F-fluoride to bone mineral has been found to be three times greater at metastatic sites compared with adjacent bone in one study (3) and five to ten times greater in another (6). However, in a further study, using lesion-to-normal ratios as a less complex semiquantitative index of uptake, Hoh et al. (5) were unable to differentiate benign from malignant lesions. It remains to be seen whether dynamic kinetic parameters measured by ^{18}F-fluoride PET, reflecting mineralization and regional blood flow, will be more successful. Because the mechanisms of uptake of ^{18}F-fluoride are thought to be similar to other bone agents such as ^{99m}Tc methylene diphosphonate (MDP)—that is, depending on bone reaction rather than tumor viability—this may not be possible. The superior quantitative accuracy inherent in PET may be useful for following the effects of therapy for bone metastases, although this remains unexplored.

There is early evidence suggesting that ^{18}F-fluoride PET may be more sensitive and possibly more specific than conventional bone scintigraphy with ^{99m}Tc-MDP. Schirrmeister et al. (8) reported 44 patients with a mixture of primary cancers, including lung, prostate, and thyroid cancer, who had both ^{18}F-fluoride PET and ^{99m}Tc-MDP bone scans. Results from computed tomography (CT), magnetic resonance imaging (MRI), and iodine-131 (^{131}I)-iodine scintigraphy were used as references (8). Fluorine-18-fluoride PET resulted in the detection of all known bone metastases and nearly twice as many benign and malignant lesions overall, compared to ^{99m}Tc-MDP. The superior spatial resolution and three-dimensional (3D) localization enabled a significantly larger number of lesions to be correctly classified as benign or malignant (97% vs. 80.5%), with the advantages of PET being particularly noticeable in the spine. The cost-effectiveness of ^{18}F-fluoride PET has not been formally assessed, but in a study of patients with breast cancer, it lead to a change in management in 4 of 34 patients (7).

It is possible that some of the apparent advantages of ^{18}F-fluoride PET are due to technologic differences, in addition to any differences that exist between ^{18}F-fluoride and ^{99m}Tc MDP. PET images have higher spatial resolution, which contributes to a higher sensitivity, and unlike with ^{99m}Tc MDP, tomographic images of the whole skeleton are routine. This leads to improved image contrast, and hence improved sensitivity and 3D localization, which should improve specificity.

^{18}F-FDG

Because tumor uptake of ^{18}F-FDG depends on the rate of glycolysis and membrane glucose transporters, both of which are known to be increased in malignant tissue, the mechanism of uptake and the information available from this tracer in the skeleton are very different from those with ^{18}F-fluoride (Fig. 5.12.1). Fluorine-18-FDG localizes to varying degrees in all metastatic sites in a patient with cancer, whether in soft tissue or bone, thereby having the potential to stage a patient in a single examination. The direct uptake of ^{18}F-FDG by tumor tissue makes the measurement of quantitative indices of uptake even more attractive than with ^{18}F-fluoride in the skeleton. It may be possible to differentiate and grade lesions, as well as to, more importantly, monitor response to therapy at an early stage. This is an area in which there are significant limitations with conventional imaging techniques. To date, this application has not been fully explored with ^{18}F-FDG, however.

When comparing FDG PET with ^{99m}Tc-MDP bone scintigraphy for the detection of skeletal metastases in 110 patients with non–small cell lung cancer, Bury et al. (9) found a similar sensitivity on a patient-by-patient basis. Both methods identified 19 of 21 subjects with proven skeletal involvement, but FDG PET was able to confirm the absence of bone metastases in a much larger fraction (87 of 89 compared with 54 of 89 patients). Further studies using FDG PET in the staging of non–small cell lung cancer have also reported a greater accuracy than other radiologic methods in the detection of bone metastases, as well as in nonskeletal sites (10,11). The most likely explanation for these observations in the skeleton is that unlike ^{99m}Tc-MDP, the uptake of FDG is more specific to malignant tissue and is hampered to a lesser degree by nonspecific uptake into coincidental benign abnormalities such as osteoarthritis.

It is possible that the improved sensitivity reported with PET is partly explained by the fact that the direct imaging of tumor metabolism is possible with FDG. Detection may occur when only bone marrow is involved and before a significant osteoblastic bone reaction has taken place, which is required for uptake of bone tracers (Fig. 5.12.2). It is also possible that observed differences might be explained by the routine use of tomography with PET, unlike conventional bone scintigraphy.

Greater accuracy for detection of skeletal metastases is not a universal finding with FDG. In breast cancer, a higher number of false-negative FDG skeletal lesions, compared with nonskeletal metastases, has been reported (12,13). A possible explanation for the apparently poorer results with FDG in breast cancer may be due to a difference in the affinity of lytic and sclerotic metastases. The detection of a significantly larger number of skeletal metastases has been described using FDG compared with ^{99m}Tc-MDP in patients with breast cancer with progressive bone disease, but only in those who had predominantly osteolytic metastases (14). Patients who had predominantly sclerotic metastases had fewer lesions identified with FDG, and standard uptake values (SUVs) were lower in visible sclerotic lesions. Patients with predominantly lytic disease were also noted to have a poorer prognosis.

It is interesting that the sensitivity for detecting bone metastases using FDG in patients with prostate cancer also appears to be less than that using conventional bone scintigraphy (15,16). This tumor nearly always produces bone metastases that are sclerotic, and it is possible that metastases that tend to produce this marked osteoblastic response have a relatively low glycolytic rate compared with metastases that result in bone resorption and lysis (17). Sclerotic metastases are relatively acellular, and lower volumes of viable tumor within the lesions may also account for the relative insensitivity of FDG, in contrast to the florid osteoblastic activity that results in uptake of nonspecific bone tracers (18). Lytic lesions may be more hypoxic because they are more aggressive tumors that could outstrip their blood supply at an earlier stage. A relationship between hypoxia and uptake of FDG has been observed in some cell lines (19), and this may be an additional factor in accumulation in bone metastases.

As in soft tissues, uptake of FDG is not specific to malig-

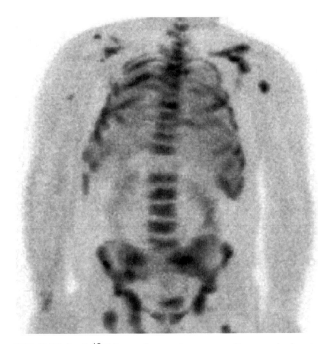

FIG. 5.12.1. A ^{18}F-fluorodeoxyglucose positron emission tomography image demonstrating widespread skeletal metastases in a male patient with an unknown primary tumor.

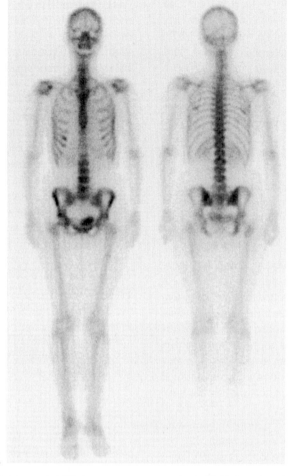

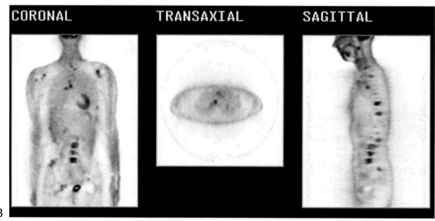

FIG. 5.12.2. A technetium-99m methylene diphosphonate bone scan **(A)** and coronal, transaxial, and sagittal ^{18}F-fluorodeoxyglucose positron emission tomography (FDG PET) images **(B)** of a woman with breast cancer. The FDG PET scan clearly demonstrates skeletal metastases that are not evident on the bone scan.

nancy in the skeleton. Increased accumulation of FDG has been described in some patients with active Paget disease [20], but fortunately, it does not appear that there is significant uptake in common causes for false-positive bone scan results, such as osteoarthritis. Inflammatory arthritides, including rheumatoid arthritis, may be positive, however.

In lymphoma, where skeletal disease is often marrow-based rather than purely osseous, a greater sensitivity for disease detection has been reported with FDG PET compared with conventional bone scintigraphy [21]. Due to the sensitivity for detecting bone marrow involvement and the ability of PET to study all skeletal areas, it has also been suggested that FDG PET might be able to replace bone marrow biopsy for staging. This procedure is most frequently

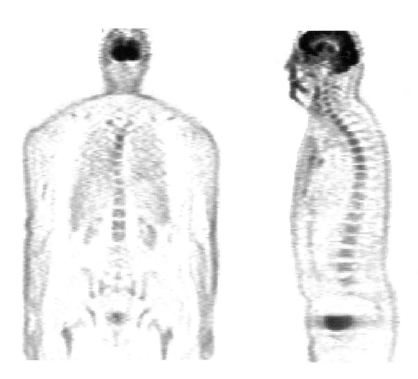

FIG. 5.12.3. There is a diffuse reactive increase in bone marrow ¹⁸F-fluorodeox-yglucose activity in a patient with lymphoma after chemotherapy.

performed at the iliac crest and therefore is limited by sampling error (22,23). The use of FDG PET to assess bone marrow disease may be less valuable after treatment with chemotherapy, because it is not uncommon to see a benign diffuse increase in activity in the bone marrow and occasionally the spleen after treatment (24) (Fig. 5.12.3). This appearance has also been reported after use of granulocyte colony-stimulating factor (25).

BONE AND SOFT-TISSUE SARCOMAS

Sarcomas are a heterogeneous group of tumors with varying grades of malignancy, and they commonly metastasize to lung and bone. A number of studies have reported the ability of FDG PET to grade tumors, although the differentiation of low-grade from benign lesions is more difficult (26–31). The differentiation of benign lesions from high-grade tumors is improved by delayed scanning, as high-grade tumors may not reach peak activity until 4 hours, whereas benign lesions plateau as early as 30 minutes (29) (Fig. 5.12.4).

By demonstrating the most metabolically active sites within a primary sarcoma, FDG may be helpful in guiding biopsies to ensure a representative sample (32) (Fig. 5.12.5). Image registration with CT or MRI should facilitate this.

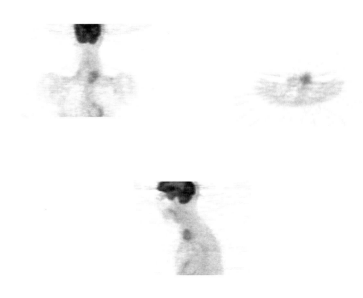

FIG. 5.12.4. Coronal, transaxial, and sagittal ¹⁸F-fluorodeoxyglucose positron emission tomography images reveal increased activity in the left lower neck of a patient with a low-grade leiomyosarcoma.

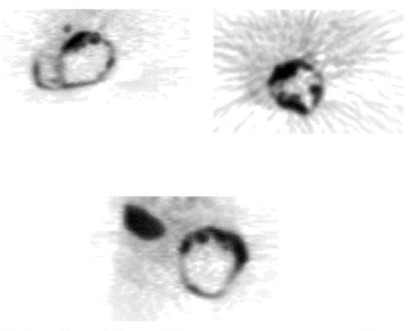

FIG. 5.12.5. Coronal **(upper left)** transaxial **(upper right)**, and sagittal **(bottom)** ¹⁸F-fluorodeoxyglucose positron emission tomographic images demonstrate a large heterogeneous mass in the right buttock, which was a high-grade sarcoma with central necrosis. FDG scans are often helpful in guiding biopsies to the most active parts of the tumor.

For the detection of metastases, FDG PET may not be quite as sensitive as CT for lung metastases or as sensitive as MRI for local recurrence, although it demonstrates good specificity and is able to detect additional distant metastases (33). It has, therefore, been suggested that all three imaging procedures may be required to accurately stage patients (Fig. 5.12.6).

Detecting local recurrence in amputation stumps may be complicated by nonspecific uptake of FDG at pressure areas and regions of skin breakdown. Diffuse activity may be seen within the stump for up to 18 months after surgery without evidence of recurrence. Focal changes, without clinical evidence of benign complications, suggest recurrent disease (34).

There are early data that suggest that FDG PET may be helpful in evaluating response to neoadjuvant therapy. In osteosarcoma, the percent decline in uptake of FDG resulting from therapy correlates well with the degree of necrosis, and with appropriate thresholds, it is possible to differentiate most responders from nonresponders (35). In a further study of mixed sarcomas, changes in uptake of FDG were again noted in responders, but reactive fibrous tissue was also noted to have prominent activity (36). Nonspecific reactive uptake has also been reported as a result of hyperthermic isolated limb perfusion therapy for soft-tissue sarcomas, making it difficult to differentiate between a complete and partial response in some cases with FDG (37).

SUMMARY

PET, particularly with FDG, is now playing a very important role in evaluating skeletal metastases of lung and other

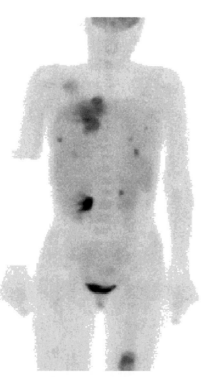

FIG. 5.12.6. The ¹⁸F-fluorodeoxyglucose positron emission tomographic image of a patient with a left thigh sarcoma shows that metastases are present in the thorax.

cancers. Although less sensitive than bone scans in blastic metastases, such as those of prostate and breast cancer, PET has a growing role in assessing primary or metastatic musculoskeletal tumors.

REFERENCES

1. Blau M, Nagler W, Bender MA. A new isotope for bone scanning. *J Nucl Med* 1962;3:332–334.
2. Blau M, Ganatra R, Bender MA. ^{18}F-fluoride for bone imaging. *Semin Nucl Med* 1972;2:31–37.
3. Hawkins RA, Choi Y, Huang SC, et al. Evaluation of the skeletal kinetics of fluorine-18-fluoride ion with PET. *J Nucl Med* 1992;33:633–642.
4. Hoegerle S, Juengling F, Otte A, et al. Combined FDG and (F-18)fluoride whole-body PET: a feasible two-in-one approach to cancer imaging? *Radiology* 1998;209:253–258.
5. Hoh CK, Hawkins RA, Dahlbom M, et al. Whole body skeletal imaging with (^{18}F)fluoride ion and PET. *J Comput Assisted Tomogr* 1993;17:34–41.
6. Petren-Mallmin M, Andreasson I, Ljunggren, et al. Skeletal metastases from breast cancer: uptake of ^{18}F-fluoride measured with positron emission tomography in correlation with CT. *Skeletal Radiol* 1998;27:72–76.
7. Schirrmeister H, Guhlmann A, Kotzerke J, et al. Early detection and accurate description of extent of metastatic bone disease in breast cancer with fluoride ion and positron emission tomography. *J Clin Oncol* 1999;17:2381–2389.
8. Schirrmeister H, Guhlmann A, Elsner K, et al. Sensitivity in detecting osseous lesions depends on anatomic localization: planar bone scintigraphy versus ^{18}F PET. *J Nucl Med* 1999;40:1623–1629.
9. Bury T, Barreto A, Daenen F, et al. Fluorine-18 deoxyglucose positron emission tomography for the detection of bone metastases in patients with non–small cell lung cancer. *Eur J Nucl Med* 1998;25:1244–1247.
10. Marom EM, McAdams HP, Erasmus JJ, et al. Staging non–small cell lung cancer with whole-body PET. *Radiology* 1999;212:803–809.
11. Pieterman RM, van Putten JWG, Meuzelaar JJ, et al. Preoperative staging of non–small cell lung cancer with positron emission tomography. *N Engl J Med* 2000;343:254–261.
12. Moon DH, Maddahi J, Silverman DH, et al. Accuracy of whole-body fluorine-18-FDG PET for the detection of recurrent or metastatic breast carcinoma. *J Nucl Med* 1998;39:431–435.
13. Wahl RL, Cody RL, Hutchins GD, et al. Primary and metastatic breast carcinoma: initial clinical evaluation with PET with the radiolabeled glucose analogue 2-(F-18)-fluoro-2-deoxy-D-glucose. *Radiology* 1991;179:765–770.
14. Cook GJ, Houston S, Rubens R, et al. Detection of bone metastases in breast cancer by [18]FDG PET: differing metabolic activity in osteoblastic and osteolytic lesions. *J Clin Oncol* 1998;16:3375–3379.
15. Shreve PD, Grossman HB, Gross MD, et al. Metastatic prostate cancer: initial findings of PET with 2-deoxy-2-(F-18)fluoro-D-glucose. *Radiology* 1996;199:751–756.
16. Yeh SD, Imbriaco M, Larson SM, et al. Detection of bony metastases of androgen-independent prostate cancer by PET-FDG. *Nucl Med Biol* 1996;23:693–697.
17. Nemoto R. New bone formation and cancer implants; relationship to tumour proliferative activity. *Br J Cancer* 1991;63:348–350.
18. Hiraga T, Mundy GR, Yoneda T. Bone metastases—morphology. In: Rubens RD, Mundy GR, eds. *Cancer and the skeleton.* London: Martin Dunitz, 2000:65–74.
19. Clavo AC, Brown RS, Wahl RL. Fluorodeoxyglucose uptake in human cancer cell lines is increased by hypoxia. *J Nucl Med* 1995;36:1625–1632.
20. Cook GJR, Maisey MN, Fogelman I. Paget's disease of bone: appearances with [18]FDG PET. *J Nucl Med* 1997;38:1495–1497.
21. Moog F, Bangerter M, Kotzerke J, et al. 18-F-fluorodeoxyglucose-positron emission tomography as a new approach to detect lymphomatous bone marrow. *J Clin Oncol* 1998;16:603–609.
22. Moog F, Kotzerke J, Reske SN. FDG PET can replace bone scintigraphy in primary staging of malignant lymphoma. *J Nucl Med* 1999;40:1407–1413.
23. Carr R, Barrington SF, Madan B, et al. Detection of lymphoma in bone marrow by whole-body positron emission tomography. *Blood* 1998;91:3340–3346.
24. Cook GJ, Fogelman I, Maisey MN. Normal physiological and benign pathological variants of 18-fluoro-2-deoxyglucose positron-emission tomography scanning: potential for error in interpretation. *Semin Nucl Med* 1996;26:308–314.
25. Hollinger EF, Alibazoglu H, Ali A, et al. Hematopoietic cytokine-mediated FDG uptake simulates the appearance of diffuse metastatic disease on whole-body PET imaging. *Clin Nucl Med* 1998;23:93–98.
26. Watanabe H, Shinozaki T, Yanagawa T, et al. Glucose metabolic analysis of musculoskeletal tumours using [18]fluorine-FDG PET as an aid to preoperative planning. *J Bone Joint Surg* 2000;82:760–767.
27. Schwarzbach MH, Dimitrakopoulou-Strauss A, Willeke F, et al. Clinical value of [18-F]fluorodeoxyglucose positron emission tomography imaging in soft tissue sarcomas. *Ann Surg* 2000;231:380–386.
28. Lucas JD, O'Doherty MJ, Cronin BF, et al. Prospective evaluation of soft tissue masses and sarcomas using fluorodeoxyglucose positron emission tomography. *Br J Surg* 1999;86:550–556.
29. Lodge MA, Lucas JD, Marsden PK, et al. A PET study of [18]FDG uptake in soft tissue masses. *Eur J Nucl Med* 1999;26:22–30.
30. Eary JF, Conrad EU, Bruckner JD, et al. Quantitative (F-18)fluorodeoxyglucose positron emission tomography in pretreatment and grading of sarcoma. *Clin Cancer Res* 1998;4:1215–1220.
31. Nieweg OE, Pruim J, van Ginkel RJ, et al. Fluorine-18-fluorodeoxyglucose PET imaging of soft-tissue sarcoma. *J Nucl Med* 1996;37:257–261.
32. Folpe AL, Lyles RH, Sprouse JT, et al. (F-18) fluorodeoxyglucose positron emission tomography as a predictor of pathologic grade and other prognostic variables in bone and soft tissue sarcoma. *Clin Cancer Res* 2000;6:1279–1287.
33. Lucas JD, O'Doherty MJ, Wong JC, et al. Evaluation of fluorodeoxyglucose positron emission tomography in the management of soft-tissue sarcomas. *J Bone Joint Surg* 1998;80:441–447.
34. Hain SF, O'Doherty MJ, Lucas JD, et al. Fluorodeoxyglucose PET in the evaluation of amputations for soft tissue sarcoma. *Nucl Med Commun* 1999;20:845–848.
35. Schulte M, Brecht-Krauss D, Werner M, et al. Evaluation of neoadjuvant therapy response of osteogenic sarcoma using FDG PET. *J Nucl Med* 1999;40:1637–1643.
36. Jones DN, McCowage GB, Sostman HD, et al. Monitoring of neoadjuvant therapy response of soft-tissue and musculoskeletal sarcoma using fluorine-18-FDG PET. *J Nucl Med* 1996;37:1438–1444.
37. van Ginkel RJ, Hoekstra HJ, Pruim J, et al. FDG-PET to evaluate response to hyperthermic isolated limb perfusion for locally advanced soft-tissue sarcoma. *J Nucl Med* 1996;37:984–990.

CHAPTER 5.13

Monitoring Treatment Response

Anthony F. Shields

Clinical imaging of many types, including x-ray, nuclear, and ultrasound techniques, is widely used to detect and stage cancer. After that is accomplished, the appropriate therapy must be chosen, and this may include a combination of surgery, radiation, chemotherapy, and biologic therapies. Evaluating the success of such treatment often requires additional imaging studies. As therapy continues to improve and more options become available for patients with cancer, the field of monitoring cancer therapy is burgeoning. For many years, the standard approach has relied on various anatomic imaging techniques to determine if the tumor has recurred, shrunk, or grown. Although cross-sectional images obtained with computed tomography (CT) and magnetic resonance imaging (MRI) have become standard in evaluating treatment response, they have a number of limitations. They only evaluate the size of the lesion, not its viability, proliferative rate, or physiologic state.

The major issues that affect the sensitivity and specificity of detecting response by measuring size include delays in shrinking of dying tumors, slow growth of tumors despite unsuccessful treatment, and the persistence of fibrotic or necrotic tumors. Positron emission tomography (PET), with its images of physiology, offers a new approach to assess tumor response. Although work in this field is still early in its exploration, studies are already demonstrating that it is becoming the new standard for some tumors and treatments. The optimal imaging approach will depend on the tumor types, treatment, and when an answer regarding the success of therapy is needed.

The measurement of the results of treatment is becoming more important as more successful treatment options become available. For example, up until the last few years, it was argued that chemotherapy had little role in the treatment of unresectable non–small lung cancer. It has now become accepted that treatment of metastatic disease can prolong survival. Thus, determining whether this treatment is successful and whether it should continue has gained importance. Knowing when to discontinue therapy is also of great importance because treatments are toxic and very costly. Recently, new second- and third-line therapies have been approved for some patients with advanced tumors resistant

to first-line treatment. This means that determining that the primary treatment has failed is more critical. New therapies, such as inhibitors of growth factors and tumor vascularity, are being extensively tested. Such agents may be cytostatic and slow tumor growth without causing extensive shrinkage in anatomic images. Finally, as therapy becomes more successful, a more common phenomenon is the persistence of fibrotic lesions, which do not contain viable tumor. All of these issues make the development of PET imaging of tumor response an area of growing interest.

The timing of response is certainly the most common issue in the assessment of response. The standard approach for patients receiving cytotoxic drugs is to have CT and/or MRI done every 2 months. The appearance of new lesions or significant growth of old lesions signals that the treatment has failed and that the patient should be offered alternative treatments or supportive care. Even when treatment is successful, it can take months to become evident. How much benefit are patients deriving from stable disease? Recent data, particularly those including cytostatic agents, suggest that stable disease provides important benefits, but it is difficult to differentiate those with slowly growing tumors in which the treatment is not helping from those in which the treatment has induced a decrease in the tumor growth rate.

TIMING OF PET IMAGING

A number of small studies have addressed the use of PET in the assessment of response and have studied a variety of times after the start of therapy. Depending on the tumor type, the treatment, and the goal of the imaging study, one can choose to image as soon as therapy starts to very late after the completion of treatment (Table 5.13.1). In assessments done within hours to days after the start of treatment, one is often looking for immediate effects on the cellular pathways targeted by the therapy. For example, has an antiangiogenesis agent really interfered with blood flow, or has tamoxifen blocked estrogen retention in the breast tumor? At this point, such uses have generally been limited to gaining a better understanding of the treatment as part of a research applica-

TABLE 5.13.1. *Possible times for imaging after the start of therapy and rationale*

Time after treatment	Imaging rationale

Immediate
  Hours to days
	Immediate effects on
	  metabolism/proliferation
	Drug pathway interference
	Blood-flow changes
	Receptor blockade

Early
  3–4 wk
  During therapy
  Cycle 1 of
  chemotherapy
	Metabolic response
	Proliferation changes

End
  2–6 mo
  (completion of
  therapy)
	Restage
	Assess residual lesions

Late Months to years	Necrosis vs. recurrence Restage

tion. Those involved in new drug development have been particularly interested in this application. In some cases, one is looking for immediate changes in proliferation or metabolism. This use blends into the next category—the early evaluation during the treatment, but after sufficient time to allow for a clear response to tumor well being. As previously discussed, anatomic imaging employed in this setting is often repeated 2 to 3 months after the start of treatment. Studies with PET early in the course of treatment are done to speed the assessment, with the idea that those without any metabolic evidence of tumor response should stop the present therapy and consider alternative treatment (1). Currently, only a limited number of studies address this use. Furthermore, third-party payers do not consistently reimburse this use. A larger number of studies have used PET at the end of a course of treatment or at later times to restage patients and to determine whether residual masses represent persistent viable tumor or fibrosis. These uses have found widespread clinical applicability and are leading to the rapidly increasing use of PET in oncology. U.S. Medicare approval of payment for such uses in a number of tumor types is likely to further spur this approach. Finally, PET is also used late after treatment to assess persistence or regrowth of the tumor compared with necrosis or fibrosis. The best example here is in the evaluation of patients after receiving treatment for brain tumors, lymphoma, and lung cancer (see below).

TRACERS FOR MEASUREMENT OF RESPONSE

FDG and Tumor Glycolysis

A wide variety of tracers have been tested in the measurement of tumor response. ^{18}F-Fluorodeoxyglucose (FDG) has become the most widely used agent for use in oncology because of its easy synthesis, moderately long half-life, and generally high tumor retention. As a result, it is very useful for detecting and staging cancer, as well as determining whether the tumor is responding to treatment. It has been commercially produced and centrally distributed, thus allowing for centers without cyclotrons to have ready access to the tracer. In some centers, it is the only tracer used, attesting to its profound importance in PET.

As with any tracer, FDG does have its limitations. The greatest limitation is that not all tumors avidly accumulate or readily retain FDG. In some cases, this reflects the fact that tumors may have mucinous or cystic areas or a high degree of fibrosis or differentiation, all of which may have limited FDG accumulation. Although the rapid renal excretion of unmetabolized FDG is generally an advantage, presence of tracer in the bladder has limited its use in the lower pelvis. This has made assessment of pelvic tumors, including bladder, prostate, and rectal tumors, more difficult. The more recent introduction of iterative reconstruction techniques has helped in this regard, by limiting streak artifacts that could potentially obscure tumors.

Methionine and Protein Synthesis

The next most commonly reported tracer in the assessment of tumor response is carbon-11 (^{11}C)-methionine. Its easy synthesis, a one-step process using methyl iodide, allows for the production of large quantities in PET centers with cyclotrons. It is readily retained in many tumors and provides high-contrast images in many sites. *In vitro* studies demonstrated that there are more rapid declines in protein synthesis than in glucose retention after successful treatment (2). This has lead to a number of promising clinical trials with this agent.

Limitations in the use of labeled methionine include the short half-life of ^{11}C and the requirement of a cyclotron on site. Although it was originally intended to provide a relative measure of protein synthesis, it has become clear that its retention also reflects the transmethylation reaction. Because of the complex pathways available for methionine retention, it is difficult to provide a simple model of kinetic analysis. Other protein synthesis tracers continue to be developed, but there have been limited studies to date.

Thymidine and Nucleoside Analogues

One of the central problems associated with cancer is the uncontrolled growth of tumor cells. The study of cell proliferation in the laboratory has been at the heart of cancer research for decades. In the clinic, measuring tumor growth has generally relied on serial size determinations, as previously discussed. More direct measurements of growth parameters have required biopsies to look for histologic evidence of proliferation (mitotic figures), nuclear antigens associated with growth, and flow cytometric measurements (S-phase fraction). In some clinical studies, direct measurements of growth have been done by injecting patients with hydrogen-3 (^{3}H)-thymidine before biopsy. The requirement of tissue samples has severely limited the studies one can do with such an approach.

Work on noninvasive imaging of cell proliferation has focused on the use of labeled nucleosides, in particular with thymidine and it analogues. The metabolic restriction of incorporation of thymidine into DNA, rather than RNA, leads to its routine use in the laboratory. Thymidine has been labeled with ^{11}C, both in the methyl group and in ring-2 positions. Although a small number of trials have demonstrated the utility of labeled thymidine in clinical studies, the short half-life of ^{11}C, the relatively difficult synthesis of the tracers, and the substantial metabolite signals in tumor have limited its widespread use. This has lead investigators to begin to explore a number of analogues that can be labeled with fluorine-18 (^{18}F), such as 3'-fluorothymidine (FLT) and iododeoxyuridine, which can be labeled with iodine-124 (3, 4).

Blood Flow

PET has been widely used to measure blood flow in the brain and heart. Initial work relied on the use of H$_2$^{15}O and many academic PET centers became very adept at using this very short half-life (2-minute) radiotracer. Repeated brain activation studies have been done, allowing just a few minutes for radioactive decay between injections. The recent introduction of tumor antivascular agents into clinical trials has led to a growing interest in the use of H$_2$^{15}O blood-flow studies. Because one may not see clear evidence of tumor shrinkage with such agents, primary disruption of the blood supply is eagerly sought by investigators to demonstrate efficacy. Furthermore, the optimal dose of the antivascular agents may be determined best by measuring the lowest dose that is needed to decrease tumor blood flow. Early trials have found changes in tumor blood flow 30 minutes after the injection of agents such as combretastatin (5). PET provides data complementary to those obtained with MRI (dynamic contrast enhanced), which measures a combination of permeability and flow. Although it is not likely that this will become a common clinical use, PET is playing a valuable role in helping to develop these new drugs.

Labeled Drugs

One particularly interesting application of PET is in the evaluation of labeled anticancer agents. The injection of such labeled compounds allows one to measure the clearance from the blood, as well as the uptake and retention into tumors. For example, studies have been done comparing the uptake of nitrogen-13-cisplatin into brain tumors and have demonstrated that intraarterial injection results in higher tumor uptake than simple intravenous delivery (6). The uptake of labeled drugs has also been used to predict whether a patient is likely to be susceptible to a given agent; that is, low uptake and retention may predict resistance to the drug.

This has been demonstrated using ^{18}F-5-fluorouracil, an agent commonly used to treat patients with colorectal cancer (7). In patients with liver metastases, those with low uptake were uniformly nonresponders while the higher the uptake the greater the likelihood of response. Overall the number of labeled drugs has been small, and although such compounds are useful in measuring the pharmacology of the drugs, they are generally not useful in monitoring response. Although labeled drugs may provide important information to understand the drugs distribution and possibly predict therapeutic outcome, there are limited uses so far in monitoring or predicting response to treatment.

Quantitation of Tumor Measurements with PET

One of the critical issues in using PET to measure treatment response is how to best quantitate the imaging results (8,9). When FDG PET is used in diagnostic studies, many centers routinely evaluate the images visually to determine if there are areas of activity with more intense uptake compared with the background. A similar approach is used in the routine staging of patients. This is often supplemented with the semiquantitative evaluation using the standardized uptake value (SUV), with malignant lesions generally having a value of more than 2.0 to 3.0.

When evaluating the response to therapy, more accurate quantitation gains added importance, because although a tumor may still be visible, significant declines in tumor metabolism may indicate a favorable response (1). This has led to the use of kinetic analysis of image data obtained dynamically, along with blood input curves. This allows one to measure overall flux of the tracer into tumors, along with the individual rate constants. The relative utility of these approaches depends on the clinical setting and is likely to vary with each tumor and treatment.

For the simple answer of determining if viable tumor is present at the end of therapy or late after the completion of treatment, simple visual assessment has been successfully employed in some studies (10). In such cases, persistent tumor may be reported if activity above background for the surrounding tissues is noted. A similar approach has been employed in determining if recurrence is present rather than necrosis.

When one wishes to obtain information immediately after the start or early in the course of therapy, more quantitative approaches are more likely to be of value (11). At this point, the relative merits of using semiquantitative measurements of SUV and more detailed measurements of kinetic parameters are still open to debate. Some studies have demonstrated benefits for both approaches (12). One issue is clearly the reproducibility of such measurements. Although data are limited, most trials suggest that repeated measurements made without intervening treatment will vary from 10% to 20% (13). Until the best technique is determined, it has been suggested that data be obtained in a standardized way. This would allow various groups to compare their results and they would later have the ability to recalculate the response values.

PET EVALUATION OF TUMOR RESPONSE: CLINICAL AND RESEARCH EXPERIENCE

Brain Tumors

The use of PET in oncology began with the study of brain tumors. A number of studies have examined the course of treatment with surgery, chemotherapy, and radiation, as well as the changes seen using PET (a sample of such studies is seen in Table 5.13.2). For a long time, the primary use of PET in oncology was the determination of disease persistence versus radionecrosis in patients late after therapy for astrocytomas (14–17). This is useful in determining patient prognosis and deciding if further surgery is indicated. The limitations of this approach are the high FDG retention in the normal brain, which can make interpretation difficult at times, and the limited therapeutic options available with each diagnosis.

In one of the earliest studies looking at response at the end of treatment, Ogawa et al. (18) demonstrated that FDG retention decreased by 1 month after chemoradiotherapy, but they did not see declines in blood flow or oxygen consumption. In another study, which included scans on days 1, 7, and 30 after multiagent chemotherapy, tumor-to-normal tissue activity ratios (T : N ratio) increased 1 day after therapy by 20% to 100% (19). The activity level then declined by 1 month and varied from 22% above baseline to 35% below. In another study in patients treated with stereotactic radiosurgery, a rapid increase on tumor activity was seen 1 day after treatment, but this declined 1 week later (20). The early increase in tumor metabolism in the day after treatment, often called a "flare" reaction, was shown to correlate with survival in patients treated with carmustine (21).

In seven children with a mixture of medulloblastoma and primitive neuroectodermal tumors (PNET), imaging was done with FDG before, during, and at the completion of therapy (22). The percentage decrease in the metabolic ratio of tumor to white matter was found to correlate with tumor response based on anatomic imaging and clinical duration of response. Unfortunately, the paucity of really effective treatment options for use in adult patients with astrocytomas has limited the clinical use of FDG imaging in this group of patients. As new drugs are developed for this disease, PET is gaining a role in evaluating response to therapy. In a recent trial, nine patients with gliomas were treated with temozolomide and imaged with FDG PET before and 14 days after the start of therapy (12). The change in metabolic rate in the regions with high focal tumor uptake was found to correlate with the anatomic response at 8 weeks (Fig. 5.13.1). This analysis required the study of those areas of tumor with high focal uptake rather than the whole tumor. SUV changes also correlated with response, but the metabolic rate parameters were a better measure of treatment outcome.

Although FDG has been the primary tracer used for PET studies of the brain, methionine has also been used in some trials. For example, patients with low-grade (13) or anaplastic (1) astrocytomas were imaged with methionine before and 3, 6, 12, or more than 21 months after radiation (23). The SUV ratio in tumor to normal brain rose significantly in those who died of progressive disease, was stable in those alive with disease, and declined slightly in those without evidence of disease.

The high background of normal glucose utilization has made the use of FDG problematic in trying to determine if

TABLE 5.13.2. *Brain tumors and PET evaluation after therapy*

Tracer (no. of patients)	Treatment	Timing of PET relative to treatment	PET analysis	Clinical evaluation	Result	Author, yr (reference no.)
FDG (n = 7)	XRT	Late after	Visual	Pathology and follow-up	100% accuracy	Doyle et al., 1987 (15)
FDG (n = 33)	XRT	Late after	Visual	Pathology and follow-up	88% accuracy	Kim et al., 1992 (17)
FDG (n = 11)	XRT and chemotherapy	24 d after end	Kinetic	CT	FDG decrease	Ogawa et al., 1988 (18)
FDG (n = 6)	Chemotherapy	During days 1, 7, and 30	T:N Kinetic	CT	Increase T:N day 1	Rozental et al., 1989 (19)
FDG (n = 11)	Chemotherapy	1 d after start	Kinetic	Survival	Correl survival and day 1 increase	De Witte et al., 1994 (21)
FDG (n = 7)	Chemotherapy	1 d after start	Kinetic	CT/MRI survival	Correl PET and clinical	Holthoff et al., 1993 (22)
FDG (n = 9)	Chemotherapy	14 d after start	Kinetic SUV	CT and follow-up	Correl PET and response	Brock et al., 2000 (12)
Methionine (n = 14)	XRT	3, 6, 12, >21 mo	T:N SUV	MRI and follow-up	Correl PET and response	Nuutinen et al., 2000 (23)

XRT, radiation therapy; T:N, tumor to normal tissue ratio; kinetic, metabolic rate calculation; correl, correlates PET with the indicated evaluation.

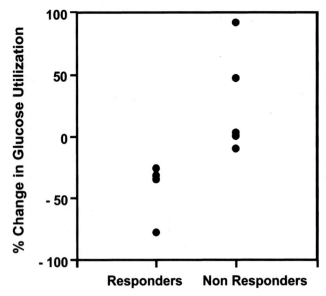

FIG. 5.13.1. Treatment results in patients with high-grade gliomas treated with temozolomide. The change in metabolic rate for ^{18}F-fluorodeoxyglucose in the highest uptake areas of the tumor was compared with objective response at 8 weeks. PET was able to separate responders from nonresponders ($p < .02$). (Adapted from Brock CS, Young H, O'Reilly SM, et al. Early evaluation of tumour metabolic response using [^{18}F]fluorodeoxyglucose and positron emission tomography: a pilot study following the phase II chemotherapy schedule for temozolomide in recurrent high-grade gliomas. *Br J Cancer* 2000;82:608–615.)

patients have small areas of persistent or recurrent disease. Proliferative tracers of metabolism have also been developed to assist in monitoring brain tumor therapy including thymidine and its analogues. Agents such as thymidine, FLT, or iododeoxyuridine may assist in this assessment (24, 25) (Fig. 5.13.2).

Lymphoma

FDG PET imaging of lymphoma is already done clinically in many centers. It is commonly used in staging, but its greatest role is in the assessment of treatment response at the end of therapy. Chemotherapy can be curative in most patients with both Hodgkin disease (HD) and non-Hodgkin lymphoma (NHL). A major problem in these patients is that they are often left with residual masses at the end of chemotherapy and this may represent persistent disease or fibrosis. Knowledge of persistent disease is critical, because alternative treatments are available including radiation, other chemotherapies, and even high-dose therapy with stem-cell rescue. Gallium-67 scintigraphy was used to assist in this problem but has been variable in its acceptance. Furthermore, recent trials have demonstrated that FDG PET is superior to gallium single-photon emission tomography in the staging of lymphoma (26,27). A number of studies have been completed that demonstrate the utility of FDG PET for evaluating patients at the end of their treatment (Table 5.13.3).

Although most studies have concentrated on imaging patients at the conclusion of treatment, Romer et al. (28) im-

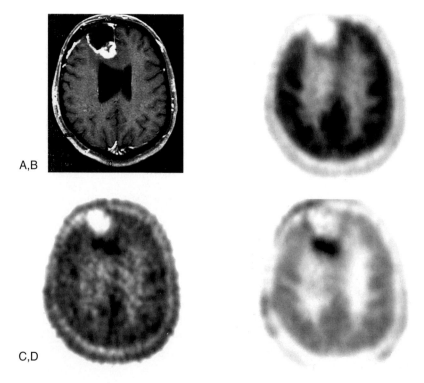

FIG. 5.13.2. Images of a patient with recurrent glioma as imaged with **(A)** magnetic resonance imaging, **(B)** ^{18}F-fluorodeoxyglucose positron emission tomography, **(C)** carbon-11-thymidine (TdR) PET imaged from 20 to 60 minutes, and **(D)** parametric image of thymidine flux constant. The later image **(D)** best shows the area of recurrent tumor in the area posterior to the previous resection. (From Eary JF, Mankoff DA, Spence AM, et al. 2-[C-11]thymidine imaging of malignant brain tumors. *Cancer Res* 1999;59:615–621, with permission.)

TABLE 5.13.3. *Lymphoma and PET evaluation after chemotherapy*

Tracer (no. of patients)	Disease	Timing of PET relative to treatment	PET analysis	Clinical evaluation	Result	Author, yr (reference no)
FDG (n = 11)	NHL	1 and 6 wk after start	SUV kinetic	Follow-up and CT	81% PET accuracy	Romer et al., 1998 (28)
FDG (n = 22)	HD	During and after	Visual	Follow-up and CT	77% PET accuracy	Weidmann et al., 1999 (29)
FDG (n = 37)	HD	After	Visual	Follow-up and CT	74% PET accuracy	de Wit et al., 2001 (30)
FDG (n = 54)	HD = 19 NHL = 85	1–3 mo after end	Visual	Follow-up and CT	85% PET accuracy	Jerusalem et al., 1999 (31)
FDG (n = 72)	HD = 29 NHL = 41	After	Visual	Follow-up and pathology	85% PET accuracy	Cremerius et al., 1999 (32)
FDG (n = 54)	HD = 43 NHL = 11	After	Visual	Follow-up and CT	93% PET accuracy	Stumpe et al., 1998 (33)

^{18}F-FDG, fluorodeoxyglucose; HD, Hodgkin disease; NHL, non-Hodgkin lymphona; SUV, standard uptake value.

aged 11 patients with NHL before and at 1 and 6 weeks after the start of therapy (Fig. 5.13.3). When measured using SUV quantitation, they noted a 60% decrease in tumor FDG uptake at 1 week and an average overall decline of 79% by 6 weeks. Although the decline at 1 week was significant, there was too much overlap between those attaining a long-term complete response (CR) and relapsing patients to be of routine clinical use. In analyzing the 6-week images, an SUV cutoff of 2.5 was able to differentiate those maintaining a CR from failing patients with an 81% accuracy (Fig. 5.13.4). All three patients with a high SUV relapsed. The problem in assessment came from patients with apparent CR by PET who went on to relapse (two patients). This is an expected

limitation with any imaging technology because it will fail to detect microscopic disease that can lead to eventual relapse.

Weidmann et al. (29) performed 22 studies in patients with HD during and at the end of chemoradiotherapy. They compared the PET results with those obtained with conventional imaging and clinical follow-up. The overall accuracy of the PET evaluation was 77% in predicting the ultimate outcome. It is notable that in three of the five patients with discrepant PET results, the follow-up scan was done after only two cycles of therapy, so imaging later may have been a better measure of ultimate outcome. One of the patients who had a false-positive FDG PET result was found to have radiation pneumonitis. This trial was also limited in that

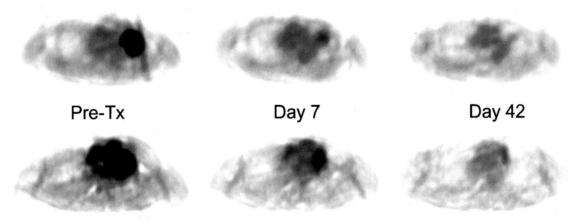

Pre-Tx   Day 7   Day 42

FIG. 5.13.3. Top row: Patient with high-grade non-Hodgkin lymphoma and a large parahilar lesion. This patient had a complete response (CR) based on PET study results and remained in CR 15 months later. **Bottom row:** A patient with extensive mediastinal involvement with high-grade lymphoma. Although the patient had a partial response to therapy, a lesion with a standard uptake value of 4.1 was still visible at day 42. The patient relapsed during the third course of chemotherapy. Images were obtained pretreatment and at days 7 and 42 after the start of therapy. (From Romer W, Hanauske A, Ziegler S, et al. Positron emission tomography in non-Hodgkin's lymphoma: assessment of chemotherapy with fluorodeoxyglucose. *Blood* 1998;91:4464–4471, with permission.)

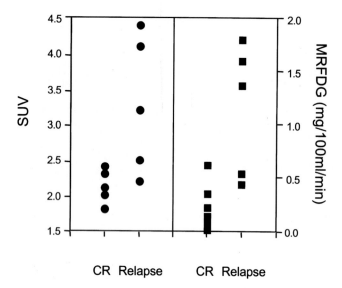

FIG. 5.13.4. Comparison of fluorodeoxyglucose (FDG) positron emission tomography and ultimate relapse or complete response in patients undergoing chemotherapy for non-Hodgkin's lymphoma. PET measurements were obtained as maximum standard uptake values (*circles*) and metabolic rate for FDG (*squares*). (From Romer W, Hanauske A, Ziegler S, et al. Positron emission tomography in non-Hodgkin's lymphoma: assessment of chemotherapy with fluorodeoxyglucose. *Blood* 1998;91:4464–4471, with permission.)

none of the patients relapsed and the investigators did not employ attenuation correction. Overall, it does demonstrate the utility of imaging at the end of the therapy to determine if a patient will remain in remission.

In a study of 37 patients with HD, imaging with FDG PET a mean of 10 weeks after treatment had a 74% accuracy in predicting relapse (30). This compared with the accuracy of 32% with CT. Only 1 of 28 patients with a negative PET scan result relapsed, whereas 12 of 22 patients with positive PET scan results did not relapse. Some patients had radiation and repeat scans done after chemotherapy. If one takes into account only the PET scans obtained after completing all therapy, the accuracy was 85% and there were only five false-positive scan results.

Jerusalem et al. (31) studied 19 patients with HD and 35 with NHL in the posttreatment evaluation of patients 1 to 3 months after chemotherapy. All 6 patients with positive posttreatment PET scan results progressed, as did 8 of 48 patients (17%) with negative scans. The overall accuracy of PET was 85% in predicting relapse, compared with 67% for CT. Although all patients with positive PET results relapsed, only 5 (26%) of 19 patients with positive CT results and negative PET results progressed, and 10% of those with both negative PET and negative CT results progressed. Similar results were found by Cremerius et al. (32) who studied 72 patients (29 with HD, 41 with NHL, and 2 unclassified) and found an accuracy of 85% for PET compared with 54% for CT. The major problem with CT is the low specificity (31%)

in those with residual masses. PET was found to be 90% accurate in predicting remission in those with moderate risk disease, but the negative predictive value of PET was only 50% to 67% in those with a high risk of relapse. Stumpe et al. (33) found an overall accuracy of 93% in a retrospective study of 54 patients with HD and NHL imaged after therapy.

In summary, the data clearly indicate the superiority of FDG PET in the restaging of both HD and NHL after the completion of therapy. The greatest advantage of PET is in the demonstration that persistent fibrotic lesions are not metabolically active. Such patients may be watched with the likelihood that they will remain in remission. Limitations of PET include the fact that even PET-negative areas may harbor microscopic tumor that may recur. Furthermore, the timing of PET is important, as studies done during or shortly after therapy may not have had time to fully resolve the tumor. This can be particularly problematic in patients who have radiation as part of their treatment. Keeping these limitations in mind, PET has been found to be an important addition to the clinical evaluation of patients being treated for lymphoma and is part of standard clinical practice.

Head and Neck Cancer

The treatment of head and neck cancers routinely employs the use of chemotherapy and radiation, often before the surgical resection of residual disease. This is a very useful setting in which to evaluate the ability of PET to measure changes resulting from treatment and to determine if viable tumor remains at the end of therapy (Table 5.13.4). In addition to the routine use of FDG, methionine has also been used in such studies. One of the early studies presented by Chaiken et al. (34) demonstrated that in patients receiving radiation therapy (XRT) with stable or increasing FDG retention, six (86%) of seven were found to have persistent or recurrent disease. All patients who achieved remission after XRT had declines in the T : N ratio after therapy.

Sakamoto et al. (35) studied 22 patients using FDG with XRT alone or with carboplatin chemotherapy. The mean SUV fell from 7.0 before therapy to 3.8 three to four weeks after the completion of therapy. In those patients going on to surgery, the SUV ranged from 8.3 to 2.9 in those with viable tumor remaining, while it was 3.3 to 1.9 if no viable tumor was present. Although there was some overlap (SUV of about 3.0), PET was clearly superior to conventional imaging techniques and the accuracy of predicting pathologic response was 73%. The results seen with conventional imaging did not correlate with those found with PET or pathologic results. Slevin et al. (36) used PET and MRI at 4 and 8 months after x-ray treatment to assess results. In almost all cases, PET and MRI were consistent and both correlated with the status of the disease and final outcome. PET was positive in four patients, of which two eventually died of the disease and two were disease free at almost 2 years. Both PET and MRI each missed one recurrence.

Imaging after treatment with chemotherapy alone has also

TABLE 5.13.4. *Head and neck cancer and PET evaluation after therapy*

Tracer (no. of patients)	Treatment	Timing of PET relative to treatment	PET analysis	Clinical evaluation	Result	Author, yr (reference no.)
FDG (n = 15)	XRT	During and 2–12 wk after	T:N	Follow-up	Positive PET results, recur in 6/7 patients	Chaiken et al., 1993 (34)
FDG (n = 22)	XRT ± chemotherapy	3–4 wk after end	SUV	Follow-up and pathology	73% PET accuracy	Sakamoto et al., 1998 (35)
FDG (n = 21)	XRT	4 mo and 8 mo after	T:N	MRI and follow-up	Result correl	Slevin et al., 1999 (36)
FDG (n = 11)	Chemotherapy	1 wk after start	SUV	CT	Change SUV correl CT	Haberkorn et al., 1993 (37)
FDG (n = 28)	Chemotherapy/XRT	1–2 wk after end	Visual SUV	Pathology	89% PET accuracy	Lowe et al., 1997 (38)
FDG (n = 6)	Chemotherapy	During and 2 yr after	T:N	Follow-up	All decrease with therapy	Berlanglieri et al., 1994 (39)
Methionine (n = 15)	XRT	During	SUV	Follow-up	No correl with outcome	Nuutinen et al., 1999 (40)
Methionine (n = 15)	XRT	3 wk after end	SUV	Pathology	84% PET accuracy	Lindholm et al., 1995 (41)

FDG, ^{18}F-fluorodeoxyglucose; XRT, radiation therapy; T:N, tumor to normal tissue ratio; SUV, standard uptake value; correl, correlates PET with the indicated evaluation.

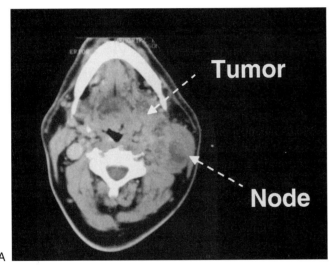

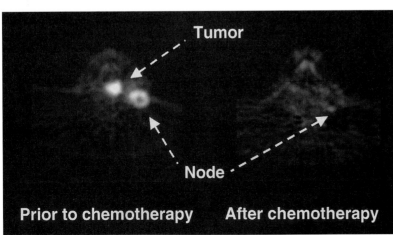

FIG. 5.13.5. A patient with head and neck cancer imaged with computed tomography before treatment **(A)** and ^{18}F-fluorodeoxyglucose positron emission tomography before and after chemotherapy **(B)**. The patient had a base of tongue lesion that resolved completely on PET and a nodal lesion with a marked decrease in metabolism. (From Lowe V, Dunphy F, Varvares M, et al. Evaluation of chemotherapy response in patients with advanced head and neck cancer using [F-18]fluorodeoxyglucose positron emission tomography. *Head Neck* 1997;19:666–674, with permission.)

demonstrated that as early as 1 week after treatment, one could see changes in FDG uptake (i.e., SUV) that correlated with changes in tumor size (37). Lowe et al. (38) also obtained images 1 to 2 weeks after chemotherapy and they were found to correlate with pathologic response to treatment (Fig. 5.13.5). The mean decline in SUV was 34% in those with residual disease and 82% in pathologic CR. PET had a 90% sensitivity for persistent pathologic disease and overall 89% accuracy. Similar results were seen at 4 weeks posttherapy by Berlangieri et al. (39).

Methionine has also been used in patients treated with radiation alone. Measurements obtained during the first 2 to 3 weeks of therapy showed declines in most of the treated patients (Fig. 5.13.6) (40). They were, however, unable to predict who would eventually relapse or remain in remission. On the other hand, methionine measurements (by SUV) obtained a median of 3 weeks after the completion of therapy were found to correlate with pathologic response at resection (41).

In summary, PET has demonstrated early declines after both radiation and chemotherapy to treat head and neck cancers. The clinical value of these images obtained during the course of treatment is unclear, given the limited number of patients studied. Images obtained at the conclusion of therapy appear to be predictive of the ultimate outcome.

Breast Cancer

Breast cancer treatment has been assessed using PET in the treatment of both metastatic and locally advanced disease (Table 5.13.5). The evaluation of both chemotherapy and hormone therapy with PET has been of interest. Wahl et al. (42) compared baseline FDG PET with up to four scans obtained during chemohormonotherapy. Metabolic changes in the tumors, determined visually and with SUVs, were documented with PET, and the kinetic parameters correlated with response as detected by mammographic shrinkage of the tumors. The response measured by PET appeared to be more prompt than declines in tumor size. Bassa et al. (43) imaged patients before, during, and at the end of neoadjuvant therapy. Visual analysis of the images obtained just before surgery were 76% accurate in determining if residual tumor was present. The greatest failing of PET was in missing small volumes of residual disease.

In a study of 30 patients with locally advanced breast cancer, the ultimate pathologic response to therapy could be predicted after the first cycle of therapy using FDG PET (44). Using a 20% decrease in SUV as a cutoff, PET had a sensitivity of 90% and a specificity of 74% (overall accuracy of 79%) in predicting the pathologic disappearance of all microscopic or macroscopic tumor (Fig. 5.13.7). A similar result was found in the study of Schelling et al. (45) who also studied patients with locally advanced breast cancer before and after the first and second cycles of chemotherapy (Fig. 5.13.8). They determined that the optimal threshold was a decrease in the SUV by at least 45% and that this had an overall accuracy of 88% in predicting that the patients would have minimal residual disease (Fig. 5.13.9). FDG PET is also gaining use in the evaluation of experimental treatment. In a study of four patients receiving stereotatic interstitial laser therapy, FDG PET was able to demonstrate that only one had no residual tumor while the other three had partial responses (46).

Methionine has also been used to monitor response to treatment in patients receiving chemotherapy for breast cancer. Jansson et al. (47) studied patients before and after the

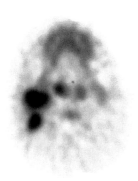
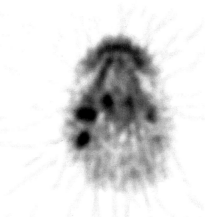

FIG. 5.13.6. Carbon-11-methionine PET images of a patient with head and neck cancer metastatic to the lymph nodes. Images were obtained before **(left)** and during radiotherapy **(right)**, and the standard uptake value decreased from 9.4 to 5.4 in the larger lymph nodes while retention in the oral mucosa increased slightly. This patient remained in remission more than 27 months after treatment. (From Nuutinen J, Jyrkkio S, Lehikoinen P, et al. Evaluation of early response to radiotherapy in head and neck cancer measured with [¹¹C]methionine-positron emission tomography. *Radiother Oncol* 1999;52: 225–232, with permission.)

TABLE 5.13.5. *Breast cancer and PET evaluation after therapy*

Tracer (no. of patients)	Treatment	Timing of PET relative to treatment	PET analysis	Clinical evaluation	Result	Author, yr (reference no.)
FDG (n = 11)	Chemotherapy, hormone	During cycles 1–3	Visual SUV	Mammogram	Correl PET and mammogram	Wahl et al., 1993 (42)
FDG (n = 16)	Chemotherapy	During and at end	SUV visual	Pathology	76% PET accuracy	Bassa et al., 1996 (43)
FDG (n = 30)	Chemotherapy	During and at end	SUV kinetic	Pathology	79% PET accuracy	Smith et al., 2000 (44)
FDG (n = 22)	Chemotherapy	During cycles 1 and 2	SUV	Pathology	88% PET accuracy	Schelling et al., 2000 (45)
FDG (n = 4)	Laser	2 wk after end	T:N	Pathology	Correl PET and pathology	Nair et al., 2000 (46)
FDG and Methionine (n = 16)	Chemotherapy	During cycles 1 and 3/4	SUV	CT and clinical	Correl PET and clinical	Jansson et al., 1995 (47)
Methioinine (n = 8)	Chemotherapy, hormone, or XRT	During 3–14 wk	SUV kinetic	Clinical	Correl PET and clinical	Huovinen et al., 1993 (48)
FES (n = 7)	Hormone	2 wk after start	Semiquantitative	Clinical	Correl PET and clinical	McGuire et al., 1991 (50)
FES and FDG (n = 11)	Hormone	7–10 d after start	Semiquantitative	Clinical	FDG 100% accurate	Dehdashti et al., 1999 (51)

SUV, standard uptake value; T:N, tumor to normal tissue ratio; correl, correlates PET with the indicated evaluation; FES, ^{18}F-fluoroestradiol.

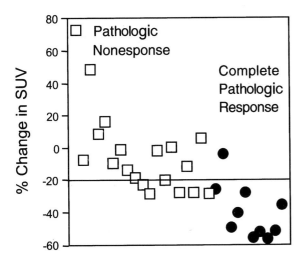

FIG. 5.13.7. ^{18}F-Fluorodeoxyglucose positron emission tomography imaging results after one cycle of treatment for primary breast cancer. The percentage change in standard uptake value was compared in those judged nonresponsive by pathology (*open squares*) or to those with at least a macroscopic pathologic response (*closed circles*). (From Smith IC, Welch AE, Hutcheon AW, et al. Positron emission tomography using [^{18}F]-fluorodeoxy-D-glucose to predict the pathologic response of breast cancer to primary chemotherapy. *J Clin Oncol* 2000;18:1676–1688, with permission.)

first and third and/or fourth cycles of chemotherapy with either FDG or methionine. Seven patients were studied with both tracers before treatment, and methionine demonstrated better contrast in five, so it was chosen for further use in repeated studies. The other patients were studied with only FDG or methionine. Out of 16 patients, 9 had repeat methionine studies and 7 FDG. Eleven of 12 patients with major clinical responses also had decreases in methionine (6 patients) or FDG (5 patients) during the first course of therapy. Methionine was also found to be useful in monitoring therapy response with both hormone therapy and chemotherapy (48).

Labeling of estrogens for the measurement of receptor status *in vivo* using PET has been employed by investigators and compared with assays made by receptor assays from pathologic specimens (49). All these studies have found that PET analysis using either labeled ^{18}F-fluorotamoxifen or 16α(^{18}F)fluoro-17β-estradiol (FES) was predictive of response to antiestrogen treatment. Imaging done before and after antiestrogen therapy showed a decline in FES uptake in all lesions (50). In a subsequent study, 11 patients with estrogen-receptor–positive breast cancer were imaged with both FDG and FES before and 7 to 10 days after the start of tamoxifen therapy (51). The responders had a greater decline in FES retention than the nonresponders, as measured by the change in SUV. Of even more scientific interest was that all the responders had a "metabolic flare" reaction, as demonstrated by an average increase in FDG retention by 1.4 SUV (minimum 0.8 in any patient). The greatest increase in FDG retention in nonresponders was 0.4 SUV.

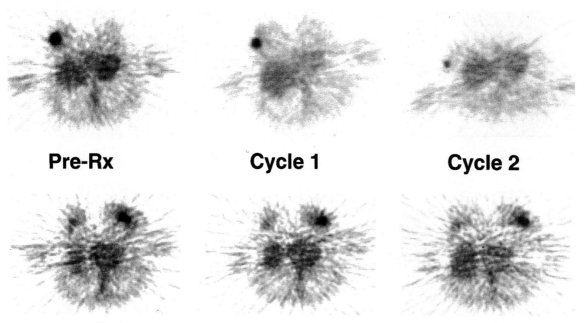

Pre-Rx   **Cycle 1**   **Cycle 2**

FIG. 5.13.8. ^{18}F-Fluorodeoxyglucose positron emission tomography images in two patients with primary breast cancer. Images were obtained before and after the first and second cycles of therapy. **Top row:** A responding patient who had minimal disease after therapy. **Bottom row:** A nonresponding patient. (From Schelling M, Avril N, Nahrig J, et al. Positron emission tomography using [^{18}F]Fluorodeoxyglucose for monitoring primary chemotherapy in breast cancer. *J Clin Oncol* 2000;18:1689–1695, with permission.)

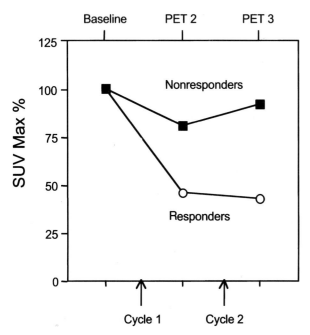

FIG. 5.13.9. Change in mean maximum standard uptake value after the treatment of breast cancer with chemotherapy. Nonresponders (17 patients) have gross residual tumor at the end of therapy while responders (7 patients) had minimal residual disease. (From Schelling M, Avril N, Nahrig J, et al. Positron emission tomography using [^{18}F]Fluorodeoxyglucose for monitoring primary chemotherapy in breast cancer. *J Clin Oncol* 2000;18:1689–1695, with permission.)

In summary, PET has been demonstrated to be useful in monitoring the response in patients being treated with breast cancer. To date, however, this has not yet entered the realm of routine clinical use. This will require enough data so oncologists are comfortable making clinical decisions based on the scan results.

Lung Cancer

PET imaging of lung cancer treatment has generally been performed after radiation, either alone or in combination with other treatments (Table 5.13.6). In patients treated with radiotherapy, Kubota et al. (52) performed PET-methionine imaging before and 2 weeks after the conclusion of therapy. They measured the change in T : N uptake with PET and change in tumor size on CT scan. Patients were divided into three response groups: those with early progression, those with late local recurrence, and those with no local recurrence. Those with no local recurrence or late recurrence had similar decreases in methionine retention (65% and 72%, respectively). This was in contrast to the early progression group, who demonstrated only a 22% decline in methionine uptake. The early and late recurrence groups could be differentiated by the lack of tumor shrinkage in the former group.

Because of the cost and difficulty of serial PET scans, few patients have been studied more than three times. In one study, two patients were imaged seven to eight times with FDG over the course of radiation therapy (53). The patient who had local control had a continuing decline over the course of treatment, as measured by $SUV_{average}$, SUV^{max},

TABLE 5.13.6. *Lung cancer and PET evaluation after therapy*

Tracer (no. of patients)	Treatment	Timing of PET relative to treatment	PET analysis	Clinical evaluation	Result	Author, yr (reference no.)
Methionine (n = 16)	XRT	2 wk after end	T:N	Follow-up and CT	Correl PET and clinical	Kubota et al. 1993 (52)
FDG (n = 12)	XRT	Variable after end	Visual SUV	Follow-up and CT	Correl CR on PET and clinical	Hebert et al. 1996 (54)
FDG (n = 56)	XRT ± chemotherapy	10 wk after end	Visual	Follow-up and CT	Correl PET and clinical	MacManus et al. 2000 (10)
FDG (n = 113)	XRT, chemotherapy surgery	Median 8 mo after end	Visual	Follow-up and CT	Correl PET and clinical	Patz et al. 2000 (55)
FDG (n = 126)	XRT, chemotherapy surgery	Every 6 mo after end	Visual SUV	Follow-up and CT	84% PET accuracy	Bury et al. 1999 (56)

XRT, radiation therapy, T:N, tumor to normal tissue ratio; SUV, standard uptake value; correl, correlates PET with the indicated evaluation.

and total tumor glycolysis. On the other hand, the patient who progressed at the conclusion of therapy had a very minor dip in tumor metabolic parameters toward the end of therapy but a rapid return to baseline. Although these data are limited, they indicate that serial studies during radiation may help to predict the ultimate outcome. Serial methionine scans over the course of therapy have also coincided with the response and regrowth of the tumors (52).

The study of Herbert et al. (54) compared the results of FDG PET before and after radiation to the local control rate in lung cancer. Four patients had CRs, as judged by PET, and none recurred locally. Of the eight patients with a partial or no response by PET, four had persistent local disease while another four remained alive and well at least 11 months after treatment. In this study, a negative PET scan result was very helpful, but a positive scan result did not predict whether the patient would relapse. It is notable that the follow-up PET scans were done at variable times after the completion of radiation, with some being performed as early as 1 month after treatment. It is this experience that has led investigators to allow more time for responses after radiation treatment.

In one recent trial of 56 patients imaged before and after radiation (with or without chemotherapy), they waited a median of 10 weeks for the second study (Fig. 5.13.10) (10). This was to allow time for inflammation in the lung, pleura, and tumor to resolve. For those visually determined to have a CR by PET, the actuarial 2-year survival was 84% while it was only 31% for those with a poorer response. Even after a multivariate analysis, PET was a significant predictor of survival. There was no difference in survival in those judged to have a CR by CT response compared to those without CR, thus demonstrating the superiority of PET for this use.

The study of Patz et al. (55) analyzed the follow-up PET scans obtained on 113 patients after treatment that could include chemotherapy, radiation, surgery, or a combination. Imaging was done a median of 8 months after treatment but ranged from 2 days to 9 years. Only 13 patients had negative PET scan results, but 11 (85%) are alive and disease free a median of 34 months after the PET scan. Of the 101 patients with positive PET scan results, the median survival was only 12 months (95% confidence interval; 9 to 15 months). Bury et al. (56) did a similar study on the follow-up of a mixed group of 126 patients imaged with PET and CT every 6 months after treatment. The accuracy of PET was 96% and that for CT was 84% in detecting residual or recurrent tumor.

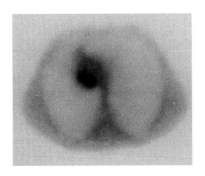

Before

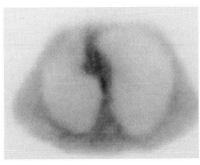

After

FIG. 5.13.10. ^{18}F-Fluorodeoxyglucose positron emission tomography images of a patient with unresectable non–small cell lung cancer before and 2 months after radiation therapy and carboplatin. Posttreatment, the tumor had the same activity level as the normal mediastinal structures and was judged a complete response. (From MacManus M, Hicks R, Wada M, et al. Early F-18 FDG-PET response to radical chemoradiotherapy correlates strongly with survival in unresectable non–small cell lung cancer. *Proc ASCO* 2000;19:483a, with permission.)

Although the specificity of both approaches were about equal in this study (92% to 95%), the sensitivity of PET in detecting tumor was 100%, and that of CT only 72%. PET had three false-positive results in patients due to radiation pneumonitis.

Other tracers have been used to evaluate the biology of tumor response in pilot trials of patients with lung cancer. In patients with small cell lung cancer treated with chemotherapy, FDG PET and ^{11}C-thymidine were imaged before and around 1 week into therapy (57). Although both imaging approaches demonstrated rapid declines in tumor metabolism, the measurements of proliferation declined more rapidly in patients with ^{11}C-thymidine. Its synthesis, its shorter half-life compared with ^{18}F, and *in vivo* degradation have limited the routine use of this approach. The more recent development of metabolically stable proliferation tracers such as FLT may allow for more routine clinical use of this approach.

The role of hypoxia in the measurement of tumor treatment response has also been evaluated with tracers such as ^{18}F-fluoromisonidazole (FMISO). In a pilot study, seven patients were imaged repeatedly during the course of radiation for non–small cell lung cancer (see Color Plate 11 following page 394) (58). The fraction of tumor volume that was judged to be hypoxic was shown to decline from a median of 58% pretreatment to 29% at mid treatment and to 22% at the end of therapy. This approach may be useful in assessing the role of tumor hypoxia on resistance to radiation. With the development of new antivascular agents, FMISO and similar compounds may find another role in determining the success of efforts to disrupt vessel perfusion.

In summary, FDG PET is gaining a role in the follow-up of patients with lung cancer, in addition to its use in initial staging. Studies indicate that it is more predictive of eventual outcome after the completion of treatment than conventional anatomic imaging with CT. Further studies are needed to evaluate the use of PET early after treatment.

Gastrointestinal Cancers

FDG PET has been used to evaluate a number of gastrointestinal tumors, but most prominently to study patients with metastatic colorectal cancer (Table 5.13.7). Findlay et al. (59) examined patients before and around 2 and 4 weeks after the start of chemotherapy. The measurement of the SUV and the T : N ratio at these times was compared with the measurements of CT obtained 12 weeks after the start of treatment. They found that a decline of at least 15% at 4 weeks in the T : N ratio was the most predictive of ultimate response (95% accurate) (Fig. 5.13.11). Although a decline was seen at 2 weeks in some patients, four lesions actually increased at 2 weeks before rapidly declining. SUVs also declined significantly by 4 weeks, but they did not separate responders and nonresponders as well as T : N ratios did.

Similar to results with other tumors, FDG PET had difficulty assessing response at the end of radiotherapy in patients with colorectal cancer (60). Patients were treated with a course of photon radiation, which was followed by neutron therapy. Imaging was done before and after the photon therapy, and then 6 weeks after completion of neutron treatment. Although all patients had evidence of clinical palliation, only 50% had a decline in FDG SUVs. The authors argue that a longer interval may be needed to assess response in these patients receiving radiation treatment.

In a study of 14 patients receiving chemotherapy for esophageal cancer, FDG PET was done before and after two to three cycles of chemotherapy (8 to 13 weeks) (61). PET results were quantitated by both T : N ratio and calculating the metabolic rate for FDG. The two approaches had a correlation coefficient of 0.87. In the six patients with a more than 30% decrease in the T : N ratio, all had clinical evidence of response while two patients with an increase in the T : N ratio had no response. Of the five patients with a 0% to 30% decrease, none had CT evidence of response, but three had clinical improvements in dysphagia.

TABLE 5.13.7. *Gastrointestinal and genitourinary cancer and PET evaluation after therapy*

Tracer (no. of patients)	Disease	Treatment	Timing of PET relative to treatment	PET analysis	Clinical evaluation	Result	Author, yr (reference no.)
FDG (n = 18)	Colon	Chemotherapy	During wk 2 and 4	SUV T:N	CT	95% PET accuracy	Findlay et al., 1996 (59)
FDG (n = 12)	Colon	Radiation	During and at end	SUV	CT	50% accuracy	Haberkom et al., 1991 (60)
FDG (n = 14)	Esophageal	Chemotherapy	During wk 13–Aug	T:N kinetics	Follow-up and CT	Correl PET and clinical	Couper et al., 1998 (61)
FDG (n = 21)	Germ cell	Chemotherapy	End	SUV kinetics	Pathology	Correl PET and clinical	Sugawara et al., 1999 (67)
FDG (n = 30)	Germ cell	Chemotherapy	6 wk	SUV	Pathology	Correl PET and clinical	Stephens et al., 1996 (66)
Methionine (n = 15)	Bladder	Chemotherapy	During wk 3 and 9	SUV kinetics	CT	Variable	Letocha et al., 1994 (68)

FDG, ^{18}F-fluorodeoxyglucose; SUV, standard uptake value; T:N, tumor to normal tissue ratio; correl, correlates PET with the indicated evaluation.

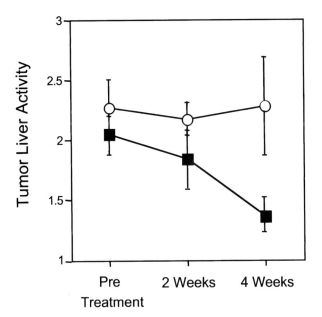

FIG. 5.13.11. ^{18}F-Fluorodeoxyglucose positron emission tomography results in patients with metastatic colorectal cancer in the liver responding (*dark squares*) or not responding (*open circles*) to chemotherapy. Patients were imaged before treatment, at 1 to 2 weeks, and at 4 to 5 weeks after the start of treatment and results expressed as the tumor-to-normal liver ratio (mean and 95% confidence intervals). (From Findlay M, Young H, Cunningham D, et al. Noninvasive monitoring of tumor metabolism using fluorodeoxyglucose and positron emission tomography in colorectal cancer liver metastases: correlation with tumor response to fluorouracil. *J Clin Oncol* 1996;14:700–708, with permission.)

Genitourinary

A limited number of studies of prostate cancer have been done with both FDG and other tracers. FDG has been somewhat limited in its use in this disease because of difficulties in detecting tumors adjacent to the bladder (62). Furthermore, even in patients with metastatic disease to the bone, FDG PET has had a relatively low sensitivity, but good specificity (63). Early trials have found a correlation between changes in FDG and blood prostate-specific antigen levels after therapy (64). Given these limitation, investigators have begun to explore other tracers such as ^{18}F-fluorocholine (65), which look promising in pilot studies, to detect and monitor tumor response.

Although chemotherapy is very successful in patients with nonseminomatous germ-cell tumors (GCTs), some patients have viable tumor remaining and can be salvaged by surgery. A proportion of the patients also have teratoma remaining in the lesions (about 40%), and this should be removed because tumor may eventually recur. Surgery is not needed in those with tumor necrosis (about 40% to 45%), but this is difficult to predict before surgery. In patients with GCT, imaging was done with FDG PET after completing chemotherapy and just before resection of residual masses (Table 5.13.7)

(66). In this study of 30 patients, the mean SUV of patients with viable tumor was 8.8, compared with 2.9 and 3.1 for those with necrosis and teratoma, respectively. Using an SUV cutoff of 5.0, PET detected all but one of the patients with active GCT. Unfortunately, PET alone could not differentiate teratoma from necrosis. It is known that those with pathologic evidence of teratoma in the primary tumor and who have rapid shrinkage of tumor on CT are at lower risk for having remaining teratoma. A negative PET scan result in this group of patients may be useful in obviating the need for surgery. A more recent study of this issue was done by Sugawara et al. (67) with similar results. They found the SUV measurement could differentiate viable tumor from necrosis or teratoma. Although SUV measurements could not distinguish necrosis from teratoma, this was possible using a kinetic analysis of k_1 rate constant for FDG. This study, which was done in a relatively small number of patients, needs confirmation.

Methionine has been used to measure the response in patients receiving neoadjuvant chemotherapy for bladder cancer (68). Patients were studied before and after cycle one of therapy, and again after cycle three for some patients. In the 11 patients studied after one cycle, all had declines in the SUV. Although those with CRs had at least a 50% decline in tumor retention, some patients with declines as high as 78% still only had partial responses. In the four patients also imaged after three cycles of therapy, two had CRs with SUV decreases of 61% and 100%, whereas those with lesser declines only had a partial response. This limited data set demonstrates that further study is needed to determine the optimal timing of imaging in this disease.

SUMMARY

It is clear that PET is the preferred imaging method for locating many cancers. It is expected that treatment monitoring will assume an important role in the practice of PET.

REFERENCES

1. Price P, Jones T. Can positron emission tomography (PET) be used to detect subclinical response to cancer therapy? The EC PET Oncology Concerted Action and the EORTC PET Study Group. *Eur J Cancer* 1995;31A:1924–1927.
2. Kubota K, Ishiwata K, Kubota R, et al. Tracer feasibility for monitoring tumor radiotherapy: a quadruple tracer study with fluorine-18-fluorodeoxyglucose or fluorine-18-fluorodeoxyuridine, L-[methyl-^{14}C]methionine, [6-^{3}H]thymidine, and gallium-67. *J Nucl Med* 1991;32: 2118–2123.
3. Tjuvajev JG, Macapinilac HA, Daghighian F, et al. Imaging of brain tumor proliferative activity with iodine-131-iododeoxyuridine. *J Nucl Med* 1994;35:1407–1417.
4. Shields A, Grierson J, Dohmen B, et al. Imaging proliferation *in vivo* with [F-18]FLT and positron emission tomography. *Nat Med* 1998;4: 1334–1336.
5. Anderson H, Jap J, Price P. Measurement of tumor and normal tissue perfusion by positron emission tomography (PET) in the evaluation of antivascular therapy: results in the phase I study of combretastatin A4 phosphate. *Proc ASCO* 2000;19:179a.
6. Ginos JZ, Cooper AJL, Dhawan V, et al. [^{13}N]Cisplatin PET to assess

pharmacokinetics of intra-arterial versus intravenous chemotherapy for malignant brain tumors. *J Nucl Med* 1987;28:1844–1852.

7. Dimitrakopoulou-Strauss A, Strauss LG, Schlag P, et al. Fluorine-18-fluorouracil to predict therapy response in liver metastases from colorectal carcinoma. *J Nucl Med* 1998;39:1197–1202.

8. Hoekstra CJ, Paglianiti I, Hoekstra OS, et al. Monitoring response to therapy in cancer using [^{18}F]-2-fluoro-2-deoxy-D-glucose and positron emission tomography: an overview of different analytical methods. *Eur J Nucl Med* 2000;27:731–743.

9. Weber WA, Schwaiger M, Avril N. Quantitative assessment of tumor metabolism using FDG-PET imaging. *Nucl Med Biol* 2000;27: 683–687.

10. MacManus M, Hicks R, Wada M, et al. Early F-18 FDG-PET response to radical chemoradiotherapy correlates strongly with survival in unresectable non–small cell lung cancer. *Proc ASCO* 2000;19:483a.

11. Young H, Baum R, Cremerius U, et al. Measurement of clinical and subclinical tumour response using [^{18}F]-fluorodeoxyglucose and positron emission tomography: review and 1999 EORTC recommendations. European Organization for Research and Treatment of Cancer (EORTC) PET Study Group. *Eur J Cancer* 1999;35:1773–1782.

12. Brock CS, Young H, O'Reilly SM, et al. Early evaluation of tumour metabolic response using [^{18}F]fluorodeoxyglucose and positron emission tomography: a pilot study following the phase II chemotherapy schedule for temozolomide in recurrent high-grade gliomas. *Br J Cancer* 2000;82:608–615.

13. Minn H, Zasadny KR, Quint LE, et al. Lung cancer: reproducibility of quantitative measurements for evaluating 2-[F-18]-fluoro-2-deoxy-D-glucose uptake at PET. *Radiology* 1995;196:167–173.

14. Barker FG II, Chang SM, Valk PE, et al. 18-Fluorodeoxyglucose uptake and survival of patients with suspected recurrent malignant glioma. *Cancer* 1997;79:115–126.

15. Doyle WK, Budinger TF, Valk PE, et al. Differentiation of cerebral radiation necrosis from tumor recurrence by [^{18}F]FDG and ^{82}Rb positron emission tomography. *J Comput Assisted Tomogr* 1987;11: 563–570.

16. Di Chiro G, Oldfield E, Wright DC, et al. Cerebral necrosis after radiotherapy and/or intraarterial chemotherapy for brain tumors: PET and neuropathologic studies. *AJR Am J Roentgenol* 1988;150:189–197.

17. Kim EE, Chung SK, Haynie TP, et al. Differentiation of residual or recurrent tumors from post-treatment changes with F-18 FDG PET. *Radiographics* 1992;12:269–279.

18. Ogawa T, Uemura K, Shishido F, et al. Changes of cerebral blood flow, and oxygen and glucose metabolism following radiochemotherapy of gliomas: a PET study. *J Comput Assisted Tomogr* 1988;12:290–297.

19. Rozental JM, Levine RL, Nickles RJ, et al. Glucose uptake by gliomas after treatment. *Arch Neurol* 1989;46:1302–1307.

20. Rozental JM, Levine RL, Mehta MP, et al. Early changes in tumor metabolism after treatment: the effects of stereotactic radiosurgery. *Int J Radiat Oncol Biol Phys* 1991;20:1053–1060.

21. De Witte O, Hildebrand J, Luxen A, et al. Acute effect of carmustine on glucose metabolism in brain and glioblastoma. *Cancer* 1994;74: 2836–2842.

22. Holthoff VA, Herholz K, Berthold F, et al. *In vivo* metabolism of childhood posterior fossa tumors and primitive neuroectodermal tumors before and after treatment. *Cancer* 1993;72:1394–1403.

23. Nuutinen J, Sonninen P, Lehikoinen P, et al. Radiotherapy treatment planning and long-term follow-up with [^{11}C]methionine PET in patients with low-grade astrocytoma. *Int J Radiat Oncol Biol Phys* 2000;48: 43–52.

24. Dohmen B, Shields A, Grierson J, et al. [^{18}F]FLT-PET in brain tumors. *J Nucl Med* 2000;41:216P.

25. Eary JF, Mankoff DA, Spence AM, et al. 2-[C-11]thymidine imaging of malignant brain tumors. *Cancer Res* 1999;59:615–621.

26. Lin P, Chu J, Pocock N. ^{18}F Fluorodeoxyglucose imaging with coincidence dual-head gamma camera (hybrid-PET) for staging of lymphoma: comparison with Ga-67 scintigraphy. *J Nucl Med* 2000;41: 118p.

27. Kostakoglu L, Leonard J, Coleman M, et al. Comparison of FDG-PET and Ga-67 SPECT in staging of lymphoma. *J Nucl Med* 2000;41:118p.

28. Romer W, Hanauske A, Ziegler S, et al. Positron emission tomography in non-Hodgkin's lymphoma: assessment of chemotherapy with fluorodeoxyglucose. *Blood* 1998;91:4464–4471.

29. Weidmann E, Baican B, Hertel A, et al. Positron emission tomography

(PET) for staging and evaluation of response to treatment in patients with Hodgkin's disease. *Leukemia Lymphol* 1999;34:545–551.

30. de Wit M, Bohuslavizki KH, Buchert R, et al. ^{18}FDG-PET following treatment as valid predictor for disease-free survival in Hodgkin's lymphoma. *Ann Oncol* 2001;12:29–37.

31. Jerusalem G, Beguin Y, Fassotte MF, et al. Whole-body positron emission tomography using ^{18}F-fluorodeoxyglucose for posttreatment evaluation in Hodgkin's disease and non-Hodgkin's lymphoma has higher diagnostic and prognostic value than classical computed tomography scan imaging. *Blood* 1999;94:429–433.

32. Cremerius U, Fabry U, Kroll U, et al. Clinical value of FDG PET for therapy monitoring of malignant lymphoma—results of a retrospective study in 72 patients. *Nuklearmedizin* 1999;38:24–30.

33. Stumpe KD, Urbinelli M, Steinert HC, et al. Whole-body positron emission tomography using fluorodeoxyglucose for staging of lymphoma: effectiveness and comparison with computed tomography. *Eur J Nucl Med* 1998;25:721–728.

34. Chaiken L, Rege S, Hoh C, et al. Positron emission tomography with fluorodeoxyglucose to evaluate tumor response and control after radiation therapy. *Int J Radiat Oncol Biol Phys* 1993;27:455–464.

35. Sakamoto H, Nakai Y, Ohashi Y, et al. Monitoring of response to radiotherapy with fluorine-18 deoxyglucose PET of head and neck squamous cell carcinomas. *Acta Otolaryngol* 1998;538[Suppl]: 254–260.

36. Slevin NJ, Collins CD, Hastings DL, et al. The diagnostic value of positron emission tomography (PET) with radiolabeled fluorodeoxyglucose (^{18}F-FDG) in head and neck cancer. *J Laryngol Otol* 1999;113: 548–554.

37. Haberkorn U, Strauss L, Dimitrakopoulou A, et al. Fluorodeoxyglucose imaging of advanced head and neck cancer after chemotherapy. *J Nucl Med* 1993;34:12–17.

38. Lowe V, Dunphy F, Varvares M, et al. Evaluation of chemotherapy response in patients with advanced head and neck cancer using [F-18]fluorodeoxyglucose positron emission tomography. *Head Neck* 1997;19:666–674.

39. Berlangieri SU, Brizel DM, Scher RL, et al. Pilot study of positron emission tomography in patients with advanced head and neck cancer receiving radiotherapy and chemotherapy. *Head Neck* 1994;16: 340–346.

40. Nuutinen J, Jyrkkio S, Lehikoinen P, et al. Evaluation of early response to radiotherapy in head and neck cancer measured with [^{11}C]methionine-positron emission tomography. *Radiother Oncol* 1999;52: 225–232.

41. Lindholm P, Leskinen-Kallio S, Grenman R, et al. Evaluation of response to radiotherapy in head and neck cancer by positron emission tomography and [^{11}C]methionine. *Int J Radiat Oncol Biol Phys* 1995; 32:787–794.

42. Wahl RL, Zasadny K, Helvie M, et al. Metabolic monitoring of breast cancer chemohormonotherapy using positron emission tomography: initial evaluation. *J Clin Oncol* 1993;11:2101–2111.

43. Bassa P, Kim EE, Inoue T, et al. Evaluation of preoperative chemotherapy using PET with fluorine-18-fluorodeoxyglucose in breast cancer. *J Nucl Med* 1996;37:931–938.

44. Smith IC, Welch AE, Hutcheon AW, et al. Positron emission tomography using [^{18}F]-fluorodeoxy-D-glucose to predict the pathologic response of breast cancer to primary chemotherapy. *J Clin Oncol* 2000; 18:1676–1688.

45. Schelling M, Avril N, Nahrig J, et al. Positron emission tomography using [^{18}F]Fluorodeoxyglucose for monitoring primary chemotherapy in breast cancer. *J Clin Oncol* 2000;18:1689–1695.

46. Nair N, Ali A, Dowlatshahi K, et al. Positron emission tomography with fluorine-18 fluorodeoxyglucose to evaluate response of early breast carcinoma treated with stereotaxic interstitial laser therapy. *Clin Nucl Med* 2000;25:505–507.

47. Jansson T, Westlin JE, Ahlstrom H, et al. Positron emission tomography studies in patients with locally advanced and/or metastatic breast cancer: a method for early therapy evaluation? *J Clin Oncol* 1995;13: 1470–1477.

48. Huovinen R, Leskinen-Kallio S, Nagren K, et al. Carbon-11-methionine and PET in evaluation of treatment response of breast cancer. *Br J Cancer* 1993:787–791.

49. Mintun MA, Welch MJ, Siegel BA, et al. Breast cancer: PET imaging of estrogen receptors. *Radiology* 1988;169:45–48.

50. McGuire AH, Dehdashti F, Siegel BA, et al. Positron tomographic

assessment of 16α-[¹⁸F]fluoro-17β-estradiol uptake in metastatic breast carcinoma. *J Nucl Med* 1991;32:1526–1531.

51. Dehdashti F, Flanagan FL, Mortimer JE, et al. Positron emission tomographic assessment of "metabolic flare" to predict response of metastatic breast cancer to antiestrogen therapy. *Eur J Nucl Med* 1999;26: 51–56.

52. Kubota K, Yamada S, Ishiwata K, et al. Evaluation of the treatment response of lung cancer with positron emission tomography and L-[methyl-¹¹C]methionine: a preliminary study. *Eur J Nucl Med* 1993; 20:495–501.

53. Erdi YE, Macapinlac H, Rosenzweig KE, et al. Use of PET to monitor the response of lung cancer to radiation treatment. *Eur J Nucl Med* 2000;27:861–866.

54. Hebert ME, Lowe VJ, Hoffman JM, et al. Positron emission tomography in the pretreatment evaluation and follow-up of non–small cell lung cancer patients treated with radiotherapy: preliminary findings. *Am J Clin Oncol* 1996;19:416–421.

55. Patz EF Jr, Connolly J, Herndon J. Prognostic value of thoracic FDG PET imaging after treatment for non–small cell lung cancer. *AJR Am J Roentgenol* 2000;174:769–774.

56. Bury T, Corhay JL, Duysinx B, et al. Value of FDG-PET in detecting residual or recurrent nonsmall cell lung cancer. *Eur Respir J* 1999;14: 1376–1380.

57. Shields AF, Mankoff DA, Link JM, et al. [¹¹C]Thymidine and FDG to measure therapy response. *J Nucl Med* 1998;39:1757–1762.

58. Koh WJ, Bergman KS, Rasey JS, et al. Evaluation of oxygenation status during fractionated radiotherapy in human nonsmall cell lung cancers using [F-18]fluoromisonidazole positron emission tomography. *Int J Radiat Oncol Biol Phys* 1995;33:391–398.

59. Findlay M, Young H, Cunningham D, et al. Noninvasive monitoring of tumor metabolism using fluorodeoxyglucose and positron emission tomography in colorectal cancer liver metastases: correlation with tumor response to fluorouracil. *J Clin Oncol* 1996;14:700–708.

60. Haberkorn U, Strauss LG, Dimitrakopoulou A, et al. PET studies of fluorodeoxyglucose metabolism in patients with recurrent colorectal tumors receiving radiotherapy. *J Nucl Med* 1991;32:1485–1490.

61. Couper GW, McAteer D, Wallis F, et al. Detection of response to chemotherapy using positron emission tomography in patients with oesophageal and gastric cancer. *Br J Surg* 1998;85:1403–1406.

62. Effert PJ, Bares R, Handt S, et al. Metabolic imaging of untreated prostate cancer by positron emission tomography with ¹⁸fluorine-labeled deoxyglucose. *J Urol* 1996;155:994–998.

63. Kao CH, Hsieh JF, Tsai SC, et al. Comparison and discrepancy of ¹⁸F-2-deoxyglucose positron emission tomography and Tc-99m MDP bone scan to detect bone metastases. *Anticancer Res* 2000;20:2189–2192.

64. Kurdziel K, Bacharach S, Carrasquillo J, et al. Using PET ¹⁸F-FDG, ¹¹CO, and ¹⁵O-water for monitoring prostate cancer during a phase II anti-angiogenic drug trial with thalidomide. *Clin Positron Imaging* 2000;3:144.

65. DeGrado TR, Coleman RE, Wang S, et al. Synthesis and evaluation of ¹⁸F-labeled choline as an oncologic tracer for positron emission tomography: initial findings in prostate cancer. *Cancer Res* 2001;61: 110–117.

66. Stephens AW, Gonin R, Hutchins GD, et al. Positron emission tomography evaluation of residual radiographic abnormalities in postchemotherapy germ cell tumor patients. *J Clin Oncol* 1996;14:1637–1641.

67. Sugawara Y, Zasadny KR, Grossman HB, et al. Germ cell tumor: differentiation of viable tumor, mature teratoma, and necrotic tissue with FDG PET and kinetic modeling. *Radiology* 1999;211:249–256.

68. Letocha H, Ahlstrom H, Malmstrom PU, et al. Positron emission tomography with L-methyl-¹¹C-methionine in the monitoring of therapy response in muscle-invasive transitional cell carcinoma of the urinary bladder. *Br J Urol* 1994;74:767–774.

Combined PET/CT Imaging

Ora Israel

Positron emission tomography (PET) of cancer images the pathophysiology and functional status of a malignant process. After many years of steady progress in the research environment, PET using fluorine-18 (^{18}F)-fluorodeoxyglucose (^{18}F-FDG) has become an important part of routine evidence-based oncologic practice. Its clinical value in the assessment of patients with cancer is now well accepted (1, 2). PET is characterized by a high sensitivity for diagnosis and staging of new or recurrent malignant disease and has a significant impact on clinical management of many malignant tumors (2–4). The limited spatial resolution and high target-to-background ratio of PET, the lack of readily identifiable anatomic structures, and different potential causes for abnormal FDG uptake reduce the specificity of the test and often make interpretation challenging (5–7).

Imaging of cancer using computed tomography (CT) assesses structural features, measured by physical characteristics such as tissue density or the atomic number in a targeted malignant tumor as compared with those of normal tissues. For decades, CT has been considered the standard procedure for evaluating cancer. Its high spatial resolution provides anatomic details that make CT a tool with excellent abilities to guide diagnostic and therapeutic procedures (8). CT, however, does not directly assess the functional or metabolic status of tumors. Modern CT scans provide extensive anatomic information, making detection of clinically relevant data potentially more difficult.

The need for complementary evaluation of the structural and functional characteristics of tumors has evolved from everyday clinical requirements. Registration of PET and CT studies provides a means to merge imaging information from both imaging techniques. The simultaneous analysis of these modalities yields complementary data on function, structure, and localization of tissues and disease (9).

THE QUEST FOR COMBINED ANATOMIC AND FUNCTIONAL DATA REGISTRATION

Combined evaluation of function and structure may potentially provide solutions for improving the specificity and accuracy of PET, a proven effective tool for measuring metabolic features of cancer (1,3). It also has the potential of improving the sensitivity of high-resolution contrast-enhanced CT in the evaluation of patients with malignancies (see Color Plate 12 following page 394).

Interpretation of PET performed with FDG, the most commonly used positron-emitting tracer in clinical oncology, may be challenging because of the physiologic distribution of the radiotracer. The variable patterns of FDG uptake must be considered in the differential diagnosis of areas with increased activity. This is a more important issue with the use of modern PET systems, characterized by improved contrast and spatial resolution. Tissues such as muscles, heart, liver, spleen, stomach, thyroid, and the brain normally take up the tracer. The kidneys and bowel excrete FDG. Knowledge of the normal distribution of FDG PET is important for correct definition of sites of increased uptake (10,11). Nevertheless, physiologic FDG uptake may be misinterpreted as a malignant lesion or mask cancer sites located in close vicinity (7).

The head and neck is a region of complex anatomy. It is also a region of multiple foci of physiologic FDG uptake such as the thyroid, the nasopharynx and oropharynx, salivary glands, and vocal cords. These sites must be differentiated from malignant lesions (12–15). In the thorax, FDG uptake in the heart, the great vessels in the mediastinum, and muscles of the chest wall may be misinterpreted as, or overlap with, malignant lesions. The most difficult diagnoses and precise definition of increased FDG uptake are in the abdomen and pelvis. Due to uptake by the stomach, liver, and spleen, tracer in the colon and the kidneys, and the presence of FDG in intestinal loops, the renal pelvis, ureter, or urinary bladder, it may be difficult to accurately diagnose abnormalities detected on PET studies (see Color Plate 13 following page 394).

Uptake of FDG is not limited to malignancy. Chemotherapy-induced thymic hyperplasia and healing bone fractures have been also reported to accumulate FDG (11). Increased metabolism and glycolysis are the reason for abnormal FDG accumulation in sites of nonmalignant pathology, such as inflammation, infection, and granulomatous diseases. Attempts to characterize areas of increased FDG uptake based on their intensity and patterns of distribution have only partially improved the specificity of this procedure (16,17). By correct definition and localization of FDG uptake to normal organs or sites unrelated to cancer, fused tomographic landmarks of CT provide the anatomic framework that may potentially facilitate interpretation of FDG PET.

Combined evaluation of structure and function may improve assessment of cancer at different stages of disease. At the time of initial diagnosis, PET detects areas with increased tumor metabolism. CT detects organomegaly or masses with changes in x-ray attenuation. Registration of data obtained from both modalities increases the confidence in diagnosis of suspicious lesions as cancer related and simplifies the differential diagnosis of equivocal sites. Multiple lesions seen on PET or CT, sometimes in close vicinity to each other, may be of potentially different etiology and can be discriminated using fused images (see Color Plate 14 following page 394) (6).

Registration of PET and CT images improves staging of cancer. Classically, enlarged lymph nodes have been considered highly suggestive of malignancy (18–22). Lymphadenopathy, however, may also be of benign etiology (23,24). On the other hand, it has been previously reported that more than 50% of metastatic lymph nodes in patients with lung cancer may be of normal size (24–26). There is a significant overlap in size between malignant and benign lymph nodes (23). PET may show abnormal FDG uptake in normal-size malignant lymph nodes allowing for detection of small tumors (20,27).

Localization of lesions detected by PET with no corresponding anatomic site is difficult and often only an approximation. Fused images may provide precise topographic coordinates for nodal involvement suspected by PET (see Color Plate 15 following page 394). This may guide further diagnostic and therapeutic procedures and lead to less invasive biopsy and surgery.

PET is the ideal whole-body technique for diagnosis of distant metastases. Registration combines a high detectability rate of metastases by PET with their precise localization by CT (see Color Plate 16 following page 394). Also, sites of increased FDG uptake suspected of being metastases can be excluded if the abnormal activity is accurately defined as unrelated to cancer. Fused images may make it possible to correctly define the N (nodal) and M (metastases) status of the tumor at hand and, by establishing tumor resectability, has a significant impact on further management of patients with cancer. Patients who are correctly downstaged may be referred for curative therapy. Patients in whom cancer is in a more advanced stage than initially suspected may be spared unnecessary surgery and consideration given to other therapeutic options (see Color Plate 17 following page 394).

Precise localization of regional lymph node and distant metastases is also a prerequisite for treatment planning. The surgical approach, radiation treatment fields or type, and dosage of chemotherapy can be modified according to information provided by fused images.

Registration of anatomic and functional data is of value for monitoring cancer response to treatment and for early diagnosis of recurrence. Response to treatment is defined on CT by changes in size and structure of tumors (8,28). Although functional changes may precede morphologic changes, for the lack of better criteria, even recent efforts to standardize the definition of response to treatment still rely in part on the size of the lesion determined, as a rule, by CT (5,29,30).

During or immediately after treatment, there is an equilibrium between the effect of treatment on sensitive malignant cells, the growth of resistant cell clones, and the presence of fibrotic and necrotic tissue. A mass shown on CT can potentially contain only nonviable, fibrotic, and necrotic tissue. On the contrary, a mass may decrease in size after treatment and still contain significant viable cancer cells (31–33). Localization of cancer inside a tumor mass may help in adequate histologic sampling for diagnosis and, if indicated, further treatment planning.

Fused images may play an important role in guiding biopsy for tissue diagnosis of cancer, by providing additional functional information for CT-guided invasive procedures. The percent of sampling error, at least partially due to misleading or insufficient information obtained from morphologic studies, should subsequently decrease. On follow-up of patients during continuous clinical remission, fused images may increase the certainty of diagnosing relapse in a previous site of disease, as is the case in about 30% of patients with recurrent lymphoma (34). Localizing the focus of abnormal metabolism inside a large residual mass will guide tissue confirmation in inconclusive cases. A combined imaging survey is even more important in suspected new sites of recurrences, particularly when changes in size or tissue density have not occurred yet (see Color Plate 15 following page 394) (29,35). Although biopsy is difficult to perform on the basis of abnormal scintigraphy without specific localization on CT, clinicians need tissue samples to make a certain diagnosis of relapse and start new treatment (36).

CO-REGISTRATION OF SEPARATELY PERFORMED PET AND CT

Image registration refers to the process of determining the geometric relationship of multiple imaging techniques. Information obtained from one modality is used in the context of a second diagnostic study (9,37). Registration can be performed as an interactive operator-matching process, may rely on automatic surface matching of organ contours and limits, or may depend on other approaches such as maximizing mutual information between two studies, among others. A number of basic criteria should be met for a registration technique to be practical and used routinely in a clinical setting. Some image-fusion algorithms may be too computationally intense for routine clinical implementation. The length of the computation time should be appropriate for the time and resource constraints and of the clinical setting.

Registration techniques are validated using a number of parameters. Precision of registration is defined as the system error measured when the registration algorithm is supplied with idealized input (i.e., phantom measurements). Precision values can be related to the entire registration system or applied to features related to the patient, acquisition protocols, the paradigm, or the optimization method used (38). Accuracy is a more direct measure, referring to the actual error occurring at a specific image location (39). Although precision is a system-related characteristic, accuracy applies to specific registration situations and can be measured using qualitative and quantitative indices. Robustness or stability of the technique measures the relationship between input and output image variations. Reliability measures the results as compared with data expected from a theoretical model (38).

Registration methods are classified as extrinsic, intrinsic, or nonimage based. Extrinsic registration methods rely on fiducial markers placed on or attached to the patient, artificial objects designed to be accurately detectable in all modalities. This makes registration relatively easy. The decision to register must be made before the acquisition of the two modalities and this is the main disadvantage of the technique. Also, markers are often invasive objects, such as the commonly used stereotactic frame screwed rigidly to the patient's skull, a device that until recently provided the ''gold standard'' for accurate brain registration (39,40). Noninvasive objects such as markers glued to the skin or larger devices that can be fitted snugly to the patient, such as individualized foam molds, head holder frames, and dental adapters, are as a rule less accurate (38). Because extrinsic methods cannot include by definition patient-related image information, the nature of the registration is restricted to rigid transformation, limited to three-dimensional (3D) translation and rotation (38).

Intrinsic registration methods are based on patient-generated image content. This technique identifies a limited set of landmarks (surface method), relies on alignment of segmented binary structures (segmentation-based method), or is based on directly computer-measured image gray values (voxel-property–based method) (38). Anatomic landmarks with clearly defined morphology can be actively identified by the operator while geometric landmarks located at the optimum of some geometric property, such as extreme local curvature or distinct corners, are generally localized in an automatic fashion (41).

Segmentation-based registration methods may use a rigid model, in which identical anatomic structures (mostly surfaces) are extracted from both images to be registered and used as the input for the alignment procedure (42,43). Rigid-model–based approaches are probably among the most popular methods currently in clinical use (44). Segmentation-based registration can be also based on deformable models in which an extracted structure, surface, or curve from one image is elastically deformed to fit the second image (45).

Although theoretically, segmentation-based registration is applicable to many areas of the body, its practical use has been largely limited to imaging of the brain (45). Voxel-property–based registration methods operate directly on the image gray values. Although developed many years ago, their extensive use in 3D clinical applications has been limited primarily to realignment of cardiac studies because of the considerable computational time and costs (46).

A number of studies have assessed the value of co-registering separately performed PET and CT of the whole body for clinical purposes. The limitations of relative low resolution and contrast of camera-based and to some degree dedicated PET systems, combined with both low and high tumor-to-background ratios, justify the need for fusion. Lesions with high tumor-to-background uptake can be very difficult to localize. Registered images may correctly define and discriminate areas of increased FDG uptake. When matched by a known anatomic location on CT that normally accumulates FDG, there is a decreased likelihood of active malignant disease in that area of FDG uptake.

Wahl et al. (41) reported their first attempt to fuse separately performed PET and CT studies using fiducial and internal markers. The method was technically satisfactory in 9 of the 10 evaluated patients with cancer. Realignment precision was up to 6.0 mm. Correct fusion was technically more difficult in the abdomen and pelvis, due to a paucity of anatomic landmarks. Misalignment was caused by changing of patient position, respiratory motion, changes in bowel and urine content, and different marker localization on the two imaging modalities performed on separate days. Long computation processes, up to 2 hours, may have been one of the reasons for the limited number of patients evaluated. Even with those suboptimal results, fusion showed the potential value of discriminating FDG uptake in normal organs and tumors involving soft tissue or bone (41). The authors concluded by predicting that in the future, after overcoming technical problems, fused images ''may well become the standard'' for PET evaluation of cancer patients (41).

The same group assessed the value of fused images for correct localization of regional lymph node involvement at presentation in staging of 23 patients with non–small cell lung cancer (47). Although PET with FDG was more sensitive and specific than CT for staging of lung cancer, fused images showed a sensitivity and specificity similar to visual side-by-side comparison of PET and CT (47). The use of co-registered images, however, improved the confidence of PET interpretation (47,48).

Fusion was of value in assessing the technical quality of PET studies, in correctly localizing physiologic FDG activity to the myocardium or sternum or in defining processes with high uptake of the radiotracer as nonmalignant (47). Fusion also provided better characterization of primary and metastatic tumors. The role of registered images in determining resectability of lung tumors was evaluated in 56 patients at staging (49). The N stage was correctly identified in 50% of patients by CT, 64% by PET, and 73% by fused images (49).

Registration of separately performed PET and CT has been used in a small group of patients with lung cancer for radiotherapy planning (50). Although a time-consuming matching method was used, it showed the potential value of fusion for correct planning of radiotherapy to a precisely delineated target volume of viable cancer and in minimizing the dose to surrounding structures (50).

Only a few studies have evaluated co-registration of anatomic and functional imaging data in regions other than the chest. An attempt to register PET and magnetic resonance imaging (MRI) in the region of the head and neck in 33 subjects was made using internal landmarks (14). Algorithms required approximately 1 hour for performing the fusion process. Alignment of large primary tumors showed good accuracy. However, more than half of metastatic lymph nodes were misregistered, with an error exceeding 15.0 mm (14). The authors attribute these results to changes in flexion and rotation of the neck on the different scanning tables of the two devices. Their proposed solutions for improved alignment include the use of a rigid cast or immobilization mask (14).

Fusion of PET and CT in the abdominopelvic region was performed in 19 patients with cancer (51). Topographic landmarks visible on both modalities were used for registration. Fusion improved localization of malignant sites in 20% of suspected lesions seen on PET, particularly in the retroperitoneum and the abdominal wall (51). A 3D registration method using internal markers such as the apex of the heart, the circumference of the liver, and the spinous process of vertebrae has been described in seven patients (52). PET was performed twice, early and at 1 hour after the injection of FDG. Registration was performed using a five-step process. Rotation error between PET and CT was less than three degrees and the translation error ranged between 4.0 and 16.0 mm (52).

Registration of PET and CT is also suggested as a good technique for evaluating patients with suspected cancer of the pancreas (53). With the use of fiducial point and line markers, performing a manual reorientation of the PET study and using the kidneys and liver as control organs, co-registration, although technically very complex, showed a good correlation between hypermetabolic lesions on PET and morphologic masses on CT in patients with pancreatic neoplasms (53).

These studies have stressed the potential value of and have underscored the need for optimizing fusion techniques. Clinical practice has not, however, recognized any of these various methods as a tool that can be routinely used in the assessment of individual patients with cancer. Retrospective co-registration of separately performed procedures is difficult, due in part to the different technical features of the two devices (5–7). The different design of beds used for PET and CT often leads to changes in patient positioning, with differences in body curvature or rotation. CT studies performed in various institutions do not always use the same standards, can be processed with different displays, and are available in a digital format only for a limited number of examinations.

There are also inherent differences in patient positioning of the two modalities. For CT, the patient lies, as a rule, with the hands above the head, whereas for PET, which is a much longer procedure, the patient often lies with the hands along the torso. Routine CT is a breath-holding procedure while PET is performed with the patient breathing normally. This may impair co-registration of chest examinations.

Misalignment caused by respiration and cardiac motion is somewhat less of a problem in the abdomen (5). When a patient is repositioned for a second test, shifting of organs can occur. Changes in the shape of the skin may lead to misplacement of external fiducial markers. Shifting of internal organs may misplace the internal anatomic markers used for registration. The temporal distance between the two tests, even only a few hours apart, may lead to misregistration due to changes in the filling of the stomach or a different urinary bladder or colon content (5,7,54). Even when fusion is considered prospectively, before the two tests are done, careful positioning cannot overcome all these limitations. Special devices recommended for rigorous repositioning put a heavy burden both on patients and on the technical staff (14,40).

After acquisition of data, processing and analysis for registration purposes are cumbersome. There may be differences in the partial volume effect between PET and CT (52). External markers may not be included in the field of view (FOV) (41). Algorithms performing warped geometric deformation may be inaccurate for the abdomen and pelvis (5). Mathematic models and computation methods are, as a rule, complex and difficult to perform (55).

Co-registration of separately performed CT and PET requires highly trained personnel and is time consuming, with processing time ranging from approximately 20 minutes to 2 hours. This in turn makes it a costly procedure (41,47,52, 55,56). For these reasons, research reports present series that do not include more than a few dozen patients. After a decade of performing such studies, there are only very limited reports on the impact of these co-registration methods on patient management and outcome.

Ideal fusion requires performing both the anatomic and functional tests within temporal and geographic proximity.

Hybrid Imaging—Dedicated and Camera-based PET/CT

Paradoxically, registration of multimodality imaging can be nonimage based. This is achieved through calibration of the imaging coordinate systems of the two involved scanners (38). Earlier work has lead to the development of a few prototypes that allow for simultaneous combined modality acquisition (57,58). The technique requires both modalities to be in the same physical location and assumes that the patient remains motionless between both acquisitions.

The advantages of using a single device for acquisition of both structural and metabolic patient data are multiple.

Positioning is identical, provided that the patient has been properly instructed and does not move between the two parts of the acquisition. The relatively similar stomach, bladder, and bowel content over the 35 to 50 minutes of data acquisition should improve the quality and precision of hybrid images of the abdomen and pelvis. Because the patient lies on the same bed, there is no shifting of organs, no change in body curvature, and no differences in angles of body axis. Sequential temporal and spatial acquisition of both modalities facilitates the fusion protocol, with no need for fiducial markers, no need for the use of complicated mathematic algorithms, and no need for long computation times and sophisticated software.

Hybrid imaging emerged from research on new ways that would provide rapid good-quality transmission studies to improve attenuation and scatter correction of PET (5). The prerequisites for such an optimal technique include the need for only a small increase in scanning time, noise-free scatter and attenuation correction, and no segmentation errors (59, 60). Besides allowing for correct and precise fusion of anatomic and functional patient information, CT images are also used for PET scatter and attenuation correction, by conversion of the CT Hounsfield units into 511 keV attenuation coefficients (61,62).

The future potential of hybrid imaging appears of even greater clinical significance with the prospective development of more specific probes for molecular imaging, which will increase the need for anatomic landmarks (27,63).

Nonimage-based registration of functional images using positron-emitting radiotracers and anatomic images has now been applied on a number of systems. One device for hybrid imaging is the dedicated PET/CT scanner. A few commercially available instruments are based on the combination of a spiral CT and a dedicated PET system (64–66). Different machine configurations have been designed to meet the needs of centers with different types of patient throughput and research interests, to achieve the optimal balance between clinical and academic benefits and cost. These devices differ in performance capabilities in regard to both the CT and the PET portion of the combined system. The PET and CT components are mounted back to back on the same assembly axially offset by a short distance. The common table for both systems, installed at the front of the combined gantry, permits 1.0 to 2.0 meters of common (PET and CT) scannable FOV. The mechanical alignment capabilities of the gantries, with respect to each other, are within the limits of a few millimeters, in up to six dimensions (three translations and three rotations).

Substituting PET transmission scanning with CT significantly reduces the acquisition time of a typical whole-body PET examination by up to one third, depending on the type of CT device and protocol available in the hybrid device, and this fact also induces direct cost savings. In at least some of the presently available devices, PET FOVs are reconstructed prospectively while being acquired, using CT data for attenuation correction of the corresponding patient segment. As a result, PET attenuation-corrected and fused hybrid images may be available a short time after completion of the PET acquisition. No degradation in quality of images of either PET or CT has been reported with the use of the combined device (64,66). Using CT images with a high data density, one may perform measured attenuation correction (instead of using approximations of segmented attenuation) with lesser partial volume effect at the borders of tissue-density changes. This may also potentially improve the precision of quantitative measurements of FDG uptake.

Another system that has been developed is a camera-based coincidence PET/CT imaging device (61,62,67). The hybrid image is performed using a nuclear medicine dual-head, variable angle, gamma camera with coincidence acquisition capabilities equipped with a low-power CT. The CT system is composed of an x-ray tube and a set of detectors fixed on opposite sides of the gamma camera gantry. The CT rotates around the patient along with the gamma camera detectors. Multiple slices are obtained by moving the table by a slice step before acquiring the next slice. Transmission data of the patient are corrected and reconstructed using filtered back-projection to produce cross-sectional attenuation images in which each pixel represents the attenuation of the imaged tissue. X-ray images are reconstructed and transmission data are integrated into the PET database. Matching pairs of images are fused, and images fusing the CT and camera-based PET data are generated (6,61,62). Because both CT and coincidence PET acquisition are performed with the patient breathing normally, respiratory motion is averaged in both images and misregistration is avoided. This CT mode is, however, characterized by low resolution and the presence of image artifacts (61,62). Radiation doses for the x-ray system added to the gamma camera are provided in the literature. They range from 130 to 336 mrad per slice at the center of a 16.0-cm-diameter tissue equivalent phantom and 425 to 500 mrad per slice surface (skin) dose. The dose from scattered radiation at the distance of 1.0 meter from the phantom is 1 mrad per slice. For a typical FOV, 40 CT slices are acquired (61,62).

There are a number of open and still controversial issues when discussing this very new technology (at the time this chapter was written). Most of these questions will probably find their solution in the near future. Positioning of the patient with arms beside the body accentuates beam-hardening effects, with some influence on the attenuation-correction factors (68). Normal breathing during both imaging procedures solves part of misalignment problems in the lungs. This will further improve with the use of breath-gating techniques, a novel procedure that minimizes the already reduced errors in fusion (69). Finding the optimal risk (and cost) to benefit ratio between producing a clinically diagnostic CT and reducing radiation doses is still under evaluation.

Another set of technical issues related to the use of contrast agents, contrast dose timing, and impact of contrast on attenuation-corrected PET images, are now in the initial steps of evaluation (70). Intravascular contrast, when given as a bolus, can lead to attenuation during the CT acquisition, which may inadvertently scale to resemble higher attenuation tissues like bone rather than soft tissue, creating attenuation-correction errors in the PET study (5). One possible solution to at least part of these open issues may be a repeated small-FOV, high-resolution, contrast-enhanced CT study done at the end of the PET/CT acquisition, allowing for better problem-oriented evaluation of small regions of interest.

Limited initial clinical reports are available on the assessment of hybrid imaging using combined devices for sequential acquisition of FDG studies and CT in the management of patients with cancer. In one study of 32 patients using PET/CT, hybrid imaging indicated the increased FDG uptake to be in sites of physiologic activity and thus excluded the presence of malignancy in one third of patients (71). In 24% of lesions, it allowed for better localization of pathology with PET (71).

Reports including small study populations have described changes in patient management with special emphasis on the differential diagnosis of FDG uptake in the region of the head and neck, abdomen, and pelvis (7,15,72). Correct localization and discrimination of areas of increased FDG affected surgical and radiation planning, as well as the correct assessment of tumor response to treatment (7,15,64).

Preliminary reports also indicate the potential value of PET/CT for improved image interpretation accuracy in about 50% of patients, again with special emphasis on precise localization in the region of the head and neck and the abdomen (54,66,72). Data published in an editorial suggested that combined imaging resulting in "true" registration may improve patient management in about 20% of patients in whom whole-body PET is performed (5). These assumptions correlate well with preliminary reports of data in 167 patients using the combined camera-based PET/CT device (73,74). Camera-based PET/CT using FDG improved the accuracy of PET or CT interpretation in 45% of patients. With PET, it was useful in correct localization of malignant lesions and in excluding cancer as the cause of FDG uptake. It retrospectively identified sites of disease missed on the initial CT reports in 7% of the patients. Combined acquisition of FDG and CT had an impact on clinical management in 29 patients (17%). Restaging and early detection of recurrence led to a change in treatment planning, referral to previously unplanned surgery, sparing of unnecessary surgery, and administration of additional chemotherapy or radiotherapy.

Initial results using combined simultaneous FDG and CT imaging techniques further prove that there is a principal difference between the presence of a mass and viable cancer in suspected lesions of patients with known malignancies. In a study of 75 patients, 25% of the suspected sites showing only an abnormal mass with no FDG uptake were malignant. In contrast, 70% of lesions showing only FDG uptake without a mass were viable cancer sites (75). This study was using a coincidence camera PET detection device.

The incremental value of hybrid imaging using a camera-based PET/CT device for lesion detectability was evaluated in 35 patients using dedicated PET as its standard of reference (76). Attenuation-corrected hybrid images obtained using an iterative reconstruction algorithm detected 78% of lesions depicted by dedicated PET. Iterative reconstruction using an algorithm based on ordered subsets–expectation maximization and attenuation correction particularly improved the detectability rate of lesions smaller than 1.5 cm in diameter and increased the confidence of interpreting the imaging studies (76). Hybrid images provided clinically relevant data in 31% of patients, correctly localizing lesions in the skeleton, separating FDG uptake in the colon from the liver, and precisely localizing lesions in the head and neck (76).

SUMMARY

PET/CT imaging provides simultaneous assessment of functional parameters of tumors using FDG PET and of anatomic data using CT. This enhances the inherent clinical potential of both techniques and provides synergistic knowledge that is as a rule greater than the sum of information provided by each modality alone. Although still under intensive study, PET/CT imaging is expected to become a frequently applied solution to many of the present diagnostic challenges in the analysis of oncologic imaging studies.

ACKNOWLEDGMENTS

The author acknowledges the help of Drs. Zohar Keidar, Rachel Bar-Shalom, Alex Frenkel, and Diana Gaitini, as well as Mr. Hernan Altman in the preparation of the manuscript. Special thanks to Dr. Gerald M. Kolodny for his many useful suggestions.

REFERENCES

1. Bar-Shalom R, Valdivia AY, Blaufox MD. PET imaging in oncology. *Semin Nucl Med* 2000;30:150–185.
2. Tucker R, Coel M, Ko J, et al. Impact of fluorine-18 fluorodeoxyglucose positron emission tomography on patient management: first year's experience in a clinical center. *J Clin Oncol* 2001;19:2504–2508.
3. Delbeke D. Oncological applications of FDG PET imaging: brain tumors, colorectal cancer, lymphoma and melanoma. *J Nucl Med* 1999;40:591–603.
4. Gambhir SS, Hoh GK, Phelps ME, et al. Decision tree sensitivity analysis for cost-effectiveness of FDG-PET in the staging and management of non–small-cell lung carcinoma. *J Nucl Med* 1996;37:1428–1436.
5. Shreve PD. Adding structure to function. *J Nucl Med* 2000;41:1380–1382.
6. Israel O, Keidar Z, Iosilevsky G, et al. The fusion of anatomic and physiologic imaging in the management of patients with cancer. *Semin Nucl Med* 2001;31:191–205.
7. Kluetz PG, Meltzer CC, Villemagne VL, et al. Combined PET/CT imaging in oncology: impact on patient management. *Clin Positron Imaging* 2000;3:223–230.
8. Hopper KD, Singapuri K, Finkel A. Body CT and oncologic imaging. *Radiology* 2000;215:27–40.
9. Weber DA, Ivanovic M. Correlative image registration. *Semin Nucl Med* 1994;24:311–323.
10. Cook GI, Maisey MN, Fogelman I. Normal variants, artifacts and interpretive pitfalls in PET imaging with 18-fluoro-deoxyglucose and carbon-11 methionine. *Eur J Nucl Med* 1999;26:1363–1378.
11. Shreve PD, Anzai Y, Wahl RL. Pitfalls in oncologic diagnosis with FDG-PET imaging: physiologic and benign variants. *Radiographics* 1999;19:61–69.

12. Strauss LG. Fluorine-18 deoxyglucose and false-positive results: a major problem in the diagnostics of oncological patients. *Eur J Nucl Med* 1996;23:1409–1415.

13. Engel H, Steinert H, Buck A, et al. Whole-body PET: physiological and artifactual fluorodeoxyglucose accumulations. *J Nucl Med* 1996; 37:441–446.

14. Uematsu H, Sadato N, Yoshiharu Y, et al. Coregistration of FDG PET and MRI of the head and neck using normal distribution of FDG. *J Nucl Med* 1998;39:2121–2127.

15. Heller MT, Meltzer CC, Fukui MB, et al. Superphysiologic FDG uptake in the non-paralyzed vocal cord: resolution of a false positive PET result with combined PET-CT imaging. *Clin Positron Imaging* 2000; 3:207–211.

16. Jabour BA, Choi Y, Hoh CK, et al. Extracranial head and neck: PET imaging with 2-[F-18] fluoro-2-deoxy-D-glucose and MR imaging correlation. *Radiology* 1993;186:27–35.

17. Keyes JW. SUV: Standard uptake or silly useless value? *J Nucl Med* 1995;36:1836–1839.

18. Eubank WB, Mankoff DA, Schmiedl UP, et al. Imaging of oncologic patients: benefit of combined CT and FDG PET in the diagnosis of malignancy. *AJR Am J Roentgenol* 1998;171:1103–1110.

19. Freeny PC, Mark WM, Ryan JA, et al. Colorectal carcinoma evaluation with CT: preoperative staging and detection of postoperative recurrence. *Radiology* 1986;158:347–353.

20. McCloud TC, Bourgouin PM, Greenberg RW, et al. Bronchogenic carcinoma: analysis of staging in the mediastinum with CT by correlative lymph node mapping and sampling. *Radiology* 1992;182:319–323.

21. Quint LE, Francis IR, Wahl RL, et al. Preoperative staging of non–small cell carcinoma of the lung: imaging methods. *AJR Am J Roentgenol* 1995;164: 1349–1359.

22. Ito K, Kato T, Tadokoro M, et al. Recurrent rectal cancer and scar: differentiation with PET and MR imaging. *Radiology* 1992;182: 549–552.

23. Studer UE, Schertz S, Scheidegger J, et al. Enlargement of regional lymph nodes in renal cell carcinoma is often not due to metastases. *J Urol* 1990;144:243–245.

24. Arita T, Mastumoto T, Kuramitsu T, et al. Is it possible to differentiate malignant mediastinal nodes from benign nodes by size? *Chest* 1996; 110:1004–1008.

25. Medina Gallardo JF, Borderas Naranjo F, Torres Cansino M, et al. Validity of enlarged mediastinal nodes as markers of involvement by non–small cell lung cancer. *Am Rev Respir Dis* 1992;146:1210–1212.

26. Goldstraw P, Mannan GM, Kaplan D, et al. Surgical management of non–small cell lung cancer with mediastinal node metastases (N2 disease). *J Thorac Cardiovasc Surg* 1994;107:19–28.

27. Phelps ME. PET: The merging of biology and imaging into molecular imaging. *J Nucl Med* 2000;41:661–681.

28. Quiox E, Wolkove N, Hanley J, et al. Problems in radiographic estimation of response to chemotherapy and radiotherapy in small cell lung cancer. *Cancer* 1988;62:489–493.

29. Front D, Bar-Shalom R, Epelbaum R, et al. Early detection of lymphoma recurrence with Gallium-67 scintigraphy. *J Nucl Med* 1993;34: 2101–2104.

30. Strauss LG, Conti PS. The application of PET in clinical oncology. *J Nucl Med* 1991;32:623–648.

31. Iosilevsky G, Front D, Bettman L, et al. Uptake of Gallium-67 citrate and [2-H$_3$] deoxyglucose in the tumor model, following chemotherapy and radiotherapy. *J Nucl Med* 1985;26:278–282.

32. Israel O, Front D, Lam M, et al. Gallium-67 imaging in monitoring lymphoma response to treatment. *Cancer* 1988;61:2439–2443.

33. Canellos GP. Residual mass in lymphoma may not be residual disease. *J Clin Oncol* 1988;6:931–933.

34. Weeks JC, Yeap BY, Canellos GP, et al. Value of follow-up procedures in patients with large-cell lymphoma who achieve a complete remission. *J Clin Oncol* 1991;9:1196–1203.

35. Spaepen K, Stroobants S, Dupont P, et al. Prognostic value of positron emission tomography (PET) with fluorine-18 fluorodeoxyglucose ([^{18}F] FDG) after first-line chemotherapy in non-Hodgkin's lymphoma: is [^{18}F]FDG-PET a valid alternative to conventional diagnostic methods? *J Clin Oncol* 2001;19: 414–419.

36. Cooper DL, Neumann RD, Caride VJ. A critical assessment of the prognostic value of Gallium-67 scintigraphy in lymphoma. In: Freeman L, ed. *Nuclear medicine annual 2000.* Philadelphia: Lippincott Williams & Wilkins, 2000:211–232.

37. Maisey MN, Hawkes DJ, Lukawiecki-Vydelingum AM. Synergistic imaging. *Eur J Nucl Med* 1992;19: 1002–1005.

38. Maintz JB, Viergever MA. A survey of medical image registration. *Med Image Anal* 1998;2:1–36.

39. Turkington TG, Jaszczak RJ, Pelizzari CA, et al. Accuracy of PET, SPECT and MR images of a brain phantom. *J Nucl Med* 1993;34: 1587–1594.

40. Pietrzyk U, Herholz K, Fink G, et al. An interactive technique for three-dimensional image registration: validation for PET, SPECT, MRI and CT brain studies. *J Nucl Med* 1994;35:2011–2018.

41. Wahl R, Quint LER, Cieslak RD, et al. "Anatometabolic" tumor imaging: fusion of FDG PET with CT or MRI to localize foci of increased activity. *J Nucl Med* 1993;34:1190–1197.

42. Anderson JLR. A rapid and accurate method to realign PET scans utilizing image edge information. *J Nucl Med* 1995;36:657–669.

43. Anderson JLR, Sundin A, Valind S. A method for coregistration of PET and MR images. *J Nucl Med* 1995;36:1307–1315.

44. Levin DN, Pelizzari CA, Chen GTY, et al. Retrospective geometric correlation of MR, CT and PET images. *Radiology* 1988;169:817–823.

45. Davatzikos C. Spatial normalization of 3D-brain images using deformable models. *J Comput Assisted Tomogr* 1996;20:656–665.

46. Slomka PJ, Hurwitz GA, Stephenson J, et al. Automated alignment and sizing of myocardial stress and rest scans to three-dimensional normal templates using an image registration algorithm. *J Nucl Med* 1995;36:1115–1122.

47. Wahl RL, Quint LE, Greenough RL, et al. Staging of mediastinal non–small cell lung cancer with FDG PET, CT, and fusion images: preliminary prospective evaluation. *Radiology* 1994;191:371–377.

48. Berlangieri SU, Scott AM. Metabolic staging of lung cancer [Editorial]. *N Engl J Med* 2000;343:290–292.

49. Vansteenkiste JF, Stroobants SG, Dupont PJ, et al. FDG-PET scan in potentially operable non–small cell lung cancer: do anatometabolic PET-CT fusion images improve the localization of regional lymph node metastases? *Eur J Nucl Med* 1998;25:1495–1501.

50. Cai J, Chu JCH, Recine D, et al. CT and PET lung image registration and fusion in radiotherapy treatment planning using the chamfer-matching method. *Int J Radiat Oncol Biol Phys* 1999;43:883–891.

51. Schaffler GJ, Groell R, Schoellnast H, et al. Digital image fusion of CT and PET data sets—clinical value in abdominal/pelvic malignancies. *J Comput Assisted Tomogr* 2000;24:644–647.

52. Inagaki H, Kato T, Tadokoro M, et al. Interactive fusion of three-dimensional images of upper abdominal CT and FDG PET with no body surface markers. *Radiat Med* 1999;17:155–163.

53. Zimny M, Buell U. F-18 FDG positron emission tomography in pancreatic cancer. *Ann Oncol* 1999;10[Suppl 4]:S28–S32.

54. Meltzer CC, Martinelli MA, Beyer T, et al. Whole-body FDG PET imaging in the abdomen: value of combined PET/CT. *J Nucl Med* 2001; 42[Suppl]:35(abst).

55. Scott AM, Macapinlac H, Zhang JJ, et al. Clinical applications of fusion imaging in oncology. *Nucl Med Biol* 1994;21:775–784.

56. Ketai L, Hartshorne M. Potential uses of computed tomography-SPECT and computed tomography-coincidence fusion images of the chest. *Clin Nucl Med* 2001;26:433–441.

57. Lang TF, Hasegawa BH, Liew SC, et al. Description of a prototype emission-transmission computed tomography imaging system. *J Nucl Med* 1992;33:1881–1887.

58. Hasegawa BH, Lang TF, Brown EL, et al. Object specific attenuation correction of SPECT with correlated dual-energy x-ray CT. *IEEE Trans Nucl Sci* 1993;40:1242–1252.

59. Akhurst T, Chisin R. Hybrid PET/CT machines: optimized PET machines for the new millennium [Letter]? *J Nucl Med* 2000;41:961–962.

60. Townsend DW. A combined PET/CT scanner: the choices [Letter]. *J Nucl Med* 2001;42:533–534.

61. Bocher M, Balan A, Krausz Y, et al. Gamma camera-mounted anatomical x-ray tomography: technology, system characteristics and first images. *Eur J Nucl Med* 2000;27:619–627.

62. Patton JA, Delbeke D, Sandler MP. Image fusion using an integrated, dual-head coincidence camera with x-ray tube–based attenuation maps. *J Nucl Med* 2000;41:1364–1368.

63. Coleman RE. Predictions for nuclear medicine in the next decade: commentary. *Radiology* 1998;208:6–7.

64. Beyer T, Townsend DW, Brun T, et al. A combined PET/CT scanner for clinical oncology. *J Nucl Med* 2000;41:1369–1379.

65. Kinahan PE, Townsend DW, Beyer T, et al. Attenuation correction for a combined 3D PET/CT scanner. *Med Phys* 1998;25:2046–2053.

66. Bar-Shalom R, Keidar Z, Engel A, et al. A new combined dedicated PET/CT system in the evaluation of cancer patients. *J Nucl Med* 2001; 42[Suppl]:34(abst).

67. Even-Sapir E, Keidar Z, Sachs J, et al. The new technology of combined transmission and emission tomography in evaluation of endocrine neoplasms. *J Nucl Med* 2001;42:998–1004.

68. Carney J, Townsend DW, Kinahan PE, et al. CT-based attenuation correction: the effects of imaging with the arms in the field of view. *J Nucl Med* 2001;42[Suppl]:56(abst).

69. Mijailovich SM, Treppo S, Venegas JG. Effects of lung motion and tracer kinetics corrections on PET imaging of pulmonary function. *J Appl Physiol* 1997;82:1154–1162.

70. Beyer T, Townsend DW. Dual-modality PET/CT imaging: CT-based attenuation correction in the presence of CT contrast agents. *J Nucl Med* 2001;42[Suppl]:56(abst).

71. Charron M, Beyer T, Bohnen NN, et al. Image analysis in patients with cancer studied with a combined PET and CT scanner. *Clin Nucl Med* 2000;25:905–910.

72. Meltzer CC, Snyderman CH, Fukui MB, et al. Combined FDG PET/CT imaging in head and neck cancer: impact on cancer patient management. *J Nucl Med* 2001;42[Suppl]:36(abst).

73. Front D, Israel O, Mor M, et al. A new technology of combined transmission (CT) and F-18 fluorodeoxyglucose (FDG) emission tomography (TET) in the evaluation of cancer patients. *J Nucl Med* 2000;41:284(abst).

74. Israel O, Mor M, Guralnik L, et al. The new technology of transmission and emission F-18 FDG tomography (FDG-TET) in the diagnosis and management of cancer patients. Paper presented at: 2000 ICP Meeting; October 16–19, 2000; Washington, DC.

75. Israel O, Mor M, Gaitini D, et al. A new technology for combined transmission and emission tomography (TET) in the diagnosis of tumor mass and tumor cancer. *Radiology* 2000(abst).

76. Delbeke D, Martin WH, Patton J, et al. Value of iterative reconstruction, attenuation correction and image fusion in the interpretation of FDG PET images with an integrated dual-head coincidence camera and X-ray–based attenuation maps. *Radiology* 2001;218:163–171.

CHAPTER 6

Neurologic Applications

Nicolaas I. Bohnen

Lesion-based anatomic imaging, such as computed tomography (CT) and magnetic resonance imaging (MRI), has revolutionized the diagnosis and management of the neurologic patient. However, a brain lesion may be present functionally, rather than structurally. For example, anatomic imaging in early idiopathic Parkinson's disease may not reveal disease-specific changes, whereas positron emission tomography (PET) has clearly demonstrated the dopaminergic abnormality in this disorder.

PET is a molecular imaging technique that uses radiolabeled molecules to image molecular interactions of biologic processes *in vivo*. Low doses of positron-emitting radioisotopes are used to radiolabel molecules or drugs that have binding sites in the brain, such as receptors, to measure regional cerebral blood flow (rCBF), or are metabolized by cerebral enzymes. PET can be used to perform neurochemical and functional brain imaging studies of CBF or glucose metabolism.

Neurochemical imaging studies allow assessment of the regional distribution and quantitative measurement of neurotransmitters, enzymes, or receptors in the living brain. Neurochemical imaging studies are mainly performed for research purposes.

Functional brain imaging studies can measure rCBF or glucose metabolism. These studies may be performed in the resting state or after a specific intervention (e.g., a mental task, sensory stimulus, or motor task) to "activate" specific regions in the brain.

Resting glucose metabolic and blood-flow brain studies represent the major clinical applications of PET in neurology and are mainly discussed in this chapter. PET studies of specific neurochemical markers are discussed when clinically useful or promising.

GENERAL PRINCIPLES OF CEREBRAL BLOOD FLOW AND METABOLIC IMAGING: FUNCTIONAL COUPLING AND PHYSIOLOGIC CORRELATES

The energy metabolism of the adult human brain depends almost completely on the oxidation of glucose (1). Because the brain is unable to store either oxygen or glucose, it is thought that rCBF is continuously regulated to supply these substrates locally. The functional coupling of rCBF and local cerebral glucose metabolism has been established in a wide range of experiments using autoradiographic techniques in animals, as well as double-tracer techniques in humans. Increased function of the central neurons results in increased neuronal metabolism, and as a consequence, increased concentration of metabolic end products (H^+, K^+, adenosine) results in increased rCBF (2). A model has been proposed in which neurogenic stimuli coming through perivascular nerve endings may act as rapid initiators responsible for moment-to-moment dynamic adjustment of rCBF to the metabolic demands (2). Functional activation of the brain (e.g., motor or visual activity) is accompanied by increases in rCBF and glucose consumption, but only minimal increases in oxygen consumption (3,4). Therefore, large changes in blood flow are required to support small changes in the oxygen metabolic rate during neuronal stimulation (5). Increased oxygen consumption may result from a combined effect of increased blood flow and increased oxygen diffusion capacity in the region of brain activation (6).

$H_2^{15}O$ is the most commonly used PET tracer for the measurement of rCBF. CBF can also be assessed by the inhalation of $C^{15}O_2$. The very short half-life of ^{15}O (123 seconds) allows repeated and rapid rCBF assessments in the same individual. Fluorine-18-fluorodeoxyglucose (^{18}F-FDG) is a PET tracer used for the study of regional cerebral glucose metabolism. Most of the glucose in the brain is needed for maintenance of membrane potentials and restoration of ion gradients. Although the FDG PET signal represents neuronal and more specifically synaptic activity (7), glutamate-mediated uptake of the radioligand into astrocytes appears to be a major mechanism of FDG uptake (8).

READING BRAIN PET IMAGES: NORMAL VARIANTS, AGING, AND OTHER FACTORS THAT MAY AFFECT BLOOD FLOW OR GLUCOSE METABOLISM

The spatial resolution of the PET camera determines the extent of the partial volume effect that causes the edges of small brain structures to blur each other due to averaging of radioactivity. The size of the imaged structure determines the recovery of counts by the camera from a specific structure (9). A structure must have dimensions greater than twice the reconstructed resolution of the PET camera at full width half maximum, to recover 100% of true tissue activity from that structure. Partial volume effects reduce the contrast and detectability of small brain structures, atrophied gyri, and smaller brain volumes, such as the inferior orbitofrontal and inferior temporal regions. Conversely, a cerebral sulcus, where two gray matter gyri face each other closely, may show relatively higher activity when a scanner does not have sufficient spatial resolution to resolve the two gyri (10). For instance, the precentral and postcentral gyri opposed at the central sulcus may form a single apparent focus of relatively high activity (10). Similarly, the adjacent areas of insular cortex and superior temporal gyral cortex generate sufficiently similar FDG activity that they may appear as one lateral mass at certain levels of scanning (11).

It should be noted that a normal individual brain is not completely symmetric. For example, the sylvian fissure in right-handed individuals is longer and more horizontal in the left hemisphere. Normal irregularity of gyral convolutions may give a heterogeneous scan appearance. Therefore, a commonly observed rule of visual PET analysis is the requirement that an area of apparent functional alteration of a brain structure should be seen on at least several adjacent slices to be deemed significant (11). Studies of left-to-right hemispheric asymmetries in normal subjects are limited and have not been conclusive. A rCBF PET study reported a slightly higher mean right hemispheric flow compared with the left-side values (12). A recent rCBF single-photon emission computed tomography (SPECT) study demonstrated consistent hemispheric asymmetry (right side greater than left side) in the cuneus, occipital cortex, occipital pole, middle temporal gyrus, and posterior middle frontal gyrus in 83% to 100% of individuals (13). FDG PET studies have indicated that hemispheric asymmetries may depend on

whether subjects are studied with open versus closed eyes or ears (14). For example, studies performed on subjects with eyes and ears closed demonstrated greater hemispheric glucose metabolism in the left than in the right. Subjects studied with closed eyes and ears also had a progressive overall decrease in glucose metabolism, reflecting general sensory deprivation (14).

Normal Variants

Several normal variants should be recognized when interpreting cerebral metabolic or blood-flow PET scans. Some normal brain regions have focally more prominent metabolic or flow activity. These include the frontal eye fields (which can be asymmetric), posterior cingulate cortex, the Wernicke region, the visual cortex (when subjects are injected with the eyes open), and an area of more intense uptake in the posterior parietal lobe (Fig. 6.1) (15).

The frontal eye fields have an approximate dimension of about 1 cm and are located a few centimeters anterior to the primary motor cortex (15). The Wernicke region is defined as an area of moderately intense activity measuring a few centimeters in size and is located in the posterosuperior temporal lobe. The posterior cingulate cortex is situated superior and anterior to the occipital cortex. An area of focally intense activity in the posterior parietal region is seen in about 50% of the normal population and appears mostly symmetric (Table 6.1) (15). Basal ganglia-to-cortex ratios are greater than unity, indicating relatively higher activity in the basal ganglia compared with the average cortex (15). Some brain regions, such as the very anterior aspect of the frontal poles, may have less prominent or decreased tracer uptake (15).

Normal Aging: From Infancy to Adulthood

CBF PET studies in children have shown lower flow values in neonates compared with older children (16). rCBF will reach adult values during adolescence (16). No major

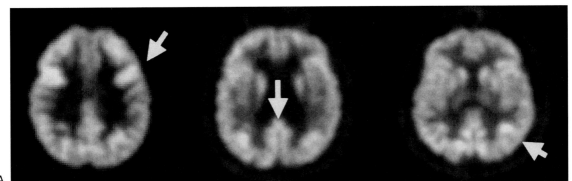

FIG. 6.1. Positron emission tomography images showing normal glucose metabolic variants in healthy volunteers. Examples of more prominent uptake in the **(A)** frontal eye fields and in the **(B)** posterior cingulate cortex, as well as **(C)** an area of more intense uptake in the posterior parietal lobe are shown (*arrows*).

TABLE 6.1. *Frequency of prominent normal fluorodeoxyglucose brain PET variants in the general population*

	Right	Left
Frontal eye field	84%	77%
Wernicke area	80%	85%
Posterior parietal lobe	58%	46%

From Loessner A, Alavi A, Lewandrowski KU, et al. Regional cerebral function determined by FDG-PET in healthy volunteers: normal patterns and changes with age. *J Nucl Med* 1995;36:1141–1149.

difference in rCBF has been observed between the basal ganglia and the cortical gray matter in children, with the exception of more prominent occipital flow.

FDG metabolic studies in infants and children have shown that infants younger than 5 weeks have highest metabolic activity in the sensorimotor cortex, thalamus, brainstem, and cerebellar vermis. By 3 months, metabolic activity increases in parietal, temporal, and occipital cortices, basal ganglia, and cerebellar cortex (17). Frontal and dorsolateral occipital cortical regions display a maturational rise in glucose metabolic activity by approximately 6 to 8 months.

Absolute values of glucose metabolic rate for various gray matter regions are low at birth (13 to 25 μmol per minute per 100 g), and rapidly rise to reach adult values (19 to 33 μmol per minute per 100 g) by 2 years. Glucose metabolic rates continue to rise until, by 3 to 4 years, reaching values of 49 to 65 μmol per minute per 100 g in most regions (17). These high rates are maintained until approximately age 9 years, at which point they begin to decline, and reach adult rates again by the latter part of the second decade of life.

The highest increases over adult values have been noted in cerebral cortical structures. Lesser increases have been found to be present in the basal ganglia and cerebellum. This time course of metabolic changes matches the process describing initial overproduction and subsequent elimination of excessive neurons, synapses, and dendritic spines known to occur in the developing brain.

A recent statistical brain mapping study of metabolic aging from 6 to 38 years found greatest age-associated changes in the thalamus and anterior cingulate cortex (18). These findings were explained by a relative increase of synaptic activity in the thalamus, possibly as a consequence of improved corticothalamic connections. Knowledge of the changing metabolic patterns during normal brain development is a necessary prelude to the study of abnormal brain development.

Normal Aging: From Adulthood to the Elderly

Postmortem studies have shown relatively stable neuronal numbers but a loss in cell size and decreased number of glial cells with advancing age (19). However, it remains a matter of controversy as to whether cerebral perfusion declines with healthy aging.

$H_2^{15}O$ rCBF PET studies have shown a negative correlation between age and rCBF in the mesial frontal cortex, involving the anterior cingulate region (20). Age-related flow decreases have also been reported for the cingulate, parahippocampal, superior temporal, medial frontal, and posterior parietal cortices bilaterally, and in the left insular and left posterior prefrontal cortices (21). It should be realized that the affected areas represent limbic or neocortical association areas, and therefore, bias from possible preclinical dementia cannot be excluded. It has also been suggested that a lack of partial volume correction for the dilution effect of age-related cerebral volume loss on PET measurements may be another reason for the observed age-related decline. For example, a recent study found a significant difference in mean cortical CBF between young life and midlife (age range, 19 to 46 years; mean $\pm$ SD, 56 $\pm$ 10 mL/100 mL per minute) and elderly (age range, 60 to 76 years; mean $\pm$ SD, 49 $\pm$ 2.6 mL/100 mL per minute) subgroups before correcting for partial volume effects (22). This group difference resolved after partial volume correction (young/midlife: mean $\pm$ SD, 62 $\pm$ 10 mL/100 mL per minute; elderly: mean $\pm$ SD, 61 $\pm$ 4.8 mL/100 mL per minute).

FDG PET imaging studies have shown decreased cortical metabolism with normal aging, particularly in the frontal lobes (15). Temporal, parietal, and occipital lobe metabolism varied considerably among subjects within the same age group, as well as over decades (15). Basal ganglia, hippocampal area, thalami, cerebellum, posterior cingulate gyrus, and visual cortex remained metabolically unchanged with advancing age (15). A recent FDG PET study found bilateral medial prefrontal, including anterior cingulate cortices, and dorsolateral prefrontal reductions with normal aging (23). Brain scans of the aging and atrophied brain demonstrate widened cerebral sulci, increased separation of the caudate nuclei and thalami, and widening of the anterior fissure.

Factors That May Affect Resting Cerebral Blood Flow or Glucose Metabolic Studies

A number of other factors must be considered when interpreting brain PET images. Metabolism or blood-flow activity will be most prominent in gray matter when compared with white matter (about four times higher). It should be realized that brain glucose metabolic or blood-flow PET images are functional in nature. For example, if a patient is moving or talking around the time of injection, increased activity in specific brain regions such as the basal ganglia, motor cortex, or language centers may be present. Subjects studied with eyes open will have increased metabolic activity in the visual cortex when compared to a baseline with the eyes closed (14). A recent FDG PET study found that passive audiovisual stimulation (watching a movie) led to significant glucose metabolic increases in visual and auditory cortical areas but significant decreases in frontal areas in normal volunteers (24).

Metabolic factors such as hyperglycemia may impair cortical FDG uptake (25). Therefore, knowledge of the clinical or behavioral state of the patient at the time of the injection and study is critical for proper image interpretation. As with any nuclear medicine study, better image quality will depend on improved count statistics. Because PET images are an average of radioactivity over a certain period of time, FDG acquisitions taken for more than 10 or 30 minutes will lead to better image quality compared with short-lasting (1 to 2 minutes) H$_2$^{15}O CBF studies.

Drugs are also well known to induce CBF or glucose metabolic changes. For example, diazepam sedation has been found to reduce cerebral glucose metabolism globally by about 20% (26). A study by Wang et al. (27) found that lorazepam significantly decreased whole-brain metabolism more than 10%. However, the regional effects of lorazepam were largest in the thalamus and occipital cortex (about 20% reduction). Similarly, antiepileptic drugs have been found to reduce glucose metabolism and rCBF. Studies of valproate have shown global FDG (about 9% to 10%) and global CBF (about 15%) reductions, with greatest regional reductions in the thalamus (28). Phenytoin has been found to cause an average reduction of cerebral glucose metabolism of 13% (29). Cerebellar metabolism may also be reduced by phenytoin, although the effect of the drug is probably less than that due to early onset of uncontrolled epilepsy (Fig. 6.2) (30,31).

Studies using the barbiturate phenobarbital and measuring cerebral glucose metabolism have shown very prominent global reductions of about 37% (32). Neuroleptic drugs can cause differential regional metabolic effects. For example, haloperidol caused cerebellar and putaminal glucose metabolic increases, whereas significant reductions were evident in the frontal, occipital, and anterior cingulate cortex in normal volunteers (33).

Diaschisis: Remote Functional Effects of Focal Brain Lesions

The functional nature of PET images may reveal metabolic or blood-flow changes as a result of focal disturbance

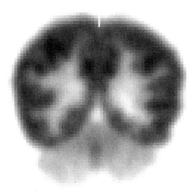

FIG. 6.2. A ^{18}F-fluorodeoxyglucose positron emission tomography image of a patient with epilepsy shows bilateral cerebellar hypometabolism. Cerebellar hypometabolism may be caused by phenytoin therapy, although the effect of the drug is probably less than that due to early onset of uncontrolled epilepsy.

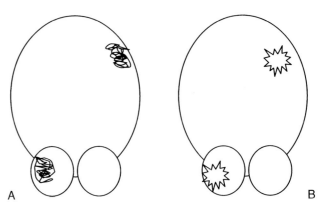

FIG. 6.3. **A:** A diagrammatic representation of crossed cerebrocerebellar diaschisis shows cerebellar hypoperfusion contralateral to a supratentorial structural lesion. **B:** Reverse crossed cerebrocerebellar diaschisis can be observed during ictal seizure activity in which a supratentorial ictal focus of hyperperfusion is associated with contralateral cerebellar hyperperfusion.

in another remote but functionally connected brain region. This phenomenon is called diaschisis and was originally recognized by Von Monakow in 1914 (34,35). Diaschisis in the cerebellum was first described by Baron et al. (36) in a patient whose PET study showed cerebellar hypoperfusion contralateral to a supratentorial stroke. Remote metabolic depression is characterized by coupled reductions in perfusion and metabolism in brain structures remote from, but connected with, the area damaged by a structural lesion. This effect has been explained as depressed synaptic activity as a result of disconnection (either direct or transneural) (37). Thus, remote effects allow mapping of the disruption in distributed networks as a result of a focal brain lesion.

Diaschisis may also occur as subcortical-cortical effects. Subcortico-cortical effects may lead to clinical symptoms, such as subcortical aphasia due to thalamic or thalamocapsular stroke. Right-sided subcortical lesions may present with left hemineglect ("subcortical neglect") (36). Small thalamic infarcts may induce metabolic depression of the ipsilateral cortical mantle (thalamocortical diaschisis) (38). Striatal and thalamic hypometabolism ipsilateral to cortical-subcortical stroke is a frequent finding. Thalamic hypometabolism may develop a few days after a stroke and presumably represents retrograde degeneration of damaged thalamocortical neurons, whereas striatal hypometabolism probably reflects loss of glutamatergic input from the cortex (36).

SPECT studies performed as ictal studies during seizure activity have demonstrated a pattern called "reverse" crossed cerebrocerebellar diaschisis where a supratentorial ictal seizure focus of hyperperfusion is associated with contralateral cerebellar hyperperfusion (Fig. 6.3) (39).

STROKE

Current management of patients with acute stroke is centered on CT and MRI. CT has a prominent role by detecting the presence of hemorrhage. MRI blood oxygen level–dependent functional imaging is playing a key role in the very early diagnosis of ischemic stroke (40).

Multitracer PET imaging has allowed major new insights into the pathophysiology of stroke in humans and may provide important guidance to the development of therapeutic strategies (41,42). Determinations of CBF, cerebral blood volume (CBV), and cerebral metabolic rate of oxygen (CMRO$_2$) permit the discrimination of various compensatory mechanisms in occlusive vascular disease. For example, compensatory changes in the CBF/CBV ratio (indicating a perfusional reserve) and increases in the oxygen extraction fraction (OEF), a marker of metabolic reserve, may prevent ischemic tissue damage during graded flow decreases (42).

Measurement of Cerebral Oxygen Metabolism, Cerebral Blood Volume, and Oxygen Extraction Fraction Using PET

PET measurements of rCBF, CBV, oxygen extraction, and oxygen and glucose consumption permit a detailed investigation of the pathophysiology of stroke (43). The short-lived PET tracer ^{15}O (half-life of 123 seconds) was first used to study CBF and cerebral oxygen utilization in humans by Ter-Pogossian et al. (44,45). Jones et al. (46) described a noninvasive inhalational method using steady-state kinetics to measure the distribution of CBF and OEF in the human brain. The continuous inhalation of either molecular ^{15}O or C^{15}O$_2$ produces complementary images in that they relate to regional oxygen uptake and blood flow, which offers direct insight to the regional demand-to-supply relationships within the brain (47).

The method of quantitative measurement of rCBF and CMRO$_2$ has been described in detail by Frackowiak et al. (48). OEF reflects the arteriovenous oxygen difference divided by the arterial oxygen content. Reliable OEF estimates can be obtained by combining dynamic C^{15}O and ^{15}O$_2$ scans (49). An expression for OEF can be obtained by dividing the cerebral activity obtained during ^{15}O inhalation by that obtained during C^{15}O$_2$ inhalation with some additional computations (48). The CMRO$_2$ can be derived from the following relationship (48):

$$CMRO_2 = CBF \times OEF \times \text{total blood oxygen count}$$
$$\text{(from arterial blood sample)}$$

Using these methods, Frackowiak et al. (48) found normal values of CMRO$_2$ of 1.81 $\pm$ 0.22 mL of O$_2$/100 mL per minute in mean white matter and 5.88 $\pm$ 0.57 mL of O$_2$/100 mL per minute in mean temporal gray matter. Corresponding values for CBF were 21.4 $\pm$ 1.9 mL/100 mL per minute in mean white matter and 65.3 $\pm$ 7.0 mL of O$_2$/100 mL per minute in mean temporal lobe gray matter (48).

Methods other than the steady-state inhalational method have been developed to measure CBF and CMRO$_2$, such as the autoradiographic CBF method using intravenous H$_2$^{15}O and newer dynamic methods (50). CBV can be measured by inhalation of C^{15}O (51). Quantitative imaging of the OEF

TABLE 6.2. *Different pathophysiologic conditions in stroke*

Condition	CBF	CMRO$_2$	OEF
Ischemia	Low	Low	Very high
Oligemia	Moderately low	Normal	High
Luxury perfusion	Low/normal/high	Low	Low

CBF, cerebral blood flow; CMRO$_2$, cerebral metabolic rate of oxygen; OEF, oxygen extraction fraction.
From Baron JC, Frackowiak RS, Herholz K, et al. Use of PET methods for measurement of cerebral energy metabolism and hemodynamics in cerebrovascular disease. *J Cereb Blood Flow Metab* 1989;9:723–742.

has been shown to be of invaluable help in the assessment of the pattern of CBF–CMRO$_2$ coupling (52). Ideally, glucose utilization should be measured simultaneously with CMRO$_2$, to provide an accurate assessment of regional energy metabolism because glucose utilization and oxygen use may become uncoupled in acute stroke and this uncoupling may go in two opposite directions: either aerobic glycolysis with relatively increased glucose consumption or use of substrates for oxidation other than glucose (52). Table 6.2 summarizes different pathophysiologic conditions in stroke (52).

Acute Ischemic Stroke

Brain tissue infarction may follow a critical reduction in rCBF and may lead to neurologic deficits. The more severe the drop in perfusion, the higher the chance of irreversible brain tissue damage (53). The development of methods for determining rCBF has made possible the determination of thresholds for the appearance of cerebral ischemia (Table 6.3). These thresholds vary depending on the method used for assessing cerebral ischemia. It should be noted that not only the level of residual CBF, but also the duration of is-

TABLE 6.3. *Ischemic thresholds and regional cerebral blood flow in human and nonhuman primates*

Cerebral blood flow threshold	Clinical correlates
20 mL per 100 g/min	Electroencephalogram (EEG) and evoked cortical potential abnormalities appear, paralysis seen in waking monkeys
15 mL per 100 g/min	EEG and evoked cortical potentials are lost
12 mL per 100 g/min	Flow values at this level in excess of 120 min produce infarction in waking animals
6 mL per 100 g/min	Massive loss of intracellular potassium

From Morawetz RB, Crowell RH, DeGirolami U, et al. Regional cerebral blood flow thresholds during cerebral ischemia. *Fed Proc* 1979;38:2493–2494.

chemia will determine the presence of irreversible infarction.

A prerequisite for the successful treatment of acute ischemic stroke is the existence of viable tissue that is morphologically intact but functionally impaired due to flow decreases below a certain threshold. The ischemic penumbra is defined as tissue with flow falling within the thresholds for maintenance of function and of morphologic integrity (54). Early in the course of acute ischemia, CBF and $CMRO_2$ levels falling below certain thresholds may lead to irreversible tissue damage, whereas preservation of $CMRO_2$ with decreased flow resulting in increased OEF ("misery" perfusion) still suggests viable tissue ("penumbra") (55).

Identification of viable or penumbra tissue is the key target for interventional therapy in acute ischemic stroke. Rapid restoration of blood flow to the penumbra even in the presence of a fixed deficit at the center of the stroke may improve stroke outcome. Identification of penumbra tissue can be achieved by multitracer PET. Multitracer PET imaging permits the assessment of acute changes in rCBF, CBV, $CMRO_2$, and glucose metabolism that may guide therapeutic decisions and predict the severity of permanent deficits (42).

Subacute Changes in Ischemic Stroke

In subacute states of cerebral ischemia, reduced blood flow can be compensated by increased blood volume, and when perfusional reserve is exhausted, OEF may increase up to 48 hours after stroke onset (42). This condition, also called misery perfusion, implies that blood flow is inadequate relative to energy metabolic tissue demand for oxygen (42). Penumbra tissue cannot be seen as a stable rim of tissue surrounding the core of infarction and it may also change in time as a dynamic phenomenon, involving new adjacent tissue compartments while others are becoming permanently necrotic (42). Therefore, studies identifying penumbra tissue could be of value in the development of effective therapeutic strategies, even in the subacute stage of stroke (42).

Some patients may have postischemic reactive hyperemia that occurs within hours or days after stroke onset. This phenomenon is called luxury perfusion and is seen in the periphery of an ischemic stroke. Unlike misery perfusion, luxury perfusion is seen as increased CBF and a low oxygen extraction ratio (OER) (42,52). Luxury perfusion may reflect recanalization of an occluded artery (52).

Chronic Arterial Occlusive Disease and Hemodynamic Reserve

Hemodynamic factors may play an important role in the pathogenesis of ischemic stroke in patients with cerebrovascular disease (56). Patients with arterial occlusive disease are protected against ischemic episodes to a certain extent by compensatory mechanisms, which may help to prevent ischemia when perfusion pressure drops (42). Severe atherosclerotic disease of the carotid and vertebral arteries may

lead to reduced perfusion pressure (57). This may cause hemodynamic impairment of the distal cerebral circulation. It should be noted that CBF studies alone do not adequately assess cerebral hemodynamic status, because CBF may be maintained by autoregulatory vasodilation and even low CBF values may not correlate with perfusion pressures (56).

Functional imaging techniques can be used to assess two basic categories of hemodynamic impairment. The first category reflects a state of autoregulatory vasodilation secondary to reduced perfusion pressure that can be assessed by the measurement of either increased CBV or an impaired CBF response to a vasodilatory stimulus. The second category is defined on the basis of OEF measurements (increased OEF) (56).

Compensatory regional vasodilation may manifest itself as a focal increase in CBV in the supply territory of the occluded artery (42,58). Here, the ratio of CBF to CBV has been used as an indicator of local perfusion pressure or perfusion reserve (normally 10) (42). The lower the value, the lower the flow velocity (42). When the perfusion pressure is exhausted (i.e., at maximal vasodilatation), any further decrease in arterial input pressure will produce a proportional decrease in both CBF and the CBF/CBV ratio (42). In this type of hemodynamic decompensation, the brain will exploit oxygen carriage reserve to prevent energy failure and loss of function, as evidenced by an increase in OEF (57, 58).

The relative importance of hemodynamic factors in the pathogenesis of stroke in patients with carotid arterial occlusive disease has been investigated in the St. Louis Carotid Occlusion Study (59). This study demonstrated that increased cerebral OEF detected by PET scanning predicted future stroke in patients with symptomatic carotid occlusion. Consequently, a trial of extracranial-to-intracranial (EC/IC) arterial bypass for this group of patients has been proposed (59). Unlike symptomatic carotid artery occlusion, patients with asymptomatic carotid arterial occlusive disease were found to have a much lower incidence of hemodynamic impairment as measured by increased OEF and thereby a very low risk of subsequent ischemic stroke (60). These data support the importance of hemodynamic factors in the pathogenesis of ischemic stroke in patients with carotid arterial occlusion. Increased OEF in symptomatic patients is associated with a high risk of subsequent stroke, whereas normal OEF is associated with a low risk. A simplified count-based PET measurement of OEF may increase the clinical utility of PET for this purpose (61).

Correlation between different methods to assess impaired blood-flow response to a vasodilatory stimulus with each other and with methods that assess OEF is quite variable (56). Vasodilatory hemodynamic stress testing relies on paired blood-flow measurements, with the initial measurement obtained at rest and the second measurement obtained after a cerebral vasodilatory stimulus (56).

A comparison of the rest–stress perfusion may provide an estimate of cerebrovascular reserve. Acetazolamide or inhaling CO_2 has been used as a vasodilatory stimulus (56).

Acetazolamide is a carbonic anhydrase inhibitor that increases the carbon dioxide in the brain. Each vasodilatory stimulus will result in a significant increase in CBF in normal persons. If the CBF response is muted or absent, preexisting autoregulatory cerebral vasodilatation due to reduced cerebral perfusion pressure is inferred (56). The blood-flow responses to vasodilatory stress have been categorized into several grades of hemodynamic impairment: (a) reduced augmentation (relative to the contralateral hemisphere or normal controls); (b) absent augmentation (same as baseline); and (c) paradoxical reduction in rCBF (steal phenomenon) (56). Although commonly applied, there is a lack of well-controlled prognostic studies on the use of these vasodilator rest–stress techniques in patients with cerebrovascular disease (56).

Hemorrhagic Stroke

Multitracer PET studies of patients with subarachnoid hemorrhage but without vasospasm have shown a significant reduction in global $CMRO_2$ with no significant change in global OEF, suggesting a primary reduction in $CMRO_2$ in the absence of vasospasm (62). However, subarachnoid hemorrhage complicated by vasospasm has been found to be associated with significantly increased regional OEF with unchanged $CMRO_2$, indicative of cerebral ischemia without infarction (62). PET studies of patients with intracerebral intraparenchymal hemorrhage have shown reduced CBF surrounding the primary bleeding site (63).

Estimation of Prognosis After Stroke

The degree of functional recovery after a stroke is related to the location and size of the lesion, the presence of remaining neurons in the neighborhood of the lesion, and the presence of compensatory mechanisms in functionally connected networks (42). Although the regional cerebral metabolic rate of glucose in early ischemia is often not coupled to flow or $CMRO_2$ and might even be increased, regional cerebral glucose metabolism is the best indicator of permanent impairment of tissue function (42). A normal FDG PET result or the presence of a mild metabolic abnormality has been strongly associated with good clinical outcome or complete reversal of the neurologic dysfunction (64). In contrast, patients with poor clinical outcome had more severe glucose metabolic deficits (64).

The presence of early luxury perfusion in the context of little or no metabolic alteration may also indicate a favorable prognosis (65). A recent study comparing early and delayed PET studies in patients with stroke found that in hyperperfused regions, the acute-stage perfusion, blood volume, and oxygen consumption were significantly increased, and the OEF was significantly reduced, whereas all these variables had significantly returned toward normality in the chronic-stage PET study. The ultimately infarcted area did not exhibit significant hyperperfusion in the acute stage (65).

These data indicate that early reperfusion into metabolically active tissue is beneficial. Flow and metabolic studies during the performance of specific tasks (so-called activation studies) are now being carried out to detect the presence of compensatory mechanisms in functionally connected networks and may also yield prognostic information after stroke (42).

New Emerging Clinical Applications of PET in Stroke

CBF and FDG PET studies of patients with stroke may not only show the local effects caused by the primary stroke lesion but also demonstrate remote effects because of diaschisis. Central benzodiazepine-receptor ligands, such as ^{11}C-flumazenil, are markers of neuronal integrity and therefore may be useful in the differentiation of functionally and morphologically damaged tissue in stroke. Carbon-11-flumazenil PET imaging has the potential to depict damaged brain tissue by directly assessing neuronal loss. A recent study demonstrated the feasibility of ^{11}C-flumazenil PET imaging in distinguishing between irreversibly damaged and viable penumbra tissue early after acute stroke (66). New tracers, such as receptor ligands or hypoxia markers, may further improve the identification of penumbra tissue in the future (54). Clinical application of such techniques may permit the extension of the critical time period for inclusion of patients for aggressive stroke management strategies.

COGNITIVE DISORDERS AND DEMENTIA

Alzheimer's disease is the most common type of dementia. Accurate diagnosis of early Alzheimer's disease is becoming increasingly important at a time when new therapeutic agents are emerging (67,68). New treatments are likely to be more effective when given early in the course of the disease, rather than late. Therefore, identification of early disease has become crucial to select patients for treatments that may slow down the progression of the dementing illness or even reverse its pathologic schema.

A definitive diagnosis of Alzheimer's disease relies on tissue diagnosis and is not readily available. Functional or volumetric neuroimaging has the potential to detect early changes of Alzheimer's disease *in vivo* (68). For example, FDG PET brain imaging and volumetric MRI assessment of hippocampal atrophy are sensitive tools for the early diagnosis of Alzheimer's disease. However, hippocampal atrophy may not be specific for Alzheimer's disease because this abnormality can also be seen in other disorders. FDG PET has the advantage of being not only sensitive, but also more specific in the diagnosis of dementia.

Alzheimer's Disease

The neuropathologic model of Braak and Braak (69) suggests the "spread" of Alzheimer's pathology through six stages of disease propagation on the basis of the location of tangle-bearing neurons that progress from transentorhinal to limbic and then to neocortical locations. Cortical neuropathologic changes in Alzheimer's disease are heterogeneous topographically but are not randomly distributed. It has been demonstrated that primary somatosensory and motor cortical regions are relatively spared, whereas association cortices are more severely involved (69). In the brain of a patient with Alzheimer's disease, FDG PET imaging reveals characteristic hypometabolism in neocortical structures, particularly in parietal, temporal, and frontal association cortices, the same locations where coexisting cortical neuronal degeneration is also found in postmortem studies (70,71). Evidence is accumulating that the metabolic reduction in Alzheimer's disease likely follows regional synaptic loss or dysfunction (72,73).

Glucose metabolic reductions in the parietotemporal association cortices have been widely recognized as a diagnostic marker for Alzheimer's disease and facilitated the use of PET in clinical settings to evaluate patients with dementia (Fig. 6.4) (74–78). These regional cortical reductions in the brain with Alzheimer's disease occur in the context of relative preservation of glucose metabolism in primary neocortical structures, such as the sensorimotor and primary visual cortex, as well as subcortical structures like the thalamus, basal ganglia, and brainstem (77–79). Metabolic reduction in the mesial temporal cortex is more variable in Alzheimer's disease (80), and frontal involvement becomes particularly more prominent with advancing disease. FDG PET studies of patients with mild or very early Alzheimer's disease can show asymmetric or unilateral parietal rather than biparietal hypometabolism (81,82). Predominant left-sided or right-sided involvement may correlate with the presence of specific cognitive or neurobehavioral symptoms. Rarely, patients with Alzheimer's disease may present with a frontal predominant syndrome (frontal variant Alzheimer's disease) (83).

Parkinson's Disease with Dementia and Dementia with Lewy Bodies

Disturbances of cognition are frequent findings in patients with Parkinson's disease, with prevalence estimates of dementia ranging up to 40% of patients (84,85). Dementia in Parkinson's disease has often been attributed to coexistent Alzheimer's pathology (86). Recently, a new entity called dementia with Lewy bodies has been identified, which may account for many cases of Parkinson's disease with dementia (87). Clinically, dementia with Lewy bodies appears to be a subset of demented patients with Parkinson's disease who have marked neuropsychiatric disturbances, such as prominent visual hallucinations, depression, and variability in arousal and attention (87).

Vander Borght et al. (79) compared metabolic differences between Alzheimer's disease and Parkinson's disease with dementia matched for severity of dementia and found similar glucose metabolic reductions globally, and regionally involving the lateral parietal, lateral temporal, lateral frontal association cortices, and posterior cingulate gyrus when compared with controls. However, patients with Parkinson's disease and dementia had greater metabolic reductions in the primary visual cortex and relatively preserved metabolism in the medial temporal lobe. In contrast, patients with Alzheimer's disease showed only mild reductions in the visual cortex but relatively more pronounced reduction in the medial temporal lobe (Table 6.4). Metabolic reduction in the posterior cingulate cortex demonstrated in Alzheimer's disease has also been found in Parkinson's disease with dementia (79). An FDG PET study of autopsy-proven patients with dementia with Lewy bodies demonstrated significant meta-

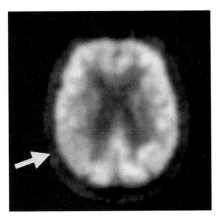

FIG. 6.4. A ¹⁸F-fluorodeoxyglucose positron emission tomography image of a patient with early Alzheimer's disease shows right parietal hypometabolism (*arrow*). There is relative preservation of metabolism in the left parietal, bilateral frontal, and occipital cortices. It is not uncommon for Alzheimer's disease to present with an asymmetric pattern of reduced uptake in the parietotemporal region.

TABLE 6.4. *Metabolic differences between Alzheimer's disease and Parkinson's disease with dementia*[a]

	Alzheimer's disease	Parkinson's disease with dementia
Lateral parietal cortex	↓	↓
Lateral temporal cortex	↓	↓
Lateral frontal cortex	↓	↓
Posterior cingulate cortex	↓	↓
Medial temporal cortex	↓	"sparing"
Visual cortex	"sparing"	↓

[a] There are similar glucose metabolic reductions globally and regionally involving the lateral parietal, lateral temporal, lateral frontal association cortices, and posterior cingulate gyrus when compared with controls. However, patients with Parkinson's disease and dementia have greater metabolic reductions in the primary visual cortex and relatively preserved metabolism in the medial temporal lobe. In contrast, patients with Alzheimer's disease showed only mild reductions in the visual cortex but relatively more pronounced hypometabolism in the medial temporal lobe.
From Vander Borght T, Minoshima S, Giordani B, et al. Cerebral metabolic differences in Parkinson's and Alzheimer's disease matched for dementia severity. *J Nucl Med* 1997;38:797–802.

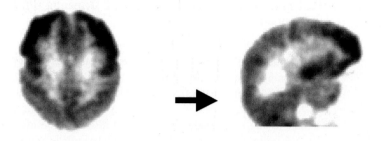

Fig. 6.5. A ^{18}F-fluorodeoxyglucose positron emission tomography study of a patient with dementia with Lewy bodies reveals occipital metabolism is reduced (*arrow*), in addition to biparietal hypometabolism.

bolic reductions in the primary occipital and occipital association cortices (Fig. 6.5) (88).

Although occipital hypometabolism may distinguish Alzheimer's disease from Parkinson's disease with dementia, it may not help the differentiation between patients with Parkinson's disease with dementia but without major neuropsychiatric disturbances from the subgroup of patients who have dementia with Lewy bodies and more prominent neuropsychiatric disturbances on this occipital finding alone.

Subcortical Dementias

Traditionally, this group includes neurodegenerative disorders, such as progressive supranuclear palsy (PSP), Parkinson's disease with dementia, Huntington's disease, thalamic dementia, or human immunodeficiency virus (HIV)–associated dementia. A major feature of this group of disorders is the pathologic involvement of subcortical structures such as the basal ganglia or thalami. Clinical features include psychomotor slowing, apathy, and general mental slowing. It should be realized that a distinction between a pure subcortical type of dementia versus a pure cortical type is rather artefactual. For example, the basal ganglia and thalami participate in important nonmotor or cognitive cerebral circuits, involving the cerebral cortex, via the existence of so-called basal ganglia–thalamus–cortical pathways (89). Although a disorder may primarily involve the basal ganglia in an early stage of the disease, progression to more severe disease, particularly when associated with dementia, will also lead to increasing cortical involvement. For example, Parkinson's disease with dementia has been found to be associated with widespread cortical reductions in glucose metabolism that partially overlap with Alzheimer's disease (79). Cortical hypometabolism may result not only from direct cortical pathologic changes but also from functional cortical deafferentation in the presence of primary subcortical lesions (90).

HIV-infected individuals are at risk of developing dementia (AIDS dementia complex). FDG PET studies have shown relative basal ganglia and thalamic glucose hypermetabolism in HIV-infected persons (91,92). Although the presence of dementia has been shown to correlate with temporal lobe glucose metabolism (91), cortical changes can be very variable. An FDG PET study of patients with familial fatal in-

somnia (which is an example of thalamic dementia) reported severely reduced glucose metabolism of the thalamus, with mild decreases in the cingulate cortex and more variable hypometabolism in the basal and lateral frontal cortex, the caudate nucleus, and the middle and inferior temporal cortex (93). PET studies of patients with PSP and Huntington's disease are discussed in the section on movement disorders, later in this chapter.

Frontotemporal Dementia

Frontotemporal dementia is a dementia syndrome characterized by peculiar behavioral changes arising from frontotemporal involvement. This is a heterogeneous group of disorders encompassing different neuropathologic entities. Although Pick's disease is most known for this type of dementia, recent advances in neurogenetics have identified other frontotemporal syndromes as more common subtypes within this group that are characterized by tau protein abnormalities (94). Functional neuroimaging studies may be able to identify a frontal or frontotemporal pattern of abnormal blood flow or glucose metabolism but lack the specificity to aid in the differential diagnosis of these different disorders, causing a similar pattern frontal or frontotemporal dementia.

FDG PET analysis of patients with frontotemporal dementia have shown metabolic reductions in dorsolateral and ventrolateral prefrontal cortices and in frontopolar and anterior cingulate regions (23). Bilateral anterior temporal, right inferior parietal, and bilateral striatal hypometabolic changes have also been reported (23).

Another FDG PET study reported decreased glucose metabolic activity in the hippocampi, orbital gyri, anterior temporal lobes, anterior cingulate gyri, basal ganglia, thalami, middle and superior frontal gyri, and left inferior frontal gyrus (95). Glucose metabolic activity was preserved in the occipital lobes. Although the metabolic abnormality in frontotemporal dementia is predominant in the frontal and anterior temporal lobes and the subcortical structures, it is more widespread than has been previously assumed (95).

Asymmetric Cortical Degeneration Syndromes

Asymmetric cortical degeneration syndromes encompass most of the atypical cortical dementia patterns that may present with early and prominent aphasia, perceptual motor, or visual-perceptual clinical syndromes (96). New insights suggest that this group is genetically heterogeneous. Debate continues over whether individual syndromes are points along a continuum or represent distinct nosologic entities. Examples in this group include primary progressive aphasia and corticobasal degeneration. Patients with primary progressive aphasia are at greater risk of developing Alzheimer's disease. An FDG PET study of a patient with primary progressive aphasia demonstrated hypometabolism in the left supramarginal gyrus and its surrounding areas (97). Corticobasal degeneration is discussed in the section on movement disorders later in this chapter.

Vascular Dementia

Vascular dementia is a poorly understood concept. Vascular dementia is an entity in which multiple ischemic brain lesions result in progressive cognitive impairment. There is significant overlap between vascular dementia and Alzheimer's disease because ischemic brain lesions may also aggravate the neuropsychologic deficit of Alzheimer's disease (98). Traditionally, this group includes patients with large vessel cerebral infarctions (also called multiinfarct dementia). However, multiple subcortical lacunar infarctions or extensive white matter ischemic disease (so-called leukoaraiosis) may also lead to dementia. Subcortical ischemic vascular disease may lead to dementia because of cortical deafferentation, atrophy of cortical gray matter, and hippocampal atrophy (99,100). Unlike regional cortical differences in patients with Alzheimer's disease, MRI volumetric studies have shown that cortical gray matter volumes are affected more diffusely in patients with subcortical ischemic vascular disease (100).

FDG PET studies of patients with vascular dementia have shown scattered areas with reduction of glucose hypometabolism typically extending over cortical and subcortical structures (101). Careful correlation with anatomic imaging studies will be important to correlate the presence of large vessel strokes with corresponding regional metabolic changes. An FDG PET study of patients with vascular dementia who had no cortical abnormalities on MRI but had significant subcortical lesions (periventricular hyperintensities, deep white matter hyperintensities, and subcortical lacunar infarcts) demonstrated overall reduced cortical metabolism (102). Although the cortical hypometabolism was generally associated with the severity of subcortical pathologic changes, there was substantial heterogeneity in the relationship between subcortical lesions and cortical metabolic activity (102). Mean global cortical metabolism was lower in patients with periventricular hyperintensities in anterior subcortical regions than in those without such lesions, whereas frontal glucose metabolism was lower in patients with lacunar infarcts of the basal ganglia or thalamus (102).

Oxygen-15–labeled PET studies have shown decreased CBF, oxygen metabolism, and oxygen extraction in affected cortical and subcortical brain regions in patients with large vessel multiinfarct dementia (103). In contrast, demented patients with subcortical lacunes and leukoaraiosis demonstrated decreased CBF and oxygen metabolism, but a relatively increased OER. This pattern suggests a state of misery perfusion not only in the deep subcortical structures but also in the cerebral cortex in patients with subcortical vascular disease (103). Therefore, there appear to be at least two possible mechanisms that can explain the occurrence of dementia in patients with stroke.

FDG PET Imaging in the Differential Diagnosis of Dementia

A prerequisite required for discriminating Alzheimer's disease with FDG PET is that the pattern of regional cerebral glucose metabolic activity should show certain stereotypical features that are distinguishable from those of normal subjects and patients with other cognitive or dementing disorders (68). Although the finding of hypometabolism of the temporoparietal association cortices has been associated with Alzheimer's disease, the specificity of this finding is not high. A recent study comparing the presence of bilateral temporoparietal glucose hypometabolism in patients with dementia to the gold standard of pathologic diagnosis reported a high sensitivity of 93% for Alzheimer's disease but a specificity of only 63% (104).

The posterior (i.e., parietal) cerebral involvement frequently differentiates Alzheimer's disease from other causes of dementia, which primarily involve the frontal lobe, such as frontotemporal dementia, including Pick's disease. In contrast, a number of other dementing illnesses may share the feature of biparietal hypometabolism, such as Parkinson's disease with dementia. Therefore, the specificity of the FDG PET diagnosis of dementia will not depend on involvement of a single (e.g., parietal) brain region, but rather on the differential pattern of involved versus preserved brain regions.

It is the complete pattern of metabolic impairment of the temporoparietal more than the frontal cortices, together with the relative preservation of the primary sensorimotor and visual cortices, basal ganglia, and cerebellum, that make up the distinct metabolic phenotype of Alzheimer's disease. There is recent evidence suggesting that reduced occipital metabolic activity may distinguish patients with dementia with Lewy bodies from those with prototypical Alzheimer's disease (79,88,105).

It must be emphasized that functional imaging studies of the brain should be interpreted in conjunction with structural imaging studies, such as brain CT or MRI scans. For example, deep focal brain lesions, such as stroke, or subcortical white matter lesions may lead to deafferentation, and hence reduced glucose metabolism, of connected cortical brain regions (99).

Other causes of false-positive PET diagnosis of Alzheimer's disease include patients with a history of alcoholism or prior traumatic brain injury. Patients with depressive

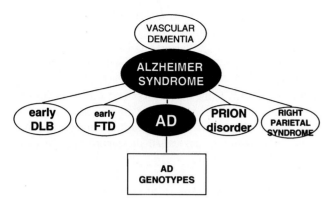

Fig. 6.6. Heterogeneity of the Alzheimer's syndrome. Patients who present in an early stage of an emerging dementia syndrome may have mild cognitive symptoms consistent with an early Alzheimer's type of clinical phenotype (Alzheimer's syndrome) but may not have prototypical Alzheimer's disease. These disorders include vascular dementia, right parietal stroke, prion disorders, early frontotemporal dementia, or early dementia with Lewy bodies. New genotypic differentiation of patients with Alzheimer's disease may also increase the heterogeneity of the Alzheimer's syndrome.

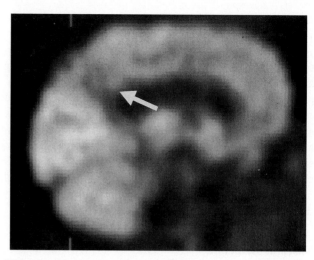

FIG. 6.7. The sagittal view of a ^{18}F-fluorodeoxyglucose positron emission tomographic study of patient with Alzheimer's disease shows glucose hypometabolism in the posterior cingulate cortex and cinguloparietal transitional area (*arrow*). There is preservation of glucose metabolism in the occipital cortex.

mood may have bilateral inferior frontal metabolic changes (106). Conversely, patients who present in an early stage of an emerging dementia syndrome may have mild cognitive symptoms indicative of an early Alzheimer's type of clinical phenotype (Alzheimer's syndrome) but may not have Alzheimer's disease per se. These etiologies include vascular dementia, right parietal stroke, prion disorders, early frontotemporal dementia, or early dementia with Lewy bodies (Fig. 6.6). More specific clinical symptoms may become transparent with progression of disease. Combined interpretation of results from genotypic laboratory testing, neuropsychologic evaluation, and functional and anatomic imaging may aid the differential diagnostic process.

FDG PET Imaging in Patients with Mild Cognitive Impairment

Early Alzheimer's disease may manifest itself as isolated forgetfulness, but it is difficult to determine in an individual patient whether initial mild and isolated memory complaints are part of a more benign aging process or may herald the onset of a dementing disorder. FDG PET imaging has the potential to detect very early neocortical dysfunction well before neuropsychologic performance becomes abnormal (107). Using FDG PET, Minoshima et al. (67,108) first reported decreased glucose metabolism in the posterior cingulate cortex and cinguloparietal transitional area in patients with Alzheimer's disease that was more prominent than typical parietotemporal cortical reductions (Fig. 6.7).

Detection of metabolic reduction in the posterior cingulate cortex has also been observed in patients with isolated forgetfulness who have very early dementia before a clinical diagnosis of Alzheimer's disease can be made (109,110). Therefore, posterior cingulate cortical metabolic reductions

may herald the first glucose metabolic changes of the dementia process. Reduced glucose metabolism in the posterior cingulate cortex may correspond to postmortem findings of cortical synaptic loss in this region in patients with dementia (73). The relative lack of extensive neurofibrillary tangles in the posterior cingulate cortex in early Alzheimer's disease relative to the medial and inferior temporal cortex also raises the possibility of functionally, but not structurally altered neuronal circuitry in the posterior cingulate cortex (67). Very early metabolic changes in Alzheimer's disease probably reflect a significant impairment of metabolic activities in the corticocortical glutamatergic systems in a preclinical stage of the disease (111).

FDG PET studies have also demonstrated cortical abnormalities in cognitively normal individuals who are at risk of dementia. For example, Small et al. (81,82) reported that relatives of patients with Alzheimer's disease who carried the apolipoprotein E (apoE) ε4 allele had lower parietal cortical metabolism than those without this allele (81,82). These nondemented relatives carrying the allele also manifested increased metabolic asymmetry in the parietal cortex. Reduced posterior cingulate cortical metabolism has also been observed in cognitively normal subjects who were homozygote for the apoE ε4 alleles (107). PET studies of a pedigree of familial Alzheimer's disease with an amyloid precursor protein mutation have also showed biparietal and bitemporal hypometabolism in asymptomatic at risk individuals (112).

Novel Trends in Dementia Imaging

Identification of early symptomatic patients is important at a time when new therapeutic or even secondarily preventive treatment modalities for dementia are emerging. FDG PET appears to correlate with the regional distribution and extent of cortical neuropathologic changes in Alzheimer's disease. FDG PET is not only useful for the very early or preclinical diagnosis of Alzheimer's disease but also for the differential diagnosis once a dementing disorder has developed. FDG PET may be able to distinguish dementia with Lewy bodies from prototypical Alzheimer's disease based on occipital metabolic reduction.

The challenge for new imaging techniques in the diagnosis of dementia is to achieve high sensitivity and specificity in the very early stage of the disease. Once a patient has been selected for treatment, functional neuroimaging can be used to predict or monitor the patient's individual response to specific therapeutic agents. New techniques for image processing and statistical brain mapping analysis using databases of normal control persons may aid the clinical utility of FDG PET in the evaluation of patients with cognitive or neurobehavioral disturbances (113).

Since the initial report by Davies and Maloney (114) of a profound cortical reduction of choline acetyltransferase in patients with Alzheimer's disease, a great deal of evidence has accumulated to support the significance of cholinergic hypofunction in this disorder. The recent development of PET technology for measuring cerebral cholinesterase activity *in vivo* offers the prospect of identifying biologic correlates of clinical or behavioral features that may help predict treatment responsiveness to anticholinesterase drugs and allows optimal monitoring of therapeutic effects.

Imaging of cholinesterase activity can be performed using a radiolabeled lipophilic acetylcholine analogue that diffuses into the brain, where it is metabolized by cholinesterase to produce a hydrophilic metabolite that is trapped at the site of its production (115). Cholinesterase activity in the human brain has been mapped using PET and ^{11}C-methylpiperadinyl propionate (PMP) (116,117) and ^{11}C-MP4A (118). Kuhl et al. (116) using ^{11}C-PMP found a distribution of acetylcholinesterase activity in normal volunteers that closely correlated with postmortem histochemical distribution. Patients with Alzheimer's disease had an average reduction of 25% to 33% of mean cortical cholinesterase activity (117). The cortical reductions in cholinesterase activity in Alzheimer's disease did correlate with imaging findings of cholinergic terminal deficits.

MOVEMENT DISORDERS

PET imaging of CBF, metabolic pathways, or neurotransmission systems has contributed to our understanding of the pathophysiology of movement disorders. PET measurements of dopaminergic pathways in the brain have confirmed the importance of dopamine and the basal ganglia in the pathophysiology of movement disorders, such as Parkinson's disease. Brain activation studies can be performed using CBF or FDG PET. These studies compare regional brain activity during specific motor or mental tasks compared with control conditions.

Activation studies have shown that the basal ganglia are activated whenever movements are performed, planned, or imagined (119). These studies support the existence of func-

TABLE 6.5. *Examples of disorders or conditions with altered glucose metabolism of the basal ganglia*

Increased fluorodeoxyglucose metabolic activity in the basal ganglia	Early Parkinson's disease Hepatocerebral degeneration Neuroleptic drug effects Human immunodeficiency virus infection
Decreased fluorodeoxyglucose metabolic activity in the basal ganglia	Atypical parkinsonism, such as progressive supranuclear palsy, multiple system atrophy, or corticobasal degeneration Wilson's disease

tionally independent distributed basal ganglia–frontal loops. The caudate–prefrontal loop appears to mediate novel sequence learning, problem solving, and movement selection while the putamen–premotor loop may facilitate automatic sequential patterns of limb movement and implicit acquisition of motor skills (119).

Although most PET studies in patients with movement disorders consist of neurochemical or functional activation studies performed for research purposes, this section focuses on resting FDG or CBF studies. Patients with movement disorders may have abnormal blood flow or metabolism in the basal ganglia (Table 6.5). Cortical changes may represent primary cortical abnormalities or deafferentation effects because of subcortical abnormalities. Patients with movement disorders who also develop dementia typically will show more widespread cortical metabolic or blood-flow changes.

Parkinson's Disease

Parkinson's disease is a clinical syndrome consisting of a variable combination of symptoms of tremor, rigidity, postural imbalance, and bradykinesia (120,121). Although Parkinson's disease accounts for most patients who have parkinsonian symptoms, parkinsonism can be seen with neurodegenerative disorders other than Parkinson's disease, such as PSP or multiple system atrophy (MSA) (120). Idiopathic Parkinson's disease distinguishes itself from other parkinsonian syndromes by marked left-to-right asymmetry in symptom severity and good symptomatic response to L-DOPA therapy (120,121). The additional presence of certain clinical findings may raise the clinical suspicion for an atypical parkinsonian syndrome, such as prominent autonomic dysfunction, cerebellar symptoms, or abnormal eye movements (120).

The clinical features of Parkinson's disease result from loss of nigrostriatal nerve terminals in the striatum secondary to the degeneration of dopamine-producing pigmented neurons in the substantia nigra in the brainstem (122,123). The greater the neuronal loss in the substantia nigra, the lower the concentration of dopamine in the striatum, and the more severe the parkinsonian symptoms. It should be noted that the cellular component of nigrostriatal nerve terminals within the striatum is far less than the number of intrinsic striatal interjection and projection neurons. Therefore, resting glucose metabolic studies primarily reflect the synaptic activity of interneurons and only to a lesser extent afferent projections.

Resting glucose metabolic and CBF studies of patients with early Parkinson's disease have shown increased striatal activity contralateral to the clinically most affected body side, which may represent a compensatory mechanism of intrinsic striatal cells (124,125). However, striatal glucose metabolism may decrease with advancing disease and regional cortical hypometabolism will occur, particularly in patients who also develop dementia (79,126).

FDG PET studies of patients with Parkinson's disease and dementia have shown a similar metabolic pattern as that seen in Alzheimer's disease, with the exception of decreased occipital metabolism (79). Decreased occipital metabolism has also been observed in nondemented patients with Parkinson's disease (127). FDG PET studies of patients with Parkinson's disease and dementia and dementia with Lewy bodies are discussed in more detail in the previous section on cognitive disorders and dementia.

FDG PET studies have also been used to predict L-DOPA response in parkinsonian patients. A recent study found that relatively increased FDG activity in the striatum contralateral to the clinically most affected body side was associated with a good L-DOPA response. In contrast, relatively decreased striatal FDG uptake was associated with poor L-DOPA responsiveness (128).

Progressive Supranuclear Palsy

PSP or Steele–Richardson–Olszewski syndrome is an atypical parkinsonian syndrome characterized by severe gait and balance disturbances, abnormal eye movements (particularly vertical supranuclear gaze palsy), and pseudobulbar palsy. More advanced disease is often associated with a frontal lobe type of dementia. Pathologic changes consist of neurofibrillary tangle formation and neuronal loss in the superior colliculi, brainstem nuclei, periaqueductal gray matter, and basal ganglia (129).

PET studies of patients with PSP have shown reduced glucose metabolism in the caudate nucleus, putamen, thalamus, pons, and cerebral cortex, but not in the cerebellum (130). There are significant metabolic reductions in most regions throughout the cerebral cortex, but they are more prominent in the frontal lobe (131). Although frontal metabolism decreases with increasing disease duration, relative frontal hypometabolism has been found to be already present in the early stages of the disease (132). Statistical brain mapping studies have demonstrated decreased glucose metabolism in the anterior cingulate, adjacent supplementary motor area, precentral cortex, middle prefrontal cortex, midbrain tegmentum, globus pallidus, and ventrolateral and dorsomedial nuclei of the thalamus (133). Clinical parkinsonian motor scores have been reported to correlate with caudate

and thalamic glucose metabolic values (132). The coupling between blood flow and metabolism has been found to be preserved even in regions showing decreased blood flow and hypometabolism (134). These data highlight predominant metabolic impairment in subcortical-cortical connections in PSP.

Corticobasal Degeneration

Corticobasal degeneration is an atypical parkinsonian syndrome characterized by clinical marked asymmetric limb rigidity with apraxia. Patients may also exhibit alien limb phenomenon, cortical sensory loss, and myoclonus. Cognitive functions are relatively well preserved in most patients. Neuropathologic findings consist of swollen, achromatic, tau-staining Pick's bodies that may be present in the inferior parietal, posterior frontal, and superior temporal lobes, as well as the dentate nucleus and substantia nigra (135). FDG PET studies have shown significantly reduced cerebral glucose metabolism in the hemisphere contralateral to the clinically most affected side. The reductions can occur in the dorsolateral frontal, medial frontal, inferior parietal, sensorimotor, and lateral temporal cortex, as well as in the corpus striatum and the thalamus in patients with corticobasal degeneration (136,137).

Statistical brain mapping analysis of patients with corticobasal degeneration have confirmed the asymmetric glucose metabolic impairment in the putamen, thalamus, precentral, lateral premotor and supplementary motor areas, dorsolateral prefrontal cortex, and the anterior part of the inferior parietal lobe including the intraparietal sulcus (138). These results confirm the marked asymmetric cerebral involvement, particularly in the contralateral motor cortex and thalamus, in patients with corticobasal degeneration (139,140).

Multiple System Atrophy

MSA is an atypical parkinsonian syndrome covering a clinical spectrum of parkinsonism in variable combination with symptoms of cerebellar ataxia or dysautonomia. This group of disorders includes Shy–Drager syndrome (MSA of the dysautonomia type), olivopontocerebellar atrophy (OPCA) (i.e., MSA of the cerebellar type), and striatonigral degeneration, which resembles Parkinson's disease but does not respond to dopaminergic drugs. The pathology of MSA is distinct from Parkinson's disease and consists of neuronal loss in the substantia nigra, striatum, cerebellum, brainstem, and spinal cord with argyrophilic and glial inclusions (141).

An FDG PET study found reduced caudate, putaminal, cerebellar, brainstem, frontal, and temporal cortical glucose metabolism in patients with MSA compared with normal controls (142). Reductions of cerebellar and brainstem glucose metabolism have been reported to be most prominent in patients with OPCA (143). Although cerebellar and brainstem glucose metabolism correlated with severity of MRI-measured atrophy, some patients who had no MRI evidence of tissue atrophy still showed decreased glucose metabolism in these regions (144). Patients with the striatonigral degeneration subtype had relatively preserved brainstem and cerebellar glucose metabolic rates (144).

Essential Tremor

Essential tremor represents a variable combination of postural and kinetic tremor. It most commonly affects the hands but also occurs in the head, voice, face, trunk, and lower extremities (145). A PET study found significant glucose hypermetabolism of the medulla and thalami, but not of the cerebellar cortex in patients with essential tremor during resting conditions (146). CBF PET studies using $H_2^{15}O$ in patients with essential tremor demonstrated abnormally increased bilateral cerebellar, red nuclear, and thalamic blood flow during tremor (147–150). Therefore, the cerebellum and thalamus appear to play important roles as part of a cerebral circuitry that is abnormally activated during tremor.

Huntington's Disease and Choreiform Movement Disorders

Huntington's disease is an autosomal-dominant neurodegenerative disorder with complete penetrance (151). The gene for Huntington's disease, containing an amplified number of CAG trinucleotide repeats, is located on the short arm of chromosome 4 (152). Chorea is the most commonly recognized involuntary movement abnormality in adult patients with Huntington's disease, but psychiatric symptoms and dementia may present variably (153). Pathologically, Huntington's disease is characterized by marked neuronal loss and atrophy in the caudate nucleus and putamen (154, 155). Glucose metabolic PET studies in Huntington's disease have demonstrated decreased glucose utilization in the caudate nucleus and putamen even before striatal atrophy is apparent on brain CT or MRI scans (156–158).

Chorea as a hyperkinetic movement disorder can also be seen with other disorders, such as dentatorubral-pallidoluysian atrophy (DRPLA), neuroacanthocytosis, or Sydenham chorea. Striatal, particularly caudate, glucose hypometabolism has been demonstrated in DRPLA and neuroacanthocytosis. This is similar to the findings in Huntington's disease, but striatal glucose metabolism has been found to be increased in a patient with Sydenham chorea and in a patient with antiphospholipid antibody syndrome and chorea (159–163).

Emerging Clinical Applications of Dopaminergic Neurochemical Imaging

The basal ganglia and the neurotransmitter dopamine have been key targets for research exploring the pathophysiology underlying movement disorders. Dopaminergic neurons from the substantia nigra project as nigrostriatal nerve terminals to the striatum where they have synaptic connections with striatal interjection or projection neurons. Presynaptic nigrostriatal dopaminergic activity can be imaged using PET radiotracers such as ^{18}F-fluoro-DOPA or dopamine transporter protein ligands, such as the cocaine analogue ^{11}C-WIN-35428 (164–166). Postsynaptic dopamine D_2-receptor binding can be imaged using the PET tracer ^{11}C-raclopride (Fig. 6.8) (167).

PET studies using presynaptic dopaminergic tracers have objectively demonstrated nigrostriatal nerve terminal loss in Parkinson's disease, even at a very early or preclinical stage of the disease (168). Reductions are more severe in the posterior putamen (when compared with those in the anterior putamen and caudate nucleus) and contralateral to the clinically most affected body side (169,170). Putaminal fluoro-DOPA uptake is also correlated with clinical measures of disease severity, particularly bradykinesia (125,171–173). Therefore, these techniques can provide neurochemical markers to follow progression of disease or evaluate the effects of therapeutic or neurorestorative interventions. Nigrostriatal denervation is not specific for Parkinson's disease, as presynaptic dopaminergic denervation has also been demonstrated in patients with MSA, PSP, or corticobasal degeneration (174–176).

In addition to presynaptic changes in the nigrostriatal neurons, striatal dopamine receptors are altered in Parkinson's disease. For instance, in early idiopathic Parkinson's disease, uptake of ^{11}C-raclopride, which is a selective dopamine D_2-receptor ligand, increases in the striatum contralateral to the predominant parkinsonian symptoms, compared with uptake in the ipsilateral striatum (177). This upregulation may disappear 3 to 5 years later (178). Studies of the postsynaptic D_2 status have demonstrated normal or increased D_2-receptor density in early Parkinson's disease and decreased receptor density in patients with advanced Parkinson's disease or atypical parkinsonism, as with MSA and PSP. Therefore, combined presynaptic and postsynaptic dopaminergic imaging may distinguish idiopathic early Parkinson's disease from atypical parkinsonian disorders (Table 6.6). It should be noted, however, that combined presynaptic and postsynaptic dopaminergic imaging may not be able to distinguish atypical Parkinsonian disorders from one another or from advanced idiopathic Parkinson's disease.

Dopaminergic PET studies should not be used as a substitute for the clinical diagnosis of Parkinson's disease. However, neurochemical and functional activation studies may play an important clinical role in the selection of patients with abnormal movements who may benefit from electrical deep brain stimulation. Dopaminergic studies may have a limited clinical role in the diagnosis of patients with symptoms suggestive of Parkinson's disease yet do not respond to typical anti-Parkinson drugs. Neurochemical studies will also allow objective monitoring of neuroprotective and neurorestorative treatments in Parkinson's disease. Although most imaging research in movement disorders has focused on the dopamine system, it is expected that the study of other

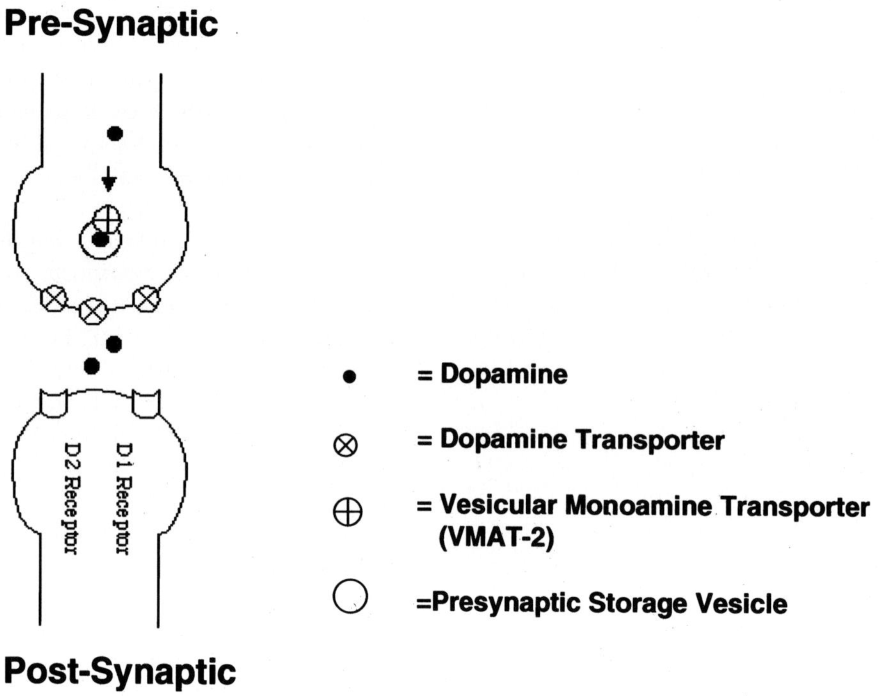

Pre-Synaptic

● = Dopamine

⊗ = Dopamine Transporter

⊕ = Vesicular Monoamine Transporter (VMAT-2)

○ = Presynaptic Storage Vesicle

Post-Synaptic

FIG. 6.8. A schematic overview of the nigrostriatal dopamine nerve terminal and a postsynaptic dopamine neuron. Dopamine metabolism (dopa decarboxylase enzyme activity), vesicular monoamine transporter type 2 (VMAT2), synaptic membrane dopamine transporter, and postsynaptic dopamine receptor type 1 and 2 activity can be studied by PET neurochemical imaging with use of the appropriate radiotracers.

neurotransmitter systems will further aid the understanding of cerebral mechanisms underlying movement disorders.

EPILEPSY

Epileptic syndromes are classified in generalized and partial types of seizures. Primary generalized epilepsy is associated with diffuse and bilateral epileptiform discharges on electroencephalography (EEG) without evidence for focal brain lesions. In contrast, partial epilepsy is thought to arise from a focal gray matter lesion. Partial-onset seizures may remain partial or may secondarily generalize. Medically refractory epilepsy is defined by seizure syndromes that are not effectively controlled by antiepileptic drugs. The management of medically refractory partial epilepsy has been revolutionized by neurosurgical techniques aimed at the resection of the epileptogenic brain focus. Therefore, precise seizure localization is the prime goal of presurgical workup. EEG monitoring and structural brain imaging using MRI are part of the standard workup of epileptic patients undergoing presurgical evaluation. FDG PET performed interictally can provide additional localizing information in patients with nonlocalizing surface ictal EEG and can reduce the number of patients requiring intracranial EEG studies (179). Even when intracranial EEG is required, FDG PET can be helpful in guiding placement of subdural grids or depth electrodes

TABLE 6.6. *Presynaptic and postsynaptic dopaminergic activity in idiopathic Parkinson's disease and atypical parkinsonian disorders*

	Presynaptic dopaminergic nigrostriatal activity	Postsynaptic striatal dopamine receptor activity
Early idiopathic Parkinson's disease	↓ (particularly posterior putamen)	↑ (upregulation)
Advanced Parkinson's disease	↓	normal or ↓
Atypical parkinsonism (e.g., progressive supranuclear palsy or multiple system atrophy)	↓	↓

before surgical ablative therapy. PET imaging should always be performed before intracranial EEG, as prior depth electrode insertion can cause small hypometabolic regions that may lead to false-positive PET interpretations (180). Patients with primary generalized epilepsy have no interictal abnormalities on CBF or FDG PET studies (181).

Regional Glucose Hypometabolism as Interictal Expression of Epileptogenic Foci

Interictal FDG PET studies can identify epileptogenic foci on the basis of regional cortical glucose hypometabolism (182). It should be noted that FDG PET may show more widespread hypometabolism than suspected on the basis of the scalp-recorded EEG (179). The pathophysiology of interictal cortical hypometabolism in partial epilepsy is poorly understood. Areas of interictal hypometabolism in epileptogenic cortex appear to be partially uncoupled from blood flow, with metabolic reductions being greater relative to flow (183). Although there are significant correlations between hippocampal volume and inferior mesial and lateral temporal lobe cerebral metabolic rates in patients with temporal lobe epilepsy (184), studies have failed to find a significant correlation between cortical metabolism on preoperative FDG PET imaging and neuronal density of resected hippocampi (185). Therefore, hippocampal neuronal loss cannot fully account for the regional interictal hypometabolism of temporal lobe epilepsy. Children with new onset of seizures are less likely to have hypometabolism (181). Therefore, it is uncertain whether hypometabolism reflects the effects of repeated seizures on the brain, the underlying pathologic process, or an initial insult such as early status epilepticus (181). It is possible that synaptic mechanisms, rather than cell loss, may contribute to the observed hypometabolism (186).

Regional Glucose Hypometabolism in Temporal Lobe Epilepsy

Mesial temporal lobe epilepsy is the most common type of partial epilepsy and is commonly associated with hippo-

campal atrophy. FDG PET has a high sensitivity in detecting temporal hypometabolic foci and can be visualized as significant left-to-right asymmetry in temporal cortical tracer uptake. It should be noted that false lateralization is rare but may occur. For example, unrecognized epileptic activity can make the contralateral temporal lobe appear spuriously depressed (180). For this reason, it is not uncommon to perform EEG recordings during the period of FDG uptake, to be certain a subclinical seizure does not result in a "false localization." Furthermore, normal right-to-left asymmetry between temporal lobes should not be interpreted as pathologic hypometabolism. Although FDG PET images can be analyzed visually, additional information can be obtained by semiquantitative analysis, such as left-to-right asymmetry indices. Semiquantitative analysis using the asymmetry index is generally considered significant when a difference of 15% or greater exists between the affected and contralateral sides (187). Quantitative asymmetry indices should reduce potential error due to misinterpreting these normal left-to-right variations (188). Registration programs can be used to align structural MRI and PET for more precise anatomic localization of the hypometabolic area.

Although regional hypometabolism is typically present in the temporal lobe ipsilateral to EEG seizure onset, other brain regions may also show patterns of glucose hypometabolism. For example, an FDG PET study of patients with temporal lobe epilepsy demonstrated hypometabolic regions ipsilateral to seizure onset that included lateral temporal (in 78% of patients), mesial temporal (70%), thalamic (63%), basal ganglia (41%), frontal (30%), parietal (26%), and occipital (4%) regions (189). The prevalence of thalamic hypometabolism suggests a pathophysiologic role for the thalamus in initiation or propagation of temporal lobe seizures (189). Cerebellar hypometabolism may be ipsilateral, contralateral, or bilateral, depending on the distribution and spread of ictal activity and possible effects of phenytoin therapy (Fig. 6.9) (30,180). Bilateral cerebellar hypometabolism, which often is present, cannot be fully explained by the effects of phenytoin (30). Unilateral temporal hypometabolism predicts good surgical outcome from temporal lobectomy. The greater the metabolic asymmetry, the greater the chance

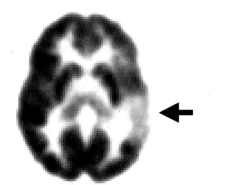
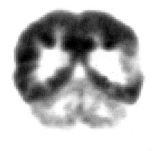

FIG. 6.9. An interictal ^{18}F-fluorodeoxyglucose positron emission tomography study of a patient with a left lateral and posterior temporal seizure focus shows an extensive area of hypometabolism (*arrow*) in addition to bilateral thalamic and cerebellar hypometabolic changes.

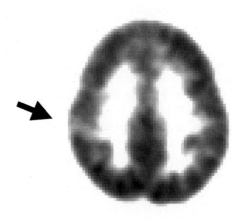

FIG. 6.10. An interictal ^{18}F-fluorodeoxyglucose positron emission tomography study of patient with partial epilepsy shows a focus of right parietal hypometabolism (*arrow*).

of becoming seizure-free (180). Bilateral temporal hypometabolism may represent a relative contraindication for surgery (180).

Extratemporal Epilepsy

FDG PET may not be as valuable in the evaluation of patients with extratemporal seizures, such as frontal lobe epilepsy, because of limited sensitivity (188,190). Areas of hypometabolism in frontal lobe epilepsy have been found to be focal, regional, or hemispheric (Fig. 6.10) (191).

Furthermore, large zones of extrafrontal, particularly temporal, hypometabolism are commonly observed ipsilateral to frontal hypometabolism in frontal lobe epilepsies (11). Recent data show that observer-independent automatic statistical brain mapping techniques may increase the usefulness of FDG PET in patients with extratemporal lobe epilepsy. For example, a study using an automated brain mapping method found a significantly higher sensitivity in detecting the epileptogenic focus (67%) than visual analysis (19% to 38%) in patients with extratemporal epilepsy (192).

Hypometabolic regions in partial epilepsies of neocortical origin have usually been associated with structural imaging abnormalities (190). Therefore, PET data should always be interpreted in the context of high-quality anatomic MRI, providing a structural-functional correlation. Interictal hypometabolism may be uncommon in the absence of a co-localized structural imaging abnormality in frontal lobe epilepsy (11). Interictal FDG PET studies will have limited usefulness in the presence of multiple hypometabolic regions in patients with multifocal brain syndromes, such as in children with tuberous sclerosis.

Interictal H$_2$^{15}O CBF PET Studies

It should be noted that interictal H$_2$^{15}O CBF PET studies when compared with FDG PET studies have reduced sensi-

tivity in localizing epileptogenic zones and sometimes may even be false lateralizing (193). Furthermore, CBF PET scans are more noisy compared with FDG PET, which may increase partial volume effects and make detection of a hypoperfused area more difficult. Therefore, interictal CBF PET studies are unreliable markers for epileptic foci and should not be used in the presurgical evaluation of patients with epilepsy (183).

Ictal PET

Although not always practical, FDG PET can also be used for ictal studies in patients who have frequent seizures (Fig. 6.11) (194). However, FDG PET may be less accurate for ictal, compared with interictal, glucose metabolic measurements because seizures may alter the lumped constant, which describes the relationship between FDG and its physiologic substrate glucose (180). Furthermore, a typical seizure is much shorter than the average 30-minute FDG uptake period. Therefore, an ictal scan may include interictal, ictal, and postictal metabolic changes with combinations of hypermetabolic and hypometabolic regions (180). H$_2$^{15}O PET imaging has been used to study quantitative alterations in rCBF accompanying seizures induced by pentylenetetrazole (195). Patients with generalized tonic-clonic seizures demonstrated asymmetric flow increases. One patient with a complex partial seizure demonstrated 70% to 80% increases in bitemporal flow. Thalamic flow increased during both complex partial and generalized seizures, indicating the importance of this subcortical structure during ictal activation (195).

Mapping of Language, Cognitive or Language Functions

Changes in the functional activity of the brain (e.g., motor activity, language, or cognitive tasks) are accompanied by

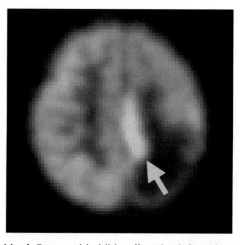

FIG. 6.11. A 5-year-old child suffered a left parietooccipital stroke caused by left thalamic and intraventricular hemorrhage and had subsequent seizure onset. An ictal PET study demonstrates metabolic activation of the left posterior cinguloparietal cortex (*arrow*) adjacent to the hypometabolic stroke lesion.

increases in rCBF and can be mapped to specific brain regions (3,4). Language-based PET activation studies have shown good correlation with the Wada language lateralization test (196). More detailed cortical mapping can be performed to better delineate the motor cortex from the epileptogenic zone. Cortical mapping using PET activation studies have shown comparable results to electrical stimulation mapping of the cortex using subdural electrodes (197).

Emerging Clinical Applications of Benzodiazepine Neuroreceptor Imaging in Epilepsy

The inhibitory neurotransmitter γ-aminobutyric acid (GABA) has anticonvulsant properties. Benzodiazepine-receptor ligands, such as ^{11}C-flumazenil, have been used to study the regional cerebral distribution of benzodiazepine-receptor binding sites that are related to GABA receptors. A regional decrease in benzodiazepine-receptor binding has been associated with the presence of a possible epileptogenic focus. When compared with FDG studies, ^{11}C-flumazenil PET studies have been reported to demonstrate less extensive cortical involvement. For example, a study comparing FDG and ^{11}C-flumazenil PET imaging in patients with temporal lobe epilepsy found a wide range of mesial temporal, lateral temporal, and thalamic glucose hypometabolism ipsilateral to ictal EEG changes, as well as extratemporal hypometabolism. In contrast, each patient demonstrated decreased benzodiazepine-receptor binding in the ipsilateral anterior mesial temporal region, without neocortical changes. Thus, interictal metabolic dysfunction can be variable and usually is extensive in temporal lobe epilepsy, whereas decreased central benzodiazepine-receptor density appears to be more restricted to mesial temporal areas (198).

Similar benzodiazepine-receptor findings have been reported for patients with extratemporal lobe seizures caused by focal cortical dysplasia (199). Unlike the more widespread glucose hypometabolic patterns, benzodiazepine-receptor changes may reflect localized neuronal loss that is more specific to the epileptogenic zone (198). Therefore, ^{11}C-flumazenil imaging may be useful in the presurgical evaluation of patients with epilepsy. However, focal increases of benzodiazepine-receptor binding have also been reported in the temporal lobe, as well as extratemporal sites in patients with temporal lobe epilepsy when statistical brain mapping analysis is performed (200). This may lead to false-localizing information when attention is only paid to areas of decreased uptake.

The development of radioligands that are specific for excitatory amino acids and selected opioid-receptor subtypes may help to better explore the pathophysiology of epileptic syndromes.

SUMMARY

PET is a method for quantitative and qualitative imaging of regional physiologic and biochemical parameters. With the tomographic principle of the PET scanner, the quantitative distribution of the administered radiopharmaceutical can be determined in the brain and images can be provided, as well as dynamic information on blood flow, metabolism, and neuroreceptor function. Glucose metabolic and blood-flow studies have been used for the study of patients with brain disorders, such as epilepsy, stroke, or dementia. It is expected that new techniques for quantitative image processing and statistical brain mapping analysis using normative databases will aid the clinical utility of brain PET. Measurement of receptors or neurotransmitter metabolism is a unique ability of PET that has not achieved its full potential in the study of patients with neurologic disorders. PET has the ability to visualize and quantify key pathophysiologic processes underlying specific brain disorders and may serve as a tool not only for diagnosis but also for the assessment of effects of therapeutic interventions.

ACKNOWLEDGMENTS

The author would like to thank Dr. Subhash Chander and the technologists of the University of Pittsburgh PET center for their assistance with the PET images.

REFERENCES

1. Siesjo BK. *Brain energy metabolism.* New York: Wiley, 1978: 101–110.
2. Sandor P. Nervous control of the cerebrovascular system: doubts and facts. *Neurochem Int* 1999;35:237–259.
3. Raichle ME. Circulatory and metabolic correlates of brain function in normal humans. In: Mountcastle VB, Plum F, eds. *Handbook of physiology. The nervous system,* vol 5. Bethesda: American Physiological Society, 1987:643–674.
4. Raichle ME. The metabolic requirements of functional activity in the brain. In: Vranic M, Efendie S, Hollenberg CH, eds. *Fuel homeostasis and the nervous system.* New York: Plenum Publishing, 1991:1–4.
5. Buxton RB, Frank LR. A model for the coupling between cerebral blood flow and oxygen metabolism during neural stimulation. *J Cereb Blood Flow Metab* 1997;17:64–72.
6. Vafaee MS, Gjedde A. Model of blood–brain transfer of oxygen explains nonlinear flow-metabolism coupling during stimulation of visual cortex. *J Cereb Blood Flow Metab* 2000;20:747–754.
7. Jueptner M, Weiller C. Review: does measurement of regional cerebral blood flow reflect synaptic activity? Implications for PET and fMRI. *Neuroimage* 1995;2:148–156.
8. Magistretti PJ, Pellerin L. Cellular mechanisms of brain energy metabolism and their relevance to functional brain imaging. *Philos Trans R Soc Lond B Biol Sci* 1999;354:1155–1163.
9. Hoffman EJ, Huang SC, Phelps ME. Quantitation in positron emission computed tomography, 1: effect of object size. *J Comput Assisted Tomogr* 1979;3:299–308.
10. Minoshima S, Koeppe RA, Frey KA, et al. Stereotactic PET atlas of the human brain: aid for visual interpretation of functional brain images. *J Nucl Med* 1994;35:949–954.
11. Henry TR, Mazziotta JC, Engel JJ. The functional anatomy of frontal lobe epilepsy studied with PET. *Adv Neurol* 1992;57:449–463.
12. Perlmutter JS, Powers WJ, Herscovitch P, et al. Regional asymmetries of cerebral blood flow, blood volume, and oxygen utilization and extraction in normal subjects. *J Cereb Blood Flow Metab* 1987;7: 64–67.
13. Lobaugh NJ, Caldwell CB, Black SE, et al. Three brain SPECT region-of-interest templates in elderly people: normative values, hemispheric asymmetries, and a comparison of single- and multihead cameras. *J Nucl Med* 2000;41:45–56.
14. Mazziotta JC, Phelps ME, Carson RE, et al. Tomographic mapping

of human cerebral metabolism: sensory deprivation. *Ann Neurol* 1982; 12:435–444.

15. Loessner A, Alavi A, Lewandrowski KU, et al. Regional cerebral function determined by FDG-PET in healthy volunteers: normal patterns and changes with age. *J Nucl Med* 1995;36:1141–1149.

16. Takahashi T, Shirane R, Sato S, et al. Developmental changes of cerebral blood flow and oxygen metabolism in children. *Am J Neuroradiol* 1999;20:917–922.

17. Chugani HT, Phelps ME, Mazziotta JC. Positron emission tomography study of human brain functional development. *Ann Neurol* 1987; 22:487–497.

18. Van Bogaert P, Wikler D, Damhaut P, et al. Regional changes in glucose metabolism during brain development from the age of 6 years. *Neuroimage* 1998;8:62–68.

19. Terry RD, DeTeresa R, Hansen LA. Neocortical cell counts in normal human adult aging. *Ann Neurol* 1987;21:530–539.

20. Schultz SK, O'Leary DS, Boles Ponto LL, et al. Age-related changes in regional cerebral blood flow among young to mid-life adults. *Neuroreport* 1999;10:2493–2496.

21. Martin AJ, Friston KJ, Colebatch JG, et al. Decreases in regional cerebral blood flow with normal aging. *J Cereb Blood Flow Metab* 1991;11:684–689.

22. Meltzer CC, Cantwell MN, Greer PJ, et al. Does cerebral blood flow decline in healthy aging? A PET study with partial-volume correction. *J Nucl Med* 2000;41:1842–1848.

23. Garraux G, Salmon E, Degueldre C, et al. Comparison of impaired subcortico-frontal metabolic networks in normal aging, subcortico-frontal dementia, and cortical frontal dementia. *Neuroimage* 1999;10: 149–162.

24. Pietrini P, Alexander GE, Furey ML, et al. Cerebral metabolic response to passive audiovisual stimulation in patients with Alzheimer's disease and healthy volunteers assessed by PET. *J Nucl Med* 2000; 41:575–583.

25. Ishizu K, Nishizawa S, Yonekura Y, et al. Effects of hyperglycemia on FDG uptake in human brain and glioma. *J Nucl Med* 1994;35: 1104–1109.

26. Foster NL, VanDerSpek AF, Aldrich MS, et al. The effect of diazepam sedation on cerebral glucose metabolism in Alzheimer's disease as measured using positron emission tomography. *J Cereb Blood Flow Metab* 1987;7:415–420.

27. Wang GJ, Volkow ND, Overall J, et al. Reproducibility of regional brain metabolic responses to lorazepam. *J Nucl Med* 1996;37: 1609–1613.

28. Gaillard WD, Zeffiro T, Fazilat S, et al. Effect of valproate on cerebral metabolism and blood flow: an ^{18}F-2-deoxyglucose and ^{15}O water positron emission tomography study. *Epilepsia* 1996;37:515–521.

29. Theodore WH, Bairamian D, Newmark ME, et al. Effect of phenytoin on human cerebral glucose metabolism. *J Cereb Blood Flow Metab* 1986;6:315–320.

30. Theodore WH, Fishbein D, Dietz M, et al. Complex partial seizures: cerebellar metabolism. *Epilepsia* 1987;28:319–323.

31. Seitz RJ, Piel S, Arnold S, et al. Cerebellar hypometabolism in focal epilepsy is related to age of onset and drug intoxication. *Epilepsia* 1996;37:1194–1199.

32. Theodore WH. Antiepileptic drugs and cerebral glucose metabolism. *Epilepsia* 1988;29[Suppl 2]:S48–S55.

33. Bartlett EJ, Brodie JD, Simkowitz P, et al. Effects of haloperidol challenge on regional cerebral glucose utilization in normal human subjects. *Am J Psychiatry* 1994;151:681–686.

34. Von Monakow C. Die Lokalisation im grosshirn und der abbau der funktion durch kortikale herde. Weisbaden: J.F. Bergman, 1914: 26–34.

35. Meyer JS, Obara K, Muramatsu K. Diaschisis. *Neurol Res* 1993;15: 362–366.

36. Baron JC, Marchal G. Functional imaging in vascular disorders. In: Mazziotta JC, Toga AW, Frackowiak RSJ, eds. *Brain mapping: the disorders.* Academic Press, 2000:299–316.

37. Baron JC, Bonsser MG, Comar D, et al. Crossed cerebellar diaschisis in human supratentorial brain infarction. *Trans Am Neurol Assoc* 1980;105:459–461.

38. Baron JC, D'Antona R, Pantano P, et al. Effects of thalamic stroke on energy metabolism of the cerebral cortex. A positron tomography study in man. *Brain* 1986;109:1243–1259.

39. Park CH, Kim SM, Streletz LJ, et al. Reverse crossed cerebellar dias-

chisis in partial complex seizures related to herpes simplex encephalitis. *Clin Nucl Med* 1992;17:732–735.

40. Baird AE, Warach S. Imaging developing brain infarction. *Curr Opin Neurol* 1999;12:65–71.

41. Powers WJ. Hemodynamics and metabolism in ischemic cerebrovascular disease. *Neurol Clin* 1992;10:31–48.

42. Heiss WD, Herholz K. Assessment of pathophysiology of stroke by positron emission tomography. *Eur J Nucl Med* 1994;21:455–465.

43. Powers WJ, Raichle ME. Positron emission tomography and its application to the study of cerebrovascular disease in man. *Stroke* 1985; 16:361–376.

44. Ter-Pogossian MM, Eichling JO, Davis DO, et al. The determination of regional cerebral blood flow by means of water labeled with radioactive oxygen-15. *Radiology* 1969;93:31–40.

45. Ter-Pogossian MM, Eichling JO, Davis DO, et al. The measure *in vivo* of regional cerebral oxygen utilization by means of oxyhemoglobin labeled with radioactive oxygen-15. *J Clin Invest* 1970;49:381–391.

46. Jones T, Chesler DA, Ter-Pogossian MM. The continuous inhalation of oxygen-15 for assessing regional oxygen extraction in the brain of man. *Br J Radiol* 1976;49:339–343.

47. Lenzi GL, Jones T, McKenzie CG, et al. Study of regional cerebral metabolism and blood flow relationships in man using the method of continuously inhaling oxygen-15 and oxygen-15 labeled carbon dioxide. *J Neurol Neurosurg Psychiatry* 1978;41:1–10.

48. Frackowiak RS, Lenzi GL, Jones T, et al. Quantitative measurement of regional cerebral blood flow and oxygen metabolism in man using ^{15}O and positron emission tomography: theory, procedure, and normal values. *J Comput Assisted Tomogr* 1980;4:727–736.

49. Lammertsma AA, Frackowiak RSJ, Hoffman JM, et al. Simultaneous measurement of regional cerebral blood flow and oxygen metabolism: a feasibility study. *J Cereb Blood Flow Metab* 1987;7[Suppl 1]:S587.

50. Herscovitch P, Markham J, Raichle ME. Brain blood flow measured with intravenous H$_2$^{15}O, I: theory and error analysis. *J Nucl Med* 1983; 24:782–789.

51. Grubb RLJ, Raichle ME, Higgins CS, et al. Measurement of regional cerebral blood volume by emission tomography. *Ann Neurol* 1978; 4:322–328.

52. Baron JC, Frackowiak RS, Herholz K, et al. Use of PET methods for measurement of cerebral energy metabolism and hemodynamics in cerebrovascular disease. *J Cereb Blood Flow Metab* 1989;9:723–742.

53. Jones TH, Morawetz RB, Crowell RM, et al. Thresholds of focal cerebral ischemia in awake monkeys. *J Neurosurg* 1981;54:773–782.

54. Heiss WD. Ischemic penumbra: evidence from functional imaging in man. *J Cereb Blood Flow Metab* 2000;20:1276–1293.

55. Heiss WD, Graf R, Grond M, et al. Quantitative neuroimaging for the evaluation of the effect of stroke treatment. *Cerebrovasc Dis* 1998; 8[Suppl 2]:23–29.

56. Derdeyn CP, Grubb RLJ, Powers WJ. Cerebral hemodynamic impairment: methods of measurement and association with stroke risk. *Neurology* 1999;53:251–259.

57. Powers WJ, Press GA, Grubb RLJ, et al. The effect of hemodynamically significant carotid artery disease on the hemodynamic status of the cerebral circulation. *Ann Intern Med* 1987;106:27–34.

58. Gibbs JM, Wise RJ, Leenders KL, et al. Evaluation of cerebral perfusion reserve in patients with carotid-artery occlusion. *Lancet* 1984;1: 310–314.

59. Grubb RLJ, Derdeyn CP, Fritsch SM, et al. Importance of hemodynamic factors in the prognosis of symptomatic carotid occlusion. *JAMA* 1998;280:1055–1060.

60. Powers WJ, Derdeyn CP, Fritsch SM, et al. Benign prognosis of never-symptomatic carotid occlusion. *Neurology* 2000;54:878–882.

61. Derdeyn CP, Videen TO, Simmons NR, et al. Count-based PET method for predicting ischemic stroke in patients with symptomatic carotid arterial occlusion. *Radiology* 1999;212:499–506.

62. Carpenter DA, Grubb RLJ, Tempel LW, et al. Cerebral oxygen metabolism after aneurysmal subarachnoid hemorrhage. *J Cereb Blood Flow Metab* 1991;11:837–844.

63. Videen TO, Dunford-Shore JE, Diringer MN, et al. Correction for partial volume effects in regional blood flow measurements adjacent to hematomas in humans with intracerebral hemorrhage: implementation and validation. *J Comput Assisted Tomogr* 1999;23:248–256.

64. Kushner M, Reivich M, Fieschi C, et al. Metabolic and clinical correlates of acute ischemic infarction. *Neurology* 1987;37:1103–1110.

65. Marchal G, Furlan M, Beaudouin V, et al. Early spontaneous hyper-

perfusion after stroke. A marker of favorable tissue outcome? *Brain* 1996;119:409–419.

66. Heiss WD, Kracht L, Grond M, et al. Early [^{11}C]flumazenil/H$_2$O positron emission tomography predicts irreversible ischemic cortical damage in stroke patients receiving acute thrombolytic therapy. *Stroke* 2000;31:366–369.

67. Minoshima S, Giordani B, Berent S, et al. Metabolic reduction in the posterior cingulate cortex in very early Alzheimer's disease. *Ann Neurol* 1997;42:85–94.

68. Bohnen NI, Minoshima S, Kuhl DE, et al. The roles of FDG PET and MRI in the diagnosis of Alzheimer's disease. *Neurosci News* 1998;1:26–33.

69. Braak H, Braak E. Staging of Alzheimer's disease-related neurofibrillary changes. *Neurobiol Aging* 1995;16:271–284.

70. Friedland RP, Brun A, Budinger TF. Pathological and positron emission tomographic correlations in Alzheimer's disease. *Lancet* 1985;1:228.

71. Mielke R, Schroder R, Fink GR, et al. Regional cerebral glucose metabolism and postmortem pathology in Alzheimer's disease. *Acta Neuropathol* 1996;91:174–179.

72. Sokoloff L. *Brain work and mental activity.* Copenhagen: Munskgaard, 1991.

73. Liu X, Erikson C, Brun A. Cortical synaptic changes and gliosis in normal aging, Alzheimer's disease and frontal lobe degeneration. *Dementia* 1996;7:128–134.

74. Benson DF, Kuhl DE, Hawkins RA, et al. The fluorodeoxyglucose ^{18}F scan in Alzheimer's disease and multi-infarct dementia. *Arch Neurol* 1983;40:711–714.

75. Kuhl DE. Imaging local brain function with emission computed tomography. *Radiology* 1984;150:625–631.

76. Foster NL, Chase TN, Mansi L, et al. Cortical abnormalities in Alzheimer's disease. *Ann Neurol* 1984;16:649–654.

77. Herholz K, Adams R, Kessler J, et al. Criteria for the diagnosis of Alzheimer's disease with PET. *Dementia* 1990;1:156–164.

78. Minoshima S, Frey KA, Koeppe RA, et al. A diagnostic approach in Alzheimer's disease using three-dimensional stereotactic surface projections of fluorine-18-FDG PET. *J Nucl Med* 1995;36:1238–1248.

79. Vander Borght T, Minoshima S, Giordani B, et al. Cerebral metabolic differences in Parkinson's and Alzheimer's disease matched for dementia severity. *J Nucl Med* 1997;38:797–802.

80. Jagust WJ, Eberling JL, Richardson BC, et al. The cortical topography of temporal lobe hypometabolism in early Alzheimer's disease. *Brain Res* 1993;629:189–198.

81. Small GW, La Rue A, Komo S, et al. Predictors of cognitive change in middle-aged and older adults with memory loss. *Am J Psychiatry* 1995;152:1757–1764.

82. Small GW. Neuroimaging and genetic assessment for early diagnosis of Alzheimer's disease. *J Clin Psychiatry* 1996;57[Suppl 14]:9–13.

83. Johnson JK, Head E, Kim R, et al. Clinical and pathological evidence for a frontal variant of Alzheimer disease. *Arch Neurol* 1999;56:1233–1239.

84. Mayeux R, Stern Y, Rosenstein R, et al. An estimate of the prevalence of dementia in idiopathic Parkinson's disease. *Arch Neurol* 1988;45:260–262.

85. Marder K, Tang M-X, Côté L, et al. The frequency and associated risk factors for dementia in patients with Parkinson's disease. *Arch Neurol* 1995;52:695–701.

86. Lieberman A, et al. Dementia in Parkinson's disease. *Ann Neurol* 1979;6:355–359.

87. McKeith IG, et al. Consensus guideline for the clinical and pathological diagnosis of dementia with Lewy bodies (LBD): report of the Consortium on DLB International Workshop. *Neurology* 1996;47:1113–1124.

88. Albin RL, Minoshima S, D'Amato CJ, et al. Fluoro-deoxyglucose positron emission tomography in diffuse Lewy body disease. *Neurology* 1996;47:462–466.

89. Alexander GE, DeLong MR, Strick PL. Parallel organization of functionally segregated circuits linking basal ganglia and cortex. *Annu Rev Neurosci* 1986;9:357–381.

90. Baron JC. Consequences des lesions des noyaux gris centraux sur l'activite metabolique cerebrale: implications cliniques. *Rev Neurol* 1994;150:599–604.

91. van Gorp WG, Mandelkern MA, Gee M, et al. Cerebral metabolic dysfunction in AIDS: findings in a sample with and without dementia. *J Neuropsychiatry Clin Neurosci* 1992;4:280–287.

92. Rottenberg DA, Sidtis JJ, Strother SC, et al. Abnormal cerebral glucose metabolism in HIV-1 seropositive subjects with and without dementia. *J Nucl Med* 1996;37:1133–1141.

93. Cortelli P, Perani D, Parchi P, et al. Cerebral metabolism in fatal familial insomnia: relation to duration, neuropathology, and distribution of protease-resistant prion protein. *Neurology* 1997;49:126–133.

94. Zhukareva V, Vogelsberg-Ragaglia V, Van Deerlin VM, et al. Loss of brain tau defines novel sporadic and familial tauopathies with frontotemporal dementia. *Ann Neurol* 2001;49:165–175.

95. Ishii K, Sakamoto S, Sasaki M, et al. Cerebral glucose metabolism in patients with frontotemporal dementia. *J Nucl Med* 1998;39:1875–1878.

96. Caselli RJ. Asymmetric cortical degeneration syndromes. *Curr Opin Neurol* 1996; 9:276–280.

97. Hachisuka K, Uchida M, Nozaki Y, et al. Primary progressive aphasia presenting as conduction aphasia. *J Neurol Sci* 1999;167:137–141.

98. Vinters HV, Ellis WG, Zarow C, et al. Neuropathologic substrates of ischemic vascular dementia. *J Neuropathol Exp Neurol* 2000;59:931–945.

99. Foster NL, Hickenbottom SL. When do strokes cause dementia? Effects of subcortical cerebral infarction on cortical glucose metabolism and cognitive function. *Arch Neurol* 1999;56:778–779.

100. Fein G, Di Sclafani V, Tanabe J, et al. Hippocampal and cortical atrophy predict dementia in subcortical ischemic vascular disease. *Neurology* 2000;55:1626–1635.

101. Mielke R, Heiss WD. Positron emission tomography for diagnosis of Alzheimer's disease and vascular dementia. *J Neural Transm* 1998;53[Suppl]:237–250.

102. Sultzer DL, Mahler ME, Cummings JL, et al. Cortical abnormalities associated with subcortical lesions in vascular dementia. Clinical and position emission tomographic findings. *Arch Neurol* 1995;52:773–780.

103. De Reuck J, Decoo D, Marchau M, et al. Positron emission tomography in vascular dementia. *J Neurol Sci* 1998;154:55–61.

104. Hoffman JM, Welsh-Bohmer KA, Hanson M, et al. FDG PET imaging in patients with pathologically verified dementia. *J Nucl Med* 2000;41:1920–1928.

105. Minoshima S, Foster NL, Frey KA, et al. Metabolic differences in Alzheimer's disease with and without cortical Lewy bodies as revealed by PET. *J Cereb Blood Flow Metab* 1997;17[Suppl 1]:S437.

106. Bromfield EB, Altshuler L, Leiderman DB, et al. Cerebral metabolism and depression in patients with complex partial seizures. *Arch Neurol* 1992;49:617–623.

107. Reiman E, Caselli R, Yun L, et al. Preclinical evidence of Alzheimer's disease in persons homozygous for the ε4 allele for apolipoprotein E. *N Engl J Med* 1996;334:752–758.

108. Minoshima S, Foster NL, Kuhl DE. Posterior cingulate cortex in Alzheimer's disease. *Lancet* 1994;344:895.

109. Minoshima S, Giordani B, Berent S, et al. [F-18]FDG PET predicts the development of Alzheimer's disease in memory impaired patients without dementia. *J Nucl Med* 1998;39[Suppl]:96P.

110. Berent S, Giordani B, Foster N, et al. Neuropsychological function and cerebral glucose utilization in isolated memory impairment and Alzheimer's disease. *J Psychiatr Res* 1999;33:7–16.

111. Minoshima S, Cross DJ, Foster NL, et al. Discordance between traditional pathologic and energy metabolic changes in very early Alzheimer's disease. Pathophysiological implications. *Ann N Y Acad Sci* 1999;893:350–352.

112. Rossor MN, Kennedy AM, Frackowiak RSJ. Clinical and neuroimaging features of familial Alzheimer's disease. *Ann N Y Acad Sci* 1996;777:49–56.

113. Signorini M, Paulesu E, Friston K, et al. Rapid assessment of regional cerebral metabolic abnormalities in single subjects with quantitative and nonquantitative [^{18}F]FDG PET: a clinical validation of statistical parametric mapping. *Neuroimage* 1999;9:63–80.

114. Davies P, Maloney A. Selective loss of central cholinergic neurons in Alzheimer's disease. *Lancet* 1976;2:1403.

115. Irie T, Fukushi K, Akimoto Y, et al. Design and evaluation of radioactive acetylcholine analogs for mapping brain acetylcholinesterase (AChE) *in vivo. Nucl Med Biol* 1994;21.

116. Kuhl D, Koeppe R, Snyder S, et al. Mapping acetylcholinesterase

activity in human brain using PET and *N*-[¹¹C]methylpiperidinyl propionate (PMP). *J Nucl Med* 1996;37[Suppl]:21P.

117. Kuhl DE, Koeppe RA, Minoshima S, et al. *In vivo* mapping of cerebral acetylcholinesterase activity in aging and Alzheimer's disease. *Neurology* 1999;52:691–699.

118. Iyo M, Namba H, Fukushi K, et al. Measurement of acetylcholinesterase by positron emission tomography in the brain of healthy controls and patients with Alzheimer's disease. *Lancet* 1997;349:1805–1809.

119. Brooks DJ. Imaging basal ganglia function. *J Anat* 2000;196:543–554.

120. Quinn N. Parkinsonism-recognition and differential diagnosis. *BMJ* 1995;310:447–452.

121. Gelb DJ, Oliver E, Gilman S. Diagnostic criteria for Parkinson disease. *Arch Neurol* 1999;56:33–39.

122. Hughes AJ. Clinicopathological aspects of Parkinson's disease. *Eur Neurol* 1997;38[Suppl 2]:13–20.

123. Hughes AJ, Daniel SE, Blankson S, et al. A clinicopathologic study of 100 cases of Parkinson's disease. *Arch Neurol* 1993;50:140–148.

124. Wolfson LI, Leenders KL, Brown LL, et al. Alterations of regional cerebral blood flow and oxygen metabolism in Parkinson's disease. *Neurology* 1985;35:1399–1405.

125. Antonini A, Vontobel P, Psylla M, et al. Complementary positron emission tomographic studies of the striatal dopaminergic system in Parkinson's disease. *Arch Neurol* 1995;52:1183–1190.

126. Eidelberg D, Moeller JR, Dhawan V, et al. The metabolic topography of parkinsonism. *J Cereb Blood Flow Metab* 1994;14:783–801.

127. Bohnen NI, Minoshima S, Giordani B, et al. Motor correlates of occipital glucose hypometabolism in Parkinson's disease without dementia. *Neurology* 1999;52:541–546.

128. Dethy S, Van Blercom N, Damhaut P, et al. Asymmetry of basal ganglia glucose metabolism and dopa responsiveness in parkinsonism. *Move Disord* 1998;13:275–280.

129. Steele JC, Richardson JC, Olszewski J. Progressive supranuclear palsy: a heterogeneous degeneration involving the brainstem, basal ganglia, and cerebellum, with vertical gaze and pseudobulbar palsy. *Arch Neurol* 1964;10:333–359.

130. Foster NL, Gilman S, Berent S, et al. Cerebral hypometabolism in progressive supranuclear palsy studied with positron emission tomography. *Ann Neurol* 1988;24:399–406.

131. D'Antona R, Baron JC, Samson Y, et al. Subcortical dementia. Frontal cortex hypometabolism detected by positron tomography in patients with progressive supranuclear palsy. *Brain* 1985;108:785–799.

132. Blin J, Baron JC, Dubois B, et al. Positron emission tomography study in progressive supranuclear palsy. Brain hypometabolic pattern and clinicometabolic correlations. *Arch Neurol* 1990;47:747–752.

133. Salmon E, Van der Linden MV, Franck G. Anterior cingulate and motor network metabolic impairment in progressive supranuclear palsy. *Neuroimage* 1997;5:173–178.

134. Otsuka M, Ichiya Y, Kuwabara Y, et al. Cerebral blood flow, oxygen and glucose metabolism with PET in progressive supranuclear palsy. *Ann Nucl Med* 1989;3:111–118.

135. Feany MB, Ksiezak-Reding H, Liu WK, et al. Epitope expression and hyperphosphorylation of tau protein in corticobasal degeneration: differentiation from progressive supranuclear palsy. *Acta Neuropathol (Berl)* 1995;90:37–43.

136. Eidelberg D, Dhawan V, Moeller JR, et al. The metabolic landscape of cortico-basal ganglionic degeneration: regional asymmetries studied with positron emission tomography. *J Neurol Neurosurg Psychiatry* 1991;54:856–862.

137. Nagahama Y, Fukuyama H, Turjanski N, et al. Cerebral glucose metabolism in corticobasal degeneration: comparison with progressive supranuclear palsy and normal controls. *Movement Disord* 1997;12:691–696.

138. Garraux G, Salmon E, Peigneux P, et al. Voxel-based distribution of metabolic impairment in corticobasal degeneration. *Movement Disord* 2000;15:894–904.

139. Blin J, Vidailhet MJ, Pillon B, et al. Corticobasal degeneration: decreased and asymmetrical glucose consumption as studied with PET. *Movement Disord* 1992;7:348–354.

140. Lutte I, Laterre C, Bodart JM, et al. Contribution of PET studies in diagnosis of corticobasal degeneration. *Eur Neurol* 2000;44:12–21.

141. Papp MI, Lantos PL. The distribution of oligodendroglial inclusions in multiple system atrophy and its relevance to clinical symptomatology. *Brain* 1994;117:235–243.

142. Otsuka M, Kuwabara Y, Ichiya Y, et al. Differentiating between multiple system atrophy and Parkinson's disease by positron emission tomography with ¹⁸F-dopa and ¹⁸F-FDG. *Ann Nucl Med* 1997;11:251–257.

143. Gilman S, Koeppe RA, Junck L, et al. Patterns of cerebral glucose metabolism detected with positron emission tomography differ in multiple system atrophy and olivopontocerebellar atrophy. *Ann Neurol* 1994;36:166–175.

144. Otsuka M, Ichiya Y, Kuwabara Y, et al. Glucose metabolism in the cortical and subcortical brain structures in multiple system atrophy and Parkinson's disease: a positron emission tomographic study. *J Neurol Sci* 1996;144:77–83.

145. Gerstenbrand F, Klingler D, Pfeiffer B. Der essentielle tremor. Phänomenologie und epidemiologie. *Nervenarzt* 1983;43:46–53.

146. Hallett M, Dubinsky RM. Glucose metabolism in the brain of patients with essential tremor. *J Neurol Sci* 1993;114:45–48.

147. Colebatch JG, Findley LJ, Frackowiak RS, et al. Preliminary report: activation of the cerebellum in essential tremor. *Lancet* 1990;336:1028–1030.

148. Jenkins IH, Bain PG, Colebatch JG, et al. A positron emission tomography study of essential tremor: evidence for overactivity of cerebellar connections. *Ann Neurol* 1993;34:82–90.

149. Wills AJ, Jenkins IH, Thompson PD, et al. Red nuclear and cerebellar but no olivary activation associated with essential tremor: a positron emission tomographic study. *Ann Neurol* 1994;36:636–642.

150. Wills AJ, Jenkins IH, Thompson PD, et al. A positron emission tomography study of cerebral activation associated with essential and writing tremor. *Arch Neurol* 1995;52:299–305.

151. Albin RL, Tagle DA. Genetics and molecular biology of Huntington's disease. *Trends Neurosci* 1995;18:11–14.

152. Huntington's Disease Collaborative Research Group. A novel gene containing a trinucleotide repeat that is expanded and unstable on Huntington's disease chromosomes. *Cell* 1993;72:971–983.

153. Vonsattel J-P, DiFiglia M. Huntington's disease. *J Neuropathol Exp Neurol* 1998;57:369–384.

154. Bernheimer H, Birkmayer W, Hornykiewicz O, et al. Brain dopamine and the syndromes of Parkinson and Huntington. Clinical, morphological and neurochemical correlations. *J Neurol Sci* 1973;20:415–455.

155. Vonsattel J-P, Meyers R, Stevens T, et al. Neuropathological classification of Huntington's disease. *J Neuropathol Exp Neurol* 1985;44:559–577.

156. Kuhl DE, Phelps ME, Markham CH, et al. Cerebral metabolism and atrophy in Huntington's disease determined by ¹⁸FDG and computed tomographic scan. *Ann Neurol* 1982;12:425–434.

157. Kuhl DE, Metter EJ, Riege WH, et al. Patterns of cerebral glucose utilization in Parkinson's disease and Huntington's disease. *Ann Neurol* 1984;15[Suppl]:S119–S125.

158. Maziotta JH, Phelps ME, Pahl JJ, et al. Reduced cerebral glucose metabolism in asymptomatic subjects at risk for Huntington's disease. *N Engl J Med* 1987;316:357–362.

159. Hosokawa S, Ichiya Y, Kuwabara Y, et al. Positron emission tomography in cases of chorea with different underlying diseases. *J Neurol Neurosurg Psychiatry* 1987;50:1284–1287.

160. Dubinsky RM, Hallett M, Levey R, et al. Regional brain glucose metabolism in neuroacanthocytosis. *Neurology* 1989;39:1253–1255.

161. Weindl A, Kuwert T, Leenders KL, et al. Increased striatal glucose consumption in Sydenham's chorea. *Movement Disord* 1993;8:437–444.

162. Bohlega S, Riley W, Powe J, et al. Neuroacanthocytosis and a prebetalipoproteinemia. *Neurology* 1998;50:1912–1914.

163. Sunden-Cullberg J, Tedroff J, Aquilonius SM. Reversible chorea in primary antiphospholipid syndrome. *Movement Disord* 1998;13:147–149.

164. Garnett ES, Firnau G, Chan PKH, et al. [¹⁸F]fluoro-dopa, an analogue of dopa, and its use in direct measurement of storage, degeneration, and turnover of intracerebral dopamine. *Proc Natl Acad Sci U S A* 1978;75:464–467.

165. Garnett ES, Firnau G, Nahmias C. Dopamine visualized in the basal ganglia of living man. *Nature* 1983;305:137–138.

166. Frost JJ, Rosier AJ, Reich SG, et al. Positron emission tomographic imaging of the dopamine transporter with ¹¹C-WIN 35,428 reveals marked declines in mild Parkinson's disease. *Ann Neurol* 1993;34:423–431.

167. Antonini A, Schwarz J, Oertel WH, et al. [¹¹C]raclopride and positron

emission tomography in previously untreated patients with Parkinson's disease: influence of L-dopa and lisuride therapy on striatal dopamine D_2-receptors. *Neurology* 1994;44:1325–1329.

168. Brooks D. The early diagnosis of Parkinson's disease. *Ann Neurol* 1998; 44[Suppl 1]:S10–S18.

169. Frey KA, Koeppe RA, Kilbourn MR, et al. Presynaptic monoaminergic vesicles in Parkinson's disease and normal aging. *Ann Neurol* 1996;40:873–884.

170. Bohnen N, Meyer P, Albin RL, et al. Clinical correlates of striatal (+)-[C-11]DTBZ binding to VMAT2 in Parkinson's disease. *J Nucl Med* 1998;39[Suppl]:15P.

171. Eidelberg D, Moeller JR, Dhawan V, et al. The metabolic anatomy of Parkinson's disease: complementary [^{18}F]fluorodeoxyglucose and [^{18}F]fluorodopa positron emission tomographic studies. *Movement Disord* 1990;5:203–213.

172. Morrish PK, Sawle GV, Brooks DJ. An [^{18}F]dopa-PET and clinical study of the rate of progression in Parkinson's disease. *Brain* 1996; 119:585–591.

173. Vingerhoets FJG, Schulzer M, Calne DB, et al. Which clinical sign of Parkinson's disease best reflects the nigrostriatal lesion? *Ann Neurol* 1997;41:58–64.

174. Brooks DJ, Ibanez V, Sawle GV, et al. Striatal D_2 receptor status in patients with Parkinson's disease, striatonigral degeneration, and progressive supranuclear palsy, measured with ^{11}C-raclopride and positron emission tomography. *Ann Neurol* 1992;31:184–192.

175. Gilman S, Frey KA, Koeppe RA, et al. Decreased striatal monoaminergic terminals in olivopontocerebellar atrophy and multiple system atrophy demonstrated with positron emission tomography. *Ann Neurol* 1996;40:885–892.

176. Pirker W, Asenbaum S, Bencsits G, et al. [^{123}I]beta-CIT SPECT in multiple system atrophy, progressive supranuclear palsy, and corticobasal degeneration. *Movement Disord* 2000;15:1158–1167.

177. Rinne UK, Laihinen A, Rinne JO, et al. Positron emission tomography demonstrates dopamine D_2 receptor supersensitivity in the striatum of patients with early Parkinson's disease. *Movement Disord* 1990;5: 55–59.

178. Antonini A, et al. Long-term changes of striatal dopamine D_2 receptors in patients with Parkinson's disease: a study with positron emission tomography and [^{11}C]raclopride. *Movement Disord* 1997;12:33–38.

179. Theodore WH, Newmark ME, Sato S, et al. [^{18}F]fluorodeoxyglucose positron emission tomography in refractory complex partial seizures. *Ann Neurol* 1983;14:429–437.

180. Theodore WH. Positron emission tomography in the evaluation of seizure disorders. *Neurosci News* 1998;1:18–22.

181. Theodore WH. Cerebral blood flow and glucose metabolism in human epilepsy. In: *Advances in neurology*, vol 79. Philadelphia: Lippincott Williams & Wilkins, 1999:873–881.

182. Kuhl DE, Engel J, Phelps ME, et al. Epileptic patterns of local cerebral metabolism and perfusion in humans determined by emission computed tomography of ^{18}FDG and ^{13}NH$_3$. *Ann Neurol* 1980;8:348–360.

183. Gaillard WD, Fazilat S, White S, et al. Interictal metabolism and blood flow are uncoupled in temporal lobe cortex of patients with complex partial epilepsy. *Neurology* 1995;45:1841–1847.

184. Gaillard WD, Bhatia S, Bookheimer SY, et al. FDG-PET and volumetric MRI in the evaluation of patients with partial epilepsy. *Neurology* 1995;45:123–126.

185. Henry TR, Babb TL, Engel J Jr, et al. Hippocampal neuronal loss and regional hypometabolism in temporal lobe epilepsy. *Ann Neurol* 1994;36:925–927.

186. Hajek M, Wieser HG, Khan N, et al. Preoperative and postoperative glucose consumption in mesiobasal and lateral temporal lobe epilepsy. *Neurology* 1994;44:2125–2132.

187. Delbeke D, Lawrence SK, Abou-Khalil BW, et al. Postsurgical outcome of patients with uncontrolled complex partial seizures and temporal lobe hypometabolism on ^{18}FDG-positron emission tomography. *Invest Radiol* 1996;31:261–266.

188. Theodore WH, Sato S, Kufta CV, et al. FDG-positron emission tomography and invasive EEG: seizure focus detection and surgical outcome. *Epilepsia* 1997;38:81–86.

189. Henry TR, Mazziotta JC, Engel J. Interictal metabolic anatomy of mesial temporal lobe epilepsy. *Arch Neurol* 1993;50:582–589.

190. Henry TR, Sutherling WW, Engel J, et al. Interictal cerebral metabolism in partial epilepsies of neocortical origin. *Epilepsy Res* 1991;10: 174–182.

191. Swartz BE, Halgren E, Delgado-Escueta AV, et al. Neuroimaging in patients with seizures of probable frontal lobe origin. *Epilepsia* 1989; 30:547–558.

192. Drzezga A, Arnold S, Minoshima S, et al. ^{18}F-FDG PET studies in patients with extratemporal and temporal epilepsy: evaluation of an observer-independent analysis. *J Nucl Med* 1999;40:737–746.

193. Leiderman DB, Balish M, Sato S, et al. Comparison of PET measurements of cerebral blood flow and glucose metabolism for the localization of human epileptic foci. *Epilepsy Res* 1992;13:153–157.

194. Meltzer CC, Adelson PD, Brenner RP, et al. Planned ictal FDG PET imaging for localization of extratemporal epileptic foci. *Epilepsia* 2000;41:193–200.

195. Theodore WH, Balish M, Leiderman D, et al. Effect of seizures on cerebral blood flow measured with ^{15}O-H$_2$O and positron emission tomography. *Epilepsia* 1996;37:796–802.

196. Hunter KE, Blaxton TA, Bookheimer SY, et al. ^{15}O water positron emission tomography in language localization: a study comparing positron emission tomography visual and computerized region of interest analysis with the Wada test. *Ann Neurol* 1999;45:662–665.

197. Bookheimer SY, Zeffiro TA, Blaxton T, et al. A direct comparison of PET activation and electrocortical stimulation mapping for language localization. *Neurology* 1997;48:1056–1065.

198. Henry TR, Frey KA, Sackellares JC, et al. *In vivo* cerebral metabolism and central benzodiazepine-receptor binding in temporal lobe epilepsy. *Neurology* 1993;43:1998–2006.

199. Arnold S, Berthele A, Drzezga A, et al. Reduction of benzodiazepine receptor binding is related to the seizure onset zone in extratemporal focal cortical dysplasia. *Epilepsia* 2000;41:818–824.

200. Koepp MJ, Hammers A, Labbe C, et al. 11C-flumazenil PET in patients with refractory temporal lobe epilepsy and normal MRI. *Neurology* 2000;54:332–339.

201. Morawetz RB, Crowell RH, DeGirolami U, et al. Regional cerebral blood flow thresholds during cerebral ischemia. *Fed Proc* 1979;38: 2493–2494.

CHAPTER 7

Psychiatric Disorders

Marc Laruelle, Peter Talbot, Diana Martinez, and Anissa Abi-Dargham

Psychiatric conditions once qualified as "functional" illnesses—that is, disorders in which no major abnormalities of brain integrity such as tumors, inflammation, or infection could be detected by neuropathologic examination. Indeed, after a century of postmortem studies, only subtle abnormalities have been found at autopsy in brains of patients who suffered from major psychiatric illnesses, and few of these have been consistently replicated. These observations led to the impression that these illnesses were due to "functional," rather than "structural," brain abnormalities. Computed tomography (CT) and magnetic resonance imaging (MRI) studies have consistently observed abnormalities in brain structures in many psychiatric disorders, but these abnormalities remain for the most part within the limits of normal variability. None of them is pathognomonic or diagnostic. Therefore, the advent of positron emission tomography (PET) and single-photon emission computed tomography (SPECT) held enormous promise for the field of psychiatry, because for the first time living brain functions were directly accessible to clinical investigation.

Using PET and SPECT, a large body of studies have documented that psychiatric disorders are associated with regional alterations in blood flow and glucose metabolism under both resting and activation conditions. In this regard, PET and SPECT have played a major role in unraveling alterations in brain function associated with these conditions. Today these techniques have largely been replaced by functional MRI (fMRI), which offers clear advantages in terms of spatial and temporal resolution, not to mention the lack of radiation exposure. It is foreseeable that the role of PET and SPECT studies of flow and metabolism in psychiatric research will be greatly reduced in the future.

On the other hand, the ability of nuclear medicine techniques to image specific biomolecules is unmatched by any other noninvasive imaging method currently available to clinical investigators. Studies of receptors, transporters, enzymes, and other processes such as transmitter release clearly constitute the best use of PET for current and future psychiatric research. These techniques have already yielded a number of fundamental observations. So far none of these findings has led to clinical applications useful in the diagnosis or treatment of individuals with these disorders. However, it is anticipated that specific applications may surface from this line of research in the near future.

This chapter describes the major findings stemming from this line of research and their implications for our understanding of the pathophysiology and treatment of major psychiatric illnesses. For the reasons already discussed, we focus this review on imaging studies of specific biomolecules (a field we refer to as *molecular imaging*), as opposed to the study of flow and metabolism. Nonetheless, important flow and metabolism studies are discussed, particularly when molecular imaging studies provide clues to the pathophysiology underlying their observations. We include here both PET and SPECT studies, as it would not be feasible to provide a comprehensive review of this field without describing the important contributions of SPECT.

Technical considerations critical to the discussion of the findings are included when appropriate, but for an overview of the sophisticated technical background of these studies, the reader is referred to the Chapters 2, 3, and 4. In line with the clinical orientation of this chapter, we review the studies by clinical disorder (schizophrenia, mood, anxiety, personality, and conduct and substance abuse disorders), rather than by transmitter system.

The main neurotransmitter systems that have been studied with PET or SPECT in relation to psychiatric disorders and their treatment include dopamine (DA), serotonin (5-HT), γ-aminobutyric acid (GABA), and opiate systems. Radiotracers most frequently used include those for the DA D_2 receptor (^{11}C-N-methylspiperone, ^{11}C-raclopride, ^{123}I-iodobenzamide [IBZM], ^{123}I-epidipride, ^{18}F-fallypride, ^{11}C-FLB-457), D_1 receptors (^{11}C-SCH-23390, ^{11}C-NNC-112), DA transporters (DATs) (^{11}C-cocaine, ^{11}C-methylphenidate, ^{123}I-β-CIT, ^{11}C/^{18}F-CFT, ^{99m}Tc-TRODAT-1), DOPA decarboxylase (^{18}F/^{11}C-DOPA), monoamine oxidase (^{11}C-deprenyl and ^{11}C-clorgyline), 5-HT$_2$ receptors (^{18}F-altanserin, ^{18}F-setoperone, ^{11}C-MDL-100907), 5-HT$_{1A}$ receptors (^{11}C-WAY-100635), 5-HT transporters (^{123}I-β-CIT, ^{11}C-McN-5652, ^{11}C-DASB), benzodiazepine receptors (^{123}I-iomazenil, ^{11}C-flumazenil [FMZ]), and mu opiate receptors (^{11}C-carfentanil, ^{18}F-cyclofoxy).

SCHIZOPHRENIA

Dopamine Transmission

The classical DA hypothesis, formulated more than 30 years ago, proposed that schizophrenia is associated with hyperactivity of dopaminergic neurotransmission (1,2). This hypothesis was essentially based on the observation that all effective antipsychotic drugs provided at least some degree of D$_2$-receptor blockade, an observation that is still true today (3,4). As D$_2$-receptor blockade is most effective against positive symptoms (delusions and hallucinations), the DA hyperactivity model appeared to be most relevant to the pathophysiology of these symptoms. This idea was further supported by the fact that sustained exposure to DA agonists such as amphetamine can induce a psychotic state characterized by some features of schizophrenia-positive symptomatology (emergence of paranoid delusions and hallucinations in the context of a clear sensorium) (5,6). These pharmacologic effects suggest, but do not establish, a dysregulation of DA systems in schizophrenia.

On the other hand, negative and cognitive symptoms are generally resistant to treatment by antipsychotic drugs. Functional brain imaging studies have suggested that these symptoms are associated with prefrontal cortex (PFC) dysfunction (7). Studies in nonhuman primates have demonstrated that deficits in DA transmission in the PFC produce cognitive impairments similar to those observed in schizophrenic patients (8), suggesting that a deficit in DA transmission in the PFC may be implicated in the cognitive impairments associated with schizophrenia (9,10).

A contemporary view of the role of DA in schizophrenia is that subcortical mesolimbic DA projections may be hyperactive (resulting in positive symptoms) and that the mesocortical DA projections to the PFC may be hypoactive (resulting in negative symptoms and cognitive impairment). These two abnormalities may be related, because the cortical DA system generally exerts an inhibitory action on subcortical DA systems (11,12). The advent in the early 1980s of techniques based on PET and SPECT to measure indices of DA activity in the living human brain opened the possibility of direct investigation of these hypotheses.

Striatal DA Transmission

Studies of striatal DA transmission in schizophrenia examined both postsynaptic (D$_2$ receptors and D$_1$ receptors) and presynaptic (DOPA decarboxylase activity, stimulant-induced DA release, baseline DA release, and DAT) functions. These studies are summarized in Tables 7.1 and 7.2, respectively.

D$_2$ Receptors

Striatal D$_2$-receptor density in schizophrenia has been extensively studied with PET and SPECT imaging. In a recent metaanalysis (13), we identified 17 imaging studies comparing D$_2$-receptor parameters in patients with schizophrenia

TABLE 7.1. *Imaging studies of striatal D$_2$ receptor parameters in drug-naive and drug-free patients with schizophrenia*

Class radiotracer	Radiotracer	Study	Controls (n)	Patients (n) (DN/DF)[a]	Method	Outcome	Controls (normalized) mean ± SD[a]	Patients (normalized) mean ± SD[a]	p	Effect size[b]	Ratio SD
Butyrophenones	^{11}C-NMSP	(14)	11	15 (10/5)	Kinetic	Bmax	100 ± 50	253 ± 105	< .05	3.06	2.10
	^{76}Br-SPI	(15)	8	16 (12/4)	Ratio	S/C	100 ± 14	111 ± 12	< .05	0.79	0.86
	^{76}Br-SPI	(16)	8	8 (0/8)	Ratio	S/C	100 ± 14	104 ± 14	ns	0.28	1.00
	^{76}Br-SPI	(17)	12	12 (0/12)	Ratio	S/C	100 ± 11	101 ± 15	ns	0.14	1.41
	^{11}C-NMSP	(18)	17	10 (8/2)	Kinetic	Bmax	100 ± 80	173 ± 143	.08	0.91	1.79
	^{11}C-NMSP	(19)	7	7 (7/0)	Kinetic	Bmax	100 ± 25	133 ± 63	ns	1.33	2.50
	^{11}C-NMSP	(20)	18	17 (10/7)	Kinetic	k_3	100 ± 21	104 ± 16	ns	0.19	0.74
Benzamides	^{11}C-raclopride	(21)	20	18 (18/0)	Equilibrium	Bmax	100 ± 29	107 ± 18	ns	0.23	0.63
	^{11}C-raclopride	(22)	10	13 (0/13)	Equilibrium	Bmax	100 ± 22	112 ± 43	ns	0.55	1.99
	^{123}I-IBZM	(23)	20	20 (17/3)	Ratio	S/FC	100 ± 8	99 ± 7	ns	−0.07	0.82
	^{123}I-IBZM	(24)	15	15 (1/14)	Equilibrium	BP	100 ± 26	115 ± 33	ns	0.56	1.25
	^{123}I-IBZM	(25)	16	21 (1/20)	Equilibrium	BP	100 ± 29	97 ± 38	ns	−0.12	1.31
	^{11}C-raclopride	(26)	12	11 (6/5)	Equilibrium	BP	100 ± 18	100 ± 30	ns	0.02	1.69
	^{123}I-IBZM	(27)	15	15 (2/13)	Equilibrium	BP	100 ± 20	102 ± 49	ns	0.09	2.50
	^{123}I-IBZM	(28)	18	18 (8/10)	Equilibrium	BP	100 ± 13	104 ± 14	ns	0.33	1.11
Ergot Alk.	^{76}Br-lisuride	(29)	14	19 (10/9)	Ratio	S/C	100 ± 10	104 ± 12	ns	0.45	1.21
	^{76}Br-lisuride	(30)	10	10 (2/8)	Ratio	S/C	100 ± 10	100 ± 13	ns	0.00	1.29

DN, drug naive; DF, drug free; BP, binding potential.
[a] Mean normalized to mean of control subjects.
[b] Effect size calculated as (mean patients − mean controls)/SD controls.

TABLE 7.2. *Imaging studies of striatal presynaptic dopamine parameters in drug naive and drug free patients with schizophrenia*

Parameter	Study	Controls (n)	Patients (n) (DN/DF)	Radiotracer (challenge)	Method	Outcome	Controls (mean ± SD)[a]	Patients (mean ± SD)[a]	p	Effect size[b]	Ratio SD
DOPA decarboxylase activity	(35)	13	5 (4/1)	^{18}F-DOPA	Kinetic	k_3	100 ± 23	120 ± 15	<0.05	0.91	0.68
	(36)	7	7 (7/0)	^{18}F-DOPA	Graphical	K_i	100 ± 11	117 ± 20	<0.05	1.54	1.82
	(37)	7	6 (2/4)	^{18}F-DOPA	Graphical	K_i	100 ± 11	103 ± 40	ns	0.30	3.80
	(39)	10	12 (10/2)	^{11}C-DOPA	Graphical	K_i	100 ± 17	113 ± 12	<0.05	0.77	0.70
	(38)	13	10 (10/0)	^{18}F-DOPA	Graphical	K_i	100 ± 14	115 ± 28	<0.05	1.09	1.25
Amphetamine-induced DA release	(24)	15	15 (2/13)	^{123}I-IBZM/ amphetamine	Equilibrium	Delta BP	100 ± 113	271 ± 221	<0.05	1.51	1.95
	(26)	18	18 (8/10)	^{11}C-raclopride/ amphetamine	Equilibrium	Delta BP	100 ± 43	175 ± 82	<0.05	1.73	1.90
	(27)	16	21 (1/20)	^{123}I-IBZM/ amphetamine	Equilibrium	Delta BP	100 ± 88	194 ± 145	<0.05	1.07	1.64
Baseline DA concentration	(28)	18	18 (8/10)	^{123}I-IBZM/ α-MPT	Equilibrium	Delta BP	100 ± 78	211 ± 122	<0.05	1.43	1.57
DAT density	(48)	9	9 (9/0)	^{18}F-CFT	Ratio	S/C	100 ± 12	101 ± 13	<0.05	0.11	1.06
	(47)	22	22 (2/20)	^{123}I-β-CIT	Equilibrium	BP	100 ± 17	93 ± 20	<0.05	−0.43	1.21

BP, binding potential; DA, dopamine; DAT, dopamine transporters; DN, drug naive; DF, drug free.
[a] Mean normalized to mean of control subjects.
[b] Effect size calculated as (mean patients—mean controls)/SD controls.

(included a total of 245 patients, 112 neuroleptic naive, and 133 neuroleptic free) with those in controls (n = 231), matched for age and sex (14–30). Radiotracers included butyrophenones (^{11}C-*N*-methyl-spiperone, ^{11}C-NMSP [n = 4], and ^{76}Br-bromospiperone [n = 3]), benzamides (^{11}C-raclopride [n = 3] and ^{123}I-IBZM [n = 5]), or the ergot derivative ^{76}Br-lisuride (n = 2). Only 2 of 17 studies detected a significant elevation of D_2-receptor density parameters. However, metaanalysis revealed a small (12%) but significant elevation of striatal D_2 receptors in patients with schizophrenia.

No clinical correlates of increased D_2-receptor binding parameters have been reliably identified. Studies performed with butyrophenones (n = 7) show an effect size of 0.96 ± 1.05, significantly larger than the effect size observed with other ligands (benzamides and lisuride, n = 10, 0.20 ± 0.26, p = .04). This difference might be due to differences in vulnerability of the binding of these tracers to competition by endogenous DA and elevation of endogenous DA in schizophrenia (31,32). Regarding striatal D_1 receptors, three imaging studies (20,33,34) have confirmed the results of postmortem studies of unaltered levels of these receptors in the striatum of patients with schizophrenia.

DOPA Decarboxylase Activity

Five studies reported rates of DOPA decarboxylase activity in patients with schizophrenia, using ^{18}F-DOPA (35–38) or ^{11}C-DOPA (39) (Table 7.2). Four out of five studies reported increased accumulation of DOPA in the striatum of patients with schizophrenia, and the combined analysis yielded a significant effect size of 0.92 ± 0.45 (p = .01).

Several of these studies reported the observation of high DOPA accumulation in psychotic paranoid patients and low accumulation in patients with negative or depressive symptoms and catatonia. Although the relationship between DOPA decarboxylase and the rate of DA synthesis is unclear (DOPA decarboxylase is not the rate-limiting step of DA synthesis), these observations are compatible with higher DA synthesis activity of DA neurons in schizophrenia, at least in subjects experiencing psychotic symptoms.

Amphetamine-induced DA Release

D_2-receptor imaging, combined with pharmacologic manipulation of DA release, enables more direct evaluation of DA presynaptic activity. Numerous groups have demonstrated that an acute increase in synaptic DA concentration is associated with decreased *in vivo* binding of ^{11}C-raclopride and ^{123}I-IBZM. These interactions have been demonstrated in rodents, nonhuman primates, and humans, using various methods to increase synaptic DA (40). It has also been consistently observed that the *in vivo* binding of spiperone and other butyrophenones is not as affected by acute fluctuations in endogenous DA levels as the binding of benzamides (40).

The decrease in ^{11}C-raclopride and ^{123}I-IBZM *in vivo* binding after acute amphetamine challenge has been well validated as a measure of the change in D_2-receptor stimulation by DA due to amphetamine-induced DA release. Manipulations that are known to inhibit amphetamine-induced DA release, such as pretreatment with the DA synthesis inhibitor α-methyl-*p*-tyrosine (α-MPT) or with the DAT blocker GR12909 also inhibit the amphetamine-induced decrease in ^{123}I-IBZM or ^{11}C-raclopride binding (41,42). Combined microdialysis and imaging experiments in primates demonstrated that the magnitude of the decrease in ligand binding was correlated with the magnitude of the increase in extracellular DA induced by the challenge (26,42), suggesting that this noninvasive technique provides an appropriate measure of the changes in synaptic DA levels.

Three out of three studies demonstrated that the amphetamine-induced decrease in ^{11}C-raclopride or ^{123}I-IBZM binding was elevated in untreated patients with schizophrenia compared with well-matched controls (24,26,27). A significant relationship was observed between the magnitude of DA release and transient induction or deterioration of positive symptoms. The increased amphetamine-induced DA release was observed in both first-episode/drug-naive patients and patients previously treated by antipsychotic drugs (43). Patients who were experiencing an episode of illness exacerbation (or a first episode of illness) at the time of the scan showed elevated amphetamine-induced DA release, whereas patients in remission showed DA release values not different from those of controls (43). These findings were generally interpreted as reflecting a larger DA release after amphetamine administration in the schizophrenic group. Another interpretation of these observations is that schizophrenia is associated with increased affinity of D_2 receptors for DA. Development of D_2-receptor imaging with radiolabeled agonists is needed to settle this issue (44).

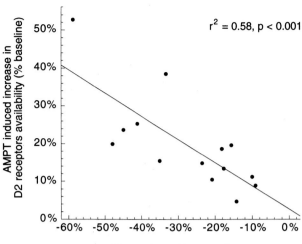

FIG. 7.1. Imaging dopamine transmission and prediction of therapeutic response in schizophrenia. There is a relationship between dopamine synaptic levels at intake, as estimated by the α-methyl-*p*-tyrosine (α-MPT) effect on iodine-123-iodobenzamide (^{123}I-IBZM) binding potential and the decrease in positive symptoms measured after 6 weeks of antipsychotic treatments. Patients with high dopamine (DA) synaptic levels showed a larger decrease in positive symptoms after treatment than patients with DA levels similar to those of controls (effect of α-MPT on ^{123}I-IBZM BP in control subjects was 9% ± 7%).

Baseline DA Release

A limitation of the amphetamine challenge imaging studies is that they measure changes in synaptic DA transmission after a nonphysiologic challenge (i.e., amphetamine) and do not provide any information about synaptic DA levels at baseline, that is, in the unchallenged state. Several laboratories have reported that acute depletion of synaptic DA in rodents is associated with an acute increase in the *in vivo* binding of ^{11}C-raclopride or ^{123}I-IBZM to D_2 receptors (40). The increased binding was observed *in vivo* but not *in vitro*, indicating that it was not due to receptor upregulation (45), but to removal of endogenous DA and unmasking of D_2 receptors previously occupied by DA. The acute DA-depletion technique was developed in humans using α-MPT to assess the degree of occupancy of D_2 receptors by DA (45, 46). Using this technique, one study (28) reported higher occupancy of D_2 receptors by DA in patients with schizophrenia experiencing an episode of illness exacerbation, compared with healthy controls. Again, assuming normal affinity of D_2 receptors for DA, the data are consistent with higher DA synaptic levels in patients with schizophrenia. Interestingly, increased D_2-receptor stimulation by DA at intake as measured with the α-MPT paradigm was predictive of rapid clinical response to antipsychotic drugs (28). This finding illustrates the potential of PET or SPECT molecular imaging to predict treatment response (Fig. 7.1).

DA Transporters

The data reviewed above are consistent with higher DA output in the striatum of patients with schizophrenia, which could be explained by increased density of DA terminals. Because striatal DATs are exclusively localized on DA terminals, this question was investigated by measuring binding of ^{123}I-β-CIT (47) or ^{18}F-CFT (48) in patients with schizophrenia. Both studies reported no differences in DAT binding between patients and controls. In addition, Laruelle et al. (47) reported no association between amphetamine-induced DA release and DAT density. Thus, the increased presynaptic output suggested by the studies reviewed above does not appear to be due to higher terminal density, an observation consistent with postmortem studies that failed to identify alterations in striatal DAT binding in schizophrenia (47).

Taken together, studies of striatal DA transmission in schizophrenia have provided support for the time-honored DA hypothesis of schizophrenia. Because animal data suggest that the antipsychotic effect of D_2-receptor antagonism is mediated by blockade of D_2 receptors in the mesolimbic as opposed to the nigrostriatal DA system (49–51), future studies will focus on studying striatal subsystems. Recent progress in PET instrumentation has provided the resolution necessary to differentiate the signal from ventral (i.e., limbic) and dorsal (i.e., motor) regions of the anterior striatum (52,53) (see Color Plate 18 following page 394). Moreover, the development of radiotracers suitable for imaging extra-striatal D_2 receptors such as ^{11}C-FLB-497 (54) and ^{18}F-fallypride (55) will enable the study of D_2-receptor transmission in other critical limbic regions such as the amygdala, the hippocampus, and the cingulate cortex.

Prefrontal DA Transmission

Most of the DA receptors in the PFC are of the D_1 subtype (56,57). A PET study with ^{11}C-SCH-23390 reported decreased density of D_1 receptors in younger patients with schizophrenia (20). In addition, low PFC D_1 density was associated with the severity of negative symptoms and poor performance on the Wisconsin Card Sorting Test. In contrast, a more recent study using the superior radiotracer ^{11}C-NNC-112 reported increased D_1-receptor availability in the dorsolateral PFC (DLPFC) of patients with schizophrenia (34). Furthermore, increased ^{11}C-NNC-112 binding was associated with poor performance on the "n-back" test of working memory (34).

The reason for the discrepancy in the results obtained with ^{11}C-SCH-23390 and ^{11}C-NNC-112 remains to be elucidated, but it is interesting to note that the binding of both radiotracers is differentially affected by endogenous DA competition and receptor trafficking (40). For example, chronic DA depletion in rodents is associated with decreased and increased *in vivo* binding of ^{11}C-SCH-23390 and ^{11}C-NNC-112, respectively (34). Thus, the contradictory observations of decreased ^{11}C-SCH-23390 binding (20) and increased ^{11}C-NNC-112 binding (34) observed in the PFC in patients with schizophrenia might in fact represent consequences of sustained deficit in prefrontal DA function. Much work remains to be done to validate this hypothesis. However, this point illustrates that the *in vivo* binding of radiotracers is affected by several factors that are not present in the typical *in vitro* situation, such as the impact of receptor trafficking on ligand affinity (40). This situation represents both a challenge, because the interpretation of the results is less straightforward, and an opportunity, because more information can be gained on the functions of the living neurons.

Serotonin Transmission

Abnormalities of 5-HT transporters (SERTs), $5-HT_{2A}$ receptors, and more consistently, $5-HT_{1A}$ receptors have been described in postmortem studies in schizophrenia, and these alterations might play a role in the pathophysiology of negative symptoms (58). Given the relatively recent development of radiotracers to study 5-HT receptors, only a limited number of imaging studies have been published. The concentration of SERT in the midbrain measured by ^{123}I-β-CIT is unaltered in patients with schizophrenia (47). Studies with more specific SERT ligands are warranted to assess the distribution of SERT in other brain areas, such as the PFC, where their density has been reported to be reduced in three out of four postmortem studies (58). A decrease in $5-HT_{2A}$ receptors has been reported in the PFC in four out of eight

postmortem studies (58). Three PET studies in drug-naive or drug-free patients with schizophrenia reported normal cortical $5-HT_{2A}$–receptor binding (59–61), although one study reported a significant decrease in PFC $5-HT_{2A}$ binding in a small group (n = 6) of drug-naive schizophrenic patients (62). The most consistent abnormality of 5-HT parameters reported in postmortem studies in schizophrenia is an increase in the density of $5-HT_{1A}$ receptors in the PFC, reported in seven out of eight studies (58). Several groups are currently evaluating the binding of this receptor *in vivo* with PET and ^{11}C-WAY-100907.

GABA-ergic Transmission

A robust body of findings suggests deficiency of GABA-ergic function in the PFC in schizophrenia (63,64). *In vivo* evaluation of GABA-ergic systems in schizophrenia has so far been limited to evaluation of benzodiazepine-receptor densities with SPECT and ^{123}I-iomazenil, and three of three studies comparing patients with schizophrenia and controls reported no significant regional differences (65–67). Although significant correlations between symptom clusters and regional benzodiazepine densities have been observed in some studies, these relationships have not been replicated. Thus, taken together, these studies are consistent with an absence of marked abnormalities of benzodiazepine-receptor concentration in the cortex of patients with schizophrenia. Alterations of GABA-ergic systems in schizophrenia might not involve benzodiazepine receptors (68) or might be restricted to certain cortical layers or classes of GABA-ergic cells that are beyond the resolutions of current radionuclide-based imaging techniques, which are in the 3.0- to 6.0-mm range with modern PET devices.

Antipsychotic Drug Occupancy Studies

Perhaps the most widespread use of neuroreceptor imaging in schizophrenia over the last decade has been the assessment of receptor occupancy achieved by typical and atypical antipsychotic drugs, a topic that has been the subject of recent reviews (69,70). The main focus has been on D_2-receptor occupancy, but $5-HT_{2A}$ and D_1 receptors have also been studied.

Studies have repeatedly confirmed the existence of a threshold of occupancy of striatal D_2 receptors (about 80%) above which extrapyramidal side effects (EPSs) are likely to occur (71). In general, studies have failed to observe a relationship between the degree of D_2-receptor occupancy and clinical response (72,73). However, most studies were performed at doses achieving more than 50% occupancy, and the minimum occupancy required for a therapeutic response remains undefined. Two studies performed with low doses of relatively selective D_2-receptor antagonists (haloperidol and raclopride) suggested that 50% to 60% occupancy was required to observe a rapid clinical response (74, 75). Clozapine, at clinically therapeutic doses, has been found to achieve only 40% to 60% D_2-receptor occupancy

(71,73,76), which in conjunction with its anticholinergic properties may account for its low risk for EPSs. Occupancy of 5-HT$_{2A}$ receptors by "5-HT$_{2A}$/D$_2$ balanced antagonists" such as risperidone does not confer protection against EPSs, because the threshold of D$_2$-receptor occupancy associated with EPSs is not markedly different between these drugs and drugs devoid of 5-HT$_{2A}$ antagonism (77–80). Studies with quetiapine suggest that at least with this agent, transient high occupancy of D$_2$ receptors might be sufficient to elicit clinical response (81,82).

An interesting question relates to putative differences in the degree of occupancy achieved by atypical antipsychotic drugs in striatal and extrastriatal areas. Pilowsky et al. (83) reported lower occupancy of striatal D$_2$ receptors compared with temporal cortex D$_2$ receptors in seven patients treated with the atypical antipsychotic drug clozapine, using the high-affinity SPECT ligand ^{123}I-epidipride. In contrast, typical antipsychotics were reported to achieve similar occupancy in striatal and extrastriatal areas, as measured with ^{11}C-FLB-457 (84) or ^{123}I-epidipride (85). It should be noted, however, that these very-high-affinity ligands do not allow accurate determination of D$_2$-receptor availability in the striatum (86). Conversely, ^{18}F-fallypride enables accurate determination of D$_2$-receptor availability in both striatal and extrastriatal areas (87), and preliminary PET experiments in primates with ^{18}F-fallypride indicate that clozapine and risperidone achieve similar D$_2$-receptor occupancy in striatal and extrastriatal regions (88). A recent study combining ^{11}C-FLB-457 imaging for extrastriatal D$_2$-receptor receptors and ^{11}C-raclopride imaging for striatal D$_2$ receptors suggested similar occupancy of D$_2$ receptors in both regions for both typical and atypical antipsychotic drugs (89). Finally, it is important to point out that the most robust evidence relative to the site of therapeutic effect of antipsychotic drugs in rodents points toward the nucleus accumbens (50,90), whereas the imaging studies reviewed above contrasted striatal versus mesotemporal D$_2$-receptor binding. Improved resolution of PET cameras now allows the dissociation of signals from the ventral and dorsal striatum (52,53), and it is now feasible to specifically study the clinical correlates of D$_2$-receptor occupancy in the ventral striatum in humans.

Another unresolved question is the discrepancy in the value of D$_2$-receptor occupancy obtained with ^{11}C-raclopride versus that obtained with ^{11}C-N-methyl spiperone (NMSP). The haloperidol plasma concentration associated with 50% inhibition of ^{11}C-NMSP binding (3 to 5 mg/mL) (91) is 10 times higher than that associated with 50% inhibition of ^{11}C-raclopride binding (0.32 ng/mL) (92). Quetiapine, at a dose of 750 mg, decreased ^{11}C-raclopride–specific binding by 51% but failed to affect ^{11}C-NMSP–specific binding (93). These observations contribute to the debate regarding differences between benzamide and butyrophenone binding to D$_2$ receptors.

AFFECTIVE DISORDERS

Numerous abnormalities of regional cerebral blood flow (rCBF) and metabolism have been demonstrated in affective disorders using SPECT and PET. These studies have implicated anatomic circuits involving subregions of PFC, striatum, amygdala, and hippocampus in the pathophysiology of these disorders (94,95). From a neurochemical perspective, abnormalities in several neurotransmitter systems may be relevant to the pathophysiology of depression. The 5-HT system has been the most extensively implicated, in part because of the antidepressant effect of medications that inhibit the synaptic reuptake of serotonin, as well as a wealth of postmortem, preclinical, and clinical data suggesting that reduced serotonergic function may be associated with depression (96). The recent availability of suitable PET radioligands for 5-HT$_{2A}$ receptors, 5-HT$_{1A}$ receptors, and SERT has allowed the in vivo investigation of their putative abnormalities in depression. These studies are summarized in Table 7.3. In addition, a number of studies have evaluated potential alterations in DA systems in major depression.

Major Depressive Disorders

Serotonin Transmission

5-HT$_2$ Receptors

The earliest PET study of 5-HT$_2$ receptors and depressive symptoms used ^{11}C-NMSP to investigate binding in patients with poststroke depression and reported increased binding (97). It is still not clear how this finding can be generalized to more common clinical presentations of depression. Another early study using 2-^{123}I-ketanserin and SPECT reported increased and asymmetric cortical uptake of the tracer in depressed patients when compared with controls (98). However, 2-^{123}I-ketanserin has significant limitations due to high nonspecific binding.

Since then, five PET studies have used newer 5-HT$_2$ PET radiotracers, ^{18}F-setoperone (99) and ^{18}F-altanserin (100), to investigate cortical 5-HT$_{2A}$–receptor binding in drug-free depressed patients (Table 7.3). Using ^{18}F-altanserin, Biver et al. (101) reported reduced tracer uptake in a region of the right hemisphere, including the orbitofrontal cortex and the anterior insular cortex. However, one limitation of ^{18}F-altanserin is that it produces radioactive lipophilic metabolites that probably cross the blood–brain barrier and contribute activity in the nondisplaceable compartment (102).

Two studies investigated midlife depression using ^{18}F-setoperone and concluded that there is no major change or asymmetry in 5-HT$_{2A}$ receptors (103,104). In both studies, the great majority of patients had been free of antidepressant medication for more than 6 months. A fourth study supported these negative findings and reported no significant alteration in 5-HT$_{2A}$–receptor binding in an untreated group of patients with late-life depression without cognitive impairment (105). Finally, the largest of the five studies (106) found a widespread reduction in 5-HT$_{2A}$–receptor binding potential and concluded that brain 5-HT$_{2A}$ receptors are decreased in patients with major depression. However, 40% of the patients in this study had been drug free for only 2 weeks

TABLE 7.3. *Imaging 5-HT system in major depression*

Target	Study	Patient (n)	Mean age (yr)	Antidepressant-free duration	Method of measuring BP	Receptor binding	Radioligand
5-HT$_2$	(101)	8 (2 men, 6 women)	48	≥3 wk Possibly confounded by effects of other medications and withdrawal from BZD	SPM on normalized regional counts at pseudo-equilibrium, with *post hoc* ratio (cortex-to-cerebellum) in identified regions	↓ 5-HT$_{2A}$ in orbitofrontal and anterior insular cortical regions	^{18}F-altanserin
	(104)	7 (3 men, 4 women)	40	≥2 wk (BZD permitted) All but one were antidepressant free >1 yr	Estimation by subtraction (cortex minus cerebellum as %id/L) at pseudo-equilibrium ROI	Slight (<5%) ↓ 5-HT$_{2A}$ in frontal region only Concluded there was no major change	^{18}F-setoperone
	(103)	14 (12 men, 2 women)	32	≥2 weeks (BZD permitted) All but one were antidepressant free >6 mo	Estimation by ratio (cortex-to-cerebellum) at pseudo-equilibrium ROI	No change or asymmetry of 5-HT$_{2A}$	^{18}F-setoperone
	(105)	11 (4 men, 7 women)	65	Untreated No concomitant medication	Kinetic modeling (graphical method of Logan et al. with arterial input function) ROI	No change in 5-HT$_{2A}$	^{18}F-altanserin
	(106)	20 (9 men, 11 women)	40	≥2 wk No concomitant medication	Estimation by ratio (cortex-to-cerebellum) at pseudo-equilibrium. SPM plus ROI	Widespread ↓ 5-HT$_{2A}$	^{18}F-setoperone
5-HT$_{1A}$	(118)	15 (all men)	38	≥12 wk (seven were drug naive, eight were drug free for 12–1196 wk)	Simplified reference tissue (cerebellum) kinetic modeling. ROI and SPM	Modest widespread ↓ cortical 5-HT$_{1A}$	^{11}C-WAY-100635
	(110)	12 (5 men, 7 women)	36	≥2 wk (≥8 wk for fluoxetine) Range, 2–130 wk	Simplified reference tissue (cerebellum) kinetic modeling. ROI	↓ 5-HT$_{1A}$ in raphe and medial temporal cortex	^{11}C-WAY-100635
SERT	(137)	15 (7 men, 8 women)	44	≥3 wk (six were drug naive, nine were drug free for 3 wk to 7 yr)	Estimation by ratio [(brainstemoccipital)/occipital] at equilibrium ROI	↓ SERT in brainstem	^{123}I-β-CIT
	(138)	11 (2 men, 9 women) Depressed SAD patients	30	≥6 mo (six were drug naive, five were drug free for 6–42 mo)	Estimation by ratio [(ROI-cerebellum)/cerebellum] at equilibrium ROI	↓ SERT inthalamus-hypothalamus. No ↓ in pons-midbrain.	^{123}I-β-CIT

BZD, benzodiazepine; BP, binding potential; %id/L, expressed as percentage of injected dose per liter of brain tissue; ROI, region of interest; SPM, statistical parametric mapping; SAD, seasonal affective disorder; SERT, 5-HT transporters.

before scanning. This factor may be significant, because most antidepressants downregulate 5-HT$_{2A}$ receptors (104, 107,108).

In summary, three studies reported no significant alteration in 5-HT$_{2A}$–receptor binding in major depression, and two studies found reduced 5-HT$_{2A}$ receptors. Differences between studies might stem from methodologic issues, illness heterogeneity, and medication effects. None of the recent studies confirmed the earlier findings of increased binding (97,98). Similarly, the increase in 5-HT$_{2A}$ receptors found in some, but not all, postmortem studies of depressed suicidal victims (109) has not been confirmed by *in vivo* investigations. Therefore, there is currently no strong evidence supporting the hypothesis that depression per se is associated with marked alterations of 5-HT$_{2A}$–receptor density.

5-HT$_{1A}$ Receptors

Two lines of evidence have implicated the 5-HT$_{1A}$ receptors in depression. The first is the finding that depressed patients have blunted neuroendocrine responses to 5-HT$_{1A}$–receptor agonists *in vivo* and the second is the dense distribution of these receptors in the hippocampus. Recent theories have implicated interactions between stress, corticosteroids, growth factors, and hippocampal 5-HT$_{1A}$ receptors in depression (110–112). Postmortem studies of 5-HT$_{1A}$ receptors in suicide and depression have been inconsistent, showing increased, decreased, and unchanged 5-HT_{1A}–receptor levels in various regions (113–117). These discrepancies may reflect the possible confounding effects of suicidality, antemortem medications, differences between radioligands, and differences in the regulation of 5-HT_{1A} receptors by corticosteroids and local levels of 5-HT in different brain regions. The results of *in vivo* PET imaging of 5-HT_{1A} receptors in depressed patients are therefore of interest.

Two PET studies have investigated 5-HT_{1A} receptors in unmedicated depressed subjects using carbonyl-^{11}C-WAY-100635 and both have reported reductions in receptor binding (Table 7.3). The first study (118) found modest (approximately 10%) but significant widespread reductions in binding potential in cortical regions, including the medial temporal cortex (hippocampus and amygdala) in a group of 15 men with major depression. Subsequently, Drevets et al. (110) reported reductions in the medial temporal cortex (27%) and raphe (41%) in a study that limited its primary hypothesis to these two regions. This group of subjects included both unipolar and bipolar depressed patients. All subjects had first-degree relatives with mood disorders. Interestingly, the differences found were largely accounted for by the subjects with bipolar disorder and those with unipolar depression who had relatives with bipolar disorder.

Additional studies are warranted to confirm these findings of a generalized decrease in 5-HT_{1A} receptors in depression. Because a major depressive episode is associated with hyperactivity of the hypothalamic–pituitary–adrenal axis and increased cortisol levels might be associated with 5-HT_{1A}–receptor downregulation (119–122), these findings might be secondary to the neuroendocrine dysregulation associated with depression.

5-HT Transporter

Reductions in SERT levels in depressed patients have been reported in numerous postmortem studies (109). The first ligand used to image SERT *in vivo* was the SPECT radiotracer ^{123}I-β-CIT. β-CIT binds to both DAT and SERT with comparable affinity ($K_i = 1.4$ and 2.4 nmol/L for DAT and SERT, respectively) (123,124). The lack of DAT versus SERT selectivity is not a problem for measuring DAT in the striatum, as the density of SERT in striatum is much lower than that of DAT (124). However, in the midbrain, this proportion is reversed, and the β-CIT midbrain uptake mostly corresponds to SERT binding (125,126). Studies in nonhuman primates and humans have shown that in the midbrain, ^{123}I-β-CIT is selectively displaced by administration of selective serotonin reuptake inhibitors (SSRIs) (but not by DAT-selective drugs) (125,127). Iodine-123-β-CIT has been extensively used in clinical studies both for striatal DAT (47,128–133) and for midbrain SERT evaluation (47, 134–136).

In depression, findings from two SPECT studies using ^{123}I-β-CIT were in agreement with postmortem results

(Table 7.3). A reduction in SERT binding was found in the midbrain in patients with unipolar depression (137), and in the thalamus–hypothalamus region in depressed patients with seasonal affective disorder (138).

A selective SERT radiotracer is required to investigate SERT density in other regions of the brain. The first PET radiotracer available to measure SERT in humans was ^{11}C-McN-5652 (139). The usefulness of ^{11}C-McN-5652 as a PET tracer for SERT was validated in primates (140) and humans (141–143). However, ^{11}C-McN-5652 has many limitations, which include high nonspecific binding, poor signal-to-noise ratio, nonmeasurable free fraction in the plasma, and slow clearance from the brain (144). Therefore, studies using ^{11}C-McN-5652 require a long scanning time (up to 120 minutes), and this ligand can provide reliable quantification of SERT only in regions of relatively high SERT density (midbrain, thalamus, and striatum).

More recently, compounds from the phenylamine class have emerged as promising targets for both SPECT and PET tracer development. Iodine-123-ADAM (145) is a highly selective SPECT imaging agent for SERT. Its ^{11}C-labeled counterpart, ^{11}C-ADAM, was recently reported (146). Another compound in this series, ^{11}C-DASB, was recently introduced and has been evaluated in rats (147) and humans (148). Thus, it is anticipated that several studies will be performed to evaluate SERT density with PET in patients with major depression. If the results obtained with ^{123}I-β-CIT are confirmed, the reduction in SERT density might provide a useful biomarker for this disorder.

Dopamine Transmission

The critical role of DA in brain-reward systems, the reports of low cerebrospinal fluid homovanillic acid levels in depressed patients, the association of major depression with Parkinson disease, and the enhancement of dopaminergic activity by several antidepressant treatments suggest that a deficiency of dopaminergic function might be associated with major depression (149–152). Five studies used ^{123}I-IBZM to compare striatal D_2-receptor availability in patients with major depression and control subjects. Two of the five studies reported higher ^{123}I-IBZM–specific binding in the striatum of depressed subjects compared with controls (153, 154), whereas three studies reported no change (155–157). Amphetamine-induced DA release was also assessed in patients with major depression and was found to be unchanged (157).

Two studies examined ^{123}I-β-CIT striatal binding in patients with major depression and yielded conflicting results: one study reported normal levels of striatal DAT in patients with major depression (134), whereas the other one reported increased DAT levels (158). Finally, ^{18}F-DOPA uptake in the left caudate was observed to be significantly lower in depressed patients with psychomotor retardation than in depressed patients with high impulsivity and in comparison subjects (159). Thus, major depression per se does not appear to be consistently associated with alteration of the dopaminergic parameters at the level of the whole striatum. However, DA might play a role in the neurobiology underlying some clinical features of depression, such as psychomotor retardation.

Antidepressant Drug Occupancy Studies

Given that ligands suitable to label SERT were only developed recently, a limited number of studies assessing the occupancy of SERT achieved by antidepressant drugs have been published so far. Pirker et al. (127) compared ^{123}I-β-CIT midbrain-specific binding to SERT in a group of 12 depressed patients treated with 20 to 60 mg per day of citalopram for a minimum of 1 week and a group of control subjects. The reduction in ^{123}I-β-CIT binding in the midbrain of the citalopram-treated patients was reported to be approximately 50% of controls. In contrast, Meyer et al. (160), using ^{11}C-DASB, reported 77% SERT occupancy during treatment with 20 mg per day of citalopram. Kent et al. (161), using ^{11}C-McN-5652, and Meyer et al. (160), using ^{11}C-DASB, reported near-complete (more than 80%) occupancy of SERT by paroxetine at therapeutic doses (20 to 40 mg/kg). Thus, the minimal occupancy of SERT associated with therapeutic response to SSRIs is still not defined, but it appears that at least with citalopram and paroxetine, high SERT occupancies are achieved after administration of these drugs at therapeutic doses.

The time lag (typically 1 to 2 weeks) in the onset of therapeutic effect of several classes of antidepressant medications may be related to the need for downregulation of 5-HT$_{1A}$ somatodendritic autoreceptors in the raphe before a net increase in forebrain 5-HT neurotransmission can occur (162). Because of this phenomenon, several groups have investigated whether the concomitant use of pindolol (antagonist at 5-HT$_{1A}$ receptor and β-adrenoceptor) with an SSRI antidepressant might accelerate the onset of an improvement in mood. The results of clinical trials were inconsistent (163, 164). Most clinical studies have used a dose of 7.5 mg daily of pindolol. Several PET centers have recently conducted human occupancy studies of pindolol at the postsynaptic and somatodendritic 5-HT$_{1A}$ receptor (165–167) (see Color Plate 19 following page 394). The consensus from these studies is that the dose used in clinical studies was too low to provide appropriate and reliable blockade of 5-HT$_{1A}$ receptors and that this factor might explain the limited success of this strategy in previous clinical trials. These studies provide another illustration of the potential of PET neuroreceptor imaging to facilitate drug development.

Bipolar Disorder

In comparison with major depressive disorder, only limited radioligand PET studies have been reported in patients with bipolar disorders. As discussed above, it may be significant that the findings of reduced 5-HT$_{1A}$–receptor binding in the medial temporal cortex and raphe of depressed patients

(110) were largely accounted for by the subjects with bipolar disorder and those with unipolar depression who had relatives with bipolar disorder.

Because of the relationship between mania and psychosis, a number of PET studies have investigated the DA system in bipolar disorders. D$_1$-receptor binding in the frontal cortex was reported to be decreased in a study of 10 symptomatically heterogeneous, drug-free bipolar patients (168). Increases in D$_2$-like (i.e., D$_2$, D$_3$, and D$_4$) receptor density in the striatum were found in 7 psychotic patients with bipolar disorder when compared with 7 nonpsychotic patients with bipolar disorder and 24 control subjects. The authors concluded that an increase in D$_2$-like receptors is associated with the state of psychosis, rather than with a diagnosis of bipolar disorder (169). As part of the same studies, Gjedde and Wong (170) also reported findings consistent with an elevated concentration of synaptic DA in bipolar patients with psychosis, but not in nonpsychotic bipolar patients. On the other hand, amphetamine-induced DA release was reported to be normal in euthymic patients with bipolar disorders (171).

In conclusion, few investigations have been reported using PET molecular imaging techniques in patients with bipolar disorders, and the findings reported so far might be related to clinical states (depression, mania with psychosis), rather than to the bipolar condition per se.

ANXIETY DISORDERS

A number of PET studies have investigated rCBF changes associated with induced anxiety in healthy volunteers (172–177). Although there is considerable variability in the findings, a number of para–limbic-cortical regions have been consistently implicated, including medial PFC, anterior cingulate cortex, orbital PFC, anterior temporal cortex, parahippocampal gyrus, and the claustrum–insular–amygdala region. In contrast to this abundant functional literature, anxiety disorders have been less studied with PET molecular imaging techniques.

Generalized Anxiety Disorder

Because benzodiazepines are the prototypical anxiolytic drugs, evaluation of potential abnormalities in the benzodiazepine-receptor distribution is of interest in anxiety disorders. An initial study in generalized anxiety disorder (GAD) with ^{123}I-NNC-13-8241 reported reduced binding in the left temporal pole in 10 drug-naive female patients with GAD compared with age- and sex-matched healthy controls (178). However, this was not confirmed in a PET study using ^{11}C-FMZ, which found no differences in drug-free patients (179).

Panic Disorder

Two studies using ^{123}I-iomazenil SPECT reported decreased uptake in the lateral temporal region (180) and increased binding in the right orbitofrontal cortex in benzodiazepine-naive patients (181). A third ^{123}I-iomazenil SPECT study, using a more quantitative measurement of regional binding potential, reported decreased binding in left hippocampus and precuneus in patients with panic disorder relative to controls. Interestingly, patients who had a panic attack at the time of the scan had a relative decrease in binding in the PFC, suggesting that benzodiazepine function in the PFC may be involved in changes in state-related panic (182). In a fully quantitative PET study using ^{11}C-FMZ in medication-free patients, Malizia et al. (183) found a global reduction in benzodiazepine binding throughout the brain in patients with panic disorder compared with controls. The largest regional decreases were in the right orbitofrontal cortex and right insula (183). Thus, there is relatively consistent evidence that panic disorder might be associated with alterations in the GABA-ergic system, the primary "endogenous" anxiolytic system. Nevertheless, the anatomic localization of these changes and their relationship with illness states remain to be clarified.

Social Phobia (Social Anxiety Disorder)

Neurobiologic mechanisms underlying social phobia, including neuroimaging findings, have been reviewed recently (184–186). One SPECT study using ^{123}I-β-CIT to label DATs in the striatum reported that densities were markedly lower in patients with social phobia than in age- and gender-matched controls (187). Another study using ^{123}I-IBZM reported a significant decrease in D_2-receptor binding potential in patients with social phobia compared with controls (188). Together, these studies suggest that the DA system might play a role in the pathophysiology of this illness. A recent study using ^{11}C-McN-5652 failed to find marked alterations in SERT in patients with social phobia, despite an excellent response to SSRI treatment (161).

Obsessive-compulsive Disorder

Obsessive-compulsive disorder (OCD) has been extensively studied by SPECT and PET metabolic studies. These studies have generated remarkably consistent results—that is, increased metabolism in the orbitofrontal cortex and striatum in symptomatic patients, which normalizes with successful treatment (189–195). These findings have implicated abnormalities in the PFC–basal ganglia–thalamic circuits, which originate from the orbitofrontal cortex in the pathophysiology of OCD and the related neuropsychiatric disorder Gilles de la Tourette syndrome. Lower pretreatment metabolism in the orbitofrontal cortex has been found to predict greater improvement on SSRI medication (193); however, different treatment modalities may have different predictive levels of pretreatment metabolism (195).

Abnormalities of serotonergic neurotransmission in OCD have been hypothesized on the basis of the therapeutic efficacy of medications that selectively increase synaptic 5-HT levels (including SSRIs and clomipramine) in nondepressed

OCD patients, and the high level of comorbid depression in OCD. No neuroreceptor PET studies have so far been reported in OCD, but studies of the regional binding of 5-HT$_{1A}$ and 5-HT$_{2A}$ receptors and the SERTs are currently under investigation in several PET centers.

Posttraumatic Stress Disorder

The results of functional neuroimaging and other studies in posttraumatic stress disorder (PTSD) have recently been reviewed in depth (196,197). It has been hypothesized that symptoms of PTSD are mediated by a dysfunction of the anterior cingulate, with a failure to inhibit amygdalar activation and/or an intrinsic lower threshold of amygdalar response to fearful stimuli. The model further proposes that hippocampal atrophy is a result of the chronic hyperarousal symptoms mediated by amygdalar activation (196). Only one neuroreceptor imaging study has been reported in this population showing lower ^{123}I-iomazenil binding in the PFC of patients with PTSD compared with comparison subjects, suggesting that this condition is associated, like panic disorder and perhaps GAD, with low benzodiazepine-receptor levels (198).

PERSONALITY DISORDERS

Personality disorders (PDs) are characterized by stable patterns of maladaptive behavior. Some, such as paranoid, schizoid, schizotypal, avoidant, and obsessive-compulsive PDs, have stable patterns of behavior reminiscent of their corresponding clinical disorders but do not reach a sufficient severity, and their response to medication is generally poor. It might therefore be expected that some PDs might be associated with neurobiologic abnormalities similar to, but less marked than, the disorders described in this chapter. Functional imaging studies have now begun to address the issue of how neurochemical brain functions may be associated with normal and pathologic personality traits.

A number of studies have investigated differences within the normal range of personality traits or temperaments in healthy subjects. Most receptor PET studies have so far investigated dopaminergic neurotransmission. Studies using ^{11}C-raclopride report that the traits of depression and personal detachment are related to low D_2-receptor density in the striatum (199,200). However, the relationship is not evident on all measures of detachment (201,202). Detachment was also found to be associated with low DAT binding in the putamen (203). These findings are also interesting in view of the association between social phobia and low DAT and D_2 receptor levels (187,188), and it has been argued that these neurobiologic findings might underlie a commonality between detachment and social phobia (204).

Beyond the DA system, a significant negative correlation has recently been reported between cortical 5-HT$_{1A}$ binding potential and trait anxiety (205). The authors report that this is consistent both with animal models that have shown higher anxiety in mice lacking 5-HT$_{1A}$ receptors and clinical trials demonstrating anxiolytic properties of partial 5-HT$_{1A}$ agonists (206).

Abnormalities of serotonergic neurotransmission are implicated in the pathophysiology of impulsive-aggressive behaviors, and PET studies have contributed to this body of evidence. ^{18}F-fluorodeoxyglucose studies of the effects of fenfluramine-stimulated serotonin release report a significantly blunted response in areas of PFC associated with regulation of impulsive behavior in patients with impulsive-aggressive personality difficulties (207,208). Moreover, serotonin synthesis has been shown to be low in this region in patients with borderline PD (209).

CONDUCT DISORDER

Interesting findings have been recently reported in the study of attention deficit hyperactivity disorder (ADHD). In a preliminary study of six adults with ADHD, Dougherty et al. (210) observed a large increase in DAT availability (70%) compared with controls. This finding was replicated in a larger sample by Dresel et al. (211), using ^{99m}Tc-TRODAT-1, the first ^{99m}Tc-labeled DAT SPECT ligand. If confirmed, these findings could lead to a clinical application, because the diagnosis of this condition can be difficult. Furthermore, the availability of a ^{99m}Tc-labeled SPECT ligand might enhance the practicality of such an investigation.

The DAT blocker methylphenidate is the treatment of choice of ADHD, and oral therapeutic doses induce a significant decrease in ^{11}C-raclopride binding (212), presumably due to increased synaptic DA levels. This method might provide a tool to monitor the biological effectiveness (increased synaptic DA) of the treatment and be useful in the evaluation of nonresponders.

SUBSTANCE ABUSE

Cocaine

Cocaine abuse has been extensively studied using PET-based molecular neuroimaging techniques. Most of the work has focused on changes in striatal DA that occur with chronic cocaine use.

D_2 Receptors

A reduction in striatal DA D$_2$ receptors has been demonstrated by Volkow et al. (213–216) using both ^{18}F-N-methylspiroperidol and ^{11}C-raclopride. The decreases reported in these studies are 35%, 14%, 20%, and 11%, respectively. In addition, this group has shown that these decreases correlate with years of use and appear to be long lasting in a group of subjects rescanned after 3 months of inpatient rehabilitation (214). Of note, studies of D$_2$-receptor availability using PET have also shown a reduction in D$_2$ receptors in heroin abuse (217) and alcoholism (218,219).

The results of these studies raise the question of whether a decrease in D$_2$ receptors is the result of years of drug abuse or represents a neurochemical risk factor for developing substance abuse. Volkow et al. (220) investigated this question in a study of healthy controls who were administered methylphenidate and asked to describe their subjective effects as pleasant, unpleasant, or neutral. Subjects who rated their experience as pleasant were found to have lower measures of D$_2$-receptor availability (14%) than subjects who reported an unpleasant experience. Nader et al. (221,222) more definitively addressed this question in a study of rhesus monkeys who were scanned before and after becoming exposed to a social stress and before cocaine self-administration studies. The monkeys, who had been reared in individual cages, were placed in social groups so a social hierarchy was established. After this change, the authors reported that the monkeys who were lowest in the social hierarchy had 20% lower D$_2$-receptor availability than monkeys who were highest in social order. Furthermore, the monkeys who were lower were found to self-administer cocaine more readily than the high-ranking monkeys. This is a study of critical importance because it demonstrates that low D$_2$-receptor levels may be a risk factor for developing substance dependence. Furthermore, this risk factor is not static, in that it is affected by environment, which has strong implications in the development of treatment and prevention strategies.

Stimulant-induced DA Release

As described above, PET and SPECT studies can be used to measure changes in subcortical DA transmission in the human brain after psychostimulant administration. In control subjects, a stimulant-induced decrease in D$_2$-receptor availability has been well characterized and is on the order of 10% to 20 % (26,27,216,223–228).

Studies of healthy controls have shown that the percentage decrease in radioligand binding (i.e., the increase in DA release) is positively correlated with pleasurable subjective effects (224,226,228). DA transmission in the ventral striatum mediates the reinforcing effects of drugs of abuse (229–231). PET studies showed a greater decrease in ^{11}C-raclopride binding in the ventral versus the dorsal striatum in healthy controls in response to an amphetamine challenge (228) and in response to a monetary reward (232). Collectively, these studies suggest that an excess in subcortical DA would correlate with increased reward value and might mediate the reinforcing effects of drugs of abuse.

However, cocaine abusers have been shown to have a blunted DA response to psychostimulants. A study of Volkow et al. (216) used ^{11}C-raclopride to measure the change in D$_2$-receptor availability before and after an intravenous dose of 0.5 mg/kg methylphenidate in healthy controls and cocaine abusers who had been abstinent for 3 to 6 weeks. The authors reported a 9% decrease in ^{11}C-raclopride binding in the cocaine abusers compared with a 21% decrease in healthy controls. Malison et al. (233) performed a similar study in abstinent cocaine abusers and controls using ^{123}I-IBZM and an amphetamine challenge (0.3 mg/kg intravenously) and reported a 1% change in binding in the cocaine abusers compared with a 10% decrease in controls.

DOPA Decarboxylase

The findings above of blunted presynaptic DA function in cocaine abusers are supported by the study of Wu et al. (234), showing a reduction in the rate of uptake of ^{18}F-6-fluoro-DOPA in abstinent cocaine abusers.

Dopamine Transporter

Three *in vivo* studies of DAT in cocaine abusers have been published, and this body of work has failed to provide a clear picture of the status of DAT in cocaine abusers. Using ^{11}C-cocaine, no changes in DAT were observed in detoxified (more than 1 month) cocaine abusers (215). We should, however, mention that in this study a decrease in ^{11}C-cocaine total distribution volume (V_t)was seen in both the striatum and the cerebellum (215). When normalizing striatal V_t by cerebellum V_t (i.e., using the distribution volume ratio), no differences were apparent between cocaine abusers and controls, and the authors concluded that DAT availability was unchanged. Yet, another interpretation of these data could be that cocaine abusers show a decrease in DAT density and a decrease in ^{11}C-cocaine nonspecific binding. The same group also studied ^{11}C-cocaine uptake in currently abusing subjects (235) and found no differences between these subjects and controls in DAT availability. However, 15 out of the 20 currently abusing subjects had a urine test positive for cocaine at the time of scan, which is expected to affect the results of the imaging study. Finally, Malison et al. (133) showed a significant upregulation of DATs, measured with SPECT and ^{123}I-β-CIT, in the striatum of recently detoxified (less than 96 hours) cocaine abusers. Such upregulation was not observed after prolonged abstinence.

On the other hand, studies of DAT occupancy by cocaine have generated critical information. Volkow et al. (236) reported that a DAT occupancy of at least 47% is needed to produce the subjective effects of cocaine. These data suggest that any treatment approach to cocaine abuse in which the transporter is blocked would need to produce somewhere between 60% and 90% occupancy of the transporters. This issue was addressed in an occupancy study of mazindol, a nonselective catecholamine reuptake inhibitor (237). This study showed that the clinical dosage generally used produced only a modest occupancy of 16% to 23% and would therefore not be expected to have sufficient efficacy.

Serotonin Transporter

Jacobsen et al. (238) reported increased serotonin transporter (SERT) availability in the diencephalon and midbrain (17% and 32%, respectively) using ^{123}I-β-CIT, suggesting that chronic cocaine abuse affects the serotonin system as well.

Mu Opiate Receptors

Zubieta et al. (239) reported an increase in mu-receptor availability using ^{11}C-carfentanil in the caudate, thalamus, cingulate, frontal, and temporal cortices (239). This finding is of particular interest given the interaction between the dopaminergic and opioid systems in the direct and indirect pathways of the striatum (240,241).

Overall, the studies in cocaine abuse demonstrate a dysregulation of the DA system in this disorder. The findings of decreased ^{18}F-DOPA accumulation, decreased amphetamine-induced and methylphenidate-induced DA release, and decreased D_2-receptor density suggest a functional deficit in D_2-receptor transmission at the level of the whole striatum in cocaine abusers. The reduction in D_2 receptors appears to be a risk factor for cocaine abuse (or addiction in general), rather than a consequence of the disorder.

Methamphetamine

Two imaging studies in methamphetamine abusers have demonstrated a significant decrease in the DAT using PET. McCann et al. (242) reported the results of six methamphetamine abusers and four methcathinone users using ^{11}C-WIN-35428. The methamphetamine abusers had a decrease in DAT availability of about 25% in the putamen and caudate compared with controls, and a similar reduction was seen in the methcathinone abusers (242). Volkow et al. (243) studied 15 methamphetamine abusers who had 2 weeks of monitored abstinence before scanning with ^{11}C-D-*threo*-methylphenidate. Compared with controls, the methamphetamine abusers had a 28% decrease in DAT availability in the caudate and a 21% decrease in the putamen (243). The authors also found that the decrease in DAT availability correlated with years of abuse and with impairment in motor and memory tasks. Both studies are in agreement with a postmortem report of reduced DAT density in the striatum of chronic methamphetamine abusers, as well as decreases in DA and tyrosine hydroxylase (244).

Evidence from studies of Parkinson disease supports the hypothesis that the reduction in DAT availability reflects a loss of DA neurons that is detectable with functional imaging (245–247). Based on this interpretation, these studies raise the issue of whether this decrease is reversible or whether methamphetamine abuse results in neurotoxicity to the dopaminergic neurons. PET and postmortem studies in nonhuman primates have shown that methamphetamine exposure results in decreased DAT and other markers of dopaminergic transmission, suggesting a frank loss of dopaminergic neurons (248,249). However, one study suggested that this reduction might be reversible after prolonged abstinence (250). Overall, the PET data demonstrate that methamphetamine abuse in humans results in a reduction in the DAT level and raise concerns about the neurotoxicity associated with this addiction.

Ecstasy

PET and SPECT were also used to evaluate the potential neurotoxic effects of methylenedioxymethamphetamine (MDMA, ecstasy). McCann et al. (251) used the radioligand ^{11}C-McN-5652 to measure SERT availability in 14 subjects who had abused MDMA on at least 25 occasions. In this study, the authors used the inactive enantiomer $(-)^{11}$C-McN-5652 as a measure of nonspecific binding. They reported a significant global decrease in specific binding, including in the cerebellum, in abstinent MDMA abusers. However, Parsey et al. (142) reported that the use of $(-)^{11}$C-McN-5652 to measure nonspecific binding resulted in an overestimation of specific binding, specifically in cortical regions.

Two other studies have imaged MDMA abusers with the SPECT radioligand ^{123}I-β-CIT (252,253). Both studies have serious methodologic problems. The authors report results in cortical regions using ^{123}I-β-CIT, yet the suitability of ^{123}I-β-CIT to quantify SERT in cortical regions has not been established (125,254,255). Neither study measured binding in the midbrain, which is the only region in which the SERT can be reliably measured with this radioligand. One study presented ^{123}I-β-CIT binding in the striatum as a measure of SERT density, despite the fact that ^{123}I-β-CIT–specific binding in the striatum corresponds to DAT binding (125, 127,255). Thus, these studies did not contribute dependable information regarding the potential serotonergic toxicity of ecstasy.

Two studies used SPECT and the radioligand ^{123}I-R93274 to measure 5-HT$_{2A}$ receptors in MDMA abusers (256,257) but reported conflicting results. Although the specific binding of ^{123}I-R93274 is selective for the 5-HT$_{2A}$ receptor, the ratio of specific binding to nonspecific binding is very low in the cortex (258,259), making a reliable measurement of this receptor problematic (258).

Overall, the data regarding MDMA neurotoxicity for serotonergic neurons in human abusers are still inconclusive. At this point, it is critical to replicate the study of McCann et al. (251), preferably with the newer generation of SERT radioligands that allow reliable measurement of this transporter in both cortical and subcortical regions (145–148).

Heroin

Surprisingly few radioligand imaging studies have been conducted in opiate-dependent subjects despite the clear indication from decades of treatment studies of a significant change in brain chemistry in this disorder.

Two groups have measured opioid-receptor occupancy in heroin-dependent subjects undergoing treatment. Kling et al. (260) reported on heroin-dependent subjects maintained on methadone using ^{18}F-cyclofoxy, a mu and kappa opioid an-tagonist (261). A decrease in receptor availability of 19% to 32% was seen in methadone-treated subjects compared with healthy volunteers. Zubieta et al. (262) reported on the occupancy of buprenorphine, a mu partial agonist soon to be approved as an alternative to methadone. Subjects were given 2-mg and 16-mg sublingual doses and were scanned using the radioligand ^{11}C-carfentanil, which is selective for the mu opioid receptor (263). The 2-mg dose resulted in 36% to 50% occupancy and the 16-mg dose resulted in 79% to 95% occupancy of the mu receptors across brain regions. Behavioral pharmacology studies show that doses of 8 to 16 mg of buprenorphine are needed to reduce heroin self-administration (264,265). Therefore, the study of Zubieta et al. (262) suggests that a higher occupancy of the mu receptor than that reported by Kling et al. (260) may be necessary for a therapeutic effect.

Zubieta et al (262) reported marked increases in mu-receptor availability in detoxified heroin-dependent subjects compared with healthy controls. However, this study included only three heroin-dependent subjects. Lastly, reductions in D$_2$-receptor availability of 18% in the putamen and 13% in the caudate were reported in the opiate-dependent subjects compared with healthy controls (217). This study is of particular interest given the reduction in D$_2$-receptor availability associated with other addictions, including cocaine dependence (213,214,216), alcoholism (218,219), and even obesity (266).

Nicotine

PET studies have investigated alterations in the dopaminergic system in the basal ganglia in cigarette smoking and demonstrated some interesting findings. In a series of studies, Fowler et al. (267–270) investigated levels of monoamine oxidase A (MAO-A) and MAO-B in smokers and showed marked and global decreases in both enzymes. MAO-A and MAO-B exist in neurons and glial cells and both enzymes degrade DA. MAO-B activity was measured using ^{11}C-L-deprenyl (271). Smokers were found to have a 42% decrease in global MAO-B activity compared with controls (267,270). Interestingly, a study in former smokers showed that levels of MAO-B activity returned to baseline after smoking cessation (269). In a later study, this same group demonstrated a decrease in MAO-A activity in the brains of cigarette smokers using ^{11}C-clorgyline (268). In this study, smokers had an average reduction of 28% in MAO-A activity across brain regions, with a 22% decrease in the basal ganglia (268). Decreased activities of MAO-A and MAO-B are expected to be associated with increased DA availability.

Salokangas et al. (272) used ^{18}F-fluoro-DOPA to measure presynaptic DA and reported higher uptake in the striatum in smokers, a finding that could be explained by an increase in DOPA decarboxylase activity or a decrease in MAO activity. A study by Dagher et al. (273) reported a reduction in D$_1$-receptor availability using ^{11}C-SCH-23390 in the striatum. The authors reported a greater decrease in the ventral striatum (15.6%) compared with the caudate and putamen (9.5% and 10.1%, respectively). Lastly, Staley et al. (274) investigated DAT and SERT density in the striatum and midbrain, respectively, in smokers and healthy controls using ^{123}I-β-CIT. No difference was seen in DAT availability between these groups, but there was a trend toward increased ^{123}I-β-CIT binding in the midbrain.

Overall, these findings are consistent with the hypothesis of alterations of the DA system in nicotine smokers, but much work remains to be done to better understand the potential role of this dysregulation in the maintenance of nicotine addiction.

Alcohol

The dopaminergic system has been the most investigated neurochemical system using SPECT and PET in alcohol research, due to the wealth of preclinical data suggesting a role for DA in the reward system and clinical data suggesting alterations in DA function in alcoholic patients.

Genetic studies have suggested, although not conclusively, an association between a nonencoding polymorphism of the D_2 receptor and alcoholism. An initial postmortem study by Noble et al. (275) described a lower D_2-receptor density in A1 carriers, but not in the alcoholic group per se. This was followed by two PET studies in small samples of alcoholic patients, which found low striatal D_2-receptor binding potential in alcoholics. A study performed with ^{11}C-raclopride reported a 20% decrease in D_2-receptor binding potential in nine abstinent (1 to 60 weeks) alcoholics and eight age-matched controls (276). Similar findings have been reported by Volkow et al. (277) in a group of 10 alcoholic subjects. An interesting study attempting to relate relapse and D_2 density found an increased density of D_2 receptors as measured with ^{123}I-IBZM and SPECT. This was interpreted by the authors as suggesting that low levels of DA could be related to early relapse in alcohol-dependent patients (278). However, information about DA levels cannot be derived from measurements of D_2-receptor availability, as endogenous DA levels do not significantly account for the variance in baseline D_2-receptor availability in humans (45).

Most of the preclinical data do not indicate that chronic alcohol exposure affects D_2-receptor density (279–283), but conflicting results have been published that suggest that the effects of chronic alcohol on DA receptors might vary according to the dose and duration of exposure (284–287). Such differences in duration of exposure, as well as interspecies differences in the response of D_2 receptors to alcohol, may undermine the relevance of rodent studies in answering the question of whether decreased D_2-receptor binding potential measured with PET in chronic alcoholics is a risk factor for, or an effect of, chronic alcohol intake. Studies targeting a nonalcoholic population at increased risk of developing alcoholism (e.g., children of alcoholics) are needed

to resolve this issue. Another important question is whether the alterations in D_2-receptor density in recently detoxified alcoholics are transient or permanent—that is, if this abnormality persists with a prolonged period of abstinence.

Few studies have reported DAT measurements in chronic alcoholics. Tiihonen et al. (288) compared the binding of ^{123}I-β-CIT to DAT in habitually violent alcoholics, nonviolent alcoholics, and controls. These authors reported, firstly, a significant reduction in ^{123}I-β-CIT binding in nonviolent alcoholics versus controls (n = 9 per group), and secondly, no change in ^{123}I-β-CIT binding in habitually violent alcoholics versus controls (n = 19 per group). More recently, the same group reported that reduced DAT binding was correlated with severity of depression in 24 recently detoxified alcoholic subjects (289). In contrast, Volkow et al. (277) measured DAT density in a group of five alcoholics abstinent for variable intervals (5 to 180 days) and found no differences compared with controls. Similarly, Heinz et al. (136) found no differences in DAT density in 20 alcoholics compared with controls. One study showed reduced DAT levels that normalized to the levels of the healthy controls after 4 weeks of abstinence (290). The most substantial recovery in DAT binding was reported to occur during the first 4 days of abstinence. This study suggests the time course of withdrawal and duration of abstinence has effects on the measurements of the DAT.

Despite the availability of PET tracers for different 5-HT receptors, to date no PET studies of serotonergic transmission have been reported in this population. Heinz et al. (135), using ^{123}I-β-CIT SPECT in male alcoholics, found decreased binding in the midbrain, an area where specific binding of this tracer is associated with the SERT. However, no information could be obtained about the levels of the transporter in other regions with ^{123}I-β-CIT due to its lack of specificity and the low sensitivity of SPECT.

Finally, PET imaging has contributed to the study of alterations in brain GABA-ergic function related to alcoholism. A blunted metabolic response to lorazepam in the thalamus, basal ganglia, and orbitofrontal cortex has been described in alcoholic subjects (291) and in the cerebellum of subjects at risk for alcoholism (292). Initial in vivo studies of benzodiazepine-receptor density failed to demonstrate abnormalities in ^{11}C-FMZ binding in limited samples of patients (293–295). However, a larger study reported a significant decrease in ^{11}C-FMZ V_T in the medial frontal lobes and cingulate gyrus in nine alcoholic subjects and a decrease in the same regions, as well as in the cerebellum, in eight alcoholic subjects with alcoholic cerebellar degeneration (296).

Another study, using SPECT and ^{123}I-iomazenil, found lower receptor levels in patients compared with controls in the frontal, anterior cingulate, and cerebellar cortices (297). These alterations have also been reported by a third group (298). Another study examined the issue of gender differences and found a trend toward reduced GABA-benzodiazepine–receptor levels in alcohol-dependent women. However, this did not reach significance (299). Lower levels were seen primarily in the cerebellum, occipital lobes, and parietal cortex but not in the frontal cortex. Gray matter atrophy, a well-documented finding in the brains of alcoholics, has not been found to play a role in these measured reductions of receptor levels in general (298).

Taken together, these studies suggest that alcoholism might be associated with a decrease in the benzodiazepine-$GABA_a$–receptor complex in some brain regions such as the frontal cortex, the cingulate cortex, the hippocampus, and the cerebellum. However, the studies do not all agree on which regions are implicated. The heterogeneity of the alcoholic patients, including the presence of neurologic impairment in some, might have contributed to the discrepancies between studies in the regions involved.

SUMMARY

This chapter has reviewed findings from PET and SPECT molecular imaging studies that have contributed to our understanding of the pathophysiology and treatment of psychiatric disorders. Since 1986, the year of publication of the seminal paper of Wong et al. (14), this field has undergone a major expansion. Figure 7.2 plots clinical studies discussed in this chapter as a function of the year of publication (excluding 2001) and illustrates the exponential growth in this field. So far, it is clear that these techniques have already provided unique insights into the neurochemical imbalances underlying some of these conditions and the pharmacologic mechanisms involved in their treatment. It is foreseeable that this contribution will continue to expand in the future.

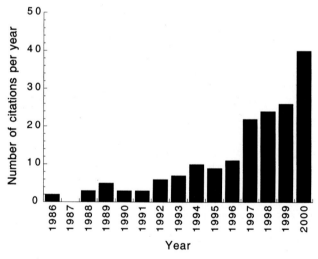

FIG. 7.2. Increase in number of psychiatric clinical studies using PET or single-photon emission computed tomography biomolecular imaging techniques as a function of year of publication (from 1986 to 2000). Studies included here are limited to clinical studies in psychiatric disorders that are cited in this review. Studies were selected based on their perceived impact and relevance to the topic. Regardless of this bias, the figure illustrates the vitality and growth of this field of investigation.

Psychiatric conditions are generally characterized by clinical heterogeneity. It is likely that a number of illnesses with different etiologies and neurobiologic mechanisms are currently subsumed under the same name by our diagnostic classifications. Despite this, a number of findings have been remarkably consistent and replicated across studies, suggesting that the clinical commonality underlying our diagnostic syndromes might be associated with unique and perhaps specific final common pathophysiologic pathways. However, as suggested by Wagner (300), the examination of the biologic processes involved in clinical conditions with nuclear medicine techniques also provides an opportunity for redefining illnesses.

For example, one study reported that elevated DA synaptic levels in acute schizophrenia were predictive of rapid symptomatic response to antipsychotic (i.e., antidopaminergic) treatment (28). A subgroup of patients showed no detectable abnormality of striatal DA function, despite frank psychotic symptoms, and failed to respond to treatment. It is possible that in these patients, the psychotic state is not driven by excess DA activity and that the antidopaminergic treatment fails because the problem being treated does not exist in these patients. This result has led to the concept of dopaminergic- versus nondopaminergic-driven psychotic states in schizophrenia (28). This biologic, rather than clinical, classification might prove useful in the evaluation of nondopaminergic antipsychotic pharmacologic strategies.

Another example is the constellation of conditions that have been reliably shown to be associated with low D_2-receptor availability in the striatum. This finding has been associated with a personality trait (detachment), anxiety disorder (social phobia), and addiction to a variety of substances, including cocaine, heroin, alcohol, and even food. These conditions are not similar but are frequently overlapping or comorbid. Therefore, imaging studies might reveal common biologic processes across conditions that were hitherto unsuspected and might help to delineate psychopathologic features more directly related to altered biologic brain functions than our current diagnostic classifications.

Despite these successes, a substantial number of studies yielded discordant results, and it is important to examine potential sources of discrepancies. An important drawback of this literature is the generally low number of subjects included in studies (typically fewer than 20 patients per group). In conditions characterized by marked heterogeneity, such as major depressive disorders, this factor is bound to yield divergent results across studies. Small samples are obviously due to the cost of these investigations, but also, in some instances, to the difficulty in recruiting appropriate clinical subjects (such as drug-free patients with schizophrenia). Another source of discrepancy is the variety of technical approaches to data acquisition and analysis. For example, analytic methods range from ''empiric'' or ''semiquantitative'' methods (typically a region of interest to a region of reference ratio measured at one time point) to model-based methods using an arterial input function. The limitations associated with empiric analytic methods are discussed in other chapters of this book and might account for artifactual results, particularly when the effect size of the between-group difference and the number of subjects are small (301).

In addressing these limitations, it will be important to increase the availability of these techniques beyond a few academic centers, to promote multicenter studies in well-characterized populations and to standardize analytic methods. Until recently, SPECT was the only widely available technique, and SPECT studies have so far provided a substantial contribution to this field. With the current increase in PET camera availability, the development of ^{18}F-based molecular imaging probes will provide unique opportunities for further dissemination of these techniques.

The greatest challenge facing this field is to develop molecular imaging probes suitable for imaging neurochemical processes beyond those currently available. Basically, four transmitter systems (DA, 5-HT, GABA, and opiates) dominate the psychiatric PET and SPECT molecular imaging literature. These systems are clearly involved in a very critical way in the mechanisms of action of psychiatric medications and drugs of abuse. However, a large number of other critical transmitter systems have not been investigated.

Radiotracers suitable for studying transmitter systems as important as the glutamatergic or adrenergic systems in the brain are still not available. Our ability to image brain chemistry beyond neurotransmission itself, to examine growth factors or intracellular signaling pathways, is still in its infancy. A sustained collaboration between industry, governmental, and private funding agencies and academic institutions will be required to expand the study of brain biomolecular processes beyond our current, and still relatively limited, arsenal.

In conclusion, this chapter has reviewed seminal findings obtained with PET and SPECT molecular imaging of psychiatric conditions. These techniques do not yet play a major clinical role in the diagnosis and treatment of these disorders and remain essentially research tools. However, the results produced by this field suggest that PET will significantly contribute to unraveling the biologic bases of these conditions and might play an increasing role in their clinical management. Moreover, it is foreseeable that PET will become more and more involved in the development and patient-specific dosing of new psychiatric medications. Expanding the availability of PET and the current radiopharmaceutical portfolio will be critical for these predictions to become reality.

ACKNOWLEDGMENTS

This work was supported by the National Alliance for Research on Schizophrenia and Depression (NARSAD and Lieber Center) and grants by the National Institute of Mental Health (K02 MH01603-01) and the National Institute of Drug Abuse (K08 DA00483-01).

REFERENCES

1. Rossum V. The significance of dopamine receptor blockade for the mechanism of action of neuroleptic drugs. *Arch Int Pharmacodyn Ther* 1966;160:492–494.
2. Carlsson A, Lindqvist M. Effect of chlorpromazine or haloperidol on formation of 3-methoxytyramine and normetanephrine in mouse brain. *Acta Pharmacol Toxicol* 1963;20:140–144.
3. Seeman P, Lee T. Antipsychotic drugs: direct correlation between clinical potency and presynaptic action on dopamine neurons. *Science* 1975;188:1217–1219.
4. Creese I, Burt DR, Snyder SH. Dopamine receptor binding predicts clinical and pharmacological potencies of antischizophrenic drugs. *Science* 1976;19:481–483.
5. Connell PH. *Amphetamine psychosis.* London: Chapman and Hill, 1958.
6. Angrist BM, Gershon S. The phenomenology of experimentally induced amphetamine psychosis—preliminary observation. *Biol Psychiatry* 1970;2:95–107.
7. Weinberger DR, Berman KF. Prefrontal function in schizophrenia: confounds and controversies. *Philos Trans Royal Soc London Series B Biol Sci* 1996;351(1346):1495–503.
8. Goldman-Rakic PS, Selemon LD. Functional and anatomical aspects of prefrontal pathology in schizophrenia. *Schizophr Bull* 1997;23: 437–458.
9. Weinberger DR. Implications of the normal brain development for the pathogenesis of schizophrenia. *Arch Gen Psychiatry* 1987;44: 660–669.
10. Knable MB, Weinberger DR. Dopamine, the prefrontal cortex and schizophrenia. *J Psychopharmacol* 1997;11(2):123–131.
11. Deutch AY. Prefrontal cortical dopamine systems and the elaboration of functional corticostriatal circuits: implications for schizophrenia and Parkinson's disease. *J Neural Transm Gen Sect* 1993;91(2-3): 197–221.
12. Wilkinson LS. The nature of interactions involving prefrontal and striatal dopamine systems. *J Psychopharmacol* 1997;11(2):143–150.
13. Weinberger DR, Laruelle M. Neurochemical and neuropharmacological imaging in schizophrenia, in neuropharmacology. In: Davis KL, Charney DS, Coyle JT, et al, eds. *The fifth generation of progress.* Philadelphia: Lippincott Williams & Wilkins, 2001.
14. Wong DF, Wagner HN, Tune LE, et al. Positron emission tomography reveals elevated D$_2$ dopamine receptors in drug-naive schizophrenics. *Science* 1986;234:1558–1563.
15. Crawley JC, Owens DG, Crow TJ, et al. Dopamine D$_2$ receptors in schizophrenia studied *in vivo. Lancet* 1986;2(8500):224–225.
16. Blin J, Baron JC, Cambon H, et al. Striatal dopamine D$_2$ receptors in tardive dyskinesia: PET study. *J Neurol Neurosurg Psychiatry* 1989; 52(11):1248–1252.
17. Martinot J-L, Peron-Magnan P, Huret J-D, et al. Striatal D$_2$ dopaminergic receptors assessed with positron emission tomography and 76-Br-bromospiperone in untreated patients. *Am J Psychiatry* 1990;147: 346–350.
18. Tune LE, Wong DF, Pearlson G, et al. Dopamine D$_2$ receptor density estimates in schizophrenia: a positron emission tomography study with ^{11}C-*N*-methylspiperone. *Psychiatry Res* 1993;49(3):219–237.
19. Nordstrom AL, Farde L, Eriksson L, et al. No elevated D$_2$ dopamine receptors in neuroleptic-naive schizophrenic patients revealed by positron emission tomography and [^{11}C]N-methylspiperone [see Comments]. *Psychiatry Res* 1995;61(2):67–83.
20. Okubo Y, Suhara T, Suzuki K, et al. Decreased prefrontal dopamine D$_1$ receptors in schizophrenia revealed by PET. *Nature* 1997; 385(6617):634–636.
21. Farde L, Wiesel F, Stone-Elander S, et al. D$_2$ dopamine receptors in neuroleptic-naive schizophrenic patients. A positron emission tomography study with [^{11}C]raclopride. *Arch Gen Psychiatry* 1990;47: 213–219.
22. Hietala J, Syvälahti E, Vuorio K, et al. Striatal D$_2$ receptor characteristics in neuroleptic-naive schizophrenic patients studied with positron emission tomography. *Arch Gen Psychiatry* 1994;51:116–123.
23. Pilowsky LS, Costa DC, Ell PJ, et al. D$_2$ dopamine receptor binding in the basal ganglia of antipsychotic-free schizophrenic patients. An I-123-IBZM single photon emission computerized tomography study. *Br J Psychiatry* 1994;164:16–26.
24. Laruelle M, Abi-Dargham A, van Dyck CH, et al. Single photon

emission computerized tomography imaging of amphetamine-induced dopamine release in drug free schizophrenic subjects. *Proc Natl Acad Sci U S A* 1996;93:9235–9240.

25. Knable MB, Egan MF, Heinz A, et al. Altered dopaminergic function and negative symptoms in drug-free patients with schizophrenia. [123I]-iodobenzamide SPECT study. *Br J Psychiatry* 1997;171: 574–577.

26. Breier A, Su TP, Saunders R, et al. Schizophrenia is associated with elevated amphetamine-induced synaptic dopamine concentrations: evidence from a novel positron emission tomography method. *Proc Natl Acad Sci U S A* 1997;94(6):2569–2574.

27. Abi-Dargham A, Gil R, Krystal J, et al. Increased striatal dopamine transmission in schizophrenia: confirmation in a second cohort. *Am J Psychiatry* 1998;155:761–767.

28. Abi-Dargham A, Rodenhiser J, Printz D, et al. Increased baseline occupancy of D2 receptors by dopamine in schizophrenia. *Proc Natl Acad Sci U S A* 2000;97(14):8104–8109.

29. Martinot JI, Paillère-Martinot ML, Loc'h C, et al. The estimated density of D2 striatal receptors in schizophrenia. A study with positron emission tomography and 76Br-bromolisuride. *Br J Psychiatry* 1991; 158:346–350.

30. Martinot JL, Paillère-Martinot ML, Loch'H C, et al. Central D2 receptors and negative symptoms of schizophrenia. *Br J Pharmacol* 1994; 164:27–34.

31. Seeman P, Guan H-C, Niznik HB. Endogenous dopamine lowers the dopamine D2 receptor density as measured by [3H]raclopride: implications for positron emission tomography of the human brain. *Synapse* 1989;3:96–97.

32. Seeman P. Brain dopamine receptors in schizophrenia: PET problems. *Arch Gen Psychiatry* 1988;45:598–560.

33. Karlsson P, Farde L, Halldin C, et al. D1-dopamine receptors in schizophrenia examined by PET. *Schizophr Res* 1997;24:179.

34. Abi-Dargham A, Gil R, Mawlawi O, et al. Selective alteration in D1 receptors in schizophrenia: a PET *in vivo* study. *J Nucl Med* 2001; 42:17P.

35. Reith J, Benkelfat C, Sherwin A, et al. Elevated dopa decarboxylase activity in living brain of patients with psychosis. *Proc Natl Acad Sci U S A* 1994;91:11651–11654.

36. Hietala J, Syvalahti E, Vuorio K, et al. Presynaptic dopamine function in striatum of neuroleptic-naive schizophrenic patients. *Lancet* 1995; 346(8983):1130–1131.

37. Dao-Castellana MH, Paillere-Martinot ML, Hantraye P, et al. Presynaptic dopaminergic function in the striatum of schizophrenic patients. *Schizophr Res* 1997;23(2):167–174.

38. Hietala J, Syvalahti E, Vilkman H, et al. Depressive symptoms and presynaptic dopamine function in neuroleptic-naive schizophrenia. *Schizophr Res* 1999;35(1):41–50.

39. Lindstrom LH, Gefvert O, Hagberg G, et al. Increased dopamine synthesis rate in medial prefrontal cortex and striatum in schizophrenia indicated by L-(beta-11C) DOPA and PET. *Biol Psychiatry* 1999; 46(5):681–688.

40. Laruelle M. Imaging synaptic neurotransmission with *in vivo* binding competition techniques: a critical review. *J Cereb Blood Flow Metab* 2000;20(3):423–451.

41. Villemagne VL, Wong DF, Yokoi F, et al. GBR12909 attenuates amphetamine-induced striatal dopamine release as measured by [11C]raclopride continuous infusion PET scans. *Synapse* 1999;33(4): 268–273.

42. Laruelle M, Iyer RN, Al-Tikriti MS, et al. Microdialysis and SPECT measurements of amphetamine-induced dopamine release in nonhuman primates. *Synapse* 1997;25:1–14.

43. Laruelle M, Abi-Dargham A, Gil R, et al. Increased dopamine transmission in schizophrenia: relationship to illness phases. *Biol Psychiatry* 1999;46(1):56–72.

44. Hwang D, Kegeles LS, Laruelle M. (−)-N-[11C]propyl-norapomorphine: a positron-labeled dopamine agonist for PET imaging of D2 receptors. *Nucl Med Biol* 2000;27(6):533–539.

45. Laruelle M, DSouza CD, Baldwin RM, et al. Imaging D-2 receptor occupancy by endogenous dopamine in humans. *Neuropsychopharmacology* 1997;17(3):162–174.

46. Fujita M, Verhoeff NP, Varrone A, et al. Imaging extrastriatal dopamine D2 receptor occupancy by endogenous dopamine in healthy humans. *Eur J Pharmacol* 2000;387(2):179–188.

47. Laruelle M, Abi-Dargham A, van Dyck C, et al. Dopamine and seroto-

nin transporters in patients with schizophrenia: an imaging study with [123I]beta-CIT. *Biol Psychiatry* 2000;47(5):371–379.

48. Laakso A, Vilkman H, Alakare B, et al. Striatal dopamine transporter binding in neuroleptic-naive patients with schizophrenia studied with positron emission tomography. *Am J Psychiatry* 2000;157(2): 269–271.

49. Robertson G, Fibiger H. Neuroleptics increase C-*fos* expression in the forebrain: contrasting effects of haloperidol and clozapine. *Neuroscience* 1992;46:315–328.

50. Robertson GS, Matsumura H, Fibiger HC. Induction patterns of *Fos*-like immunoreactivity in the forebrain as predictors of atypical antipsychotic activity. *J Pharmacol Exp Ther* 1994;271(2):1058–1066.

51. Deutch A, Moghadam B, Innis R, et al. Mechanisms of action of atypical antipsychotic drugs. Implication for novel therapeutic strategies for schizophrenia. *Schizophr Res* 1991;4:121–156.

52. Mawlawi O, Martinez D, Slifstein M, et al. Imaging human mesolimbic dopamine transmission with positron emission tomography, I: accuracy and precision of D2 receptor parameter measurements in ventral striatum. *J Cereb Blood Flow Metab* 2001;21(9):1034–1057.

53. Drevets WC, Gautier C, Price JC, et al. Amphetamine-induced dopamine release in human ventral striatum correlates with euphoria. *Biol Psychiatry* 2001;49(2):81–96.

54. Halldin C, Farde L, Hogberg T, et al. Carbon-11-FLB 457: a radioligand for extrastriatal D2 dopamine receptors. *J Nucl Med* 1995;36(7): 1275–1281.

55. Mukherjee J, Yang ZY, Das MK, et al. Fluorinated benzamide neuroleptics, III: development of (S)-N-[(1-allyl-2-pyrrolidinyl)methyl]-5-(3-[18F]fl uoropropyl)-2,3-dimethoxybenzamide as an improved dopamine D-2 receptor tracer. *Nucl Med Biol* 1995;22(3):283–296.

56. De Keyser J, Ebinger G, Vauquelin G. Evidence for a widespread dopaminergic innervation of the human cerebral neocortex. *Neurosci Lett* 1989;104:281–285.

57. Hall H, Sedvall G, Magnusson O, et al. Distribution of D1- and D2-dopamine receptors, and dopamine and its metabolites in the human brain. *Neuropsychopharmacology* 1994;11:245–256.

58. Abi-Dargham A, Krystal J. Serotonin receptors as target of antipsychotic medications. In: Lidow MS, ed. *Neurotransmitter receptors in actions of antipsychotic medications*. Boca Raton, FL: CRC Press, 2000:79–107.

59. Lewis R, Kapur S, Jones C, et al. Serotonin 5-HT2 receptors in schizophrenia: a PET study using [18F]setoperone in neuroleptic-naive patients and normal subjects. *Am J Psychiatry* 1999;156(1):72–78.

60. Trichard C, Paillere-Martinot ML, Attar-Levy D, et al. No serotonin 5-HT2A receptor density abnormality in the cortex of schizophrenic patients studied with PET. *Schizophr Res* 1998;31(1):13–17.

61. Okubo Y, Suhara T, Suzuki K, et al. Serotonin 5-HT2 receptors in schizophrenic patients studied by positron emission tomography. *Life Sci* 2000;66(25):2455–2464.

62. Ngan ET, Yatham LN, Ruth TJ, et al. Decreased serotonin 2A receptor densities in neuroleptic-naive patients with schizophrenia: a PET study using [18F]setoperone. *Am J Psychiatry* 2000;157(6): 1016–1018.

63. Lewis DA. GABAergic local circuit neurons and prefrontal cortical dysfunction in schizophrenia. *Brain Res Rev* 2000;31(2-3):270–276.

64. Benes FM. Emerging principles of altered neural circuitry in schizophrenia. *Brain Res Rev* 2000;31(2-3):251–269.

65. Busatto GF, Pilowsky LS, Costa DC, et al. Correlation between reduced *in vivo* benzodiazepine receptor binding and severity of psychotic symptoms in schizophrenia. *Am J Psychiatry* 1997;154(1): 56–63.

66. Verhoeff NP, Soares JC, D'Souza CD, et al. [123I]Iomazenil SPECT benzodiazepine receptor imaging in schizophrenia. *Psychiatry Res* 1999;91(3):163–173.

67. Abi-Dargham A, Laruelle M, Krystal J, et al. No evidence of altered *in vivo* benzodiazepine receptor binding in schizophrenia. *Neuropsychopharmacology* 1999;20(6):650–661.

68. Benes FM, Wickramasinghe R, Vincent SL, et al. Uncoupling of GABAA and benzodiazepine receptor binding activity in the hippocampal formation of schizophrenic brain. *Brain Res* 1997;755(1): 121–129.

69. Kapur S, Zipursky RB, Remington G. Clinical and theoretical implications of 5-HT2 and D2 receptor occupancy of clozapine, risperidone, and olanzapine in schizophrenia. *Am J Psychiatry* 1999; 156(2): 286–293.

70. Nyberg S, Nilsson U, Okubo Y, et al. Implications of brain imaging for the management of schizophrenia. *Int Clin Psychopharmacol* 1998; 13[Suppl 3]:S15–S20.

71. Farde L, Nordström AL, Wiesel FA, et al. Positron emission tomography analysis of central D_1 and D_2 dopamine receptor occupancy in patients treated with classical neuroleptics and clozapine. *Arch Gen Psychiatry* 1992;49:538–544.

72. Wolkin A, Barouche F, Wolf AP, et al. Dopamine blockade and clinical response: evidence for two biological subgroups of schizophrenia. *Am J Psychiatry* 1989;146(7):905–908.

73. Pilowsky LS, Costa DC, Ell PJ, et al. Clozapine, single photon emission tomography, and the D_2 dopamine receptor blockade hypothesis of schizophrenia. *Lancet* 1992;340:199–202.

74. Nordstrom AL, Farde L, Wiesel FA, et al. Central D_2-dopamine receptor occupancy in relation to antipsychotic drug effects: a double-blind PET study of schizophrenic patients. *Biol Psychiatry* 1993;33(4): 227–235.

75. Kapur S, Zipursky R, Jones C, et al. Relationship between dopamine D_2 occupancy, clinical response, and side effects: a double-blind PET study of first-episode schizophrenia. *Am J Psychiatry* 2000;157(4): 514–520.

76. Nordstrom AL, Farde L, Nyberg S, et al. D_1, D_2, and 5-HT_2 receptor occupancy in relation to clozapine serum concentration: a PET study of schizophrenic patients. *Am J Psychiatry* 1995;152(10):1444–1449.

77. Nyberg S, Farde L, Eriksson L, et al. 5-HT_2 and D_2 dopamine receptor occupancy in the living human brain. A PET study with risperidone. *Psychopharmacology* 1993;110:265–672.

78. Kapur S, Remington G, Zipursky RB, et al. The D_2 dopamine receptor occupancy of risperidone and its relationship to extrapyramidal symptoms: a PET study. *Life Sci* 1995;57(10):L103–L107.

79. Knable MB, Heinz A, Raedler T, et al. Extrapyramidal side effects with risperidone and haloperidol at comparable D_2 receptor occupancy levels. *Psychiatry Res Neuroimaging* 1997;75(2):91–101.

80. Kapur S, Zipursky RB, Remington G, et al. 5-HT_2 and D_2 receptor occupancy of olanzapine in schizophrenia: a PET investigation. *Am J Psychiatry* 1998;155(7):921–928.

81. Gefvert O, Bergstrom M, Langstrom B, et al. Time course of central nervous dopamine-D_2 and 5-HT_2 receptor blockade and plasma drug concentrations after discontinuation of quetiapine (Seroquel) in patients with schizophrenia. *Psychopharmacology (Berl)* 1998;135(2): 119–126.

82. Kapur S, Zipursky R, Jones C, et al. A positron emission tomography study of quetiapine in schizophrenia: a preliminary finding of an antipsychotic effect with only transiently high dopamine D_2 receptor occupancy. *Arch Gen Psychiatry* 2000;57(6):553–559.

83. Pilowsky LS, Mulligan RS, Acton PD, et al. Limbic selectivity of clozapine. *Lancet* 1997;350(9076):490–491.

84. Farde L, Suhara T, Nyberg S, et al. A PET study of [C-11]FLB 457 binding to extrastriatal D-2-dopamine receptors in healthy subjects and antipsychotic drug-treated patients. *Psychopharmacology* 1997; 133(4):396–404.

85. Bigliani V, Mulligan RS, Acton PD, et al. *In vivo* occupancy of striatal and temporal cortical D_2/D_3 dopamine receptors by typical antipsychotic drugs. [^{123}I]epidepride single photon emission tomography (SPET) study. *Br J Psychiatry* 1999;175:231–238.

86. Olsson H, Farde L. Potentials and pitfalls using high affinity radioligands in PET and SPECT determinations on regional drug induced D_2 receptor occupancy—a simulation study based on experimental data. *Neuroimage* 2001;14(4):936–945.

87. Abi-Dargham A, Hwang DR, Huang Y, et al. Reliable quantification of both striatal and extrastriatal D_2 receptors in humans with [^{18}F]fallypride. *J Nucl Med* 2000;41:139P.

88. Mukherjee J, Christian BT, Narayanan TK, et al. Measurement of striatal and extrastriatal D-2 receptor occupancy by clozapine and risperidone using [^{18}F]fallypride and PET. *Neuroimage* 2000;11:S53.

89. Talvik M, Nordstrom AL, Nyberg S, et al. No support for regional selectivity in clozapine-treated patients: a PET study with [^{11}C]raclopride and [^{11}C]FLB 457. *Am J Psychiatry* 2001;158(6):926–930.

90. Deutch AY, Lee MC, Iadarola MJ. Regionally specific effects of atypical antipsychotic drugs on striatal *Fos* expression: the nucleus accumbens shell as a locus of antipsychotic action. *Molecular Cellular Neurosci* 1992;3:332–341.

91. Wolkin A, Brodie JD, Barouche F, et al. Dopamine receptor occu-

92. Fitzgerald PB, Kapur S, Remington G, et al. Predicting haloperidol occupancy of central dopamine D_2 receptors from plasma levels. *Psychopharmacology (Berl)* 2000; 149(1):1–5.

93. Hagberg G, Gefvert O, Bergstrom M, et al. N-[^{11}C]methylspiperone PET, in contrast to [^{11}C]raclopride, fails to detect D_2 receptor occupancy by an atypical neuroleptic. *Psychiatry Res* 1998; 82(3): 147–160.

94. Drevets WC. Neuroimaging studies of mood disorders. *Biol Psychiatry* 2000; 48:813–829.

95. Mayberg HS, Liotti M, Brannan SK, et al. Reciprocal limbic-cortical function and negative mood: converging PET findings in depression and normal sadness. *Am J Psychiatry* 1999;156(5):675–682.

96. Blier P, de Montigny C, Chaput Y. A role for the serotonin system in the mechanism of action of antidepressant treatments: preclinical evidence. *J Clin Psychiatry* 1990;51[Suppl]:14–21.

97. Mayberg H, Robinson R, Wong D, et al. PET imaging of cortical S_2 serotonin receptors after stroke: lateralized changes and relationship to depression. *Am J Psychiatry* 1988;145(8):937–943.

98. D'haenen H, Bossuyt A, Mertens J, et al. SPECT imaging of serotonin-2 receptors in depression. *Psychiatry Res Neuroimaging* 1992; 45(4):227–237.

99. Blin J, Pappata S, Kijosawa M, et al. [^{18}F]setoperone: a new high-affinity ligand for positron emission tomography study of the serotonin-2 receptors in baboon brain *in vivo*. *Eur J Pharmacol* 1988;147: 73–82.

100. Lemaire C, Cantineau R, Guillaume M, et al. Fluorine-18-altanserin: a radioligand for the study of serotonin receptors with PET: radiolabeling and *in vivo* biologic behavior in rats. *J Nucl Med* 1991;32(12): 2266–2272.

101. Biver F, Wikler D, Lotstra F, et al. Serotonin 5-HT_2 receptor imaging in major depression: focal changes in orbito-insular cortex. *Br J Psychiatry* Nov 1997;171:444–448.

102. Tan PZ, Baldwin RM, Van Dyck CH, et al. Characterization of radioactive metabolites of 5-HT_{2A} receptor PET ligand [^{18}F]altanserin in human and rodent. *Nucl Med Biol* 1999;26(6):601–608.

103. Meyer JH, Kapur S, Houle S, et al. Prefrontal cortex 5-HT_2 receptors in depression: an [^{18}F]setoperone PET imaging study. *Am J Psychiatry* 1999;156(7):1029–1034.

104. Attar-Levy D, Martinot J-L, Blin J, et al. The cortical serotonin-2 receptors studied with positron-emission tomography and [^{18}F]-setoperone during depressive illness and antidepressant treatment with clomipramine. *Biol Psychiatry* 1999;45(2):180–186.

105. Meltzer CC, Price JC, Mathis CA, et al. PET imaging of serotonin type 2A receptors in late-life neuropsychiatric disorders. *Am J Psychiatry* 1999;156(12):1871–1878.

106. Yatham LN, Liddle PF, Shiah I-S, et al. Brain serotonin-2 receptors in major depression: a positron emission tomography study. *Arch Gen Psychiatry* 2000;57(9):850–858.

107. Meyer JH, Kapur S, Eisfeld B, et al. The effect of paroxetine on 5-HT_{2A} receptors in depression: an [^{18}F]setoperone PET imaging study. *Am J Psychiatry* 2001;158(1):78–85.

108. Yatham LN, Liddle PF, Dennie J, et al. Decrease in brain serotonin 2 receptor binding in patients with major depression following desipramine treatment: a positron emission tomography study with fluorine-18-labeled setoperone. *Arch Gen Psychiatry* 1999;56(8): 705–711.

109. Mann JJ. Role of the serotonergic system in the pathogenesis of major depression and suicidal behavior. *Neuropsychopharmacology* 1999; 21[Suppl 2]:99S–105S.

110. Drevets WC, Frank E, Price JC, et al. PET imaging of serotonin 1A receptor binding in depression. *Biol Psychiatry* 1999;46(10): 1375–1387.

111. Fujita M, Charney DS, Innis RB. Imaging serotonergic neurotransmission in depression: hippocampal pathophysiology may mirror global brain alterations. *Biol Psychiatry* 2000;48(8):801–812.

112. Duman RS, Heninger GR, Nestler EJ. A molecular and cellular theory of depression. *Arch Gen Psychiatry* 1997;54(7):597–606.

113. Lowther S, DePaermentier F, Cheetham SC, et al. 5-HT_{1A} receptor binding sites in post-mortem brain samples from depressed suicides and controls. *J Affective Disord* 1997;42(2-3):199–207.

114. Dillon KA, Gross-Isseroff R, Israeli M, et al. Autoradiographic analy-

sis of serotonin 5-HT$_{1A}$ receptor binding in the human brain postmortem: effects of age and alcohol. *Brain Res* 1991;554(1-2):56–64.

115. Matsubara S, Arora RC, Meltzer HY. Serotonergic measures in suicide brain: 5-HT$_{1A}$ binding sites in frontal cortex of suicide victims. *J Neural Transm Gen Sect* 1991;85(3):181–194.

116. Arranz B, Eriksson A, Mellerup E, et al. Brain 5-HT$_{1A}$, 5-HT$_{1D}$, and 5-HT$_2$ receptors in suicide victims. *Biol Psychiatry* 1994;35(7): 457–463.

117. Arango V, Underwood MD, Gubbi AV, et al. Localized alterations in pre- and postsynaptic serotonin binding sites in the ventrolateral prefrontal cortex of suicide victims. *Brain Res* 1995;688(1-2): 121–133.

118. Sargent PA, Kjaer KH, Bench CJ, et al. Brain serotonin(1A) receptor binding measured by positron emission tomography with [^{11}C]WAY-100635: effects of depression and antidepressant treatment. *Arch Gen Psychiatry* 2000;57(2):174–180.

119. Porter RJ, McAllister-Williams RH, Jones S, et al. Effects of dexamethasone on neuroendocrine and psychological responses to L-tryptophan infusion. *Psychopharmacology (Berlin)* 1999;143(1):64–71.

120. Lopez JF, Liberzon I, Vazquez DM, et al. Serotonin 1A receptor messenger RNA regulation in the hippocampus after acute stress. *Biol Psychiatry* 1999;45(7):934–937.

121. Lopez JF, Vazquez DM, Chalmers DT, et al. Regulation of 5-HT receptors and the hypothalamic–pituitary–adrenal axis. Implications for the neurobiology of suicide. *Ann N Y Acad Sci* 1997;836:106–134.

122. Chaouloff F. Regulation of 5-HT receptors by corticosteroids: where do we stand? *Fundam Clin Pharmacol* 1995;9(3):219–233.

123. Wang S, Gao Y, Laruelle M, et al. Enantioselectivity of cocaine recognition sites: binding of (1S)- and (1R)-2 beta-carbomethoxy-3 beta-(4-iodophenyl)tropane (beta-CIT) to monoamine transporters. *J Med Chem* 1993;36(13):1914–1917.

124. Laruelle M, Giddings SS, Zea-Ponce Y, et al. Methyl 3 beta-(4-[^{125}I]iodophenyl)tropane-2 beta-carboxylate *in vitro* binding to dopamine and serotonin transporters under ''physiological'' conditions. *J Neurochem* 1994;62(3):978–986.

125. Laruelle M, Baldwin RM, Malison RT, et al. SPECT imaging of dopamine and serotonin transporters with [^{123}I]beta-CIT: pharmacological characterization of brain uptake in nonhuman primates. *Synapse* 1993;13(4):295–309.

126. Brücke T, Kornhuber J, Angelberger P, et al. SPECT imaging of dopamine and serotonin transporters with [^{123}I]β-CIT. Binding kinetics in the human brain. *J Neural Transm Gen Sect* 1993;94(2): 137–146.

127. Pirker W, Asenbaum S, Kasper S, et al. beta-CIT SPECT demonstrates blockade of 5HT-uptake sites by citalopram in the human brain *in vivo. J Neural Transm Gen Sect* 1995;100(3):247–256.

128. Seibyl JP, Marek KL, Quinlan D, et al. Decreased single-photon emission computed tomographic [^{123}I]beta-CIT striatal uptake correlates with symptom severity in Parkinson's disease. *Ann Neurol* 1995; 38(4):589–598.

129. Marek KL, Seibyl JP, Zoghbi SS, et al. [^{123}I] beta-CIT/SPECT imaging demonstrates bilateral loss of dopamine transporters in hemi-Parkinson's disease. *Neurology* 1996;46(1):231–237.

130. Eising EG, Muller TT, Zander C, et al. SPECT-evaluation of the monoamine uptake site ligand [I-123](1R)-2-beta-carbomethoxy-3-beta-(4-iodophenyl)-tropane ([I-123]beta-CIT) in untreated patients with suspicion of Parkinson disease. *J Invest Med* 1997;45(8): 448–452.

131. Seibyl JP, Marek K, Sheff K, et al. Iodine-123-beta-CIT and iodine-123-FPCIT SPECT measurement of dopamine transporters in healthy subjects and Parkinson's patients. *J Nucl Med* 1998;39(9):1500–1508.

132. Muller U, Wachter T, Barthel H, et al. Striatal [^{123}I]beta-CIT SPECT and prefrontal cognitive functions in Parkinson's disease. *J Neural Transm* 2000;107(3):303–319.

133. Malison RT, Best SE, van Dyck CH, et al. Elevated striatal dopamine transporters during acute cocaine abstinence as measured by [^{123}I] beta-CIT SPECT. *Am J Psychiatry* 1998;155(6):832–834.

134. Malison RT, Price LH, Berman R, et al. Reduced brain serotonin transporter availability in major depression as measured by [^{123}I]-2 beta-carbomethoxy-3 beta-(4-iodophenyl)tropane and single photon emission computed tomography. *Biol Psychiatry* 1998;44(11): 1090–1098.

135. Heinz A, Ragan P, Jones DW, et al. Reduced central serotonin transporters in alcoholism. *Am J Psychiatry* 1998;155(11):1544–1549.

136. Heinz A, Knable MB, Wolf SS, et al. Tourette's syndrome: [I-123]beta-CIT SPECT correlates of vocal tic severity. *Neurology* 1998; 51(4):1069–1074.

137. Malison RT, Price LH, Berman R, et al. Reduced brain serotonin transporter availability in major depression as measured by [^{123}I]-2 beta-carbomethoxy-3 beta-(4-iodophenyl)tropane and single photon emission computed tomography. *Biol Psychiatry* 1998;44(11): 1090–1098.

138. Willeit M, Praschak-Rieder N, Neumeister A, et al. [^{123}I]-beta-CIT SPECT imaging shows reduced brain serotonin transporter availability in drug-free depressed patients with seasonal affective disorder. *Biol Psychiatry* 2000;47(6):482–489.

139. Suehiro M, Scheffel U, Ravert HT, et al. [^{11}C](+)McN5652 as a radiotracer for imaging serotonin uptake sites with PET. *Life Sci* 1993; 53(11):883–892.

140. Szabo Z, Scheffel U, Suehiro M, et al. Positron emission tomography of 5-HT transporter sites in the baboon brain with [^{11}C]McN5652. *J Cereb Blood Flow Metab* 1995;15(5):798–805.

141. Szabo Z, Scheffel U, Mathews WB, et al. Kinetic analysis of [^{11}C]McN5652: a serotonin transporter radioligand. *J Cereb Blood Flow Metab* 1999;19(9):967–981.

142. Parsey RV, Kegeles LS, Hwang DR, et al. *In vivo* quantification of brain serotonin transporters in humans using [^{11}C]McN 5652. *J Nucl Med* 2000;41(9):1465–1477.

143. Buck A, Gucker PM, Schonbachler RD, et al. Evaluation of serotonergic transporters using PET and [^{11}C](+)McN-5652: assessment of methods. *J Cereb Blood Flow Metab* 2000;20(2):253–262.

144. Parsey RV, Kegeles LS, Hwang DR, et al. *In vivo* quantification of brain serotonin transporters in humans using [^{11}C]McN5652. *J Nucl Med* 2000; 41(9):1465–1477.

145. Oya S, Choi SR, Hou C, et al. 2-((2-((dimethylamino)methyl)phenyl)thio)-5-iodophenylamine (ADAM): an improved serotonin transporter ligand. *Nucl Med Biol* 2000;27(3):249–254.

146. Vercouillie J, Tarkiainen J, Halldin C, et al. Precursor synthesis and radiolabeling of [^{11}C]ADAM: a potent radioligand for the serotonin transporter exploration by PET. *J Labelled Compounds Radiopharm* 2001;44:113–120.

147. Wilson AA, Ginovart N, Schmidt M, et al. Novel radiotracers for imaging the serotonin transporter by positron emission tomography: synthesis, radiosynthesis, and *in vitro* and *ex vivo* evaluation of (11)C-labeled 2-(phenylthio)araalkylamines. *J Med Chem* 2000;43(16): 3103–3110.

148. Houle S, Ginovart N, Hussey D, et al. Imaging the serotonin transporter with positron emission tomography: initial human studies with [^{11}C]DAPP and [^{11}C]DASB [In Process Citation]. *Eur J Nucl Med* 2000;27(11):1719–1722.

149. Kapur S, Mann JJ. Role of the dopaminergic system in depression. *Biol Psychiatry* 1992;32(1):1–17.

150. Brown AS, Gershon S. Dopamine and depression. *J Neural Transm Gen Sect* 1993;91(2-3):75–109.

151. Diehl DJ, Gershon S. The role of dopamine in mood disorders. *Compr Psychiatry* 1992;33(2):115–120.

152. Willner P, Muscat R, Papp M. Chronic mild stress-induced anhedonia: a realistic animal model of depression. *Neurosci Biobehav Rev* 1992; 16(4):525–534.

153. D'Haenen HA, Bossuyt A. Dopamine D$_2$ receptors in depression measured with single photon emission computed tomography. *Biol Psychiatry* 1994;35(2):128–132.

154. Shah PJ, Ogilvie AD, Goodwin GM, et al. Clinical and psychometric correlates of dopamine D$_2$ binding in depression. *Psychol Med* 1997; 27(6):1247–1256.

155. Ebert D, Feistel H, Loew T, et al. Dopamine and depression—striatal dopamine D$_2$ receptor SPECT before and after antidepressant therapy. *Psychopharmacology (Berl)* 1996;126(1):91–94.

156. Klimke A, Larisch R, Janz A, et al. Dopamine D$_2$ receptor binding before and after treatment of major depression measured by [^{123}I]IBZM SPECT. *Psychiatry Res* 1999;90(2):91–101.

157. Parsey RV, Oquendo MA, Zea-Ponce Y, et al. Dopamine D$_2$ receptor availability and amphetamine-induced dopamine release in unipolar depression. *Biol Psychiatry* 2001;50(5):313–322.

158. Laasonen-Balk T, Kuikka J, Viinamaki H, et al. Striatal dopamine transporter density in major depression. *Psychopharmacology (Berl)* 1999;144(3):282–285.

159. Martinot M, Bragulat V, Artiges E, et al. Decreased presynaptic dopa-

mine function in the left caudate of depressed patients with affective flattening and psychomotor retardation. *Am J Psychiatry* 2001;158(2): 314–316.

160. Meyer JH, Wilson AA, Ginovart N, et al. Occupancy of serotonin transporters by paroxetine and citalopram during treatment of depression: a [^{11}C]DASB PET imaging study. *Am J Psychiatry* 2001; 158(11):1843–1849.

161. Kent JM, Coplan JD, Lombardo I, et al. Imaging the serotonin transporter in social phobia with (+)[C-11]McN5652. *J Nucl Med* 2000; 41:200P.

162. Blier P, de Montigny C. Possible serotonergic mechanisms underlying the antidepressant and anti–obsessive-compulsive disorder responses. *Biol Psychiatry* 1998;44(5):313–323.

163. Martinez D, Broft A, Laruelle M. Pindolol augmentation of antidepressant treatment: recent contributions from brain imaging studies. *Biol Psychiatry* 2000; 48(8):844–853.

164. Artigas F, Celada P, Laruelle M, et al. How does pindolol improve antidepressant action? *Trends Pharmacol Sci* 2001;22(5):224–228.

165. Martinez D, Hwang D, Mawlawi O, et al. Differential occupancy of somatodendritic and postsynaptic 5-HT$_{1A}$ receptors by pindolol. A dose-occupancy study with [^{11}C]WAY 100635 and positron emission tomography in humans. *Neuropsychopharmacology* 2001;24(3): 209–229.

166. Andree B, Thorberg SO, Halldin C, et al. Pindolol binding to 5-HT$_{1A}$ receptors in the human brain confirmed with positron emission tomography. *Psychopharmacology* 1999;144(3):303–305.

167. Rabiner EA, Gunn RN, Castro ME, et al. Beta-blocker binding to human 5-HT$_{1A}$ receptors *in vivo* and *in vitro*: implications for antidepressant therapy. *Neuropsychopharmacology* 2000;23(3):285–293.

168. Suhara T, Nakayama K, Inoue O, et al. D$_1$ dopamine receptor binding in mood disorders measured by positron emission tomography. *Psychopharmacology* 1992;106(1):14–18.

169. Wong WF, Pearlson GD, Tune LE, et al. Quantification of neuroreceptors in the living human brain, IV: effect of aging and elevations of D$_2$-like receptors in schizophrenia and bipolar illness. *J Cereb Blood Flow Metab* 1997;17(3):331–342.

170. Gjedde A, Wong DF. Quantification of neuroreceptors in living human brain, V: endogenous neurotransmitter inhibition of haloperidol binding in psychosis. *J Cereb Blood Flow Metab* 2001;21(8): 982–994.

171. Anand A, Verhoeff P, Seneca N, et al. Brain SPECT imaging of amphetamine-induced dopamine release in euthymic bipolar disorder patients. *Am J Psychiatry* 2000;157(7):1108–1114.

172. Benkelfat C, Bradwejn J, Meyer E, et al. Functional neuroanatomy of CCK4-induced anxiety in normal healthy volunteers [see Comments]. *Am J Psychiatry* 1995;152(8):1180–1184.

173. Javanmard M, Shlik J, Kennedy SH, et al. Neuroanatomic correlates of CCK-4-induced panic attacks in healthy humans: a comparison of two time points. *Biol Psychiatry* 1999;45(7):872–882.

174. Chua P, Krams M, Toni I, et al. A functional anatomy of anticipatory anxiety. *Neuroimage* 1999;9[Suppl 6, Pt 1]:563–571.

175. Simpson JR Jr, Drevets WC, Snyder AZ, et al. Emotion-induced changes in human medial prefrontal cortex, II: during anticipatory anxiety. *Proc Natl Acad Sci U S A* 2001;98(2):688–693.

176. Kimbrell TA, George MS, Parekh PI, et al. Regional brain activity during transient self-induced anxiety and anger in healthy adults. *Biol Psychiatry* 1999;46(4):454–465.

177. Liotti M, Mayberg HS, Brannan SK, et al. Differential limbic—cortical correlates of sadness and anxiety in healthy subjects: implications for affective disorders. *Biol Psychiatry* 2000;48(1):30–42.

178. Tiihonen J, Kuikka J, Rasanen P, et al. Cerebral benzodiazepine receptor binding and distribution in generalized anxiety disorder: a fractal analysis. *Mol Psychiatry* 1997;2(6):463–471.

179. Abadie P, Boulenger JP, Benali K, et al. Relationships between trait and state anxiety and the central benzodiazepine receptor: a PET study. European *J Neurosci* 1999;11(4):1470–1478.

180. Kaschka W, Feistel H, Ebert D. Reduced benzodiazepine receptor binding in panic disorders measured by iomazenil SPECT. *J Psychiatr Res* 1995;29(5):427–434.

181. Brandt CA, Meller J, Keweloh L, et al. Increased benzodiazepine receptor density in the prefrontal cortex in patients with panic disorder. *J Neural Transm (Budapest)* 1998;105(10-12):1325–1333.

182. Bremner JD, Innis RB, White T, et al. SPECT [I-123]iomazenil measurement of the benzodiazepine receptor in panic disorder. *Biol Psychiatry* 2000;47(2):96–106.

183. Malizia AL, Cunningham VJ, Bell CJ, et al. Decreased brain GABA$_a$-benzodiazepine receptor binding in panic disorder: preliminary results from a quantitative PET study. *Arch Gen Psychiatry* 1998;55(8): 715–720.

184. Dewar KM, Stravynski A. The quest for biological correlates of social phobia: an interim assessment. *Acta Psychiatrica Scandinavica* 2001; 103(4):244–251.

185. Bell CJ, Malizia AL, Nutt DJ. The neurobiology of social phobia [Review]. *Eur Arch Psychiatry Clin Neurosci* 1999;249[Suppl 1]: S11–S18.

186. Nutt DJ, Bell CJ, Malizia AL. Brain mechanisms of social anxiety disorder [Review]. *J Clin Psychiatry* 1998;59[Suppl 17]:4–11.

187. Tiihonen J, Kuikka J, Bergstrom K, et al. Dopamine reuptake site densities in patients with social phobia. *Am J Psychiatry* 1997;154(2): 239–242.

188. Schneier FR, Liebowitz MR, Abi-Dargham A, et al. Low dopamine D$_2$ receptor binding potential in social phobia. *Am J Psychiatry* 2000; 157(3):457–459.

189. Perani D, Colombo C, Bressi S, et al. [^{18}F]FDG PET study in obsessive-compulsive disorder. A clinical/metabolic correlation study after treatment. *Br J Psychiatry* 1995;166(2):244–250.

190. Biver F, Goldman S, Francois A, et al. Changes in metabolism of cerebral glucose after stereotactic leukotomy for refractory obsessive-compulsive disorder: a case report. *J Neurol Neurosurg Psychiatry* 1995;58(4):502–505.

191. Rauch SL, Savage CR, Alpert NM, et al. Probing striatal function in obsessive-compulsive disorder: a PET study of implicit sequence learning. *J Neuropsychiatry Clin Neurosci* 1997;9(4):568–573.

192. Mallet L, Mazoyer B, Martinot JL. Functional connectivity in depressive, obsessive-compulsive, and schizophrenic disorders: an explorative correlational analysis of regional cerebral metabolism. *Psychiatry Res* 1998;82(2):83–93.

193. Saxena S, Brody AL, Maidment KM, et al. Localized orbitofrontal and subcortical metabolic changes and predictors of response to paroxetine treatment in obsessive-compulsive disorder. *Neuropsychopharmacology* 1999;21(6):683–693.

194. Baxter LR Jr. Positron emission tomography studies of cerebral glucose metabolism in obsessive compulsive disorder [Review]. *J Clin Psychiatry* 1994;55[Suppl]:54–59.

195. Brody AL, Saxena S, Schwartz JM, et al. FDG-PET predictors of response to behavioral therapy and pharmacotherapy in obsessive compulsive disorder. *Psychiatry Res* 1998;84(1):1–6.

196. Villarreal G, King CY. Brain imaging in posttraumatic stress disorder. *Semin Clin Neuropsychiatry* 2001;6(2):131–145.

197. Bremner JD. Alterations in brain structure and function associated with post-traumatic stress disorder. *Semin Clin Neuropsychiatry* 1999; 4(4):249–255.

198. Bremner JD, Innis RB, Southwick SM, et al. Decreased benzodiazepine receptor binding in prefrontal cortex in combat-related posttraumatic stress disorder. *Am J Psychiatry* 2000;157(7):1120–1126.

199. Farde L, Gustavsson JP, Jonsson E. D$_2$ dopamine receptors and personality traits. *Nature* 1997;385(6617):590.

200. Breier A, Kestler L, Adler C, et al. Dopamine D$_2$ receptor density and personal detachment in healthy subjects. *Am J Psychiatry* 1998; 155(10):1440–1442.

201. Breier A, Kestler L, Adler C, et al. Dopamine D$_2$ receptor density and personal detachment in healthy subjects. *Am J Psychiatry* 1998; 155(10):1440–1442.

202. Kestler LP, Malhotra AK, Finch C, et al. The relation between dopamine D$_2$ receptor density and personality: Preliminary evidence from the NEO Personality Inventory-Revised. *Neuropsychiatry Neuropsychol Behav Neurol* 2000;13(1):48–52.

203. Laakso A, Vilkman H, Kajander J, et al. Prediction of detached personality in healthy subjects by low dopamine transporter binding. *Am J Psychiatry* 2000;157(2):290–292.

204. Schneier FR, Liebowitz MR, Laruelle M. Detachment and generalized social phobia. *Am J Psychiatry* 2001;158(2):327.

205. Tauscher J, Bagby RM, Javanmard M, et al. Inverse relationship between serotonin 5-HT$_{1A}$ receptor binding and anxiety: a [^{11}C]WAY-100635 PET investigation in healthy volunteers. *Am J Psychiatry* 2001;158(8):1326–1328.

206. Zhuang X, Gross C, Santarelli L, et al. Altered emotional states in knockout mice lacking 5-HT$_{1A}$ or 5-HT$_{1B}$ receptors. *Neuropsychopharmacology* 1999;21[Suppl 2]:52S–60S.

207. Soloff PH, Meltzer CC, Greer PJ, et al. A fenfluramine-activated FDG-PET study of borderline personality disorder. *Biol Psychiatry* 2000;47(6):540–547.

208. Siever LJ, Buchsbaum MS, New AS, et al. D,L-Fenfluramine response in impulsive personality disorder assessed with [^{18}F]fluorodeoxyglucose positron emission tomography. *Neuropsychopharmacology* 1999;20(5):413–423.

209. Leyton M, Okazawa H, Diksic M, et al. Brain regional [alpha]-[^{11}C]methyl-L-tryptophan trapping in impulsive subjects with borderline personality disorder. *Am J Psychiatry* 2001;158(5):775–782.

210. Dougherty DD, Bonab AA, Spencer TJ, et al. Dopamine transporter density in patients with attention deficit hyperactivity disorder. *Lancet* 1999;354(9196):2132–2133.

211. Dresel S, Krause J, Krause KH, et al. Attention deficit hyperactivity disorder: binding of [^{99m}Tc]TRODAT-1 to the dopamine transporter before and after methylphenidate treatment. *Eur J Nucl Med* 2000; 27(10):1518–1524.

212. Volkow ND, Wang GJ, Fowler JS, et al. Therapeutic doses of oral methylphenidate significantly increase extracellular dopamine in the human brain. *J Neurosci* 2001;21(2):RC121.

213. Volkow ND, Fowler JS, Wolf AP, et al. Effects of chronic cocaine abuse on postsynaptic dopamine receptors. *Am J Psychiatry* 1990; 147(6):719–724.

214. Volkow ND, Fowler JS, Wang GJ, et al. Decreased dopamine D$_2$ receptor availability is associated with reduced frontal metabolism in cocaine abusers. *Synapse* 1993;14(2):169–177.

215. Volkow ND, Wang GJ, Fowler JS, et al. Cocaine uptake is decreased in the brain of detoxified cocaine abusers. *Neuropsychopharmacology* 1996;14(3):159–168.

216. Volkow ND, Wang GJ, Fowler JS, et al. Decreased striatal dopaminergic responsiveness in detoxified cocaine-dependent subjects. *Nature* 1997;386:830–833.

217. Wang GJ, Volkow ND, Fowler JS, et al. Dopamine D$_2$ receptor availability in opiate-dependent subjects before and after naloxone-precipitated withdrawal. *Neuropsychopharmacology* 1997;16(2):174–182.

218. Hietala J, West C, Syvalahti E, et al. Striatal D$_2$ dopamine receptor binding characteristics *in vivo* in patients with alcohol dependence. *Psychopharmacology (Berl)* 1994;116(3):285–290.

219. Volkow ND, Wang JG, Fowler JS, et al. Decreases in dopamine receptors but not in dopamine transporters in alcoholics. *J Nucl Med* 1996; 37:33P.

220. Volkow ND, Wang GJ, Fowler JS, et al. Prediction of reinforcing responses to psychostimulants in humans by brain dopamine D$_2$ receptor levels. *Am J Psychiatry* 1999;156(9):1440–1443.

221. Nader MA, Gage HD, Moore T, et al. Rapid down-regulation of dopamine D$_2$ receptors in a rhesus monkey model of cocaine abuse. *J Nucl Med* 2000;41:104P.

222. Nader MA, Gage HD, Mach RH, et al. *The use of PET imaging to examine the effects of cocaine and environmental context on dopamine D$_2$ receptors in monkeys.* Washington, DC: US Government Printing Office, 2001.

223. Volkow ND, Wang G-J, Fowler JS, et al. Imaging endogenous dopamine competition with [^{11}C]raclopride in the human brain. *Synapse* 1994;16:255–262.

224. Laruelle M, Abi-Dargham A, van Dyck CH, et al. SPECT imaging of striatal dopamine release after amphetamine challenge. *J Nucl Med* 1995;36:1182–1190.

225. Laruelle M, Abi-Dargham A, van Dyck CH, et al. Single photon emission computerized tomography imaging of amphetamine-induced dopamine release in drug free schizophrenic subjects. *Proc Natl Acad Sci U S A* 1996;93:9235–9240.

226. Volkow ND, Wang GJ, Fowler JS, et al. Reinforcing effects of psychostimulants in humans are associated with increases in brain dopamine and occupancy of D$_2$ receptors. *J Pharmacol Exp Ther* 1999; 291(1):409–415.

227. Kegeles LS, Zea-Ponce Y, Abi-Dargham A, et al. Stability of [^{123}I]IBZM SPECT measurement of amphetamine-induced striatal dopamine release in humans. *Synapse* 1999;31(4):302–308.

228. Drevets WC, Gautier C, Price JC, et al. Amphetamine-induced dopamine release in human ventral striatum correlates with euphoria. *Biol Psychiatry* 2001;49(2):81–96.

229. Wise R, Romprè P. Brain dopamine and reward. *Annu Rev Psychol* 1989;40:191.

230. Di Chiara G, Imperato A. Drugs abused by humans preferentially

231. Le Moal M, Simon H. Mesocorticolimbic dopamine network: functional and regulatory role. *Physiol Rev* 1991;71:155–324.

232. Koepp MJ, Gunn RN, Lawrence AD, et al. Evidence for striatal dopamine release during a video game. *Nature* 1998;393(6682):266–268.

233. Malison RT, Mechanic KY, Klummp H, et al. Reduced amphetamine-stimulated dopamine release in cocaine addicts as measured by [^{123}I]IBZM SPECT. *J Nucl Med* 1999;40[Suppl 5]:110P.

234. Wu JC, Bell K, Najafi A, et al. Decreasing striatal 6-FDOPA uptake with increasing duration of cocaine withdrawal. *Neuropsychopharmacology* 1997;17(6):402–409.

235. Wang GJ, Volkow ND, Fowler JS, et al. Cocaine abusers do not show loss of dopamine transporters with age. *Life Sci* 1997;61(11): 1059–1065.

236. Volkow ND, Wang GJ, Fischman MW, et al. Relationship between subjective effects of cocaine and dopamine transporter occupancy. *Nature* 1997;386(6627):827–830.

237. Malison RT, McCance E, Carpenter LL, et al. [^{123}I]beta-CIT SPECT imaging of dopamine transporter availability after mazindol administration in human cocaine addicts. *Psychopharmacology (Berl)* 1998; 137(4):321–325.

238. Jacobsen LK, Staley JK, Malison RT, et al. Elevated central serotonin transporter binding availability in acutely abstinent cocaine-dependent patients. *Am J Psychiatry* 2000;157(7):1134–1140.

239. Zubieta JK, Gorelick DA, Stauffer R, et al. Increased mu opioid receptor binding detected by PET in cocaine-dependent men is associated with cocaine craving. *Nat Med* 1996;2(11):1225–1229.

240. Hurd YL, Herkenham M. Molecular alterations in the neostriatum of human cocaine addicts. *Synapse* 1993;13(4):357–369.

241. Steiner H, Gerfen CR. Role of dynorphin and enkephalin in the regulation of striatal output pathways and behavior. *Exp Brain Res* 1998; 123(1-2):60–76.

242. McCann UD, Wong DF, Yokoi F, et al. Reduced striatal dopamine transporter density in abstinent methamphetamine and methcathinone users: evidence from positron emission tomography studies with [^{11}C]WIN-35428. *J Neurosci* 1998;18(20):8417–8422.

243. Volkow ND, Wang G, Fowler JS, et al. Therapeutic doses of oral methylphenidate significantly increase extracellular dopamine in the human brain. *J Neurosci* 2001;21(2):RC121.

244. Wilson JM, Kalasinsky KS, Levey AI, et al. Striatal dopamine nerve terminal markers in human, chronic methamphetamine users. *Nat Med* 1996;2(6):699–703.

245. Wilson JM, Levey AI, Rajput A, et al. Differential changes in neurochemical markers of striatal dopamine nerve terminals in idiopathic Parkinson's disease. *Neurology* 1996;47(3):718–726.

246. Seibyl JP, Marek K, Sheff K, et al. Test/retest reproducibility of iodine-123-betaCIT SPECT brain measurement of dopamine transporters in Parkinson's patients. *J Nucl Med* 1997;38(9):1453–1459.

247. Guttman M, Burkholder J, Kish SJ, et al. [^{11}C]RTI-32 PET studies of the dopamine transporter in early dopa-naive Parkinson's disease: implications for the symptomatic threshold. *Neurology* 1997;48(6): 1578–1583.

248. Villemagne V, Yuan J, Wong DF, et al. Brain dopamine neurotoxicity in baboons treated with doses of methamphetamine comparable to those recreationally abused by humans: evidence from [^{11}C]WIN-35428 positron emission tomography studies and direct *in vitro* determinations. *J Neurosci* 1998;18(1):419–427.

249. Melega WP, Lacan G, Harvey DC, et al. Dizocilpine and reduced body temperature do not prevent methamphetamine-induced neurotoxicity in the vervet monkey: [^{11}C]WIN 35428 positron emission tomography studies. *Neurosci Lett* 1998;258(1):17–20.

250. Harvey DC, Lacan G, Tanious SP, et al. Recovery from methamphetamine induced long-term nigrostriatal dopaminergic deficits without substantia nigra cell loss. *Brain Res* 2000;871(2):259–270.

251. McCann UD, Szabo Z, Scheffel U, et al. Positron emission tomographic evidence of toxic effect of MDMA ("ecstasy") on brain serotonin neurons in human beings. *Lancet* 1998;352(9138):1433–1437.

252. Semple DM, Ebmeier KP, Glabus MF, et al. Reduced *in vivo* binding to serotonin transporter in the cerebral cortex of MDMA ("ecstasy") users. *Br J Psychiatry* 1999;175:63–69.

253. Reneman L, Lavalaye J, Schmand B, et al. Cortical serotonin transporter density and verbal memory in individuals who stopped using

3,4-methylenedioxymethamphetamine (MDMA or "ecstasy"): preliminary findings. *Arch Gen Psychiatry* 2001;58(10):901–906.

254. Heinz A, Jones DW. Serotonin transporters in ecstasy users. *Br J Psychiatry* 2000;176:193–195.

255. Laruelle M, Wallace E, Seibyl JP, et al. Graphical, kinetic, and equilibrium analyses of in vivo [^{123}I] beta-CIT binding to dopamine transporters in healthy human subjects. *J Cereb Blood Flow Metab* 1994;14(6):982–994.

256. Reneman L, Booij J, Schmand B, et al. Memory disturbances in "ecstasy" users are correlated with an altered brain serotonin neurotransmission. *Psychopharmacology (Berl)* 2000;148(3):322–324.

257. Reneman L, Habraken JB, Majoie CB, et al. MDMA ("ecstasy") and its association with cerebrovascular accidents: preliminary findings. *AJNR Am J Neuroradiol* 2000;21(6):1001–1007.

258. Abi-Dargham A, Zea-Ponce Y, Terriere D, et al. Preclinical evaluation of [I-123]R93274 as a SPECT radiotracer for imaging serotonin 5-HT$_{2A}$ receptors. *Eur J Pharmacol* 1997;321:285–293.

259. Busatto GF, Pilowsky LS, Costa DC, et al. Initial evaluation of ^{123}I-5-I-R91150, a selective 5-HT$_{2A}$ ligand for single-photon emission tomography, in healthy human subjects. *Eur J Nucl Med* 1997;24(2):119–124.

260. Kling MA, Carson RE, Borg L, et al. Opioid receptor imaging with positron emission tomography and [^{18}F]cyclofoxy in long-term, methadone-treated former heroin addicts. *J Pharmacol Exp Ther* 2000;295(3):1070–1076.

261. Carson RE, Channing MA, Blasberg RG, et al. Comparison of bolus and infusion methods for receptor quantitation: application to [^{18}F]cyclofoxy and positron emission tomography. *J Cereb Blood Flow Metab* 1993;13(1):24–42.

262. Zubieta J, Greenwald MK, Lombardi U, et al. Buprenorphine-induced changes in mu-opioid receptor availability in male heroin-dependent volunteers: a preliminary study. *Neuropsychopharmacology* 2000;23(3):326–334.

263. Frost JJ, Douglass KH, Mayberg HS, et al. Multicompartmental analysis of [^{11}C]-carfentanil binding to opiate receptors in humans measured by positron emission tomography. *J Cereb Blood Flow Metab* 1989;9(3):398–409.

264. Mello NK, Mendelson JH, Kuehnle JC. Buprenorphine effects on human heroin self-administration: an operant analysis. *J Pharmacol Exp Ther* 1982;223(1):30–39.

265. Comer SD, Collins ED, Fischman MW. Buprenorphine sublingual tablets: effects on IV heroin self-administration by humans. *Psychopharmacology (Berl)* 2001;154(1):28–37.

266. Wang GJ, Volkow ND, Logan J, et al. Brain dopamine and obesity. *Lancet* 2001;357(9253):354–357.

267. Fowler JS, Volkow ND, Wang GJ, et al. Inhibition of monoamine oxidase B in the brains of smokers. *Nature* 1996;379(6567):733–736.

268. Fowler JS, Volkow ND, Wang GJ, et al. Brain monoamine oxidase A inhibition in cigarette smokers. *Proc Natl Acad Sci U S A* 1996;93(24):14065–14069.

269. Fowler JS, Volkow ND, Wang GJ, et al. Neuropharmacological actions of cigarette smoke: brain monoamine oxidase B (MAO B) inhibition. *J Addict Dis* 1998;17(1):23–34.

270. Fowler JS, Wang GJ, Volkow ND, et al. Maintenance of brain monoamine oxidase B inhibition in smokers after overnight cigarette abstinence. *Am J Psychiatry* 2000;157(11):1864–1866.

271. Logan J, Fowler JS, Volkow ND, et al. Reproducibility of repeated measures of deuterium substituted [^{11}C]L-deprenyl ([^{11}C]L-deprenyl-D$_2$) binding in the human brain. *Nucl Med Biol* 2000;27(1):43–49.

272. Salokangas RK, Vilkman H, Ilonen T, et al. High levels of dopamine activity in the basal ganglia of cigarette smokers. *Am J Psychiatry* 2000;157(4):632–634.

273. Dagher A, Bleicher C, Aston JA, et al. Reduced dopamine D$_1$ receptor binding in the ventral striatum of cigarette smokers. *Synapse* 2001;42(1):48–53.

274. Staley JK, Krishnan-Sarin S, Zoghbi S, et al. Sex differences in [^{123}I]beta-CIT SPECT measures of dopamine and serotonin transporter availability in healthy smokers and nonsmokers. *Synapse* 2001;41(4):275–284.

275. Noble EP, Blum K, Ritchie T, et al. Allelic association of the D$_2$ dopamine receptor gene with receptor-binding characteristics in alcoholism. *Arch Gen Psychiatry* 1991;48(7):648–654.

276. Hietala J, West C, Syvälahti E, et al. Striatal D$_2$ dopamine receptor binding characteristics in vivo in patients with alcohol dependence. *Psychopharmacology* 1994;116:285–290.

277. Volkow ND, Wang GJ, Fowler JS, et al. Decreases in dopamine receptors but not in dopamine transporters in alcoholics. *Alcohol Clin Exp Res* 1996;20(9):1594–1598.

278. Guardia J, Catafau AM, Batlle F, et al. Striatal dopaminergic D$_2$ receptor density measured by [(^{123})I]iodobenzamide SPECT in the prediction of treatment outcome of alcohol-dependent patients. *Am J Psychiatry* 2000;157(1):127–129.

279. Tabakoff B, Hoffman P. Development of functional dependence on ethanol in dopaminergic systems. *J Pharmacol Exp Ther* 1979;208:216–222.

280. Muller P, Britton R, Seman P. The effects of long term ethanol on brain receptors for dopamine, acetylcholine, serotonin and noradrenaline. *Eur J Pharmacol* 1980;65:31–37.

281. Rabin RA, Wolfe BB, Dibner MD, et al. Effects of ethanol administration and withdrawal on neurotransmitter receptor systems in C57 mice. *J Pharmacol Exp Ther* 1983;213:491–496.

282. Fuchs V, Coper H, Rommelspacher H. The effects of ethanol and haloperidol on dopamine receptors (D$_2$) density. *Neuropharmacology* 1987;26:1231–1233.

283. Hietala J, Salonen I, Lappalainen J, et al. Ethanol administration does not alter dopamine D$_1$ and D$_2$ receptor characteristic in rat brain. *Neurosci Lett* 1990;108:289–294.

284. Lai H, Carino MA, Hrita A. Effects of ethanol on central dopamine function. *Life Sci* 1980;27:299–304.

285. Hruska RE. Effects of ethanol administration on striatal D$_1$ and D$_2$ receptors. *J Neurochem* 1988;50:1929–1933.

286. Lucchi L, Moresco RM, Govoni S, et al. Effect of chronic ethanol treatment on dopamine receptor subtypes in rat striatum. *Brain Res* 1988;449(1-2):347–351.

287. Hamdi A, Prasad C. Bidirectional changes in striatal D$_2$-dopamine receptor density during chronic ethanol intake. *Alcohol* 1993;93:203–206.

288. Tiihonen J, Kuikka J, Bergström K, et al. Altered striatal dopamine re-uptake site densities in habitually violent and non-violent alcoholics. *Nat Med* 1995;1:654–657.

289. Laine TP, Ahonen A, Rasanen P, et al. Dopamine transporter availability and depressive symptoms during alcohol withdrawal [In Process Citation]. *Psychiatry Res* 1999;90(3):153–157.

290. Laine TP, Ahonen A, Torniainen P, et al. Dopamine transporters increase in human brain after alcohol withdrawal. *Mol Psychiatry* 1999;4(2):104–105,189–191.

291. Volkow ND, Wang GJ, Hitzemann R, et al. Decreased cerebral response to inhibitory neurotransmission in alcoholics. *Am J Psychiatry* 1993;150(3):417–422.

292. Volkow ND, Wang GJ, Begleiter H, et al. Regional brain metabolic response to lorazepam in subjects at risk for alcoholism. *Alcohol Clin Exp Res* 1995;19(2):510–516.

293. Pauli S, Liljequist S, Farde L, et al. PET analysis of alcohol interaction with the brain disposition of [^{11}C]flumazenil. *Psychopharmacology* 1992;107:180–185.

294. Litton J-E, Neiman J, Pauli S, et al. PET analysis of [^{11}C]flumazenil binding to benzodiazepine receptors in chronic alcohol-dependent men and healthy controls. *Psychiatry Res Neuroimaging* 1992;50:1–13.

295. Farde L, Pauli S, Litton JE, et al. PET-determination of benzodiazepine receptor binding in studies on alcoholism. *EXS* 1994;71:143–153.

296. Gilman S, Koeppe RA, Adams K, et al. Positron emission tomographic studies of cerebral benzodiazepine-receptor binding in chronic alcoholics. *Ann Neurol* 1996;40:163–171.

297. Abi-Dargham A, Krystal JH, Anjilvel S, et al. Alterations of benzodiazepine receptors in type II alcoholic subjects measured with SPECT and [^{123}I]iomazenil. *Am J Psychiatry* 1998;155(11):1550–1555.

298. Lingford-Hughes AR, Acton PD, Gacinovic S, et al. Reduced levels of GABA-benzodiazepine receptor in alcohol dependency in the absence of grey matter atrophy. *Br J Psychiatry* 1998;173:116–122.

299. Lingford-Hughes AR, Acton PD, et al. Levels of gamma-aminobutyric acid-benzodiazepine receptors in abstinent, alcohol-dependent women: preliminary findings from an ^{123}I-iomazenil single photon emission tomography study. *Alcohol Clin Exp Res* 2000;24(9):1449–1455.

300. Wagner HW Jr. Highlights 2001 lecture. *J Nucl Med* 2001;42:12N–30N.

301. Laruelle M. The role of model-based methods in the development of single scan techniques. *Nucl Med Biol* 2000;27(7):637–642.

CHAPTER 8.1

Myocardial Perfusion

Nagara Tamaki, Terrence D. Ruddy, Robert deKemp, and Rob S. B. Beanlands

Coronary artery disease (CAD) continues to be a major cause of death in modern industrialized societies. Techniques for evaluating myocardial blood flow have an important role to play in the identification of patients with CAD and determination of their prognosis. Patients at high risk for subsequent cardiac events can be treated with aggressive interventional therapy and low-risk patients can be managed medically. Measurement of regional myocardial perfusion permits measurement of coronary flow reserve and the evaluation of the physiologic significance of coronary lesions and the adequacy of collateral supply. These myocardial blood-flow measures are often essential for characterizing the functional significance of CAD and are complementary to coronary angiography. Positron emission tomography (PET) measurements of myocardial blood-flow reserve are also useful for the serial evaluation of patients with the goals of determining the response to therapy and progression or regression of disease. Although the present clinical use of PET is somewhat limited by the high cost of the technology, the development of less-expensive PET cameras and greater reimbursement for cardiac PET will result in wider clinical application. PET is uniquely suited to be a quantitative research tool for studies evaluating myocardial perfusion *in vivo* in humans.

PET is accepted as the most accurate noninvasive imaging technique for measurement of regional myocardial blood flow. Tissue perfusion in milliliters per minute per gram can be measured *in vivo* by relating myocardial tracer kinetics to arterial tracer input. The accuracy of these noninvasive measurements requires (a) a radiotracer with retention or clearance kinetics related to myocardial blood flow during normal and pathophysiologic states, (b) accurate measurement of the arterial blood and myocardial activity of the radiotracer with adequate temporal resolution to define the tracer kinetics, and (c) established methods of modeling of the tracer kinetics to permit calculation of regional flow measurements. Current PET technology has high spatial resolution of 4.0 to 6.0 mm and accurate attenuation correction, permitting measurement of myocardial radiotracer concentration at frequent time intervals. Suitable kinetic modeling has been developed for several PET flow tracers and makes possible the accurate measurement of tissue blood flow (1–4).

MYOCARDIAL BLOOD-FLOW TRACERS

The commonly used PET blood-flow tracers can be divided into (a) inert freely diffusible tracers such as $H_2^{15}O$ and (b) physiologically retained tracers such as nitrogen-13 (^{13}N)-ammonia and rubidium-82 (^{82}Rb). The commonly used PET myocardial blood-flow tracers are listed in Table 8.1.1 in order of increasing half-life.

Diffusible tracers such as $H_2^{15}O$ pass freely across membranes, resulting in a distribution of tracer between vascular and extravascular space related to the partition coefficient. The partition coefficient for $H_2^{15}O$ is stable over a wide range of flow rates so that uptake of $H_2^{15}O$ is not diffusion limited. Conversely, the extraction fraction of physiologically retained radiotracers decreases with increasing blood flow and results in underestimation of myocardial blood flow based on the measurement of tissue uptake. These physiologic properties are incorporated into the kinetic models for determination of myocardial blood flow.

^{13}N-ammonia

Nitrogen-13-ammonia is the most commonly used myocardial perfusion tracer in PET centers with an on-site cyclotron. Nitrogen-13 is produced with a cyclotron and a water target via the oxygen-16 ^{16}O $(p,\alpha)^{13}N$ nuclear reaction to yield the radionuclide. Ammonium ions can be readily converted to ammonia with reducing agents.

After intravenous administration of ^{13}N-ammonia, ^{13}N-ammonia crosses capillary and cell membranes via passive diffusion and is retained in myocardial tissue by the incorporation of the label into the amino acid pool as glutamine. The synthesis of glutamine is the rate-limiting step for tissue retention of ^{13}N-ammonia. Nitrogen-13-ammonia in blood is in an equilibrium state with ionic ^{13}N-ammonium (5,6). The first-pass extraction fraction is nearly 100%, because

TABLE 8.1.1. *PET myocardial blood-flow tracers*

Radioisotope	Pharmaceutical	Half-life	Positron energy (MeV)
Rubidium-82 (^{82}Rb)	Rubidium	76 sec	3.15
Oxygen-15 (^{15}O)	Water	110 sec	1.72
Potassium-38 (^{38}K)	Potassium	7.6 min	2.7
Copper-62 (^{62}Cu)	PTSM	9.8 min	2.94
Nitrogen-13 (^{13}N)	Ammonia	10 min	1.19
Carbon-11 (^{11}C)	Acetate butanol	20 min	0.96

PTSM, pyruvaldehyde methylthiosemicarbazone.

^{13}N-ammonia diffuses freely across membranes (6). In the myocardium, ^{13}N-ammonia either is incorporated into the synthesis of ^{13}N-glutamine or back-diffuses into the vascular space (7). The net extraction fraction is approximately 80% in the resting flow range but decreases with higher flow rates.

Studies in normal volunteers showed a slight heterogeneity of regional tracer retention (8). Nitrogen-13-ammonia retention was decreased by 10% in the lateral wall of the left ventricle as compared with the septum. The underlying mechanism of this phenomenon is poorly understood. However, this mild heterogeneity must be recognized when interpreting ^{13}N-ammonia perfusion images. Changes in the metabolic and hemodynamic environment within physiologic ranges do not significantly alter the retention of ^{13}N-ammonia (6,7). Other factors to consider with ^{13}N-ammonia imaging include intense liver activity, which can interfere with the evaluation of the inferior wall and increased lung activity in patients with pulmonary disease or pulmonary congestion. Overall, these imaging problems are uncommon. The image quality achieved with ^{13}N-ammonia is considered to be the best among all of the PET perfusion tracers due to the relatively long physical half-life, relatively high extraction fraction, and low background and low positron energy (Fig. 8.1.1).

To quantify myocardial blood flow, several tracer kinetic models of ^{13}N-ammonia have been described. The most common approach assumes a three-compartment model, with the compartments being the vascular, extravascular, and metabolic spaces (9). The first-pass extraction is assumed to be 100%. K_1 represents the transport of the tracer from

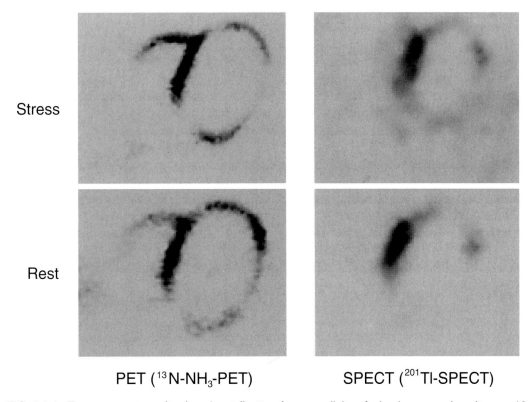

Stress

Rest

PET (^{13}N-NH$_3$-PET)   SPECT (^{201}Tl-SPECT)

FIG. 8.1.1. Transverse stress **(top)** and rest **(bottom)** myocardial perfusion images using nitrogen-13-ammonia PET **(left)** and thallium-201 single-photon emission computed tomography **(right)** acquired in a patient with an inferior wall myocardial infarction. The perfusion defect in the posterolateral region is well demonstrated by both studies, but the stress-induced perfusion abnormality in the apex is more clearly seen in the PET perfusion study.

the vascular space into the extravascular space is an estimate of myocardial blood flow. These PET measurements have been well validated with microsphere measurements in experimental preparations and confirm that regional myocardial blood flow can be quantitatively measured over a wide blood-flow range with ^{13}N-ammonia and this three-compartment approach (10–12).

A number of simplified approaches have been used to quantify regional myocardial blood flow with ^{13}N-ammonia. The simplest method is the microsphere model, which requires one static scan, an arterial input function, and correction for the net extraction fraction (13–15). However, the quantitative value is quite variable and depends on the time of measurement after tracer administration. To minimize this effect, the Patlak graphical analysis of the early uptake phase has recently been applied for the quantitative estimate of myocardial blood flow (16,17). With the use of any of these approaches, accurate quantification of regional myocardial blood flow can be achieved with ^{13}N-ammonia at rest and during stress conditions (18). Automated analysis is required to facilitate rapid processing with minimal interobserver variability (19).

For relative perfusion imaging, ^{13}N-ammonia is injected as a bolus of 15 to 25 mCi and static images are acquired 2 to 6 minutes after tracer administration for an imaging time of 5 to 20 minutes. Myocardial perfusion can be evaluated with either exercise or pharmacologic stress. Because imaging starts shortly after tracer administration, pharmacologic stress is preferred. However, ^{13}N-ammonia can be used in conjunction with treadmill or bicycle exercise tests. The tracer is administrated at peak exercise and exercise is continued for an additional 30 to 60 seconds. The patient is then repositioned in the PET scanner to start the acquisition within 4 to 6 minutes (20–22). Accurate repositioning is important to minimize artifacts due to incorrect attenuation correction. A bicycle ergometer can be attached to the PET bed, making this approach more feasible.

Pharmacologic stress is usually performed with either dipyridamole or adenosine. These agents increase myocardial blood flow and permit measurement of myocardial blood-flow reserve. Dobutamine infusion can also be used and increases cardiac work and subsequently myocardial blood flow. The increase in myocardial blood flow with dobutamine may be submaximal depending on the increase in cardiac workload and results in an underestimation of maximal myocardial blood-flow reserve.

For quantitative measurement of myocardial blood flow, serial dynamic PET imaging begins simultaneously with tracer administration. From the dynamic images, time-activity curves (TACs) are generated for the myocardium and the blood pool. Global and regional myocardial blood flow can be measured with the use of compartmental tracer kinetic modeling to fit the myocardial activity data and correct it for the arterial input function. Previously, the arterial input function was measured by sequential arterial blood sampling. However, blood-pool time-activity data provide an accurate measurement without the use of arterial cannulation, which makes acquisitions more feasible and easier for the patient.

Rubidium-82

This tracer is produced from a strontium-82 (^{82}Sr)/^{82}Rb generator, which can be eluted every 10 minutes (23). Rubidium-82 is a widely used PET perfusion tracer in centers without access to an on-site cyclotron. The half-life of the parent isotope is 25.5 days and results in a generator life of about 4 to 6 weeks. Not requiring a cyclotron is a major advantage of this radiotracer. Although the commercial generator is expensive, a high volume of cardiac studies significantly reduces the cost of radiotracer per examination. The short physical half-life of 76 seconds makes ^{82}Rb suitable for repeated and sequential perfusion studies (Fig. 8.1.2). The short half-life necessitates rapid image acquisition shortly after tracer administration. The relatively high positron energy of ^{82}Rb (3.15 MeV) is associated with a positron range averaging 7.5 mm and results in lower spatial resolution than seen with ^{13}N-ammonia with a positron range of 2.5 mm.

Rubidium-82 is an analogue of potassium and has similar biologic activity to thallium-201 (^{201}Tl) (24,25). Rubidium-82 is rapidly extracted from the blood and concentrated by the myocardium. In animal models, the first-pass extraction fraction is 50% to 60% at rest and decreases to 25% to 30% at peak flow (24,26,27). In addition, the extraction fraction may remain reduced in myocardium recovering from transient ischemia (28). This radiotracer is retained in the myocardium and equilibrates in the potassium pool. Thus, cell membrane disruption may cause rapid tissue loss of radioactivity and ^{82}Rb kinetics can be used as a marker of tissue viability (29).

For quantitative assessment of regional myocardial blood flow, a two-compartment model has been used, and it includes activity in the vascular space and within the tissue compartment (30). After bolus injection of the tracer, predominantly unidirectional transport is assumed from the vascular space into the tissue space. In the canine model, regional myocardial blood flow can be accurately estimated using ^{82}Rb (30). A simplified approach using a summed late image corrected for the input function similar to that described for ^{13}N-ammonia has also been used. This approach allows reasonable quantification of perfusion and may be easier to apply in the clinical setting (31,32).

A large amount of tracer can be administered to the patient because of the short physical half-life of ^{82}Rb. Approximately 50 to 60 mCi of ^{82}Rb can be injected as a bolus, followed by serial dynamic acquisition using a PET camera with a high count rate and high sensitivity with a short acquisition time (24,26). Alternatively, the newer generation of PET cameras can acquire data in three-dimensional (3D) modes and without septa, which results in higher sensitivity and the use of smaller doses of ^{82}Rb (31).

A small and mobile generator infusion system is used

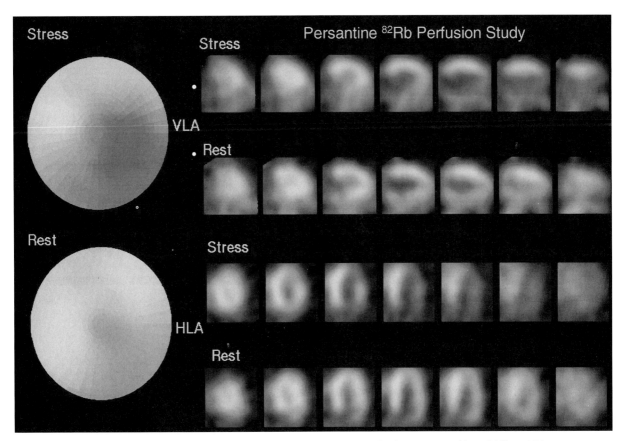

FIG. 8.1.2. Severe ischemia of the apical, lateral, and inferior walls demonstrated by rubidium-82 images acquired at rest and during dipyridamole stress and reoriented in the vertical long axis and horizontal long axis planes. The transient ischemic dilatation of the left ventricle is consistent with multivessel ischemia.

for eluting ^{82}Rb every 10 to 15 minutes with low radiation exposure to personnel or patient. Quantitative assessment of myocardial blood flow and flow reserve is feasible and clinically practical with this generator and has advantages compared with cyclotron-produced compounds (31–34).

Copper-62-PTSM

Copper-62 (^{62}Cu)-pyruvaldehyde-methylthiosemicarbazone (PTSM) is another generator-produced PET perfusion tracer and is produced from a zinc-62 (^{62}Zn)/^{62}Cu generator (35–41). The ^{62}Zn/^{62}Cu generator is inexpensive because ^{62}Zn can be easily produced with a medium-energy cyclotron and ^{82}Sr requires a high-energy cyclotron. Copper-62-PTSM is quite suitable for serial measurement of myocardial blood flow, because the half-life of 9.7 minutes is short (42). Unfortunately, the relatively short half-life of 9.2 hours of the parent, ^{62}Zn, results in the need for a fresh generator on a daily basis.

After intravenous administration of ^{62}Cu-PTSM, the radiotracer clears rapidly from blood, with high tracer uptake in the myocardium. The uncharged lipophilic copper-PTSM rapidly diffuses across cell membranes. Within the cell, the

^{62}Cu-PTSM is susceptible to reductive decomposition by reaction with ubiquitous intracellular enzymes. As a result, an effectively irreversible deposition of ionic copper occurs in the cells.

Copper-62-PTSM is a promising tracer for the evaluation of myocardial and cerebral perfusion. High-quality myocardial perfusion images can be obtained shortly after tracer administration in both animal and human studies (42–44). Approximately 5% to 10% of the injected dose remains in the circulation due to binding to red blood cells. Therefore, the quantitative measurement of regional myocardial blood flow using the microsphere model requires correction of the arterial blood TAC for blood-pool binding (45). A significant reduction in the extraction fraction is observed in the high-flow range and requires correction to express data as absolute myocardial blood flow (45). The extraction fraction is reduced in the occlusion-reperfusion model, suggesting that this tracer can be used as a functional marker (46).

Myocardial contrast was high in myocardial perfusion images acquired at rest and during pharmacologic stress in normal volunteers, although liver uptake interfered with the evaluation of the inferior wall (8,42). Coronary stenotic lesions were identified as areas of reduced coronary flow reserve. Reduced contrast of perfusion defects were observed in studies with ^{62}Cu-PTSM compared with that in studies using ^{13}N-ammonia, presumably due to the significantly lower extraction fraction of ^{62}Cu-PTSM in the high-flow range (47).

$H_2{}^{15}O$

The $H_2{}^{15}O$ was one of the first radiopharmaceuticals developed for PET use and is considered the gold standard for quantitation of myocardial perfusion. $H_2{}^{15}O$ is usually obtained from $^{15}O_2$ gas combined with hydrogen gas. The ^{15}O gas is produced either by the $^{14}N(d,n)^{15}O$ reaction or the $^{15}N(p,n)^{15}O$ method. Because the physical half-life of $^{15}O^-$ is only 2 minutes, an in-house cyclotron is required to use $H_2{}^{15}O$.

One of the major advantages of $H_2{}^{15}O$ is the feasibility for quantitative assessment of myocardial blood flow. Because water is freely diffusible in the myocardium without dependence on metabolism, the biological behavior of $H_2{}^{15}O$ can be modeled with a simple one-compartment model, as originally described by Kety (48) and Bermann et al. (49). Rapid sequential image acquisition is needed after tracer administration. Because of the short physical half-life, a large amount of activity is administrated, which requires a high-count rate and high-sensitivity PET camera for quantitation of radioactivity concentration after dead-time correction.

Tomographic visualization of the $H_2{}^{15}O$ perfusion images requires correction of blood-pool activity. A separate scan is acquired after inhalation of ^{15}O-carbon monoxide, which labels erythrocytes and delineates the vascular blood pool. High-contrast myocardial perfusion images can be obtained after subtraction of the blood-pool images from the $H_2{}^{15}O$ images (Fig. 8.1.3) (49,50). Principal component analysis has been used to define the blood and myocardial signals, without the need for an additional blood-pool scan. Patient motion between the two scans can introduce significant error into the subtraction images. The kinetic model used in the determination of myocardial blood flow accounts for partial volume and blood-to-tissue spillover effects.

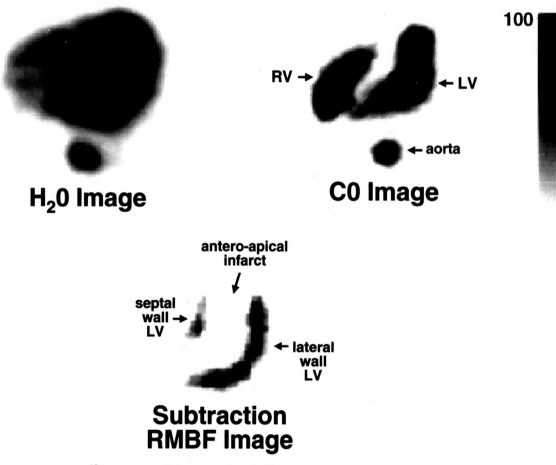

FIG. 8.1.3. $H_2{}^{15}O$ perfusion transverse slice ($H_2{}^{15}O$ image) demonstrates myocardial and blood-pool activity. A corresponding ^{15}O-carbon monoxide image (CO image) delineates the vascular blood pool and was acquired after inhalation of ^{15}O-carbon monoxide and subsequent labeling of erythrocytes. The myocardial perfusion image (subtraction RMBF image) was obtained after subtraction of the blood-pool image from the $H_2{}^{15}O$ image and shows a large infract.

Iida et al. (51) proposed a mathematic model to correct the input function for the tissue-to-blood spillover (52) and partial volume effect (53). This model permits estimation of the perfusable tissue fraction, defined as the water-perfusable tissue, divided by total extravascular anatomic tissue. This parameter is independent of the size of the region of interest and may discriminate water-perfusable viable tissue from nonperfusable infarcted tissue, assuming that irreversibly damaged tissue cannot exchange water rapidly (54,55).

^{11}C-butanol

Radiolabeled aliphatic alcohols have been evaluated in the search for better blood-flow tracers. Butanol seems to be a nearly optimal flow tracer because it has a better partition coefficient than $H_2^{15}O$. Carbon-11-butanol can be produced with a simple synthesis with a high yield (56,57). However, this tracer has been mainly used for cerebral perfusion studies and it is not yet well evaluated for measurement of myocardial blood flow.

CLINICAL APPLICATIONS

Diagnosis and Prognosis in Coronary Artery Disease

Nitrogen-13-ammonia PET perfusion imaging can identify reduced perfusion associated with a coronary artery lesion with less than 50% stenosis in an animal model (58). Schelbert et al. (59) first demonstrated the clinical value of ^{13}N-ammonia PET perfusion imaging with pharmacologic stress for the accurate detection of CAD. Table 8.1.2 summarizes published data on the sensitivity and specificity of PET stress perfusion imaging for detection of CAD (60–67). PET stress perfusion imaging has high diagnostic accuracy for detection of CAD, with a sensitivity of 94% and a specificity of 95%. In a community hospital study of more than 1,400 patients, PET stress perfusion imaging with ^{82}Rb had a sensitivity of 87% and a specificity of 88% for detecting larger than 67%-diameter stenoses and a sensitivity of 92% for detecting larger than 90%-diameter stenoses (68).

The diagnostic accuracy for detecting CAD with PET stress perfusion imaging has been compared with results with conventional single-photon emission computed tomography (SPECT) stress perfusion imaging in the same patient population (Table 8.1.3). The first report from Tamaki et al. (69) showed a similar high diagnostic accuracy for both techniques, although the image quality of the PET perfusion images was superior with better delineation of stress-induced ischemia than observed with ^{201}Tl SPECT (Fig. 8.1.1). The other two studies included a greater number of patients with suspected CAD and reported higher sensitivity and specificity of PET perfusion imaging (66,67). In addition, the localization of CAD was more accurate with PET than thallium SPECT (67). Overall, the accuracy for detection of CAD from the pooled data was greater for PET versus SPECT, with a greater sensitivity of 93% versus 85%, specificity of 82% versus 67%, and diagnostic accuracy of 91% versus 81% (Table 8.1.3). MacIntyre et al. (70) studied the clinical outcome of patients with a false-negative ^{201}Tl SPECT but true-positive ^{82}Rb-PET and observed that the majority were recommended for revascularization procedures.

Myocardial perfusion imaging using PET has several advantages over the conventional single-photon perfusion imaging. (a) The higher sensitivity of the PET camera provides more photons from the myocardium and higher quality myocardial images. (b) Accurate correction of photon attenuation can be performed with PET, which reduces attenuation artifacts and makes precise quantitative analysis of myocardial perfusion possible. In the future, SPECT perfusion imaging with new attenuation-correction methods may also provide higher specificity and accuracy for detection of CAD. (c) The commonly used perfusion tracers, such as ^{13}N-ammonia and the generator-produced agent, ^{82}Rb, have relatively high extraction fractions, which may permit detection of mild degrees of ischemia. This advantage of PET may be particularly important for the comparison of perfusion imaging with PET versus SPECT using technetium-99m perfusion agents that have a lower extraction fraction than ^{201}Tl. (d) The short physical half-lives of the PET tracers make repetitive PET perfusion studies feasible over short time intervals. (e) Although stress perfusion abnormalities can be identified with conventional SPECT in most cases, the interpretation of PET perfusion images provides greater confidence due to the better quality images.

With the rapid development of computer software mainly

TABLE 8.1.2. *Detection of coronary artery disease with stress perfusion PET imaging*

Reference (no.)	N	Stress	Sensitivity (%)	Specificity (%)	Accuracy (%)
Schelbert et al. (60)	32	Pharmacologic	97	100	98
Tamaki et al. (61)	46	Exercise	98	—	—
Yonekura et al. (62)	49	Exercise	97	100	—
Gould et al. (63)	50	Pharmacologic	95	100	—
Williams et al. (64)	146	Pharmacologic	98	100	96
Demer et al. (65)	193	Pharmacologic	82	95	88
Go et al. (66)	135	Pharmacologic	95	82	95
Stewart et al. (67)	81	Pharmacologic	84	88	85
Total	732		94	95	92

TABLE 8.1.3. *Detection of coronary artery disease with stress perfusion PET versus SPECT imaging*

	Year	N	Sensitivity (%)		Specificity (%)		Accuracy (%)	
			PET	SPECT	PET	SPECT	PET	SPECT
Tamaki et al. (69)	1988	51	98	96	100	100	98	98
Go et al. (66)	1990	132	95[a]	79	82	76	92[a]	78
Stewart et al. (67)	1991	81	87	87	82[a]	52	85	78
Total		264	93[a]	85	82[a]	67	91[a]	81

[a] $p < .05$ vs. SPECT.

used for myocardial perfusion SPECT, automated image analysis of perfusion PET can be applied to assist the visual interpretation (71,72). This automated image-analysis approach had a diagnostic accuracy of 91%, 79%, and 88% for localization of disease to the left anterior descending artery, circumflex, and right coronary artery distributions, respectively (73).

Defining prognosis in patients with suspected or known coronary artery disease is important in clinical care. In a large series of 685 patients, PET perfusion imaging results were independent predictors of cardiac death and total cardiac events (74). Within a mean follow-up period of 41 months, patients with a normal PET scan result had an event-free survival of 90%; whereas those with a mild defect had a survival rate of 87%, which fell to 75% for those with severe defects. The results of PET perfusion imaging added incremental prognostic information in comparison to clinical and angiographic findings alone. This incremental prognostic value is most likely due to the additional value of assessment of the physiologic severity of abnormalities of myocardial perfusion and perfusion reserve by stress perfusion PET. Similar results have been observed with SPECT stress perfusion imaging.

Cost-effectiveness

The higher cost of PET studies compared to echocardiography or SPECT raises questions about the cost-effectiveness of PET perfusion imaging. Patterson et al. (75) used a straightforward mathematic model based on the Bayes theorem to compare the cost-effectiveness and utility of four diagnostic strategies using exercise ECG, stress SPECT, stress PET, and coronary angiography for the diagnosis of CAD. The risk, cost, and diagnostic accuracy of each test were calculated based on literature data and were fitted using a management algorithm for each diagnostic strategy. PET stress imaging had the lowest cost per effect or cost per utility unit in patients with a pretest probability of less than 70%, whereas coronary angiography had the lowest cost per effect in patients, with a pretest probability of more than 70%. The relative savings of PET perfusion imaging were related to the high specificity. Using the PET strategy may reduce unnecessary coronary angiography. Furthermore, a high fraction of stress treadmill tests had undetermined re-

sults, which may lead to greater number of unnecessary coronary angiograms. PET perfusion imaging appears to be the method of choice for detection of CAD in centers with access to (and reimbursement for) both PET and SPECT. However, improved specificity for detecting CAD may be possible with SPECT imaging due to the recent development of attenuation correction and the addition of functional assessment with gated acquisitions.

Subsequent cost-benefit studies have been conflicting. Garber and Solomon (76), in spite of a wide range of sensitivity (40% to 100%) for stress echocardiography, suggested this modality was the most cost-effective noninvasive approach (76). This study, however, only included three PET studies in the analysis, made assumptions about clinical practice that did not consider current surgical techniques, intervention, and new medical therapies, and did not consider the decreasing cost of PET. On the other hand, in a decision-analysis study including a comprehensive literature review, Maddahi and Gambhir (77) showed that exercise ECG, followed by PET or SPECT if the stress test result was positive, was the most cost-effective approach for patients with low pretest likelihood of disease. For intermediate-risk patients, performing PET or SPECT first was the most cost-effective approach, whereas in high-risk patients, direct angiography was the best first test [similar to Patterson et al. (75)].

Thus, PET appears in some, but not all, studies to be a cost-effective approach. Cost analyses can be complex. Often, many variables are considered and others are overlooked. None of the cost analyses have considered the potential prognostic information that PET imaging can provide. Further studies of cost-effectiveness will be necessary as competing technologies evolve and as PET costs decrease.

Quantitative Measurement of Myocardial Blood-flow Reserve

PET imaging is an excellent technique for quantifying regional tracer concentration *in vivo*. With use of appropriate tracer kinetic models, PET imaging permits quantitative measurement of regional myocardial blood flow and flow reserve (ratio of maximal blood flow vs. control resting blood flow). Myocardial blood flow can be measured with PET and ^{13}N-ammonia, ^{82}Rb, or $H_2{}^{15}O$ over a wide range of blood flows (9–17,31,49,51).

After experimental validation, several studies have employed PET imaging to establish the normal range of myocardial blood flow and flow reserve in healthy volunteers. The mean normal value of flow reserve ranged from 3.5 to 4.7 with dipyridamole or adenosine administration and there was no regional heterogeneity (9,49,78,79). Myocardial blood-flow reserve with exercise and dobutamine was 1.9 ± 0.8 and 2.9 ± 0.8, respectively (19,80). Despite varying methodology, the magnitude of the increase of myocardial blood flow during pharmacologic stress was reproducible among different centers (81,82). The PET myocardial blood-flow values obtained at rest and with pharmacologic stress and flow reserve correlated well with data estimated by invasive measurement with Doppler wire studies (83).

Assessment of Myocardial Blood-flow Reserve in Coronary Artery Disease

Quantitative measurements of myocardial blood-flow reserve with PET provide a noninvasive means to estimate the functional severity of coronary stenosis. Although coronary angiography defines stenosis severity on the basis of morphologic alterations, the measurement of myocardial blood flow or flow reserve represents a more physiologic evaluation of cellular perfusion as the net result of antegrade epicardial coronary flow and collateral circulation.

Gould et al. (84,85) described the value of myocardial blood-flow reserve as a measure of the functional severity of CAD. Although myocardial blood flow at rest remains normal during the progression of coronary lesions until they reach an 80%- to 85%-diameter stenosis, coronary flow reserve begins to decrease with a 40%- to 50%-diameter stenosis (86). In contrast to coronary flow measurement by invasive Doppler wire, PET provides 3D information about myocardial blood flow and flow reserve and facilitates easy assessment of the extent of perfusion abnormalities.

Demer et al. (65) first reported a significant relationship between the severity of relative perfusion abnormalities on PET perfusion images and coronary reserve measurements from quantitative coronary angiography. Uren et al. (87) showed a relationship between coronary artery stenosis seen on angiography and coronary flow reserve data obtained with $H_2^{15}O$ PET perfusion studies. A similar relationship was also described with ^{13}N-ammonia PET perfusion data (88,89). Despite a significant correlation between the severity of coronary stenosis and coronary flow reserve in these studies, there was considerable scatter between the two parameters. A quantitative measurement of coronary stenosis may possibly provide closer correlation. On the other hand, there seem to be inherent differences between the anatomic stenosis on angiography and functional coronary flow reserve on PET, such as accounting for collateral flow. In a study of patients with single-vessel disease, coronary flow and flow reserve were significantly decreased in the remote areas supplied by arteries with no significant stenosis in patients compared with normal subjects. Quantitative measurement of myocardial blood flow by PET may be a more sensitive and accurate method than coronary angiography to detect altered coronary flow dynamics in patients with CAD (90). Conversely, quantitative measurements of myocardial blood flow with PET may provide high sensitivity but low specificity for detecting CAD when coronary stenosis is used as a gold standard in the study of high-risk CAD. Because myocardial flow reserve reflects the functional status of tissue flow, this parameter may be discordant with the anatomic stenosis of major coronary arteries (91).

A number of other factors, such collateral circulation (92, 93) and endothelial modulation of vascular smooth-muscle tone (94,95), may play major roles in the determination of the coronary flow reserve measured by PET studies. Atherosclerosis may introduce potential variability in the behavior of both the epicardial coronary vessels and the coronary resistance vessels. A coronary stenosis in a patient may not produce a fixed degree of anatomic narrowing of the epicardial artery, and the resistance vessels may not predictably undergo maximal vasodilatation in the response to pharmacologic vasodilators. Thus, interpretation of coronary flow reserve may require consideration of the dynamic characteristics of both epicardial arteries and resistance vessels.

Altered myocardial blood flow and flow reserve may be much more extensive than angiographic documentation of regional CAD. Accordingly, PET has been used to detect the early stages of vascular alterations and to monitor response to therapy. VanTosh et al. (96), using ^{82}Rb PET imaging and dipyridamole stress, reported regions of abnormal flow reserve in the areas of restenosis after angioplasty. PET perfusion imaging has also been used to delineate the efficacy of interventional therapies (32,97,98). Thus, PET can be used to objectively identify the patients who recover or ameliorate the functional flow reserve after the treatment.

Coronary Flow Reserve In Relation To Coronary Risk Factors

A number of risk factors associated with atherosclerosis may cause a reduction of coronary flow reserve despite angiographically normal coronary arteries. PET has been extensively used to investigate the relationship of coronary flow reserve and risk factors for CAD, including hypercholesterolemia, diabetes, smoking, and hypertension.

Coronary flow reserve is a complex physiologic parameter influenced by many factors other than coronary artery stenosis. For example, coronary flow reserve may slightly decrease with age, mainly due to an increased workload at rest rather than abnormal vasodilator capacity (99,100). PET perfusion studies have demonstrated a reduction of flow reserve in many cardiac disorders without evidence of CAD. About 10% to 30% of patients with chest pain who undergo cardiac catheterization are found with angiography to have normal coronary arteries. However, PET perfusion studies indicated about 40% to 50% of those patients showed high flow at rest and impaired flow reserve in response to dipyridamole (101,102).

Dayanikli et al. (103) first described a linear relationship between coronary flow measurement and serum cholesterol levels in asymptomatic patients at high risk of developing CAD. Yokoyama et al. (104,105) confirmed these results by describing reduction of coronary flow reserve in asymptomatic patients with familial hypercholesterolemia. A significant inverse correlation was demonstrated between total cholesterol and coronary flow reserve in individual patients. Pitkanen et al. (106,107) showed a significant reduction of coronary flow reserve in patients younger than 40 years with familial hypercholesterolemia in comparison to an age-matched control population. The baseline myocardial blood flow was similar between the two groups, but the flow at maximal vasodilatation was 29% lower in patients with hypercholesterolemia than in healthy control subjects. Reduction of coronary flow reserve was related to lipid phenotype (107). Kaufmann et al. (108) showed a reduction of coronary flow reserve in patients with hypercholesterolemia and demonstrated that low-density lipoprotein (LDL) cholesterol, but not total cholesterol, correlated inversely with coronary flow reserve in these patients. Mellwig et al. (109) showed the acute improvement of coronary vasodilatation capacity by single LDL apheresis.

Gould et al. (110) showed that short-term cholesterol-lowering therapy decreased the size and severity of PET perfusion abnormalities in patients with CAD. Guthlin et al. (111) evaluated the coronary flow reserve before and at 3 months and 6 months after initiation of therapy with fluvastatin. All patients showed significant reductions of cholesterol, LDL, and triglycerides early after therapy. Coronary flow reserve did not increase with 3 months of therapy but increased only after 6 months of therapy. These findings are in agreement with a recent report evaluating endothelial function with quantitative coronary angiography and acetylcholine injection (112). Similar improvement in coronary flow reserve has been reported after cholesterol-lowering treatment using simvastatin (113–115). Czernin et al. (116) evaluated the effect of short-term cardiovascular conditioning and low-fat diet on myocardial blood flow and flow reserve in 13 patients. Myocardial blood flow reserve increased in association with an improvement in exercise capacity and serum lipid profiles.

Alteration of coronary flow reserve has also been demonstrated in patients with diabetes. Yokoyama et al. (117,118) showed a significant reduction of coronary flow reserve in patients with non–insulin-dependent diabetes compared with age-matched control subjects. The coronary flow reserve values were comparable between the diet and medication therapy groups. Coronary flow reserve was inversely correlated with average hemoglobin A_{Ic} and hyperglycemia for 5 years but not lipid fractions or insulin resistance. Di-Carli et al. (119) confirmed the reduction of coronary flow reserve in diabetic patients and showed that the decrease in myocardial flow response to cold pressor in diabetics with

sympathetic nerve dysfunction was greater than that in those without dysfunction. These results are consistent with previous reports showing a reduction of angiographic coronary vasodilatory capacity in human diabetes (120,121).

Czernin et al. (122) evaluated the acute effect of smoking on myocardial vasculature reactivity to vasodilatory stimulation. Short-term smoking markedly reduced coronary flow reserve from 3.4 ± 0.8 at baseline to 2.3 ± 0.3 after smoking in smokers. On the other hand, myocardial blood flow and flow reserve were similar in young, long-term smokers, and age-matched healthy nonsmokers. Short-term smoking may increase coronary vasomotor tone during dipyridamole-induced hyperemia and thus reduce myocardial flow reserve. Campisi et al. (123) demonstrated an altered response of myocardial blood flow during a cold presser test despite normal coronary flow reserve in long-term smokers, suggesting abnormal coronary vasomotion but normal vasodilator capacity in the smokers. Because significant correlations were obtained between the vasomotor responses to intracoronary administration of acetylcholine and cold presser testing in human coronary angiographic studies, cold presser testing has been used for probing endothelium-dependent coronary vasomotion (124). These results support the reports of endothelial dysfunction in brachial and coronary arteries in long-term smokers and even passive smokers (125–127).

Because coronary dysfunction is partly caused by increased oxidative stress, a number of trials have been attempted to improve coronary vasomotion by use of antioxidants. Vitamin C, a water-soluble antioxidant, has been shown to improve endothelium-dependent vasomotion of epicardial coronary arteries (128). Kaufmann et al. (128) recently demonstrated that vitamin C restored coronary microcirculatory responsiveness and impaired coronary flow reserve in smokers, suggesting that the altered coronary circulation in smokers may be partly accounted for by an increased oxidative stress.

Arterial hypertension often causes reduced coronary flow reserve. Hypertension with and without left ventricular hypertrophy reduces coronary flow reserve by altering the coronary vasculature and resistance (130–132). Laine et al. (133) showed reduced coronary flow reserve in young borderline hypertensives with no clinical signs of angina or hypertrophy. Because resting myocardial blood flow was unchanged, this reduction of coronary flow reserve may be dependent on impaired maximal vasodilatory capacity. Gistri et al. (134) reported improvement in the altered flow reserve after verapamil treatment of hypertension, indicating reversible reduction of coronary flow reserve in these patients.

PET Perfusion Imaging in Nonatherosclerotic Heart Disease

In patients with hypertrophic cardiomyopathy, Camici et al. (135) showed decreased coronary flow reserve with dipyridamole stress not only in the hypertrophic septal wall but also in the lateral free wall, suggesting that reductions in coronary flow reserve were not a consequence of hypertrophy. They also described subendocardial hypoperfusion after dipyridamole administration (136). Treatment with calcium channel blockers can result in a more homogenous transmural flow distribution without an increase in total flow (137).

In patients with dilated cardiomyopathy, Parodi et al. (138) reported a global reduction of coronary flow reserve with dipyridamole infusion. This coronary flow reduction is seen in the subclinical stage of cardiomyopathy and may be due to a microvascular abnormality in these patients. Neglia et al. (139) reported lower resting flow with decreased flow reserve in patients with dilated cardiomyopathy without overt heart failure.

In patients with cardiac transplantation, Rechavia et al. (140) demonstrated higher resting myocardial blood flow with reduction of coronary flow reserve. Senneff et al. (141) reported similar results. Chan et al. (142) described a decrease in hyperemic flow, with an increase in resting flow in excess of cardiac work in patients with transplant rejection. During a follow-up study after successful treatment, patients with transplant rejection had significant improvement, suggesting the role and possible importance of serial noninvasive flow measurements by PET.

Syndrome X is defined as a heart disease associated with chest pain with ischemic ECG changes but normal coronary arteries. Camici et al. (143) first reported the reduction of coronary flow reserve in 30% of patients with syndrome X, with no correlation of alteration of coronary blood flow with ECG or other signs of ischemia. Buus et al. (144) also supported their findings about reduction of coronary flow reserve. Botthcher et al. (145) found preserved microcirculatory endothelial function but markedly attenuated hyperemic flow in these patients. Conversely, Rosen et al. (146) studied 29 patients with syndrome X and 20 age-matched normal controls and found no differences of coronary flow reserve after correction of rate pressure product.

Muzik et al. (147) found reduced hyperemic flow and coronary flow reserve but normal resting blood flow in patients with a history of Kawasaki disease and normal epicardial coronary arteries. This reduction of coronary flow reserve may be the result of inflammation of the coronary arteries.

Coronary flow reserve has also been assessed in long-term survivors of repair of an anomalous left coronary artery from the pulmonary artery. This rare congenital disorder is associated with poor left ventricular function due to inadequate coronary flow, resulting in myocardial infarction or ischemic cardiomyopathy. After surgical repair to establish blood flow to the left coronary arteries from the aorta, dramatic improvement in left ventricular function is seen. However, PET perfusion imaging has shown reduced coronary flow reserve in these patients after the repair, which may contribute to impaired exercise performance by limited cardiac output reserve (148).

Singh et al. (149) studied the coronary flow reserve in long-term survivors with transposition of great arteries after the atrial switch operation (Mustard operation). Coronary flow reserve was reduced in these patients compared with healthy control subjects, suggesting possible systemic ventricular dysfunction in these patients. Hauser et al. (150) compared myocardial blood flow and flow reserve in the patients who received the atrial switch operation to patients with pulmonary autograft aortic valve replacement (Ross operation). Patients with the atrial switch operation had stress-induced perfusion defects with attenuated coronary flow reserve. Although the long-term prognosis remains unclear in these patients after surgery of the congenital heart disease, PET may provide important information about myocardial perfusion and flow reserve and may predict cardiac dysfunction.

Assessment of New Therapies

The recent development of new treatments for improving impaired myocardial perfusion has created the need for noninvasive and quantitative measurements of myocardial blood flow using PET to confirm the improvement with these therapies. One of the most exciting areas is gene therapy for neovascularization in severe CAD. A number of studies have been focused on imaging of reporter gene expression (151, 152). In addition to the imaging of the genotype expression, the actual improvement in myocardial perfusion has been well demonstrated by SPECT imaging (153,154). To date, gene therapy studies in cardiac disease have not taken advantage of the quantification capabilities of PET. PET has significant potential application in this area because it is a very sensitive means to define the changes in flow over time.

Transmyocardial laser revascularization is another new technique to treat patients with severe angina who are not amenable to conventional revascularization. Despite significant symptomatic improvement, the exact mechanism of the action of this treatment remains unclear. Rimoldi et al. (155) measured myocardial blood flow using $H_2^{15}O$ and PET imaging in seven patients and demonstrated no significant improvement in myocardial perfusion at 7 and 35 weeks after transmural laser revascularization. Al-Sheikh et al. (156) also showed no improvement in relative perfusion by ^{13}N-ammonia PET but demonstrated cardiac sympathetic denervation by PET imaging of ^{11}C-hydroxyephedrine after transmural laser revascularization.

SUMMARY

PET myocardial perfusion imaging provides accurate evaluation of regional myocardial blood flow at rest and during stress. The role of PET myocardial perfusion imaging is well established for diagnosis and prognosis of CAD. In the past, widespread clinical use has been limited by the cost of the technology and access to the radiotracers. However, clinical use is increasing as the expense of PET instrumentation decreases and both cyclotrons and generator-produced radiotracers become more widely available. This trend is expected to continue.

PET perfusion imaging is the most validated noninvasive method for quantification of absolute myocardial blood flow and flow reserve. The ability of PET to quantify absolute perfusion provides a new dimension in addition to the traditional applications of standard perfusion imaging. PET is an ideal research tool for the study of the pathophysiology of CAD and other cardiac diseases. PET is also well suited for the evaluation of treatment, both acutely and longitudinally, and will be very useful as new therapies continue to develop.

REFERENCES

1. Schwaiger M, Ziegler SI, Bengel FM. Assessment of myocardial blood flow with positron emission tomography. In: Pohost GM, O'Rourke RA, Bermna DS, et al., eds. *Radionuclide-based methods/nuclear cardiology.* Philadelphia: Lippincott Williams & Wilkins, 2000: 195–212.
2. Tamaki N. PET perfusion tracers. In: Taille R, Tamaki N, eds. New radiotracers in cardiac imaging: principles and applications. Stanford, CT: Appleton & Lange, 1999:213–227.
3. Bergmann SR. Cardiac positron emission tomography. *Semin Nucl Med* 1998;28:320–340.
4. Schelbert HR. Current status and prospects of new radionuclide and radiopharmaceuticals for cardiovascular nuclear medicine. *Semin Nucl Med* 1987;17:145–181.
5. Schelbert HR, Phelps ME, Hottman EJ, et al. Regional myocardial perfusion assessed with N-13 labeled ammonia and positron emission computerized axial tomography. *Am J Cardiol* 1979;43:209–218.
6. Schelbert HR, Phelps ME, Huang S-C, et al. N-13 ammonia as an indicator of myocardial blood flow. *Circulation* 1981;63:1259–1272.
7. Krivokapich J, Huang S, Phelps M, et al. Dependence of $^{13}NH_3$ myocardial extraction and clearance on flow and metabolism. *Am J Physiol* 1982;242:H536–H542.
8. Beanlands R, Muzik O, Hutchins G, et al. Heterogeneity of regional nitrogen 13-labeled ammonia tracer distribution in the normal heart: comparison with rubidium 82 and copper-62–labeled PTSM. *J Nucl Cardiol* 1994;35:1122–1124.
9. Hutchins GD, Schwaiger M, Rosenspire KC, et al. Noninvasive quantification of regional myocardial blood flow in the human heart using N-13 ammonia and dynamic positron emission tomography imaging. *J Am Coll Cardiol* 1990;15:1032–1042.
10. Bol A, Melin JA, Vanoverschelde J-L, et al. Direct comparison of ^{13}N ammonia and ^{15}O water estimates of perfusion with quantification of regional myocardial blood flow by microspheres. *Circulation* 1993; 87:512–525.
11. Kuhle WG, Porenta G, Huang SC, et al. Quantification of regional myocardial blood flow using N-13 ammonia and reoriented dynamic positron emission tomographic imaging. *Circulation* 1993;86: 1004–1017.
12. Muzik O, Beanlands RSB, Hutchins GD, et al. Validation of nitrogen-13-ammonia tracer kinetic model for quantification of myocardial blood flow using PET. *J Nucl Med* 1993;34:83–91.
13. Shah A, Schelbert HR, Schwaiger M, et al. Measurement of regional myocardial blood flow with N-13 ammonia and positron-emission tomography in intact dogs. *J Am Coll Cardiol* 1985;5:92–100.
14. Bellina CR, Parodi O, Camici P, et al. Simultaneous *in vitro* and *in vivo* validation of nitrogen-13-ammonia for the assessment of regional myocardial blood flow. *J Nucl Med* 1990;31:1335–1343.
15. Nienaber CA, Ratib O, Gambhir SS, et al. A quantitative index of regional blood flow in canine myocardium derived noninvasively with N-13 ammonia and dynamic positron emission tomography. *J Am Coll Cardiol* 1991;17:260–269.
16. Choi Y, Huang SC, Hawkins RA, et al. A simplified method for quantification of myocardial blood flow using nitrogen-13-ammonia and dynamic PET. *J Nucl Med* 1993;34:488–497.
17. Tadamura E, Tamaki N, Yonekura Y, et al. Assessment of coronary vasodilator reserve by N-13 ammonia PET using the microsphere method and Patlak plot analysis. *Ann Nucl Med* 1995;9:109–118.
18. Choi Y, Huang SC, Hawkins RA, et al. Quantification of myocardial blood flow using ^{13}N-ammonia and PET: comparison of tracer models. *J Nucl Med* 1999;40:1045–1055.
19. Muzik O, Beanlands RSB, Wolfe E, et al. Automated region definition for cardiac nitrogen-13-ammonia PET imaging. *J Nucl Med* 1993;34: 336–344.
20. Krivokapich J, Smith G, Huang S, et al. ^{13}N-ammonia myocardial imaging at rest and with exercise in normal volunteers. Quantification of absolute myocardial perfusion with dynamic positron emission tomography. *Circulation* 1989;80:1328–1337.
21. Tamaki N, Yonekura Y, Senda M, et al. Myocardial positron computed tomography with ^{13}N-ammonia at rest and during exercise. *Eur J Nucl Med* 1985;11:246–251.
22. Yonekura Y, Tamaki N, Senda M, et al. Detection of coronary artery disease with ^{13}N-ammonia and high resolution positron-emission computed tomography. *Am Heart J* 1987;113:645–654.
23. Yano Y, Budinger TF, Chiange G. Evaluation and application of alumina-based Rb-82 generators charged with high levels of Sr-82/85. *J Nucl Med* 1979;20:961–966.
24. Mullani N, Gould K. First pass regional blood flow measurements with external detectors. *J Nucl Med* 1983;24:577–581.
25. Nishiyama H, Sodd V, Adolph R, et al. Intercomparison of myocardial imaging agents: ^{201}Tl, ^{129}Cs, ^{43}K, and ^{81}Rb. *J Nucl Med* 1976;17: 880–889.
26. Mullani N, Goldstein R, Gould K, et al. Myocardial perfusion with rubidium-82, I: measurement of extraction fraction and flow with external detectors. *J Nucl Med* 1983;24:898–906.
27. Ziegler H, Goresky C. Kinetics of rubidium uptake in the working dog heart. *Circ Res* 1971;29:208–220.
28. Wilson RA, Shea M, DeLandsheere C, et al. Rubidium-82 myocardial uptake and extraction after transient ischemia: PET characteristics. *J Comput Assisted Tomogr* 1987;11:60–66.
29. Gould KL, Yoshida K, Hess M, et al. Myocardial metabolism of fluorodeoxyglucose compared to cell membrane integrity for the potassium analogue rubidium-82 for assessing infarct size in man by PET. *J Nucl Med* 1991;32:10–12.
30. Herrero P, Markham J, Shelton ME, et al. Noninvasive quantification of regional myocardial perfusion with rubidium-82 and positron emission tomography. *Circulation* 1990;82:1377–1386.
31. deKemp R, Ruddy TD, Hewitt T, et al. Detection of serial changes in absolute myocardial perfusion with Rb-82 PET. *J Nucl Med* 2000; 41:1426–1435.
32. Scott NS, Le May MR, deKemp R, et al. Evaluation of myocardial perfusion using Rb-82 PET after myocardial infarction in patients receiving primary stent implantation or thrombolytic therapy. *Am J Cardiol* 2001;88:886–889.
33. Yoshida K, Mullani N, Gould K. Coronary flow and flow reserve by PET simplified for clinical applications using rubidium-82 or nitrogen-13 ammonia. *J Nucl Med* 1996;37:1701–1712.
34. Williams BR, Mullani NA, Jansen DE, et al. A retrospective study of the diagnostic accuracy of a community hospital-based PET center for the detection of coronary artery disease using rubidium-82. *J Nucl Med* 1994;35:1586–1592.
35. Green MA. A potential copper radiopharmaceutical for imaging the heart and brain: copper-labeled pyruvaldehyde *bis*(N14-methylthiosemicarbazone). *Nucl Med Biol* 1987;14:89.
36. Green MA, Klippenstein DR, Tennison JR. Copper(II)*bis*(thiosemicarbazone)complexes as potential tracers for evaluation of cerebral and myocardial blood flow with PET. *J Nucl Med* 1988;29: 1549–1557.
37. Green MA, Mathias CJ, Welch MJ, et al. Copper-62–labeled pyruvaldehyde bis(N4-methylthiosemicarbazonato)copper(II): synthesis and evaluation as a positron emission tomography tracer for cerebral and myocardial perfusion. *J Nucl Med* 1990;31:1989–1996.
38. Sheton ME, Green MA, Green MA, et al. Kinetics of copper-PTSM in isolated heart: a novel tracer for measuring blood flow with positron emission tomography. *J Nucl Med* 1989;30:1843–1847.
39. Shelton ME, Mathias CJ, Welch MJ, et al. Assessment of regional myocardial and renal blood flow with copper-PTSM and positron emission tomography. *Circulation* 1990;82:990–997.
40. Fujibayashi Y, Matsumoto K, Yonekura Y, et al. A new zinc-62/copper-62 generator as a copper-62 source for PET radiopharmaceuticals. *J Nucl Med* 1989;30:1838–1842.
41. Matsumoto K, Fujibayashi Y, Yonekura Y, et al. Application of the

new zinc-62/copper-62 generator: an effective labeling method for ^{62}Cu-PTSM. *Nucl Med Biol* 1992;19:39–44.

42. Beanlands RSB, Music O, Minute M, et al. The kinetics of copper-62-PTSM in the normal human heart. *J Nucl Med* 1992;33:684–690.

43. Herrero P, Markham J, Weinheimer CJ, et al. Quantification of regional myocardial perfusion with generator-produced ^{62}Cu-PTSM and positron emission tomography. *Circulation* 1993;87:173–183.

44. Marthias CJ, Welch MJ, Green MA, et al. *In vivo* comparison of copper blood-pool agents: potential radiopharmaceuticals for use with copper-62. *J Nucl Med* 1991;32:475–480.

45. Mathias CJ, Bergmann SR, Green MA. Development and validation of a solvent extraction technique for determination of Cu-PTSM in blood. *Nucl Med Biol* 1993;20:343–349.

46. Wada K, Fujibayashi Y, Taniuchi H, et al. Effects of ischemia-reperfusion injury on myocardial single pass extraction and retention of Cu-PTSM in perfused rat heart. *Nucl Med Biol* 1994;21:613–617.

47. Tadamura E, Tamaki N, Okazawa H, et al. Generator-produced copper-62-PTSM as a myocardial PET perfusion tracer compared with nitrogen-13-ammonia. *J Nucl Med* 1996;37:729–735.

48. Kety S. The theory and applications of the exchange of inert gas at the lungs and tissues. *Pharmacol Rev* 1951;3:1–41.

49. Bergmann SR, Fox KAA, Rand AL, et al. Quantification of regional myocardial blood flow *in vivo* with $H_2^{15}O$. *Circulation* 1984;70:724–733.

50. Walsh NM, Bergmann SR, Steele RL, et al. Delineation of impaired regional myocardial perfusion by positron emission tomography with $H_2^{15}O$. *Circulation* 1988;78:612–620.

51. Iida H, Kanno I, Takahashi A, et al. Measurement of absolute myocardial blood flow with $H_2^{15}O$ and dynamic positron emission tomography: strategy for quantification in relation to the partial-volume effect. *Circulation* 1988;78:104–115.

52. Henze E, Huang SC, Ratib O, et al. Measurement of regional tissue and blood radiotracer concentrations from serial tomographic images of the heart. *J Nucl Med* 1983;24:987–996.

53. Hoffman EJ, Huang S-C, Phelps ME. Quantitation in positron emission computed tomography, 1: effect of object size. *J Comput Assisted Tomogr* 1979;3:299–408.

54. Iida H, Rhodes CG, deSilva R, et al. Myocardial tissue fraction: correction for partial volume effects and measure of tissue viability. *J Nucl Med* 1991;32:2169–2175.

55. Yamamoto Y, deSilva R, Rhodes CG, et al. A new strategy for the assessment of viable myocardium and regional myocardial blood flow using ^{15}O-water and dynamic positron emission tomography. *Circulation* 1992;86:167–178.

56. Herscovitch P, Raichle ME, Kilbourn MR, et al. Positron emission tomographic measurement of cerebral blood flow and permeability-surface area product of water using ^{15}O-water and ^{11}C-butanol. *J Cereb Blood Flow Metab* 1987;7:527–542.

57. Kaballka GW, Lmbrecht RM, Sajjad M, et al. Synthesis of ^{15}O-labeled butanol via organoborane chemistry. *Appl Radiat Isot* 1985;36:853–855.

58. Gould K, Schelbert H, Phelps M, et al. Noninvasive assessment of coronary stenoses with myocardial perfusion imaging during pharmacologic coronary vasodilatation. *Am J Cardiol* 1979;43:200–208.

59. Schelbert H, Wisenberg G, Phelps M, et al. Noninvasive assessment of coronary stenoses by myocardial imaging during pharmacologic coronary vasodilation, VI: detection of coronary artery disease in man with intravenous 13-NH$_3$ and positron computed tomography. *Am J Cardiol* 1982;49:1197–1207.

60. Schelbert HR, Phelps ME, Huang S-C, et al. N-13 ammonia as an indicator of myocardial blood flow. *Circulation* 1981;63:1259–1272.

61. Tamaki N, Yonekura Y, Senda M, et al. Myocardial positron computed tomography with ^{13}N-ammonia at rest and during exercise. *Eur J Nucl Med* 1985;11:246–251.

62. Yonekura Y, Tamaki N, Senda M, et al. Detection of coronary artery disease with ^{13}N-ammonia and high resolution positron-emission computed tomography. *Am Heart J* 1987;113:645–654.

63. Gould K, Goldstein R, Mullani N. Economic analysis of clinical positron emission tomography of the heart with rubidium-82. *J Nucl Med* 1989;30:707–717.

64. Williams B, Jansen D, Wong L, et al. Positron emission tomography for the diagnosis of coronary artery disease: a nonuniversity experience and correlation with coronary angiography. *J Nucl Med* 1989;30:845.

65. Demer LL, Gould KL, Goldstein RA, et al. Assessment of coronary artery disease severity by positron emission tomography: comparison with quantitative arteriography in 193 patients. *Circulation* 1989;79:825–835.

66. Go R, Marwick T, MacIntyre W, et al. A prospective comparison of rubidium-82 PET and thallium-201 SPECT myocardial perfusion imaging utilizing a single dipyridamole stress in the diagnosis of coronary artery disease. *J Nucl Med* 1990;31:1899–1905.

67. Stewart RE, Schwaiger M, Molina E, et al. Comparison of rubidium-82 positron emission tomography and thallium-201 SPECT imaging for detection of coronary artery disease. *Am J Cardiol* 1991;67:1303–1310.

68. Williams BR, Mullani NA, Jansen DE, et al. A retrospective study of the diagnostic accuracy of a community hospital-based PET center for the detection of coronary artery disease using rubidium-82. *J Nucl Med* 1994;35:1586–1592.

69. Tamaki N, Yonekura Y, Senda M, et al. Value and limitation of stress thallium-201 single photon emission computed tomography: comparison with nitrogen-13 ammonia positron tomography. *J Nucl Med* 1988;29:1181–1188.

70. MacIntyre WJ, Go RT, King JL, et al. Clinical outcome of cardiac patients with negative thallium-201 SPECT and positive rubidium-82 PET myocardial perfusion imaging. *J Nucl Med* 1993;34:400–404.

71. Hicks K, Ganiti G, Mullani N, et al. Automated quantitation of three-dimensional cardiac positron emission tomography for routine clinical use. *J Nucl Med* 1989;30:1787–1797.

72. Porenta G, Kuhle W, Czernin J, et al. Semiquantitative assessment of myocardial blood flow and viability using polar map display of cardiac PET images. *J Nucl Med* 1992;33:1628–1636.

73. Laubenbacher C, Rothley J, Sitomer J, et al. An automated analysis program for the evaluation of cardiac PET studies: initial results in the detection and localization of coronary artery disease using nitrogen-13-ammonia. *J Nucl Med* 1993;34:968–978.

74. Marwick T, Shan K, Patel S, et al. Incremental value of rubidium-82 positron emission tomography for prognostic assessment of known or suspected coronary artery disease. *Am J Cardiol* 1997;80:865–870.

75. Patterson RP, Eisner RL, Horowitz SF. Comparison of cost-effectiveness and utility of exercise ECG, single photon emission computed tomography, positron emission tomography, and coronary angiography for diagnosis of coronary artery disease. *Circulation* 1995;91:54–65.

76. Garber AM, Solomon NA. Cost-effectiveness of alternative test strategies for the diagnosis of coronary disease. *Ann Intern Med* 1999;130:719–728.

77. Maddahi J, Gambhir SS. Cost-effective selection of patients for coronary angiography. *J Nucl Cardiol* 1997;4:S141–S151.

78. Geltman E, Henes C, Senneff M, et al. Increased myocardial perfusion at rest and diminished reserve in patients with angina and angiographically normal coronary arteries. *J Am Coll Cardiol* 1990;16:586–595.

79. Czernin J, Muller P, Chan S, et al. Influence of age and hemodynamics on myocardial blood flow and flow reserve. *Circulation* 1993;88:62–69.

80. Krivokapich J, Czernin J, Schelbert HR. Dobutamine positron emission tomography: absolute quantitation of rest and dobutamine myocardial blood flow and correlation with cardiac work and percent diameter stenosis in patients with and without coronary artery disease. *J Am Coll Cardiol* 1996;28:565–572.

81. Sawada S, Muzik O, Beanlands RSB, et al. Interobserver and interstudy variability of myocardial blood flow and flow-reserve measurement with nitrogen 13-ammonia–labeled positron emission tomography. *J Nucl Cardiol* 1995;2:413–422.

82. Nagamach S, Czernin J, Kim A, et al. Reproducibility of measurements of regional resting and hyperemic myocardial blood flow assessed with PET. *J Nucl Med* 1996;37:1626–1631.

83. Merlet P, Mazoyer B, Hittinger L, et al. Assessment of coronary reserve in man: comparison between positron emission tomography with oxygen-15 labeled water and intracoronary Doppler technique. *J Nucl Med* 1993;34:1899–1904.

84. Gould K, Lipscomb K, Hamilton G. Physiologic basis for assessing critical coronary stenosis. *Am J Cardiol* 1974;33:87–94.

85. Gould K, Kirkeeide RL, Buchi M. Coronary flow reserve as a physiologic measure of stenosis severity. *J Am Coll Cardiol* 1990;15:459–474.

86. Gould KL. Quantification of coronary artery stenosis *in vivo*. *Circ Res* 1985;57:341–353.

87. Uren NG, Melin JA, DeBruyne B, et al. Relation between myocardial blood flow and the severity of coronary artery stenosis. *N Engl J Med* 1994;330:1782–1788.

88. Beanlands RSB, Melon P, Muzik O, et al. N-13 ammonia PET identifies reduced perfusion reserve in angiographically normal regions of patients with CAD. *Circulation* 1992;86:1–184.

89. DiCarli M, Czernin J, Hoh CK, et al. Relation among stenosis severity, myocardial blood flow, and flow reserve in patients with coronary artery disease. *Circulation* 1995;91:1944–1951.

90. Beanlands RB, Muzik O, Melon P, et al. Noninvasive quantification of regional myocardial flow reserve in patients with atherosclerosis using nitrogen-13 ammonia positron emission tomography. *J Am Coll Cardiol* 1995;26:1465–1475.

91. Wilson RF, Marcus ML, White CW, et al. Prediction of the physiologic significance of coronary arterial lesions by quantitative lesion geometry in patients with limited coronary artery disease. *Circulation* 1987;75:723–732.

92. Demer LL, Gould KL, Goldstein RA, et al. Noninvasive assessment of coronary collaterals in man by PET perfusion imaging. *J Nucl Med* 1990;31:259–270.

93. Holmvang G, Fry S, Skopicki HA, et al. Relation between coronary "steal" and contractile function at rest in collateral-dependent myocardium of humans with ischemic heart disease. *Circulation* 1999; 99:2510–2516.

94. Maseri A, Crea F, Cianflone D. Myocardial ischemia caused by distal coronary vasoconstriction. *Am J Cardiol* 1992;70:1602–1605.

95. Zeiher A, Drezler H, Wollchlager H, et al. Endothelial dysfunction of the coronary microvasculature is associated with impaired coronary blood flow regulation in patients with early atherosclerosis. *Circulation* 1991;84:1984–1991.

96. VanTosh A, Garza D, Roberti R, et al. Serial myocardial perfusion imaging with dipyridamole and rubidium-82 to assess restenosis after angioplasty. *J Nucl Med* 1995;36:1553–1560.

97. Stewart RE, Miller DD, Bowers TR, et al. PET perfusion and vasodilator function after angioplasty for acute myocardial infarction. *J Nucl Med* 1997;38:770–777.

98. Walsh MN, Geltman EM, Steele RL, et al. Augmented myocardial perfusion reserve after angioplasty quantified by positron emission tomography with $H_2^{15}O$. *J Am Coll Cardiol* 1990;15:119–127.

99. Czernin J, Muller P, Chan S, et al. Influence of age and hemodynamics on myocardial blood flow and flow reserve. *Circulation* 1993;88: 62–69.

100. Uren N, Camici PG, Melin JA, et al. Effect of age on myocardial perfusion reserve. *J Nucl Med* 1995;36:2032–2036.

101. Camici P, Gistri R Lorenzoni R, et al. Coronary reserve and exercise ECG in patients with chest pain and normal coronary angiograms. *Circulation* 1992;86:179–186.

102. Geltman E, Henes C, Senneff M, et al. Increased myocardial perfusion at rest and diminished perfusion reserve in patients with angina and angiographically normal coronary arteries. *J Am Coll Cardiol* 1990; 16:586–595.

103. Dayanikli F, Grambow D, Muzik O, et al. Early detection of abnormal coronary flow reserve in asymptomatic men at high risk for coronary artery disease using positron emission tomography. *Circulation* 1994; 90:808–817.

104. Yokoyama I, Ohtake T, Momomura S, et al. Reduced coronary flow reserve in hypercholesterolemic patients without overt coronary stenosis. *Circulation* 1996;94:3232–3238.

105. Yokoyama I, Murakami T, Ohtake T, et al. Reduced coronary flow reserve in familial hypercholesterolemia. *J Nucl Med* 1996;37: 1937–1942.

106. Pitkanen O, Raitakari O, Niinikoski H, et al. Coronary flow reserve is impaired in young men with familial hypercholesterolemia. *J Am Coll Cardiol* 1996;28:1705–1711.

107. Pitkanen O, Nuutila P, Raitakari O, et al. Coronary flow reserve in young men with familial combined hyperlipidemia. *Circulation* 1999; 99:1678–1684.

108. Kaufmann PA, Gnecchi-Ruscone T, Schafers KP, et al. Low density lipoprotein cholesterol and coronary microvascular dysfunction in hypercholesterolemia. *J Am Coll Cardiol* 2000;36:103–109.

109. Mellwig K, Baller D, Gleichmann U, et al. Improvement of coronary vasodilatation capacity through single LDL apheresis. *Atherosclerosis* 1998;139:173–178.

110. Gould KL, et al. Short-term cholesterol lowering decreases size and severity of perfusion abnormalities after dipyridamole in patients with coronary artery disease. A potential noninvasive marker of healing coronary endothelium. *Circulation* 1994;89:1530–1538.

111. Guethlin M, Kasel A, Coppenrath K, et al. Delayed response of myocardial flow reserve to lipid lowering therapy with fluvastatin. *Circulation* 1999;99:475–481.

112. Huggins GS, Pasternak RC, Alpert NM, et al. Effects of short-term treatment of hyperlipidemia on coronary vasodilator function and myocardial perfusion in regions having substantial impairment of baseline dilator reserve. *Circulation* 1998;98:1291–1296.

113. Baller D, Notohamiprodjo GN, Gleichmann U, et al. Improvement in coronary flow reserve determined by positron emission tomography after 6 months of cholesterol-lowering therapy in patients with early stages of coronary atherosclerosis. *Circulation* 1999;99:2871–2875.

114. Treasure C, Klein J, Weintraub W, et al. Beneficial effects of cholesterol-lowering therapy on the coronary endothelium in patients with coronary artery disease. *N Engl J Med* 1995;332:481–487.

115. Yokoyama I, Momomura S, Ohtake T, et al. Improvement of impaired myocardial vasodilatation due to diffuse coronary atherosclerosis in hypercholesterolemics after lipid lowering therapy. *Circulation* 1999; 100:117–122.

116. Czernin J, Barnard R, Sun K, et al. Effect of short-term cardiovascular conditioning and low-fat diet on myocardial blood flow and flow reserve. *Circulation* 1995;91:2891–2897.

117. Yokoyama I, Momomura S, Ohtake T, et al. Reduced myocardial flow reserve in non-insulin dependent diabetes mellitus. *J Am Coll Cardiol* 1997;30:1472–1477.

118. Yokoyama I, Ohtake T, Momomura S, et al. Hyperglycemia rather than insulin resistance is related to reduced coronary flow reserve in NIDDM. *Diabetes* 1998;47:119–124.

119. DiCarli MF, Bianco-Batlles D, Landa ME, et al. Effects of autonomic neuropathy on coronary blood flow in patients with diabetes mellitus. *Circulation* 1999;100:813–819.

120. Nitenberg A, Valensi P, Sachs R, et al. Impairment of coronary vascular reserve and ACh-induced coronary vasodilation in diabetic patients with angiographically normal coronary arteries and normal ventricular systolic function. *Diabetes* 1993;32:1017–1023.

121. Nahser PJ Jr, Brown RE, Oskarsson H, et al. Maximal coronary flow reserve and metabolic coronary vasodilation in patients with diabetes mellitus. *Circulation* 1995;91:635–640.

122. Czernin J, Sun K, Brunken R, et al. Effect of acute and long-term smoking on myocardial blood flow and flow reserve. *Circulation* 1995;91:2891–2897.

123. Campici R, Czernin J, Schoder H, et al. Effects of long-term smoking on myocardial blood flow, coronary vasomotion and vasodilator capacity. *Circulation* 1998;98:119–125.

124. Zeiher A, Drexler H, Wollschlaeger H, et al. Coronary vasomotion in response to sympathetic stimulation in humans; importance of the functional integrity of the endothelium. *J Am Coll Cardiol* 1989;14: 1181–1190.

125. Celermajer DS, Sorensen KE, Georgakopoulos D, et al. Cigarette smoking is associated with dose-related and potentially reversible impairment of endothelium-dependent dilation in healthy young adults. *Circulation* 1993;88:2149–2155.

126. Zeiher AM, Schachinger V, Minners J, et al. Long-term cigarette smoking impairs endothelium-dependent coronary arterial vasodilator function. *Circulation* 1995;92:1094–1100.

127. Celermajer DS, Adams MR, Clarkson P, et al. Passive smoking and impaired endothelium-dependent arterial dilation in healthy young adults. *N Engl J Med* 1996;334:150–154.

128. Solzbach U, Horning B, Jeserich M, et al. Vitamin C improves endothelial dysfunction of epicardial coronary arteries in hypertensive patients. *Circulation* 1997;96:1513–1519.

129. Kaufmann PA, Gnecchi T, diTerlizzi M, et al. Coronary heart disease in smokers; vitamin C restores coronary microcirculatory function. *Circulation* 2000;102:1233–1238.

130. Opherk D, Mall G, Zebe H, et al. Reduction of coronary reserve: a mechanism for angina pectoris in patients with arterial hypertension and normal coronary arteries. *Circulation* 1984;69:1–7.

131. Treasure CB, Klein JL, Vita JA, et al. Hypertension and left ventricular hypertrophy are associated with impaired endothelium-mediated reali-

zation in human coronary resistance vessels. *Circulation* 1993;87: 86–93.

132. Kozakova M, Palombo C, Pratali L, et al. Mechanisms of coronary flow reserve impairment in human hypertension. *Hypertension* 1997; 29:551–559.

133. Laine H, Raitakari OT, Niinikoski H, et al. Early impairment of coronary flow reserve in young men with borderline hypertension. *J Am Coll Cardiol* 1998;32:147–153.

134. Gistri R, Genovesi-Ebert R, Palombo C, et al. Effect of chronic lowering of blood pressure on coronary vasodilator reserve in arterial hypertension. *Cardiovasc Drugs Ther* 1994;8:169–171.

135. Camici P, Chiriatti G, Lorenzori R, et al. Coronary vasodilation is impaired in both hypertrophied and nonhypertrophied myocardium of patients with hypertrophic cardiomyopathy: a study with nitrogen-13 ammonia and positron emission tomography. *J Am Coll Cardiol* 1991;17:879–886.

136. Camici PG, Cecchi F, Gistri R, et al. Dipyridamole-induced subendocardial underperfusion in hypertrophic cardiomyopathy assessed by positron emission tomography. *Coron Artery Dis* 1991;2:837–841.

137. Gistri R, Cecchi F, Choudhury L, et al. Effect of verapamil on absolute myocardial blood flow in hypertrophic cardiomyopathy. *Am J Cardiol* 1994;74:363–368.

138. Parodi O, Maria R, Oltrona L, et al. Myocardial blood flow distribution in patients with ischemic heart disease or dilated cardiomyopathy undergoing heart transplantation. *Circulation* 1993;88:509–522.

139. Neglia D, Parodi O, Gallopin M, et al. Myocardial blood flow response to pacing tachycardiac and to dipyridamole infusion in patients with dilated cardiomyopathy without overt heart failure. *Circulation* 1995; 92:796–804.

140. Rechavia A, Araujo L, DeSilva R, et al. Dipyridamole vasodilator response after human orthotopic heart transplantation: quantification by oxygen-15–labeled water and positron emission tomography. *J Am Coll Cardiol* 1992;19:100–106.

141. Senneff M, Hartman J, Sobel B, et al. Persistence of coronary vasodilator responsivity after cardiac transplantation. *Am J Cardiol* 1993; 71:333–338.

142. Chan SY, Kobashigawa J, Stevenson W, et al. Myocardial blood flow at rest and during pharmacological vasodilation in cardiac transplants during and after successful treatment of rejection. *Circulation* 1994; 90:204–212.

143. Camici P, Gistri R Lorenzoni R, et al. Coronary reserve and exercise ECG in patients with chest pain and normal coronary angiograms. *Circulation* 1992;86:179–186.

144. Buus NH, Bottcher M, Botker HE, et al. Reduced vasodilator capacity in syndrome X related to structure and function resistance arteries. *Am J Cardiol* 1999;83:149–154.

145. Bottcher M, Botker HE, Sonne H, et al. Endothelium-dependent and -independent perfusion reserve and the effect of L-arginine on myocardial perfusion in patients with syndrome X. *Circulation* 1999;99: 1795–1801.

146. Rosen SD, Uren NG, Kaski JC, et al. Coronary vasodilator reserve, pain perception, and sex in patients with syndrome X. *Circulation* 1994;90:50–60.

147. Muzik O, Paridon SM, Singh TP, et al. Quantification of myocardial blood flow and flow reserve in children with a history of Kawasaki disease and normal coronary arteries using positron emission tomography. *J Am Coll Cardiol* 1996;28:757–762.

148. Singh TP, DiCarli MF, Sullivan NM, et al. Myocardial flow reserve in long-term survivors of repair of anomalous left coronary artery from pulmonary artery. *J Am Coll Cardiol* 1998;31:437–443.

149. Singh TP, Humes RA, Muzik O, et al. Myocardial flow reserve in patients with a systemic right ventricle after atrial switch repair. *J Am Coll Cardiol* 2001;37:2120–2125.

150. Hauser M, Bengel FM, Kuhn A, et al. Myocardial blood flow and flow reserve after coronary reimplantation in patients after arterial switch and Ross operation. *Circulation* 2001;103:1875–1880.

151. Gambhir SS, Barrio JR, Phelps ME, et al. Imaging adenoviral-directed reporter gene expression in living animals with positron emission tomography. *Proc Natl Acad Sci U S A* 1999;96:2333–2338.

152. Iyer M, Barrio JR, Namavari M, et al. 8-[^{18}F]fluoropenciclovir: an improved reporter probe for imaging HSV1-tk reporter gene expression *in vivo* using PET. *J Nucl Med* 2001;42:96–105.

153. Losordo DW, Vale PR, Symes JF, et al. Gene therapy for myocardial angiogenesis: initial clinical results with direct myocardial injection of phVEGF165 as sole therapy for myocardial ischemia. *Circulation* 1998;98:2800–2804.

154. Udelson JE, Dilsizian V, Laham RJ, et al. Therapeutic angiogenesis with recombinant fibroblast growth factor-2 improves stress and rest myocardial perfusion abnormalities in patients with severe symptomatic chronic coronary artery disease. *Circulation* 2000;102: 1605–1610.

155. Rimoldi O, Burns SM, Rosen SD, et al. Measurement of myocardial blood flow with positron emission tomography before and after transmyocardial laser revascularization. *Circulation* 1999;100: II134–II138.

156. Al-Sheikh T, Allen KB, Straka SP, et al. Cardiac sympathetic denervation after transmural laser revascularization. *Circulation* 1999;100: 135–140.

CHAPTER 8.2

Myocardial Viability

Rob S.B. Beanlands, Terrence D. Ruddy, and Jamshid Maddahi

Heart failure resulting from impaired left ventricular (LV) function is associated with significant morbidity and mortality. The leading cause of heart failure is coronary artery disease (CAD). Among patients with coronary disease and severe ventricular dysfunction, mortality rates range from 10% to 60% at 1 year (1–5). The inverse relationship of ventricular function with mortality is well established (3,6). In recent years, advances in medical therapy have improved the outcome for patients with heart failure (7–10). However, mortality rates remain high (11% to 36% for patients with class IV heart failure) (8,10). With limited access to transplantation, revascularization is often considered because this may improve outcome in some patients (3,11,12). However, bypass surgery in such patients can have high perioperative risk (13–15). Hence, a need arose for *diagnostic techniques that could better define and select the high-risk patients with ventricular dysfunction most likely to benefit from revascularization.* The definition of viable myocardium has become pivotal in this regard. Although several approaches have been developed, the identification of preserved metabolic activity in the myocardium using ^{18}F-fluorodeoxyglucose (FDG) positron emission tomography (PET) imaging is the most well-established approach.

GLUCOSE METABOLISM

The primary substrate for energy metabolism in the normal myocardium depends on the substrate that is most available for oxidative metabolism. Most of the time, this is fatty acids. However, after a glucose load, there is an increase in insulin levels. This leads to an increase in glucose metabolism and inhibition of lipolysis. Thus, in the fed state, the preferred substrate becomes glucose (16,17).

In ischemic myocardium, oxidative metabolism is reduced. There is shift from aerobic to anaerobic metabolism. The primary substrate for energy metabolism becomes glucose to support adenosine triphosphate (ATP) production from glycolysis. With ischemia, glucose is the preferred substrate regardless of the availability of other fuels (16,17).

Imaging techniques that can track myocardial glucose utilization are useful in defining the state of viability in the myocardium.

Glucose is transported across the myocyte membrane by the glucose transporters (GLUTs), primarily GLUT-4 and GLUT-1 (18,19). Once in the cell, it undergoes phosphorylation to glucose 6-phosphate, which is further used for glycolysis, glucose oxidation, or glycogen synthesis. FDG is a glucose analogue that enters the myocyte in proportion to glucose uptake and undergoes phosphorylation (20,21). Unlike glucose, however, the resulting FDG-6-phosphate becomes metabolically trapped by the myocyte. The rate of exogenous glucose utilization can be reflected by FDG uptake. Because radiolabeled fluorine-18-FDG myocardial uptake reflects glucose utilization, it is used to identify viable myocardium (22,23).

VIABILITY, STUNNING, AND HIBERNATION

When flow is reduced to the myocardium, metabolic cellular changes occur due to ischemia. This ischemia results in reduced contractile function of the myocardium. When ischemia is acute, severe, and sufficiently prolonged (more than 20 to 30 minutes in the acute setting), infarction may result, leading to irreversible cell injury, cell death, and subsequent myocardial scar formation. Once irreversibly injured or if scar tissue has formed, this myocardium is no longer viable and cannot recover even if adequately revascularized.

However, the metabolic derangements in the myocyte after short bouts of ischemia may result in more prolonged reduction in myocardial contractile function that can eventually recover. This *postischemic ventricular dysfunction* has been termed "stunned myocardium" (24,25). More prolonged sustained reductions in flow may also lead to myocardial dysfunction. Some investigators have referred to this *ischemic but viable myocardium* as "hibernating myocardium" (26,27). Hibernating myocardium can recovery if adequate nutrient flow is restored.

Myocardial Stunning

The myocardial dysfunction that results after an episode of ischemia (24,25,28) is a form of reperfusion injury that may result from calcium influx, which hinders the myocyte contractile function (29). It has been well described in animal models and in patients, particularly in the setting of acute myocardial infarction after reperfusion therapy, in acute coronary syndromes, and less frequently after severe exercise-induced ischemia (24–26,28,29). When blood flow is restored, the recovery of function may take minutes to days or even weeks depending on the severity of the initial ischemic episode. However, it is considered completely reversible. On the other hand, if repeated episodes of ischemia occur, the resulting postischemic dysfunction may become more persistent. The latter may be an important cause of chronic LV dysfunction in patients with severe ischemic heart disease (28,30–32). This stunned myocardium is viable and has the potential to recover after adequate revascularization (31, 32).

Hibernating Myocardium

Hibernating myocardium is the term applied to dysfunctional myocardium with reduced myocardial perfusion at rest but preserved cell viability (26,27). The resulting reduction in myocardial function has been thought to be a protective chronic downregulation mechanism to reduce myocardial oxygen utilization and ensure myocyte survival (26–28). The classic perfusion-metabolism mismatch pattern seen on perfusion-weighted FDG PET imaging supported this hypothesis of sustained reduction in flow with maintained viability (and therefore, glucose utilization). This perfusion-metabolism mismatch is considered to represent hibernating (ischemic viable) myocardium.

Recent data suggest that the pathophysiology may be more complex than chronic low-flow ischemia alone. Reductions in flow have been demonstrated in some studies but not in others (30,33–38), suggesting that repeated stunning leading to a more persistent reduction in function also plays a role in the LV dysfunction in these patients. Ischemia from reduction in flow may not be the only factor contributing to the perfusion-metabolism mismatch pattern observed on imaging (30–32,38–43). These recent data suggest that there may be a continuing degenerative process from stunned to hibernating myocardium (see Color Plate 20 following page 394). This is discussed further in the ''Image Interpretation'' section later in this chapter. Despite this complexity, the accuracy of the PET ''mismatch'' pattern has been well demonstrated and is associated with recovery after revascularization (5,28,31,32,44–52).

IMAGE ACQUISITION, ANALYSIS, AND INTERPRETATION

Cardiac FDG PET Imaging Protocols

Several approaches for FDG imaging have been developed. However, because myocardial substrate metabolism can be quite variable, most centers use some form of glucose loading and/or insulin protocol to optimize FDG uptake in viable tissue. In addition, because there can also be regional variability, normalization to the perfusion-weighted imaging is often required. Knowledge of the regional perfusion also helps to better characterize the state of the myocardium. Most of the existing accuracy studies have used combined perfusion/FDG uptake imaging protocols using qualitative relative imaging. Accurate detection of myocardial viability, particularly in patients with severely impaired ventricular function, is best achieved by the evaluation of both perfusion and metabolism (5,28,47).

Transmission imaging is required to obtain measured attenuation correction. This is particularly important in cardiac studies because of the significant problems of attenuation in the thorax. Transmission imaging to measure attenuation correction may be acquired before the perfusion or before FDG (if perfusion is done at a separate time). More recently post–emission transmission has been used. This can significantly shorten scanner time for the patient by allowing the patient to enter the camera after FDG is injected and just before the image acquisition begins.

Perfusion-weighted imaging is important to define the relative state of blood flow in the myocardium at rest. This is usually performed at rest and is compared with FDG uptake. Stress perfusion-weighted imaging may also be required in the assessment of some patients with ischemic heart disease to rule out stress-induced ischemia.

Several agents have been used as PET perfusion tracers, including rubidium-82 (^{82}Rb), nitrogen-13 (^{13}N)-ammonia, and H$_2$^{15}O. In centers without access to a cyclotron or strontium-82/^{82}Rb generators, technetium-99m (^{99m}Tc)–based agents or thallium-201 (^{201}Tl) single-photon emission computed tomography (SPECT) imaging can be used for the assessment of perfusion (49,50,53–55). This approach carries a limitation of having perfusion-weighted images without attenuation correction while having FDG imaging with attenuation correction. This must be considered when interpreting the images.

FDG imaging can be either static or dynamic. Static imaging typically is a 20- to 30-minute image that begins 40 to 50 minutes after injection of FDG. This is usually sufficient time for myocardial uptake to be well visualized while the blood-pool activity is low. Dynamic imaging begins simultaneously with FDG injection and continues for 60 to 70 minutes, so time-activity data for blood pool and myocardium can be determined (36 frames: 12 × 10 seconds, 6 × 20 seconds, 6 × 60 seconds, 12 × 300 seconds). The dynamic data are necessary for quantitative analysis of the rate of myocardial glucose utilization.

Patient Preparation

Oral glucose loading has become the most widely used approach for preparing patients for FDG imaging. FDG is administered 60 to 90 minutes after a 50-g oral glucose load

(5,46,47,51,53–57). This switches the primary substrate for myocardial metabolism from free fatty acids to glucose. This is facilitated by the release of insulin. Thus, viable myocardium will preferentially take up glucose and hence FDG. However, oral glucose loading can result in suboptimal image quality in 2% to 30% of patients (57–61). After the oral load, blood glucose values often unmask glucose intolerance. In such patients and those with frank diabetes, supplemental insulin is necessary (47,57). Even with such glucose-loading protocols with bolus insulin, images are often suboptimal in patients with diabetes (57,61).

In many centers, the hyperinsulinemic-euglycemic clamp has been used to improve image quality (37,58,61–67). This approach can be more time consuming and cumbersome for the patient and staff.

Some centers have modified the hyperinsulinemic glucose clamp with front loading to reduce the time required to reach steady state. However, this clamp approach still requires monitoring of glucose levels every 5 minutes until stable, and then every 5 to 10 minutes. Glucose infusion rates are adjusted accordingly, aiming to maintain baseline glucose levels (67). Patients with diabetes whose blood glucose has not been well controlled before the study may present with high baseline glucose values. In these cases, a supplemental insulin bolus may be required in addition to the clamp, with careful monitoring of glucose. Because FDG and glucose compete for the same uptake mechanism, lowering the blood glucose level to the normal or near-normal range may reduce the competition for FDG uptake and improve image quality.

Practically speaking, the oral glucose-loading protocol is technically easier to perform and requires less nursing and technology resources than the insulin clamp approach. The insulin clamp approach is often preferred for patients with diabetes who are likely to have poor imaging quality.

Newer approaches use nicotinic acid derivatives (niacin in North America; acipimox in Europe). The antilipolytic effect of these agents leads to a reduction of competing free fatty acids, which facilitates glucose utilization by the myocardium. These agents have been successful for improving image quality in some studies but not all (61,68,69). The approach is simple, making it an attractive alternative. There may be some flushing, but this can usually be minimized by administration of acetylsalicylic acid (ASA) before the niacin. One recent study in patients with CAD, *severe* LV dysfunction, and diabetes suggested that only the clamp approach significantly improved uptake of FDG in this patient population (61). Further studies on the role of nicotinic acid derivatives are needed.

Because the administration of glucose and insulin can also lead to the influx of K^+ into cells, hypokalemia could theoretically result. In the author's experience the K^+ may drop by up to 0.5 mEq/L after insulin clamp. Supplemental K^+ may be necessary, but generally, this is only a problem in patients who already have hypokalemia, often due to the use of diuretics, and those who undergo the insulin clamp or receive multiple insulin boluses.

Image Interpretation

Accurate tissue characterization and detection of myocardial viability, particularly in patients with severely impaired ventricular function, is best achieved by evaluation of both perfusion and metabolism (5,31,47). Perfusion/FDG imaging has become the standard approach for PET viability imaging and is the focus of the discussion later in this chapter.

After the usual evaluation of image quality, interpretation should begin with a view of the perfusion-weighted images to identify regions of maintained or reduced perfusion. Then FDG imaging should be viewed relative to the maximal zones of perfusion (see Color Plate 21 following page 394). Because FDG uptake may actually be greater than normal in ischemic or hibernating zones, it may be necessary to normalize the FDG uptake to the zones of maximal perfusion. This can be achieved by scale adjustments or by semi-quantitative analysis (see Color Plate 22 following page 394).

It is also important to consider regional and global ventricular function to identify the regions where viability is in question and to determine the potential impact on overall LV function.

Several patterns of uptake may be observed and are discussed.

Reduced Perfusion/Maintained or Increased FDG (Mismatch)

The (low) perfusion-(preserved) metabolism mismatch in a dysfunctional myocardial segment is considered the *sine qua non* of hibernating myocardium (see Color Plate 21A following page 394). Typically, this has been viewed as representing regions with reduced flow that have been rendered ischemic but are still viable (5,22,28,30,33–36). As the term hibernating implies, this has been viewed as a downregulation and a protective mechanism (26,27). More recent data suggest that the pathophysiology of the mismatch pattern may be more complex. Ischemia from reduction in flow may be only one of many contributing factors. Even though perfusion tracer uptake appears reduced, absolute flow may or may not be reduced (30,33–38).

Stunning from recurrent stress-induced ischemia may occur and alter the uptake of the perfusion tracer or FDG. Wall thinning and reduced motion may, in part, account for apparent defects on the perfusion-weighted image (30). The mixture of ischemic and necrotic tissue may add to the complexity. Reduction in fatty acid oxidation has also been demonstrated in hibernating myocardium (38). Alteration in the GLUT-1 and GLUT-4 transporter expression has been proposed for hibernating and ischemic tissue (39,40,70), and glycogen accumulation has been observed, which may not be expected in the presence of ischemia alone (30–32,42, 43). In addition, the extensive depletion of sarcomeres, loss of sarcoplasmatic reticulum, and the observed cellular sequestration suggest that this is a progressive process that

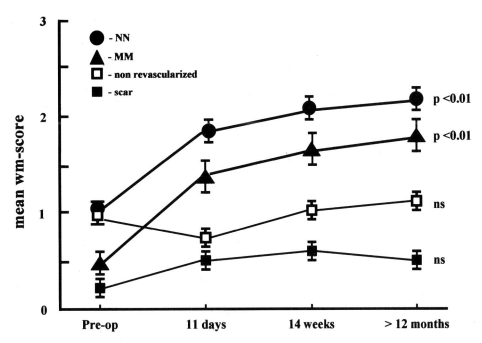

FIG. 8.2.1. Time course of recovery of regional wall motion (*wm*) scores after revascularization in mismatched myocardium (*MM*), normally perfused myocardium (*NN*), and scar tissue (mean ± SEM). In contrast to viable tissue (MM and NN), no significant changes were observed for scar tissue. ns, not significant. (From Haas F, Augustin N, Holper K, et al. Time course and extent of improvement of dysfunctioning myocardium in patients with coronary artery disease and severely depressed left ventricular function after revascularization: correlation with positron emission tomography. *J Am Coll Cardiol* 2000;36:1927–1934, with permission.)

may quickly become irreversible injury if not corrected by adequate revascularization (30–32,42,43) (see Color Plate 20 following page 394).

Hibernating myocardium may represent the limits of viability when adaptive processes have been exhausted (31,42). It may also take several months after revascularization for recovery of function, which may be incomplete (31,32). This concept of a progressive process of injury is further supported by studies showing increased mortality and impaired recovery of function when revascularization is delayed in patients with viable myocardium (54).

Regardless of the mechanism, the accuracy of PET ''mismatch'' as a marker for hibernating myocardium has been well demonstrated and is associated with recovery after revascularization (5,28,31,32,44–52,54). Furthermore, the extent of mismatch is related to the degree of recovery (5, 28,46). Regional recovery may, however, be incomplete or delayed (Fig. 8.2.1) due to the extent of cellular disruption or coexisting subendocardial infarction, ventricular remodeling, or incomplete revascularization (31,32) (Table 8.2.1).

Reduced Perfusion/Reduced FDG (Match)

A matched reduction in perfusion and metabolism indicates scar tissue formation. When severe, this usually indicates transmural scar and the absence of any significant via-

ble tissue. Typically, such regions will not recover after revascularization (see Color Plate 21B following page 394).

When the perfusion/FDG defect is mild, this indicates that the scar is ''non-transmural.'' Both scar tissue and viable tissue are in the defect zone, but there is no hibernating tissue. The negative predictive value (NPV) for mild defects is not as high as that for more severe defects (47), probably because of the residual viable myocardium. The dysfunction in such segments is in part related to the non-transmural scar, but if the wall motion abnormality is more severe than expected, there may also be stunned myocardium. Stress perfusion-weighted imaging may be helpful in defining the

TABLE 8.2.1. *Factors contributing to the MISMATCH pattern on perfusion ^{18}F-fluorodeoxyglucose imaging*

- Reduced perfusion
- Impaired perfusion reserve plus repeated ischemia (stunning)
- Wall thinning
- Mixture of tissue (normal; ischemia and necrosis)
- Increased anaerobic metabolism (ischemia)
- Reduced fatty acid oxidation
- Altered glucose transporter messenger RNA expression (altered GLUT 1/GLUT 4 ratio)
- Glycogen deposition
- Sarcomere depletion

presence of stress-induced ischemia, which leads to the recurrent stunning and dysfunction.

Recent data indicate that the extent of scar may be as important in predicting overall LV function recovery as the extent of hibernating myocardium, with a smaller scar predicting a greater degree of recovery (71,72).

Reduced Perfusion/Partly Reduced FDG (Partial Mismatch)

This is observed when FDG uptake is reduced but not as severely as the perfusion defect. This finding indicates the presence of scar mixed with hibernating myocardium. In these defects, the relative extent of the "match" portion and the intensity of the "mismatch" portion may be helpful in predicting the degree of recovery. Recovery would be expected to be incomplete, because there is some scar tissue present (see Color Plate 21C following page 394).

Normal Perfusion/Normal FDG ("Normal Pattern")

In the absence of a wall motion abnormality, such segments are normal at rest and therefore viable. Because the standard perfusion/FDG images are acquired at rest, it is still possible that such regions are supplied by a stenotic coronary vessel. Stress perfusion-weighted imaging would be required to rule out stress-induced ischemia. In the presence of a wall motion abnormality, however, the "normal pattern" may indicate repetitive stunning, which would be expected to improve if adequately revascularized. Clinical information, angiography, and stress perfusion-weighted imaging may all help in this setting (see Color Plate 21D following page 394).

Recent data indicate that in dysfunctional segments, the "normal" pattern is more common than mismatch (70% vs. 24% of dysfunctional segments), has less associated tissue injury, and is more likely to demonstrate complete recovery than mismatched segments (31% vs. 18%, respectively) (see Color Plate 22 following page 394) (31,32). Lack of complete recovery in these segments may be due to incomplete revascularization or the effect of remodeling.

When the normal pattern is more global in patients with LV dysfunction, this may indicate a more global process such as a nonischemic dilated cardiomyopathy or balanced severe proximal three-vessel CAD or left main coronary artery disease with right coronary artery disease. In a nonischemic dilated cardiomyopathy, the perfusion and FDG pattern may be patchy, which is consistent with patchy areas of fibrosis (73) while ischemic heart disease often (but not always) has at least one moderate or severe regional perfusion defect. Correlation with coronary angiography may be necessary, because these patients will typically do well if they have coronary disease amenable to revascularization. Recovery will depend on the extent of scar, "normal pattern," and mismatch (5,31,32,46,71,72).

Normal Perfusion/Reduced FDG ("Reverse Mismatch")

A pattern of normal perfusion with a relative reduction in FDG uptake is often observed with perfusion/FDG viability imaging. Some studies have associated this with recent (less than 2 weeks after) myocardial infarction and the presence of multivessel disease (74). In most circumstances, however, this finding should be viewed with caution. Often it is related to a lack of normalization of FDG uptake to the zone of most normal perfusion zone (75).

With severe mismatch where FDG uptake may be greater than normal, a reverse mismatch occurs on the opposite wall if the FDG is not normalized correctly (see Color Plate 21E following page 394). Increased uptake in the lateral wall relative to the septum may occur in the presence of a left bundle–branch block where resting perfusion is maintained but metabolism is decreased because of the decreased workload in the septum. We have also observed reverse mismatch in patients who have undergone bypass surgery, possibly because flow has been restored to regions that have nontransmural scar. This may be due to a mechanism similar to reverse redistribution observed with ^{201}Tl imaging (76).

In patients with diabetes, nonischemic viable tissue can have relative reductions in FDG due to impairment of glucose transport. This could lead to regions of reverse mismatch. The use of an insulin clamp may reduce this by increasing glucose uptake in the healthy myocardium in patients with diabetes (61,63,66).

Thus, when reverse mismatch is observed, it is important to consider why it may have occurred, to ensure that a normalization error has not underestimated the degree of mismatch in another territory. Importantly, however, perfusion is usually maintained in these segments. With normal resting perfusion, these regions usually represent viable myocardium that is not ischemic at rest.

Right Ventricular Uptake

With many cardiac radiotracers, when right ventricular hypertrophy (RVH) develops due to pulmonary hypertension, the tracer uptake in the right ventricle (RV) is increased. FDG is no exception. We have most often observed increased RV uptake in patients with greatly impaired LV function where secondary pulmonary hypertension was known or suspected. Recently, interest in RV FDG uptake has increased, particularly as it relates to the LV. Whether RV FDG uptake will have independent prognostic significance is currently being investigated (77).

Image Reporting

The patterns of perfusion/FDG uptake, the extent of hibernating scar and normal tissue, and the LV cavity size must all be considered. When interpreting and reporting perfusion/FDG image results, one must understand the clinical information available, angiographic data (if available), and stress imaging results, and one must be in contact with the referring cardiologist or surgeon.

Determining the presence or extent of viable myocardium and whether there is adequate viable tissue to warrant revascularization is challenging and imaging issues are important to managing this very difficult patient population. Key management decisions are required, which in any given patient depend on integrating the clinical data with the PET findings. Reporting styles differ for individual physicians and their referral base, but when conveying a message regarding viability, one must characterize all the LV tissue. Reporting only the area of the perfusion defect as scar or mismatch may be incomplete information and can sometimes be misleading to the referring physician or surgeon. We have found that defining all three types of tissue: mismatch (ischemic but viable hibernating myocardium), match (scar), and normal (viable and not ischemic at rest) should encompass the whole myocardium. This helps to emphasize to the referring physician the true extent of viability and the potential for recoverable tissue.

A note of caution is worth mention in considering patients early after myocardial infarction. Overestimation of FDG uptake in the myocardium may occur due to uptake from the intense glycolytic activity of leukocytes in the necrotic zones of the infarct (78). This can lower the predictive accuracy of FDG PET viability imaging (75,79). Alternatively, FDG uptake may appear less than perfusion (reverse mismatch) (74) or uptake may be less than expected in the first week after thrombolysis (80). The accuracy of FDG PET in the subacute phase of myocardial infarction may be impaired compared with the usual patient with chronic CAD in which FDG PET has been much more widely applied (75).

Patients with Poor Image Quality

Image quality may occasionally hinder interpretation. Standard quality control issues should always be considered. Was sufficient glucose administered; was insulin administered if needed; was a sufficient dose of FDG administered; was there patient motion or other technical reasons for poor quality? Poor quality is most often due to poor myocardial FDG uptake. Images may appear as a blood-pool image when FDG has not been adequately taken up by the heart. This most often occurs in patients with diabetes or glucose intolerance. When this occurs, several options are available. The perfusion-weighted image should be examined to determine whether there is sufficient information about viability to assist in decision making for the patient. If not, FDG imaging can be continued for an additional 20 minutes to allow for the slower rate of myocardial glucose (and FDG) uptake. If the blood glucose remains elevated, additional insulin can be administered. If this is not successful, the rates of glucose and FDG uptake are even slower. It may be necessary to remove the patient from the camera and have him or her return an hour later. This approach is possible now with posttransmission imaging. If the study was done

with oral loading, repeating the study on a separate day with the "clamp" approach may be considered. These approaches will solve the poor image quality problem in most patients. For the remaining few, other modalities to assess viability could be considered.

Quantification of the Rate of Myocardial FDG Uptake and Glucose Utilization

The rate of myocardial FDG uptake (K) can be calculated using the Patlak graphical analysis. This mathematic model uses the tissue time-activity curves to determine a combined rate constant, K, for FDG myocardial entry and phosphorylation (81). This approach defines the relationship between (a) myocardial activity, $C_m(t)$, corrected for blood-pool activity, $C_b(t)$, and (b) the integral of $C_b(t)$ from time equals 0 to a time t corrected for the blood activity at that time t ($\int C_b dt / C_b[t]$).

This relationship becomes linear after equilibration of tissue FDG (around 5 minutes). K is the slope of the linear portion of this relationship. To determine the rate of myocardial glucose utilization (rMGU), K is multiplied by the mean of three to five blood glucose samples taken after FDG injection and divided by the lumped constant (LC), which corrects for differences in rates of FDG uptake compared with glucose (81) (a value of 0.67 has been used as the LC) (82).

$$rMGU = K \times [Glu] \div LC$$

In comparison to the standard approach, quantification of the rMGU requires a 70-minute dynamic scan to determine the time-activity data for FDG uptake. This technique allows an estimate of myocardial glucose utilization. Because FDG uptake stops at the hexokinase reaction (i.e., FDG 6-phosphate accumulates), the rMGU does not reflect a single metabolic pathway alone, but rather exogenous myocardial glucose utilization.

The rMGU quantification requires the assumption that the LC is fixed. A fixed LC approach has been applied in many previous studies (61,63,65,68,69). However, recent studies (83,84) suggest that the rMGU in non–steady-state conditions may be less accurate because of a varying LC. Regardless, the rMGU provides a tool to measure exogenous glucose utilization, which reflects FDG uptake. This approach has been extremely useful in understanding myocardial glucose utilization and metabolism. Although some centers have applied this approach to measure viability (71,85), in comparative studies, the quantitative methods have not been shown to improve viability determination but have been shown to add time and complexity to the studies (86).

APPLICATION AND UTILITY OF FDG PET

Ischemic Cardiomyopathy

The following clinical endpoints have been used to assess the utility of FDG PET and to relate it to the recovery of LV dysfunction: (a) recovery of regional LV dysfunction, (b) recovery of LV ejection fraction (LVEF), (c) improvement in heart failure symptoms, and (d) improvement in survival. Myocardial metabolic imaging with FDG PET is an established method for assessing myocardial viability using these four clinical endpoints (87). Several additional studies have shown that myocardial metabolic imaging with FDG PET significantly influences management of patients with LV dysfunction. The literature in support of FDG PET myocardial imaging for the assessment of myocardial viability is summarized below.

Prediction of Recovery of Regional LV Dysfunction after Revascularization

The positive predictive value (PPV) and the NPV of FDG PET to detect improvement in regional contractile function after revascularization in a total of 598 patients in 20 studies have recently been reported in a review by Bax et al. (52); these results are summarized in Fig. 8.2.2.

With the increasing number of studies using FDG PET, the NPV has remained high in most reports. In particular, the NPV is highest in patients with lower LV function (47). The PPV for regional recovery has decreased somewhat compared with earlier reviews (5). This likely reflects wider use of FDG PET in patients with more severely impaired LV function where recovery may be delayed (31) and where the benefit of revascularization may be to improve outcome,

with or without improved regional LV function (discussed further below).

Prediction of Improvement in Left Ventricular Ejection Fraction After Revascularization

Literature reports on the value of PET for predicting improvement in the LVEF are predominantly presented as a comparison between pre-revascularization and post-revascularization LVEFs in patients with and those without significant perfusion/FDG-metabolism mismatch (i.e., PET evidence of myocardial viability). In a study by Tillisch et al. (46), the average LVEF significantly increased from pre-revascularization to post-revascularization in patients who had the PET pattern of myocardial viability (LVEF pre-revascularization was 30% ± 11% and LVEF post-revascularization was 45% ± 14%). This observation has been supported by subsequent studies (5,28,49,88,89).

In studies in which the LVEF was also determined in patients who did not have the PET pattern of viability, the LVEF remained unchanged or decreased after revascularization (5,46,88).

Many studies have used mismatch as the viability indicator to predict improved function after revascularization. Recent data indicate that total FDG (71) or its inverse (the extent of scar) (72) is also important in predicting recovery (Fig. 8.2.3) (71). In addition, clinical parameters have been incorporated into prediction models along with PET parameters. In one preliminary study, extent of scar and extent of mismatch were the important PET predictors, whereas age, diabetes, previous coronary artery bypass graft, and time

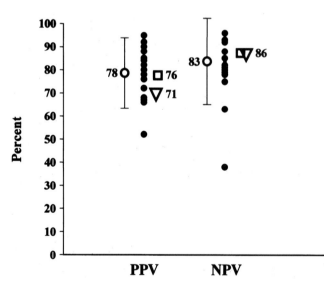

FIG. 8.2.2. Positive predictive value (PPV) and negative predictive value (NPV) for wall motion recovery from 20 studies (n = 598) using 18F-fluorodeoxyglucose positron emission tomography. Individual study PPV and NPV (*solid circles*), mean (*open circles*), mean weighted by number of patients (*open square*), and mean weighted by number of segments (*open triangle*). Both the PPV and the NPV for wall motion recovery are quite high. (From Bax JJ, Poldermans D, Elhendy A, et al. Sensitivity, specificity, and predictive accuracies of various noninvasive techniques for detecting hibernating myocardium. *Curr Probl Cardiol* 2001;26:141–186, with permission.)

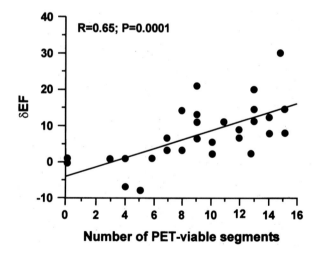

FIG. 8.2.3. Correlation between the number of viable dysfunctional left ventricular (LV) segments and the absolute change in the LV ejection fraction (LVEF) (δEF) after revascularization. $Y = 1.2X \pm 3.97$. (From Pagano D, Townend J, Littler W, et al. Coronary artery bypass surgery as treatment for ischemic heart failure: the predictive value of viability assessment with quantitative positron emission tomography for symptomatic and functional outcome. *J Thorac Cardiovasc Surg* 1998;115:791–799, with permission.)

to surgery were important clinical parameters in predicting recovery of function (72).

Prediction of Improvement in Heart Failure Symptoms After Revascularization

Because most patients with poor LV function suffer from symptoms of heart failure, an important goal in assessing myocardial viability is to predict recovery of heart failure symptoms after myocardial revascularization. Eitzman et al. (90) used PET to assess myocardial viability in 82 patients with poor LV function (average LVEF = 34%). Improvement in heart failure, by at least one class, was related to the PET pattern (presence or absence of mismatch) and type of treatment (revascularization or medical therapy). More patients in the subgroup with mismatch who underwent revascularization had improvement in heart failure class compared with the other subgroups.

Di Carli et al. (91) performed perfusion/FDG-metabolic PET studies in 93 patients with LV dysfunction (average LVEF = 25%) who were followed up for an average of 13.6 months. Sixty-six patients had severe heart failure symptoms. In the medically treated patients as a group, the severity of heart failure symptoms did not change significantly during the follow-up. In contrast, a significant improvement in heart failure symptoms was observed only in the subgroup of patients with mismatch who underwent revascularization. Stated differently, in the 34 patients with heart failure who underwent revascularization, 71% of the subgroup with a PET mismatch pattern before surgery had improvement in heart failure symptoms, whereas only 31% of patients without a PET mismatch pattern had improvement in heart failure symptoms.

In a subsequent study by Di Carli et al. (92), 36 patients with ischemic cardiomyopathy (mean LVEF = 28%) who were undergoing revascularization were studied. Preoperative extent and severity of flow-metabolism mismatch were assessed by quantitative analysis of PET images with ^{13}N-ammonia and FDG. The patients' functional status was determined before and after revascularization using a specific activity scale. The total extent of a PET mismatch before surgery correlated linearly and significantly, with a percent improvement in functional state after CABG ($r = 0.87$; $p < .0001$). A blood-flow–metabolism mismatch of more than 18% was associated with a sensitivity of 76% and a specificity of 78% for predicting a change in functional state after revascularization. Patients with large mismatches (more than 18%) achieved a significantly higher functional state compared with those with minimal or no PET mismatch (less than 5%).

These data indicate that the PET pattern of myocardial viability not only predicts recovery of regional and global LV dysfunction after myocardial revascularization but also identifies the subgroup of patients with poor LV function and heart failure who are most likely to show relief of heart failure symptoms as a result of revascularization. Furthermore, in patients with ischemic cardiomyopathy, the magnitude of improvement in heart failure symptoms after coronary bypass surgery is related to the preoperative extent and magnitude of myocardial viability as assessed by PET imaging. Patients with large perfusion-metabolism mismatches (i.e., greatest magnitude of ischemic viable myocardium by PET) appear to exhibit the greatest clinical benefit after revascularization.

Prediction of Improvement in Survival After Revascularization

A major goal of noninvasive diagnostic procedures in the assessment of CAD is to evaluate prognosis and to assess the potential of survival benefit from a treatment plan. Because survival of patients with LV dysfunction relates to the resting LVEF, it may be implied that perfusion/FDG-metabolic PET imaging, by predicting improvement in LVEF, also predicts survival after myocardial revascularization. This hypothesis has been addressed by four retrospective reports using perfusion/FDG-metabolic PET imaging in 339 patients (90,91, 93,94). The weighted average results indicate that in the subgroup of 61 patients with viable myocardium by FDG PET imaging who were on medical therapy, the event rate (death or myocardial infarction) was 48% (Figs. 8.2.4 and 8.2.5). Importantly, in the subgroup of 121 patients with viable myocardium who underwent revascularization, the event rate was significantly lower at 13%. In 157 patients without FDG PET evidence of myocardial viability, medical therapy (101 patients) and revascularization (56 patients) had similar event rates (15% vs. 13%, respectively). These data suggest that in patients with ischemic cardiomyopathy, revascularization should be recommended only in those with FDG PET evidence of myocardial viability.

In a more recent study, Di Carli et al. (95) evaluated the long-term (median follow-up of 4 years) benefit of FDG PET myocardial viability assessment in 93 consecutive patients with low LVEFs (median of 25%) for stratifying risk and predicting outcome after revascularization. In patients with PET perfusion/FDG-metabolism mismatch who were revascularized, 4-year survival was significantly better as compared with those on medical therapy (75% vs. 30%; $p = .007$). Furthermore, in revascularized patients with PET mismatch, significant improvement in angina and heart failure symptoms was noted as compared with those with PET mismatch who underwent medical therapy. In patients without PET mismatch, revascularization did not significantly improve survival and symptoms as compared with medical therapy. These data corroborate the findings of the above-mentioned four studies and indicate that PET perfusion/FDG-metabolic assessment of myocardial viability may predict long-term survival as a benefit of revascularization.

Influence of FDG PET Metabolism Evaluation of Myocardial Viability on Clinical Decision Making and Patient Management

Cardiac transplantation has been the ultimate therapy for end-stage heart failure; however, because of its limited avail-

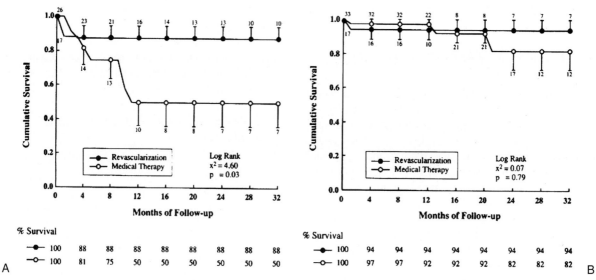

FIG. 8.2.4. A: Mismatch and **(B)** no mismatch cumulative survival of patients, by presence or absence of positron emission tomographic mismatch and mode of treatment (i.e., medical therapy or revascularization). (From Di Carli MF, Davidson M, Little R, et al. Value of metabolic imaging with positron emission tomography for evaluating prognosis in patients with coronary artery disease and left ventricular dysfunction. *Am J Cardiol* 1994;73:527–533, with permission.)

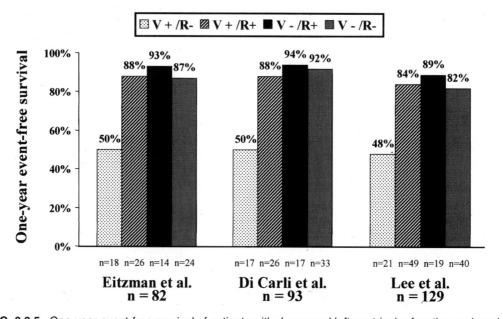

FIG. 8.2.5. One-year event-free survival of patients with depressed left ventricular function undergoing medical therapy or revascularization by presence or absence of viable myocardium on PET imaging. V+, presence of perfusion-metabolism PET mismatch; R+, revascularization [from three outcome studies (90,91,94)]. (From Di Carli M. Predicting improved function after myocardial revascularization. *Curr Opin Cardiol* 1998;13:415–424, with permission.)

ability, the waiting period for a heart transplant by eligible recipients has been prolonged and ranges from 8 months to well over a year. By detecting the presence of a sufficient amount of viable myocardium, potential candidates for myocardial revascularization in place of transplantation may be identified. Such an approach not only lowers the number of patients who are waiting for a transplant but also reduces the overall cost of patient care by offering CABG to patients who would otherwise undergo cardiac transplantation, which is more costly.

Duong et al. (96) evaluated 112 candidates for cardiac transplantation with ischemic cardiomyopathy (LVEF ≤ 35%) who also underwent PET perfusion/FDG-metabolic imaging for the assessment of the presence and extent of myocardial viability; 30 of the 112 patients were found to have evidence of mismatch in at least two regions of the myocardium and have suitable coronary targets. All 30 of these patients were subsequently taken off the transplant list and underwent CABG. The operative mortality rate was 10% and two more patients died later in the follow-up period, for an overall mortality rate of 16.7%. Of the remaining 82 patients who had either minimal or no evidence of PET mismatch, 33 patients underwent cardiac transplantation and 49 continued medical therapy. The perioperative mortality rate for cardiac transplantation was 6.1% and four additional patients died during the follow-up period, for an overall mortality rate of 18.2% for patients undergoing transplantation. Of the 49 patients who underwent medical therapy, 22 patients died, a 44.9% mortality rate. The 5-year actuarial survival rates for the CABG, transplant, and medical therapy groups were 71.4%, 80.1%, and 42.2%, respectively. Therefore, in this study, PET assessment of myocardial viability in cardiac transplant candidates allowed the identification of adequate hibernating tissue in 27% of the patients, who were subsequently referred for CABG and had similar perioperative and long-term survival rates as those who were referred for cardiac transplantation.

In these 112 patients, use of a PET-based algorithm for the management of ischemic cardiomyopathy resulted in $3.8 million in savings in overall patient care, primarily by identifying candidates in whom coronary artery graft surgery could be offered as an alternative to the more costly cardiac transplantation procedure. Similar findings have been observed on a smaller scale among patients referred for transplant assessment for heart failure (97).

In a subsequent study, Beanlands et al. (53) evaluated the influence of PET perfusion/FDG-metabolic imaging in the management of 87 patients with low LVEFs. Before knowledge of the PET data, the physicians were asked to indicate their intended management among the four choices of workup for (a) cardiac transplantation, (b) medical therapy, (c) revascularization, or (d) uncertain. The same questions were repeated after PET data were made available to the physicians. Assessment of myocardial viability by PET imaging redirected therapy from transplantation workup to revascularization in 7 (63%) of 11 patients, medical therapy to revascularization in 8 (44%) of 18 patients, and from revascularization to medical therapy in 16 (42%) of 38 patients; 50 (57%) of 87 patients had their management influenced by PET data.

Among the subgroup of patients with an ejection fraction (EF) less than 30%, 29 (71%) of 41 had their management influenced by PET data. They concluded that the definition of myocardial viability by PET perfusion/FDG-metabolic imaging has a significant impact on difficult therapy decisions in patients with impaired ventricular function and CAD.

In another study from Beanlands et al. (54), 46 patients with coronary disease and an LVEF of less than or equal to 35% were considered candidates for revascularization based on perfusion/FDG-metabolic PET imaging; 35 of 46 patients were subsequently accepted for revascularization. Patients were divided into two groups based on median waiting time after PET: an early group (less than 35 days; n = 18) and a late group (≥35 days; n = 17). Perioperative mortality rates were significantly increased in the late group (24% vs. 0%; $p < .05$). The LVEF increased after early revascularization (24% ± 7% to 29% ± 8%; $p < .001$) but not in the late group (27% ± 5% to 28% ± 6%; $p = $ NS). They concluded that preoperative perfusion/FDG-metabolic PET imaging can be used to identify a high-risk group of patients who may benefit from early revascularization.

A long waiting time for revascularization is associated with a high mortality rate and suggests that early revascularization is desirable after the identification of hibernating viable myocardium. Further studies have also shown an effect of FDG PET on decision making, as shown in Table 8.2.2.

The impact of FDG PET on therapy decisions may also affect outcome. Haas et al. (101), in a cohort design study

TABLE 8.2.2. *Decision making studies: revascularization rates for patients with viable myocardium (PET viable) or predominantly matched defects (PET scar)*

Author, year (ref. no.)	No. of patients	PET viable % revascularized (patients)	PET scar % revascularized (patients)
Vom Dahl, 1997 (55)	161	80 (57/71)	30 (27/90)
Auerbach, 1999 (98)	110	62 (37/60)	36 (18/50)
Akinboboye, 1998 (99)	33	65 (11/17)	13 (2/16)
Calhoun, 1996 (100)	59	84 (29/34)	0 (0/25)
Beanlands, 1998 (54)	46	76 (35/46)	N/A

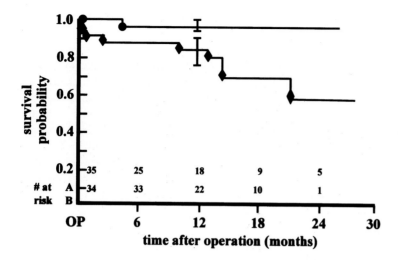

FIG. 8.2.6. Actuarial survival curve (±SE) with the hospital mortality rate included for patients undergoing surgical revascularization. The decision for surgery was based on coronary angiography and clinical data (group A; *diamonds*) compared with patients in whom the decision was based on coronary angiography, clinical data, and ¹⁸F-fluorodeoxyglucose positron emission tomographic viability data (group B; *circles*). Survival was significantly improved in group B ($p < .01$). (From Haas F, Haehnel C, Picker W, et al. Preoperative positron emission tomographic viability assessment and perioperative and postoperative risk in patients with advanced ischemic heart disease. *J Am Coll Cardiol* 1997;30: 1693–1700, with permission.)

of 69 patients, showed that the patients who had FDG PET imaging data used in decisions for surgery had better outcomes after surgical revascularization than patients whose decision was based on coronary angiography and clinical data alone. Mortality rates after revascularization in patients with FDG and without FDG PET were 0% and 11%, respectively, at 30 days. This difference was maintained at 1 year when mortality rates were 3% and 14%, respectively (Fig. 8.2.6).

Comparisons to Other Methods to Assess Myocardial Viability

Several modalities have been used clinically for the detection of myocardial viability. Although many of these can be applied in patients with mild or moderate LV dysfunction, FDG PET appears to be preferred in patients with more severe LV dysfunction. Previous studies and reviews have indicated a greater impact of FDG PET over ²⁰¹Tl viability imaging (5,99,102). Other studies have shown that severe ⁹⁹ᵐTc-methoxyisobutyl isonitrile (MIBI) defects underestimate viability on FDG imaging (103–105). A recent extensive review of the literature has demonstrated that FDG PET

myocardial metabolic imaging is superior to SPECT imaging for the assessment of improvement in regional LV dysfunction after myocardial revascularization (52).

In this same review, FDG PET was found to be significantly more sensitive for predicting regional recovery of function than any of the other viability techniques, whereas dobutamine echocardiography was the most specific (52). However, 45% (9 of 20 patients) of the FDG studies included patient populations with a mean EF less than 35%, while 28% (9 of 32) of dobutamine echocardiography studies included such patients (52).

Four studies that have directly compared FDG imaging [three PET (85,106,107) and one SPECT (108)] to dobutamine echocardiography are summarized in Table 8.2.3. The overall mean PPVs are similar, but FDG PET has a superior NPV.

Another study by Sambuceti et al. (109) reported that dobutamine detected 55% of stunned and only 16% of hibernating myocardium. Recently, a key finding in the study by Pagano et al. (85) was the superiority of FDG PET over dobutamine echocardiography in a group of patients with severe LV dysfunction (EF = 23% ± 7%). This was even greater in the worst functioning (akinetic) segments (PPV/

TABLE 8.2.3. *Predictive values for regional recovery of function in studies including both FDG imaging and dobutamine echocardiography*

Author, year (ref. no.)	No. of patients	Mean EF	PPV % (segments)		NPV % (segments)	
			FDG	DBT	FDG	DBT
Gerber, 1996 (106)	39	33 ± 10	78 (18/23)	89 (17/19)	63 (10/16)	65 (13/20)
Baer, 1996 (107)	42	40 ± 13	92 (24/26)	83 (25/30)	88 (14/16)	92 (11/12)
Bax, 1996ᵃ (108)	17	36 ± 11	62 (24/39)	49 (23/47)	94 (47/50)	91 (41/45)
Pagano, 1998 (71)	30	23 ± 7	66 (190/286)	68 (117/171)	96 (48/50)	55 (90/165)
Total	128					
Weighted Mean			68 (256/374)	68 (182/267)	90 (119/132)	64 (155/242)
Mean			75 ± 14	72 ± 18	85 ± 15	75 ± 18

ᵃ FDG SPECT.

EF, ejection fraction; PPV, positive predictive valve; NPV, negative predictive valve; FDG, ¹⁸F-fluorodeoxyglucose; DBT, dobutamine.

NPV of FDG PET: 80%/94%; dobutamine echocardiography: 73%/41%).

Many of the current myocardial imaging techniques have clinical value in assessment of viability. However, when considering the patients with severely impaired LV function where viability is most relevant, FDG PET appears to be more useful.

A recent randomized controlled trial compared FDG PET to ^{99m}Tc-MIBI-SPECT and observed no significant differences in outcome between the two techniques (110). Unfortunately, the study was probably too small (n = 103) as a prospective outcome study to detect a significant difference. In addition, the patients were a relatively low-risk population with predominately mild to moderate LV dysfunction, who waited a long time for revascularization (115 days). Event rates were low, making it too difficult to demonstrate differences (111). Larger randomized controlled trials are needed to further support the utility of PET in patients with severe LV dysfunction. Such studies are ongoing.

FDG SPECT using single-photon imaging with high-energy collimation or coincidence imaging with dual-head systems has recently been evaluated as a potential alternative to FDG PET imaging (60,108,112–114). Although studies assessing LV function, recovery, and outcome have been limited, this technique does hold promise. Positron imaging with SPECT has a lower count sensitivity (in particular, high-energy collimator SPECT) than PET, which could make imaging more difficult, particularly in patients with obesity or diabetes (59,60,115). The lack of attenuation correction is also problematic, but correction approaches are under development. Currently, SPECT imaging does not allow quantification of FDG and glucose utilization rates, but this is less critical with standard clinical imaging in which visual analysis is used (60). Larger comparative and long-term follow-up studies are needed.

Other PET Viability Methods

In addition to FDG, other methods using PET perfusion or metabolic imaging have been used to define myocardial viability. The utility of perfusion tracers alone in viability detection is threefold: (a) Tracer uptake or kinetics measured at stress and rest can define flow reserve. This provides insight into potential regions of stress-induced ischemia that may contribute to myocardial stunning and possibly hibernation; (b) resting flow provides insight into tissue perfusion, and there is a level of perfusion below which viability may not be sustainable; and (c) as with perfusion/FDG imaging, the characterization of viability is often best achieved through techniques that can define both perfusion and cell integrity (5,31,47). The kinetics of some perfusion tracers depends on both delivery to the tissue (or flow) and retention in intact viable cells, and both perfusion and cell viability information can be obtained with one study.

H$_2$^{15}O and the Perfusable Tissue Index

H$_2$^{15}O is freely diffusible. Its kinetics are related directly to flow. This has allowed measurement of the perfusable

tissue fraction (PTF), which is the fraction of tissue in a given region that can rapidly exchange water (116). Such tissue is presumed to be viable. The method then corrects for the anatomic tissue fraction (ATF), which represents the extravascular tissue density defined from transmission data and the C^{15}O blood-pool images. The perfusable tissue index (PTI) is the PTF/ATF and quantifies the amount of tissue that is freely perfusable with water (and therefore viable) within the given myocardial segment. Normal PTI is 1.0. A PTI higher than 0.7 defines viable tissue and predicts functional recovery after revascularization (117).

^{13}N-ammonia: Flow and Retention

Mathematic modeling of ^{13}NH$_3$ kinetics allows quantification of absolute myocardial blood flow. Gewirtz et al. (118) have used this approach and demonstrated that there is a threshold blood flow (less than 0.25 mL per minute per gram), below which viable recoverable myocardium is unlikely. This finding certainly fits with observations that very severe perfusion defects are less likely to have viable myocardium. However, when flow is reduced but above the threshold, the likelihood of recovery may be less certain. Metabolic or cell integrity information may help tissue characterization in these circumstances.

Nitrogen-13-ammonia retention in the cell is due to conversion to ^{13}N-glutamine, which is an energy-requiring process and therefore depends on cell integrity. In one study, a combined approach of flow data and the volume of distribution of ^{13}NH$_3$ was shown to be an accurate measure of viability (119). More recently ^{13}NH$_3$ uptake alone has been shown to more accurately predict recovery of function than flow measurements alone (120).

Rubidium-82 Washout Kinetics

As a potassium analogue, ^{82}Rb uptake is dependent on flow and cell membrane integrity. In the presence of necrotic tissue, ^{82}Rb uptake may be reduced due to more rapid washout. This differential washout has been used as a marker of viability (121,122). However, studies evaluating recovery post-revascularization and long-term outcome are limited.

Carbon-11-acetate Washout Kinetics

The clearance kinetics of carbon-11 (^{11}C)-acetate directly correlate with rates of oxidative metabolism and myocardial oxygen consumption. In addition, ^{11}C-acetate PET yields quantitative data on myocardial blood flow. Not surprisingly, it also can be used for defining viability. In experienced centers, it has been found to be a reliable and accurate approach (51,123–126). The addition of dobutamine with ^{11}C-acetate offers significant potential for defining metabolic reserve and recovery of function. This approach is discussed in greater detail in Chapter 8.3.

All of these methods are promising, but studies evaluating LV function recovery and long-term outcome are limited.

An on-site cyclotron is required for ^{11}C-acetate, ^{13}N-ammonia, and H$_2$^{15}O production, which has limited their application in the past in comparison to FDG. Rubidium-82 is generator produced and more widely available in North America but has limited availability in other parts of the world. With the worldwide growth in PET imaging, these tracers will become more accessible. Large clinical trials are needed to determine the potential role of these techniques in the determination of viability.

OTHER APPLICATIONS OF FDG PET AND FUTURE DIRECTIONS

Dilated Cardiomyopathy

FDG PET imaging may have a role in the diagnosis of dilated nonischemic cardiomyopathy; however, its usefulness is not well established (87). Mody et al. (73) demonstrated that patients with nonischemic dilated cardiomyopathy had fewer defects and more homogeneity than those with ischemic cardiomyopathy. Although there was some overlap with the visual method, a quantitative approach was quite accurate for defining ischemic etiology (sensitivity of 100% and specificity of 80% in 21 patients). Despite these data, this approach has not been widely applied, because subsequent studies have been limited and there are often other clinical parameters that assist in differentiating etiologies of cardiomyopathy.

Stress-induced Ischemia

Although FDG imaging alone has been used in the detection of stress-induced ischemia (127), perfusion imaging is still required to properly interpret the FDG uptake stress images. This approach may, in the end, be better suited to FDG SPECT imaging, where dual-isotope techniques could allow simultaneous measurement of a perfusion tracer and FDG administered during stress (114).

Gated FDG PET Imaging

Gated FDG PET imaging is also under development. Several centres have been able to produce accurate measures of global and regional ventricular function (128–133) (Fig. 8.2.7). Although further studies are needed, there is significant promise in this area. Gating of PET images will allow better tissue characterization of perfusion, metabolism, and function without the problems of image registration that occur between PET and radionuclide angiography or echocardiography. This approach may also permit evaluation of wall motion and thickening at rest and with dobutamine stress, thus taking advantage of both metabolic and contractile reserve data (128). Advances in image registration between PET and other modalities are ongoing. Co-registration of data from coronary angiography and magnetic resonance imaging may allow highly comprehensive tissue characteri-

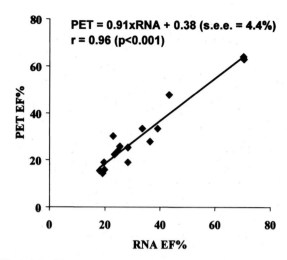

FIG. 8.2.7. There is excellent agreement between left ventricular ejection fraction measured with gated fluorodeoxyglucose positron emission tomography and QGS versus planar-gated radionuclide angiography in 16 patients. (From de-Kemp R, Van Kriekinge SD, Germano G, et al. LV ejection fraction with gated FDG studies on a partial-ring rotating PET scanner. *J Nucl Med* 2000;41:88P(abst), with permission.)

zation with coronary anatomy, flow, metabolism, myocardial structure, and function.

Viability Imaging for Alternatives to Revascularization

The role of FDG PET in directing patients to revascularization, transplantation, or medical therapies is well established, but viability imaging is also used in newer alternatives to traditional revascularization including transmyocardial laser and angiogenesis. In these approaches, viable tissue that has potential to recover must be defined so therapy can be targeted to these regions. More recently, FDG PET has been used in cellular cardiomyoplasty (use of skeletal myoblasts or stem cells in regions of injury), to define regions of scar and then to demonstrate the differentiation of skeletal myoblasts into viable myocytes (134) (see Color Plate 23 following page 394). The definition of appropriate target sites for these new therapy approaches is critical to their success and potential future application.

SUMMARY

The role of FDG PET viability imaging in patients with poor LV function has been widely evaluated. This approach is an established accurate method for determining the diagnosis of viable myocardium and the prognosis of recovery after adequate revascularization. Although defining mismatch is important, the extent of scar or total viable myocardium is also relevant because stunned myocardium may also play an important role in LV dysfunction. The greatest impact is in patients with severe LV dysfunction, although recovery of the viable myocardium may take several months after revascularization.

FDG PET is now an integral part of clinical cardiology practice in centers where the technology is available. Data from FDG PET images clearly alter clinical decision making, identify patients at high risk of subsequent events who would benefit from revascularization, and do this in a potentially cost-effective manner. Proper identification of such patients for treatment has an impact on optimizing patient outcome. Although FDG PET is an established technique in ischemic heart disease, ongoing studies, including randomized controlled trials, continue to evaluate its evolving role in patients with severe LV dysfunction and heart failure. FDG PET will also be valuable in the future evaluation of new therapies that can improve the integrity and function of the myocardium.

ACKNOWLEDGMENTS

The authors thank Sherri Nipius, Linda Garrard, May Aung, and Rob deKemp for their help in preparing this chapter. Rob Beanlands is a research scientist supported by the Canadian Institute for Health Research.

REFERENCES

1. McKee PA, Castelli WP, McNamara PM, et al. The natural history of congestive heart failure: the Framingham study. *N Engl J Med* 1971;285:1441–1446.
2. Yateau RF, Peter RH, Behar VS, et al. Ischemic cardiomyopathy: the myopathy of coronary artery disease. Natural history and results of medical versus surgical treatment. *Am J Cardiol* 1974;34:520–525.
3. Alderman EL, Fisher LD, Litwin P, et al. Results of coronary artery surgery in patients with poor left ventricular function (CASS). *Circulation* 1983;68:785–795.
4. Franciosa JA, Wilen M, Ziesche S, et al. Survival in men with severe chronic left ventricular failure due to either coronary heart disease or idiopathic dilated cardiomyopathy. *Am J Cardiol* 1983;51:831–836.
5. Maddahi J, Schelbert H, Brunken R, et al. Role of thallium-201 and PET imaging in evaluation of myocardial viability and management of patients with coronary artery disease and left ventricular dysfunction. *J Nucl Med* 1994;35:707–715.
6. Serruys PW, Simoons ML, Suryapranata H, et al. Preservation of global and regional left ventricular function after early thrombolysis in acute myocardial infarction. *J Am Coll Cardiol* 1986;7:729–742.
7. Cohn J, Archibald D, Ziesche S, et al. Effect of vasodilator therapy on mortality in chronic congestive heart failure. Results of a veterans administration cooperative study. *N Engl J Med* 1987; 314: 1547–1552.
8. CONSENSUS Trial Study Group. Effects of enalapril on mortality in severe congestive heart failure: results of the cooperative North Scandinavian Enalapril Survival Study. *N Engl J Med* 1987;316: 1429–1435.
9. Packer MD, Bristow MR, Cohn JN, et al. The effect of carvedilol on morbidity and mortality in patients with chronic heart failure. *N Engl J Med* 1996;334:1349–1355.
10. Packer M, Coats AJ, Fowler MB, et al. Effect of carvedilol on survival in severe chronic heart failure. *N Engl J Med* 2001;344:1651–1658.
11. Evans R, Manninen DL, Garrison LP, et al. Donor availability as the primary determinant of the future of heart transplantation. *JAMA* 1986;255:1892–1898.
12. Baker DW, Jones R, Hodges J, et al. Management of heart failure, III: the role of revascularization in the treatment of patients with moderate or severe left ventricular systolic dysfunction. *JAMA* 1994;272: 1528–1534.
13. Louie HW, Laks H, Milgalter E, et al. Ischemic cardiomyopathy: criteria for coronary revascularization and cardiac transplantation. *Circulation* 1991;84:III290–III295.
14. Hochberg MS, Parsonnet V, Gielchinsky I, et al. Coronary artery bypass grafting in patients with ejection fractions below forty percent: early and late results in 466 patients. *J Thorac Cardiovasc Surg* 1983; 86:519–527.
15. Kron IL, Flanagan TL, Blackbourne LH, et al. Coronary revascularization rather than cardiac transplantation for chronic ischemic cardiomyopathy. *Ann Surg* 1989;210:348–352.
16. Opie LH. Substrate and energy metabolism of the heart. In: Sperelakis N, ed. *Function of the heart in normal and pathological states,* 2nd ed. Boston: Kluwer Academic Publishers, 1989:327–359.
17. Camici P, Ferrannini E, Opie LH. Myocardial metabolism in ischemic heart disease: basic principles and application to imaging by positron emission tomography. *Prog Cardiovasc Dis* 1989;XXXII:217–238.
18. Kolter T, Uphues I, Wichelhaus A, et al. Contraction-induced translocation of the glucose transporter GLUT4 in isolated ventricular cardiomyocytes. *Biochem Biophys Res Commun* 1992;189:1207–1214.
19. Lopaschuk GD, Stanley W. Glucose metabolism in the ischemic heart. *Circulation* 1997;95:415–422.
20. Phelps ME, Hoffman EJ, Selin CE, et al. Investigation of [18-F]2-fluoro-2-deoxyglucose for the measure of myocardial glucose metabolism. *J Nucl Med* 1978;19:1311–1319.
21. Choi Y, Brunken RC, Hawkins RA, et al. Factors affecting myocardial 2-[^{18}F]fluoro-2-deoxy-D-glucose uptake in positron emission tomography studies of normal humans. *Eur J Nucl Med* 1993;20:308–318.
22. Marshall RC, Tillisch JH, Phelps ME, et al. Identification and differentiation of resting myocardial ischemia and infarction in man with positron computed tomography, ^{18}F-labeled fluorodeoxyglucose and N-13 ammonia. *Circulation* 1983;67:766–778.
23. Schwaiger M, Schelbert HR, Ellison D, et al. Sustained regional abnormalities in cardiac metabolism after transient ischemia in the chronic dog model. *J Am Coll Cardiol* 1985;6:336–347.
24. Braunwald E, Kloner RA. The stunned myocardium: prolonged, postischemic ventricular dysfunction. *Circulation* 1982;66:1146–1149.
25. Bolli R. Myocardial ''stunning'' in man. *Circulation* 1992;86: 1671–1691.
26. Rahimtoola SH. From coronary artery disease to heart failure: role of the hibernating myocardium. *Am J Cardiol* 1995;75:16E–22E.
27. Rahimtoola SH. The hibernating myocardium. *Am Heart J* 1989;117: 211–221.
28. Di Carli M. Predicting improved function after myocardial revascularization. *Curr Opin Cardiol* 1998;13:415–424.
29. Kloner RA. Does reperfusion injury exist in humans? *J Am Coll Cardiol* 1993;21:537–545.
30. Vanoverschelde J-LJ, Wijns W, Borgers M, et al. Chronic myocardial hibernation in humans. From beside to bench. *Circulation* 1997;95: 1961–1971.
31. Haas F, Augustin N, Holper K, et al. Time course and extent of improvement of dysfunctioning myocardium in patients with coronary artery disease and severely depressed left ventricular function after revascularization: correlation with positron emission tomography. *J Am Coll Cardiol* 2000;36:1927–1934.
32. Haas F, Jennen L, Heinzmann U, et al. Ischemically compromised myocardium displays different time-courses of functional recovery: correlation with morphological alterations? *Eur J Cardiothorac Surg* 2001;20:290–298.
33. Shivalkar B, Maes A, Borgers M, et al. Only hibernating myocardium invariably shows early recovery after coronary revascularization. *Circulation* 1996;94:308–315.
34. Berman M, Fischman AJ, Southern J, et al. Myocardial adaptation during and after sustained, demand-induced ischemia: observations in closed-chest, domestic swine. *Circulation* 1996;94:755–762.
35. Schulz R, Guth BD, Peiper K, et al. Recruitment of an inotropic reserve in moderately ischemic myocardium at the expense of metabolic recovery: a model of short-term hibernation. *Circ Res* 1992;70: 1282–1295.
36. Fallavollita JA, Perry BJ, Canty JM. 18-F-2-deoxyglucose deposition and regional flow in pigs with chronically dysfunctional myocardium. Evidence for transmural variations in chronic hibernating myocardium. *Circulation* 1997;95:1900–1909.
37. Marinho NVS, Keogh BE, Costa DC, et al. Pathophysiology of chronic left ventricular dysfunction: new insights from the measure-

ment of absolute myocardial blood flow and glucose utilization. *Circulation* 1996;93:737–744.

38. Liedtke AJ, Renstrom B, Nellis SH, et al. Mechanical and metabolic functions in pig hearts after 4 days of chronic coronary stenosis. *J Am Coll Cardiol* 1995;26:815–825.

39. Depre C, Vanoverschelde JL, Grillenberger K, et al. Correlation of glucose transporter messenger RNA expression with morphological pattern and glucose uptake in chronically dysfunctional myocardium. *Circulation* 1995;92:I651(abst).

40. Brosius FC, Sun DQ, England R, et al. Altered glucose transporter mRNA levels in cardiac ischemia. *Circulation* 1993;88:I-542-2923(abst).

41. Doenst T, Taegtmeyer H. Profound underestimation of glucose uptake by [18-F]2-deoxy-2-fluoroglucose in reperfused rat heart muscle. *Circulation* 1998;97:2454–2462.

42. Schwarz ER, Schaper J, vom Dahl J, et al. Myocyte degeneration and cell death in hibernating human myocardium. *J Am Coll Cardiol* 1996; 27:1577–1585.

43. Borgers M, Thone F, Wouters L, et al. Structural correlates of regional myocardial dysfunction in patients with critical coronary artery stenosis: chronic hibernation. *Cardiovasc Pathol* 1993;2:237–245.

44. Tamaki N, Yonekura Y, Yamashita K, et al. Positron emission tomography using fluorine-18-deoxyglucose in evaluation of coronary artery bypass grafting. *Am J Cardiol* 1989;64:860–865.

45. Tamaki N, Ohtani H, Yamashita K, et al. Metabolic activity in the areas of new fill-in after thallium-201 reinjection: comparison with positron emission tomography using fluorine-018-deoxyglucose. *J Nucl Med* 1991;32:673–678.

46. Tillisch J, Brunken R, Marshall R, et al. Reversibility of cardiac wall-motion abnormalities predicted by positron tomography. *N Engl J Med* 1986;314:884–888.

47. vom Dahl J, Eitzman DT, Al-Aouar ZR, et al. Relation of regional function, perfusion, and metabolism in patients with advanced coronary artery disease undergoing surgical revascularization. *Circulation* 1994;90:2356–2365.

48. Carrel T, Jenni R, Haubold-Reuter S, et al. Improvement of severely reduced left ventricular function after surgical revascularization in patients with preoperative myocardial infarction. *Eur J Nucl Med* 1992;6:479–484.

49. Lucignani G, Paolini G, Landoni C, et al. Presurgical identification of hibernating myocardium by combined use of technetium-99m hexakis 2-methoxyisobutyl isonitrile single photon emission tomography and fluorine-18 fluoro-2-deoxy-D-glucose positron emission tomography in patients with coronary artery disease. *Eur J Nucl Med* 1992; 19:874–881.

50. Altehoefer C, Kaiser H-J, Dorr R, et al. Fluorine-18 deoxyglucose PET for assessment of viable myocardium in perfusion defects in 99mTc-MIBI SPECT: a comparative study in patients with coronary artery disease. *Eur J Nucl Med* 1992;19:334–342.

51. Gropler RJ, Geltman EM, Sampathkumaran K, et al. Comparison of carbon-11-acetate with fluorine-18-fluorodeoxyglucose for delineating viable myocardium by positron emission tomography. *J Am Coll Cardiol* 1993;22:1597.

52. Bax JJ, Poldermans D, Elhendy A, et al. Sensitivity, specificity, and predictive accuracies of various noninvasive techniques for detecting hibernating myocardium. *Curr Probl Cardiol* 2001;26:141–186.

53. Beanlands RSB, deKemp RA, Smith S, et al. F-18-Fluorodeoxyglucose PET imaging alters clinical decision making in patients with impaired ventricular function. *Am J Cardiol* 1997;79:1092–1095.

54. Beanlands RS, Hendry P, Masters R, et al. Delay in revascularization is associated with increased mortality rate in patients with severe LV dysfunction and viable myocardium on fluorine-18-fluorodeoxyglucose positron emission tomography imaging. *Circulation* 1998;98: II51–II56.

55. vom Dahl J, Altehoefer C, Sheehan FH, et al. Effect of myocardial viability assessed by technetium-99m-sestamibi SPECT and fluorine-18-FDG PET on clinical outcome in coronary artery disease. *J Nucl Med* 1997;38:742–748.

56. Fallen EL, Nahmias C, Scheffel A, et al. Redistribution of myocardial blood flow with topical nitroglycerin in patients with coronary artery disease. A PET study. *Circulation* 1995;91:1381–1388.

57. Rothley J, Weeden ARJ. Clinical PET protocols. In: Schwaiger M, ed. *Cardiac positron emission tomography*. Boston: Kluwer Academic Publishers, 1996:357.

58. Pirich C, Schwaiger M. The clinical role of positron emission tomography in management of the cardiac patient. *Rev Port Cardiol* 2000; 19:89–98.

59. Arrighi JA, Dilsizian V. Myocardial viability. Radionuclide-based methods. (radionuclide-based methods/nuclear cardiology). In: Pohost GM, et al, eds. *Imaging in cardiovascular disease*. Philadelphia: Lippincott Williams & Wilkins, 2000:213–232.

60. Sandler MP, Bax JJ, Patton JA, et al. Fluorine-18-fluorodeoxyglucose cardiac imaging using a modified scintillation camera. *J Nucl Med* 1998;39:2035–2043.

61. Vitale G, deKemp R, Ruddy TD, et al. Myocardial glucose utilization and the optimization of F-18 FDG PET imaging in patients with non–insulin-dependent diabetes mellitus, coronary artery disease and left ventricular dysfunction. *J Nucl Med* 2001;42:1730–1736.

62. vom Dahl J, Herman WH, Hicks RJ, et al. Myocardial glucose uptake in patients with insulin-dependent diabetes mellitus assessed quantitatively by dynamic positron emission tomography. *Circulation* 1993; 88:395–404.

63. Ohtake T, Yokoyama I, Watanabe T, et al. Myocardial glucose metabolism in noninsulin-dependent diabetes mellitus patients evaluated by FDG-PET. *J Nucl Med* 1995;36:456–463.

64. Maki M, Luotolahti M, Nuutila P, et al. Glucose uptake in the chronically dysfunctional but viable myocardium. *Circulation* 1996; 93: 1658–1666.

65. Knuuti MJ, Nuutila P, Ruotsalainen U, et al. Euglycemic hyperinsulinemic clamp and oral glucose load in stimulating myocardial glucose utilization during positron emission tomography. *J Nucl Med* 1992; 33:1255–1262.

66. Voipio-Pulkki LM, Nuutila P, Knuuti J, et al. Heart and skeletal muscle glucose disposal in type 2 diabetic patients as determined by PET. *J Nucl Med* 1993;34:2064–2067.

67. DeFronzo RA, Tobin JD, Andres R. Glucose clamp technique: a method for quantifying insulin secretion and resistance. *Am J Physiol* 1979;273:E214–E223.

68. Knuuti JM Y-JH, Voipio-Pulkki LM, et al. Enhancement of myocardial FDG uptake by a nicotinic acid derivative. *J Nucl Med* 1994;35: 989–998.

69. Stone CK, Holden JE, Stanley W, et al. Effect of nicotinic acid on exogenous myocardial glucose utilization. *J Nucl Med* 1995;36: 996–1002.

70. Sun D, Nguyen N, deGrado TR, et al. Ischemia induced translocation of the insulin-responsive glucose transporter GLUT4 to the plasma membrane of cardiac myocytes. *Circulation* 1994;89:793–798.

71. Pagano D, Townend J, Littler W, et al. Coronary artery bypass surgery as treatment for ischemic heart failure: the predictive value of viability assessment with quantitative positron emission tomography for symptomatic and functional outcome. *J Thorac Cardiovasc Surg* 1998;115: 791–799.

72. Beanlands R, deKemp R, Ruddy TD, et al. A quantitative method for defining scar with F-18-FDG PET predicts the degree of recovery of LV function post-revascularization. *Circulation* 2000;102:II-724-3500(abst).

73. Mody FV, Brunken RC, Stevenson LW, et al. Differentiating cardiomyopathy of coronary artery disease from nonischemic dilated cardiomyopathy utilizing positron emission tomography. *J Am Coll Cardiol* 1991;17:373–383.

74. Yamagishi H, Akioka K, Hirata K, et al. A reverse flow-metabolism mismatch pattern on PET is related to multivessel disease in patients with acute myocardial infarction. *J Nucl Med* 1999;40:1492–1498.

75. Schwaiger M, Pirich C. Reverse flow-metabolism mismatch: what does it mean? *J Nucl Med* 1999;40:1499–1502.

76. Langer A, Burns RJ, Freeman MR, et al. Reverse distribution on exercise thallium scintigraphy: relationship to coronary patency and ventricular function after myocardial infarction. *Can J Cardiol* 1992; 9:709–715.

77. Khin MM, Panza JA, Ernst IR, et al. Right ventricular fluorodeoxyglucose uptake in patients with chronic ischemic heart disease: relation to severity of left ventricular dysfunction. *J Nucl Med* 2001;42:171P-744(abst).

78. Wijns W, Melin JA, Leners N, et al. Accumulation of polymorphonuclear leucocytes in reperfused ischemic canine myocardium: relation with tissue viability assessed by 18F fluorodeoxyglucose uptake. *J Nucl Med* 1988;29:1826–1832.

79. Schwaiger M, Brunken R, Grover-McKay M, et al. Regional myocar-

dial metabolism in patients with acute myocardial infarction assessed by positron emission tomography. *J Am Coll Cardiol* 1986;8: 800–808.

80. Maes A, Van de Werf F, Mesotten LV, et al. Early assessment of regional myocardial blood flow and metabolism in thrombolysis in myocardial infarction flow grade 3 reperfused myocardial infarction using carbon-11-acetate. *J Am Coll Cardiol* 2001;37:30–36.

81. Patlak CS, Blasberg RG. Graphical evaluation of blood-to-brain transfer constants from multiple-time uptake data: generalizations. *J Cereb Blood Flow Metab* 1985;5:584–590.

82. Ratib O, Phelps ME, Huang SC, et al. Positron tomography with deoxyglucose for estimating local myocardial glucose metabolism. *J Nucl Med* 1982;23:577–586.

83. Hariharan R, Bray M, Ganim R, et al. Fundamental limitations of [^{18}F]2-deoxy-2-fluoro-D-glucose for assessing myocardial glucose uptake. *Circulation* 1995;91:2435–2444.

84. Botker HE, Bottcher M, Schmitz O, et al. Glucose uptake and lumped constant variability in normal human hearts determined with [^{18}-F]fluorodeoxyglucose. *J Nucl Cardiol* 1997;4:125–132.

85. Pagano D, Bonser RS, Townend J, et al. Predictive value of dobutamine echocardiography and positron emission tomography in identifying hibernating myocardium in patients with postischaemic heart failure. *Heart* 1998;79:281–288.

86. Knuuti MJ, Nuutila P, Ruotsalainen U, et al. The value of quantitative analysis of glucose utilization in detection of myocardial viability by PET. *J Nucl Med* 1993;34:2068–2075.

87. ACC/AHA Task Force. Guidelines for clinical use of cardiac radionuclide imaging. Report of the American College of Cardiology/American Heart Association Task Force on Assessment of Diagnostic and Therapeutic Cardiovascular Procedures (Committee on Radionuclide Imaging), developed in collaboration with the American Society of Nuclear Cardiology. *J Am Coll Cardiol* 1995;25:521–547.

88. Depre C, Melin JA, Vanoverschelde J-LJ, et al. Assessment of myocardial viability after bypass surgery by pre-operative PET flow-metabolism measurements and ultrastructural analysis of myocardial biopsies. *Circulation* 1993;88:I-199-1062(abst).

89. Paolini G, Lucignani G, Zuccari M, et al. Identification and revascularization of hibernating myocardium in angina-free patients with left ventricular dysfunction. *Eur J Cardiothorac Surg* 1994;8:139–144.

90. Eitzman D, Al-Aouar Z, Kanter HL, et al. Clinical outcome of patients with advanced coronary artery disease after viability studies with positron emission tomography. *J Am Coll Cardiol* 1992;20:559–565.

91. Di Carli MF, Davidson M, Little R, et al. Value of metabolic imaging with positron emission tomography for evaluating prognosis in patients with coronary artery disease and left ventricular dysfunction. *Am J Cardiol* 1994;73:527–533.

92. Di Carli MF, Asgazadie F, Schelbert HR, et al. Quantitative relation between myocardial viability and improvement in heart failure symptoms after revascularization in patients with ischemic cardiomyopathy. *Circulation* 1995;92:3436–3444.

93. Yoshida K, Gould KL. Quantitative relation of myocardial infarct size and myocardial viability by positron emission tomography to left ventricular ejection fraction and 3-year mortality with and without revascularization. *J Am Coll Cardiol* 1993;22:984–997.

94. Lee KS, Marwick TH, Cook SA, et al. Prognosis of patients with left ventricular dysfunction, with and without viable myocardium after myocardial infarction: relative efficacy of medical therapy and revascularization. *Circulation* 1995;90:2687–2694.

95. Di Carli M, Maddahi J, Rokhsar S, et al. Long-term survival of patients with coronary artery disease and left ventricular dysfunction: implications for the role of myocardial viability assessment in management decisions. *J Thorac Cardiovasc Surg* 1998;116:997–1004.

96. Duong TH, Hendi P, Fonarow G, et al. Role of positron emission tomographic assessment of myocardial viability in the management of patients who are referred for cardiac transplantation. *Circulation* 1995;8:582.

97. Beanlands RSB, Nichol G, Visentin DE, et al. Potential for cost savings with FDG PET imaging in patients being considered for cardiac transplantation. *Circulation* 1997;96:I-13(abst).

98. Auerbach M, Schoder H, Hoh CK, et al. Prevalence of myocardial viability as detected by positron emission tomography in patients with ischemic cardiomyopathy. *Circulation* 1999;99:2921–2926.

99. Akinboboye OO, Idris O, Cannon P, et al. Usefulness of positron emission tomography in defining myocardial viability in patients referred for cardiac transplantation. *Am J Cardiol* 1999;83:1271–1274.

100. Calhoun WB, Mills RM, Drane WE. Clinical importance of viability assessment in chronic ischemic heart failure. *Clin Cardiol* 1996;19: 367–369.

101. Haas F, Haehnel C, Picker W, et al. Preoperative positron emission tomographic viability assessment and perioperative and postoperative risk in patients with advanced ischemic heart disease. *J Am Coll Cardiol* 1997;30:1693–1700.

102. Tamaki N, Kawamoto M, Takahashi N, et al. Prognostic value of an increase in fluorine-18 deoxyglucose uptake in patients with myocardial infarction: comparison with stress thallium imaging. *J Am Coll Cardiol* 1993;22:1621–1627.

103. Sawada S, Muzik O, Allman K, et al. Positron emission tomography detects evidence of viability in rest technetium-99m sestamibi defects. *J Am Coll Cardiol* 1994;23:92–98.

104. Soufer R, Dey H, Ng C-K, et al. Comparison of sestamibi single-photon emission computed tomography with positron emission tomography for estimating left ventricular myocardial viability. *Am J Cardiol* 1995;75:1214–1219.

105. Dilsizian V, Arrighi JA, Diodati JG, et al. Myocardial viability in patients with chronic coronary artery disease. Comparison of ^{99m}Tc-sestamibi with thallium reinjection and [^{18}F]fluorodeoxyglucose. *Circulation* 1994;89:578–587.

106. Gerber BL, Vanoverschelde J-LJ, Bol A, et al. Myocardial blood flow, glucose uptake, and recruitment of inotropic reserve in chronic left ventricular ischemic dysfunction. implications for the pathophysiology of chronic myocardial hibernation. *Circulation* 1996;94:651–659.

107. Baer FM, Voth E, Deutsch HJ, et al. Predictive value of low dose dobutamine transesophageal echocardiography and fluorine-18 fluorodeoxyglucose positron emission tomography for recovery of regional left ventricular function after successful revascularization. *J Am Coll Cardiol* 1996;23:60–69.

108. Bax JJ, Cornel JH, Visser FC, et al. Prediction of recovery of regional ventricular dysfunction following revascularization: comparison of F-18 fluorodeoxyglucose SPECT, thallium-201 stress-reinjection SPECT and dobutamine echocardiography. *J Am Coll Cardiol* 1996; 28:558–564.

109. Sambuceti G, Giorgetti L, Corsiglia L, et al. Perfusion-contraction mismatch during inotropic stimulation in hibernating myocardium. *J Nucl Med* 1998;39:396–402.

110. Siebelink H-MJ, Blanksma PK, Crijns HJGM, et al. No difference in cardiac event-free survival between positron emission tomography–guided and single-photon emission computed tomography–guided management. *J Am Coll Cardiol* 2001;37:81–88.

111. Beanlands RS, Ruddy TD, Freeman MR, et al. Patient management guided by viability imaging. *J Am Coll Cardiol* 2001;38:1271–1272.

112. Burt RW, Perkins OW, Oppenheim BE, et al. Direct comparison of fluorine-18-FDG SPECT, fluorine-18-FDG PET and rest thallium-201 SPECT for detection of myocardial viability. *J Nucl Med* 1995; 2:179.

113. Bax JJ, Visser FC, Blanksma PK, et al. Comparison of myocardial uptake of Fluorine-18-Fluorodeoxyglucose imaged with PET and SPECT in dyssynergic myocardium. *J Nucl Med* 1996;37:1631–1636.

114. Sandler MP, Videlefsky S, Delbeke D, et al. Evaluation of myocardial ischemia using a rest metabolism/stress perfusion protocol with fluorine-18 deoxyglucose/technetium-99m MIBI and dual-isotope simultaneous-acquisition single-photon emission computed tomography. *J Am Coll Cardiol* 1995;26:870–878.

115. Bailey DL, Young H, Bloomfiled PM, et al. ECAT ART—a continuously rotating PET camera: performance characteristics, initial clinical studies, in a nuclear medicine department. *Eur J Nucl Med* 1997;24: 6–15.

116. Iida H, Kanno I, Takahashi A, et al. Measurement of absolute myocardial blood flow with H$_2$-^{15}O and dynamic positron emission tomography. Strategy for quantification in relation to the partial-volume effect. *Circulation* 1988;78:104–115.

117. deSilva R, Yamamoto Y, Rhodes CG, et al. Preoperative prediction of the outcome of coronary revascularization using positron emission tomography. *Circulation* 1992;86:1738–1742.

118. Gewirtz H, Fischman AJ, Abraham S, et al. Positron emission tomographic measurements of absolute regional myocardial blood flow permits identification of nonviable myocardium in patients with chronic myocardial infarction. *J Am Coll Cardiol* 1994;23:851–859.

119. Beanlands RSB, deKemp R, Scheffel A, et al. Can nitrogen-13 ammonia kinetic modeling define myocardial viability independent of fluorine-18 fluorodeoxyglucose? *J Am Coll Cardiol* 1997;29:537–543.

120. Kitsiou AN, Bacharach SL, Bartlett ML, et al. ^{13}N-ammonia myocardial blood flow and uptake: relation to functional outcome of asynergic regions after revascularization. *J Am Coll Cardiol* 1999;33:678–686.

121. Gould KL, Yoshida K, Hess MJ, et al. Myocardial metabolism of fluorodeoxyglucose compared to cell membrane integrity for the potassium analogue rubidium-82 for assessing infarct size in man by PET. *J Nucl Med* 1991;32:1–9.

122. vom Dahl J, Muzik O, Wolfe E, et al. Myocardial rubidium-82 tissue kinetics assessed by dynamic positron emission tomography as a marker of myocardial cell membrane integrity and viability. *Circulation* 1996;93:238–245.

123. Gropler RJ, Siegel BA, Sampathkumaran K, et al. Dependence of recovery of contractile function on maintenance of oxidative metabolism after myocardial infarction. *J Am Coll Cardiol* 1992;19:989–997.

124. Hata T, Nohara R, Fujita M, et al. Noninvasive assessment of myocardial viability by positron emission tomography with 11-C acetate in patients with old myocardial infarction. *Circulation* 1996;94:1834–1841.

125. Gropler RJ, Geltman EM, Sampathkumaran K, et al. Functional recovery after coronary revascularization for chronic coronary artery disease is dependent on maintenance of oxidative metabolism. *J Am Coll Cardiol* 1992;20:569–577.

126. Wolpers HG, Burshert W, van den Hoff J, et al. Assessment of myocardial viability by use of ^{11}C-acetate and positron emission tomography. Threshold criteria of reversible dysfunction. *Circulation* 1997;95:1417–1424.

127. Abramson B, Ruddy TD, deKemp R, et al. Stress perfusion/metabolism imaging: a pilot study for a potential new approach to the diagnosis of coronary disease in women. *J Nucl Cardiol* 2000;7:205–212.

128. Yamagishi H, Akioka K, Hirata K, et al. Dobutamine-stress electrocardiographically gated positron emission tomography for detection of viable but dysfunctional myocardium. *J Nucl Cardiol* 1999;6:626–632.

129. Hor G, Kranert WT, Maul FD, et al. Gated metabolic positron emission tomography (GAPET) of the myocardium: ^{18}F-FDG-PET to optimized recognition of myocardial hibernation. *Nucl Med Commun* 1998;19:535–545.

130. Willemsen ATM, Siebelink H-MJ, Blanksma PK, et al. Automated ejection fraction determined from gated myocardial FDG-PET data. *J Nucl Cardiol* 1999;6:577–582.

131. Hattori N, Bengel FM, Mehilli J, et al. Global and regional functional measurements with gated PET in comparison with left ventriculography. *Eur J Nucl Med* 2001;28:221–229.

132. deKemp R, Van Kriekinge SD, Germano G, et al. LV ejection fraction with gated FDG studies on a partial-ring rotating PET scanner. *J Nucl Med* 2000;41:88P(abst).

133. Saab G, deKemp R, Ukkonen H, et al. Technical advances in assessing perfusion, function, and metabolism with radionuclide imaging. *Presented at the 51st Annual Scientific Presentation Poster Session.* American College of Cardiology, Bethesda, MD, 2002.

134. Menasche P, Hagege AA, Scorsin M, et al. Myoblast transplantation for heart failure. *Lancet* 2001;37:279–280(abst).

Oxidative Metabolism and Cardiac Efficiency

Heikki Ukkonen and Rob S.B. Beanlands

Oxidative metabolism of fuels provides the heart with the energy required for contraction and basal metabolism. Impaired myocardial energy transfer plays an important role in the development of contractile dysfunction in many clinical syndromes, including ischemic heart disease. Positron emission tomography (PET) provides a unique tool for noninvasive quantitative characterization of myocardial metabolic processes *in vivo*, and it has been widely used for the detection of viable myocardium in ischemic heart disease. However, the capabilities of PET to define myocardial metabolism have not been used to their fullest extent. Currently, the efficacy of therapy is monitored primarily by evaluating patients' functional capacity, ventricular function, and hemodynamics. By combining the functional data with PET-derived metabolic data, the treatment effects can be more physiologically assessed. This approach has been applied to measure myocardial efficiency (i.e., myocardial work related to myocardial oxygen consumption) to evaluate cardiac disease and its therapies.

This chapter focuses on myocardial metabolism, particularly the application of oxidative metabolism and oxygen consumption imaging with PET, in cardiac disease and treatment. The role of PET in the determination of myocardial efficiency is also emphasized; application of this methodology in the optimization of therapy is expected to increase as PET becomes more widely available.

MYOCARDIAL METABOLISM

The heart requires a constant supply of energy to sustain contractile function. This energy is supplied by hydrolysis of adenosine triphosphate (ATP), which is primarily derived from aerobic metabolism of fatty acids and carbohydrates and to a significantly lesser extent from aerobic metabolism of amino acids and ketone bodies (Fig. 8.3.1). Although the mechanisms that connect the mechanical work and energy production of the heart are not fully understood, it has been suggested that intracellular calcium plays a regulatory role in the link between cardiac mechanics and energy production (1).

Oxygen is the final electron acceptor in all pathways of aerobic metabolism in the myocardium. Therefore, under steady-state conditions, myocardial oxygen consumption provides an accurate measure of overall myocardial metabolism (2). However, the relative predominance of different energy substrates depends mainly on the concentration of these substrates in the afferent blood vessels, on hormonal influences, workload, blood flow, and oxygen demand (3).

ATP is the immediate and quantitatively by far the most important substance that fuels most myocellular processes. Because the myocardium relies predominantly on aerobic metabolism for its energy requirements, myocardial oxygen consumption ultimately reflects the rate of mitochondrial metabolism and ATP production.

The processes of the heart requiring ATP (and therefore oxygen) may be divided into three main categories: basal metabolism, excitation–contraction coupling (ion movements against electrochemical gradients), and force generation by the actin and myosin molecules (4). In clinical terms, the major determinants of myocardial oxygen consumption are basal metabolism of the heart, heart rate, and myocardial wall stress and contractility. Wall stress and contractility are the principal components of "force generation" that results from the actin–myosin interaction.

Approximately 65% to 80% of the total energy produced is converted to heat and the rest is available for the force generation and basal metabolism. Basal metabolic energy is required for protein synthesis and maintenance of cellular membrane integrity. The energy needed for excitation–contraction coupling, that is, energy for calcium cycling, is at most 20% to 25% of the total ATP consumption during the isovolumetric contraction phase (5,6). Cross-bridge activation by actin and myosin molecules (myosin adenosine triphosphatase), which lead to myocardial contraction, uses approximately 65% of the energy available for all mechanical processes of the heart.

Fatty Acid Oxidation

Free fatty acids (FFAs) are considered the preferred substrate for myocardial metabolism (7). In the fasted state and

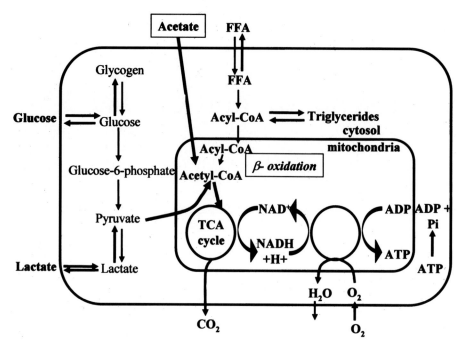

FIG. 8.3.1. Schematic diagram for myocardial substrate metabolism. The tricarboxylic acid *(TCA)* cycle is linked to myocardial oxygen consumption via the electron transport chains, which supply most of the energy (adenosine triphosphate; *ATP*) of the heart.

after a meal rich in fat, the level of blood FFAs is high and FFAs become the major source of energy, accounting for up to 90% of myocardial oxygen consumption (8). In addition, myocardial workload influences substrate metabolism. FFAs are preferred over glucose up to a moderate level of exercise (9,10). When fatty acids are oxidized, glucose oxidation is inhibited and the glucose is shuttled into glycogen synthesis (3). Myocardial uptake of albumin-bound FFAs is related to the level of FFA in the blood and to the FFA/albumin ratio. Once inside the myocardial cell, fatty acids are activated to long-chain acyl-coenzyme A (acyl-CoA) by an acyl-CoA synthetase (Fig. 8.3.1). Long-chain acyl-CoA is oxidized to produce acetyl-coenzyme A (acetyl-CoA) (so-called beta-oxidation). Each molecule of acetyl-CoA that is oxidized by beta-oxidation produces one molecule of NADH and one molecule of $FADH_2$. Acetyl-CoA then enters the tricarboxylic acid (TCA) cycle and produces two molecules of CO_2, three of NADH, and one of $FADH_2$ for each molecule of acetyl-CoA (see later discussion).

Carbohydrate Oxidation (Glucose, Lactate)

Besides FFA, the other main source of acetyl-CoA for the TCA cycle is oxidation of carbohydrates, particularly glucose and lactate. When the organism is in a carbohydrate-fed state, lipolysis is inhibited by insulin and subsequently carbohydrate oxidation increases (11). In this case, carbohydrates can account for 100% of the myocardial oxygen consumption (glucose, 70%; lactate, 30%). During heavy dynamic exercise (65% of an individual's maximal oxygen

uptake), the production of lactate increases and lactate becomes the major fuel of the heart, accounting for up to 60% to 70% of the myocardial oxygen consumption (3,12).

During ischemia, the metabolism of glucose to lactate is the main source of energy for the heart. With the lack of a sufficient oxygen supply, glucose uptake, glycogenolysis, glycolytic flux and ATP hydrolysis are all stimulated (13).

Glucose is transported into the myocardial cell by the glucose transporters GLUT-4 and GLUT-1 (14). Intracellularly, glucose is rapidly phosphorylated to glucose 6-phosphate, which is further used for glycolysis or glycogen synthesis (Fig. 8.3.1). In glycolysis, glucose 6-phosphate is metabolized to pyruvate. Pyruvate is also formed from lactate taken up by the heart. Under aerobic conditions, most of the pyruvate is converted to acetyl-CoA, which enters the TCA cycle (see later discussion). A minor portion of glucose and lactate is converted to oxaloacetate, which enters the TCA cycle at a different site than acetyl-CoA (13).

Tricarboxylic Acid Cycle

The metabolic pathways for energy substrates transform the major fuels into acetyl-CoA, which then enters the TCA cycle. One molecule of acetyl-CoA produces three molecules of NADH, one of $FADH_2$, and one of guanosine triphosphate (GTP), which is also a high-energy compound. NADH and $FADH_2$ are oxidized in the respiratory electron-transport chain and ultimately yield 11 molecules of ATP. Mitochondrial respiration appears to be regulated by nitrous oxide (NO), at least *in vitro,* and thus NO might have a regulatory role in the myocardial metabolic rate of oxygen ($MMRO_2$) *in vivo* (15).

The rate at which the TCA cycle operates is the major factor that controls the rate of production of ATP by the heart. The TCA cycle activity increases when myocardial work increases. Reduced ATP/adenosine diphosphate or $NAD/NADH_2$ ratios may be the major determinants of the rate at which the TCA cycle operates (16), but this has been disputed (17).

Efficiency

In the healthy heart, myocardial metabolism and contraction are closely linked by ATP production and consumption. However, in certain clinical conditions such as ischemic heart disease, in which oxygen supply is restricted, and in heart failure, this close connection can be lost. The overloaded failing heart is characterized by an imbalance between energy production and utilization (18). The overload itself increases energy expenditure by increasing wall stress in the dilated heart. The energy deficit of the myocardium may further aggravate both systolic and diastolic dysfunction (18).

Myocardial metabolism can be related to myocardial work to further evaluate cardiac physiology. The concept of efficiency has been used for decades for this purpose (19) and was originally described by Starling and Visshcr (20) in isolated heart preparations. Efficiency is defined as the ratio between the energy created by a system and the energy put into the system. Because most of the energy (approximately 65% to 80%) consumed by the heart is converted to heat, experimental thermodynamic studies are important for assessing the total efficiency of the heart (21,22). However, *in vivo* (in animal and human studies), efficiency is usually defined as the ratio of mechanical work performed relative to the myocardial oxygen consumption (mechanical efficiency). It has been claimed that the efficiency is maximized under physiologic conditions both in the right ventricle (RV) and in the left ventricle (LV) (19,23). However, the question whether the heart was built to operate at maximum efficiency or at maximum stroke work is still a matter of controversy.

In 1979, Suga et al. (24) introduced a comprehensive time-varying elastance model. In this model, the area of the pressure–volume relationship (PVA) is a measure of the total work performed by the ventricle during one cardiac cycle. The PVA concept includes both the external or stroke (pressure–volume) work of the heart and an internal component, termed potential energy. The PVA correlates closely with invasively measured $MMRO_2$ per beat (24). The method allows the assessment of contractile efficiency, as well as the cost of basal and activation metabolism. The PVA is the only one of the mechanical variables that can be used to assess myocardial efficiency without a need to separately measure myocardial oxygen consumption. The PVA method to measure oxygen consumption is highly invasive, requiring catheterization with LV micromanometers and conductance catheters. Therefore, the applicability of the method in human studies is limited.

Other approaches require a measure or estimate of both external work and oxygen consumption to determine efficiency. There are several applicable approaches for noninvasive measurement of external cardiac work, which usually employ measurement of blood pressure and heart rate with or without stroke volume (25,26). External work can be assessed with the pressure work index, a product of systolic (or mean) pressure, heart rate, and stroke volume (27), which covers both pressure and flow work. Energy is used for building and maintaining tension, which is needed for contractility and wall stress. Systolic contraction of the ventricle is enhanced by preload and is opposed by afterload, which are both oxygen-requiring processes (28). When related to $MMRO_2$, the pressure work index gives a measure of useful forward mechanical efficiency. The pressure work index and its modifications are readily assessed noninvasively *in vivo*, which improves the applicability of this method in human studies (29–33).

ASSESSMENT OF MYOCARDIAL ENERGY METABOLISM

In Vitro Methods

A common way to study the energy metabolism of the heart is to measure the intracellular levels of metabolic intermediates or the activity of enzymes involved in the various pathways of energy metabolism. With these techniques, the levels of intermediates are measured from frozen or lyophilized tissue samples by spectrophotometry, radiometry, or high-performance liquid chromatography. Although these methods have formed the basis of our understanding of myocardial metabolism, they require tissue samples and are not clinically practical. These methods are also limited in that they can give relevant information about the energy status of the heart, but not information about the rate of the production or utilization of ATP (i.e., oxygen consumption) (34).

Invasive Methods

Percutaneous catheterization of the coronary sinus and blood sampling allow the measurement of cardiac metabolism *in vivo*. Simultaneous measurements of the concentration of energy substrates (carbohydrates, fatty acids) or oxygen in the coronary sinus and in the arterial blood and coronary blood flow allow calculation of net rates of carbohydrate and lipid metabolism and myocardial oxygen consumption (35). The net substrate metabolism can be calculated more accurately if specific substrates labeled with carbon-14 (^{14}C) or tritium (^3H) are used. Despite improved accuracy, *regional* myocardial metabolism cannot be assessed with such methods. Furthermore, coronary sinus catheterization is a highly invasive and sometimes difficult procedure, which limits the use of this approach.

Noninvasive Methods

Nuclear Magnetic Resonance

Nuclear magnetic resonance (NMR) spectroscopy allows assessment of molecular structure and substrate concentration. The two most common nuclides measured in studies involving energy metabolism are phosphate-31 (^{31}P) and carbon-13 (^{13}C). The use of ^{31}P NMR provides information about the levels of ATP, creatinine phosphate, inorganic phosphate, and sugar phosphates, all of which play a role in the myocardial energy system (34). Various intermediates of metabolism can be labeled with ^{13}C. NMR spectroscopy allows quantitative detection of these intermediates in the tissue, an approach that has been used to assess TCA cycle activity. Fluorine-19 (^{19}F)–labeled compounds that bind calcium have been used with NMR to measure intracellular calcium.

Phosphate-31 NMR provides information about the concentration of high-energy phosphate compounds, but not about the rate of ATP production or utilization, which limits the usefulness of this method. Carbon-13 NMR can be used to detect the fate of a predefined substrate in the chain of oxidative metabolism (TCA cycle) (36). However, TCA cycle intermediates and the ^{13}C label are quickly equilibrated, and as a consequence, ^{13}C NMR mainly measures incorporation of ^{13}C into the glutamate pool (37). Carbon-13 NMR is further limited by difficulties in kinetic analysis of metabolite labeling (34).

Magnetic Resonance Imaging

Recent technical advances in cardiac magnetic resonance imaging (MRI) have made it possible to accurately study cardiac morphology and function, as well as myocardial perfusion in humans (38). T2-weighted fast spin-echo imaging, combined with perfusion-sensitive spin labeling, has also been used to measure myocardial perfusion and oxygen concentration in isolated blood-perfused rabbit hearts (39). However, MRI does not allow quantification of myocardial oxygen consumption.

PET

Regional myocardial metabolism, blood flow, and oxygen consumption can be readily studied with PET using radiolabeled metabolite analogues. The advantages of PET over other radionuclide methods are the unique ability to quantitatively measure tracer concentrations in selected tissue volumes with better spatial and temporal resolution and better sensitivity due to multiple detectors.

Measurement of Glucose and Fatty Acid Metabolism with PET

PET can be used to measure the initial steps of glucose metabolism (fluorine-18 [^{18}F]–fluorodeoxyglucose [FDG])

(40) and the rate of fatty acid metabolism (^{11}C-palmitate, ^{18}F-FTHA) (41,42). The clearance of ^{11}C-palmitate represents beta-oxidation and oxidation in the TCA cycle. Because the rapid *washout* of ^{11}C-palmitate from myocardium partly represents the TCA cycle activity, it correlates to some extent with myocardial oxygen consumption. However, the method is sensitive to levels of tissue oxygenation and arterial fatty acids, as well as to the pattern of substrate use (43–46). Fluorine-18-FTHA is a false long-chain fatty acid substrate and inhibitor of fatty acid metabolism. After transport into the mitochondria, it undergoes initial steps of beta-oxidation and is thereafter trapped in the cell. The rate of radioactivity accumulation in the myocardium would, therefore, directly reflect the beta-oxidation rate of long-chain fatty acids. The uptake rate constant of ^{18}F-FTHA correlates well with the rate–pressure product in healthy volunteers (47).

It has to be kept in mind that the rate of metabolism of one single-energy substrate may reflect only a portion of the overall oxidative metabolism of the heart and depends on prevailing metabolic circumstances. Mitochondrial oxidation of intermediary substrates can also be impaired in specific conditions such as myocardial ischemia (48). The overall oxidative metabolism can, however, be quantitatively assessed with ^{11}C-acetate and $^{15}O_2$ PET.

ASSESSMENT OF MYOCARDIAL OXYGEN CONSUMPTION WITH PET

Carbon-11-acetate PET

FFAs and carbohydrates share the TCA cycle for oxidative metabolism (Fig. 8.3.1). The turnover rate of the TCA cycle reflects the rate of overall oxidative metabolism, and therefore, it is an ideal site for assessing myocardial oxidative metabolism. Carbon-11-acetate is readily metabolized to CO_2 almost exclusively by oxidative metabolism through the TCA cycle.

First-pass extraction of acetate into the myocardium is inversely related to the myocardial blood flow (MBF) (49). In a steady state, the reported myocardial extraction fraction (EF) of radiolabeled acetate in animal models is 60% to 70% for healthy myocardium and up to 95% for ischemic myocardium (50,51). In humans, the EF of acetate is approximately 30% to 40% (52). Acetate is converted to acetyl-CoA in mitochondria, which then enters the TCA cycle. In the TCA cycle, the radiolabel in the carboxyl (C-1) position of acetate undergoes two cycle turns before the label is released as CO_2 (or bicarbonate in tissue) (53). Nearly all (80% to 90%) of the acetate extracted by myocardium is oxidized. The major alternative route is transamination of acetate to glutamate and aspartate via the TCA cycle intermediates (54). Therefore, the elimination rate of radiolabeled acetate reflects the overall TCA cycle flux and consequently overall oxygen consumption over a wide range of cardiac workloads (50,54).

Preparation of the Tracer

The production of ^{11}C-acetate is based on a method developed by Pike et al. (55). In short, ^{11}C-carbon dioxide is produced by the [14]N(p,α)[11]C reaction with medical cyclotron. Methyl magnesium bromide in diethyl ether is carbonated under nitrogen with ^{11}C-labeled carbon dioxide. After this, hydrochloric acid is added to the reaction during vigorous stirring and then the phases are allowed to separate. Sodium bicarbonate (10 mL) is added to the solution and the solution is heated under a stream of nitrogen and finally sterilized by filtration.

Imaging Protocols

The imaging protocol for ^{11}C-acetate is simple. A short rectilinear scan (e.g., a 5-minute transmission scan) is performed with a removable source (such as germanium-68) to confirm the location of the heart (this may not be necessary with larger field-of-view [FOV] PET cameras). To correct the data for tissue photon attenuation, 15- to 20-minute transmission imaging with a removable source is also performed before the emission scanning. Carbon-11-acetate is administered as an intravenous bolus over 30 to 60 seconds (29,56). The target dose varies according to camera properties and the dose is usually 10 to 20 mCi. The length of dynamic scanning in clinical studies varies between 20 and 49 minutes (30,57). To detect the early part of the clearance curve, the early time frames are short and the frames get longer toward the end of the study; for example, 10×10 seconds, 1×60 seconds, 5×100 seconds, 5×120 seconds, and 7×240 seconds (30).

Analysis of the Data

Regional Analysis

In clinical practice, several different approaches have been used to assess regional myocardial oxygen consumption. Most commonly the regions of interest (ROIs) have been placed on transaxial slices (see Color Plate 24 following page 394) or short-axis slices (58) of the LV and in some cases on the RV simultaneously (30,59,60).

Regional analysis of the data is of special interest in coronary artery disease (CAD), particularly after a myocardial infarction (MI) when there are likely to be regional differences in myocardial function and metabolism (33). Regional differences can also exist in nonischemic cardiomyopathy (61). An important clinical application of ^{11}C-acetate PET has been in assessing myocardial viability (57). To facilitate the comparison between PET and echocardiographic studies, one must use the same segmental division in both modalities (29,30,61–64).

Modeling of the Data

In most clinical studies, ^{11}C-acetate data have been analyzed by monoexponential fitting of the clearance portion of the time-activity curve (TAC) (Fig. 8.3.2) (29,30,32,33, 60,65–68).

Biexponential fitting of the data (Fig. 8.3.2) has been used less frequently because the second part of the curve might be less reliable in clinical studies (69). The conventional exponential fitting analysis does not account for the distribution of arterial input function, the recirculating ^{11}C-acetate, the spillover, or the presence of metabolites. Therefore, more sophisticated compartmental and kinetic models have been introduced for estimation of myocardial oxygen consumption with ^{11}C-acetate PET.

Because only a fraction of injected ^{11}C-acetate is delivered to the heart during the first pass, a recirculating amount of the tracer can be considerable and may therefore affect the shape of tissue TACs. Using computer simulations, it has been shown that the shape of the arterial input function can significantly alter the monoexponential fitting of the myocardial TAC. Buck et al. (70) introduced a two-compartment

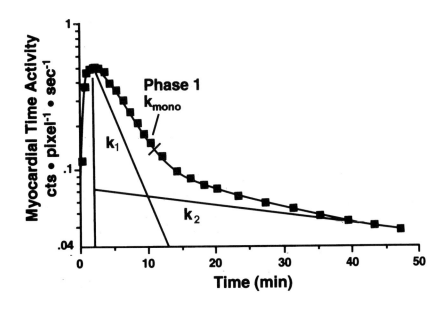

FIG. 8.3.2. Diagrammatic representation of the monoexponential and biexponential fitting of myocardial time-activity curves of carbon-11-acetate to obtain rate constants k_1, k_2, and k_{mono}. (From Armbrecht JJ, Buxton DB, Brunken R, et al. Regional myocardial oxygen consumption determined noninvasively in humans with [1-^{11}C] acetate and dynamic positron emission tomography. *Circulation* 1989;80:863–872, with permission.)

model for ^{11}C-acetate kinetics that accounts for tracer recirculation. The model requires assessment of an input function and correction for tracer metabolites and spillover effects. The model-derived parameter k_2 correlated closely with directly measured MMRO$_2$. This method has been successfully used in patients with congestive heart failure (CHF) (33) and patients with acute MI (71). Usually data from a single ROI are analyzed at a time. Raylman et al. (72) were able to improve the accuracy of the fitted k_2 parameter by simultaneously fitting data from multiple ROIs. Sun et al. (73) tested a comprehensive tracer kinetic model (six-compartment model) for ^{11}C-acetate kinetics in dogs, which takes into account differences in input function. This model yielded accurate MMRO$_2$ measurements compared with invasive measurements. However, this model has not been validated in humans. The same is true for the compartmental model introduced by Ng et al. (74).

Although these models are theoretically more accurate than the traditional fitting methods, their complexity and

the need for additional assessments, such as arterial blood sampling, limit their feasibility in clinical studies.

Experimental Studies and Validation of the Method

The detected TAC reflecting the clearance of ^{11}C-acetate from the myocardium can be either monoexponential or biexponential depending on the level of oxidative metabolism. The curve is usually monoexponential at rest, during hypoxia, and ischemia, and it is usually biexponential during increased metabolic demands such as during dobutamine infusion (51,69). The decay constant of the initial component of the clearance curve has been shown to be linearly related to myocardial oxygen consumption. The accuracy of ^{11}C-acetate PET in measuring myocardial oxygen consumption in the LV has been validated in experimental studies in isolated perfused rabbit hearts, rat hearts, and dogs (50,51,54, 75) (Fig. 8.3.3). In humans, the elimination rate of ^{11}C-acetate has been shown to correlate with indirect estimates of

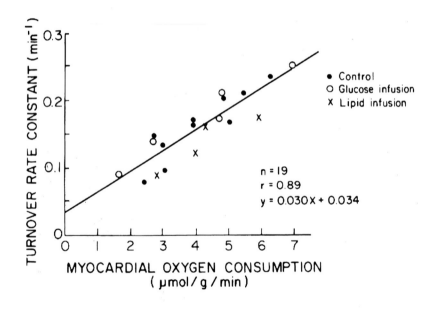

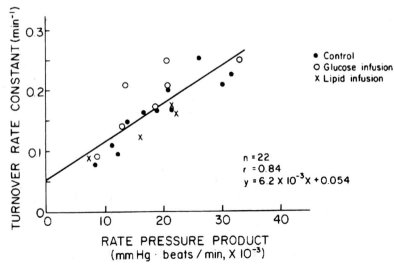

FIG. 8.3.3. **Top:** Correlation between the rate constant of the rapid phase of clearance and directly measured myocardial oxygen consumption. There is no significant difference between the control, post–glucose administration and post–lipid administration imaging studies. **Bottom:** Correlation between the rate constant of the rapid phase of clearance and the rate pressure product, which is an index of total myocardial work. There are no significant differences between the control, post–glucose administration and post–lipid administration studies. (From Brown MA, Myears DW, Bergmann SR. Validity of estimates of myocardial oxidative metabolism with carbon-11 acetate and positron emission tomography despite altered patterns of substrate utilization. *J Nucl Med* 1989;30:187–193, with permission.)

myocardial oxygen consumption both in the LV (60,68) and in the RV (59). The elimination rate of ^{11}C-acetate also correlates well with directly (invasively) measured myocardial oxygen consumption in healthy volunteers (76,77) and patients with dilated cardiomyopathy (33,78). Although variations in the pattern of substrate utilization can alter the ratio of TCA cycle flux to oxygen consumption, the magnitude of the change is insignificant (75).

Potential Sources of Error and Limitations of ^{11}C-acetate PET

The accuracy of ^{11}C-acetate PET in assessing $MMRO_2$ may be reduced in specific conditions. In experimental prolonged low-flow ischemia in pigs, the myocardial clearance rate constant (k_{mono}) of ^{11}C-acetate may overestimate the myocardial oxygen consumption (79). Correction for a decrease in peak ^{11}C activity and a reduced amino acid pool observed with the prolonged ischemia restores the relationship with $MMRO_2$. The ratio of ^{11}C-acetate clearance rate to myocardial oxygen consumption in ischemic canine hearts has also been reported to be higher than that in nonischemic canine hearts (51). It has been suggested that ^{11}C-acetate could overestimate myocardial oxygen consumption in myocardial segments containing infarcted myocardium, compared with the $^{15}O_2$-based method (80).

To date, the clinical application of ^{11}C-acetate PET has been established by using the rate constant indices of oxidative metabolism and not absolute quantification of $MMRO_2$. The assessment of treatment efficacy has also been based on relative changes in myocardial oxidative metabolism and not absolute quantification of $MMRO_2$. Therefore, in clinical practice, it is usually not necessary to correct for the changes in the oxidative metabolism/$MMRO_2$ relationship mentioned above. However, when assessment of absolute myocardial oxygen consumption is needed, correction for these factors should be considered.

$^{15}O_2$ PET

It has been possible to label molecular oxygen with ^{15}O and to detect the fate of the tracer with PET for over 20 years (81). Yet, the assessment of $MMRO_2$ of the LV with $^{15}O_2$ PET has only recently been achieved in humans. A new PET technique employing $^{15}O_2$ inhalation was introduced by Iida et al. (82) for the direct quantification of regional $MMRO_2$ ($rMMRO_2$). This steady-state method takes into account the systematic underestimation of tissue signals caused by the small transmural wall thickness and contractile wall motion (partial volume effect). It also allows the assessment of $rMMRO_2$ in absolute terms (i.e., in milliliters per minute per gram).

Preparation of the Tracer

Production of ^{15}O compounds with a low-energy accelerator on-site improves the feasibility of this method in the

assessment of $rMMRO_2$ because it provides excellent flexibility for the timetable in clinical studies. Radiochemical purity of $^{15}O_2$ is high (up to 97%). $H_2^{15}O$ is produced using a dialysis technique (83). Sterility and pyrogen tests must be performed daily to verify the purity of the product. Oxygen-15 is processed to $C^{15}O$ in a charcoal oven at 950°C. Gas chromatographic analysis is regularly performed to verify the purity of the product.

Scanning Protocol

The measurement of $rMMRO_2$ with $^{15}O_2$ is based on a series of PET scans that are used for the calculation of functional images. Special attention must be paid to avoid patient movement during the study. The sequence of PET scans does not have any effect on $rMMRO_2$ values, and therefore, the sequence can be modified according to the local practice. All PET data are corrected for dead time, decay, and photon attenuation. The emission data of ^{15}O studies are reconstructed either by a conventional filtered back-projection (FBP) method (82,84) or with a new iterative reconstruction algorithm using median root prior (MRP) reconstruction (85). The MRP reconstruction method provides higher reproducibility and lower variability in the quantitative myocardial parameters when compared with the FBP method (86).

Rectilinear Scan

The optimal imaging position is determined by a 5-minute rectilinear scan after exposure to an external $^{68}Ge/^{68}Ga$ ring source. (In scanners with a larger FOV, this step may not always be necessary.)

Transmission Scan

To correct for tissue photon attenuation, 20-minute transmission imaging with a removable source (such as ^{68}Ge) is performed before the emission scanning to allow correction for attenuation.

Blood-pool Scan

To obtain blood volume data, the subject's nostrils are closed and he or she inhales $C^{15}O$ for 2 minutes through a three-way inhalation flap valve (0.14% CO mixed with room air). After the inhalation, 2 minutes are allowed for carbon monoxide to combine with hemoglobin in red blood cells before a static scan for 4 minutes is started. During the scan period, three blood samples are drawn at 2-minute intervals and blood radioactivity is measured immediately with an automatic gamma counter.

Myocardial Blood Flow

Before the flow measurements, 10 minutes is allowed for $C^{15}O$ radioactive decay. In clinical practice, blood flow is measured either with slow $H_2^{15}O$ infusion or with slow $C^{15}O_2$ inhalation (87). In a slow $H_2^{15}O$ infusion protocol, the tracer is injected intravenously during 2 minutes and dynamic scanning of the thoracic region, for 6 minutes (with time frames of 6 × 5 seconds, 6 × 15 seconds, 8 × 30 seconds), is started when radioactivity appears in the FOV. In a slow $C^{15}O_2$ inhalation protocol, subjects inhale the tracer for 2 minutes and dynamic scanning is started simultaneously with $C^{15}OCO_2$ inhalation.

Dynamic $O_2^{15}O$ Scan

Ten minutes after the infusion of $H_2^{15}O$ or inhalation of $C^{15}O_2$, continuous inhalation of $^{15}O_2$ is started for 16 minutes and PET imaging is performed under steady-state conditions (4 × 30 seconds, 6 × 60 seconds, 1 × 600 (or 480) seconds, 9 × 30 seconds) (82). Minor modifications in steady-state framing may also be used depending on scanner properties. The steady-state image of myocardial $^{15}O_2$ uptake is determined from normalized subtractions of blood volume and lung gas volume from the 10-minute (8-minute) data acquisition obtained during steady-state conditions.

Finally, a short 5-minute transmission scan is usually performed at the end, to rule out patient movement during the study.

Processing and Modeling of the Data

The measurement of rMMRO$_2$ and regional oxygen extraction fraction (rOEF) with this method is based on the inhalation of $^{15}O_2$ gas. The compartmental model describing $^{15}O_2$ behavior in the myocardium is illustrated in Fig. 8.3.4. The model requires a correction for spillover of activity from the vascular pools of the heart chambers and lungs and from the pulmonary airways. The spillover of activity from the vascular pools is corrected by the blood volume measurement using $C^{15}O$, and the spillover of activity from the pulmonary airways is corrected with an indirect measurement of gas volume obtained from the transmission scan.

$^{15}O_2$ is carried as ^{15}O-hemoglobin by blood and it diffuses to myocardium, where it is converted to water ($H_2^{15}O$). This diffusion process is explained by OEF. The $H_2^{15}O$ equilibrates instantaneously and its washout rate is proportional to prevailing MBF. The recirculating $H_2^{15}O$, produced by other tissues, also contributes to the observed activity in the myocardium and correction for this is required. Sophisticated mathematic modeling of the data yields the quantified rOEF. Iida et al. (82) described the relationship between rOEF and rMMRO$_2$ as

$$rMMRO_2 = [O_2]_a \times rOEF \times rMBF$$

where $[O_2]_a$ is the total oxygen content of the arterial blood (milliliters of O_2 per milliliter of blood) and rMBF is regional MBF assessed by $C^{15}O_2$ inhalation (88) or $H_2^{15}O$ infusion (87). The $[O_2]_a$ is assessed as

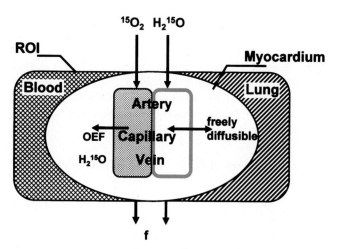

FIG. 8.3.4. A compartmental model to measure the regional oxygen extraction fraction (rOEF) and the regional myocardial metabolic rate of oxygen by the use of PET and $^{15}O_2$ inhalation. The myocardial region of interest includes radioactivity in the myocardial tissue, spillover from the radioactivity of blood occupying the cardiac chamber, and spillover from radioactivity in the lung. The myocardial compartment consists of the tissue component and a vascular component (which includes arterial, capillary, and venous volumes). The hemoglobin-bound $^{15}O_2$ is supplied to the capillary and diffuses into the tissue space, where it is instantaneously converted into labeled water of metabolism ($H_2^{15}O$-met). This diffusion process is assumed to be explained by an OEF. There is another input of radioactivity with a different chemical form, circulating $H_2^{15}O$, which is assumed to be freely diffusible across the capillary membrane. This radioactivity is assumed to distribute in the same tissue space as $H_2^{15}O$-met and is washed out in proportion to the blood flow divided by the partition coefficient of water. (From Iida H, Rhodes CG, Araujo LI, et al. Noninvasive quantification of regional myocardial metabolic rate of oxygen by use of 15-O_2 inhalation and positron emission tomography. Theory, analysis and application in humans. *Circulation* 1996;94: 792–807, with permission.)

$$[O_2]_a = \frac{1.39 \times Hb \times \%Sat}{100}$$

where *Hb* is the hemoglobin concentration of the blood (grams per milliliter), *%Sat* represents the percentage saturation of oxygen in arterial blood, and 1.39 denotes the maximum binding capacity of oxygen per unit mass of hemoglobin (milliliters of O_2 per gram of hemoglobin). The value of 94% was assigned to *%Sat*.

Analysis of the Data

The myocardial ROIs can be placed on extravascular density images according to anatomic segments (80,84,89,90). To avoid spillover from the RV, septal ROIs are placed on the LV side of the septum. A large ROI (input function for rMBF) and a small ROI (for calculation of rOEF) are also placed on the LV on blood volume images. A lung ROI,

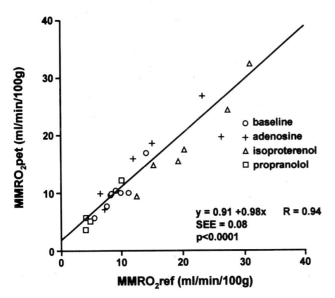

FIG. 8.3.5. Comparison of $MMRO_2$ measured by $^{15}O_2$ PET ($MMRO_2$-pet) and invasive arteriovenous sampling and $MMRO_2$ microspheres ($MMRO_2$-ref) shows a close correlation between the two methods despite pharmacologic provocation ($MMRO_2$-pet = 0.98 $MMRO_2$-ref + 0.91; r = 0.94). (From Yamamoto Y, de Silva R, Rhodes CG, et al. Noninvasive quantification of regional myocardial metabolic rate of oxygen by $^{15}O_2$ inhalation and positron emission tomography: experimental validation. *Circulation* 1996;94:808–816, with permission.)

needed for rOEF calculation, is also placed on gas volume images. All the ROIs are projected onto blood and gas volume images and the dynamic $^{15}O_2$ and $H_2{}^{15}O$ data sets to generate arterial and myocardial tissue TACs that are subsequently used for calculation of rMMRO$_2$ (82).

Validation and Experimental Studies

A linear relationship has been established between $^{15}O_2$ PET–derived and directly measured $MMRO_2$ in animal studies. Studies with dogs (90–92) using various pharmacologic interventions with isoprenaline, adenosine, propranolol, and morphine demonstrated that OEF and $MMRO_2$ values obtained by this technique agreed closely with those obtained by direct measurement of OEF with arteriovenous (AV) sampling (Fick method) and MBF with the microsphere technique (Fig. 8.3.5). There is also a close linear correlation between $^{15}O_2$ PET–derived rMMRO$_2$ and k_{mono} of ^{11}C-acetate in patients with CAD and old MI (r = 0.89; $p < .001$). (Fig. 8.3.6) (80).

Potential Sources of Error and Limitations of $^{15}O_2$ PET

Although $^{15}O_2$ PET has great potential in noninvasive assessment of myocardial oxygen consumption, there are certain limitations to this method (82). Calculation of regional myocardial oxygen consumption with $^{15}O_2$ PET is based on sophisticated modeling requiring a series of PET studies. The complexity of the scanning procedure increases the vulnerability of the method. The mean intersubject variability for rMMRO$_2$ has varied from 21% to 32% (82), and this variation is mainly due to the variation in rMBF and to a lesser degree due to the variation in rOEF. However, a lower variability and higher reproducibility of the quantitative parameters can be achieved if an iterative reconstruction method based on median root prior reconstruction is used instead of the traditional FBP method (85,86). In particular, the reproducibility of the septal rMMRO$_2$ values, which have previously been problematic, has significantly improved with the MRP reconstruction method. The main practical problem of the method is, nevertheless, the sensitivity of the

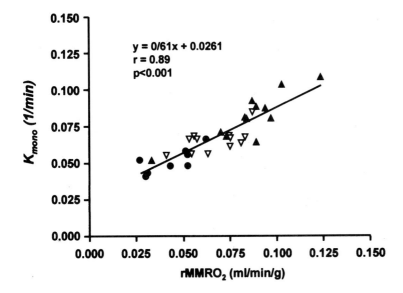

FIG. 8.3.6. A close linear correlation between k_{mono} and rMMRO$_2$ exists from low to normal myocardial blood flow (MBF) (r = 0.89; $p < .001$; y = 0.61x + 0.026). (▲, group A, normal segments; ▽, group B, segments with moderately reduced MBF; •, group C, segments with low MBF.) (From Ukkonen H, Knuuti J, Katoh C, et al. Use of [^{11}C]acetate and [^{15}O]O$_2$ PET for the assessment of myocardial oxygen utilization in patients with chronic myocardial infarction. *Eur J Nucl Med* 2001;28:334–339, with permission.)

subject to movement. This can be particularly problematic in critically ill patients. Due to the complex logistics associated with the use of $^{15}O_2$, at the moment ^{11}C-acetate is still preferred for the estimation of rMMRO$_2$ using PET.

Special Features of PET in Assessing Myocardial Oxygen Consumption

The invasive approach to measure cardiac oxygen balance and efficiency carries, apart from an inherent risk to the patient, important methodologic drawbacks, particularly if the patient has significant heart disease. Invasively achieved estimates of MMRO$_2$ usually apply to the left anterior descending coronary artery territory only but are extrapolated to the entire LV muscle mass. Measurements of myocardial oxygen consumption by PET are necessary to evaluate cardiac efficiency by noninvasive methods. Because cardiac catheterization is not required, this approach facilitates pharmacodynamic studies in both healthy volunteers and patients with disease and makes repeated patient studies more feasible. Moreover, PET allows assessment of myocardial perfusion and metabolism directly at the tissue level. The method assigns accurate topographical data to all vascular beds, even to the RV.

CLINICAL APPLICATIONS

Applications of ^{11}C-acetate PET in Coronary Artery Disease and Viability Assessment

The heart metabolizes a wide variety of substrates such as FFAs, glucose, lactate, pyruvate, ketone bodies, and amino acids, but under normal conditions, FFAs and glucose are the major sources of energy. In contrast, with ischemia, oxidative metabolism of FFAs is decreased and exogenous glucose becomes the preferred substrate. The production of energy mainly depends on anaerobic glycolysis. In clinical practice, assessment of ^{18}F-FDG PET has been used as the gold standard in assessing myocardial viability in dysfunctional myocardium. The role of oxidative metabolism in ischemic heart disease, particularly in MI, has been studied with ^{11}C-acetate PET.

PET has provided evidence of decreased myocardial perfusion reserve in patients with risk factors for CAD before clinical signs or symptoms of ischemia (93). The perfusion reserve is further decreased in territories of stenosed coronary arteries (94). The oxidative metabolism assessed with ^{11}C-acetate at rest and during dobutamine stimulation is intact regardless of impaired flow reserve, suggesting perfusion-MMRO$_2$ mismatch during myocardial ischemia (95). Oxidative metabolism is also preserved in reperfused but dysfunctional (stunned) myocardium after percutaneous transluminal coronary angioplasty (96).

The natural history of MI has changed tremendously in the era of new revascularization therapies with thrombolysis

and stents. Instead of having an infarcted area with only necrotic tissue, there is an area at risk that has a mixture of viable and nonviable tissue. The functional outcome of these regions relies on the amount of the viable tissue within the infarcted area (97).

Carbon-11-acetate PET has been shown to have prognostic value with regard to the recovery of LV function after MI. Maes et al. (71) assessed myocardial oxidative metabolism in 18 patients with acute MI within 24 hours of the onset of symptoms. All the patients received thrombolytic therapy with subsequent Thrombolysis in Myocardial Infarction (TIMI) flow grade 3 in the infarct-related artery. $^{13}NH_3$ and ^{18}F-FDG PET were performed on day five to assess conventional PET viability. A radionuclide angiogram was performed on day five and 3 months later to assess LV function. Oxidative metabolism was comparable in PET-viable and nonviable segments, which is in keeping with previously published data (98). This could be partly due to the inconsistency of NH$_3$ and FDG in defining myocardial viability in the very early stage after infarction and reperfusion therapy. There was a linear correlation between oxidative metabolism and LV ejection fraction at 3 months. Multivariate analysis found the oxidative metabolism of the reperfused myocardium to be the only predictor of LV function at 3 months. This prognostic information concerning LV function could potentially be used to identify the patients with patent infarct-related arteries but poor recovery of LV function (TIMI flow grade 3) who would potentially benefit from more aggressive medical therapy.

Infarcted areas of the myocardium often contain a mixture of viable and necrotic tissue. The recovery of wall motion abnormality after revascularization therefore depends on metabolic activity and amount of scar tissue within the segment. Traditionally, ^{18}F-FDG PET in combination with a flow tracer has been used to detect viable myocardium. Flow-metabolism mismatch accurately predicts functional recovery after revascularization. Preservation of oxidative metabolism is also necessary for recovery of function after revascularization (99). Carbon-11-acetate PET yields quantitative data both on MBF and oxidative metabolism and therefore can be applied for detecting viability.

Gropler et al. (100) studied 34 patients, comparing ^{11}C-acetate and ^{18}F-FDG in detecting myocardial viability. All patients had LV wall motion abnormalities due to CAD (21 patients had a history of previous MI). Dysfunctional myocardium was defined as viable if myocardial oxidative metabolism (assessed by k_1) or regional utilization of glucose were within 2 SD of normal or if glucose utilization normalized to flow was more than 2 SD of the mean value for a control group. Carbon-11-acetate was able to identify viable myocardium in 67% and nonviable in 89% of the cases. The corresponding predictive values for ^{18}F-FDG were 52% and 81%. However this FDG accuracy is below the mean predictive accuracies of 71% and 86% reported from a pooled data analysis of 20 previous studies (101). In severely dysfunctional segments, both methods had better predictive accuracy. Positive predictive values for viable myocardium were 85% with ^{11}C-acetate and 72% with ^{18}F-FDG. Negative predictive values (NPVs) were 87% and 82%, respectively.

Wolpers et al. (58) studied 30 post-MI patients and found the positive predictive accuracy of ^{11}C-acetate PET to be 62% and negative predictive accuracy to be 65%. It is important to keep in mind, however, that the resting level of myocardial oxidative metabolism can significantly overlap between nonviable and viable segments (57).

The presence of contractile reserve on the dobutamine stress echocardiogram has been shown to be accurate in predicting recovery after reperfusion (102,103). However, the method may have reduced the NPV in certain clinical settings in comparison with conventional metabolic imaging (104–106). Lee et al. (107) studied 19 patients with dysfunctional myocardial segments due to CAD with dobutamine stress echocardiograms, as well as H$_2$^{15}O and ^{11}C-acetate PET. Myocardial oxidative metabolism reserve and blood-flow reserve were lower, both in contractile negative and positive groups compared with normal. In contractile reserve–positive segments, both reserves were higher than in contractile reserve–negative segments. Of the segments defined as viable by PET, 54% were contractile reserve negative and exhibited blunted MBF response to dobutamine. Percent reduction in coronary artery diameter was more severe in the contractile reserve–negative group than in other groups. This also shows the blood-flow dependency of the contractile reserve phenomenon.

Hata et al. (57) validated dobutamine stress ^{11}C-acetate PET in 28 patients with old Q-wave anterior MI. Segmental wall motion assessment was performed after coronary revascularization with echocardiography. The clearance rate constant k_{mono} of ^{11}C-acetate at rest was significantly higher in viable segments $0.052 \pm 0.010\ min^{-1}$ versus $0.033 \pm 0.010\ min^{-1}$. However, there was considerable overlap between the groups, with COVs of $18.2\% \pm 6.6\%$ and $27.4\% \pm 10.1\%$, respectively. The baseline k_{mono} of the viable segment was $70.7\% \pm 15.8\%$ and the nonviable segment $43.1\% \pm 13.0\%$ of that of normal myocardium. The k_{mono} response to low-dose dobutamine was directionally different between the groups, allowing the detection of viable myocardium. In viable segments, normalized k_{mono} increased ($70.7\% \pm 15.8\%$ to $83.2\% \pm 9.9\%$) and decreased in nonviable segments ($43.1\% \pm 13.0\%$ to $26.9\% \pm 10.3\%$) during dobutamine infusion.

Carbon-11-acetate PET also yields a measure of relative myocardial perfusion. Relative myocardial perfusion was significantly different between the viable and nonviable segments without overlap ($67.9\% \pm 9.6\%$ vs. $32.7\% \pm 5.8\%$). During dobutamine administration, relative myocardial perfusion increased slightly in viable segments (to $70.4\% \pm$

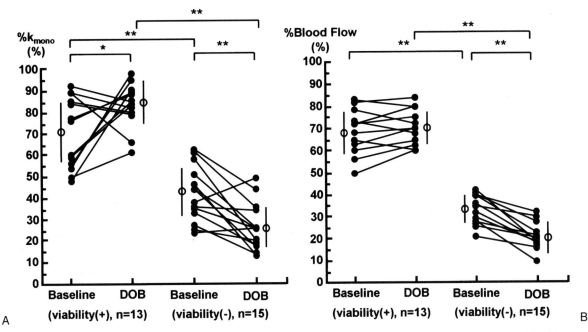

FIG. 8.3.7. Noninvasive assessment of myocardial viability using carbon-11-acetate in patients with old myocardial infarction. **A:** Changes in normalized oxidative metabolism (% k_{mono}) of the infarct region before and during dobutamine infusion in the two groups. **B:** Changes in normalized blood flow (% blood flow) of the infarct area before and during dobutamine (DOB) infusion in the two groups. (*$p < .05$; **$p < .001$.) (From Hata T, Nohara R, Fujita M, et al. Noninvasive assessment of myocardial viability by positron emission tomography with 11-C acetate in patients with old myocardial infarction. *Circulation* 1996;94:1834–1841, with permission.)

7.5%) but decreased significantly in nonviable segments (to 21.1% ± 5.3%) (Fig. 8.3.7).

Myocardial Efficiency

Oxidative metabolism is providing the heart with ATP needed for myocardial work and other energy-requiring processes. To understand the overall energy metabolism in different disease states, one should relate myocardial metabolism to myocardial work. Myocardial efficiency can be noninvasively indexed with the work metabolic index (WMI), as follows:

$$WMI = \frac{SVI \times PSP \times HR}{k}$$

where *SVI* is the noninvasively (usually by echocardiography) assessed stroke volume index, *PSP* is peak systolic pressure, *HR* is heart rate, and *k* is the clearance rate constant of ^{11}C-acetate (29,30,32,33). PSP may be replaced by systolic or mean blood pressure. $^{15}O_2$ PET yields an absolute level of myocardial oxygen consumption and therefore efficiency (%) can be calculated as follows:

$$Efficiency(\%) = \frac{SV \times MAP \times HR \times 0.0136}{MMRO_2 \times c}$$

where *MAP* is mean arterial pressure, *SV* stroke volume, and $MMRO_2$ is metabolic rate of oxygen of whole heart (89, 108). The number 0.0136 represents the constant with units g/m/mL/mm Hg, and *c* is a conversion factor representing energy equivalent per milliliter of oxygen metabolized, equaling 2.059 kg/m/mL oxygen consumed.

Hypertension and Efficiency

Hypertension is a common and well-known risk factor for CAD and heart failure. If hypertension is not well controlled, increased workloads over the years finally result in structural adaptive hypertrophy of the myocardium. The mechanisms that further lead to the development of heart failure are poorly understood. Laine et al. (89) used $^{15}O_2$ PET and echocardiography to study myocardial oxygen consumption and efficiency in 9 hypertensive patients with LV hypertrophy and in 8 hypertensive patients without hypertrophy and compared the results with the data from 10 healthy controls. Myocardial workload, MBF (0.84 ± 0.16 vs. 1.06 ± 0.22 mL/g/min), and oxygen consumption (0.09 ± 0.02 vs. 0.14 ± 0.03 mL/g/min) were increased in patients with hypertension without LV hypertrophy compared with healthy volunteers. After structural adaptation, LV hypertrophy, workload, MBF, and oxygen consumption were again at the level observed in healthy volunteers. However, myocardial efficiency was significantly reduced in these patients (13.5% ± 1.9% vs. 18.1% ± 4.1%; *p* < .05).

In hypertrophic cardiomyopathy, regional myocardial oxidative metabolism and efficiency are also both lower in hypertrophic myocardium compared with nonhypertrophic myocardium (109). These data suggest that structural adapta-

tion in LV hypertrophy is aiming more at preserving the LV oxygen consumption than efficiency. This structural adaptation is known to predict adverse outcome in cardiac patients. On the other hand, hypertrophy and increased myocardial mass in endurance athletes' hearts are usually considered a benign process. It also appears to be different with regard to the myocardial energetics.

Takala et al. (110) studied oxygen consumption in 9 endurance athletes and 11 sedentary men with $^{15}O_2$ PET. Athletes had 27% lower $MMRO_2$ than controls (8.8 ± 2.3 vs. 12.0 ± 3.8 mL/min/100 g; *p* = .044). However, myocardial efficiency was comparable between the athletes and sedentary men (16% ± 4% and 14% ± 4%, respectively).

Myocardial Efficiency in Congestive Heart Failure

The level of myocardial oxidative metabolism of the failing LV is often comparable to or even lower than that of the normal LV at rest (30,111). Patients with ischemic heart failure and myocardial scarring due to old MI are expected to have regional heterogeneity in both function and metabolism (112). Heterogeneity of regional function and oxidative metabolism also exists in nonischemic dilated cardiomyopathy (61). Myocardial efficiency, assessed with the WMI, is lower in the failing heart compared with the healthy heart (111, 113). Recent data also indicate that the transplanted human heart is comparable to the healthy heart in terms of myocardial efficiency (114).

Evaluation of Drug Therapy in Heart Failure

In the ideal situation, "mechanism of action" would be the primary basis for decision making in drug development (115). Modern techniques such as gene therapy technology provide numerous new potential mechanisms of action and targets for drug development. Surrogate endpoints, such as myocardial efficiency, allow the testing of *in vitro* hypotheses in these phase I-II clinical studies before starting large-scale clinical phase III-IV trials. This approach potentially saves both time and research costs (116). In addition, these approaches may allow improved selection of drug therapy for a given patient.

Dobutamine is one of the most commonly used β-adrenergic agonists in the clinical setting. It exerts its inotropic effect mainly through β_1-receptor stimulation. Dobutamine increases contractility in the LV and RV and reduces preload and afterload. It has been used as a reference drug for numerous inotropic agents. On the other hand, sodium nitroprusside can be used as a model agent of vasodilator therapy.

Beanlands et al. (33) noninvasively studied the energetic effects of dobutamine in eight patients with nonischemic cardiomyopathy (mean LV ejection fraction of 22%) and CHF. Myocardial oxidative metabolism was measured with ^{11}C-acetate PET and myocardial performance by echocardiography during steady-state infusion of dobutamine (mean dose of 13.2 ± 9.2 μg/kg per minute. The WMI increased by 30%, but this happened at the expense of myocardial oxidative metabolism, because k_2, a clearance rate constant of ^{11}C-acetate, increased by 48%. Systemic vascular resistance and mitral regurgitation were significantly reduced, which contributed to the observed increase in myocardial efficiency.

The investigators used the same methodology to study the effects of nitroprusside in patients with CHF (117). These patients were characterized by elevated systemic vascular resistance (SVR) and pulmonary capillary wedge pressure (PCWP). As expected, nitroprusside infusion (mean dose of 2.3 ± 1.4 μg/kg per minute) resulted in marked reductions in PCWP (48%) and SVR (53%). The k_{mono} of acetate decreased from 0.064 ± 0.012 to 0.055 ± 0.010 min^{-1} (-14%) during nitroprusside infusion. Furthermore, a 61% increase in myocardial efficiency was observed, which highlights the importance of afterload reduction as an energetically favorable treatment modality for CHF. Understanding the energetics with these model drugs provides a framework for understanding the evaluation of new drugs.

Long-term use of β-adrenergic drugs in patients with heart failure has resulted in an increase in mortality. On the other hand, the antagonists of the β-adrenergic system, such as bisoprolol, carvedilol, and metoprolol, have improved the prognosis of patients with heart failure, which further emphasizes the deleterious effect of long-term β-adrenergic activation (118–120). Interestingly metoprolol, a selective β$_1$-receptor antagonist, has also been shown to improve myocardial energetics after long-term use (32). In this study, 40 patients with LV dysfunction (mean LV ejection fraction of 31% and New York Heart Association [NYHA] functional classification II) were randomized to placebo or metoprolol. Nineteen patients in the placebo arm and 14 patients in the metoprolol arm completed the protocol. In the placebo group, there was no change in either k_{mono} (0.061 ± 0.022 vs. 0.054 ± 0.012 min^{-1}; $p = $ ns) or efficiency measured as the WMI ($5.29 \pm 2.46 \times 10^6$ vs. $5.14 \pm 2.06 \times 10^6$ mm Hg/mL/m^2; $p = $ NS). However, in the metoprolol group, a significant decrease in k_{mono} (0.062 ± 0.024 vs. 0.045 ± 0.015 min^{-1}; $p = .002$) and a significant increase in WMI were observed ($5.31 \pm 2.15 \times 10^6$ vs $7.08 \pm 2.36 \times 10^6$ mm Hg/mL/m^2; $p < .001$) (Fig. 8.3.8). These changes were also significant between treatment groups. Heart rate decreased significantly (from 73 ± 10 to 68 ± 11 beats per minute; $p = .02$) in the metoprolol group, but there were no significant changes in blood pressure or echocardiographic parameters. These improvements in myocardial energetics suggest that β-blockade therapy has an energy-sparing effect in patients with heart failure. This may account for some of the outcome benefits observed in this patient population in other studies.

Due to the known problems of the drugs acting via cyclic adenosine monophosphate to increase intracellular calcium (β-agonists and phosphodiesterase inhibitors), other treatment modalities have been tested for the treatment of heart failure. Calcium sensitizers increase myocardial contractility

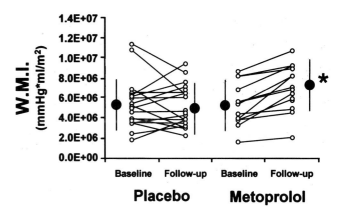

FIG. 8.3.8. The effect of β$_1$-blockade on oxygen cost of ventricular work in patients with left ventricular dysfunction. Work metabolic index is an estimate of myocardial efficiency in patients receiving placebo (n = 19) or metoprolol (n = 13). ($^*p < .02$ vs. baseline and placebo). (From Beanlands RSB, Nahmais C, Gordon E, et al. The effects of β$_1$-blockade on oxidative metabolism and the metabolic cost of ventricular work in patients with left ventricular dysfunction. A double-blind, placebo-controlled, positron-emission tomography study. *Circulation* 2000;102:2021–2160, with permission.)

by generating more force for the prevailing level of intracellular calcium, unlike other cardiotonic drugs that simply increase the level of intracellular calcium (121). In theory, this mechanism could result in an energy-saving effect during enhanced contractility.

The myocardial energetics effects of levosimendan, a new calcium-sensitizing drug with vasodilatory properties, were first assessed in healthy volunteers using ^{11}C-acetate PET and echocardiography (29). The effects of levosimendan on myocardial oxidative metabolism (k_{mono}) and cardiac efficiency were neutral, whereas the hemodynamic profile was consistent with a balanced inotropic effect and vasodilation. Low-dose dobutamine (5 g/kg per minute) enhanced cardiac efficiency at the expense of an increased oxygen requirement, but the effects of nitroprusside on k_{mono} and cardiac efficiency were neutral. The study also showed the feasibility of PET in phase I pharmacodynamic studies.

In a phase II study, the effects of levosimendan on biventricular energetics were studied in eight hospitalized patients with decompensated (NYHA class III and IV) chronic heart failure (30). In this double-blind crossover comparison (levosimendan vs. placebo), PET with ^{11}C-acetate was used to assess myocardial oxygen consumption, H$_2$^{15}O to measure MBF, and cardiac performance was assessed by pulmonary artery catheterization. During administration of levosimendan, cardiac output increased by 32% ($p = .002$), mainly because of higher stroke volume. Coronary resistance, pulmonary resistance, and SVR values were significantly reduced. Mean MBF increased from 0.76 to 1.02 mL per minute per gram ($p = .033$). Levosimendan did not affect myocardial oxygen consumption (LV k_{mono} 0.066 ± 0.003 vs. 0.061 ± 0.004 min^{-1}; $p = .15$ and RV k_{mono} $0.053 \pm$

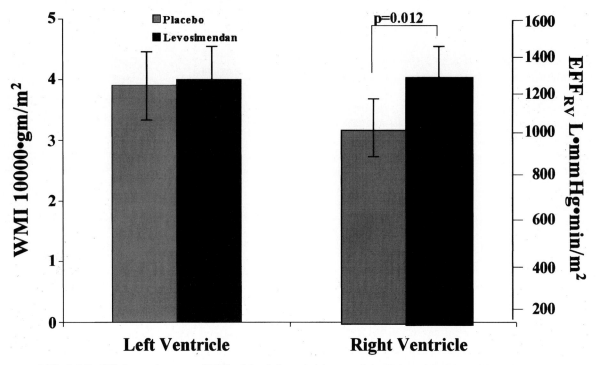

FIG. 8.3.9. Efficiency (mean ± SEM) of the left and right ventricle during placebo and levosimendan. Levosimendan, a novel calcium sensitizer, had no effect on myocardial efficiency in the left ventricle (work metabolic index; *WMI*) but improved right ventricular efficiency by 24% (*p* = .012). (From Ukkonen H, Saraste M, Akkila J, et al. Myocardial efficiency during levosimendan infusion in congestive heart failure. *Clin Pharmacol Ther* 2000;68:522–531, with permission.)

0.004 vs. 0.055 ± 0.005 min^{-1}; p = NS) and LV efficiency, but it improved RV mechanical efficiency by 24% (p = .012) (Fig. 8.3.9). This study suggests that levosimendan has an energetically favorable short-term profile in the treatment of CHF because it enhances cardiac output without oxygen wasting, particularly by improving efficiency in the RV.

Right Ventricular Oxygen Consumption

The monoexponential elimination rate of ^{11}C-acetate (k_{mono}) correlates with indirect estimates of myocardial oxygen consumption in the RV (59), which offers an intriguing opportunity to quantitate myocardial oxidative metabolism simultaneously in the LV and RV. This approach has been used in healthy volunteers (60), patients with aortic valve disease (122), and those with CHF (30). However, the validation of the method is limited and requires further study.

Measurement of Myocardial Oxidative Metabolism in Other Diseases

Carbon-11-acetate PET has been used to understand the mechanisms of disease in other cardiac conditions. In hypertrophic cardiomyopathy, impairment in regional efficiency has been identified. Ishiwata et al (109) demonstrated that the septum had reduced oxidative metabolism compared with the lateral wall There was an increase in the k_{mono}/regional work (effectively the inverse of regional efficiency) for the whole heart in patients with hypertrophic cardiomyopathy. This was greater in the septum. Thus, impaired regional metabolism and reduced regional and overall LV efficiency may play a role in the pathophysiology of hypertrophic cardiomyopathy.

Nony et al. (123) used ^{11}C-acetate PET and echocardiography to evaluate anthracycline cardiotoxicity. Although the investigators detected a small but significant decrease in LV systolic function, myocardial oxidative metabolism was preserved. They concluded that myocardial oxidative metabolism does not contribute to the mechanism of disease in anthracycline cardiotoxicity.

Carbon-11-acetate PET has also been used to study myocardial involvement in endocrine disorders. Investigators have demonstrated regional heterogeneity in myocardial oxidative metabolism in patients with non–insulin-dependent diabetes mellitus (124). In another study, excessive myocardial oxidative metabolism was observed in hyperthyroid patients despite β-blocker therapy with propranolol (65).

SUMMARY

To date, according to the American College of Cardiology/American Heart Association guidelines, the use of PET in clinical cardiology has primarily focused on myocardial perfusion and viability imaging. Although ^{11}C-acetate PET can be applied for both flow and viability imaging, its greatest potential probably lies in the evaluation of oxidative metabolism and cardiac efficiency. Both [15]O$_2$ and ^{11}C-acetate PET have been demonstrated to be feasible in assessing global and regional myocardial oxygen consumption in healthy volunteers and patients with heart disease of various etiologies. This technique offers a unique opportunity to evaluate the myocardial energetic effects of new and established treatments to better direct therapies in cardiac conditions such as CHF.

ACKNOWLEDGMENTS

The authors are grateful to Linda Garrard, May Aung, and Sherri Nipius for their help in preparing the manuscript and figures. Dr. Ukkonen is funded by the Academy of Finland.

REFERENCES

1. Kojima S, Wu ST, Parmley W, et al. Relationship between intracellular calcium and oxygen consumption: effects of perfusion pressure, extracellular calcium, dobutamine and nifedipine. *Am Heart J* 1994; 127:386–391.
2. Braunwald E. Control of myocardial oxygen consumption: physiologic and clinical considerations. *Am J Cardiol* 1971;27:416
3. Opie LH. Aerobic and anaerobic metabolism. In: Opie LH, ed. *The heart: physiology from cell to circulation.* Philadelphia: Lippincott–Raven Publishers, 1998:295–342.
4. Burkoff D. Introduction—the hierarchy of cardiac function. *Basic Res Cardiol* 1993;88:3–5.
5. Takaki M, Kohzuki H, Kawatani Y, et al. Sarcoplasmic reticulum Ca^{2+} pump blockade decreases O$_2$ use of unloaded contracting rat heart slices: Thapsigardin and cyclopiazonic acid. *J Mol Cell Cardiol* 1998;30:649–659.
6. Ohgoshi Y, Goto Y, Kawaguchi O, et al. Epinephrine and calcium have similar oxygen costs of contractility. *Heart Vessels* 1992;7:123–132.
7. Neely J, Morgan H. Relationship between carbohydrate and lipid metabolism and energy balance of the heart. *Rev Physiol* 1974;36:413–459.
8. Wisneski JA, Gertz E, Neese RA, et al. Myocardial metabolism of free fatty acids: studies with ^{14}C labeled substrates in humans. *J Clin Invest* 1987;79:359–366.
9. Schelbert HR, Henze E, Sochor H, et al. Effects of substrate availability on myocardial carbon-11-palmitate kinetics by positron emission tomography in normal subjects and patients with ventricular dysfunction. *Am Heart J* 1986;111:1055–1064.
10. Neely J, Hansen CA, Lopaschuk GD, et al. Substrate utilization in the normal and diseased heart. In: Schelbert HR, Neely J, Phelps ME, et al, eds. *Advances in clinical cardiology: regional myocardial metabolism by positron emission tomography* vol 3. Foundation for Advances in Clinical Medicine Inc, Mahwah, NJ, 1987:20–31.
11. Knuuti J, Maki M, Yki-Jarvinen H, et al. The effect of insulin and FFA on myocardial glucose uptake. *J Mol Cell Cardiol* 1995;27:1359–1367.
12. Heiss HW, Barmeyer SR, Wink K, et al. Studies on the regulation of myocardial blood flow in man. Training effects on blood flow and metabolism of the healthy heart at rest and during standardized heavy exercise. *Basic Res Cardiol* 1976;71:658–675.
13. Depre C, Vanoverschelde J-LJ, Taegtmeyer H. Glucose for the heart. *Circulation* 1999:578–588.
14. Lopaschuk GD, Stanley W. Glucose metabolism in the ischemic heart. *Circulation* 1997;95:415–422.
15. Shinke T, Takaoka H, Takeuchi K, et al. Nitric oxide spares myocardial oxygen consumption through attenuation of contractile response to beta-adrenergic stimulation in patients with idiopathic dilated cardiomyopathy. *Circulation* 2000;101:1925–1930.
16. Opie LH, Owen P. Assessment of mitochondrial free NAD$^+$/NADH ratios and oxaloacetate concentrations during increased mechanical work in isolated perfused rat heart during production or uptake of ketone bodies. *Biochem J* 1975;148:403–415.
17. Heineman FW, Balaban RS. Effects of afterload and heart rate on NAD(P)H redox state in isolated rabbit heart. *Am J Physiol* 1993; 264:H433–H440
18. Katz AM. Cardiomyopathy of overload. A major determinant of prognosis in congestive heart failure. *N Engl J Med* 1990;322:100–110.
19. Schipke JD. Cardiac efficiency. *Basic Res Cardiol* 1994;89:207–240.
20. Starling EH, Vissher MB. The regulation of energy output of the heart. *J Physiol (London)* 1926;62:243.
21. Denslow S. Relationship between PVA and myocardial oxygen consumption can be derived from thermodynamics. *Am J Physiol* 1996; 270:H730–H740.
22. Backx P. Efficiency of cardiac muscle: thermodynamic and statistical mechanical considerations. *Basic Res Cardiol* 1993;88:21–27.
23. Fourier PR, Coetzee AR, Bolliger CT. Pulmonary artery compliance: its role in right ventricular-arterial coupling. *Cardiovasc Res* 1992; 26:839–844.
24. Suga H. Total mechanical energy of a ventricle model and cardiac oxygen consumption. *Am J Physiol* 1979;236:H498–H505
25. Robinson BF. Relation of heart rate and systolic blood pressure to the onset of pain in angina pectoris. *Circulation* 1967;34:1073–1083.
26. Nelson RR, Gobel F, Jorgensen CR, et al. Hemodynamic predictors of myocardial oxygen consumption during static and dynamic exercise. *Circulation* 1974;50:1179–1189.
27. Rooke GA, Feigl EO. Work as a correlate of canine left ventricular oxygen consumption and the problem of catecholamine oxygen wasting. *Circ Res* 1982;50:273–286.
28. Opie LH. Mechanisms of cardiac contraction and relaxation. In: Braunwald E, ed. *Heart disease.* Philadelphia: WB Saunders, 1997.
29. Ukkonen H, Saraste M, Akkila J, et al. Myocardial efficiency during calcium sensitization with levosimendan: a noninvasive study with positron emission tomography and echocardiography in healthy volunteers. *Clin Pharmacol Ther* 1997;61:596–607.
30. Ukkonen H, Saraste M, Akkila J, et al. Myocardial efficiency during levosimendan infusion in congestive heart failure. *Clin Pharmacol Ther* 2000;68:522–531.
31. Beanlands RSB, Muzik O, Hutchins GD, et al. Heterogeneity of regional nitrogen 13–labeled ammonia tracer distribution in the normal human heart: comparison with rubidium 82 and copper 62–labeled PTSM. *J Nucl Cardiol* 1994;1:225–235.
32. Beanlands RSB, Nahmais C, Gordon E, et al. The effects of β$_1$-blockade on oxidative metabolism and the metabolic cost of ventricular work in patients with left ventricular dysfunction. A double-blind, placebo-controlled, positron-emission tomography study. *Circulation* 2000;102:2021–2160.
33. Beanlands R, Bach D, Raylman R, et al. Acute effects of dobutamine on myocardial oxygen consumption and cardiac efficiency measured using C-11 acetate kinetics in patients with dilated cardiomyopathy. *J Am Coll Cardiol* 1993;22:1389–1398.
34. Lopaschuk GD. Advantages and limitations of experimental techniques used to measure cardiac energy metabolism. *J Nucl Cardiol* 1997;4:316–328.
35. Ganz W, Tamura K, Marcus HS, et al. Measurement of coronary sinus blood flow by continuous thermodilution in man. *Circulation* 1971; 44:181–195.
36. Weiss RG, Gloth ST, Kalik-Filho R, et al. Indexing tricarboxylic acid cycle flux intact hearts by carbon-13 nuclear magnetic resonance. *Circ Res* 1992;70:392–408.
37. Deleted in proof.
38. Koskenvuo JW, Sakuma H, Niemi P, et al. Global Myocardial blood flow and global reserve measurements by MRI and PET are comparable. *J Magn Reson Imaging* 2001;13:361–366.
39. Reeder SB, Holmes A, McVeigh ER, et al. Simultaneous noninvasive determination of regional myocardial perfusion and oxygen content in rabbits: toward direct measurement of myocardial oxygen consumption at MR imaging. *Radiology* 1999;212:739–747.
40. Gambhir SS, Schwaiger M, Huang S-C, et al. Simple noninvasive quantification method for measuring myocardial glucose utilization in humans employing positron emission tomography and fluorine-18 deoxyglucose. *J Nucl Med* 1989;30:359–366.

41. Taegtmeyer H. Energy metabolism of the heart: from basic concepts to clinical applications. *Curr Probl Cardiol* 1994;19:59–113.

42. Maki M, Haaparanta M, Nuutila P, et al. Free fatty acid uptake in the myocardium and skeletal muscle using fluorine-18-fluoro-6-heptadecanoic acid. *J Nucl Med* 1998;39:1320–1327.

43. Schelbert HR, Henze E, Schon HR, et al. Carbon-11-palmitate for the noninvasive evaluation of regional myocardial fatty acid metabolism with positron computed tomography. *In vivo* demonstration of the effects of substrate availability on myocardial metabolism. *Am Heart J* 1983;105:492–504.

44. Schelbert HR, Phelps ME, Schon HR. Normal alterations in substrate metabolism demonstrated by positron emission tomography. In: Schelbert HR, Neely J, Phelps ME, et al, eds. *Advances in clinical cardiology: regional myocardial metabolism by positron emission tomography,* vol 3. Foundation for Advances in Clinical Medicine Inc, Mahwah, NJ, 1987:205–213.

45. Rosamond TL, Abendschein DR, Sobel BE, et al. Metabolic fate of radiolabeled palmitate in ischemic canine myocardium: implications for positron emission tomography. *J Nucl Med* 1987;28:1322–1329.

46. Fox K, Abendschein DR, Amdos HD, et al. Efflux of metabolized and nonmetabolized fatty acid from canine myocardium. Implications for quantifying myocardial metabolism tomographically. *Circ Res* 1985;57:232–243.

47. Ebert A, Herzog H, Stocklin G, et al. Kinetics of 14(R,S)-fluorine-18-fluoro-6-thia-heptadecanoic acid in normal human hearts at rest, during exercise and after dipyridamole injection. *J Nucl Med* 1994; 35:51–56.

48. Liedtke AJ. Alterations of carbohydrate and lipid metabolism in the acutely ischemic heart. *Prog Cardiovasc Dis* 1981;23:321–336.

49. Chan S, Brunken RC, Phelps M, et al. Use of the metabolic tracer carbon-11 acetate for evaluation of regional myocardial perfusion. *J Nucl Med* 1991;32:665–672.

50. Brown M, Marshall DR, Sobel BE, et al. Delineation of myocardial oxygen utilization with carbon-11–labeled acetate. *Circulation* 1987; 3:687–696.

51. Armbrecht JJ, Buxton D, Schelbert H. Validation of [1-11C] acetate as a tracer for noninvasive assessment of oxidative metabolism with positron emission tomography in normal, ischemic, postischemic, and hyperemic canine myocardium. *Circulation* 1990;81:1594–1605.

52. Lindeneg O, Mellemgaard K, Fabricius J, et al. Myocardial utilization of acetate, lactate and free fatty acids after ingestion of ethanol. *Clin Sci* 1964;27:427–435.

53. Klein LJ, Visser FC, Knaapen P, et al. Carbon-11 acetate as a tracer of myocardial oxygen consumption. *Eur J Nucl Med* 2001;28:651–668.

54. Buxton D, Schwaiger M, Nguyen A, et al. Radiolabeled acetate as a tracer of myocardial tricarboxylic acid cycle flux. *Circ Res* 1988;63: 628–634.

55. Pike V, Eakins M, Allan R, et al. Preparation of [1-11C] acetate—an agent for the study of myocardial metabolism by positron emission tomography. *Int J Appl Radiat Isot* 1982;33:505–512.

56. Beanlands R, Bach D, Raylman R, et al. Acute effects of dobutamine on myocardial oxygen consumption and cardiac efficiency measured using C-11 acetate kinetics in patients with dilated cardiomyopathy. *J Am Coll Cardiol* 1993;22:1389–1398.

57. Hata T, Nohara R, Fujita M, et al. Noninvasive assessment of myocardial viability by positron emission tomography with 11-C acetate in patients with old myocardial infarction. *Circulation* 1996;94: 1834–1841.

58. Wolpers HG, Burshert W, van den Hoff J, et al. Assessment of myocardial viability by use of ^{11}C-acetate and positron emission tomography. Threshold criteria of reversible dysfunction. *Circulation* 1997; 95:1417–1424.

59. Hicks RJ, Kalff V, Savas V, et al. Assessment of right ventricular oxidative metabolism by positron emission tomography with C-11 acetate in aortic valve disease. *Am J Cardiol* 1991;67:753–757.

60. Tamaki N, Magata Y, Takahashi N, et al. Oxidative metabolism in the myocardium in normal subjects during dobutamine infusion. *Eur J Nucl Med* 1993;20:231–237.

61. Bach D, Beanlands R, Schwaiger M, et al. Regional wall motion heterogeneity and myocardial oxidative metabolism in nonischemic dilated cardiomyopathy. *J Am Coll Cardiol* 1995;1256–1262.

62. Marshall RC, Tillisch JH, Phelps ME, et al. Identification and differentiation of resting myocardial ischemia and infarction in man with positron computed tomography, ^{18}F-labeled fluorodeoxyglucose and N-13 ammonia. *Circulation* 1983;67:766–778.

63. Knuuti MJ, Nuutila P, Ruotsalainen U, et al. Euglycemic hyperinsulinemic clamp and oral glucose load in stimulating myocardial glucose utilization during positron emission tomography. *J Nucl Med* 1992; 33:1255–1262.

64. Czernin J, Porenta G, Brunken RC, et al. Regional blood flow oxidative metabolism and glucose utilization in patients with recent myocardial infarction. *Circulation* 1993;88:884–895.

65. Torizuka T, Tamaki N, Kasagi K, et al. Myocardial oxidative metabolism in hyperthyroid patients assessed by PET with carbon-11-acetate. *J Nucl Med* 1995;36:1981–1986.

66. Ohte N, Hashimoto T, Iida H, et al. Extent of myocardial damage in regions with reverse redistribution at 3h and at 24h on ^{201}Tl SPECT: evaluation based on regional myocardial oxidative metabolism. *Nucl Med Commun* 1998;19:1081–1087.

67. Bach DS, Beanlands RSB, Schwaiger M, et al. Heterogeneity of ventricular function and myocardial oxidative metabolism in nonischemic dilated cardiomyopathy. *J Am Coll Cardiol* 1995;25:1258–1262.

68. Armbrecht JJ, Buxton DB, Brunken R, et al. Regional myocardial oxygen consumption determined noninvasively in humans with [1-^{11}C] acetate and dynamic positron emission tomography. *Circulation* 1989;80:863–872.

69. Henes CG, Bergmann SR, Walsh MN, et al. Assessment of myocardial oxidative metabolic reserve with positron emission tomography and carbon-11 acetate. *J Nucl Med* 1989;30:1798–1808.

70. Buck A, Wolpers G, Hutchins GD, et al. Effect of carbon-11-acetate recirculation on estimates of myocardial oxygen consumption by PET. *J Nucl Med* 1991;32:1950–1957.

71. Maes A, Van de Werf F, Mesotten LV, et al. Early assessment of regional myocardial blood flow and metabolism in thrombolysis in myocardial infarction flow grade 3 reperfused myocardial infarction using carbon-11-acetate. *J Am Coll Cardiol* 2001;37:30–36.

72. Raylman RR, Hutchins GD, Beanlands R, et al. Modeling of C-11 acetate kinetics by simultaneously fitting data from multiple ROI's coupled by common parameters. *J Nucl Med* 1994;35:1286–1291.

73. Sun KT, Chen K, Huang S-C, et al. Compartment model for measuring myocardial oxygen consumption using [1-^{11}C] acetate. *J Nucl Med* 1997;38:459–466.

74. Ng C-K, Huang S-C, Schelbert HR, et al. Validation of a model for [1-^{11}C] acetate as a tracer of cardiac oxidative metabolism. *Am Physiol Soc* 1994:H1304–H1315.

75. Brown MA, Myears DW, Bergmann SR. Validity of estimates of myocardial oxidative metabolism with carbon-11 acetate and positron emission tomography despite altered patterns of substrate utilization. *J Nucl Med* 1989;30:187–193.

76. Gropler R, Shelton ME, Herrero P, et al. Measurement of myocardial oxygen consumption using positron emission tomography and C-11 acetate: direct validation in human subjects. *Circulation* 1993;88:I-172(abst).

77. Sun KT, Yeatman L, Buxton D, et al. Simultaneous measurement of myocardial oxygen consumption and blood flow using [1-carbon-11] acetate. *J Nucl Med* 1998;39:272–280.

78. Beanlands RSB, Schwaiger M. Changes in myocardial oxygen consumption and efficiency with heart failure therapy measured by ^{11}C acetate PET. *Can J Cardiol* 1995;11:293–300.

79. Schulz R, Kappeler C, Coenen H, et al. Positron emission tomography analysis of [1-^{11}C]acetate kinetics in short-term hibernating myocardium. *Circulation* 1998;97:1009–1016.

80. Ukkonen H, Knuuti J, Katoh C, et al. Use of [^{11}C]acetate and [^{15}O]O$_2$ PET for the assessment of myocardial oxygen utilization in patients with chronic myocardial infarction. *Eur J Nucl Med* 2001;28: 334–339.

81. Parker JA, Beller G, Hoop B, et al. Assessment of regional myocardial blood flow and regional fractional oxygen extraction in dogs, using ^{15}O-water and ^{15}O-hemoglobin. *Circulation* 1978;42:511–518.

82. Iida H, Rhodes CG, Araujo LI, et al. Noninvasive quantification of regional myocardial metabolic rate of oxygen by use of 15-O$_2$ inhalation and positron emission tomography. Theory, analysis and application in humans. *Circulation* 1996;94:792–807.

83. Crouzel C, Clark J, Brihaye C, et al. Radiochemistry automation for PET. In: Stocklin G, Pike V, eds. *Radiopharmaceuticals for positron emission tomography.* Dordrecht, The Netherlands: Kluwer Academic Publishers, 1993:45–90.

84. Agostini D, Iida H, Takahashi A, et al. Regional myocardial metabolic rate of oxygen measured by [^{15}O]O$_2$-inhalation and positron emission tomography in patients with cardiomyopathy. *Clin Nucl Med* 2001; 26:41–49.

85. Alenius S, Ruotsalainen U. Bayesian image reconstruction for emission tomography based on median root prior. *Eur J Nucl Med* 1997; 24:258–265.

86. Katoh C, Ruotsalainen U, Alenius S, et al. Iterative reconstruction based on median root prior in quantification of myocardial blood flow and oxygen metabolism. *J Nucl Med* 1999;40:862–867.

87. Iida H, Takahashi A, Tamura Y, et al. Myocardial blood flow: comparison of oxygen-15 water bolus injection, slow infusion and oxygen-15-carbon dioxide slow inhalation. *J Nucl Med* 1995;36:78–85.

88. Araujo LI, Lammerstma AA, Rhodes CG, et al. Noninvasive quantification of regional myocardial blood flow in normal volunteers and patients with coronary artery disease using oxygen-15 labeled water and positron emission tomography. *Circulation* 1991;83:875–885.

89. Laine H, Katoh C, Luotolahti M, et al. Myocardial oxygen consumption is unchanged but efficiency is reduced in patients with essential hypertension and left ventricular hypertrophy. *Circulation* 1999;100: 2425–2430.

90. Yamamoto Y, de Silva R, Rhodes CG, et al. Noninvasive quantification of regional myocardial metabolic rate of oxygen by ^{15}O$_2$ inhalation and positron emission tomography: experimental validation. *Circulation* 1996;94:808–816.

91. Bol A, Melin JA, Bahija E, et al. Assessment of myocardial oxygen reserve with PET: comparison with Fick oxygen consumption. *Circulation* 1991;84:II-425(abst).

92. Yamamoto Y, de Silva R, Rhodes CG, et al. Validation of quantification of myocardial oxygen consumption and oxygen extraction fraction using ^{15}O$_2$ and positron emission tomography. *Circulation* 1991; 84:II-47(abst).

93. Pitkanen OP, Raitakari OT, Ronnemaa T, et al. Influence of cardiovascular risk status on coronary flow reserve in healthy young men. *Am J Cardiol* 1997;79:1690–1692.

94. Uren NG, Melin JA, De Bruyne B, et al. Relation between myocardial blood flow and the severity of coronary artery stenosis. *N Engl J Med* 1994;330:1782–1788.

95. Janier MF, Andre-Fouet X, Landais P, et al. Perfusion-MVo$_2$ mismatch during inotropic stress in CAD patients with normal contractile function. *Am J Physiol (Heart Circ Physiol)* 1996;271:H59–H67.

96. Gerber B, Wijns W, Vanoverschelde J-LJ, et al. Myocardial perfusion and oxygen consumption in reperfused noninfarcted dysfunctional myocardium after unstable angina: direct evidence for myocardial stunning in humans. *J Am Coll Cardiol* 1999;34:1939–1946.

97. deSilva R, Yamamoto Y, Rhodes CG, et al. Preoperative prediction of the outcome of coronary revascularization using positron emission tomography. *Circulation* 1992;86:1738–1742.

98. Vanoverschelde J-LJ, Melin JA, Bol A, et al. Regional oxidative metabolism in patients after recovery from reperfused anterior infarction. Relation to regional blood flow and glucose uptake. *Circulation* 1992; 85:9–21.

99. Gropler RJ, Geltman EM, Sampathkumaran K, et al. Functional recovery after coronary revascularization for chronic coronary artery disease is dependent on maintenance of oxidative metabolism. *J Am Coll Cardiol* 1992;20:569–577.

100. Gropler RJ, Geltman EM, Sampathkumaran K, et al. Comparison of carbon-11-acetate with fluorine-18-fluorodeoxyglucose for delineating viable myocardium by positron emission tomography. *J Am Coll Cardiol* 1993;22:1597.

101. Bax JJ, Poldermans D, Elhendy A, et al. Sensitivity, specificity, and predictive accuracies of various noninvasive techniques for detecting hibernating myocardium. *Curr Probl Cardiol* 2001;26:141–186.

102. Cigarroa CG, deFilippi CR, Brickner ME, et al. Dobutamine stress echocardiography identifies hibernating myocardium and predicts recovery of left ventricular function after coronary revascularization. *Circulation* 1993;88:430–436.

103. LaCanna G, Alfieri O, Giubbini R, et al. Echocardiography during infusion of dobutamine for identification of reversible dysfunction in patients with chronic coronary artery disease. *J Am Coll Cardiol* 1994; 23:617–626.

104. Afridi I, Klieman NS, Raizner AE, et al. Dobutamine echocardiography in myocardial hibernation: optimal dose and accuracy in predicting recovery of ventricular function after coronary angioplasty. *Circulation* 1995;91:663–670.

105. Panza JA, Dilsizian V, Laurienzo JM, et al. Relation between thallium uptake and contractile response to dobutamine: implications regarding myocardial viability in patients with chronic coronary artery disease and left ventricular dysfunction. *Circulation* 1995:990–998.

106. Perrone-Filardi P, Pace L, Prastaro M, et al. Assessment of myocardial viability in patients with chronic coronary artery disease: rest-4-hour-24-hour ^{201}Tl tomography versus dobutamine echocardiography. *Circulation* 1996;94:2712–2719.

107. Lee H, Davila-Roman VG, Ludbrook P, et al. Dependency of contractile reserve on myocardial blood flow. Implications for the assessment of myocardial viability with dobutamine stress echocardiography. *Circulation* 1997;96:2884–2891.

108. Bing R, Hammond M, Handelsman J, et al. The measurement of coronary blood flow, oxygen consumption, and efficiency of the left ventricle in man. *Am Heart J* 1949;38:1–24.

109. Ishiwata S, Maruno H, Senda M, et al. Mechanical efficiency in hypertrophic cardiomyopathy assessed by positron emission tomography with carbon 11 acetate. *Am Heart J* 1997;133:497–503.

110. Takala TO, Nuutila P, Katoh C, et al. Myocardial blood flow, oxygen consumption and fatty acid uptake in endurance athletes during insulin stimulation. *Am J Physiol* 1999;[Suppl 4, Pt 1]:E585–E590.

111. Bengel FM, Permanetter B, Ungerer M, et al. Non-invasive estimation of myocardial efficiency using positron emission tomography and carbon-11 acetate—comparison between the normal and failing human heart. *Eur J Nucl Med* 2000;27:319–326.

112. Kalff V, Hicks RJ, Hutchins G, et al. Use of carbon-11 acetate and dynamic positron emission tomography to assess regional myocardial oxygen consumption in patients with acute myocardial infarction receiving thrombolysis or coronary angioplasty. *Am J Cardiol* 1990;71: 529–535.

113. Bengel FM, Ueberfuhr P, Ziegler S, et al. Patterns of sympathetic reinnervation after cardiac transplantation: comparison of the orthotopically transplanted with heterotopically transplanted and autotransplanted heart. *J Nucl Med* 2000;41:168P-773(abst).

114. Bengel FM, Ueberfuhr P, Schiepel N, et al. Myocardial efficiency and sympathetic reinnervation after orthotopic heart transplantation. *Circulation* 2001;103:1881–1886.

115. Frank R. Nuclear bioimaging in drug development and regulatory review. *J Clin Pharmacol* 1999;39:51S–55S.

116. Gradnik R. Drug design in cardiology: the pharmaceutical industry point of view. In: Comar D, ed. *Positron emission tomography for drug development and evaluation.* The Netherlands: Kluwer Academic Publishers, 1995:215–218.

117. Beanlands R, Armstrong WF, Hicks R, et al. The effects of afterload reduction on myocardial C-11 acetate kinetics and noninvasively estimated mechanical efficiency in patients with dilated cardiomyopathy. *J Nucl Cardiol* 1994;1:3–16.

118. CIBIS-II Investigators and Committees. The Cardiac Insufficiency Bisoprolol Study II (CIBIS-II). *Lancet* 1999;353:9–13.

119. MERIT-HF Study Group. Effect of metoprolol CR/XL in chronic heart failure: metoprolol CR/XL. Randomized Intervention Trial in Congestive Heart Failure. (MERIT-HF). *Lancet* 1999;353: 2001–2007.

120. Packer MD, Bristow MR, Cohn JN, et al. The effect of carvedilol on morbidity and mortality in patients with chronic heart failure. *N Engl J Med* 1996;334:1349–1355.

121. Haikala H, Linden IB. Mechanism of action of calcium-sensitizing drugs. *J Cardiovasc Pharmacol* 1995;26:S10–S19.

122. Hicks RJ, Savas V, Currie PJ, et al. Assessment of myocardial oxidative metabolism in aortic valve disease using positron emission tomography with C-11 acetate. *Am Heart J* 1992;123:653–664.

123. Nony P, Guastalla JP, Rebattu P, et al. *In vivo* measurement of myocardial oxidative metabolism and blood flow does not show changes in cancer patients undergoing doxorubicin therapy. *Cancer Chemother Pharmacol* 2000;45:375–380.

124. Hattori N, Tamaki N, Kudoh T, et al. Abnormality of myocardial oxidative metabolism in noninsulin-dependent diabetes mellitus. *J Nucl Med* 1998;39:1835–1840.

Myocardial Neurotransmitter Imaging

Markus Schwaiger and Ichiro Matsunari

The innervation of the heart represents an important aspect for the adaptation of cardiac performance to the hemodynamic requirements in the healthy and diseased human body. The cardiovascular work of the normal heart depends on neuronal input for its adequate response to physiologic stimuli such as exercise and mental stress. The importance of the autonomic nervous system (ANS) in the pathophysiology of various heart diseases, such as congestive heart failure (CHF) (1) and arrhythmias (2), has been increasingly recognized. In the past, evaluation of the ANS *in vivo* was limited to invasive procedures. With the introduction of tracer approaches, noninvasive functional assessment of the cardiac ANS by scintigraphic techniques has become possible and may provide important pathophysiologic information in various cardiac disease states.

Using catecholamine analogues such as iodine-123 (^{123}I) metaiodobenzylguanidine (MIBG) (3,4) has made noninvasive assessment of presynaptic neuronal function a reality in the clinical setting using single-photon emission computed tomography (SPECT). More sophisticated imaging techniques such as positron emission tomography (PET) have been developed recently to assess the sympathetic nervous system using tracers such as carbon-11 (^{11}C)–hydroxyephedrine (HED) (5,6), fluorine-18 (^{18}F)–fluorodopamine (7,8), and CGP-12177 (9). These agents permit the regional quantification of tracer concentration in presynaptic and postsynaptic sites with high spatial resolution.

This chapter describes the basic physiology of the ANS, followed by the principles of scintigraphic techniques for neurotransmitter imaging. Current applications of PET for noninvasive characterization of the presynaptic nervous system are discussed. The scintigraphic evaluation of the postsynaptic nervous system is also briefly described.

DESCRIPTION OF THE AUTONOMIC NERVOUS SYSTEM IN THE HEART

The ANS, referred to as the visceral nervous system, consists of two main divisions: sympathetic and parasympathetic innervation. The two systems have different major neurotransmitters, norepinephrine or acetylcholine (ACh),

which define the stimulatory and inhibitory physiologic effects of each system (10). Sympathetic and parasympathetic innervation of the heart facilitates electrophysiologic and hemodynamic adaptation to changing cardiovascular demands: Both sympathetic and parasympathetic tone control the rate of electrophysiologic stimulation and conduction, whereas contractile performance is primarily modulated by sympathetic neurotransmission. This functional characterization is reflected by the anatomic distribution of sympathetic and parasympathetic nerve fibers and nerve terminals.

Sympathetic nerve fibers are characterized by multiple nerve endings that are filled with vesicles containing norepinephrine. Sympathetic nerve fibers travel parallel to the vascular structures on the surface of the heart and penetrate into the underlying myocardium in much the same fashion as the coronary vessels. Based on tissue norepinephrine concentration, the mammalian heart is characterized by dense adrenergic innervation with a norepinephrine concentration gradient from the atria to the base of the heart and from the base to the apex of the ventricles (11).

In contrast to sympathetic nerve fibers, parasympathetic innervation is most prevalent in the atria of the heart, the atrioventricular node, and to a lesser degree within the ventricular myocardium. Parasympathetic fibers in the ventricles appear to travel close to the endocardial surface, in contrast to sympathetic innervation.

The enzyme choline acetyltransferase (ChAT) has been used as a reliable marker of cholinergic innervation (12). ChAT concentration is highest in the atria and decreases sharply in both the right and left ventricular myocardium. Figure 8.4.1 depicts norepinephrine and ACh synthesis in the sympathetic and parasympathetic nerve terminal, respectively.

Sympathetic Nerve Terminal

Norepinephrine, the dominant transmitter in the sympathetic nervous system, is synthesized from the amino acid tyrosine by several enzymatic steps (7). The generation of DOPA from tyrosine is the rate-limiting step in the biosynthesis of catecholamines. After DOPA conversion to dopa-

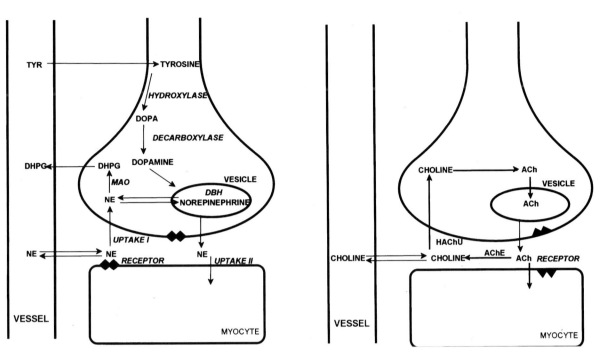

FIG. 8.4.1. Schematic display of sympathetic and parasympathetic nerve terminals. NE, norepinephrine; TYR, tyrosine; MAO, monoamine oxydase; ACh, acetylcholine; AChE, acetylcholinesterase.

mine by DOPA decarboxylase, dopamine is transported into storage vesicles by an energy-requiring mechanism. Norepinephrine is synthesized by the action of dopamine beta-hydroxylase (DBH) on dopamine within the storage vesicles. Nerve stimulation leads to norepinephrine release, which occurs as the vesicles fuse with the neuronal membrane and expel their contents by exocytosis. Single nerve stimulation, however, leads to exocytosis of only a small fraction of the many thousands of storage vesicles in the sympathetic nerve terminal.

The average adrenergic neuron has approximately 25,000 vesicles. Each vesicle contains approximately 250 pg of norepinephrine (13). Thus, although most norepinephrine is thought to be released by exocytosis, nonvesicular release also occurs. Apart from neuronal stimulation, norepinephrine release is also regulated by a number of receptor systems. α_2-Receptors on the membrane surface are thought to provide negative feedback of the exocytotic process, and thus, the exocytotic release can be inhibited by presynaptic α_2-receptor agonists such as clonidine, guanabenz, and guanfacine (14).

Muscarinic and adenosine receptors have an antiadrenergic effect in the heart. Neuropeptide Y is stored and released together with norepinephrine from the nerve terminal. Neuropeptide Y is thought to inhibit norepinephrine release by the nerve terminal (15). Presynaptic angiotensin II receptors and β-receptors, on the other hand, mediate facilitation of norepinephrine release from sympathetic nerve endings.

Therefore, some antihypertensive pharmaceuticals such as angiotensin-converting enzyme inhibitors and nonselective β-blocking agents can inhibit excessive norepinephrine release.

The complex modulation of sympathetic neurotransmission obviously involves many systems including dopamine, prostaglandin, and histamine. Only a small amount of the norepinephrine released by the nerve terminal is actually available to activate receptors on the myocyte surface. Most of the norepinephrine released undergoes reuptake in the nerve terminal (uptake-1 mechanism) and recycles into the vesicles or is metabolized in the cytosol of the nerve terminal. The uptake-1 system is characterized as saturable and sodium, temperature, and energy dependent (16). It can be inhibited by cocaine and desipramine (17). Structurally related amines such as epinephrine (EPI), guanethidine, and metaraminol are also transported by this system.

In addition to neuronal uptake via uptake-1, the uptake-2 system moves norepinephrine into nonneuronal tissue (18). Uptake-2 is characterized as nonsaturable and not sodium, temperature, or energy dependent. It can be inhibited by steroid and clonidine (19). Free cytosolic norepinephrine is degraded rapidly to dihydroxyphenylglycol by monoamine oxidase (MAO). Only a small fraction of the released norepinephrine diffuses into the vascular space where it can be measured as norepinephrine spillover in the coronary sinus venous blood.

Parasympathetic Nerve Terminal

ACh is synthesized within the parasympathetic nerve terminal. Choline is transported into the cytosol of the nerve ending via a high-affinity choline uptake system (20). In the nerve terminal, choline is rapidly acetylated by ChAT and is subsequently shuttled into storage vesicles. In contrast to amine uptake in the sympathetic nerve terminals, the choline uptake system is restrictive. Even choline analogues with very similar structures are poor substrates for this uptake mechanism. Upon nerve stimulation, ACh is released into the synaptic cleft where it interacts with muscarinic receptors. Free ACh is rapidly metabolized by acetylcholinesterase.

RADIOPHARMACEUTICALS FOR NEUROTRANSMITTER IMAGING

Presynaptic Function

Tracers for neurotransmitter imaging have been developed by either direct labeling of the physiologic neurotransmitter or labeling of their structural analogues (Fig. 8.4.2). Table 8.4.1 summarizes currently available radiopharmaceuticals for the scintigraphic evaluation of the presynaptic nervous function. Iodine-123 MIBG was developed as a norepinephrine analogue by Wieland et al. (4); it was first used in the human heart by Kline et al. (3) in the early 1980s. This compound is an analogue of guanethidine and shares a cellular uptake mechanism similar to norepinephrine at the sympathetic nerve terminals. It is transported into cells by uptake-1 and is stored in the vesicles but not catabolized by MAO or catechol-*O*-methyltransferase (COMT). This compound has a low affinity for postsynaptic adrenergic receptors and thus has little pharmacologic action. It has been shown that tissue norepinephrine concentration correlates with MIBG uptake (21).

Because PET has several advantages over SPECT (e.g., quantification of regional tracer uptake with the use of accurate attenuation correction and higher spatial resolution), efforts have been made to develop positron-emitting tracers for neurotransmitter imaging.

Fluorine-18–labeled metaraminol, which also was first synthesized by the research group of Dr. Wieland at the University of Michigan, is taken up by the sympathetic nerve terminal in a manner similar to norepinephrine but is not catabolized by MAO (22). Imaging studies in regionally denervated canine hearts indicated suitability of the tracer to quantitatively assess the integrity of myocardial sympathetic innervation. Transient myocardial ischemia, again in the canine model, resulted in reduced ^{18}F-metaraminol retention in tissue consistent with neuronal dysfunction in reversibly damaged myocardium (23). Radiopharmaceutical problems associated with low specific activity and potential pharmacologic effects, however, limited its further clinical application.

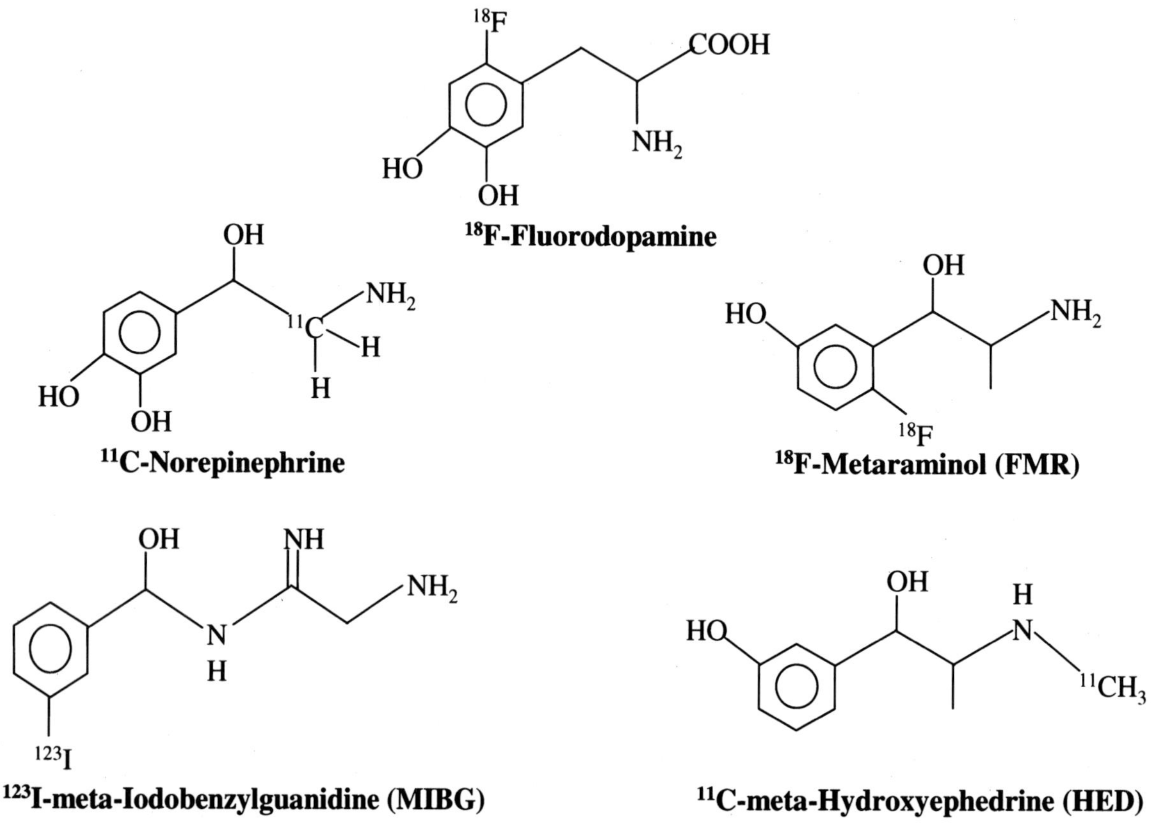

FIG. 8.4.2. Chemical structures of radiolabeled catecholamine analogues.

TABLE 8.4.1. *Radiopharmaceuticals used for neurotransmitter imaging*

	SPECT	PET
Sympathetic	^{123}I-metaiodobenzylguanidine (^{123}I-MIBG)	^{18}F-fluorometaraminol ^{11}C-hydroxyephedrine (^{11}C-HED) ^{11}C-epinephrine (^{11}C-EPI) ^{11}C-phenylephrine ^{18}F-fluorobenzylguanidine ^{18}F-fluorodopamine ^{18}F-fluoronorepinephrine
Parasympathetic		^{18}F-fluoroethoxybenzovesamicol

Carbon-11-HED, also introduced by the Michigan group, emerged as a more promising tracer because it can be synthesized with high specific activity (5). Experimental studies have indicated that there is a highly specific uptake into sympathetic nerve terminals with little nonneuronal binding (24). Carbon-11-HED is currently the most successfully used positron-emitting tracer for neurotransmitter imaging in humans (25–30). More recently, ^{11}C-EPI has been proposed as a truly physiologic tracer (31,32). It has been demonstrated that, as with norepinephrine, accumulation of ^{11}C-EPI by the heart reflects mainly vesicular storage in the sympathetic neuron. In contrast to ^{11}C-HED, free ^{11}C-EPI is metabolized in the cytosol by the MAO system. Because ^{11}C-HED is not metabolized, it diffuses out of the nerve terminal and undergoes reuptake.

Myocardial retention of ^{11}C-HED primarily reflects uptake-1 activity and to a lesser degree the storage capacity of neurons for norepinephrine (33). Therefore, ^{11}C-EPI may be the more suitable tracer for the evaluation of sympathetic vesicular function of the heart (34). Because ^{11}C-EPI is metabolized by MAO and COMT, careful consideration should be given to the influence of metabolic pathways on measurements of ^{11}C retention attributed to vesicular storage functions.

A further analogue of EPI is ^{11}C-phenylephrine, which also has been synthesized by Wieland et al. (35) at the University of Michigan. This tracer enters the nerve terminal via uptake-1 but is primarily metabolized by the MAO enzyme system. Carbon-11-phenylephrine, therefore, allows for the evaluation of the enzymatic integrity of the nerve terminal. Other potential tracers include ^{18}F-fluorodopamine (8,36) and ^{18}F-fluoronorepinephrine (37). Although the available clinical and experimental data for these tracers are still limited, the longer physical half-life of ^{18}F may allow for washout analysis to assess sympathetic nerve tone.

Other PET tracers for assessing sympathetic nerve function such as bromine-76 (^{76}Br)–labeled or ^{18}F-labeled benzyl guanidine (38), an analogue of MIBG, have also been proposed and await further experimental and clinical investigations.

To date, only a few studies have addressed myocardial parasympathetic neuronal imaging, probably because of a low specificity for neuronal uptake and storage. However, recent studies in the brain in mice (39) and rats (40) have shown that iodine-125 (^{125}I)–labeled iodobenzovesamicol

allowed scintigraphic assessment of cholinergic nerve terminals. Fluorine-18-fluoroethoxybenzovesamicol was developed for parasympathetic neurotransmitter imaging using PET (41). The myocardial retention of the tracer was low because of the low cholinergic neuron density, limiting its potential as an imaging agent. Further efforts in developing tracers for the parasympathetic nervous system are required.

Postsynaptic Receptor Imaging

The sympathetic neurotransmission in the heart primarily involves adrenoceptors of type β_1 and β_2, which are located on myocardial cells. α-Adrenoceptors are primarily associated with vascular structures. The positive inotropic and chronotropic response of the heart is mediated by β-receptors. The neurotransmitters norepinephrine and EPI have a high affinity to these receptors. Adrenoreceptors are linked to a complex second-messenger system that modifies the signal transduction (42,43). The surface density of receptors can be upregulated and downregulated in response to the extraneuronal catecholamine concentration. This downregulation of β-receptors, primarily by β_1-receptors, has been described in patients with heart failure. In addition, the treatment of patients with heart failure today includes β-receptor antagonists, which have a beneficial effect on left ventricular function. This has led to an increasing interest in the noninvasive characterization of receptor distribution by tracer techniques.

The most commonly used tracer for postsynaptic imaging is ^{11}C-CGP-12177, which represents a nonselective but hydrophilic β-receptor antagonist. Lipophilic tracers such as ^{11}C-propranolol and pindolol display a high retention in lung tissue and are, therefore, not suitable for cardiac imaging purposes.

Delforge et al. (44) developed a quantitative imaging method that includes two tracer injections with varying specific activity, yielding absolute measurements of β-receptor density in the heart. Merlet et al. (9) applied receptor imaging to various disease groups including patients with dilated cardiomyopathy. This imaging approach has emerged as the most widely used test to visualize β-receptors. The radiochemistry of ^{11}C-CGP-12177 is demanding because of the need for phosgene as a precursor for synthesis. An alternative tracer with similar biologic characteristics has been proposed by Vaalburg et al. (45). Clinical results are promising but await further careful evaluation.

Law et al. (46) reported the evaluation of ^{11}C-N-desmethyl-GB-67 as a specific α_1-receptor ligand in the heart. Rapid plasma clearance, no metabolites, and high myocardial retention yield good image quality (46). Future studies will have to document the ability of this new tracer to visualize and quantitate α-receptor density in the healthy and diseased heart.

Finally, radioactive-labeled ligands have been used to visualize the muscarinic receptors in the heart. There is a high density of these receptors in both the right and the left ventricle, which yields excellent image quality. This is surprising in the presence of very sparse cholinergic presynaptic innervation of both cardiac ventricles. The PET research group at Orsay has developed tracer approaches using ^{11}C-MQNB for the quantitative assessment of muscarinic receptors (47, 48).

IMAGING PROTOCOLS

An ^{11}C-HED PET imaging protocol typically includes dynamic PET acquisition for 40 to 60 minutes after injection and blood-flow imaging using flow tracers such as nitrogen-13 (^{13}N)-ammonia or rubidium-82 (6,25–28,30). For ^{11}C-EPI PET imaging, with which high levels of ^{11}C metabolites are detected in the blood, correction for metabolite radioactivity in the arterial input function is required for the calculation of tracer retention in the tissue (49). The use of ^{18}F-labeled tracers allows a longer imaging time, because of their longer physical half-life (110 minutes) compared with ^{11}C (20 minutes). The longer half-life of ^{18}F may obviate the necessity of an on-site cyclotron and thus may potentially allow for wide clinical use.

DATA INTERPRETATION

After intravenous injection of ^{11}C-HED or ^{11}C-EPI, there is rapid uptake of the tracers into the myocardium and clearance of the ^{11}C activity from the blood pool. The myocardial time-activity curves show a very slow clearance of ^{11}C activity with a biologic half-life of several hours for HED and EPI (49). In contrast, in the denervated heart, there is very little tracer retention, indicating low nonspecific binding in the human heart (Fig. 8.4.3). Regional myocardial tracer dis-

Normal Heart

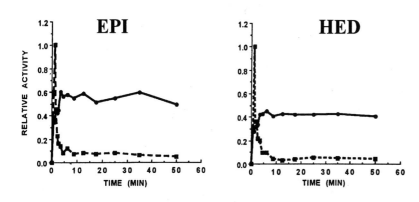

Transplant Heart

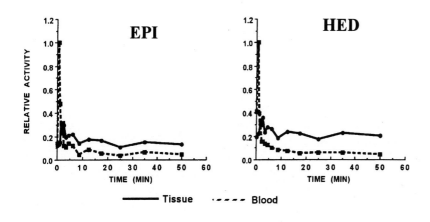

FIG. 8.4.3. Time-activity curves in blood, as well as myocardial tissue derived from regions of interest placed over the left ventricular cavity and the myocardial walls. A few minutes after injection, there is high retention of both tracers, epinephrine (EPI) and hydroxyephedrine (HED) in myocardial tissue, which remains constant over the imaging time period of 50 minutes. In contrast, the transplanted heart tissue shows very little uptake of both EPI and HED, indicating low nonspecific binding.

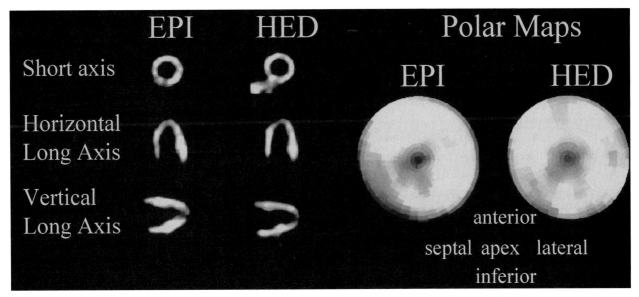

FIG. 8.4.4. PET images obtained in healthy volunteers after injection of carbon-11 (^{11}C)–labeled epinephrine and ^{11}C-labeled hydroxyephedrine. The PET images are displayed in short axis, horizontal long axis, and vertical long axis. Semiquantitative analysis reveals homogeneous distribution of tracer retention throughout the left ventricle, as displayed in the polar maps.

tribution can be visually assessed by summing imaging frames 10 to 20 minutes after tracer injection. Myocardial activity is homogeneous in the healthy heart for both ^{11}C-HED and ^{11}C-EPI, yielding excellent image quality (Fig. 8.4.4).

Several approaches have been introduced for the quantification of regional tracer retention (6,50). The most commonly used method includes the calculation of the myocardial retention fraction (liters per minute), which represents the regional myocardial activity measured between, for example, 30 and 40 minutes after injection, normalized to the integral of the arterial input function from 0 to 40 minutes after tracer injection derived by placing a region of interest over the left ventricular cavity (6). The myocardial retention fraction averaged about 0.14 for ^{11}C-HED and 0.24 for ^{11}C-EPI in the healthy heart. In patients with recent cardiac transplantation, these values were reduced to 0.04 and 0.05, respectively, consistent with denervation of the heart (49).

The Hammersmith PET research group developed a tracer kinetic model to calculate the distribution volume for ^{11}C-HED in the myocardium. Because the tissue half-life of HED is long and the physical half-life of ^{11}C only 20 minutes, this approach is methodologically quite challenging. Although the first clinical results are promising, no in-depth validation of this method has yet been published (50).

The neuronal extraction of catecholamine analogues is relatively high due to the efficient uptake-1 transport, at least under resting conditions, and absolute measurements of myocardial tracer retention must be corrected for blood flow. Although this may not pose a problem for the regional evaluation of relative tracer uptake, it may be of utmost importance for the interindividual comparison of tracer retention

fractions. Most PET studies include the measurement of regional myocardial blood flow, which allows for the regional normalization of ^{11}C activity to, for example, ^{13}N-ammonia measurements (51).

CLINICAL APPLICATIONS

Myocardial Infarction

Myocardial infarction (MI) has been shown to induce cardiac denervation exceeding the area of necrosis and/or scar (21,52–57). Minardo et al. (56) demonstrated that MIBG images in dogs after transmural MI show perfused but denervated myocardial areas apical to the infarct. Their observation was confirmed by the study of Dae et al. (21). In the latter study, they showed that non-transmural infarction also leads to regional ischemic damage of sympathetic nerves, but with minimal extension of denervation beyond the infarct.

Wolpers et al. (58) showed in the canine model of ischemia/reperfusion that the neuronal dysfunction as defined by decreased ^{11}C-HED retention correlated closely with the extent and severity of ischemia during coronary occlusion. A recent study (59) at our laboratory demonstrated that sympathetic neuronal damage measured by ^{99m}Tc-MIBG SPECT (MIBI) is closely related to risk area, as assessed by methoxyisobutyl isonitrile imaging in patients with acute MI, supporting the notion that sympathetic nerves are more sensitive to ischemia than myocardial tissue. This in turn may explain the mismatch between the extent of denervation and perfusion abnormalities in the experimental and clinical setting.

Although denervation defects extending beyond necrotic regions are commonly observed in patients after MI, the prognostic significance of this scintigraphic information remains to be elucidated. Published studies were based on relatively small patient populations, which may limit the ability to draw conclusions. Further prospective studies involving a larger patient population are necessary, to evaluate the clinical impact of autonomic imaging in terms of clinical outcome in patients after MI.

Reinnervation After Myocardial Infarction

Although inhomogeneity of cardiac sympathetic reinnervation may play an important role in the risk of arrhythmias early after MI, it remains controversial whether reinnervation after MI occurs in humans. Cardiac sympathetic reinnervation after MI has been reported in experimental canine studies (56,60). Minardo et al. (56) observed reinnervation within 14 weeks after infarction in the dog heart. Their results were confirmed by the study of Nishimura et al. (60), who observed recovery in MIBG uptake, as well as in norepinephrine content, during the first 6 weeks after infarction.

In humans, Mitrani et al. (61) reported partial sympathetic reinnervation between 1 and 8 months after MI. This was confirmed by the study of Hartikainen et al. (62), who showed partial reinnervation in the periinfarct zone between 3 and 12 months after infarction. Conversely, McGhie et al. (55) and Spinnler et al. (63) did not detect a significant change in MIBG uptake up to 30 months after infarction.

Using serial HED PET imaging, Allman et al. (25) studied the extent and reversibility of neuronal abnormalities in patients with an acute MI. They observed more extensive HED abnormalities than those for blood flow, particularly in patients with non–Q-wave infarction, but they did not observe any change in either the extent of abnormality or the tracer retention 8 ± 3 months later, suggesting persistent neuronal damage without evidence of reinnervation.

A role for the sympathetic nervous system in the generation of arrhythmias has been suggested (64–67). Different theories are proposed for the induction of arrhythmias, but *in vivo* data are limited. Therefore, scintigraphic techniques may provide unique information on the pathophysiology of arrhythmogenic heart disease.

Mitrani et al. (68) reported that abnormal MIBG uptake occurred in patients with ventricular tachycardia even in the absence of coronary artery disease. Gill et al. (69) observed reduced MIBG uptake in the septal region in patients with ventricular tachycardia. Using HED PET, Calkins et al. (27) observed a correlation between reduced HED retention and ventricular refractoriness in patients with a history of sustained ventricular tachycardia. Regional ^{11}C-HED retention and blood flow were correlated with epicardial electrophysiologic mapping during open heart surgery. Denervated myocardial segments displayed a significant prolonged relative refractory period, suggesting regional dispersion of electrophysiologic properties, which can be imaged with ^{11}C-HED.

Thus, the presence of denervated but viable myocardium, as assessed by scintigraphic techniques, may have important implications for the pathogenesis of ventricular arrhythmias.

Wichter et al. (70) studied 48 patients with arrhythmogenic right ventricular cardiomyopathy (ARVC) using MIBG scintigraphy and observed that most (83%) patients with ARVC showed reduced MIBG uptake despite normal thallium-201 study results. The location of defects on the MIBG scan correlated with the site of origin of ventricular tachycardia, which was determined by an invasive electrophysiologic study, suggesting potential utility of MIBG imaging for the noninvasive detection of localized sympathetic denervation.

The same group investigated eight patients with ARVC using PET (71). The density of β-receptors was determined and correlated with the distribution volume of ^{11}C-HED. They reported a significant global decrease of β_{max} (5.9 vs. 10.2 pmol/g of tissue), but no significant decrease of ^{11}C-HED retention. Myocardial blood flow measured with $H_2{}^{15}O$ was not altered. These PET data contradict to a certain degree the MIBG data by the same group, which demonstrated regional presynaptic abnormalities, and emphasize the need for a better understanding of the differences between MIBG and ^{11}C-HED pharmacokinetics.

Schafers et al. (50) investigated another group of patients with idiopathic arrhythmias. Eight patients with right ventricular outflow tract tachycardia underwent PET studies with ^{11}C-HED, ^{11}C-CGP-12177, and $H_2{}^{15}O$. Both the density of β-receptors and the distribution volume of ^{11}C-HED were reduced, suggesting an abnormality in presynaptic and postsynaptic function. Surprisingly, no regional differences were reported in this disease group that had a structural abnormality involving the right ventricle. Myocardial blood flow in these patients was not significantly different from that of a control group of 29 volunteers (50).

Sympathetic imbalance with decreased right cardiac sympathetic activity has been attributed to the induction of ventricular arrhythmias in long QT syndrome (72). Decreased MIBG uptake in the inferior and infero-septal wall was reported in patients with long QT syndrome (73), supporting the "sympathetic imbalance" hypothesis. Abnormalities of HED uptake, however, were not observed in the study by Calkins et al. (28).

Diabetes Mellitus

Diabetic patients often develop autonomic neuropathy, and autonomic dysfunction may be associated with increased morbidity in these patients (74). Scintigraphic techniques may allow for the objective assessment of sympathetic nervous system function in diabetic patients. Mantysaari et al. (75) reported for the first time the relationship between clinical autonomic dysfunction and myocardial MIBG uptake. They observed reduced myocardial MIBG uptake in diabetic patients, particularly those with autonomic neuropathy. Their findings were confirmed by subsequent studies (76, 77). In patients with insulin-dependent diabetes mellitus,

Kreiner et al. (78) observed more frequent abnormalities in MIBG uptake than expected by a cardiovascular reflex test.

Using HED PET, Allman et al. (26) studied diabetic patients with and without autonomic neuropathy and observed regional reduction in cardiac HED retention, predominantly in apical, inferior, and lateral regions, in patients with autonomic neuropathy, compared with healthy subjects, but not in diabetic patients without evident neuropathy (Fig. 8.4.5). They also observed a correlation between the extent of the scintigraphic abnormality and the severity of autonomic dysfunction.

Stevens et al. (79) compared regional ^{11}C-HED retention with severity of diabetic neuronal dysfunction (i.e., diabetic autonomic neuropathy [DAN]). The sensitivity of the imaging approach was demonstrated by the fact that 40% of DAN-negative diabetic patients displayed an abnormality on their ^{11}C-HED images. In subjects with mild neuropathy, defects were observed in the distal inferior wall of the left ventricle, whereas with more severe neuropathy, tracer defects extended to involve the distal anterolateral and inferior walls. The investigators also observed an increased regional blood flow by PET in the denervated myocardial segments of diabetic patients. In a subsequent study, Stevens et al. (79) compared DAN as evidenced by ^{11}C-HED imaging with measurements of regional coronary flow reserve and demonstrated a decreased vasodilatory reactivity in severely denervated segments.

Because silent myocardial ischemia is known to occur in diabetic patients and the absence of angina does not necessarily indicate a benign prognosis, several studies have focused on characterizing silent myocardial ischemia in diabetic patients using MIBG. Langer et al. (76) reported that patients with silent myocardial ischemia had more diffuse abnormalities in MIBG uptake than those without silent ischemia. Matsuo et al. (80) observed frequent inferior MIBG defects in patients with silent ischemia. These results suggest that sympathetic nervous system function may play an important role in asymptomatic ischemia in diabetic patients. To date, no data are available on HED PET in diabetic patients with silent myocardial ischemia.

Reinnervation After Heart Transplantation

In 1990, Schwaiger et al. (30) described for the first time scintigraphic evidence of reinnervation in patients after heart transplantation using HED PET. In that study, patients who had undergone transplantation more than 2 years before the PET scan showed partial sympathetic reinnervation in the proximal anterior and septal walls, whereas patients who had recently received a transplant (less than 1 year) did not show evidence of reinnervation. Figure 8.4.6 displays a representative patient 8 years after undergoing heart transplantation compared with a healthy subject. These observations were confirmed in a subsequent study by DeMarco et al. (81), who investigated the development of sympathetic reinnervation after heart transplantation using serial MIBG imaging. Sym-

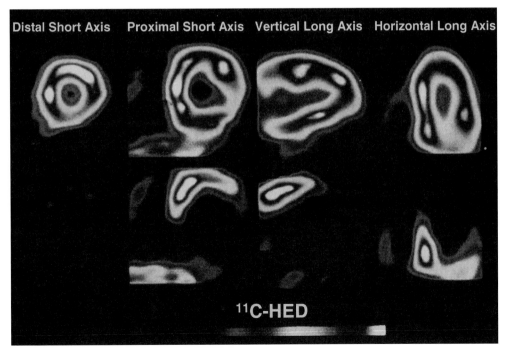

FIG. 8.4.5. PET images of myocardial perfusion with nitrogen-13-ammonia **(top row)** and sympathetic nerve function [carbon-11-hydroxyephedrine (HED)] in a patient with diabetic cardiac neuropathy. There is maintained myocardial perfusion but decreased HED retention in the inferior and apical wall of the left ventricle.

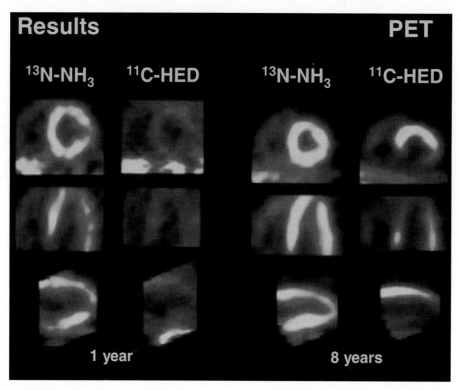

FIG. 8.4.6. PET images of two patients after cardiac transplantation. Blood-flow images were obtained after intravenous injection of nitrogen-13-ammonia and images of sympathetic nerve terminals after injection of carbon-11 (^{11}C)–hydroxyephedrine (HED). In the patient early after cardiac transplantation, there is maintained myocardial perfusion but no visible myocardial uptake of HED, documenting complete denervation. In contrast, in the patient 8 years after transplantation, there is regional reuptake of ^{11}C-HED in the anterior wall of the left ventricle, indicating reinnervation.

pathetic reinnervation from 1 to 3 years after transplantation was suggested in approximately half of those patients who had not shown any signs of sympathetic reinnervation at 1 year after transplantation. This is consistent with a study that suggested that functional autonomic reinnervation of transplanted hearts may occur more than 1 year after transplantation (82). Notably, they also reported that reinnervation after transplantation was less likely to occur in patients with a preoperative diagnosis of idiopathic cardiomyopathy than in patients with a pre-transplantation diagnosis of ischemic or rheumatic heart disease, suggesting that systemic abnormalities in sympathetic nervous function may play a role in the incidence and time course of reinnervation in such patients.

Recently, Ziegler et al. (83) performed HED PET imaging in 48 patients at various times after heart transplantation and reported that sympathetic reinnervation was a time-dependent phenomenon that paralleled electrophysiologic evidence of functional reinnervation such as an increase in heart-rate variability. Bengel et al. (84) performed serial PET studies in patients with orthotopic heart transplantation within several years. They reported little reinnervation within 18 months after transplantation but continuing reinnervation in the following years.

It is interesting to note that the reinnervation process leads only to a partial reappearance of neuronal structures limited primarily to the anterior, septal, and anterolateral segments of the left ventricle. The largest reinnervated area observed in a patient was 66% of the left ventricle. This regional heterogeneity of innervation within the transplanted heart provides a unique model to study the effect of autonomic innervation on cardiac performance.

Bengel et al. (84) correlated the pattern of innervation in transplant patients with cardiac substrate metabolism as assessed by ^{11}C-acetate and ^{18}F-fluorodeoxyglucose and PET. The data suggest that innervation has a significant impact on myocardial substrate utilization. Denervated segments displayed a higher glucose utilization rate, whereas the innervated heart most likely is dependent on free fatty acid oxidation. This observation is important with respect to myocardial energy metabolism in the failing heart, which is often associated with denervation.

The functional integrity of sympathetic nerve terminals in the transplanted heart was investigated by the comparison of ^{11}C-HED uptake and pharmacologically induced norepinephrine release (85). Both measurements were well correlated, indicating the ability of the nerve terminals to adequately respond to tyrosine.

Most recently, the clinical impact of the reinnervation on hemodynamic and cardiac performance was investigated. Schwaiblmair et al. (87) showed that transplant patients with PET evidence of reinnervation did exhibit a longer exercise time as compared with denervated patients.

Our laboratory addressed the question, "does the reappearance of innervation lead to an improved cardiac performance during exercise (87)?" Global and regional function was measured by radionuclide ventriculography at rest and during exercise in innervated and denervated transplant patients. The global left ventricular ejection fraction (LVEF) increased significantly during exercise in innervated patients and the regional response correlated with the ^{11}C-HED retention pattern in the left ventricle. These data suggest the importance of the reinnervation process for the functional recovery after cardiac transplantation.

Congestive Heart Failure

There is general agreement that increased adrenergic nervous system activity plays an important role in the pathophysiology of CHF (88). Increased plasma norepinephrine levels (88), increased spillover of norepinephrine (89), reduced cardiac stores of norepinephrine (90), and desensitization of β-adrenoreceptors (91) have been reported in patients in heart failure. This increased sympathetic nervous system activity is perhaps attributed to increased norepinephrine turnover and reduced efficiency of norepinephrine reuptake and storage (92). It has also been suggested that patients in heart failure with high plasma norepinephrine levels have an unfavorable prognosis (1). Plasma norepinephrine, however, is derived from sympathetic activity throughout the body and, thus, does not necessarily reflect cardiac sympathetic activity. Noninvasive scintigraphic techniques, therefore, may provide important knowledge of cardiac sympathetic nervous system activity, which could be of value in understanding the pathogenesis and prognosis of heart failure.

A number of studies have shown that abnormal MIBG findings in the case of heart failure typically include a reduced heart/mediastinum uptake ratio, heterogeneous distribution of MIBG within the myocardium, and increased MIBG washout from the heart (93–96). A reduced heart/mediastinum uptake ratio (less than 1.2) is reportedly a powerful predictor of poor prognosis in patients with CHF (97). It appears that these scintigraphic findings are independent of the underlying cause (98,99).

Reduced HED retention has been reported in patients with idiopathic dilated cardiomyopathy (100). Using quantitative analysis, the reduction of HED retention correlated with the severity of heart failure as expressed by the New York Heart Association functional classification (101). Vesalainen et al. (102) reported a 30% reduction of ^{11}C retention in 30 patients with moderate heart failure and correlated these findings with heart-rate variability and blood pressure control. There was no significant relationship of HED retention with heart-rate variability, but a relationship was found with blood pressure regulation during the tilt test (102). The retention of ^{11}C-HED in the failing heart is heterogeneous with more pronounced abnormalities in distal segments. This neuronal dysfunction is independent of myocardial blood flow, as shown by direct comparison with ^{13}N-ammonia distribution in the same patients (51).

Ungerer et al. (103) investigated the relationship between scintigraphic findings and myocardial tissue analysis in candidates for cardiac transplantation. Regional ^{11}C-HED retention correlated with tissue norepinephrine content and the density of catecholamine transport proteins (uptake-1). There was no significant relationship between presynaptic scintigraphic measurements and density of β-receptors (104). These quantitative PET data in patients in heart failure indicate the validity of the imaging approach to delineate neuronal dysfunction and to use PET in combination with ^{11}C-HED to monitor neuronal function during therapy.

Aside from a downregulation of β-receptor density, there are scintigraphic data suggesting an upregulation of muscarinic receptors in patients in heart failure. LeGuludec et al. reported approximately 30% upregulation of ^{11}C-MQNB binding in 22 patients with severe reduction of left ventricular function (mean LVEF of 22%) as compared with 12 healthy controls. The clinical and pathophysiologic significance of this finding remains to be elucidated.

Recently, Pietila et al. (105) published initial results on the prognostic value of ^{11}C-HED imaging in patients with advanced heart failure. Forty-six patients with impaired left ventricular function (LVEF of 8% to 35%) were monitored for 55 ± 19 months after a HED PET study. The patients were divided into two groups based on myocardial HED retention. Below the cutoff value of 0.184 for retention fraction, there was a significantly higher incidence of complications (death, cardiac transplantation) as compared with patients with maintained tracer retention. Myocardial HED retention was independent from peak oxygen uptake and end-diastolic volume as a significant predictor for complications. These initial clinical results with ^{11}C-HED confirm the prognostic experience with MIBG imaging and suggest a potentially important application of PET in patients in heart failure.

Myocardial Hypertrophy and Hypertrophic Cardiomyopathy

It has been shown that myocardial hypertrophy, secondary to mechanical overload such as valvular aortic stenosis (106, 107), essential hypertension (108), and pulmonary arterial hypertension (109), causes reduced MIBG uptake and increased washout. Interestingly, the abnormalities seen with MIBG imaging improved after medical treatment and regression of hypertensive cardiac hypertrophy (108), indicating that such neuronal dysfunction may be reversible.

Using HED PET and compartmental analysis, a significantly reduced distribution volume of HED was reported in patients with hypertrophic cardiomyopathy (110). The interesting aspect of this finding is that not only the hypertrophic segments of the heart were involved but also the free lateral wall. Schafers et al. (50) investigated presynaptic and postsynaptic function in these patients. The myocardial distribution volume for ^{11}C-HED was reduced in nine patients to 33.4 mL/g of tissue as compared with 71.0 mL/g of tissue in healthy controls. The density of β-adrenoceptors in 13 patients (6 patients had both measurements) was also decreased to 7.3 pmol/g of tissue as compared with 10.2 pmol/g of tissue for healthy controls. These findings suggest a global impairment of both presynaptic and postsynaptic function in patients with hypertrophic cardiomyopathy. Thus, neuronal imaging may provide new insights into the pathogenesis of myocardial hypertrophy, although the clinical significance of PET imaging in these disease conditions remains largely unknown.

SUMMARY

Myocardial neurotransmitter imaging has been successfully performed to assess cardiac autonomic innervation in humans under various clinical conditions. Early detection of abnormalities before there is evidence of structural changes is an important goal of these scintigraphic approaches. Monitoring of therapeutic procedures also appears to be a promising application of neurotransmitter imaging.

Several issues remain to be addressed in studies. First, controversial results have been published for healthy subjects and for various disease conditions using MIBG and HED. It is also noteworthy that a number of MIBG studies describe regional abnormalities involving the inferior wall. These differences may be attributed to technical differences between SPECT and PET (e.g., the attenuation correction and higher spatial resolution of PET compared with SPECT) and differences in tracer kinetics and characteristics between MIBG and HED, including differences in specific activity and uptake of the tracer in nerve terminals. Second, the clinical significance and prognostic value of scintigraphic techniques have not yet been fully established. More convincing data involving a large patient population are required to draw significant conclusions regarding the utility of these scintigraphic techniques in the clinical setting. Finally, future developments aimed at synthesizing new radiopharmaceuticals to discriminate different aspects of autonomic nerve function will further broaden the experimental and clinical applications of imaging approaches.

PET will provide the opportunity to quantitatively map the presynaptic and postsynaptic innervation using a combination of tracers. No other imaging technique has the sensitivity or the biologic specificity to rival tracer techniques in the delineation of cardiac neuronal tissue. PET is and will remain an attractive research tool to investigate the relationship between cardiac disease and autonomic innervation. It is hoped that this research will lead to wider clinical application and potentially new therapeutic strategies.

REFERENCES

1. Cohn JN, Levine TB, Olivari MT, et al. Plasma norepinephrine as a guide to prognosis in patients with chronic congestive heart failure. N Engl J Med 1984;311:819–823.
2. Barron HV, Lesh MD. Autonomic nervous system and sudden cardiac death. J Am Coll Cardiol 1996;27:1053–1060.
3. Kline RC, Swanson DP, Wieland DM, et al. Myocardial imaging in man with I-123 metaiodobenzylguanidine. J Nucl Med 1981;22: 129–132.
4. Wieland DM, Brown LE, Rogers WL, et al. Myocardial imaging with a radioiodinated norepinephrine storage analog. J Nucl Med 1981;22: 22–31.
5. Rosenspire KC, Haka MS, Van-Dort ME, et al. Synthesis and preliminary evaluation of carbon-11-meta-hydroxyephedrine: a false transmitter agent for heart neuronal imaging. J Nucl Med 1990;31: 1328–1334.
6. Schwaiger M, Kalff V, Rosenspire K, et al. Noninvasive evaluation of sympathetic nervous system in human heart by positron emission tomography. Circulation 1990;82:457–464.
7. Goldstein DS, Chang PC, Eisenhofer G, et al. Positron emission tomographic imaging of cardiac sympathetic innervation and function. Circulation 1990;81:1606–1621.
8. Goldstein DS, Eisenhofer G, Dunn BB, et al. Positron emission tomographic imaging of cardiac sympathetic innervation using 6-[^{18}F]fluorodopamine: initial findings in humans. J Am Coll Cardiol 1993;22: 1961–1971.
9. Merlet P, Delforge J, Syrota A, et al. Positron emission tomography with ^{11}C CGP-12177 to assess beta-adrenergic receptor concentration in idiopathic dilated cardiomyopathy. Circulation 1993;87: 1169–1178.
10. Randall W, Ardell J. Functional anatomy of the cardiac efferent innervation. In: Kulbertus H, Frank G, eds. Neurocardiology. New York: Future Publishing, 1988.
11. Pierpont GL, DeMaster EG, Reynolds S, et al. Ventricular myocardial catecholamines in primates. J Lab Clin Med 1985;106:205–210.
12. Schmid PG, Greif BJ, Lund DD, et al. Regional choline acetyltransferase activity in the guinea pig heart. Circ Res 1978;42:657–660.
13. Crout J. The uptake and release of 3H-epinephrine by guinea pig heart in vivo. Naunyn Schmiedebergs Arch Pharmacol 1964;248:85.
14. Francis GS. Modulation of peripheral sympathetic nerve transmission. J Am Coll Cardiol 1988;12:250–254.
15. Kilborn MJ, Potter EK, McCloskey DI. Neuromodulation of the cardiac vagus: comparison of neuropeptide Y and related peptides. Regul Pept 1985;12:155–161.
16. Jaques S Jr, Tobes MC, Sisson JC. Sodium dependency of uptake of norepinephrine and m-iodobenzylguanidine into cultured human pheochromocytoma cells: evidence for uptake-one. Cancer Res 1987; 47:3920–3928.
17. Schomig A. Catecholamines in myocardial ischemia. Systemic and cardiac release. Circulation 1990;82:II13–II22.
18. Russ H, Gliese M, Sonna J, et al. The extraneuronal transport mechanism for noradrenaline (uptake-2) avidly transports 1-methyl-4-phenylpyridinium (MPP+). Naunyn Schmiedebergs Arch Pharmacol 1992;346:158–165.
19. Salt PJ. Inhibition of noradrenaline uptake 2 in the isolated rat heart by steroids, clonidine and methoxylated phenylethylamines. Eur J Pharmacol 1972;20:329–340.
20. Ducis I. The high affinity choline uptake system. In: Whittaker V, ed. The cholinergic synapse. New York: Springer-Verlag New York, 1988.
21. Dae MW, Herre JM, O'Connell JW, et al. Scintigraphic assessment of sympathetic innervation after transmural versus nontransmural myocardial infarction. J Am Coll Cardiol 1991;17:1416–1423.
22. Wieland DM, Rosenspire KC, Hutchins GD, et al. Neuronal mapping of the heart with 6-[^{18}F]fluorometaraminol. J Med Chem 1990;33: 956–964.
23. Schwaiger M, Guibourg H, Rosenspire K, et al. Effect of regional myocardial ischemia on sympathetic nervous system as assessed by fluorine-18-metaraminol. J Nucl Med 1990;31:1352–1357.
24. DeGrado TR, Hutchins GD, Toorongian SA, et al. Myocardial kinetics of carbon-11-meta-hydroxyephedrine: retention mechanisms and effects of norepinephrine. J Nucl Med 1993;34:1287–1293.
25. Allman KC, Wieland DM, Muzik O, et al. Carbon-11 hydroxyephe-

drine with positron emission tomography for serial assessment of cardiac adrenergic neuronal function after acute myocardial infarction in humans. *J Am Coll Cardiol* 1993;22:368–375.

26. Allman KC, Stevens MJ, Wieland DM, et al. Noninvasive assessment of cardiac diabetic neuropathy by carbon-11 hydroxyephedrine and positron emission tomography. *J Am Coll Cardiol* 1993;22:1425–1432.

27. Calkins H, Allman K, Bolling S, et al. Correlation between scintigraphic evidence of regional sympathetic neuronal dysfunction and ventricular refractoriness in the human heart. *Circulation* 1993;88:172–179.

28. Calkins H, Lehmann MH, Allman K, et al. Scintigraphic pattern of regional cardiac sympathetic innervation in patients with familial long QT syndrome using positron emission tomography. *Circulation* 1993;87:1616–1621.

29. Pierpont GL, Francis GS, DeMaster EG, et al. Elevated left ventricular myocardial dopamine in preterminal idiopathic dilated cardiomyopathy. *Am J Cardiol* 1983;52:1033–1035.

30. Schwaiger M, Hutchins GD, Kalff V, et al. Evidence for regional catecholamine uptake and storage sites in the transplanted human heart by positron emission tomography. *J Clin Invest* 1991;87:1681–1690.

31. Chakraborty PK, Gildersleeve DL, Jewett DM, et al. High yield synthesis of high specific activity R-(−)-[^{11}C]epinephrine for routine PET studies in humans. *Nucl Med Biol* 1993;20:939–944.

32. Schwaiger M, Wieland D, Muzik O, et al. Comparison of C-11 epinephrine and C-11 HED for evaluation of sympathetic neurons of the heart. *J Nucl Med* 1993;34:13P(abst).

33. DeGrado T, Hutchins G, Toorongian S, et al. Myocardial kinetics of carbon-11-meta-hydroxyephedrine: retention mechanisms and effects of norepinephrine. *J Nucl Med* 1993;34:1287–1293.

34. Nguyen NT, DeGrado TR, Chakraborty P, et al. Myocardial kinetics of carbon-11-epinephrine in the isolated working rat heart. *J Nucl Med* 1997;38:780–785.

35. Corbett J, Chiao P-C, del Rosario R, et al. Mapping neuronal enzyme function of the human heart with C-11 phenylephrine. *J Nucl Med* 1994;35:109P.

36. Coates G, Chirakal R, Fallen EL, et al. Regional distribution and kinetics of [^{18}F]6-fluorodopamine as a measure of cardiac sympathetic activity in humans. *Heart* 1996;75:29–34.

37. Ding YS, Fowler JS, Dewey SL, et al. Comparison of high specific activity (−) and (+)-6-[^{18}F]fluoronorepinephrine and 6-[^{18}F]fluorodopamine in baboons: heart uptake, metabolism and the effect of desipramine. *J Nucl Med* 1993;34:619–629.

38. Berry CR, Garg PK, DeGrado TR, et al. Para-[^{18}F]fluorobenzylguanidine kinetics in a canine coronary artery occlusion model. *J Nucl Cardiol* 1996;3:119–129.

39. Rogers GA, Parsons SM, Anderson DC, et al. Synthesis, *in vitro* acetylcholine-storage-blocking activities, and biological properties of derivatives and analogues of trans-2-(4-phenylpiperidine)cyclohexanol (vesamicol). *J Med Chem* 1989;32:1217–1230.

40. Jung YW, Van Dort ME, Gildersleeve DL, et al. A radiotracer for mapping cholinergic neurons of the brain. *J Med Chem* 1990;33:2065–2068.

41. DeGrado TR, Mulholland GK, Wieland DM, et al. Evaluation of (−)[^{18}F]fluoroethoxybenzovesamicol as a new PET tracer of cholinergic neurons of the heart. *Nucl Med Biol* 1994;21:189–195.

42. Vatner D, Asai K, Iwase M, et al. Beta-adrenergic receptor-G protein-adenylyl cyclase signal transduction in the failing heart. *Am J Cardiol* 1999;17:80H–85H.

43. Xiao R, Cheng H, Zhou Y, et al. Recent advances in cardiac beta(2)-adrenergic signal transduction. *Circ Res* 1999;85:1092–1100.

44. Delforge J, Syrota A, Lancon JP, et al. Cardiac beta-adrenergic receptor density measured in vivo using PET, CGP 12177, and a new graphical method [published correction appears in *J Nucl Med* 1994;35(5):921]. *J Nucl Med* 1991;32:739–748.

45. De Groot T, van Waarde A, Elsinga P, et al. Synthesis and evaluation of 1'-[^{18}F] fluorometoprolol as a potential tracer for the visualization of beta-adrenoceptors with PET. *Nucl Med Biol* 1993;20:637–642.

46. Law MP, Osman S, Pike VW, et al. Evaluation of [^{11}C]GB67, a novel radioligand for imaging myocardial alpha 1-adrenoceptors with positron emission tomography. *Eur J Nucl Med* 2000;27:7–17.

47. Delforge J, LeGuludec D, Syrota A, et al. Quantification of myocardial muscarinic receptors with PET in humans. *J Nucl Med* 1993;34:981–991.

48. Valett H, Deleuze P, Syrota A, et al. Canine myocardial beta-adrenergic, muscarinic receptor densities after denervation: a PET study. *J Nucl Med* 1995;36:1727.

49. Munch G, Nguyen N, Nekolla S, et al. Evaluation of sympathetic nerve terminals using C-11 epinephrine and C-11 hydroxyephedrine and PET. *Circulation* 2000;101:516–523.

50. Schafers M, Lerch H, Wichter T, et al. Cardiac sympathetic innervation in patients with idiopathic right ventricular outflow tract tachycardia. *J Am Coll Cardiol* 1998;32:181–186.

51. Hartmann F, Ziegler S, Nekolla S, et al. Regional patterns of myocardial sympathetic denervation in dilated cardiomyopathy: an analysis using carbon-11 hydroxyephedrine and positron emission tomography. *Heart* 1999;81:262–270.

52. Barber MJ, Mueller TM, Henry DP, et al. Transmural myocardial infarction in the dog produces sympathectomy in noninfarcted myocardium. *Circulation* 1983;67:787–796.

53. Fagret D, Wolf JE, Comet M. Myocardial uptake of meta-[^{123}I]-iodobenzylguanidine [^{123}I]-MIBG) in patients with myocardial infarct. *Eur J Nucl Med* 1989;15:624–628.

54. Hartikainen J, Mantysaari M, Kuikka J, et al. Extent of cardiac autonomic denervation in relation to angina on exercise test in patients with recent acute myocardial infarction. *Am J Cardiol* 1994;74:760–763.

55. McGhie AI, Corbett JR, Akers MS, et al. Regional cardiac adrenergic function using I-123 meta-iodobenzylguanidine tomographic imaging after acute myocardial infarction. *Am J Cardiol* 1991;67:236–242.

56. Minardo JD, Tuli MM, Moch BH, et al. Scintigraphic and electrophysiological evidence of canine myocardial sympathetic denervation and reinnervation produced by myocardial infarction or phenol application. *Circulation* 1988;78:1008–1019.

57. Stanton MS, Tuli MM, Radtke NL, et al. Regional sympathetic denervation after myocardial infarction in humans detected noninvasively using I-123-metaiodobenzylguanidine. *J Am Coll Cardiol* 1989;14:1519–1526.

58. Wolpers H, Nguyen N, Rosenspire K, et al. Comparison of C-11 HED and I-131 MIBG for the assessment of ischemic neuronal injury in the canine heart. *J Nucl Med* 1990;31:725(abst).

59. Matsunari I, Schricke U, Bengel FM, et al. Extent of cardiac sympathetic neuronal damage is determined by the area of ischemia in patients with acute coronary syndromes. *Circulation* 2000;101:2579–2585.

60. Nishimura T, Oka H, Sago M, et al. Serial assessment of denervated but viable myocardium following acute myocardial infarction in dogs using iodine-123 metaiodobenzylguanidine and thallium-201 chloride myocardial single photon emission tomography. *Eur J Nucl Med* 1992;19:25–29.

61. Mitrani R, Burt RW, Klein LS, et al. Regional cardiac sympathetic denervation and reinnervation following myocardial infarction in humans. *Circulation* 1992;86[Suppl 1]:I-247.

62. Hartikainen J, Kuikka J, Mantysaari M, et al. Sympathetic reinnervation after acute myocardial infarction. *Am J Cardiol* 1996;77:5–9.

63. Spinnler MT, Lombardi F, Moretti C, et al. Evidence of functional alterations in sympathetic activity after myocardial infarction. *Eur Heart J* 1993;14:1334–1343.

64. Corr PB, Gillis RA. Autonomic neuronal influences on the dysrhythmias resulting from myocardial infarction. *Circ Res* 1978;43:1.

65. Inoue H, Zipes DP. Results of sympathetic denervation in the canine heart: supersensitivity that may be arrhythmogenic. *Circulation* 1987;75:877–887.

66. Schwartz PJ, Zaza A, Pala M, et al. Baroreflex sensitivity and its evolution during the first year after myocardial infarction. *J Am Coll Cardiol* 1988;12:629–636.

67. Wilber DJ, Baerman J, Olshansky B, et al. Adenosine-sensitive ventricular tachycardia. Clinical characteristics and response to catheter ablation. *Circulation* 1993;87:126–134.

68. Mitrani RD, Klein LS, Miles WM, et al. Regional cardiac sympathetic denervation in patients with ventricular tachycardia in the absence of coronary artery disease. *J Am Coll Cardiol* 1993;22:1344–1353.

69. Gill JS, Hunter GJ, Gane J, et al. Asymmetry of cardiac [^{123}I] meta-iodobenzyl-guanidine scans in patients with ventricular tachycardia and a "clinically normal" heart. *Br Heart J* 1993;69:6–13.

70. Wichter T, Hindricks G, Lerch H, et al. Regional myocardial sympathetic dysinnervation in arrhythmogenic right ventricular cardiomyop-

athy. An analysis using ^{123}I-meta-iodobenzylguanidine scintigraphy. *Circulation* 1994;89:667–683.

71. Wichter T, Schafers M, Rhodes C, et al. Abnormalities of cardiac sympathetic innervation in arrhythmogenic right ventricular cardiomyopathy: quantitative assessment of presynaptic norepinephrine reuptake and postsynaptic beta-adrenergic receptor density with positron emission tomography. *Circulation* 2000;101:1552–1558.

72. Schwartz P, Periti M, Malliani A. The long Q-T syndrome. *Am Heart J* 1975;89:378–390.

73. Gohl K, Feistel H, Weikl A, et al. Congenital myocardial sympathetic dysinnervation (CMSD)—a structural defect of idiopathic long QT syndrome. *Pacing Clin Electrophysiol* 1991;14:1544–1553.

74. Ewing DJ, Campbell IW, Clarke BF. The natural history of diabetic autonomic neuropathy. *Q J Med* 1980;49:95–108.

75. Mantysaari M, Kuikka J, Mustonen J, et al. Noninvasive detection of cardiac sympathetic nervous dysfunction in diabetic patients using ^{123}I]metaiodobenzylguanidine. *Diabetes* 1992;41:1069–1075.

76. Langer A, Freeman MR, Josse RG, et al. Metaiodobenzylguanidine imaging in diabetes mellitus: assessment of cardiac sympathetic denervation and its relation to autonomic dysfunction and silent myocardial ischemia. *J Am Coll Cardiol* 1995;25:610–618.

77. Wei K, Dorian P, Newman D, et al. Association between QT dispersion and autonomic dysfunction in patients with diabetes mellitus. *J Am Coll Cardiol* 1995;26:859–863.

78. Kreiner G, Wolzt M, Fasching P, et al. Myocardial m-^{123}I]iodobenzylguanidine scintigraphy for the assessment of adrenergic cardiac innervation in patients with IDDM. Comparison with cardiovascular reflex tests and relationship to left ventricular function. *Diabetes* 1995; 44:543–549.

79. Stevens M, Raffel D, Allman K, et al. Cardiac sympathetic dysinnervation in diabetes: implications for enhanced cardiovascular risk. *Circulation* 1998;98:961–968.

80. Matsuo S, Takahashi M, Nakamura Y, et al. Evaluation of cardiac sympathetic innervation with iodine-123-metaiodobenzylguanidine imaging in silent myocardial ischemia. *J Nucl Med* 1996;37:712–717.

81. DeMarco T, Dae M, Yuen-Green MS, et al. Iodine-123 metaiodobenzylguanidine scintigraphic assessment of the transplanted human heart: evidence for late reinnervation. *J Am Coll Cardiol* 1995;25:927–931.

82. Kaye DM, Esler M, Kingwell B, et al. Functional and neurochemical evidence for partial cardiac sympathetic reinnervation after cardiac transplantation in humans. *Circulation* 1993;88:1110–1118.

83. Ziegler SI, Überfuhr P, Frey A, et al. Incidence and time course of reinnervation in the orthotopic transplanted human heart. *J Nucl Med* 1996;37:70P.

84. Bengel F, Permanetter B, Ungerer M, et al. Non-invasive estimation of myocardial efficiency using positron emission tomography and carbon-11 acetate—comparison between the normal and failing human heart. *J Nucl Med* 2000;41:837–844.

85. Odaka K, von Scheidt W, Ziegler S, et al. Reappearance of cardiac presynaptic sympathetic nerve terminals in the transplanted heart: correlation between PET using ^{11}C-hydroxyephedrine and invasively measured norepinephrine release. *J Nucl Med* 2001;42:1011–1016.

86. Schwaiblmair M, von Scheidt W, Uberfuhr P, et al. Functional significance of cardiac reinnervation in heart transplant recipients. *J Heart Lung Transplant* 1999;18:838–845.

87. Bengel F, Ueberfuhr P, Schiepel N, et al. Effect of sympathetic reinnervation on allograft performance after orthotopic heart transplantation. *N Engl J Med* 2001;345:731–738.

88. Thomas JA, Marks BH. Plasma norepinephrine in congestive heart failure. *Am J Cardiol* 1978;41:233–243.

89. Hasking GJ, Esler MD, Jennings GL, et al. Norepinephrine spillover to plasma in patients with congestive heart failure: evidence of increased overall and cardiorenal sympathetic nervous activity. *Circulation* 1986;73:615–621.

90. Chidsey CA, Braunwald E, Morrow AG, et al. Myocardial norepinephrine concentration in man: effects of reserpine and of congestive heart failure. *N Engl J Med* 1963;269:653–658.

91. Bristow MR, Ginsburg R, Minobe W, et al. Decreased catecholamine sensitivity and beta-adrenergic-receptor density in failing human hearts. *N Engl J Med* 1982;307:205–211.

92. Chang PC, Szemeredi K, Grossman E, et al. Fate of tritiated 6-fluorodopamine in rats: a false neurotransmitter for positron emission tomographic imaging of sympathetic innervation and function. *J Pharmacol Exp Ther* 1990;255:809–817.

93. Henderson EB, Kahn JK, Corbett JR, et al. Abnormal I-123 metaiodobenzylguanidine myocardial washout and distribution may reflect myocardial adrenergic derangement in patients with congestive cardiomyopathy. *Circulation* 1988;78:1192–1199.

94. Glowniak JV, Turner FE, Gray LL, et al. Iodine-123 metaiodobenzylguanidine imaging of the heart in idiopathic congestive cardiomyopathy and cardiac transplants. *J Nucl Med* 1989;30:1182–1191.

95. Schofer J, Spielmann R, Schuchert A, et al. Iodine-123 meta-iodobenzylguanidine scintigraphy: a noninvasive method to demonstrate myocardial adrenergic nervous system disintegrity in patients with idiopathic dilated cardiomyopathy. *J Am Coll Cardiol* 1988;12:1252–1258.

96. Simmons WW, Freeman MR, Grima EA, et al. Abnormalities of cardiac sympathetic function in pacing-induced heart failure as assessed by ^{123}I]metaiodobenzylguanidine scintigraphy. *Circulation* 1994;89:2843–2851.

97. Merlet P, Valette H, Dubois-Rande JL, et al. Prognostic value of cardiac metaiodobenzylguanidine imaging in patients with heart failure. *J Nucl Med* 1992;33:471–477.

98. Imamura Y, Ando H, Mitsuoka W, et al. Iodine-123 metaiodobenzylguanidine images reflect intense myocardial adrenergic nervous activity in congestive heart failure independent of underlying cause. *J Am Coll Cardiol* 1995;26:1594–1599.

99. Nakajima K, Taki J, Tonami N, et al. Decreased ^{123}I-MIBG uptake and increased clearance in various cardiac diseases. *Nucl Med Commun* 1994;15:317–323.

100. Schwaiger M, Beanlands R, vom Dahl J. Metabolic tissue characterization in the failing heart by positron emission tomography. *Eur Heart J* 1994;15:14–19.

101. Hartmann F, et al. Evidence of regional myocardial sympathetic denervation in dilated cardiomyopathy: an analysis using C-11 hydroxyephedrine and positron emission tomography. *Eur Heart J* 1996;17.

102. Vesalainen R, Pietila M, Tahvanainen K, et al. Cardiac positron emission tomography imaging with (^{11}C) hydroxyephedrine, a specific tracer for sympathetic nerve endings, and its functional correlates in congestive heart failure. *Am J Cardiol* 1999;84:568–574.

103. Ungerer M, Hartmann F, Karoglan M, et al. Regional *in vivo* and *in vitro* characterization of autonomic innervation in cardiomyopathic human heart. *Circulation* 1998;97:174–180.

104. Ungerer M, Weig H, Kubert S, et al. Regional pre- and postsynaptic sympathetic system in the failing human heart—regulation of beta ARK-1. *Eur J Heart Fail* 2000;2:23–31.

104a. LeGuludec D, Cohen-Solal A, Delforge J, et al. Increased myocardial muscarinic receptor density in idiopathic dilated cardiomyopathy: an in vivo PET study. *Circulation* 1997;96(10):3416–3422.

105. Pietila M, Malminiemi K, Ukkonen H, et al. Reduced myocardial carbon-11 hydroxyephedrine retention is associated with poor prognosis in chronic heart failure. *Eur J Nucl Med* 2001;28:373–376.

106. Fagret D, Wolf JE, Vanzetto G, et al. Myocardial uptake of metaiodobenzylguanidine in patients with left ventricular hypertrophy secondary to valvular aortic stenosis. *J Nucl Med* 1993;34:57–60.

107. Rabinovitch MA, Rose CP, Schwab AJ, et al. A method of dynamic analysis of iodine-123-metaiodobenzylguanidine scintigrams in cardiac mechanical overload hypertrophy and failure. *J Nucl Med* 1993;34:589–600.

108. Morimoto S, Terada K, Keira N, et al. Investigation of the relationship between regression of hypertensive cardiac hypertrophy and improvement of cardiac sympathetic nervous dysfunction using iodine-123 metaiodobenzylguanidine myocardial imaging. *Eur J Nucl Med* 1996;23:756–761.

109. Morimitsu T, Miyahara Y, Sinboku H, et al. Iodine-123-metaiodobenzylguanidine myocardial imaging in patients with right ventricular pressure overload. *J Nucl Med* 1996;37:1343–1346.

110. Schwaiger M, Hutchins GD, Das SK, et al. C-11 hydroxy-ephedrine kinetics in patients with hypertrophic cardiomyopathy. *J Am Coll Cardiol* 1991;17:343A(abst).

CHAPTER 9

Infection and Inflammation

Yoshifumi Sugawara

As described in the previous chapters, positron emission tomography (PET) with ^{18}F-fluorodeoxyglucose (FDG) has been extensively used in oncology, and the usefulness of FDG PET for differentiating malignant from benign tumors, for tumor staging, and for evaluating treatment efficacy in patients with cancer is well recognized (1). Indeed, FDG accumulates in cancer cells due to their increased glucose metabolism (2), but it is not a tumor-specific agent.

Inflammatory cells such as activated lymphocytes, neutrophils, and macrophages have increased glucose utilization (3,4), and increased FDG uptake has been demonstrated in experimental infectious and inflammatory lesions in rodents (5–8). FDG is also known to accumulate in various inflammatory and infectious lesions in humans. Although FDG uptake in infection and inflammation may cause a dilemma when diagnosing patients with cancer (9,10) and may be a cause of false-positive results (11), FDG is recognized as an agent for the detection and localization of infection.

RODENT STUDIES

In 1990, Daley et al. (12) demonstrated in rats with a carrageenan wound model that there was increased glucose uptake in the presence of inflammatory cells (predominantly macrophages) at the site of injury. Three and 5 days after injury, glucose uptake was significantly increased in the injured hind limbs when compared with the hind limbs of pair-fed control animals. Similarly, Yamada et al. (7) from Tohoku University reported in turpentine oil–induced inflammation that the highest FDG uptake was seen in the abscess wall, which consisted of an inflammatory cell layer and granulation tissue. Micro-autoradiography of the abscess wall showed that the highest grain density was found in the marginal zone of young fibroblasts, endothelial cells of vessels, and phagocytes of neutrophils and macrophages, followed by that in the neutrophil layer and granulation tissue. Recently, Higashi et al. (13) reported in rodents that bone marrow FDG uptake transiently increased the first day after irradiation due to an increased percentage of neutrophils.

It is well known that abscess-forming bacteria use glucose as an energy source (14). After successfully creating a model of *Escherichia coli*–induced infection in rodents, the group from the University of Michigan (8) found that the necrotic center of a bacterially infected abscess showed slightly higher FDG uptake than the surrounding edematous muscle. This differed from the turpentine model described above in that its center showed very low FDG uptake (7). This difference in the location of FDG uptake could be partly attributed to bacterial FDG uptake or the presence of some living infiltrating cells in the necrotic area of the infection model.

Using the same infection model, the authors (8) performed a comparative biodistribution study of FDG, thymidine (Thy), methionine (Met), gallium-67 (^{67}Ga)-citrate and iodine-125 (^{125}I)-HSA in infections. Although fluorine-18 (^{18}F)-FDG, ^{67}Ga-citrate and ^{125}I-HSA all showed comparatively high uptake in the infected muscle, the infected muscle-to-blood ratio was much higher for ^{18}F-FDG than for ^{67}Ga-citrate or ^{125}I-HSA. FDG also showed much higher infection-to-background ratios at early time points compared with ^{67}Ga-citrate or ^{125}I-HSA. Methionine, and to a greater extent thymidine, was less actively accumulated in the infectious foci than FDG.

HUMAN STUDY

In 1989 Tahara et al. (15) reported high FDG uptake in patients with abdominal abscesses. Several reports have subsequently shown that FDG accumulates in various kinds of inflammatory and infectious lesions in almost all tissues and organs in the body (11,16–34) (Table 9.1). Although FDG uptake in infection and inflammation may be a cause of false-positive results when studying patients with cancer (9, 10), it holds promise as an infection detection agent.

CLINICAL UTILITY

Fever of Unknown Origin

Fever of unknown origin (FUO) has been defined as elevated body temperature occurring in a cyclic pattern and

TABLE 9.1 *References for FDG uptake in infectious and inflammatory lesions*

Head and neck: Brain abscess (18–20), aspergillosis (21), herpes encephalitis (22), chronic thyroiditis (62, 63), chronic sinusitis (61), inflammation after radiotherapy (23)

Chest: Breast infection and inflammation (24), tuberculosis (25, 26, 70), fungal disease (25, 27, 70), sarcoidosis (55–60), pneumonia (25, 28, 29, 70, 86), radiation pneumonitis (86), airway inflammation with bronchial asthma (74)

Abdomen: Enterocolitis (30, 31), pancreatitis (29, 32, 68, 71, 79), inflammation after radiotherapy (9), abdominal abscess 15, 70), pelvic inflammatory disease (36)

Musculoskeletal: Rheumatoid arthritis (33, 72, 73), acute fracture (34), osteomyelitis (43, 45–51), loosening (53), spondylitis (47), sarcoidosis (55, 60), synovitis (50), fasciitis (43, 50), myositis (50), abscess (43, 50)

Others: Fever of unknown origin (36, 42), vasculitis (64, 65)

lasting for at least 3 weeks (35). Localizing signs of the fever are usually lacking. Most patients with FUO have neoplasms, autoimmune diseases, or collagen diseases, although infection accounts for only 20% to 40% of cases (35,36).

The purpose of radionuclide imaging is to detect a potential focus that is causing the fever, which subsequently can be evaluated further by conventional anatomic imaging (37, 38). Although whole-body imaging using ^{67}Ga-citrate has been performed extensively, some disadvantages exist; for example, scanning usually must be done 48 to 72 hours after tracer injection, and high normal tracer uptake is observed in the liver and bowel (37,39). Although indium-111 (^{111}In)-hexamethylpropyleneamine oxime (HMPAO) or technetium-99m (^{99m}Tc)-HMPAO white blood cell (WBC) imaging could be an alternative to ^{67}Ga-citrate, particularly for abdominal imaging (38), ^{67}Ga-citrate is generally preferred in patients with FUO because of its superiority in chronic inflammatory and infectious conditions (39,40) (i.e., FUO is a process of at least 3 weeks' duration). The inconvenience and expense of labeling leukocytes with ^{111}In or ^{99m}Tc-HMPAO are also drawbacks to these agents (38,40,41).

Recent studies have shown that FDG PET can be useful for detecting the source of FUO (36,42). Meller et al. (36) reported a prospective comparison of FDG imaging with a dual-head coincidence camera (DHCC) and ^{67}Ga-citrate imaging with single-photon emission computed tomography (SPECT). FDG with DHCC was superior to ^{67}Ga SPECT for the evaluation of patients with FUO. In 18 patients who were imaged with both modalities, transaxial FDG tomography showed 81% sensitivity and 86% specificity, whereas ^{67}Ga SPECT showed 67% sensitivity and 78% specificity. This can probably be explained by the favorable tracer kinetics of FDG compared with that of ^{67}Ga and by the better spatial resolution of the DHCC system compared with SPECT imaging (36). When compared with ^{67}Ga, FDG provides a more rapid diagnosis (8,36,43).

O'Doherty et al. (42) investigated the use of PET scanning in patients with human immunodeficiency virus (HIV) infec-

tion and FUO, confusion, and/or weight loss. FDG PET enabled rapid assessment of the whole body in HIV-positive patients. A FDG PET scan with approximately half the body in the field of view had a sensitivity of 92% (23 of 25 patients) and a specificity of 94% (30 of 32 patients) for localization of focal pathology that needed treatment. High uptake of FDG (greater than liver) had a positive predictive value of 95% for disease needing treatment. Unlike labeled leukocytes, no complex labeling procedure is required, and unlike ^{67}Ga-citrate, an early result after tracer injection is possible (42).

Osteomyelitis

Osteomyelitis may be a complication of any systemic infection, but frequently it manifests as a primary solitary focus of disease (28). Accurate and prompt diagnosis is desirable for optimal treatment of osteomyelitis. However, there are some clinical situations in which a definitive diagnosis is difficult to establish using conventional radiologic or scintigraphic approaches. In contrast to acute osteomyelitis, it remains challenging to diagnose chronic osteomyelitis, which may occur insidiously after traumatic injuries or surgical procedures. In many cases of chronic osteomyelitis, the clinical symptoms and laboratory and radiologic findings are nonspecific.

Published data on FDG PET imaging of chronic osteomyelitis are encouraging (42–51). FDG PET has been reported to be more accurate [overall sensitivity and specificity are 90% to 100% and 70% to 96%, respectively (45,46, 50,51)] than other radionuclide imaging modalities, such as three-phase bone scintigraphy (sensitivity of 95%, specificity of 33%), or ^{67}Ga-citrate imaging (sensitivity of 81% and specificity of 69%) (52). WBC scintigraphy has been performed in conjunction with bone scintigraphy and has been used to overcome the limitations of ^{67}Ga-citrate, with a sensitivity of 88% and a specificity of 85% reported (52). Clear differentiation between bone infection and infections of surrounding soft tissue might be difficult with WBC scintigraphy. Such differentiation is possible with FDG PET due to the high spatial resolution of the PET technique (Fig. 9.1).

Guhlmann et al. (45) prospectively used FDG PET to evaluate 31 patients suspected of having chronic osteomyelitis. The overall sensitivity and specificity of FDG PET for detecting chronic osteomyelitis were 100% and 92%, respectively. Zhuang et al. (49) reported in 22 patients suspected of having chronic osteomyelitis that FDG PET showed a sensitivity of 100% (6 of 6 patients), a specificity of 87.5% (14 of 16 patients), and an accuracy of 90.9% (20 of 22 patients). Because there were no false-negative results, this study suggested that a negative FDG PET scan result could effectively eliminate the possibility of chronic osteomyelitis. In practice, it is rare for a technique to be 100% sensitive, although the data are encouraging.

Kalicke et al. (47) reported in 15 patients with histopathologically confirmed infectious bone diseases (acute or

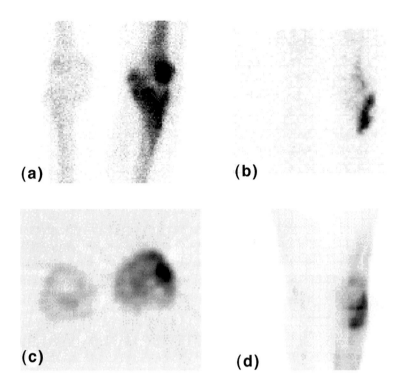

FIG. 9.1. A 28-year-old man with chronic osteomyelitis. **a:** Technetium-99m (^{99m}Tc) methylene diphosphonate bone scan, **(b)** indium-111 white blood cell scan, **(c)** transaxial fluorodeoxyglucose positron emission tomography (FDG PET), and **(d)** projection FDG PET image. Images show focal intense uptake at the left knee, indicating active chronic osteomyelitis. The FDG distribution is not identical to that of the bone scan. (From Sugawara Y, Braun DK, Kison PV, et al. Rapid detection of human infections with fluorine-18 fluorodeoxyglucose and positron emission tomography: preliminary results. *Eur J Nucl Med* 1998;25:1238–1243, with permission.)

chronic osteomyelitis or inflammatory spondylitis) that FDG PET yielded 15 true-positive results. FDG PET could differentiate osteomyelitis or inflammatory spondylitis from soft-tissue infections surrounding the bone (activity outside normal bone contours). Robiller et al. (48) reported a case of chronic osteomyelitis, in which infection of the fibular transplant was demonstrated clearly by FDG PET but not by the other methods. On magnetic resonance imaging (MRI), the fibular transplant could not be imaged well due to extensive metallic artifacts. Antigranulocyte antibody scintigraphy showed limitations in specificity when the infectious focus was in an area of hematopoietic bone marrow, due to substantial normal tracer uptake in marrow.

Unlike computed tomography (CT) and MRI, orthopedic devices such as metallic implants do not as severely affect the excellent spatial resolution and accuracy of FDG PET in detection of osteomyelitis (45,48). This advantage suggests that FDG PET is particularly suitable when an infection is suspected in the area around metal implants used for fixing fractures (47).

In follow-up of patients with osteomyelitis, FDG PET reveals normal or clearly reduced uptake after successful treatment, whereas the bone scan results often remain abnormal for a long time (Fig. 9.2) (43,47). FDG PET can be used to monitor therapeutic effects because it sensitively reflects the glucose metabolism within the infection. It remains unclear how long FDG uptake remains after a prosthesis is placed, however.

Although FDG PET is promising for diagnosing chronic osteomyelitis (accuracy of 96% [49 of 51 patients]) reported by Guhlmann et al. (46), FDG PET will probably not be able to distinguish infection from inflammation. In the early postoperative phase, it may be difficult to differentiate between postsurgical inflammatory changes and infections

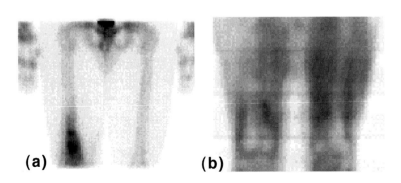

FIG. 9.2. A 24-year-old man with chronic osteomyelitis after treatment. Although technetium-99m methylene diphosphonate bone scan **(a)** results remain abnormal (intense uptake in the right distal femoral bone), fluorodeoxyglucose positron emission tomography study **(b)** shows no obvious bone uptake in the areas of increased uptake seen on the bone scan. The patient was reported to have done well clinically after treatment. (From Sugawara Y, Braun DK, Kison PV, et al. Rapid detection of human infections with fluorine-18 fluorodeoxyglucose and positron emission tomography: preliminary results. *Eur J Nucl Med* 1998;25:1238–1243, with permission.)

using FDG PET (47,49). Postsurgical inflammatory changes can cause false-positive FDG PET scan results for as long as 6 months after the procedure (49). High FDG uptake in a patient with aseptic loosening 4 years after a knee prosthesis was placed was reported (53).

On the other hand, Zhuang et al. (51) recently reported that FDG PET is promising for detecting infected lower limb prosthesis implants. FDG PET may be more accurate for detecting infections associated with hip prosthesis than for detecting infections associated with knee prosthesis (90% sensitive, 89% specific, 90% accurate for hip prosthesis infections vs. 91% sensitive, 72% specific, 78% accurate for knee prosthesis infections). Interestingly, the authors mentioned that the intensity of uptake at the bone–prosthesis interface was not important when making the diagnosis, and that just the presence of uptake was sufficient to indicate infection. If the FDG uptake was limited around the femoral head or neck and did not extend to the bone–prosthesis interface, the probability of infection was low (51). This warrants more study.

The FDG uptake in normal bone and marrow is generally low and the increased ^{18}F activity associated with infection is readily detected, even though it may show a wide range of intensity. Guhlmann et al. (10) reported that the osseous FDG uptake in proven osteomyelitis [mean standard uptake value (SUV) = 4.5 ± 2.8, range 1.9 to 10.1] was clearly higher than that in normal bone (mean SUV = 0.2 ± 0.1, range, 0.1 to 0.3 in peripheral, and mean SUV = 0.9 ± 0.2, range 0.7 to 1.2 in central bone). Differentiation of an infected from an uninfected prosthesis (such as loosening) is essential for optimal and cost-effective management of these patients. This area continues to evolve and the number of studies remains limited. Little has been reported on the FDG scan appearance of normal joint prostheses at various times after surgery.

Sarcoidosis

Sarcoidosis is a chronic inflammatory granulomatous disease of unknown etiology and many tissues and organs can be involved (54). Sarcoidosis may vary in severity and have a heterogeneous distribution, which often makes it difficult to evaluate the lesion activity and systemic location. FDG uptake is seen in sarcoidosis (55–60). Lewis and Salama (55) reported two cases of sarcoidosis in which FDG uptake was seen in both intrathoracic and extrathoracic lesions, as well as in associated erythema nodosum. Kobayashi et al. (60) reported a case of sarcoidosis in which osseous lesions clearly demonstrated FDG uptake. Thus, whole-body FDG PET is useful for the detection of the systemic distribution of sarcoidosis (Fig. 9.3).

Brudin et al. (56) reported that in seven patients with sarcoidosis, the metabolic rate of glucose measured by FDG PET may reflect disease activity in sarcoidosis. Uptake of FDG decreased after successful steroid therapy. Yamada et al. (58) reported in 31 patients with sarcoidosis that the over-

all sensitivities of FDG and methionine (Met) PET in detecting mediastinum-bilateral hilar lymphadenopathy (MBHL) were both 97% (30 of 31 patients). However, the mean FDG uptake value (SUV = 6.02 ± 0.58) was significantly higher than that of Met (SUV = 3.14 ± 0.29) (p < .01). The group with higher FDG than Met uptake showed a significantly greater incidence of remission of MBHL when compared with the group with relatively higher Met uptake (78% vs. 33%) (p < .05).

Recently, the group from Gunma University in Japan (59) reported on the feasibility of FDG PET in diagnosing cardiac sarcoidosis. All 10 patients (100%) with cardiac complications showed abnormal myocardial uptake of FDG, whereas 5 (50%) of 10 patients showed an abnormality with ^{67}Ga-citrate. Although ^{99m}Tc-methoxyisobutyl isonitrile (MIBI) SPECT had a similar sensitivity (80%), there were differences in the localization of regional abnormalities. This discrepancy may reflect inflammatory and degenerative processes in the myocardium. FDG PET is useful for evaluating the activity and the extent of cardiac sarcoidosis. By comparing a myocardial perfusion study obtained with ^{99m}Tc-MIBI SPECT with the FDG PET study, one may estimate the extent of myocardial injury due to sarcoidosis. FDG PET can be used to predict the therapeutic effects in patients with sarcoidosis, and it may be useful for monitoring patients with cardiac complications. It must be noted that myocardial uptake of FDG is variable in healthy people, so more study is needed before one should routinely recommend myocardial PET for the diagnosis or monitoring of myocardial sarcoidosis.

Detection of Subclinical or Early Phase of Inflammation

While performing studies for cancer screening, Yasuda et al. observed that FDG uptake was incidentally seen in subclinical or asymptomatic inflammatory lesions such as sarcoidosis (57), sinusitis (61), and chronic thyroiditis (62). Diffuse thyroidal FDG uptake was found in 36 (3.3%) of 1,102 healthy subjects who underwent cancer screening with whole-body FDG PET (63). The authors suggested that FDG PET might be useful for detecting subclinical inflammation such as chronic thyroiditis (Fig. 9.4).

Hara et al. (64) reported a case of early phase Takayasu arteritis in which increased FDG uptake was demonstrated in the walls of the aorta, great vessels, and pulmonary arteries. This suggests that FDG PET may be useful for diagnosing the extent and activity of disease in early phase Takayasu arteritis, and that it may prove useful for the management of patients with other types of vasculitis (64,65). Caution is in order, because it is common to see vascular uptake in the aorta of older patients.

Autoimmune Pancreatitis

Autoimmune pancreatitis (AIP) is a form of chronic pancreatitis believed to be caused by an autoimmune mechanism

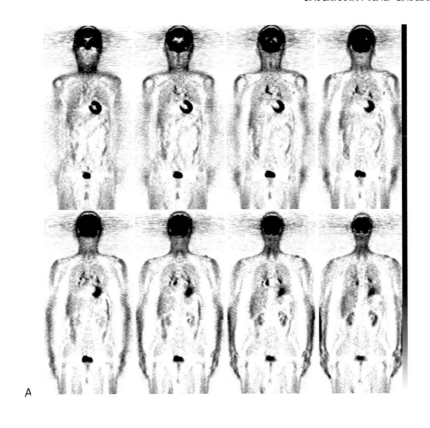

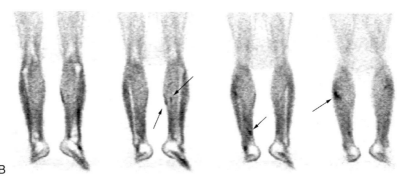

FIG. 9.3. A 70-year-old man with sarcoidosis. **A:** Coronal images from a whole-body fluorodeoxyglucose positron emission tomography (FDG PET) scan (without attenuation correction) show multiple areas of focal intense FDG uptake in the mediastinal and bilateral hilar lymph nodes. Transbronchial lung biopsy revealed characteristic sarcoid noncaseating granuloma. **B:** Coronal FDG PET images of the lower extremities of the same patient also shows focal spotty uptake (*arrows*) in areas of both calves and the right ankle. Later, subcutaneous nodules were palpated in the areas corresponding to areas of increased FDG uptake. All findings are believed to be related to active sarcoidosis. (Courtesy of Tatsuo Torizuka, MD, Positron Medical Center, Hamamatsu Medical Center, Japan.)

(66). Recognition of this disease is clinically important because it is reversible with steroid therapy. It may be difficult to reach the correct diagnosis, because patients with AIP may show no symptoms or only mild symptoms. Usually, there has not been an acute attack of pancreatitis and patient laboratory data are not specific for acute inflammation (67). Recently, Nakamoto et al. (67,68) reported in patients with AIP that intense FDG uptake was observed in the pancreas.

Histopathologically, it has been reported that the pancreas is infiltrated by activated CD4-positive lymphocytes, which can explain the abnormalities (e.g., diffuse pancreatic enlargement with segmental narrowing of the pancreatic duct) seen with CT and MRI (69). It is also speculated that these activated lymphocytes in the pancreas of patients with AIP accumulate FDG (67). In patients with positive PET scan results (five of six patients in their study), uptake of FDG

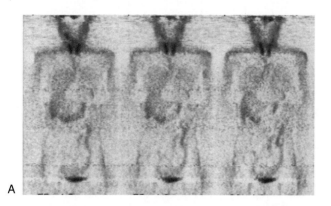

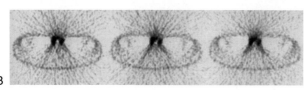

FIG. 9.4. A 55-year-old woman with chronic thyroiditis. **A:** Coronal and **(B)** transaxial images obtained with fluorodeoxyglucose positron emission tomography (without attenuation correction) show diffuse FDG uptake in the thyroid gland. (Courtesy of Seiei Yasuda, MD, HIMEDIC Imaging Center at Lake Yamanaka, Japan.)

was diffuse in four cases and focal in one (67). This may have been due to the difference in the degree of lymphocyte infiltration. Follow-up PET scans after steroid therapy, performed in three patients, showed that the FDG uptake in the pancreas clearly decreased (mostly disappeared) (Fig. 9.5). Thus, AIP is a relatively new disease entity of chronic pancreatitis and should be kept in mind when evaluating pancreatic disease, particularly when FDG PET is being used to make the differential diagnosis between pancreatic cancer and pancreatitis (67).

Assessment of the Lesion Activity in Infection/ Inflammation

FDG PET is useful not only for detection of infection, but also for assessment of lesion activity. Ichiya et al. (70) reported that acute active lesions showed higher FDG uptake than in chronic or healing lesions (lesion-to-muscle ratios were 9.8 ± 3.6, 3.6 ± 1.8, and 4.3 ± 1.7, respectively) (Fig. 9.6). Okazumi et al. (71) reported in 29 cases of abdominal inflammatory diseases that there was a significant positive correlation between the FDG uptake and the C-reactive protein (CRP) value. Palmer et al. (72) quantified the activity of joint inflammation with MRI and FDG PET. The volume of enhancing pannus (by MRI) and FDG uptake (SUV) were closely correlated ($r = 0.87$; $p < .0001$; n = 32).

Contrast-enhanced MRI and FDG PET can be valuable examinations in the quantification of joint inflammation. Treatment-related changes in the volume and metabolic activity of pannus were closely correlated. The authors believe

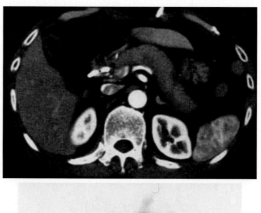

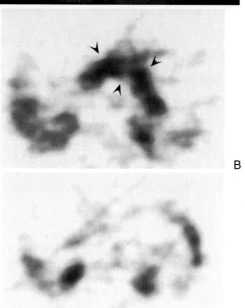

FIG. 9.5. A 66-year-old man with autoimmune pancreatitis. **A:** CT scan with contrast enhancement demonstrates enlargement of the pancreas without dilatation of the main pancreatic duct. **B:** Fluorodeoxyglucose positron emission tomography shows intense FDG uptake in the pancreas (*arrowheads*). **C:** After steroid therapy, no uptake is observed in the pancreas. (Courtesy of Yuji Nakamoto, MD, Kyoto University, Japan. Adapted from Nakamoto Y, Saga T, Ishimori T, et al. FDG-PET of autoimmune-related pancreatitis: preliminary results. *Eur J Nucl Med* 2000;27:1835–1838, with permission.)

that these quantitative imaging techniques are promising for monitoring and comparing the efficacy of antiinflammatory drugs in the treatment of inflammatory arthritis. Yasuda et al. (73) also reported a case of FDG accumulation in rheumatoid arthritis and suggested that FDG PET may be useful for evaluating treatment of inflamed joints. There have also been some reports regarding the usefulness of quantitative or semiquantitative measurements of FDG uptake in inflammatory and infectious lesions (56,65,74).

In the study discussed earlier, Ichiya et al. (70) also reported that the time-activity curve (TAC) of FDG may provide additional information for the assessment of lesion ac-

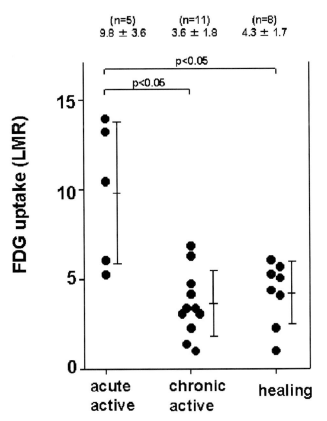

FIG. 9.6. ^{18}F-fluorodeoxyglucose uptake as a function of lesion activity. The mean lesion-to-muscle ratio *(LMR)* in the acute active lesions was higher than that in the chronic active lesions (mean ± SD: 9.8 ± 3.6 vs. 3.6 ± 1.8; p < .05). It was also higher than that in the healing lesions (the latter: 4.3 ± 1.7; p < .05). (From Ichiya Y, Kuwabara Y, Sasaki M, et al. FDG-PET in infectious lesions: the detection and assessment of lesion activity. *Ann Nucl Med* 1996;10: 185–191, with permission.)

tivity. In acute or chronic active lesions, the pattern of the TAC was either an increase (without an initial peak) or a plateau, whereas those in the healing lesions showed predominantly an increase with an initial sharp peak. The pattern of increased radiotracer (without an initial peak) was observed in the active lesions, and this is the same pattern seen in malignant tumors before therapy (75). A fast initial component represents tissue blood flow, rather than glucose metabolism, whereas the slow component reflects tissue glucose metabolism (e.g., lesion activity in both infections and tumors). The initial peak probably represents a vascular component resulting from increased blood flow due to newly formed or dilated vessels in healing lesions (76,77). This pattern may also be seen in tumors after radiotherapy (75). Special attention should be given to secondary inflammatory or infectious changes because they may cause false-positive results when interpreting FDG PET images in patients with malignant tumors.

Differentiation of Infection/Inflammation from Tumor

FDG is not a tumor-specific agent, and even within the tumor, FDG accumulates in both cancer cells and inflammatory cells (5,78). FDG uptake in inflammatory lesions results in relatively lower specificity (but higher sensitivity) in oncology (11) (Figs. 9.7 and 9.8). It may be difficult to differentiate infectious or inflammatory lesions from malignant tumors solely by the intensity of FDG uptake (i.e., the value of SUV or SUV_{lean}), because intense FDG uptake (i.e., high SUV or SUV_{lean}) is often observed in some infectious or inflammatory lesions (Figs. 9.9 and 9.10) (43). Shreve (79) reported that the focal FDG uptake (SUV ranging from 3.4 to 11.2) in pancreatitis (12 of 42 patients studied in this series with FDG PET) showed the same intensity range as those with pancreatic tumors (SUV ranging from 3.5 to 8.2 in this series). In response to the Shreve report, Zimny et al. (80) emphasized the need for appropriate preselection of patients to avoid a high incidence of false-positive results when using FDG PET in patients with cancer.

In 1983, Fukuda et al. (81) reported that in rodents with tumor- and croton oil–induced inflammation that tumor uptake was high and increased with time during 60 minutes postinjection, whereas the uptake in inflammation was relatively constant. Later, Kubota et al. (82) also reported that nonneoplastic cellular elements could be differentiated from viable cancer cells by the time course of increasing activity.

In clinical studies in humans, Nakamoto et al. (83) have shown that delayed FDG PET scanning 2 hours after injection may contribute to the differentiation between malignant and benign lesions in the pancreas (Fig. 9.11). Of 27 malignant lesions, the SUVs of 22 lesions increased 2 hours after injection, whereas the FDG uptake in 17 of 20 benign lesions decreased. Lodge et al. (84) reported that high-grade sarcomas reached a peak concentration of FDG approximately 4 hours after injection, whereas benign lesions reached a maximum within 30 minutes. Hustinx et al. (85) also reported that dual time-point imaging was helpful in differentiating malignancy from inflammation and normal tissue in the head and neck, particularly when separated by a sufficient time interval. These preliminary data suggest that assessment of the time-activity course of FDG uptake postinjection may be helpful in differentiating inflammatory lesions from malignant lesions, although this is not always possible [as previously mentioned (70,75,83)]. More extensive clinical studies are needed to confirm or refute this interesting hypothesis and initial observation.

The delineation of FDG uptake in suspicious lesions could be helpful to differentiate inflammatory lesions from tumors (Figs. 9.12 and 9.13) (11,86). Inoue et al. (86) studied patients with suspected recurrence of lung cancer and found that a curvilinear contour of increased FDG uptake was seen mostly in inflammatory lesions, whereas focal uptake was seen mostly in recurrent tumors. Of course, comparison with other available morphologic imaging modalities (such as CT

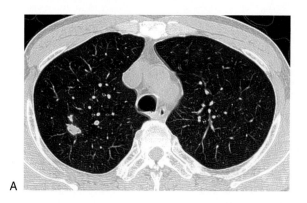

A

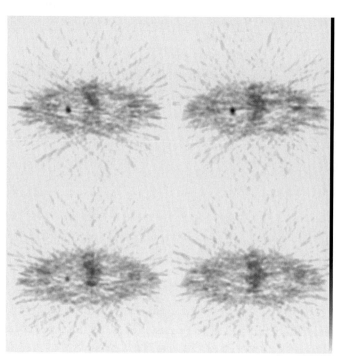

B

FIG. 9.7. A 50-year-old man with cryptococcosis. **A:** A transaxial CT image shows a small pulmonary nodule with a somewhat irregular margin in the right upper lobe. **B:** Transaxial fluorodeoxyglucose positron emission tomographic images (with attenuation correction) show intense FDG uptake in the nodule with a standard uptake value of 1.87. Open lung biopsy confirmed cryptococcal granuloma. (Courtesy of Tatsuo Torizuka, MD, Positron Medical Center, Hamamatsu Medical Center, Japan.)

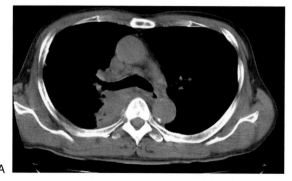

A

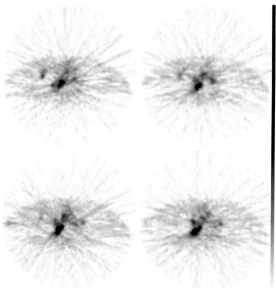

B

FIG. 9.8. A 58-year-old man with nonspecific inflammation. **A:** A transaxial CT image demonstrates well-defined areas of consolidation in the right lung and mediastinal lymphadenopathy. **B:** Transaxial fluorodeoxyglucose positron emission tomographic images show increased FDG uptake in both the right lung and the mediastinum. The maximum standard uptake value is 6.21. Although lung cancer with mediastinal lymph node metastases was considered before surgery, open lung biopsy revealed nonspecific inflammation. (Courtesy of Tatsuo Torizuka, MD, Positron Medical Center, Hamamatsu Medical Center, Japan.)

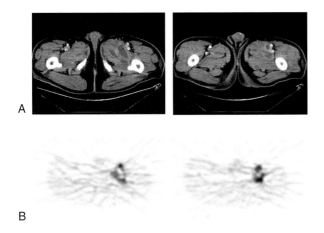

FIG. 9.9. A 60-year-old man with an inguinal abscess. **A:** CT images at the level of the inguinal region show an abscess cavity with a ring-enhanced wall and central liquefaction in the adductor compartment of the left upper thigh. **B:** Transaxial fluorodeoxyglucose positron emission tomographic images show ringlike intense FDG uptake (lean standard uptake value = 6.69) in the corresponding areas of abscess seen on the CT. (From Sugawara Y, Braun DK, Kison PV, et al. Rapid detection of human infections with fluorine-18 fluorodeoxyglucose and positron emission tomography: preliminary results. *Eur J Nucl Med* 1998;25:1238–1243, with permission.)

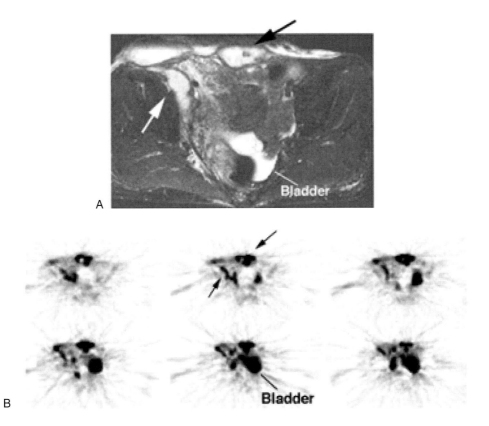

FIG. 9.10. A 51-year-old woman with pelvic inflammatory disease (PID). An intrauterine device (IUD) that had been implanted for 30 years was removed 2 months before the PET study. Her white blood cell count was high and C-reactive protein (CRP) was elevated. **A:** Transaxial T2-weighted magnetic resonance imaging (MRI) shows areas of increased signal intensity in the pelvic cavity. **B:** Transaxial fluorodeoxyglucose positron emission tomographic images show intense focal FDG uptake (*arrows*) corresponding to the areas of high intensity on MRI. The maximum standard uptake value is 8.13. Because it was difficult to differentiate PID from ovarian cancer, open abdominal surgery was performed and PID was confirmed. (Courtesy of Tatsuo Torizuka, MD, Positron Medical Center, Hamamatsu Medical Center, Japan.)

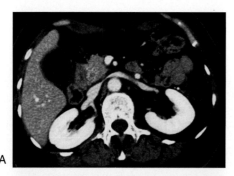

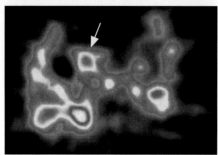

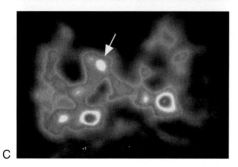

FIG. 9.11. A 49-year-old woman with autoimmune pancreatitis. **A:** CT with contrast enhancement demonstrates no definite tumor in the pancreatic head region. **B:** Fluorodeoxyglucose positron emission tomography at 1 hour postinjection shows focal uptake [standard uptake value (SUV) = 3.83] (*arrow*) in the pancreatic head. **C:** At 2 hours postinjection, the uptake was reduced (SUV = 3.14) (*arrow*). (From Nakamoto Y, Higashi T, Sakahara H, et al. Delayed (18)F-fluoro-2-deoxy-D-glucose positron emission tomography scan for differentiation between malignant and benign lesions in the pancreas. *Cancer* 2000;89(12):2547–2554, with permission.)

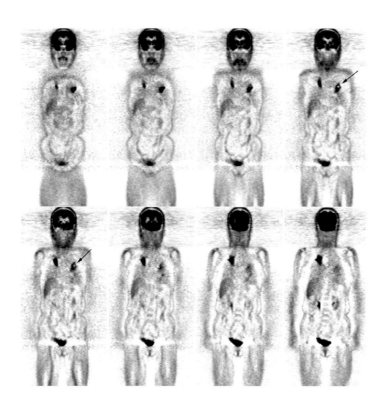

FIG. 9.12. An 82-year-old woman with tuberculosis. Coronal whole-body fluorodeoxyglucose positron emission tomographic images (without attenuation correction) show intense FDG uptake in the bilateral upper lobes and left lower lobe. The lesion has a cavitary feature that is well depicted (*arrows*). (Courtesy of Tatsuo Torizuka, MD, Positron Medical Center, Hamamatsu Medical Center, Japan.)

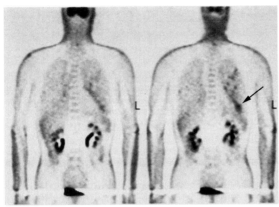

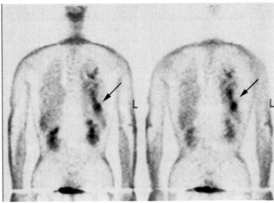

FIG. 9.13. A 54-year-old man with organizing pneumonia. The patient had a history of esophageal cancer. A pulmonary nodule in the left lower lung was detected on follow-up CT (not shown). Coronal fluorodeoxyglucose positron emission tomographic images show focal intense linear uptake in the left lower lung. (Courtesy of Yuji Nakamoto, MD, Kyoto University, Japan.)

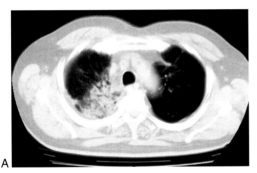

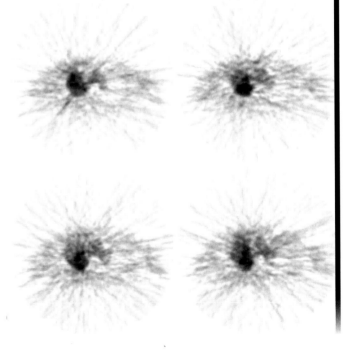

FIG. 9.14. A 70-year-old man with radiation pneumonitis. He had a history of radiotherapy (total dose of 50 Gy) to the recurrent small cell lung cancer on the right chest wall. **A:** A transaxial CT image, which was obtained 2 days before the completion of radiotherapy, demonstrates ill-defined areas of infiltration with air bronchogram in the right upper lobe compatible with radiation pneumonitis. **B:** Transaxial fluorodeoxyglucose positron emission tomographic images, which were obtained 2 weeks after completion of the radiotherapy, show increased FDG uptake in the areas corresponding to the radiation pneumonitis. (Courtesy of Tatsuo Torizuka, MD, Positron Medical Center, Hamamatsu Medical Center, Japan.)

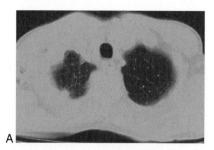

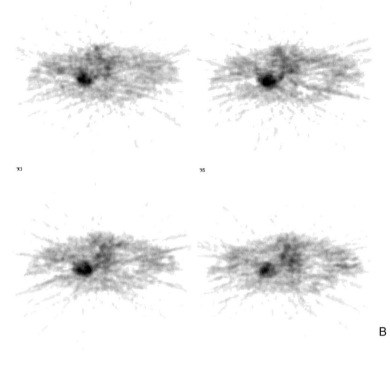

FIG. 9.15. A 65-year-old man with bronchoscopy-induced inflammatory change. **A:** A transaxial CT image demonstrates an ill-defined pleural-based nodule in the right apex. He subsequently underwent bronchoscopy, and the transbronchial lung biopsy and the brushing results were negative for malignancy. **B:** Transaxial FDG PET images, performed 4 days after bronchoscopy, show increased uptake in the right apex. Because the size of the increased area of FDG uptake was larger than that of the nodule seen on CT, this increased FDG uptake was attributed to bronchoscopy-induced inflammatory change. Open lung biopsy, performed about 1 month later, confirmed inflammatory granuloma. (Courtesy of Tatsuo Torizuka, MD, Positron Medical Center, Hamamatsu Medical Center, Japan.)

and MRI) and understanding the patients' clinical histories, including any interventions before the PET scanning, would contribute to accurate interpretations of these studies (Figs. 9.14 and 9.15).

SUMMARY

Although FDG uptake in infectious and inflammatory lesions can increase false-positive results and reduce the specificity of PET in oncology, FDG PET can be exploited for imaging infections and it shows considerable promise as a method for detecting infection and inflammation. PET provides better spatial resolution than conventional nuclear medicine modalities, and therefore, PET with FDG can better detect small and subtle changes in infections that may be missed by other techniques. Moreover, an FDG PET study can be completed within a few hours compared with the several hours or days that other nuclear medicine methods require. Accurate prompt diagnosis by FDG PET can allow appropriate treatment to be started. This is expected to result in better outcomes. FDG PET is promising as a modality for accurately diagnosing infection and inflammation, although its role is not as well established as the clear role of FDG PET in the patient with cancer.

REFERENCES

1. Wahl RL. Positron emission tomography: application in oncology. In: Murray IPC, Ell PJ, Strauss HW, eds. *Nuclear medicine in clinical diagnosis and treatment.* London: Churchill Livingstone, 1994: 801–820.
2. Warburg O. *The metabolism of tumors.* New York: Richard R. Smith Inc, 1931:129–169.
3. Fantone JC, Ward PA. Role of oxygen-derived free radicals and metabolites in leukocyte-dependent inflammatory reactions. *Am J Pathol* 1982;107:395–418.
4. Weisdorf DJ, Craddock PR, Jacob HS. Glycogenolysis versus glucose transport in human granulocytes: differential activation in phagocytosis and chemotaxis. *Blood* 1982;60:888–893.
5. Kubota R, Yamada S, Kubota K, et al. Intratumoral distribution of fluorine-18-fluorodeoxyglucose *in vivo:* high accumulation in macrophages and granulation tissues studied by microautoradiography. *J Nucl Med* 1992;33:1972–1980.
6. Jones HA, Clark RJ, Rhodes CG, et al. *In vivo* measurement of neutrophil activity in experimental lung inflammation. *Am J Respir Crit Care Med* 1994;149:1635–1639.
7. Yamada S, Kubota K, Kubota R, et al. High accumulation of fluorine-18-fluorodeoxyglucose in turpentine-induced inflammatory tissue. *J Nucl Med* 1995;36:1301–1306.
8. Sugawara Y, Gutowski TD, Fisher SJ, et al. Uptake of positron emission tomography tracers in experimental bacterial infections: a comparative biodistribution study of radiolabeled FDG, thymidine, L-methionine, ^{67}Ga-citrate, and ^{125}I-HSA. *Eur J Nucl Med* 1999;26:333–341.
9. Haberkorn U, Strauss LG, Dimitrakopoulou A, et al. PET studies of fluorodeoxyglucose metabolism in patients with recurrent colorectal tumors receiving radiotherapy. *J Nucl Med* 1991;32:1485–1490.
10. Larson SM. Cancer or inflammation? A Holy Grail for nuclear medicine [Editorial; comment]. *J Nucl Med* 1994;35:1653–1655.
11. Strauss LG. Fluorine-18 deoxyglucose and false-positive results: a major problem in the diagnostics of oncological patients. *Eur J Nucl Med* 1996;23:1409–1415.
12. Daley JM, Shearer JD, Mastrofrancesco B, et al. Glucose metabolism in injured tissue: a longitudinal study. *Surgery* 1990;107:187–192.
13. Higashi T, Fisher SJ, Brown RS, et al. Evaluation of the early effect of local irradiation on normal rodent bone marrow metabolism using FDG: preclinical PET studies. *J Nucl Med* 2000;41:2026–2035.

14. Anderson RL, Wood WA. Carbohydrate metabolism in microorganisms. *Annu Rev Microbiol* 1969;23:539–578.

15. Tahara T, Ichiya Y, Kuwabara Y, et al. High [^{18}F]-fluorodeoxyglucose uptake in abdominal abscesses: a PET study. *J Comput Assisted Tomogr* 1989;13:829–831.

16. Bakheet SM, Powe J. Benign causes of 18-FDG uptake on whole body imaging. *Semin Nucl Med* 1998;28:352–358.

17. Shreve PD, Anzai Y, Wahl RL. Pitfalls in oncologic diagnosis with FDG PET imaging: physiologic and benign variants. *Radiographics* 1999;19:61–77.

18. Sasaki M, Ichiya Y, Kuwabara Y, et al. Ringlike uptake of [^{18}F]FDG in brain abscess: a PET study. *J Comput Assisted Tomogr* 1990;14:486–487.

19. Meyer MA, Frey KA, Schwaiger M. Discordance between F-18 fluorodeoxyglucose uptake and contrast enhancement in a brain abscess. *Clin Nucl Med* 1993;18:682–684.

20. Dethy S, Manto M, Kentos A, et al. PET findings in a brain abscess associated with a silent atrial septal defect. *Clin Neurol Neurosurg* 1995;97:349–353.

21. Hanson MW, Glantz MJ, Hoffman JM, et al. FDG-PET in the selection of brain lesions for biopsy. *J Comput Assisted Tomogr* 1991;15:796–801.

22. Meyer MA, Hubner KF, Raja S, et al. Sequential positron emission tomographic evaluations of brain metabolism in acute herpes encephalitis. *J Neuroimaging* 1994;4:104–105.

23. Hautzel H, Muller-Gartner HW. Early changes in fluorine-18-FDG uptake during radiotherapy. *J Nucl Med* 1997;38:1384–1386.

24. Bakheet SM, Powe J, Kandil A, et al. F-18 FDG uptake in breast infection and inflammation. *Clin Nucl Med* 2000;25:100–103.

25. Patz EF Jr, Lowe VJ, Hoffman JM, et al. Focal pulmonary abnormalities: evaluation with F-18 fluorodeoxyglucose PET scanning. *Radiology* 1993;188:487–490.

26. Bakheet SM, Powe J, Ezzat A, et al. F-18-FDG uptake in tuberculosis. *Clin Nucl Med* 1998;23:739–742.

27. Kubota K, Matsuzawa T, Fujiwara T, et al. Differential diagnosis of lung tumor with positron emission tomography: a prospective study. *J Nucl Med* 1990;31:1927–1932.

28. Lowe VJ, Duhaylongsod FG, Patz EF, et al. Pulmonary abnormalities and PET data analysis: a retrospective study. *Radiology* 1997;202:435–439.

29. Bakheet SM, Saleem M, Powe J, et al. F-18 fluorodeoxyglucose chest uptake in lung inflammation and infection. *Clin Nucl Med* 2000;25:273–278.

30. Meyer MA. Diffusely increased colonic F-18 FDG uptake in acute enterocolitis. *Clin Nucl Med* 1995;20:434–435.

31. Bicik I, Bauerfeind P, Breitbach T, et al. Inflammatory bowel disease activity measured by positron-emission tomography [Letter]. *Lancet* 1997;350:262.

32. Inokuma T, Tamaki N, Torizuka T, et al. Evaluation of pancreatic tumors with positron emission tomography and F-18 fluorodeoxyglucose: comparison with CT and US. *Radiology* 1995;195:345–352.

33. Bakheet SM, Powe J. Fluorine-18-fluorodeoxyglucose uptake in rheumatoid arthritis-associated lung disease in a patient with thyroid cancer. *J Nucl Med* 1998;39:234–236.

34. Meyer M, Gast T, Raja S, et al. Increased F-18 FDG accumulation in an acute fracture. *Clin Nucl Med* 1994;19:13–14.

35. Petersdorf RG, Beeson PB. Fever of unexplained origin: report on 100 cases. *Medicine* 1961;40:1–30.

36. Meller J, Altenvoerde G, Munzel U, et al. Fever of unknown origin: prospective comparison of [^{18}F]FDG imaging with a double-head coincidence camera and gallium-67 citrate SPET. *Eur J Nucl Med* 2000;27:1617–1625.

37. Alazraki NP. Gallium-67 imaging in infection. In: Early PJ, Sodee DB, eds. *Principles and practice of nuclear medicine*. St. Louis: Mosby–Year Book, 1995:702–713.

38. Preston DF. Indium-111 label in inflammation and neoplasm imaging. In: Early PJ, Sodee DB, eds. *Principles and practice of nuclear medicine*. St. Louis: Mosby–Year Book, 1995:714–724.

39. Seabold JE, Palestro CJ, Brown ML, et al. Procedure guideline for gallium scintigraphy in inflammation. Society of Nuclear Medicine. *J Nucl Med* 1997;38:994–997.

40. Seabold JE, Forstrom LA, Schauwecker DS, et al. Procedure guideline for indium-111-leukocyte scintigraphy for suspected infection/inflammation. Society of Nuclear Medicine. *J Nucl Med* 1997;38:997–1001.

41. Datz FL, Seabold JE, Brown ML, et al. Procedure guideline for technetium-99m-HMPAO-labeled leukocyte scintigraphy for suspected infection/inflammation. Society of Nuclear Medicine. *J Nucl Med* 1997;38:987–990.

42. O'Doherty MJ, Barrington SF, Campbell M, et al. PET scanning and the human immunodeficiency virus-positive patient. *J Nucl Med* 1997;38:1575–1583.

43. Sugawara Y, Braun DK, Kison PV, et al. Rapid detection of human infections with fluorine-18 fluorodeoxyglucose and positron emission tomography: preliminary results. *Eur J Nucl Med* 1998;25:1238–1243.

44. Rosenberg A. Bones, joints, and soft tissue tumors. In: Cotran RS, Kumar V, Collins T, eds. *Robbins pathologic basis of disease*. Philadelphia: WB Saunders, 1999:1215–1268.

45. Guhlmann A, Brecht-Krauss D, Suger G, et al. Chronic osteomyelitis: detection with FDG PET and correlation with histopathologic findings. *Radiology* 1998;206:749–754.

46. Guhlmann A, Brecht-Krauss D, Suger G, et al. Fluorine-18-FDG PET and technetium-99m antigranulocyte antibody scintigraphy in chronic osteomyelitis. *J Nucl Med* 1998;39:2145–2152.

47. Kalicke T, Schmitz A, Risse JH, et al. Fluorine-18 fluorodeoxyglucose PET in infectious bone diseases: results of histologically confirmed cases. *Eur J Nucl Med* 2000;27:524–528.

48. Robiller FC, Stumpe KD, Kossmann T, et al. Chronic osteomyelitis of the femur: value of PET imaging. *Eur Radiol* 2000;10:855–858.

49. Zhuang H, Duarte PS, Pourdehand M, et al. Exclusion of chronic osteomyelitis with F-18 fluorodeoxyglucose positron emission tomographic imaging. *Clin Nucl Med* 2000;25:281–284.

50. Stumpe KD, Dazzi H, Schaffner A, et al. Infection imaging using whole-body FDG-PET. *Eur J Nucl Med* 2000;27:822–832.

51. Zhuang H, Duarte PS, Pourdehand M, et al. The promising role of ^{18}F-FDG PET in detecting infected lower limb prosthesis implants. *J Nucl Med* 2001;42:44–48.

52. Schauwecker DS. The scintigraphic diagnosis of osteomyelitis. *AJR Am J Roentgenol* 1992;158:9–18.

53. De Winter F, Van De Wiele C, De Clercq D, et al. Aseptic loosening of a knee prosthesis as imaged on FDG positron emission tomography. *Clin Nucl Med* 2000;25:923.

54. Kobzik L. The lung. In: Cotran RS, Kumar V, Collins T, eds. *Robbins pathologic basis of disease*. Philadelphia: WB Saunders, 1999:697–755.

55. Lewis PJ, Salama A. Uptake of fluorine-18-fluorodeoxyglucose in sarcoidosis. *J Nucl Med* 1994;35:1647–1649.

56. Brudin LH, Valind SO, Rhodes CG, et al. Fluorine-18 deoxyglucose uptake in sarcoidosis measured with positron emission tomography. *Eur J Nucl Med* 1994;21:297–305.

57. Yasuda S, Shohtsu A, Ide M, et al. High fluorine-18 labeled deoxyglucose uptake in sarcoidosis. *Clin Nucl Med* 1996;21:983–984.

58. Yamada Y, Uchida Y, Tatsumi K, et al. Fluorine-18-fluorodeoxyglucose and carbon-11-methionine evaluation of lymphadenopathy in sarcoidosis. *J Nucl Med* 1998;39:1160–1166.

59. Okumura W, Iwasaki T, Ueda T, et al. Usefulness of ^{18}F-FDG PET for diagnosis of cardiac sarcoidosis. *Kaku Igaku* 1999;36:341–348.

60. Kobayashi A, Shinozaki T, Shinjyo Y, et al. FDG PET in the clinical evaluation of sarcoidosis with bone lesions. *Ann Nucl Med* 2000;14:311–313.

61. Yasuda S, Shohtsu A, Ide M, et al. Elevated F-18 FDG uptake in plasmacyte-rich chronic maxillary sinusitis. *Clin Nucl Med* 1998;23:176–178.

62. Yasuda S, Shohsu A, Ide M, et al. Diffuse F-18 FDG uptake in chronic thyroiditis. *Clin Nucl Med* 1997;22:341.

63. Yasuda S, Shohtsu A, Ide M, et al. Chronic thyroiditis: diffuse uptake of FDG at PET. *Radiology* 1998;207:775–778.

64. Hara M, Goodman PC, Leder RA. FDG-PET finding in early-phase Takayasu arteritis. *J Comput Assisted Tomogr* 1999;23:16–18.

65. Smith GT, Wilson TS, Hunter K, et al. Assessment of skeletal muscle viability by PET. *J Nucl Med* 1995;36:1408–1414.

66. Yoshida K, Toki F, Takeuchi T, et al. Chronic pancreatitis caused by an autoimmune abnormality. Proposal of the concept of autoimmune pancreatitis. *Dig Dis Sci* 1995;40:1561–1568.

67. Nakamoto Y, Saga T, Ishimori T, et al. FDG-PET of autoimmune-related pancreatitis: preliminary results. *Eur J Nucl Med* 2000;27:1835–1838.

68. Nakamoto Y, Sakahara H, Higashi T, et al. Autoimmune pancreatitis

with F-18 fluoro-2-deoxy-D-glucose PET findings. *Clin Nucl Med* 1999;24:778–780.

69. Irie H, Honda H, Baba S, et al. Autoimmune pancreatitis: CT and MR characteristics. *AJR Am J Roentgenol* 1998;170:1323–1327.

70. Ichiya Y, Kuwabara Y, Sasaki M, et al. FDG-PET in infectious lesions: the detection and assessment of lesion activity. *Ann Nucl Med* 1996; 10:185–191.

71. Okazumi S, Enomoto K, Fukunaga T, et al. Evaluation of the cases of benign disease with high accumulation on the examination of ^{18}F-fluorodeoxyglucose PET. *Kaku Igaku* 1993;30:1439–1443.

72. Palmer WE, Rosenthal DI, Schoenberg OI, et al. Quantification of inflammation in the wrist with gadolinium-enhanced MR imaging and PET with 2-[F-18]-fluoro-2-deoxy-D-glucose. *Radiology* 1995;196: 647–655.

73. Yasuda S, Shohtsu A, Ide M, et al. F-18 FDG accumulation in inflamed joints. *Clin Nucl Med* 1996;21:740.

74. Taylor IK, Hill AA, Hayes M, et al. Imaging allergen-invoked airway inflammation in atopic asthma with [18F]-fluorodeoxyglucose and positron emission tomography. *Lancet* 1996;347:937–940.

75. Minn H, Paul R, Ahonen A. Evaluation of treatment response to radiotherapy in head and neck cancer with fluorine-18 fluorodeoxyglucose. *J Nucl Med* 1988;29:1521–1525.

76. Cotran RS, Kumar V, Collins T. Acute and chronic inflammation. In: Cotran RS, Kumar V, Collins T, eds. *Robbins pathologic basis of disease.* Philadelphia: WB Saunders, 1999:50–88.

77. Cotran RS, Kumar V, Collins T. Tissue repair: cellular growth, fibrosis, and wound healing. In: Cotran RS, Kumar V, Collins T, eds. *Robbins pathologic basis of disease.* Philadelphia: WB Saunders, 1999:89–112.

78. Brown RS, Leung JY, Fisher SJ, et al. Intratumoral distribution of tritiated fluorodeoxyglucose in breast carcinoma, I: are inflammatory cells important? *J Nucl Med* 1995;36:1854–1861.

79. Shreve PD. Focal fluorine-18 fluorodeoxyglucose accumulation in inflammatory pancreatic disease. *Eur J Nucl Med* 1998;25:259–264.

80. Zimny M, Buell U, Diederichs CG, et al. False-positive FDG PET in patients with pancreatic masses: an issue of proper patient selection? *Eur J Nucl Med* 1998;25:1352.

81. Fukuda H, Yoshioka S, Watanuki S, et al. Experimental study for cancer diagnosis with [18]FDG: differential diagnosis of inflammation from malignant tumor. *Kaku Igaku* 1983;20:1189–1192.

82. Kubota R, Kubota K, Yamada S, et al. Microautoradiographic study for the differentiation of intratumoral macrophages, granulation tissues and cancer cells by the dynamics of fluorine-18-fluorodeoxyglucose uptake. *J Nucl Med* 1994;35:104–112.

83. Nakamoto Y, Higashi T, Sakahara H, et al. Delayed ^{18}F-fluoro-2-deoxy-D-glucose positron emission tomography scan for differentiation between malignant and benign lesions in the pancreas. *Cancer* 2000; 89:2547–2554.

84. Lodge MA, Lucas JD, Marsden PK, et al. A PET study of [18]FDG uptake in soft tissue masses. *Eur J Nucl Med* 1999;26:22–30.

85. Hustinx R, Smith RJ, Benard F, et al. Dual time point fluorine-18 fluorodeoxyglucose positron emission tomography: a potential method to differentiate malignancy from inflammation and normal tissue in the head and neck. *Eur J Nucl Med* 1999;26:1345–1348.

86. Inoue T, Kim EE, Komaki R, et al. Detecting recurrent or residual lung cancer with FDG-PET. *J Nucl Med* 1995;36:788–793.

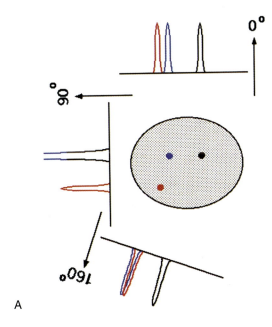

A

Projection Sinogram

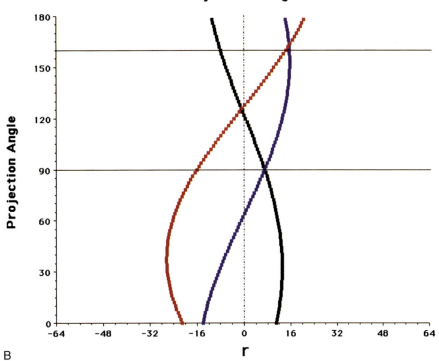

B

COLOR PLATE 1. Two-dimensional projections and projection sinogram. **A:** The top of the illustration depicts an elliptical two-dimensional object containing three discrete points of equal radioactivity (*red, blue, and black dots*). A full set of projections covers angles from 0° to 180°. Three sample projections are shown at 0°, 90°, and 160°. Due to the finite resolution of a PET system, point sources appear within a projection roughly as Gaussian distributions (*red, blue, and black curves*). If the points fall along different rays within a projection as in $p_{0°}$, the resultant curves in the projection are of equal magnitude and are separated spatially. If two of the points fall along the same ray, as seen in $p_{90°}$, only two curves are seen, the red curve representing radioactivity from one point, and the blue/black curve having twice the magnitude, representing radioactivity from the other two points. The 160° projection shows a case where two of the points are slightly offset. The resolution of the PET system determines how large a difference in r or θ is necessary to distinguish between two points within an object. Part **B** shows the projection sinogram for this object. A sinogram is a plot of all the projection rays $p(r,\theta)$, sorted as projection angle θ versus r. Note that each point of the object traces out a sinusoidal pattern in this plot, hence the name sinogram. Compare the three projections in **A** with the three horizontal lines in **B** corresponding to projection angles at 0°, 90°, and 160°. Note that the blue and black traces intersect at 90°, while the red and blue traces nearly overlap at 160°.

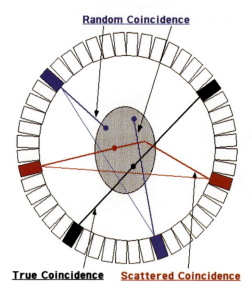

Random Coincidence

True Coincidence   Scattered Coincidence

COLOR PLATE 2. Random and scattered coincidences. One would like each detected coincidence event to correctly identify a line of response passing through the point of positron decay. For this to occur both 511 keV photons need to be detected and neither photon can be scattered in tissue. The black dot, detectors, and connecting line of response depict such a "true" coincidence event. If only one photon is detected from each of two positron decays and these are detected with the coincidence resolving time, a "random" or accidental coincidence is said to have occurred. This is depicted by the two blue dots and detectors. The two thicker blue lines indicate the path of the two detected photons, while the thinner blue line corresponds to the line of response that is recorded for this "random" coincidence event. Note that this line does not pass through either of the two points and therefore causes misplacement of the coincidence event and hence error in the reconstructed image. If both photons from a single decay are detected but one (or both) photons are scattered in the body prior to detection, the coincidence event also is misplaced as shown by the red dot, detectors, and lines. The two thicker red lines indicate the actual paths taken by the two photons, while the thinner red line indicates the line of response that is recorded for this "scattered" coincidence event. Again, the line does not pass through the point of decay and causes error in the reconstructed image.

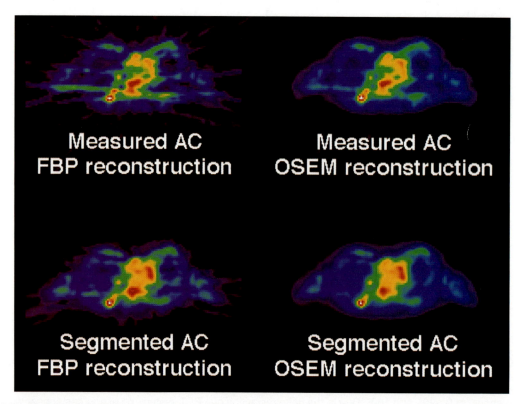

COLOR PLATE 3. Effects of segmented attenuation correction and iterative reconstruction on whole-body images. Shown are four different reconstructions of the same set of two-dimensional emission data. The **left image** is reconstructed using measured attenuation correction and filtered back-projection. The **right image** is reconstructed using measured attenuation correction and the iterative OS-EM algorithm. The **lower left image** is reconstructed using segmented attenuation correction and filtered back-projection. Finally, the **lower right image** is reconstructed using both segmented attenuation correction and OS-EM. The streak artifacts caused by back-projection are seen clearly in the upper left image. These streaks are reduced considerably either by using an iterative algorithm, or by using segmented attenuation which eliminates the majority of the noise associated with the transmission scan. The improvement when using both segmented attenuation correction and iterative reconstruction is striking.

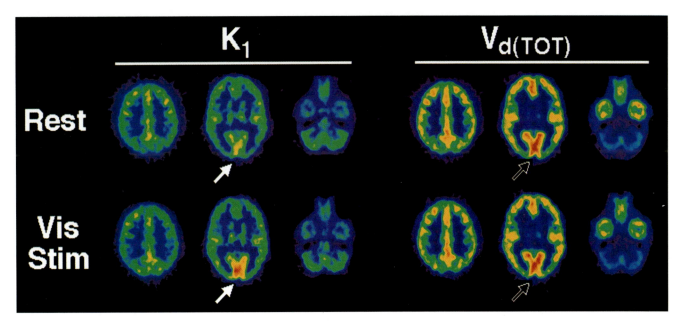

COLOR PLATE 4. Model validation: specificity of parameter estimates. Shown are functional images of two parameters, K_1 **(left)** and $V_{d(TOT)}$ **(right)**, for [^{11}C]FMZ estimated using a single tissue compartment model at three transverse levels of the brain. Calculations were performed voxel-by-voxel. The top set of images was acquired during a study with the eyes closed. The bottom set of images are from a second study on the same subject, but with visual stimulation and the eyes open. The large increase in tracer uptake due to increased flow is seen clearly in the visual cortex region of the K_1 image (*solid arrows*). In the corresponding slice there was no change in the estimate of $V_{d(TOT)}$, the index of receptor density (*open arrows*). This validation study demonstrates the specificity of the receptor density measure, $V_{d(TOT)}$, due to its insensitivity to changes in flow.

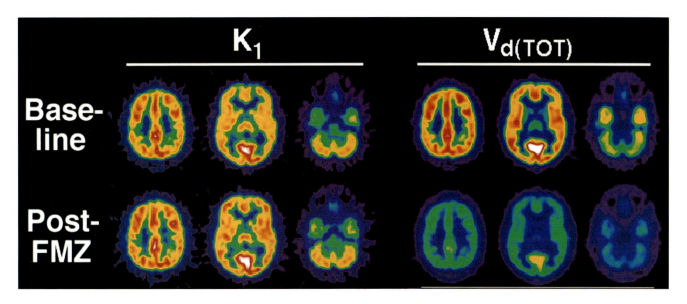

COLOR PLATE 5. Model validation: sensitivity of parameter estimates; single-tissue compartment model. Shown are a similar set of functional images from a pair of [^{11}C]FMZ studies on another individual, but with the two scans being performed before and following administration of a partial blocking dose of unlabeled FMZ. The transport estimate is nearly identical before and after administration of cold FMZ, while a global decrease of 35% to 40% is seen in the receptor density measure $V_{d(TOT)}$. This validation study demonstrates the sensitivity of the receptor measure to changes in binding site availability.

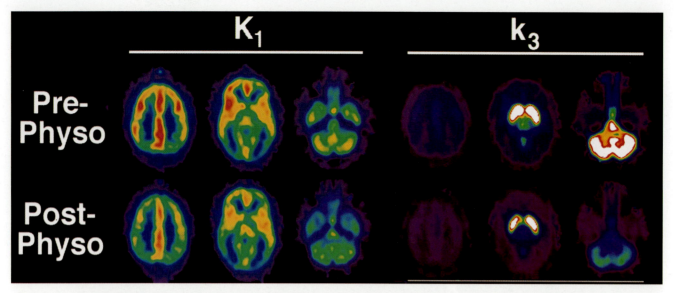

COLOR PLATE 6. Model validation: sensitivity of parameter estimates; 2-tissue compartment model. Shown are functional images from a pair of scans using N [^{11}C]methylpiperidinyl propionate (PMP), a substrate for the enzyme acetylcholinesterase (AChE). The top images were acquired at baseline while the bottom images were acquired following administration of 1.5 mg physostigmine, an AChE inhibitor. The distribution of AChE is seen to vary widely across the brain with enzyme activity being 20 to 25 times higher in basal ganglia than in cortex (making visual display of the k_3 images difficult). The brain uptake as measured by K_1 is seen to have decreased slightly, while the index of AChE activity is decreased by approximately 50% in all brain regions (most easily seen in cerebellum and brainstem). This validation study demonstrates the sensitivity of the index of AChE activity, k_3, to changes in the concentration of the enzyme.

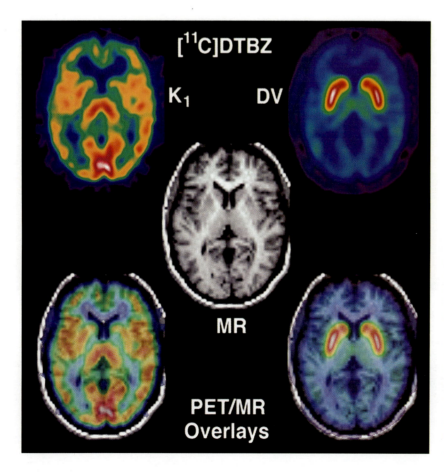

COLOR PLATE 7. Functional and anatomic image registration: PET and MR. Shown for a single transverse level of the brain are functional images of the two model parameters for [^{11}C]DTBZ, K_1 and $V_{d(TOT)}$ (**top left and right**, respectively), and the co-registered image of the corresponding brain level from an MR scan of the same subject (**middle**). The overlays of the two functional images are seen superimposed on the co-registered structural MR image in the bottom corners. PET and MR data sets were registered by maximization of their mutual information (see text).

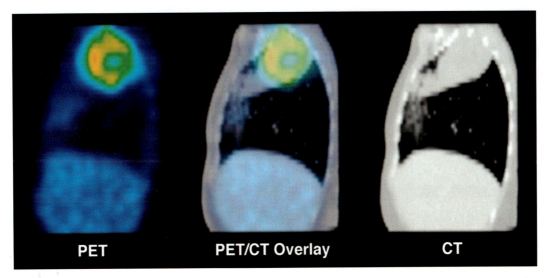

COLOR PLATE 8. Functional and anatomic image registration: PET and CT. Shown for a single sagittal section of the body are a functional image of glucose metabolism using [^{18}F]FDG, (**left**), the corresponding co-registered image from a CT scan of the same subject (**right**), and the overlay of functional and anatomic information (**middle**). PET and CT data sets were registered by maximization of their mutual information and includes non-linear warping by thin-plate splines (see text) to account for different body positions of the subject in the PET and CT gantries.

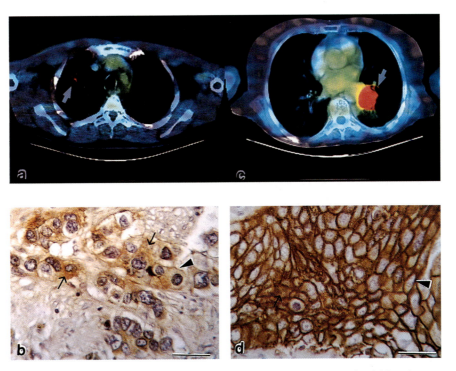

COLOR PLATE 9. FDG uptake on PET (fused with CT using computer methods) into lung cancers in different patients. The FDG avid tumor on the right has high cellularity and highly Glut-1 positive cancer cells. The tumor on the left has lower FDG uptake and lower Glut-1 positivity.

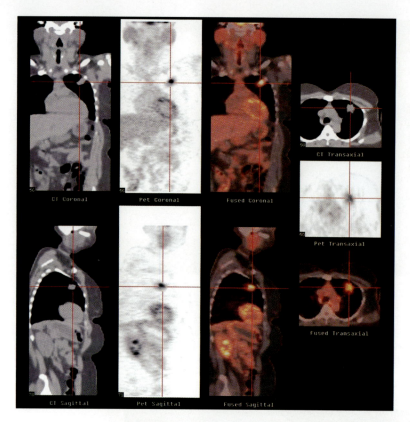

COLOR PLATE 10. "Anatomolecular" images obtained from a patient with suspected lung cancer using the Discovery LS (GE) PET/CT system. Fusion of molecular functional information with CT is achieved and demonstrates intense uptake into a left lung abnormality seen on CT, which indicates primary lung cancer.

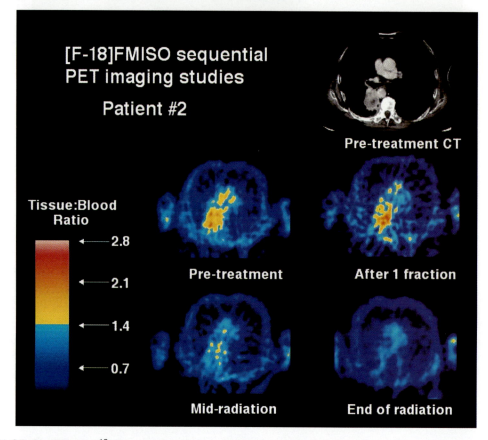

COLOR PLATE 11. [^{18}F]Fluoromisonidazole (FMISO) images from a patient with unresectable non-small cell lung cancer. The patient was imaged before, during, and at the end of a 4-week course of neutron radiation. The image intensity scale is set so that areas of hypoxia appear yellow to red and had a FMISO tumor: blood ratio greater than or equal to 1.4. (From Koh WJ, Bergman KS, Rasey JS, et al. Evaluation of oxygenation status during fractionated radiotherapy in human nonsmall cell lung cancers using [F-18]fluoromisonidazole positron emission tomography. Int J Radiat Oncol Biol Phys 1995; 33:391–398, with permission.)

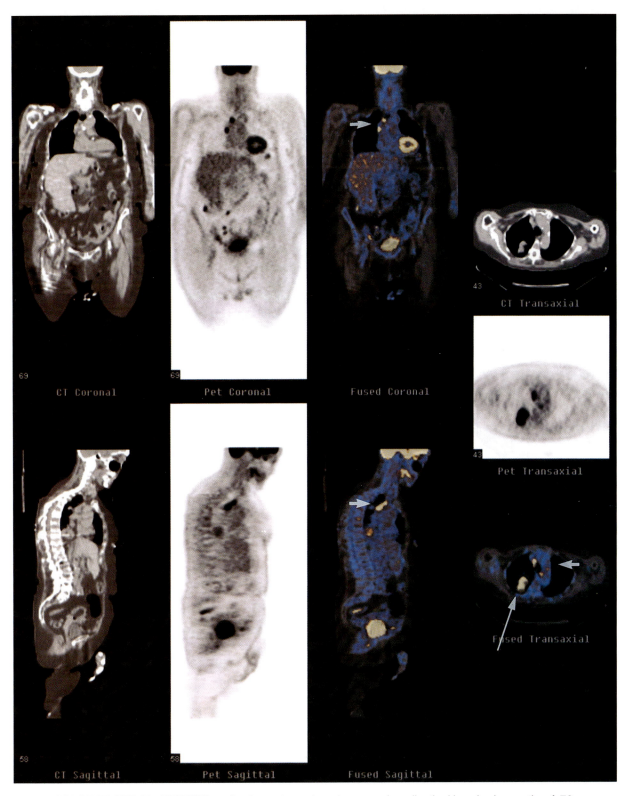

CT Coronal	Pet Coronal	Fused Coronal

CT Transaxial

Pet Transaxial

CT Saqittal	Pet Saqittal	Fused Saqittal

Fused Transaxial

COLOR PLATE 12. PET/CT imaging in a primary lung tumor and mediastinal lymphadenopathy. A 78-year-old woman had a past history of heavy smoking. The **upper three images** are coronal, whole body slices with CT on the left, PET in the center and fused PET/CT images on the right. The **lower three images** are sagittal slices in the same sequence. The three images on the right are the transaxial slices: CT at the top, PET in the center, and fused PET/CT images at the bottom. Transaxial CT shows a space occupying lesion, 5 cm in diameter, in the right upper lobe. Transaxial PET shows abnormal FDG uptake in this lesion and additional areas of increased activity in the mediastinum. Images were obtained using dedicated PET/CT (Discovery LS, GE Medical Systems) show the primary lesion (*thin arrow*) and localize additional areas of pathological uptake in the right pretracheal region and hilar lymphadenopathy (*thick arrows*).

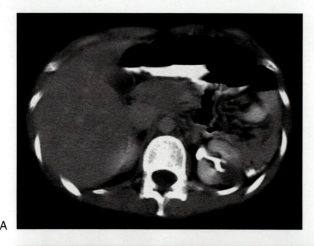

A

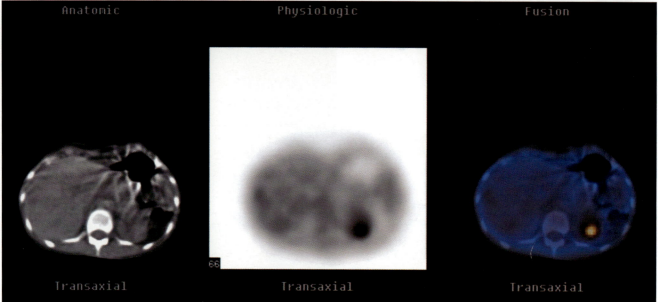

Anatomic	Physiologic	Fusion
Transaxial	Transaxial	Transaxial

B

COLOR PLATE 13. Dual head coincidence/CT imaging for exclusion of cancer in an area of increased FDG uptake and findings on CT. A 35-year-old woman with a history of aggressive non-Hodgkin's lymphoma, status post chemotherapy. The patient was referred for restaging. High resolution CT (**A**) shows a round hypodense lesion in the mid-third of the left kidney parenchyma. Camera-based PET following injection of FDG using coincidence and x-ray imaging (Hawkeye & 1″ crystal VG, GE Medical Systems) shows an area of increased uptake at the level of the left kidney (**B**, *center*). Fused images (**B**, *right*) show the localization of the area of increased FDG activity in the renal pelvis with no abnormal uptake in the renal cortical lesion. In this case fused PET/CT imaging clarified the location of normal FDG uptake.

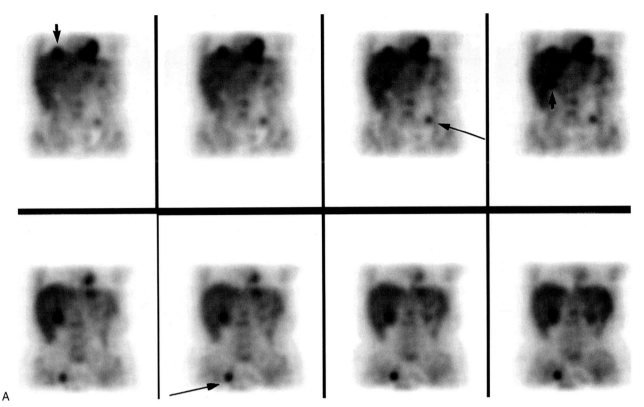

A

COLOR PLATE 14. Dual head coincidence/CT imaging for precise localization of additional sites of disease and exclusion of malignancy in areas of physiologic FDG uptake. A 55-year-old woman had a past history of ovarian cancer, and was status post surgery and chemotherapy 8 years prior to the scan. Routine laboratory examinations showed a slight but steady increase in serum marker levels. CT detected two hepatic lesions. Partial hepatectomy was considered and camera-based FDG PET and x-ray imaging (Hawkeye & 1″ crystal VG, GE Medical Systems) was performed to establish tumor resectability. FDG study (**A**) shows two areas of abnormal uptake in the liver (*thick arrows*). Two additional areas of increased activity are seen on both sides of the pelvis (*thin arrows*). *(continued)*

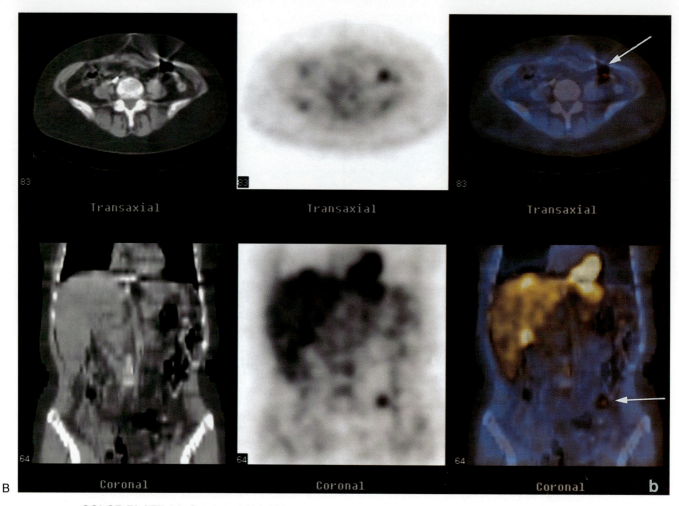

Transaxial	Transaxial	Transaxial
Coronal	Coronal	Coronal

B · b

COLOR PLATE 14 *Continued.* Hybrid images at the level of the suspected left pelvic lesion (**B**) localize the area of increased FDG uptake to physiologic colon excretion (*arrows*). *(continued)*

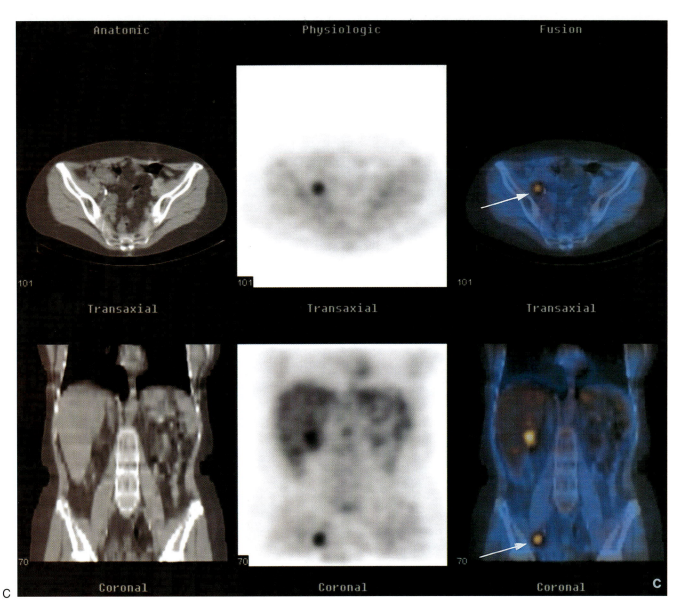

COLOR PLATE 14 *Continued.* CT (*left*), coincidence (*center*), and fused (*right*) (**C**) localize the abnormal FDG uptake to right external iliac lymphadenopathy (*arrows*). Retrospective evaluation of high resolution CT visualized a mildly enlarged right inguinal lymph node, 12 mm in diameter. Planned surgery was canceled and the patient was referred for chemotherapy.

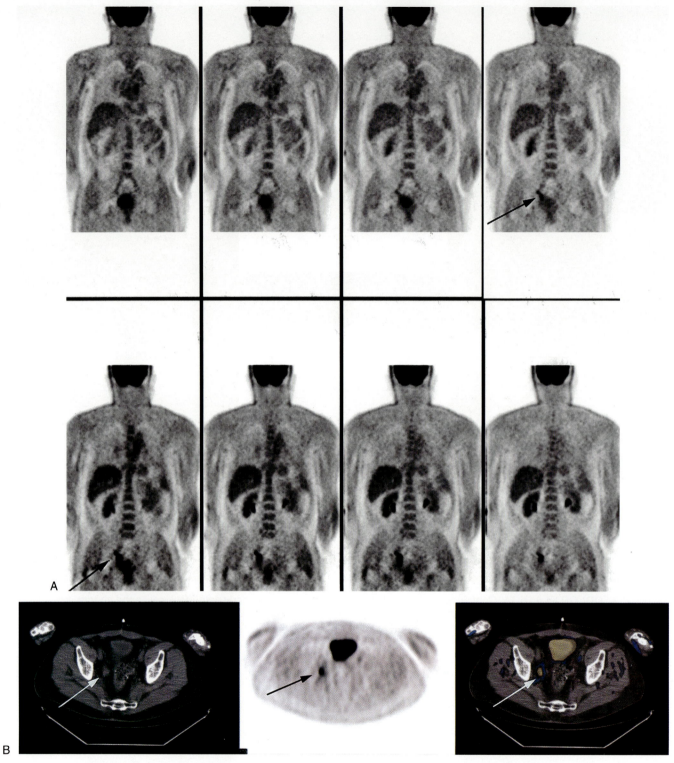

COLOR PLATE 15. PET/CT imaging for precise localization of malignancy in normal size lymph nodes. A 56-year-old man had a history of adenocarcinoma of the rectum, status post surgery, chemotherapy, and radiotherapy. The patient was referred for a PET/CT (Discovery LS, GE Medical Systems) study due to elevated CEA blood levels and a normal CT. FDG PET (**A**) shows an area of focal increased uptake in the right anatomic pelvis, adjacent to the urinary bladder (*arrows*). This abnormal uptake is localized by fusion images (**B**) to a normal sized lymph node in the perirectal fat on the right side (*arrows*), close to the prior surgical field. In retrospect there was a slight increase in the diameter of this node as compared to CT images performed 3 months earlier, indicating tumor recurrence.

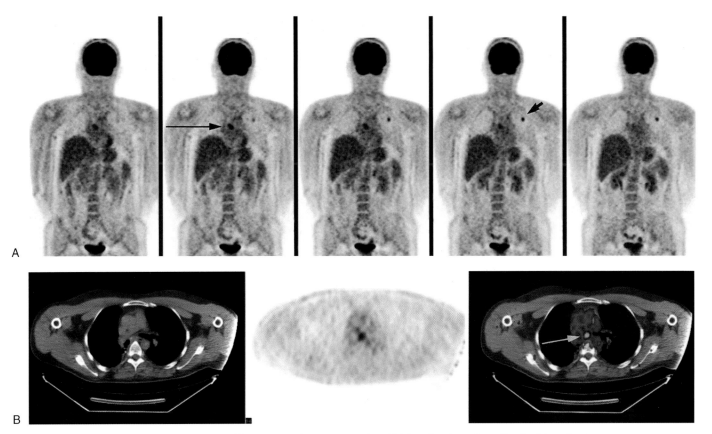

COLOR PLATE 16. PET/CT images for retrospective CT localization of mediastinal lymphadenopathy. A 36-year-old man had a history of right lung cancer, status post neoadjuvant chemotherapy and surgery, in remission for 3 years. Routine follow up showed a mass in the left upper lobe, 12 mm in diameter. PET/CT (Discovery LS, GE Medical Systems) was performed to establish a diagnosis and resectability of this new lesion. PET (**A**) shows FDG uptake in the left upper lobe (*thick arrow*), consistent with the lesion seen on CT. There is an additional area of increased uptake in the mediastinum (*thin arrow*). Fusion images (**B**) localize this mediastinal uptake to a subcarinal lymph node, 10 x 15 mm in size, only retrospectively detected on CT (*arrow*). Planned surgery was cancelled and fused imaging coordinates were used for radiotherapy planning.

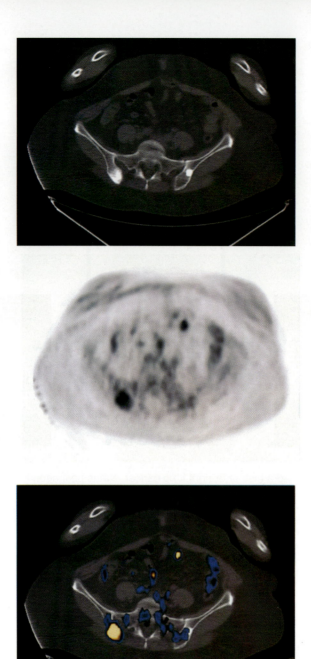

COLOR PLATE 17. PET/CT imaging for localization of distant bone metastases. A 76-year-old woman with non-small cell lung cancer, status post right upper lobectomy and radiotherapy. The patient was referred for further evaluation of a right upper lung infiltrate, with a differential diagnosis of postradiation pneumonitis or recurrence of disease. FDG-PET of the thorax showed diffuse increased uptake in the right lung, consistent with inflammatory postradiation changes. An area of abnormal FDG uptake is seen on the PET study in the right pelvis (**middle**). Fused image (**bottom**) (Discovery LS, GE Medical Systems) localizes this area of uptake to a sclerotic lesion seen on CT (**top**) in the right iliac wing, consistent with an osteoblastic bone metastasis. CT also shows a second round, sclerotic, well-circumscribed lesion in the left ilium, which has no corresponding FDG uptake and is consistent with a benign sclerotic bone island.

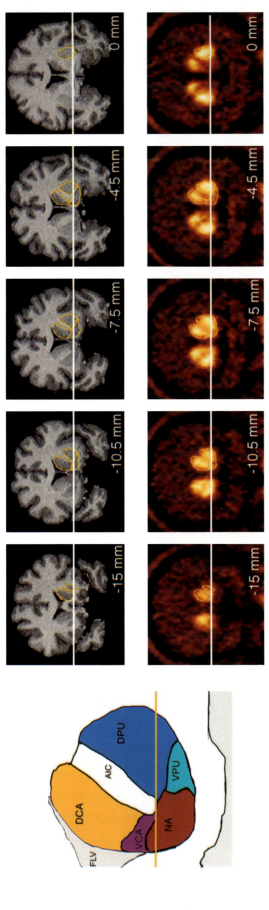

COLOR PLATE 18. PET imaging of striatal substructures. The anterior striatum includes several subregions that are involved in different brain functions. The ventral striatum, which includes the nucleus accumbens (NA), the ventral caudate (VCA) and ventral putamen (VPU), is part of the limbic system, and is involved in the reward and drives mediations. This might be the site where blockade of D_2 receptors by antipsychotic drugs is responsible for their therapeutic effects. The dorsal caudate (DCA) and dorsal putamen (DPU) are involved in the mediations of cognitive and motor functions, and might be the site where blockade of D_2 receptors by antipsychotic drug is responsible for their extrapyramidal effects. These regions were drawn on the coronal MRI slides and on coregistered [^{11}C]raclopride PET scans. Columns represent coronal sections at levels −15.0, −10.5, −7.5, −4.5, and 0 mm anterior to the plane of the anterior commissure (levels anterior to AC level are denoted by negative numbers). The horizontal solid line identifies the transaxial AC/PC plane. Modern PET technology enables the measurement of activity concentration in these subregions with a high level of reproducibility. Accuracy of these measurements requires partial volume correction (see ref. 52 in chapter 7).

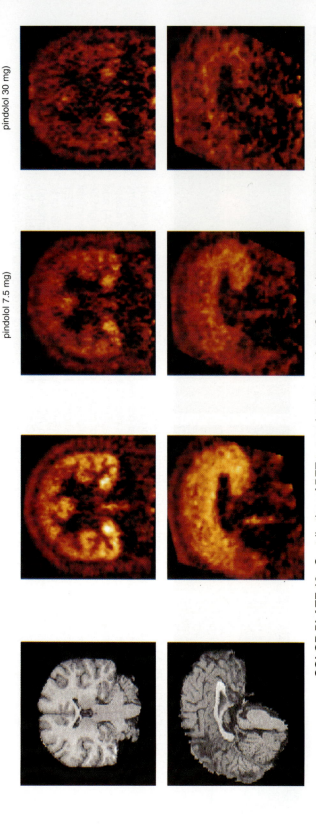

COLOR PLATE 19. Contribution of PET to psychopharmacology. Coronal (**top row**) and sagittal (**bottom row**) MRI and coregistered PET images following injection of [^{11}C]WAY 100635 in a 29-year-old male under baseline conditions, and following administration of the 5-HT1A partial agonist pindolol 7.5 mg and 30 mg. The PET image is the sum of 5 frames of 10 min duration/frame between 30 and 80 min. Activity was corrected for the injected dose and color-coded using the same scale across the three scans. At each dose, pindolol administration is associated with a decrease in specific binding of the radiotracer to 5-HT1A receptors. This study (see ref. 165 in chapter 7) revealed that the dose of pindolol used in clinical trials of augmentation of SSRI therapeutic action in depression (7.5 mg QD) induced only low and variable occupancy of 5HT1A receptors. This factor presumably accounts for the inconsistent results of these clinical studies.

MRI

Scan 1
(Baseline)

Scan 2
(4 h after
pindolol 7.5 mg)

Scan 4
(4 h after
pindolol 30 mg)

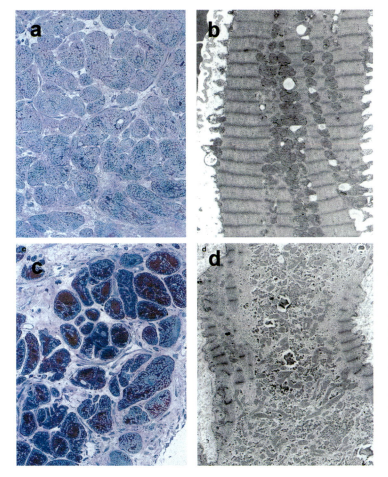

COLOR PLATE 20. a: Light micrograph of myocardium showing normal cardiomyocytes with virtually no glycogen (PAS staining in red). **b:** Transmission electron micrograph of normal cardiac myocytes. **c:** Representative light micrograph of a biopsy sample of human hibernating myocardium. Cardiac myocytes are depleted of their contractile material and filled with glycogen (PAS-positive staining). **d:** Representative transmission electron micrograph of a hibernating cardiomyocyte. Myocytic cytoplasm is devoid of sarcomeres and filled with glycogen. Original magnification: a and c, x320; b x7100; and d, x7500. (From Vanoverschelde J-L et al. *Circulation.* 1997;95:1961–1971, with permission.)

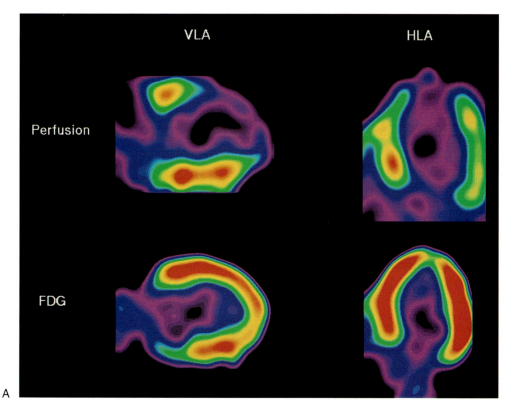

COLOR PLATE 21. Examples of perfusion/FDG imaging patterns. *Color scale:* lowest to highest radioactivity concentration = black/blue/green/yellow/red (yellow/red are normal). **A:** Perfusion/metabolism mismatch in the anterior, lateral, and anteroseptal regions indicating extensive hibernating myocardium and high risk. This patient died awaiting revascularization. *(continued)*

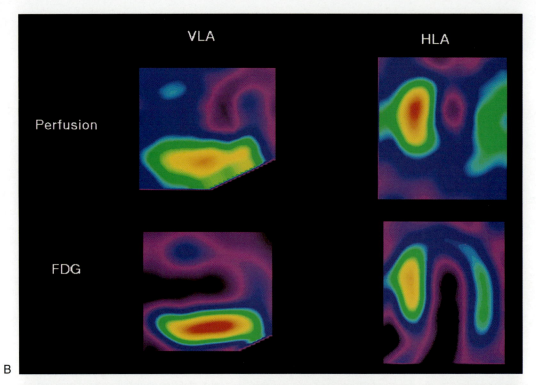

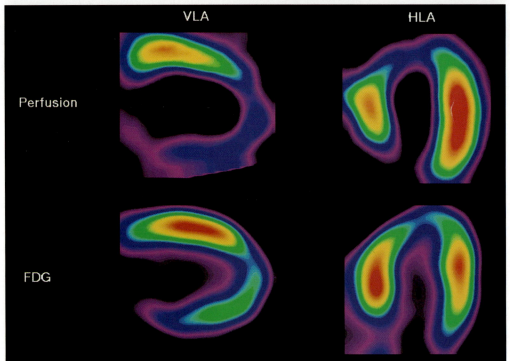

COLOR PLATE 21. *Continued.* **B:** Perfusion/metabolism matched defect in the anterior, lateral, and apical regions indicating extensive scar. This 45-year-old woman subsequently underwent cardiac transplant. **C:** Partial mismatch in the inferior wall and apex indicating a mixture of nontransmural scar and hibernating myocardium. This patient underwent revascularization and had a modest improvement in ejection fraction from 23% to 28%. *(continued)*

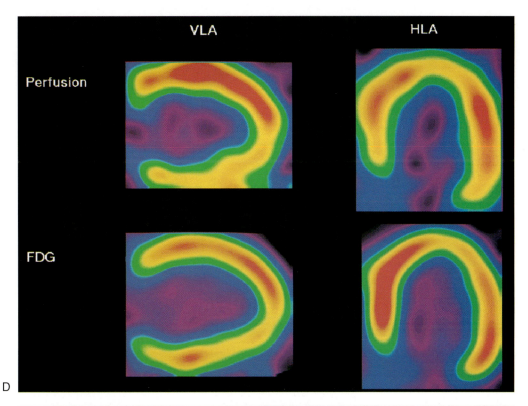

D

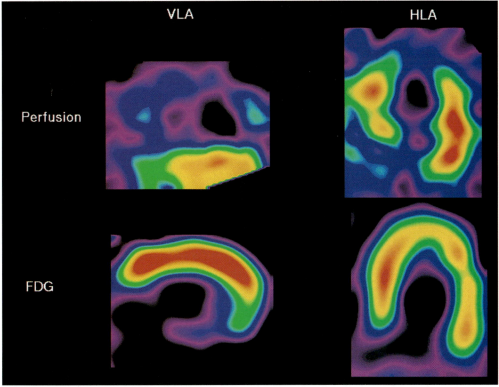

E

COLOR PLATE 21. *Continued.* **D:** "Normal" perfusion/metabolism pattern in most of the left ventricle (LV) indicating maintained relative perfusion and metabolism at rest. This patient had severe proximal 3-vessel disease and global LV dysfunction. Much of the myocardium was probably "stunned" due to prior ischemic episodes. Ejection fraction improved from 32% to 53% after revascularization. **E:** Reverse mismatch in the inferior wall. There is a large mismatch in the anterior wall and apex. In this case, the reverse mismatch is due to normalization error because of the intense FDG uptake in the contralateral anterior wall. The patient had single vessel proximal LAD disease and underwent successful PTCA with improvement in heart failure symptoms.

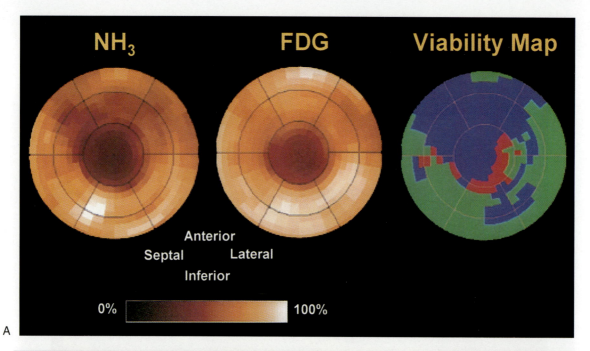

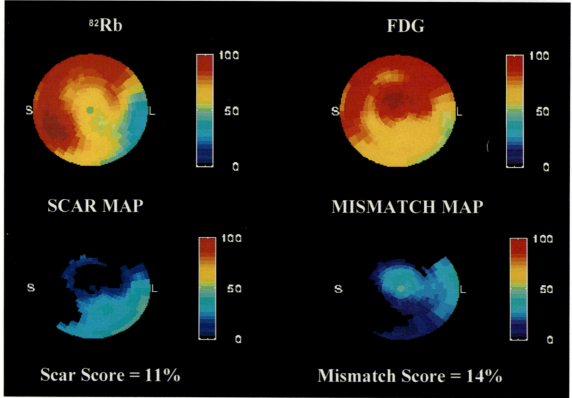

COLOR PLATE 22. Examples of semi-quantitative polar map displays. **A:** ^{13}NH-ammonia perfusion and FDG polar maps are shown. The viability map (*right*) shows the percentage of the left ventricular myocardium with "normally" perfused myocardium (green), "flow-metabolism mismatch" (blue) and "scar tissue" (red). (From Haas et al. *Eur Jour of Cardio-thoracic Surgery* 2001;20: 290–298, with permission.) **B:** ^{82}Rb perfusion and FDG polar maps are shown. The lower maps are on the same color scale to show the size and extent of the abnormal myocardium expressed as a percentage of the total LV for both scar tissue and mismatch. The advantage of **A** is the ease of interpretation of the parametric map and emphasis on the mismatch in a segment. The advantage of **B** is that when there is mixture of scar and mismatch it can be defined in the same segment.

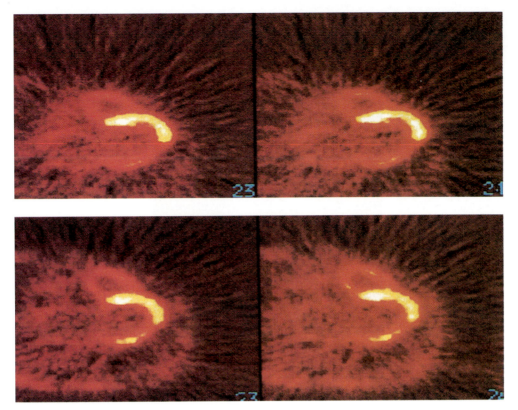

COLOR PLATE 23. FDG PET myocardial imaging (transaxial views) in a patient treated with revascularization and cellular cardiomyoplasty to an infarcted region in the posterior wall. **Upper panel:** Before treatment there is homogenous metabolic activity in the anterior and septal walls with a decrease in metabolic activity in the posterior wall. **Lower panel:** Five months after treatment FDG uptake in the posterior wall has increased suggesting the presence of metabolic activity in viable cells in the region of the previous infarct. Wall motion also improved in this region. (From Menasch P et al. *The Lancet* 2001;37, with permission.)

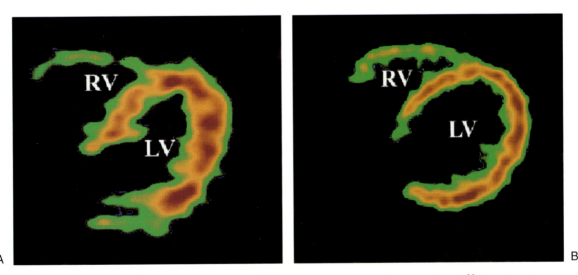

A   B

COLOR PLATE 24. Representative transaxial images showing maximal uptake of ^{11}C-acetate in a healthy volunteer (**A**) and a patient with congestive heart failure due to dilated cardiomyopathy (**B**). ^{11}C-acetate uptake is enhanced in the right ventricle (RV) of the patient with heart failure. LV, left ventricle. (From Ukkonen H. *Clin Pharmacol Ther* 2000;68:522-531, with permission.)

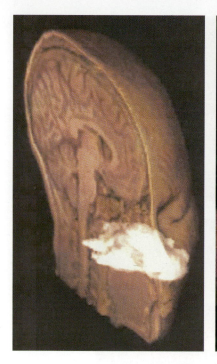
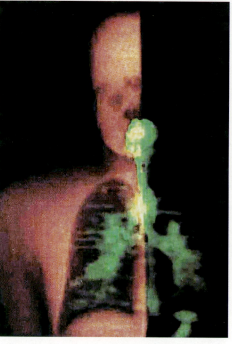

COLOR PLATE 25. Inhalation therapy. Distribution at early times within the nasal passages (**left panel**) and subsequent distribution throughout the bronchial tree. (From Berridge MS, Heald DL. In vivo characterization of inhaled pharmaceuticals using quantitative positron emission tomography. *J Clin Pharmacol* 1999; 39:25S–29S, with permission.)

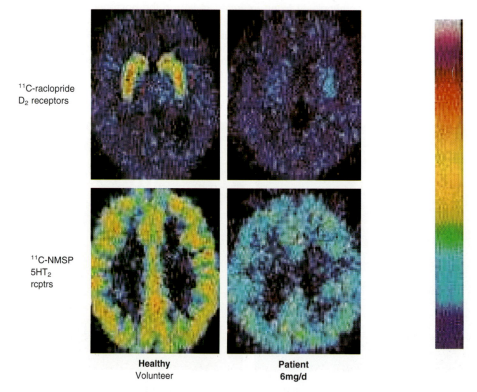

^{11}C-raclopride
D_2 receptors

^{11}C-NMSP
$5HT_2$
rcptrs

Healthy
Volunteer

Patient
6mg/d

COLOR PLATE 26. Impact of the antipsychotic drug, risperidone (6 mg/d), on D_2 and $5HT_2$ neuroreceptors. The **right panel** indicates that D_2 receptors are almost completely blocked by this dose of risperidone. In the **bottom left panel** the broad pattern of spatial distribution for $5HT_2$ receptors in the human brain can be identified as quite different from the narrower localization of D_2 receptors (**upper left**). A substantial blockage of $5HT_2$ receptors by risperidone can be observed, but the quantitative extent is lower than the drug's impact on D_2 receptors. (From Farde L, Nyberg S, Oxenstierna G, et al. Positron emission tomography studies on D_2 and 5-HT_2 receptor binding in risperidone-treated schizophrenic patients. *J Clin Psychopharmacol* 1995;15(Suppl 1):19S–23S, with permission.)

Pre-tamoxifen

day 7-tamoxifen

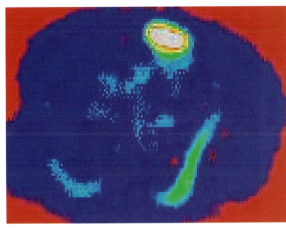
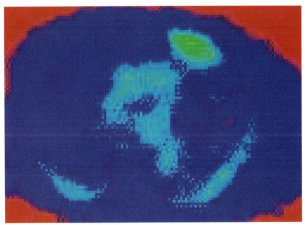

SUV = 5.0

SUV = 1.5 receptor occupied

COLOR PLATE 27. A patient with estrogen-receptor positive metastases of breast cancer in the pleural space. ^{18}F-Fluoroestradiol is the radiopharmaceutical. The PET image obtained prior to therapy clearly shows tracer uptake by the tumor (oval at top of **left panel**). The **right panel** is the same image slice after 7 days of tamoxifen therapy. A decrease in tracer uptake is apparent in the lesion. (From Dehdashti F, Flanagan FL, Mortimer JE, et al. Positron emission tomographic assessment of "metabolic flare" to predict response of metastatic breast cancer to antiestrogen therapy. *Eur J Nucl Med* 1999; 26:51–56, with permission.)

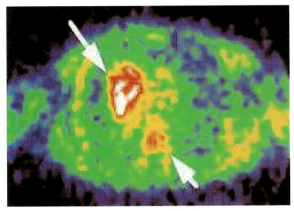
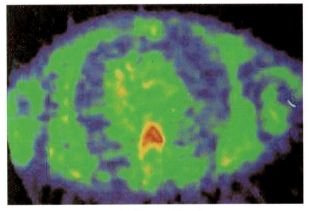

Before Therapy (day 0)

After Therapy (day 6)

COLOR PLATE 28. A patient with primary lung cancer was evaluated with ^{11}C-d-thymidine (^{11}C-dThd) as the probe. Prior to therapy (**left panel**) transverse PET images show extensive uptake of ^{11}C-dThd was observed both in the tumor (*large arrow*) and the vertebral space (*small arrow*). In the **right panel**, the same patient was evaluated on day 6 of therapy, after a dose of cisplatin on day 1 and etoposide on days 1 to 3. The tumor was still present anatomically, but it had stopped taking up ^{11}C-dThd. This tracer is used to image DNA synthesis and cell proliferation. (From Shields AF, Mankoff DA, Link JM, et al. Carbon-11-thymidine and FDG to measure therapy response. *J Nucl Med* 1998; 39:1757–1762, with permission.)

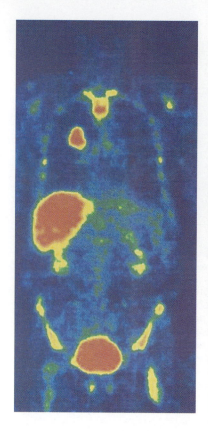
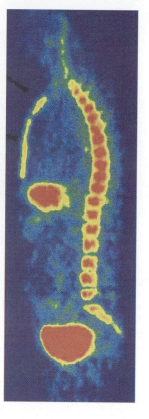

COLOR PLATE 29. Coronal (**left**) and sagittal (**right**) PET images obtained using ^{18}F-FLT, 1.3 mCi, administered to a patient with a lung tumor and imaged at 60 min. post injection. Uptake in the right upper lung, liver, bone marrow, and bladder is seen. (Adapted from Shields AF, Grierson JR, Dohmen BM, et al. Imaging proliferation in vivo with [F-18]FLT and positron emission tomography. *Nat Med* 1998; 4:1334–1336, with permission.)

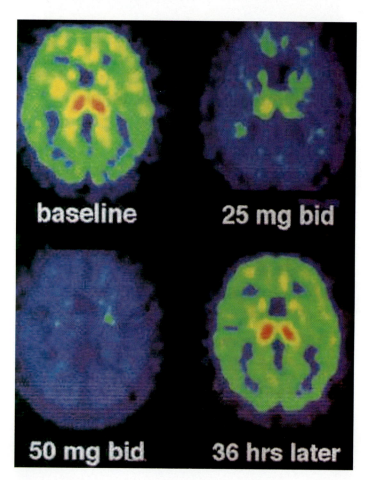

COLOR PLATE 30. Reversible dose-dependent monoamine oxidase B (MAO B) inhibition by lazabemide. (From Fowler JS, Volkow ND, Logan J, et al. MAO B inhibitor therapy in Parkinson's disease: the degree and reversibility of human brain MAO B inhibition by Ro 19 6327. *Neurology* 1993; 43:1984–1992, with permission.)

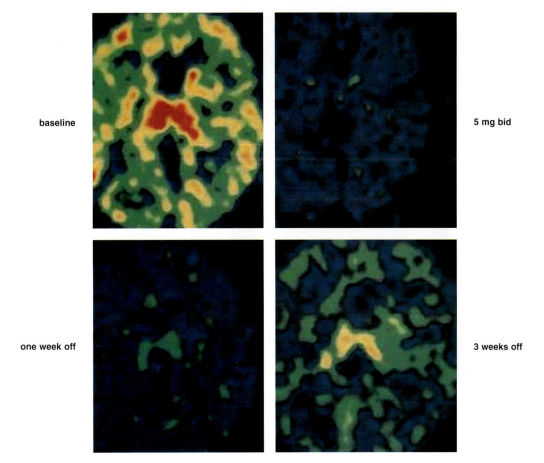

baseline

5 mg bid

one week off

3 weeks off

COLOR PLATE 31. Irreversible inhibition of monoamine oxidase B (MAO B) by selegiline. (From Fowler JS, Volkow ND, Logan J, et al. Slow recovery of human brain MAO B after L-deprenyl (selegiline) withdrawal. *Synapse* 1994; 18:86–93, with permission.)

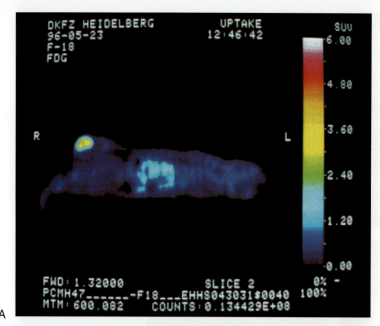

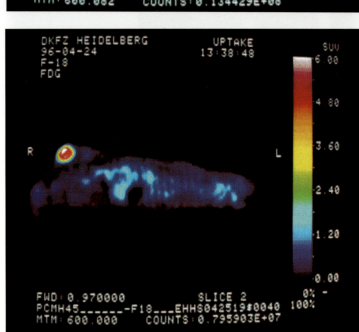

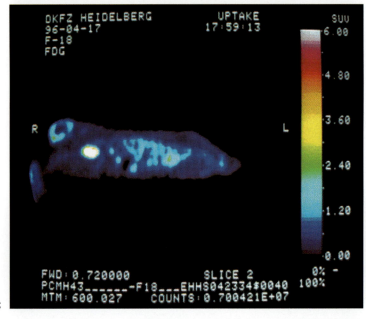

COLOR PLATE 32. FDG uptake (80–90 min *p.i.*) in animals with HSV-tk-expressing tumors after sodium chloride administration (**A**) as well as two days (**B**) and four days (**C**) after the start of treatment with 100 mg GCV/kg bw. Intense tracer activity is seen in the bladder in this image due to normal excretion of FDG. The images are standardized to the injected dose and the body weight (bw) of the animals. R, right; L, left.

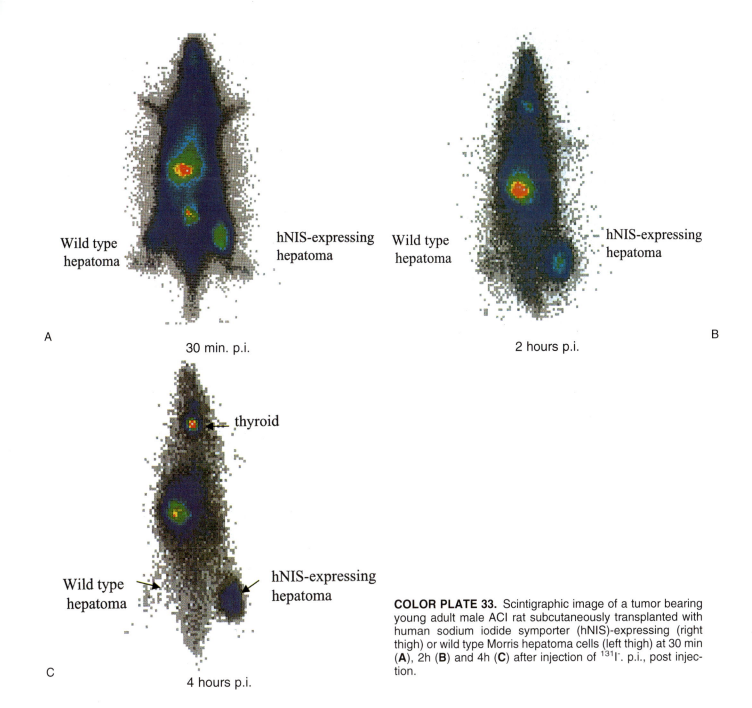

Wild type hepatoma

hNIS-expressing hepatoma

A

30 min. p.i.

Wild type hepatoma

hNIS-expressing hepatoma

B

2 hours p.i.

thyroid

Wild type hepatoma

hNIS-expressing hepatoma

C

4 hours p.i.

COLOR PLATE 33. Scintigraphic image of a tumor bearing young adult male ACI rat subcutaneously transplanted with human sodium iodide symporter (hNIS)-expressing (right thigh) or wild type Morris hepatoma cells (left thigh) at 30 min (**A**), 2h (**B**) and 4h (**C**) after injection of $^{131}I^-$. p.i., post injection.

CHAPTER 10

Pediatrics

Hossein Jadvar, Leonard P. Connolly, and Barry L. Shulkin

Experience using positron emission tomography (PET) in pediatric diseases has followed its uses in adult medicine. Reports of PET in pediatrics are fewer in number than in adults, in part because some of the conditions studied in adult patients are much less common in pediatric patients. Only about 2% of all cancers, for example, occur before age 15 years. Furthermore, currently only a few PET units are in pediatric hospitals. Nevertheless, PET is emerging as an important tool in pediatric nuclear medicine. In this chapter, we review the clinical applications of PET in pediatrics, with an emphasis on the more common applications in epilepsy and oncology. General considerations in patient preparation and radiation dosimetry are also discussed.

PATIENT PREPARATION

Preparation of children and parents for nuclear medicine imaging has been thoroughly reviewed elsewhere (1,2). As with any imaging study, gaining the trust and allaying the fears of both the patient and the parents are essential before attempting to image. Patient cooperation may be ensured by relatively simple methods. Sheets wrapped around the body, sandbags, and special holding devices are often sufficient for immobilization. Parents usually accompany their child during the course of a study to provide emotional support, although on occasion, children are more cooperative when their parents are absent.

Sedation is indicated when, on the basis of careful consideration, it is anticipated that simple methods will be inadequate to ensure acceptable image quality. Sedation protocols, particularly regarding the recommended medications and the level of sedation required for an imaging procedure, vary from institution to institution. Guidelines, such as those advanced by the Society of Nuclear Medicine (3), are useful in developing an institutional sedation program and a sedation formulary.

Also important to consider are the potential effects of sedatives on ^{18}F-fluorodeoxyglucose (FDG) tracer distribution. Many sedatives may affect cerebral metabolism. When performing FDG PET of the brain, it is preferable to withhold sedation for 30 minutes after FDG administration, because this is the period during which most of cerebral FDG uptake occurs. Sedatives are not known to cause significant changes in tumoral metabolism and can be administered at any time relative to FDG administration for studies of tumors outside the central nervous system (CNS) (4). We attempt to minimize the period of sedation and sedate children as close to the time of imaging as possible.

RADIATION DOSIMETRY

Administered doses of FDG ranging from 0.15 to 0.30 mCi/kg (5 to 10 MBq/kg) have been recommended for pediatric use (5). Special consideration must be given to neonates and infants in whom the concept of minimal total dose is applied. This is the radiopharmaceutical dose below which a study will be inadequate regardless of the body weight or surface area. For FDG PET imaging with dedicated PET scanners, a minimal dose of 1 mCi (37 MBq) may be used. The maximum dose is 20 mCi (750 MBq).

The radiation dose from an intravenous injection of FDG has been studied in adults (6). The radiation dose to infants has been reported in one study (7). The target organ is the bladder wall, which receives 3.81 ± 7.77 rad/mCi (1.03 ± 2.10 mGy/MBq), and is about fourfold higher than the absorbed dose per unit of administered activity in adults. Good hydration and voiding or early drainage of the urine reduces the absorbed bladder wall dose.

Infants also receive a higher absorbed dose to the brain (by a factor of about 10) per unit of administered dose (0.89 ± 0.18 rad/mCi or 0.24 ± 0.05 mGy/MBq) than that received by the adult brain. This is due to a slightly higher percentage of FDG uptake in the infant brain (8.8%) compared with the adult brain (6.9%) and differing cerebral tracer distribution, with higher tracer accumulation in the infant subcortical gray matter in contrast to the higher uptake by the adult cortical gray matter.

Heart, liver, and pancreas also receive a higher absorbed dose per unit of administered activity in infants than in adults. Due to the low administered FDG dose in infants, the total body absorbed radiation dose is lower than, or similar to, that of adults and that imposed by the other radiographic and scintigraphic procedures (4,7).

PET IN PEDIATRIC NEUROLOGY

Normal Brain Development

An understanding of normal brain development and evolution of cerebral glucose utilization is important when FDG PET is considered as a diagnostic functional imaging study. Glucose metabolism is initially high in the sensorimotor cortex, thalamus, brainstem, and cerebellar vermis. During the first 3 months of life, glucose metabolism gradually increases in the basal ganglia and in the parietal, temporal, calcarine, and cerebellar cortices. Maturation of the frontal cortex and the dorsolateral cortex occurs during the second 6 months of life. Cerebral FDG distribution in children older than 1 year resembles that of adults (Fig. 10.1) (8–10).

Epilepsy

Epilepsy is a relatively common neurologic condition during childhood. Its incidence in children and adolescents is between 40 and 100 per 100,000 (11). The 1990 National Institutes of Health Consensus Conference on Surgery for Epilepsy estimated that 10% to 20% of epilepsy cases prove medically intractable and that 2,000 to 5,000 epileptic patients per year can benefit from surgical resection of the seizure focus (12).

Accurate preoperative localization of the epileptogenic region is an essential but difficult task that is best accomplished by finding a concordance between results obtained with clinical examination, electroencephalography (EEG), neuropsychologic evaluation, and imaging studies. Computed tomography (CT) and magnetic resonance imaging (MRI) are used to detect anatomic lesions that may cause the seizures. However, structural lesions occur in a relatively small percentage of patients with epilepsy, and when such lesions are detected, they may not necessarily represent the epileptogenic region (13). Ictal or interictal single-photon emission tomography (SPECT) evaluation of regional cerebral blood flow (rCBF) with tracers such as technetium-99m (^{99m}Tc)-hexamethylpropyleneamine oxide (HMPAO) and ^{99m}Tc-ethyl cysteinate dimer (ECD) can localize the epileptogenic region regardless of the presence or absence of structural abnormalities. The characteristic appearance of an epileptogenic region is relative zonal hyperperfusion on ictal SPECT and relative zonal hypoperfusion on interictal SPECT. The sensitivity of ictal rCBF with SPECT may approach 90%, whereas that of interictal SPECT is in the range of 50% (14). The utility of ictal SPECT is somewhat reduced by difficulty in coordinating tracer administration with seizures. Noninvasive evaluation is often unsuccessful in precisely localizing an epileptogenic region. As a result, surgical placement of electrode grids on the brain surface or insertion of depth electrodes becomes necessary. These invasive steps carry risk to the patient.

FDG PET has proven useful in preoperative localization of the epileptogenic region (Fig. 10.2) (15). FDG PET is generally performed after an interictal injection. Although metabolic alterations might be localized better ictally than interictally, the relatively short half-life of fluorine-18 (^{18}F) limits the window of opportunity during which it can be administered ictally. Even when FDG can be administered at seizure onset, the approximately 30-minute brain uptake time of FDG means that the study may depict periictal, as well as, ictal FDG distribution. Ictal FDG studies may also show areas of seizure propagation, which could be confused with the actual seizure focus. Despite these considerations, some favorable results have been reported employing ictal PET to patients with continuous or frequent seizures (16).

For interictal PET, FDG should be administered in a set-

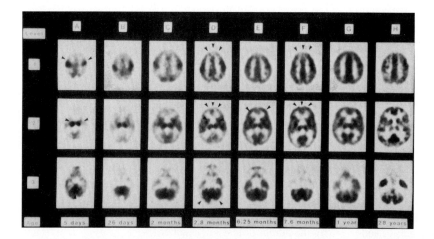

FIG. 10.1. Normal brain maturation. PET scans showing ontogenic changes in local cerebral glucose metabolism of the normal human infant. **A:** In the 5-day-old, glucose metabolism is highest in the sensorimotor cortex, thalamus, cerebellar vermis (*arrows*), and brainstem (not shown). **B, C, and D:** Glucose metabolism increases gradually in the parietal, temporal, and calcarine cortices, basal ganglia, and cerebellar cortex (*arrows*), particularly during the second and third months of life. **E:** In the frontal cortex, glucose metabolism increases first in the lateral prefrontal regions by approximately 6 months. **F:** By about 8 months, glucose metabolism also increases in the medial aspects of the frontal cortex (*arrows*), as well as in the dorsolateral occipital cortex. **G:** By 1 year, the glucose metabolic pattern resembles that of a healthy adult, although metabolic rates are twofold to threefold elevated in comparison to values expected in healthy adults **(H).** (From Chugani HT. Positron emission tomography. In: Berg BO, ed. *Principles of child neurology.* New York: McGraw-Hill, 1996:113–128, with permission.)

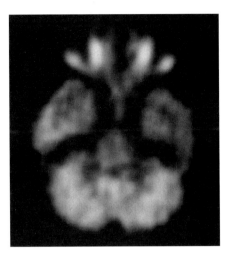

FIG. 10.2. Transaxial brain fluorodeoxyglucose positron emission tomography scan of a 14-year-old girl shows a hypometabolic epileptogenic left temporal lobe. (From Jadvar H, Connolly LP, Shulkin BL, et al. Positron-emission tomography in pediatrics. *Nucl Med Annu* 2000:53–83, with permission.)

ting where environmental stimuli are minimal, such as a quiet room and dim lights. During the 30 minutes after FDG administration, it is best to have the child remain awake with minimal parental interaction during this period. Pharmacologic sedation, if needed for imaging, is best withheld during this 30-minute interval to avoid unwanted effects of sedation on cerebral metabolism during the uptake interval. EEG monitoring during the uptake period is essential to detect seizure activity that might affect FDG distribution.

The sensitivity of interictal FDG PET approaches that of ictal rCBF SPECT in localizing the epileptogenic region, which is indicated by regional hypometabolism. Importantly, the hypometabolism may predominantly affect cortex bordering the epileptogenic focus. Epileptic activity may originate in cortical areas bordering the hypometabolic regions, rather than the hypometabolic region itself (17).

Incorporation of FDG PET into preoperative evaluation of epileptic patients significantly reduces the need for intracranial EEG monitoring and the cost of preoperative evaluation (18). The best results have been obtained in epilepsy of temporal lobe origin, for which metabolic abnormalities may be evident in as many as 90% of surgical candidates (18, 19). Extratemporal epileptogenic regions are more difficult to identify, but some success has been achieved in children with intractable frontal lobe epilepsy and normal CT or MRI study results (20).

FDG PET has been particularly helpful in the evaluation of infantile spasms, which is a subtype of seizure disorder. This entity, which has an incidence of 2 to 6 per 10,000 live births, consists of a characteristic pattern of infantile myoclonic seizures and is frequently associated with profound developmental delay despite medical treatment (11, 21). Before the availability of FDG PET, surgical intervention was attempted and successful in only isolated instances.

Incorporation of FDG PET into the evaluation of children with infantile spasms has resulted in identification of a significant number of children who benefit from cortical resection. FDG PET has revealed marked focal cortical glucose hypometabolism associated with malformative or dysplastic lesions that are not evident on anatomic imaging. There is a marked decline in seizure frequency and in some patients, reversal of developmental delay when a single metabolic abnormality that correlates with EEG findings is shown by FDG PET. Patients with bitemporal hypometabolism on FDG PET have a poor prognosis and are typically not candidates for resective surgery (22–25).

In addition to FDG, PET tracers that assess altered abundance or function of receptors, enzymes, and neurotransmitters in epileptogenic regions have been applied to localizing the epileptogenic region. Among alterations that have been observed are relatively reduced uptake of carbon-11 (^{11}C)-flumazenil, a central benzodiazepine-receptor antagonist, and ^{11}C-labeled (S)-[N-methyl]ketamine, which binds to the N-methyl D-aspartate receptor–gated ion channel (26–30). Relative increases in uptake of ^{11}C-carfentanil, a selective mu opiate–receptor agonist, and ^{11}C-deprenyl, an irreversible inhibitor of monoamine oxidase B, have also been described (31,32).

Other Neurologic Applications

PET with oxygen-labeled water ($H_2{}^{15}O$) has also been investigated in infants with intraventricular hemorrhage and hemorrhagic infarction, as well as in infants with hypoxic-ischemic encephalopathy (32,33). CBF was markedly reduced not only in the hemorrhagic areas, but also in the remainder of the involved hemisphere, suggesting that neurologic deficits may be caused by ischemia, rather than the presence of blood within the brain parenchyma or cerebral ventricles (33). In full-term infants with perinatal asphyxia, diminished blood flow to the parasagittal cortical regions suggested that injury to the brain in these infants was also ischemic in etiology (34).

PET has also been employed to study the pathophysiology of many other childhood brain disorders such as autism (35), attention deficit hyperactivity disorder (36), schizophrenia (37), sickle cell encephalopathy (38), and anorexia and bulimia nervosa (39,40). However, the exact role of PET in these clinical settings remains unclear. Further experience may result in an expanded role of PET in many childhood neurologic disorders.

PET IN PEDIATRIC CARDIOLOGY

Currently, PET plays a relatively minor role in pediatric cardiology. Quinlivan et al. (41) reviewed the cardiac applications of PET in children. PET with nitrogen-13 (^{13}N)-ammonia has been employed to measure myocardial perfusion in infants after anatomic repair of congenital heart defects and after Norwood palliation for hypoplastic left heart syndrome (42). Infants with repaired heart disease had higher resting blood flow levels and less coronary flow reserve than previously reported for adults. Infants with Norwood palliation also had less perfusion and oxygen delivery to the systemic ventricle than the infants with a repaired congenital heart lesion, explaining in part the less favorable outcome for patients with Norwood palliation. Evaluation of myocardial perfusion with ^{13}N-ammonia PET in infants after a neonatal arterial switch operation has demonstrated that patients with myocardial perfusion defects may have a more complicated postoperative course (43).

A major application of PET in adult cardiology is the assessment of myocardial viability with FDG as the tracer for glucose metabolism. A recent study evaluated the regional glucose metabolism and contractile function by gated FDG PET in seven infants and seven children after arterial switch operation and suspected myocardial infarction (44). Gated FDG PET was found to contribute pertinent information to guide additional therapy, including high-risk revascularization procedures.

In another study in children with Kawasaki disease, PET with ^{13}N-ammonia and FDG showed abnormalities in about 60% of patients during the acute and subacute stages and about 40% of patients in the convalescent stage of disease (45). PET was specifically valuable in assessing immunoglobulin therapy response at differing doses and administration schedules.

Beyond the more common assessment of myocardial perfusion and oxidative metabolism, PET has been used to study such fundamental functional abnormalities as mitochondrial dysfunction in children with hypertrophic cardiomyopathy and dilated cardiomyopathy (46). Dynamic PET with ^{11}C-acetate demonstrated a reduction in myocardial Krebs cycle activity (i.e., decreased oxidative metabolism) in children with cardiomyopathy despite normal myocardial perfusion. The diminished oxidative metabolism was associated with a compensatory increase in glycolysis activity as demonstrated on FDG PET.

PET IN PEDIATRIC ONCOLOGY

The incidence of cancer is estimated to be 133.3 per million children in the United States (47). Although cancer is much less common in children than adults, it is still an important cause of mortality in pediatrics. The approximately 10% of deaths during childhood that are attributable to cancer make it the leading cause of childhood death from disease (48).

Childhood cancers often differ from those encountered in adults. This can be appreciated from review of Table 10.1, which delineates the estimated incidence rates of the more commonly encountered cancers in American children. Of the adult cancers to which FDG PET has been most widely applied, only lymphomas and brain tumors occur with an appreciable incidence in children.

Before reviewing the applications of PET in pediatric oncology, it is important to consider potential causes of misinterpretation of FDG PET that relate to physiologic FDG dis-

TABLE 10.1. *Cancer incidence rates per million children younger than 15 years in the United States as derived from the Surveillance, Epidemiology, and End Results (SEER) program and reported in reference 47[a]*

Histology	Total[b]			Men		Women		Male: female	Whites		Blacks		White: black
	No.	Rate	(%)	No.	Rate	No.	Rate		No.	Rate	No.	Rate	
All histologic types	10,555	133.3	(100)	5,711	140.9	4,844	125.1	1.13	8,756	139.5	1,064	108.3	1.29
Acute lymphoid leukemia	2,484	30.9	(23.2)	1,383	33.7	1,101	28.0	1.20	2,092	32.9	169	16.9	1.95
All central nervous system (CNS)	2,205	27.6	(20.7)	1,195	29.3	1,010	26.0	1.13	1,847	29.3	239	23.8	1.23
Astrocytomas and gliomas	1,329	16.8	(12.6)	692	17.1	637	16.2	1.06	1,130	17.9	144	14.3	1.25
Primitive neurectodermal	532	6.6	(5.0)	311	7.7	221	5.6	1.38	433	6.8	56	5.9	1.15
Other CNS	344	4.3	(3.2)	192	4.6	152	3.9	1.18	284	4.6	37	3.6	1.28
Neuroblastoma	754	9.7	(7.3)	389	9.8	365	9.6	1.02	632	10.2	78	7.8	1.31
Non-Hodgkin's lymphoma	666	8.4	(6.3)	484	12.0	182	4.6	2.61	578	9.1	53	5.4	1.69
Wilms' tumor	638	8.1	(6.1)	287	6.9	351	8.9	0.78	520	8.3	94	9.4	0.88
Hodgkin's disease	511	6.6	(5.0)	295	7.4	216	5.6	1.32	451	7.3	46	4.7	1.55
Acute myeloid leukemia	454	5.6	(4.2)	224	5.5	230	6.0	0.92	358	5.8	47	4.8	1.21
Rhabdomyosarcoma	354	4.5	(3.4)	211	5.2	143	3.6	1.44	294	4.7	40	4.1	1.15
Retinoblastoma	306	3.9	(2.9)	144	3.6	162	4.2	0.86	234	3.9	44	4.5	0.87
Osteosarcoma	262	3.4	(2.6)	130	3.3	132	3.4	0.97	197	3.4	38	3.9	0.87
Ewing's sarcoma	208	2.8	(2.1)	109	2.8	99	2.6	1.08	194	3.3	3	0.3	11.00
All other histologic types	1,713	21.8	(16.4)	860	21.4	853	22.6	0.95	1,359	21.3	213	22.7	0.94

[a] Rates are standardized to the 1980 SEER population and reported per million children per year.
[b] Includes all races and both sexes.

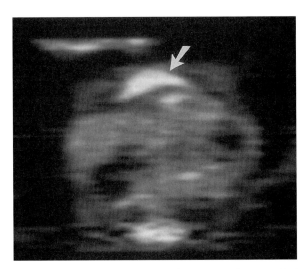

FIG. 10.3. Coronal fluorodeoxyglucose positron emission tomographic image shows physiologic uptake in the thymus. (From Jadvar H, Connolly LP, Shulkin BL, et al. Positron-emission tomography in pediatrics. *Nucl Med Annu* 2000: 53–83, with permission.)

tribution in children. High FDG uptake in the thymus (49, 50) and skeletal growth centers, particularly the long bone physes, are two important physiologic variations in FDG distribution encountered in children (Figs. 10.3 and 10.4). Other potential pitfalls, which also apply to imaging adults, include variable FDG uptake in working skeletal muscles, the myocardium, thyroid gland, and the gastrointestinal tract,

as well as accumulation of excreted FDG in the renal pelves and bladder, and possible tracer accumulation in draining lymph nodes from extravasated tracer at the time of injection (51). Diffuse high bone marrow and splenic FDG uptake after administration of hematopoietic stimulating factors may also resemble disseminated metastatic disease (Fig. 10.5) (52,53). Elevated bone marrow FDG uptake has been

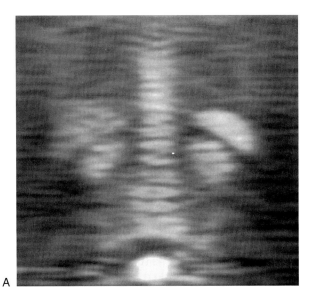

A

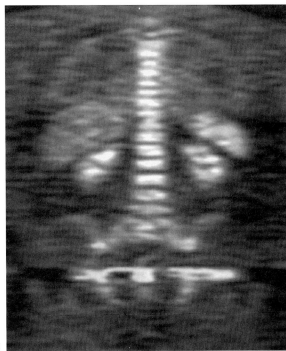

B

FIG. 10.5. A: Coronal fluorodeoxyglucose positron emission tomographic images show normal uptake in the bone marrow before chemotherapy in a patient with non-Hodgkin's lymphoma. **B:** After chemotherapy given in conjunction with granulocyte colony-stimulating factor, there is high vertebral bone marrow uptake of FDG. (From Jadvar H, Connolly LP, Shulkin BL, et al. Positron-emission tomography in pediatrics. *Nucl Med Annu* 2000:53–83, with permission.)

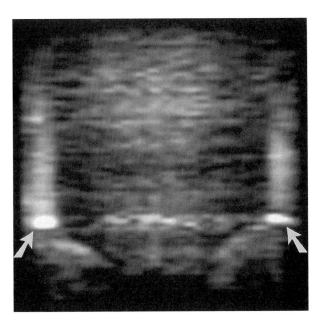

FIG. 10.4. Coronal fluorodeoxyglucose positron emission tomography of the distal upper extremities shows high physiologic uptake in the growth plates bilaterally. (From Jadvar H, Connolly LP, Shulkin BL, et al. Positron-emission tomography in pediatrics. *Nucl Med Annu* 2000:53–83, with permission.)

observed in patients as long as 4 weeks after completion of treatment with granulocyte colony-stimulating factor (G-CSF) (52). This observation is probably reflective of increased bone marrow glycolytic metabolism in response to hematopoietic growth factors. Thymic activity may also occasionally be elevated in a few young adults after chemotherapy because of reactive thymus hyperplasia (54). We have also noticed thymic uptake in younger children before chemotherapy.

CNS Tumors

Tumors of the CNS are the most common nonhematologic tumors of childhood. They account for about 20% of all pediatric malignancies. The grouping includes many histologically diverse tumors of both neuroepithelial and nonneuroepithelial origin. Most pediatric brain tumors arise from neuroepithelial tissue. CNS tumors are subclassified histopathologically by cell type and graded for degree of malignancy using criteria that include mitotic activity, infiltration, and anaplasia (55,56).

One may consider the distribution of the most common tumors according to the major anatomic compartment involved. In the posterior fossa, medulloblastoma, cerebellar astrocytoma, ependymoma, and brain stem gliomas are most common. Tumors arising in the region of the third ventricle include tumors that arise from suprasellar, pineal, and ventricular tissue. The most common neoplasms about the third ventricle are optic and hypothalamic gliomas, craniopharyngiomas, and germ-cell tumors. Supratentorial tumors are most often astrocytomas, many of which are low grade (56).

MRI and CT are the principal imaging modalities used in staging and following treatment of children with CNS tumors. Their main limitation is distinguishing viable recurrent or residual tumor from abnormalities resulting from surgery or radiation. SPECT with thallium-201 (^{201}Tl) and ^{99m}Tc-methoxyisobutyl isonitrile (MIBI) have proven valuable for this determination in a number of pediatric brain tumors (57–60). Use of FDG PET in brain tumors has been widely reported in series that predominantly include adult patients for whom FDG PET has helped distinguish viable tumor from posttherapeutic changes (61–63). High FDG uptake relative to adjacent brain indicates residual or recurrent tumor, whereas low or absent FDG uptake is observed in areas of necrosis. This distinction is most readily made with high-grade tumors that show high uptake of FDG at diagnosis. Even with high-grade tumors, the presence of microscopic tumor foci is not excluded by an FDG PET study that does not show increased uptake, however. This is particularly true after intensive radiation therapy, in which case FDG PET results may not accurately correlate with tumor progression (64). An additional stipulation is that in the immediate posttherapy period, elevated FDG uptake may persist (65).

FDG PET has been applied to tumor grading and prognostic stratification. Higher-grade aggressive tumors typically

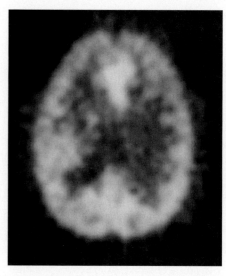

FIG. 10.6. Transaxial fluorodeoxyglucose positron emission tomographic image shows intense uptake of FDG in a high-grade astrocytoma in the left frontal lobe. (From Jadvar H, Connolly LP, Shulkin BL, et al. Positron-emission tomography in pediatrics. *Nucl Med Annu* 2000:53–83, with permission.)

have higher FDG uptake than lower grade tumors (Figs. 10.6 and 10.7) (66). Some low-grade tumors show insufficient FDG uptake to be distinguished from adjacent brain and some appear hypometabolic. The development of hypermetabolism as evidenced by increased FDG uptake in a low-grade tumor that appeared hypometabolic at diagnosis indicates transformation to a higher grade (67). The biological

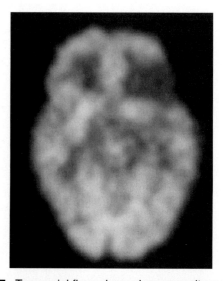

FIG. 10.7. Transaxial fluorodeoxyglucose positron emission tomographic brain image from a 4½-year-old boy with generalized tonic-clonic seizures demonstrates hypometabolism in the left frontal lobe. This area was resected and shown to be a low-grade glioma. (From Jadvar H, Connolly LP, Shulkin BL, et al. Positron-emission tomography in pediatrics. *Nucl Med Annu* 2000:53–83, with permission.)

behavior of high-grade tumors may be reflected in their appearance on FDG PET. Shorter survival times have been reported for patients whose tumors show the highest degree of FDG uptake (68). Limited available data suggest that FDG PET findings also correlate well with pathology and clinical outcome in children (69–71). A potential pediatric application of this entails a reported excellent correlation between FDG PET findings and clinical outcome in children affected by neurofibromatosis who have low-grade astrocytomas (72). In that series, high tumoral glucose metabolism shown by FDG PET was a more accurate predictor of tumor behavior than was histologic analysis.

Another positron-emitting radiotracer that has been used to study pediatric brain tumors is ^{11}C-L-methionine (^{11}C-L-Met), which localizes to only a minimal degree in healthy brain. Uptake of this labeled amino acid reflects amino acid transport and to some extent transmethylation pathways that are present in some tumors. However, similar to FDG, some low-grade gliomas may escape detection (73,74). Carbon-11-L-Met PET has been reported to be useful in differentiating viable tumor from treatment-induced changes (73,75). It is worth noting, however, that ^{11}C-L-Met is not tumor specific, because it has been shown to accumulate in some nontumoral CNS diseases, likely as a result of blood–brain barrier disruption (76). Carbon-11-L-Met, because of the relatively short 20-minute half-life of the ^{11}C label, must be produced locally for administration and is not commercially available.

Lymphoma

Non-Hodgkin's and Hodgkin's lymphomas account for between 10% and 15% of pediatric malignancies. Non-Hodgkin's lymphoma occurs throughout childhood. Lymphoblastic and small-cell tumors, including Burkitt's lymphoma, are the most common histologic types. The disease is usually widespread at diagnosis. Mediastinal and hilar involvement are common with lymphoblastic lymphoma. Burkitt's most often occurs in the abdomen. Hodgkin's disease has a peak incidence during adolescence. Nodular sclerosing and mixed cellularity are the most common histologic types. The disease is rarely widespread at diagnosis and most cases have intrathoracic nodal involvement (47,77).

Gallium-67 (^{67}Ga)-citrate scintigraphy has proven useful in staging and monitoring therapeutic response of patients with non-Hodgkin's and Hodgkin's lymphomas (78–82). In numerous studies, which have included predominantly adult patient populations, FDG has been shown to accumulate in non-Hodgkin's and Hodgkin's lymphomas (Fig. 10.8) (51, 83–102). Similar to ^{67}Ga-citrate, FDG uptake tends to be somewhat greater in higher-grade lymphomas than in lower grade lymphomas (90,92). FDG PET has been shown to reveal sites of nodal and extranodal disease that are not detected by conventional staging methods, resulting in upstaging of disease (87,88,93–95). Identification of areas of intense FDG uptake within the bone marrow can be

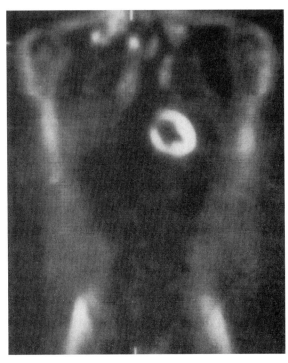

FIG. 10.8. A 16-year-old with Hodgkin's disease. A coronal image from fluorodeoxyglucose positron emission tomography shows abnormal uptake in multiple nodal groups in the upper chest and lower neck.

particularly useful in directing the site of biopsy or even eliminating the need for biopsy at staging (88,101). FDG PET is also useful for assessing residual soft-tissue masses shown by CT after therapy. Absence of FDG uptake in a residual mass is predictive of remission, whereas high uptake indicates residual or recurrent tumor (95,103). Preliminary experience with FDG coincidence imaging suggests that this technology may also be useful in the evaluation of patients with lymphoma (104–107). In adults, coincidence imaging is less sensitive than dedicated PET for the detection of small tumor foci, that is, those less than 2 cm in diameter.

FDG PET has been compared with ^{11}C-L-Met PET in a relatively small series of 14 patients with non-Hodgkin's lymphoma. Carbon-11-L-Met PET provided superior tumor-to-background contrast while FDG PET was superior in distinguishing between high- and low-grade lymphomas (86).

Neuroblastoma

Neuroblastoma is the most common extracranial solid malignant tumor in children. The mean age of patients at presentation is 20 to 30 months and it is rare after age 5 years (77). The most common location of neuroblastoma is the adrenal gland. Other sites of origin include the paravertebral and presacral sympathetic chain, the organ of Zuckerkandl, the posterior mediastinal sympathetic ganglia, and the cervical sympathetic plexuses. Gross or microscopic calcification is often present in the tumor. Two related neural crest tumors, ganglioneuroma and ganglioneuroblastoma, have been described. Some neuroblastomas spontaneously regress or mature into ganglioneuroma, which is benign. However, the unpredictability and apparent infrequency of spontaneous regression and maturation, and the consequences of delaying therapy, militate that treatment be instituted at diagnosis in most cases. Ganglioneuroblastoma is a malignant tumor that contains both undifferentiated neuroblasts and mature ganglion cells.

Disseminated disease is present in up to 70% of neuroblastoma cases at diagnosis and most commonly involves cortical bone and bone marrow. Less frequently, there is involvement of liver, skin, and lung. A primary tumor is not detected in up to 10% of children with disseminated neuroblastoma (108). The primary tumor may also go undetected in patients who present with paraneoplastic syndromes such as infantile myoclonic encephalopathy.

Surgical excision is the preferred treatment of localized neuroblastoma. When local disease is extensive, intensive preoperative chemotherapy may be used. When distant metastases are present, surgical removal is not likely to improve survival. The prognosis in these cases is poor, but high-dose chemotherapy, total-body irradiation, or bone marrow reinfusion is beneficial for some children with this presentation.

Delineation of local disease extent is achieved with MRI, CT, and scintigraphic studies. These tests are also used in localizing the primary site in children who present with disseminated disease or with a paraneoplastic syndrome. Iodine-131 (^{131}I) or iodine-123 (^{123}I) metaiodobenzylguanidine (^{131}I-MIBG or ^{123}I-MIBG) and indium-111 (^{111}In)-pentetreotide scintigraphy have been employed in these settings, with a sensitivity of more than 85% for detecting neuroblastoma. Uptake of MIBG, which is an analogue of guanethidine and norepinephrine, into neuroblastoma is by a neuronal sodium and energy-dependent transport mechanism. The localization of ^{111}In-pentetreotide in neuroblastoma reflects the presence of somatostatin type 2 receptors on some neuroblastoma cells (109).

Bone scintigraphy has been most widely used for the detection of skeletal involvement for staging. MIBG, and to a lesser extent ^{111}In-pentetreotide, imaging have also been increasingly used for detecting skeletal involvement.

Patients with residual unresected primary tumors are periodically evaluated with MRI or CT. However, these studies cannot distinguish viable tumor from treatment-related scar or tumor that has matured into ganglioneuroma. Specificity in establishing residual viable tumor can be improved with MIBG or ^{111}In-pentetreotide imaging when the primary tumor had been shown to accumulate one of these agents. These agents are also useful in assessing residual skeletal disease in patients with MIBG-avid or ^{111}In-pentetreotide–avid skeletal metastases. Bone scintigraphy, however, is unable to distinguish active disease from bony repair on the basis of tracer uptake.

Neuroblastomas are metabolically active tumors. Neuroblastomas and/or their metastases avidly concentrated FDG before chemotherapy or radiation therapy in 16 of 17 patients studied with FDG PET and MIBG imaging (110). Uptake after therapy was variable but tended to be lower. FDG and MIBG results were concordant in most instances (Fig. 10.9). However, there were occasions that one agent accumulated at a site of disease and the other did not. MIBG imaging overall was considered superior to FDG PET, particularly in delineation of residual disease. Because the patients in this series had aggressive tumors and poor prognoses, the value of FDG PET for assessing therapeutic response could not be determined. An advantage of FDG PET is the initiation of imaging 30 to 60 minutes after FDG administration, whereas MIBG imaging is performed 1 or more days after tracer administration.

FDG PET may be limited for the evaluation of the bone marrow involvement of neuroblastoma due to mild FDG accumulation by the normal bone marrow (110). Pitfalls resulting from physiologic FDG uptake in the bowel and the thymus are additional factors that may limit the role for FDG PET in neuroblastoma. Currently the primary role of FDG PET in neuroblastoma is in the evaluation of known or suspected neuroblastomas that do not demonstrate MIBG uptake.

Carbon-11-hydroxyephedrine (HED), an analogue of norepinephrine, and ^{11}C-epinephrine PET have also been used in evaluating neuroblastoma (Fig. 10.10). All seven neuroblastomas studied showed uptake of ^{11}C-HED (111) and four of five neuroblastomas studied showed uptake of ^{11}C-epinephrine (112). Uptake of these tracers is demonstrated within minutes after administration, which is an advantage over MIBG imaging. Limitations regarding cost and the need for on-site synthesis of short-lived ^{11}C (half-life of 20 minutes) suggest that neither ^{11}C-HED nor ^{11}C-epinephrine PET is likely to replace MIBG imaging. These tracers may prove useful adjuncts in difficult cases in which a primary tumor is difficult to identify with more readily available agents. They have the potential to lead to further the understanding of this disease. Compounds labeled with ^{18}F, such as fluoro-norepinephrine, fluorometaraminol, and fluorodopamine may also be useful tracers. PET using 4-[^{18}F]fluoro-3-iodobenzylguanidine (113) and iodine-124 (^{124}I)–labeled MIBG (114) has also been described.

Wilms' Tumor

Wilms' tumor is the most common renal malignancy of childhood. Wilms' tumor is predominantly seen in younger children and uncommonly encountered after the age of 5 years (47). Bilateral renal involvement occurs in about 5% of all cases and can be identified synchronously or metachronously (77,115). An asymptomatic abdominal mass is the typical mode of presentation. Nephrectomy and adjuvant chemotherapy are the treatments of choice. Radiation ther-

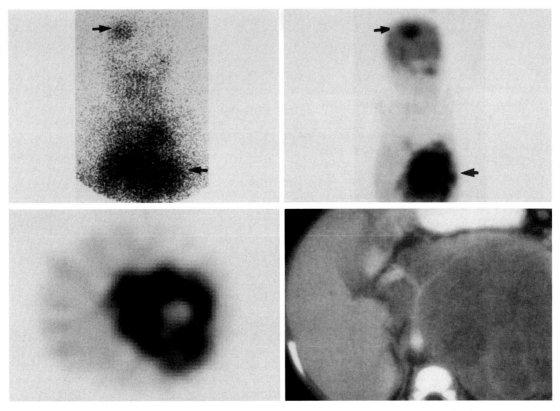

FIG. 10.9. Images of a 2-year-old girl with neuroblastoma at presentation. **Top left:** Anterior planar view of the head, neck, chest, and upper abdomen 48 hours after iodine-131 metaiodobenzylguanidine (^{131}I-MIBG) injection. An area of abnormal uptake is present in the right superior aspect of the skull (*upper arrow*). A large focus of abnormal uptake in the primary tumor (*lower arrow*) extends from the upper left abdomen medially and inferior to the liver. **Top right:** Anterior projection of the head, neck, chest, and upper abdomen approximately 1 hour after ^{18}F-fluorodeoxyglucose (FDG) injection. Increased FDG uptake in the skull (*upper arrow*) corresponding to the site of abnormal ^{131}I MIBG uptake is well visualized against the normal brain uptake of FDG. Increased FDG uptake is present in the primary tumor (*lower arrow*). There is a paucity of background activity in the chest and abdomen. **Bottom left:** Transaxial image through the mid abdomen shows marked FDG uptake in the primary tumor. A central area of decreased FDG accumulation probably represents necrosis. **Bottom right:** A large mass in the left abdomen is shown in a transaxial CT image. This set of images demonstrates that neuroblastomas are metabolically active. The primary tumor and metastases can be well visualized with FDG PET. (From Jadvar H, Connolly LP, Shulkin BL, et al. Positron-emission tomography in pediatrics. *Nucl Med Annu* 2000:53–83, with permission.)

apy is used in selected cases in which resection is incomplete.

Scintigraphy has not played an important role in imaging of Wilms' tumor. Radiography, ultrasonography, CT, and MRI are commonly employed in anatomic staging and detection of metastases, which predominantly involve lung, occasionally liver, and only rarely other sites. Anatomic imaging, however, is limited in the assessment of residual or recurrent tumor (115). Uptake of FDG by Wilms' tumor (Fig. 10.11) has been described (116), but a role for FDG PET in Wilms tumor has not been established. Normal excretion of FDG through the kidney is also a limiting factor. However, careful correlation with anatomic cross-sectional imaging usually allows distinction of tumor uptake from normal renal FDG excretion.

Bone Tumors

Osteosarcoma and Ewing's sarcoma are the two primary bone malignancies of childhood. Osteosarcoma is the more common.

Osteosarcoma predominantly affects adolescents and young adults. A second peak affects older adults, predominantly individuals with a history of prior radiation to bone or Paget disease. This tumor rarely affects children younger than 7 years. Osteosarcoma is typically a lesion of the long bones. The treatment of choice for osteosarcoma of an extremity is wide resection and limb-sparing surgery. Limb-sparing procedures entail the resection of tumor with a cuff of surrounding normal tissue at all margins, skeletal reconstruction, and muscle and soft-tissue transfers. When chemothera-

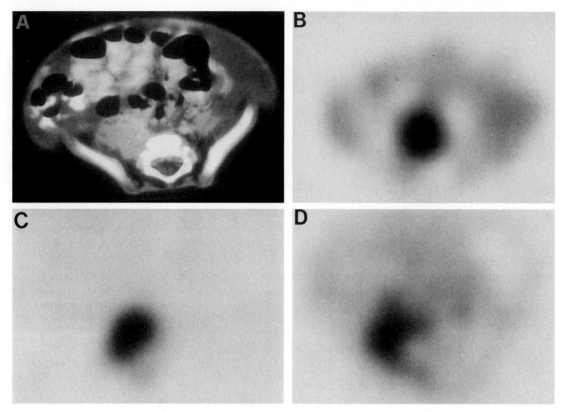

FIG. 10.10. A: CT scan of the pelvis of a 6-month-old boy after surgical debulking of an abdominopelvic neuroblastoma: There is abnormal soft tissue with speckled calcification in the right posterior pelvis. **B:** Metaiodobenzylguanidine (MIBG) single-photon emission computed tomography (SPECT) scan at 24 hours shows uptake into the tumor. **C:** Hydroxyephedrine (HED) PET scan at 20 minutes after injection: There is excellent uptake within the neuroblastoma, and the image appears similar to the MIBG SPECT examination. **D:** Fluorodeoxyglucose positron emission tomography scan at 50 minutes: There is moderate accumulation of FDG within the mass relative to surrounding background. However, the tumor appears better delineated with the more specific adrenergic tumor imaging agent HED. (From Shulkin BL, Wieland DM, Baro ME, et al. PET hydroxyephedrine imaging of neuroblastoma. *J Nucl Med* 1996; 37:16–21, with permission.)

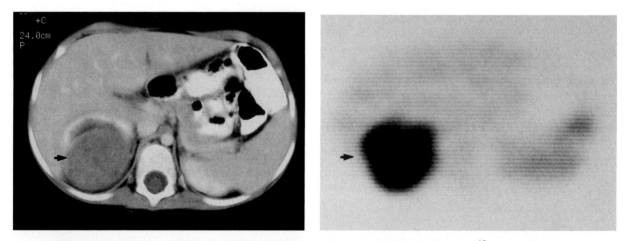

FIG. 10.11. A CT scan **(left)** and a PET scan **(right)**. Markedly increased uptake of ^{18}F-fluorodeoxyglucose (*arrow*) is present within the right-sided mass seen on CT (*arrow*). The mass was surgically removed and confirmed histologically to represent a Wilms' tumor. (From Shulkin BL, Chang E, Strouse PJ, et al. PET FDG studies of Wilms tumors. *J Pediatr Hematol/Oncol* 1997;19:334–338, with permission.)

peutic regimens are employed preoperatively and postoperatively and imaging is used to define tumor extent and tumor viability preoperatively, limb-sparing procedures can be appropriately performed in 80% of patients with osteosarcoma (117).

Almost all cases of Ewing's sarcoma occur between the ages of 5 and 30 years, with the highest incidence being in the second decade of life. In patients younger than 20 years, Ewing's sarcoma most often affects the appendicular skeleton. Beyond that age, pelvic, rib, and vertebral lesions predominate. The tumor is believed to be of neuroectodermal origin and, along with the primitive neuroectodermal tumor (PNET), to be part of a spectrum of a single biologic entity (118). Ewing's sarcoma is considered an undifferentiated variant and PNET a more differentiated peripheral neural tumor. Therapy for Ewing's sarcoma involves multiagent chemotherapy for eradication of microscopic or overt metastatic disease and irradiation and/or surgery for control of the primary lesion. Because late recurrence is not uncommon, resection of the primary tumor is gaining favor for local disease control (119).

MRI is used to define the local extent of osteosarcoma and Ewing's sarcoma in bone and soft tissue. However, signal abnormalities caused by peritumoral edema can result in an overestimation of tumor extension (120). Scintigraphy has been used primarily to detect skeletal metastases of these tumors at diagnosis and during follow-up. With osteosarcoma, skeletal scintigraphy occasionally demonstrates extraosseous metastases, most often pulmonary, due to osteoid production by the metastatic deposits.

Determination of preoperative chemotherapeutic response is important in planning limb-salvage surgery. Due to the nonspecific appearance of viable tumor on MRI, variable results have been reported for assessing chemotherapeutic response (121–126). Scintigraphy with ^{201}Tl has been shown to be useful for assessing therapeutic response in osteosarcoma (127–132) and perhaps Ewing's sarcoma (129,130). Marked decrease in tumoral ^{201}Tl uptake indicates a favorable response to chemotherapy. When tumoral ^{201}Tl uptake does not decrease within weeks of chemotherapy, a therapeutic change may be needed. Technetium-99m MIBI may also be useful in osteosarcoma but seemingly not with Ewing's sarcoma (133,134).

The exact role of FDG PET in osteosarcoma and Ewing's sarcoma is unclear (Figs. 10.12 and 10.13). However, early experience has suggested that in patients with Ewing's sar-

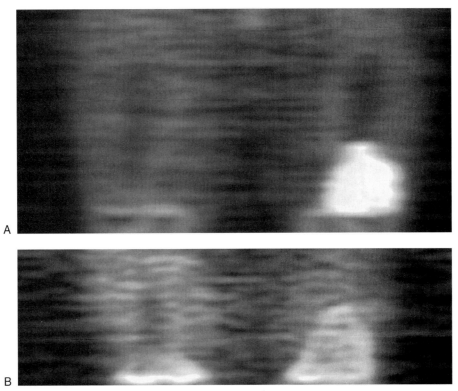

FIG. 10.12. High-grade osteoblastic osteosarcoma. **A:** Coronal image at diagnosis shows high ^{18}F-fluorodeoxyglucose (FDG) uptake in the distal left femoral tumor of a 14-year-old boy. **B:** Coronal PET after chemotherapy shows a marked decrease in the level of FDG uptake, indicative of chemotherapeutic response. The patient underwent resection of the tumor and osteoarticular graft replacement. The surgical specimen showed 95% tumor necrosis. There is physiologically increased physeal uptake in the right distal femur at diagnosis and after therapy. (From Jadvar H, Connolly LP, Shulkin BL, et al. Positron-emission tomography in pediatrics. *Nucl Med Annu* 2000:53–83, with permission.)

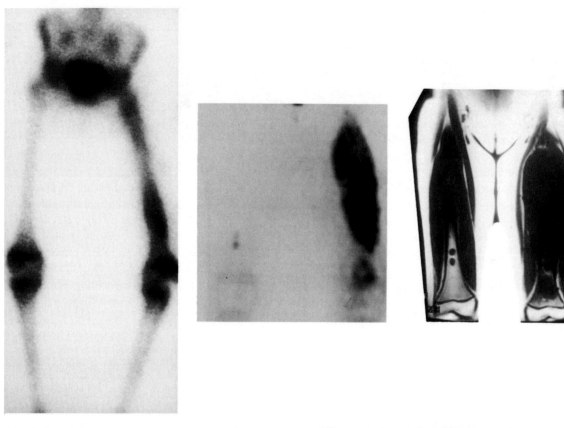

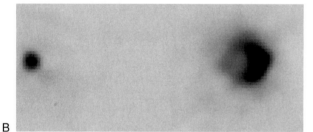

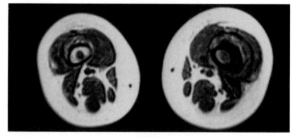

FIG. 10.13. An 11-year-old girl who complained of pain and swelling in the left thigh. Plain film radiographs showed findings suggestive of a Ewing's sarcoma, subsequently confirmed on biopsy. **A:** Bone scan **(left)** obtained 2 hours after injection of technetium-99m methylene diphosphonate. Abnormal accumulation of tracer is noted throughout the left femur; the right femur is unremarkable. Anterior projection image **(center)** from PET study shows intense irregular uptake of ^{18}F-fluorodeoxyglucose (FDG) within the soft tissues of the left thigh. Two small foci of activity are seen in the region of the distal right femur that are not present on bone scanning. T1-weighted coronal magnetic resonance imaging (MRI) **(right)** shows a soft-tissue mass in the left thigh, replacement of normal marrow of the left femur, and two focal lesions in the distal right femur. **B:** Transverse image **(left)** from a PET scan at the level of the distal femurs. Intense uptake of FDG is present in the soft tissues surrounding the left femur and focally within the right femur. T1-weighted MRI **(right)** at the same level shows the soft-tissue mass surrounding the left femur, replacement of marrow of the left femur, and a lesion in the center of the right femur. (From Shulkin BL, Mitchell DS, Ungar DR, et al. Neoplasms in a pediatric population: 2-[F-18]-fluoro-2-deoxy-D-glucose PET studies. *Radiology* 1995;194:495–500, with permission.)

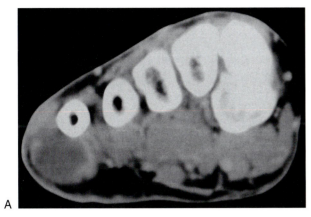

A

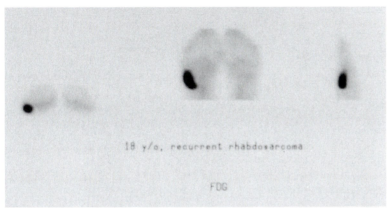

B

FIG. 10.14. Rhabdomyosarcoma. **A:** CT of the right foot of an 18-year-old girl after chemotherapy shows an abnormal residual soft-tissue mass below the right fifth metatarsal. **B:** Depicted left to right are transverse, coronal, and sagittal ^{18}F-fluorodeoxyglucose images. (From Jadvar H, Connolly LP, Shulkin BL, et al. Positron-emission tomography in pediatrics. *Nucl Med Annu* 2000:53–83, with permission.)

coma, FDG PET may play a role in monitoring response to therapy (135–137). Another potential role is in assessing patients with suspected or known pulmonary metastases, which is particularly common with osteosarcoma.

Soft-tissue Tumors

Rhabdomyosarcoma is the most common soft-tissue malignancy of childhood. The peak incidence occurs between ages 3 and 6 years. Rhabdomyosarcomas can develop in any organ or tissue. Contrary to what the name implies, this tumor does not usually arise in muscle. The most common anatomic locations are the head, particularly the orbit and paranasal sinuses, the neck, and the genitourinary tract. CT or MRI is important for establishing the extent of local disease. Radiography and CT are used for detecting pulmonary metastases and skeletal scintigraphy is employed for identifying osseous metastases. Radiation therapy and surgery are used for local disease control and chemotherapy is employed for treatment of metastases. Rhabdomyosarcomas show variable degrees of FDG accumulation. Cases showing the clinical use of FDG PET have been described, but similar to the case for osteosarcoma and Ewing's sarcoma, the exact role of FDG PET in rhabdomyosarcoma is currently unclear (Fig. 10.14) (1,135).

SUMMARY

FDG PET is increasingly being applied to study diseases of childhood, particularly in oncology patients. Because pediatric tumors are relatively rare, it will be difficult to perform well-designed prospective clinical trials at a single institution. The recent merger of the Children's Cancer Group and the Pediatric Oncology Group to form the Children's Oncology Group brings the opportunity to examine the use of FDG PET in the management of childhood tumors in multiinstitutional cooperative efforts. We expect that future data will show that FDG PET does contribute unique and useful information for the care of childhood tumors.

ACKNOWLEDGMENTS

This research was supported in part by grant no. NCI 54216 (B. S.). The authors thank Carol Kruise for secretarial expertise and Alan Fischman, MD, PhD for assistance with illustrations.

REFERENCES

1. Gordon I. Issues surrounding preparation, information, and handling the child and parent in nuclear medicine. *J Nucl Med* 1998;39: 490–494.
2. Treves ST. Introduction. In: Treves ST, ed. *Pediatric nuclear medicine,* 2nd ed. New York: Springer-Verlag, 1995:1–11.

3. Mandell GA, Cooper JA, Majd M, et al. Procedure guidelines for pediatric sedation in nuclear medicine. *J Nucl Med* 1997;38: 1640–1643.

4. Shulkin BL. PET applications in pediatrics. *Q J Nucl Med* 1997;41: 281–291.

5. Schelbert H, Hoh CK, Royal HD, et al. Procedure guideline for tumor imaging using fluorine-18-FDG. *J Nucl Med* 1998;39:1302–1305.

6. Jones SC, Alavi A, Christman D, et al. The radiation dosimetry of 2-[^{18}F]fluoro-2-deoxy-D-glucose in man. *J Nucl Med* 1982;23:613–617.

7. Ruotsalainen U, Suhonen-Povli H, Eronen E, et al. Estimated radiation dose to the newborn in FDG-PET studies. *J Nucl Med* 1996;37: 387–393.

8. Chugani HT, Phelps ME. Maturational changes in cerebral function in infants determined by ^{18}FDG positron emission tomography. *Science* 1986;231:840–843.

9. Chugani HT, Phelps ME, Mazziotta JC. Positron emission tomography study of human brain functional development. *Ann Neurol* 1987; 22:487–497.

10. Chugani HT. Positron emission tomography. In: Berg BO, ed. *Principles of child neurology*. New York: McGraw-Hill, 1996:113–128.

11. Hauser W. Epidemiology of epilepsy in children. *Neurosurg Clin North Am* 1995;6:419–428.

12. National Institutes of Health. National Institutes of Health Consensus Development Conference Statement: surgery for epilepsy. *Epilepsia* 1990;31:806–812.

13. Kuzniecky R, Suggs S, Gaudier J, et al. Lateralization of epileptic foci by magnetic resonance imaging in temporal lobe epilepsy. *J Neuroimaging* 1991;1:163–167.

14. Treves ST, Connolly LP. Single photon emission computed tomography in pediatric epilepsy. *Neurosurg Clin North Am* 1995;6:473–480.

15. Snead OC III, Chen LS, Mitchell WG, et al. Usefulness of [^{18}F]fluorodeoxyglucose positron emission tomography in pediatric epilepsy surgery. *Pediatr Neurol* 1996;14:98–107.

16. Meltzer CC, Adelson PD, Brenner RP, et al. Planned ictal FDG PET imaging for localization of extratemporal epileptic foci. *Epilepsia* 2000;41(2):193–200.

17. Juhasz C, Chugani DC, Muzik O, et al. Is epileptogenic cortex truly hypometabolic on interictal positron emission tomography? *Ann Neurol* 2000;48(1):88–96.

18. Cummings TJ, Chugani DC, Chugani HT. Positron emission tomography in pediatric epilepsy. *Neurosurg Clin North Am* 1995;6:465–472.

19. Engel J Jr, Kuhl DE, Phelps ME. Patterns of human local cerebral glucose metabolism during epileptogenic seizures. *Science* 1982;218: 64–66.

20. da Silva EA, Chugani DC, Muzik O, et al. Identification of frontal lobe epileptic foci in children using positron emission tomography. *Epilepsia* 1997;38:1198–1208.

21. Hrachovy R, Frost J. Infantile spasms. *Pediatr Clin North Am* 1989; 36:311–329.

22. Chugani HT, Shields WD, Shewmon DA, et al. Infantile spasms, I: PET identifies focal cortical dysgenesis in cryptogenic cases for surgical treatment. *Ann Neurol* 1990;27:406–413.

23. Chuagni HT, Shewmon DA, Shields WD, et al. Surgery for intractable infantile spasms: neuroimaging perspectives. *Epilepsia* 1993;34: 764–771.

24. Chugani HT, Da Silva E, Chugani DC. Infantile spasms, III: prognostic implications of bitemporal hypometabolism on positron emission tomography. *Ann Neurol* 1996;39:643–649.

25. Chugani HT, Conti JR. Etiologic classification of infantile spasms in 140 cases: role of positron emission tomography. *J Child Neurol* 1996; 11:44–48.

26. Savic I, Svanborg E, Thorell JO. Cortical benzodiazepine receptor changes are related to frequency of partial seizures: a positron emission tomography study. *Epilepsia* 1996;37:236–244.

27. Arnold S, Berthele A, Drzezga A, et al. Reduction of benzodiazepine receptor binding is related to the seizure onset zone in extratemporal focal cortical dysplasia. *Epilepsia* 2000;41(7):818–824.

28. Richardson MP, Koepp MJ, Brooks DJ, et al. ^{11}C-Flumazenil PET in neocortical epilepsy. *Neurology* 1998;51:485–492.

29. Debets RM, Sadzot B, van Isselt JW, et al. Is ^{11}C-flumazenil PET superior to ^{18}FDG PET and ^{123}I-iomazenil SPECT in presurgical evaluation of temporal lobe epilepsy? *J Neurol Neurosurg Psychiatry* 1997;62:141–150.

30. Kumlien E, Hartvig P, Valind S, et al. NMDA-receptor activity visualized with (S)-[N-methyl-11-C]ketamine and positron emission tomography in patients with medial temporal epilepsy. *Epilepsia* 1999;40: 30–37.

31. Mayberg HS, Sadzot B, Meltzer CC, et al. Quantification of mu and non-mu opiate receptors in temporal lobe epilepsy using positron emission tomography. *Ann Neurol* 1991;30:3–11.

32. Kumlien E, Bergstrom M, Lilja A, et al. Positron emission tomography with [C-11]deuterium deprenyl in temporal lobe epilepsy. *Epilepsia* 1995;36:712–721.

33. Volpe JJ, Herscovitch P, Perlman JM, et al. Positron emission tomography in the newborn: extensive impairment of regional cerebral blood flow with intraventricular hemorrhage and hemorrhagic intracerebral involvement. *Pediatrics* 1983;72(5):589–601.

34. Volpe JJ, Herscovitch P, Perlman JM, et al. Positron emission tomography in the asphyxiated term newborn: parasagittal impairment of cerebral blood flow. *Ann Neurol* 1985;17(3):287–296.

35. Zilbovicius M, Boddaert N, Belin P, et al. Temporal lobe dysfunction in childhood autism: a PET study. *Am J Psychiatry* 2000;157(12): 1988–1993.

36. Ernst M, Zametkin AJ, Matochik JA, et al. High midbrain [^{18}F]DOPA accumulation in children with attention deficit hyperactivity disorder. *Am J Psychiatry* 1999;156(8):1209–1215.

37. Jacobson LK, Hamburger SD, Van Horn JD, et al. Cerebral glucose metabolism in childhood onset schizophrenia. *Psychiatry Res* 1997; 75(3):131–144.

38. Reed W, Jagust W, Al-Mateen M, et al. Role of positron emission tomography in determining the extent of CNS ischemia in patients with sickle cell disease. *Am J Hematol* 1999;60(4):268–272.

39. Delvenne V, Lotstra F, Goldman S, et al. Brain hypometabolism of glucose in anorexia nervosa: a PET scan study. *Biol Psychiatry* 1995; 37(3):161–169.

40. Delvenne V, Goldman S, Simon Y, et al. Brain hypometabolism of glucose in bulimia nervosa. *Int J Eat Disord* 1997;21(4):313–320.

41. Quinlivan RM, Robinson RO, Maisey MN. Positron emission tomography in pediatric cardiology. *Arch Dis Child* 1998;79(6):520–522.

42. Donnelly JP, Raffel DM, Shulkin BL, et al. Resting coronary flow and coronary flow reserve in human infants after repair or palliation of congenital heart defects as measured by positron emission tomography. *J Thorac Cardiovasc Surg* 1998;115(1):103–110.

43. Yates RW, Marsden PK, Badawi RD, et al. Evaluation of myocardial perfusion using positron emission tomography in infants following a neonatal arterial switch operation. *Pediatr Cardiol* 2000;21(2): 111–118.

44. Rickers C, Sasse K, Buchert R, et al. Myocardial viability assessed by positron emission tomography in infants and children after the arterial switch operation and suspected infarction. *J Am Coll Cardiol* 2000;36(5):1676–1683.

45. Hwang B, Liu RS, Chu LS, et al. Positron emission tomography for the assessment of myocardial viability in Kawasaki disease using different therapies. *Nucl Med Commun* 2000;21(7):631–636.

46. Litvinova I, Litvinov M, Loeonteva I, et al. PET for diagnosis of mitochondrial cardiomyopathy in children. *Clin Positron Imaging* 2000;3(4):172.

47. Gurney JG, Severson RK, Davis S, et al. Incidence of cancer in children in the United States. *Cancer* 1995;75:2186–2195.

48. Robison L. General principles of the epidemiology of childhood cancer. In: Pizzo P, Poplack D, eds. *Principles and practice of pediatric oncology*. Philadelphia: Lippincott–Raven Publishers, 1997:1–10.

49. Weinblatt ME, Zanzi I, Belakhlef A, et al. False-positive FDG-PET imaging of the thymus of a child with Hodgkin's disease. *J Nucl Med* 1997;38:888–890.

50. Patel PM, Alibazoglu H, Ali A, et al. Normal thymic uptake of FDG on PET imaging. *Clin Nucl Med* 1996;21:772–775.

51. Delbeke D. Oncological applications of FDG PET imaging: colorectal cancer, lymphoma, and melanoma. *J Nucl Med* 1999;40:591–603.

52. Sugawara Y, Fisher SJ, Zasadny KR, et al. Preclinical and clinical studies of bone marrow uptake of fluorine-1-fluorodeoxyglucose with or without granulocyte colony-stimulating factor during chemotherapy. *J Clin Oncol* 1998;16:173–180.

53. Hollinger EF, Alibazoglu H, Ali A, et al. Hematopoietic cytokine-mediated FDG uptake simulates the appearance of diffuse metastatic disease on whole-body PET imaging. *Clin Nucl Med* 1998;23:93–98.

54. Brink I, Reinhardt MJ, Hoegerle S, et al. Increased metabolic activity

in the thymus gland studied with ^{18}F-FDG PET: age, dependency, and frequency after chemotherapy. *J Nucl Med* 2001;42:591–595.

55. Kleihues P, Burger P, Scheithauer B. The new WHO classification of brain tumors. *Brain Pathol* 1993;3:255–268.

56. Robertson R, Ball WJ, Barnes P. Skull and brain. In: Kirks D, ed. *Practical pediatric imaging. Diagnostic radiology of infants and children.* Philadelphia: Lippincott–Raven Publishers, 1997:65–200.

57. Maria B, Drane WB, Quisling RJ, et al. Correlation between gadolinium-diethylenetriaminepentaacetic acid contrast enhancement and thallium-201 chloride uptake in pediatric brainstem glioma. *J Child Neurol* 1997;12:341–348.

58. O'Tuama L, Janicek M, Barnes P, et al. Tl-201/Tc-99m HMPAO SPECT imaging of treated childhood brain tumors. *Pediatr Neurol* 1991;7:249–257.

59. O'Tuama L, Treves ST, Larar G, et al. Tl-201 versus Tc-99m MIBI SPECT in evaluation of childhood brain tumors. *J Nucl Med* 1993;34:1045–1051.

60. Rollins N, Lowry P, Shapiro K. Comparison of gadolinium-enhanced MR and thallium-201 single photon emission computed tomography in pediatric brain tumors. *Pediatr Neurosurg* 1995;22:8–14.

61. Valk PE, Budinger TF, Levin VA, et al. PET of malignant cerebral tumors after interstitial brachytherapy. Demonstration of metabolic activity and correlation with clinical outcome. *J Neurosurg* 1988;69:830–838.

62. Di Chiro G, Oldfield E, Wright DC, et al. Cerebral necrosis after radiotherapy and/or intraarterial chemotherapy for brain tumors: PET and neuropathologic studies. *AJR Am J Roentgenol* 1988;150:189–197.

63. Glantz MJ, Hoffman JM, Coleman RE, et al. Identification of early recurrence of primary central nervous system tumors by [18F]fluorodeoxyglucose positron emission tomograph. *Ann Neurol* 1991;29:347–355.

64. Janus T, Kim E, Tilbury R, et al. Use of [18F] fluorodeoxyglucose positron emission tomography in patients with primary malignant brain tumors. *Ann Neurol* 1993;33:540–548.

65. Rozental JM, Levine RL, Nickles RJ. Changes in glucose uptake by malignant gliomas: preliminary study of prognostic significance. *J Neurooncol* 1991;10:75–83.

66. Schifter T, Hoffman JM, Hanson MW, et al. Serial FDG-PET studies in the prediction of survival in patients with primary brain tumors. *J Comput Assisted Tomogr* 1993;17:509–561.

67. Francavilla TL, Miletich RS, Di Chiro G, et al. Positron emission tomography in the detection of malignant degeneration of low-grade gliomas. *Neurosurgery* 1989;24:1–5.

68. Patronas NJ, Di Chiro G, Kufta C, et al. Prediction of survival in glioma patients by means of positron emission tomography. *J Neurosurg* 1985;62:816–822.

69. Molloy PT, Belasco J, Ngo K, et al. The role of FDG PET imaging in the clinical management of pediatric brain tumors [Abstract]. *J Nucl Med* 1999;40:129P.

70. Holthof VA, Herholz K, Berthold F, et al. *In vivo* metabolism of childhood posterior fossa tumors and primitive neuroectodermal tumors before and after treatment. *Cancer* 1993;1394–1403.

71. Hoffman JM, Hanson MW, Friedman HS, et al. FDG-PET in pediatric posterior fossa brain tumors. *J Comput Assisted Tomogr* 1992;16:62–68.

72. Molloy PT, Defeo R, Hunter J, et al. Excellent correlation of FDG PET imaging with clinical outcome in patients with neurofibromatosis type I and low grade astrocytomas [Abstract]. *J Nucl Med* 1999;40:129P.

73. O'Tuama LA, Phillips PC, Strauss LC, et al. Two-phase [11C]L-methionine PET in childhood brain tumors. *Pediatr Neurol* 1990;6:163–170.

74. Mosskin M, von Holst H, Bergstrom M, et al. Positron emission tomography with ^{11}C-methionine and computed tomography of intracranial tumors compared with histopathologic examination of multiple biopsies. *Acta Radiol* 1987;28:673–681.

75. Lilja A, Lundqvist H, Olsson Y, et al. Positron emission tomography and computed tomography in differential diagnosis between recurrent or residual glioma and treatment-induced brain lesion. *Acta Radiol* 1989;38:121–128.

76. Mineura K, Sasajima T, Kowada M, et al. Indications for differential diagnosis of nontumor central nervous system diseases from tumors. A positron emission tomography study. *J Neuroimaging* 1997;7:8–15.

77. Cohen MD. *Imaging of children with cancer.* St. Louis: Mosby–Year Book, 1992.

78. Nadel HR, Rossleigh MA. Tumor imaging. In: Treves ST, ed. *Pediatric nuclear medicine,* 2nd edition New York: Springer-Verlag, 1995:496–527.

79. Rossleigh MA, Murray IPC, Mackey DWJ. Pediatric solid tumors: evaluation by gallium-67 SPECT studies. *J Nucl Med* 1990;31:161–172.

80. Howman-Giles R, Stevens M, Bergin M. Role of gallium-67 in management of paediatric solid tumors. *Aust Paediatr J* 1982;18:120–125.

81. Yang SL, Alderson PO, Kaizer HA, et al. Serial Ga-67 citrate imaging in children with neoplastic disease: concise communication. *J Nucl Med* 1979;20:210–214.

82. Sty JR, Kun LE, Starshak RJ. Pediatric applications in nuclear oncology. *Semin Nucl Med* 1985;15:171–200.

83. Barrington SF, Carr R. Staging of Burkitt's lymphoma and response to treatment monitored by PET scanning. *Clin Oncol* 1995;7:334–335.

84. Bangerter M, Moog F, Buchmann I, et al. Whole-body 2-[18F]-fluoro-2-deoxy-D-glucose positron emission tomography (FDG-PET) for accurate staging of Hodgkin's disease. *Ann Oncol* 1998;9:1117–1122.

85. Jerusalem G, Warland V, Najjar F, et al. Whole-body ^{18}F-FDG PET for the evaluation of patients with Hodgkin's disease and non-Hodgkin's lymphoma. *Nucl Med Commun* 1999;20:13–20.

86. Leskinen-Kallio S, Ruotsalainen U, Nagren K, et al. Uptake of carbon-11-methionine and fluorodeoxyglucose in non-Hodgkin's lymphoma: a PET study. *J Nucl Med* 1991;32:1211–1218.

87. Moog F, Bangerter M, Kotzerke J, et al. ^{18}F-Fluorodeoxyglucose positron emission tomography as a new approach to detect lymphomatous bone marrow. *J Clin Oncol* 1998;16:603–609.

88. Moog F, Bangerter M, Diederichs CG, et al. Extranodal malignant lymphoma: detection with FDG PET versus CT. *Radiology* 1998;206:475–481.

89. Moog F, Bangerter M, Diederichs CG, et al. Lymphoma: role of whole-body 2-deoxy-2-[F-18]fluoro-D-glucose (FDG) PET in nodal staging. *Radiology* 1997;203:795–800.

90. Okada J, Yoshikawa K, Imazeki K, et al. The use of FDG-PET in the detection and management of malignant lymphoma: correlation of uptake with prognosis. *J Nucl Med* 1991;32:686–691.

91. Okada J, Yoshikawa K, Itami M, et al. Positron emission tomography using fluorine-18-fluorodeoxyglucose in malignant lymphoma: a comparison with proliferative activity. *J Nucl Med* 1992;33:325–329.

92. Rodriguez M, Rehn S, Ahlstrom H, et al. Predicting malignancy grade with PET in non-Hodgkin's lymphoma. *J Nucl Med* 1995;36:1790–1796.

93. Paul R. Comparison of fluorine-18-2-fluorodeoxyglucose and gallium-67 citrate imaging for detection of lymphoma. *J Nucl Med* 1987;28:288–292.

94. Newman JS, Francis IR, Kaminski MS, et al. Imaging of lymphoma with PET with 2-[F-18]-fluoro-2-deoxy-D-glucose: correlation with CT. *Radiology* 1994;190:111–116.

95. de Wit M, Bumann D, Beyer W, et al. Whole-body positron emission tomography (PET) for diagnosis of residual mass in patients with lymphoma. *Ann Oncol* 1997;8[Suppl 1]:57–60.

96. Cremerius U, Fabry U, Neuerburg J, et al. Positron emission tomography with 18-F-FDG to detect residual disease after therapy for malignant lymphoma. *Nucl Med Commun* 1998;19:1055–1063.

97. Hoh CK, Glaspy J, Rosen P, et al. Whole-body FDG PET imaging for staging of Hodgkin's disease and lymphoma. *J Nucl Med* 1997;38:343–348.

98. Romer W, Hanauske AR, Ziegler S, et al. Positron emission tomography in non-Hodgkin's lymphoma: assessment of chemotherapy with fluorodeoxyglucose. *Blood* 1998;91:4464–4471.

99. Stumpe KD, Urbinelli M, Steinert HC, et al. Whole-body positron emission tomography using fluorodeoxyglucose for staging of lymphoma: effectiveness and comparison with computed tomography. *Eur J Nucl Med* 1998;25:721–728.

100. Lapela M, Leskinen S, Minn HR, et al. Increased glucose metabolism in untreated non-Hodgkin's lymphoma: a study with positron emission tomography and fluorine-18-fluorodeoxyglucose. *Blood* 1995;86:3522–3527.

101. Carr R, Barrington SF, Madan B, et al. Detection of lymphoma in bone marrow by whole-body positron emission tomography. *Blood* 1998;91:3340–3346.

102. Segall GM. FDG PET imaging in patients with lymphoma: a clinical perspective. *J Nucl Med* 2001;42(4): 609–610.

103. Mody R, Shulkin B, Yanik G, et al. PET FDG imaging in pediatric lymphomas. *J Nucl Med* 2001;42(5):39P.

104. Kostakoglu L, Leonard JP, Coleman M, et al. Comparison of FDG-PET and Ga-67 SPECT in the staging of lymphoma [Abstract]. *J Nucl Med* 2000;41[Suppl 5]:118P.

105. Lin PC, Chu J, Pocock N. F-18 fluorodeoxyglucose imaging with coincidence dual-head gamma camera (hybrid FDG-PET) for staging of lymphoma: comparison with Ga-67 scintigraphy [Abstract]. *J Nucl Med* 2000;41[Suppl 5]:118P.

106. Tomas MB, Manalili E, Leonidas JC, et al. F-18 FDG imaging of lymphoma in children using a hybrid PET system: comparison with Ga-67. *J Nucl Med* 2000;[Suppl 5]:96P.

107. Tatsumi M, Kitayama H, Sugahara H, et al. Whole-body hybrid PET with ^{18}F-FDG in the staging of non-Hodgkin's lymphoma. *J Nucl Med* 2001;42(4):601–608.

108. Bousvaros A, Kirks DR, Grossman H. Imaging of neuroblastoma: an overview. *Pediatr Radiol* 1986;16:89–106.

109. Briganti V, Sestini R, Orlando C, et al. Imaging of somatostatin receptors by indium-111-pentetreotide correlates with quantitative determination of somatostatin receptor type 2 gene expression in neuroblastoma tumor. *Clin Cancer Res* 1997;3:2385–2391.

110. Shulkin BL, Hutchinson RJ, Castle VP, et al. Neuroblastoma: positron emission tomography with 2-[fluorine-18]-fluoro-2-deoxy-D-glucose compared with metaiodobenzylguanidine scintigraphy. *Radiology* 1996;199:743–750.

111. Shulkin BL, Wieland DM, Baro ME, et al. PET hydroxyephedrine imaging of neuroblastoma. *J Nucl Med* 1996;37:16–21.

112. Shulkin BL, Wieland DM, Castle VP, et al. Carbon-11 epinephrine PET imaging of neuroblastoma [Abstract]. *J Nucl Med* 1999;40:129P.

113. Vaidyanathan G, Affleck DJ, Zalutsky MR. Validation of 4-[fluorine-18]fluoro-3-iodobenzylguanidine as a positron-emitting analog of MIBG. *J Nucl Med* 1995;36:644–650.

114. Ott RJ, Tait D, Flower MA, et al. Treatment planning for ^{131}I-MIBG radiotherapy of neural crest tumors using ^{124}I-MIBG positron emission tomography. *Br J Radiol* 1992;65:787–791.

115. Barnewolt CE, Paltiel HJ, Lebowitz RL, et al. Genitourinary system. In: Kirks DR, ed. *Practical pediatric imaging. Diagnostic radiology of infants and children*, 3rd ed. Philadelphia: Lippincott–Raven Publishers, 1997:1009–1170.

116. Shulkin BL, Chang E, Strouse PJ, et al. PET FDG studies of Wilms tumors. *J Pediatr Hematol/Oncol* 1997;19:334–338.

117. McDonald DJ. Limb salvage surgery for sarcomas of the extremities. *AJR Am J Roentgenol* 1994;163:509–513.

118. Triche TJ. Pathology of pediatric malignancies. In: Pizzo PA, Poplack DG, eds. *Principles and practice of pediatric oncology*, 2nd ed. Philadelphia: JB Lippincott Co, 1993:115–152.

119. O'Connor MI, Pritchard DJ. Ewing's sarcoma. Prognostic factors, disease control, and the reemerging role of surgical treatment. *Clin Orthop* 1991;262:78–87.

120. Jaramillo D, Laor T, Gebhardt M. Pediatric musculoskeletal neoplasms. Evaluation with MR imaging. *MRI Clin North Am* 1996;4:1–22.

121. Frouge C, Vanel D, Coffre C, et al. The role of magnetic resonance imaging in the evaluation of Ewing sarcoma—a report of 27 cases. *Skeletal Radiol* 1988;17:387–392.

122. MacVicar AD, Olliff JFC, Pringle J, et al. Ewing sarcoma: MR imaging of chemotherapy-induced changes with histologic correlation. *Radiology* 1992;184:859–864.

123. Lemmi MA, Fletcher BD, Marina NM, et al. Use of MR imaging to assess results of chemotherapy for Ewing sarcoma. *AJR Am J Roentgenol* 1990;155:343–346.

124. Erlemann R, Sciuk J, Bosse A, et al. Response of osteosarcoma and Ewing sarcoma to preoperative chemotherapy: assessment with dynamic and static MR imaging and skeletal scintigraphy. *Radiology* 1990;175:791–796.

125. Holscher HC, Bloem JL, Vanel D, et al. Osteosarcoma: chemotherapy-induced changes at MR imaging. *Radiology* 1992;182:839–844.

126. Lawrence JA, Babyn PS, Chan HS, et al. Extremity osteosarcoma in childhood: prognostic value of radiologic imaging. *Radiology* 1993;189:43–47.

127. Connolly LP, Laor T, Jaramillo D, et al. Prediction of chemotherapeutic response of osteosarcoma with quantitative thallium-201 scintigraphy and magnetic resonance imaging [Abstract]. *Radiology* 1996;201(P):349.

128. Lin J, Leung WT. Quantitative evaluation of thallium-201 uptake in predicting chemotherapeutic response of osteosarcoma. *Eur J Nucl Med* 1995;22:553–555.

129. Menendez LR, Fideler BM, Mirra J. Thallium-201 scanning for the evaluation of osteosarcoma and soft tissue sarcoma. *J Bone Joint Surg* 1993;75:526–531.

130. Ramanna L, Waxman A, Binney G, et al. Thallium-201 scintigraphy in bone sarcoma: comparison with gallium-67 and technetium-99m MDP in the evaluation of chemotherapeutic response. *J Nucl Med* 1990;31:567–572.

131. Rosen G, Loren GJ, Brien EW, et al. Serial thallium-201 scintigraphy in osteosarcoma. Correlation with tumor necrosis after preoperative chemotherapy. *Clin Orthop* 1993;293:302–306.

132. Ohtomo K, Terui S, Yokoyama R, et al. Thallium-201 scintigraphy to assess effect of chemotherapy to osteosarcoma. *J Nucl Med* 1996;37:1444–1448.

133. Bar-Sever Z, Connolly LP, Treves ST, et al. Technetium-99m MIBI in the evaluation of children with Ewing's sarcoma [Abstract]. *J Nucl Med* 1997;38:13P.

134. Caner B, Kitapel M, Unlu M, et al. Technetium-99m-MIBI uptake in benign and malignant bone lesions: a comparative study with technetium-99m-MDP. *J Nucl Med* 1992;33:319–324.

135. Lenzo NP, Shulkin B, Castle VP, et al. FDG PET in childhood soft tissue sarcoma [Abstract]. *J Nucl Med* 2000;41[Suppl 5]:96P.

136. Abdel-Dayem HM. The role of nuclear medicine in primary bone and soft tissue tumors. *Semin Nucl Med* 1997;27:355–363.

137. Shulkin BL, Mitchell DS, Ungar DR, et al. Neoplasms in a pediatric population: 2-[F-18]-fluoro-2-deoxy-D-glucose PET studies. *Radiology* 1995;194:495–500.

138. Jadvar H, Connolly LP, Shulkin BL, et al. Positron-emission tomography in pediatrics. *Nucl Med Annu* 2000:53–83.

CHAPTER 11

PET and Drug Development

Jerry M. Collins

Development of a drug is a process that depends heavily on knowledge of its distribution in the body and its effects on the body. As phrased in Table 11.1, we want to know where the drug goes, what it does there, and if there are apparent relationships between drug localization and drug effects. At each stage of development, more refined answers are sought to these questions.

Positron emission tomography (PET) imaging can obtain direct information about both the distribution and the functional effects of a drug. Thus, PET can provide unique, value-added contributions to the drug development process. As described elsewhere in this book, PET provides data that are unmatched for sensitivity. Perhaps even more important than its exquisite sensitivity, PET provides spatial information on drug distribution and drug effects that is virtually never attained in living humans by other means.

There are many similarities between the development of therapeutic agents and probes for PET imaging of *in vivo* functions (the term *probe* is used in this chapter to designate the radiopharmaceutical or positron-emitting compound used to image biochemical, molecular, and/or physiologic pathways). Both treatment and imaging approaches attempt to exploit differences between some process within the target and in other tissues. Another very practical characteristic for both therapeutics and probes is that the development process can be viewed as a pipeline that stretches over several years. The time at which a novel therapeutic agent enters clinical testing is far too late to decide that it would be useful to pursue imaging of its impact. Once a target for screening of new therapeutics has been identified, it also becomes a target to be considered for imaging. Even if developed from the same screening approach, the ideal probe molecule may or may not be the same as the optimal therapeutic molecule.

One of our major challenges is development of new probes. Fluorine-18 (^{18}F)-fluorodeoxyglucose (FDG) is the only functional imaging probe readily available at all PET facilities. Exploratory trials have been reported for various other potential probes, but a concerted effort is required to prioritize targets and probe development projects.

Although drug development and probe development can be interrelated, they can also be separate processes. At one level, the role of a probe is to support the development of the therapeutic. In some cases, the probe might assist in the choice of doses of the therapeutic for the pivotal trials leading to marketing approval. In such cases, the approval of the therapeutic is based on the success of the trials, not the imaging studies. The probe itself may never be used again.

In other cases, a general functional probe may be valuable for an entire class of drugs, or even many classes of drugs. The probe itself becomes a diagnostic tool that might be marketed in its own right. Fluorine-18-FDG is the most advanced example of this pattern for PET probes.

As described in the next two sections, useful probes for PET imaging can be obtained by positron labeling of either the therapeutic substance itself or the indicators (ligands, substrates, tracers) of functional status. For drug distribution studies, the most relevant information is obtained when the drug itself can be labeled with a positron-emitting atom.

Functional imaging evaluates processes occurring at the cellular or tissue/organ level: physiologic (e.g., transport carrier system), molecular (e.g., receptor binding), or biochemical (e.g., enzymatic activity). Thus, for functional imaging, the most important factor is a clear concept of the process to be probed. Focus on specific targets at these levels is part of a general shift in the paradigm of clinical diagnosis and treatment.

In addition to the value of imaging for drug development, the same tools could be used for customizing patient-specific treatment. Physicians have long sought tests that could assist in the choice of the most appropriate therapy for the individual patient. Traditional selection of therapy for individuals has relied on prognostic factors derived from large popula-

TABLE 11.1. *Question-based drug development*

1. Does the drug reach its target?
2. What does it do there?
   a. Desired impact on target?
   b. Side effects?
3. What is relationship between questions 1 and 2?

411

tions. For example, in anticancer therapy, the histology of the tumor is a key factor. Once therapy has been selected, it is generally continued until there is an obvious failure to control disease (e.g., tumor growth) or to control symptoms (e.g., pain).

By shifting emphasis toward underlying targets, functional imaging with PET has the potential to improve the selection and subsequent evaluations of therapy. PET provides the opportunity to measure several characteristics of a disease target serially and noninvasively.

For some imaging targets (e.g., enzymes, receptors, and transporters), patients can be phenotyped *before* initiation of treatment. The goal is to obtain information that can be used to optimize the match between drugs and the patient-specific characteristics of the target. In addition to the potential for improving efficacy, these procedures would be valuable for avoiding needless toxicity from treatment regimens that are inappropriate for the individual patient being assessed.

Regardless of whether pretreatment phenotyping is feasible, all potential targets should be able to provide therapeutic assessment once treatment is underway. Rather than waiting until overt failure is demonstrated, which could be many months for conditions that are difficult to assess, the goal is to determine as quickly as possible whether the particular therapy is working for a specific patient. The optimal imaging time will depend on the mechanism of action for the therapy, but the ideal situation would be immediately after the first dose so a decision can be made regarding further treatment. Positive findings would be greatly appreciated by all. Negative results would provide the opportunity to explore other therapeutic approaches before further deterioration of the patient's condition and ability to tolerate therapy.

The examples provided in the next two sections elaborate on these concepts. It is important to keep in mind that all of these examples are works in progress. There are currently very few PET imaging probes that are "accepted" for routine use by the nuclear medicine community except ¹⁸F-FDG.

ASSESSMENT OF DRUG DELIVERY WITH PET

The ultimate goal of drug delivery (pharmacokinetics) is to get the active molecule to the target site. In classic drug development, systemic exposure to the drug is assessed by serial measurements of the drug concentration in plasma. These measurements are very helpful for verifying that a drug has been absorbed or for evaluating intersubject variability in elimination rates. In general terms, we expect that the impact of the drug on the body will be related to the extent of systemic exposure. This principle is equally valid for desirable effects (therapy) and adverse events (toxicity).

Monitoring plasma concentrations to determine the systemic exposure component of drug delivery is certainly helpful, but there remain fundamental questions that can only be addressed by examining the second component of drug delivery, namely, the interaction between systemic exposure

and local transport processes. In the preclinical phases of drug development, drug distribution studies are conducted in animal species to gain confidence that the active molecules reach the target sites of interest. In contrast, once human testing begins, we no longer have access to invasive sampling of many tissue sites. Without the noninvasive tools of imaging, the second component of local drug delivery is invisible, and we can only evaluate the systemic component.

Antiinfective Drugs: Penetration to Target

The success of an antiinfective drug depends on its ability to reach bacteria, viruses, fungi, or other parasites wherever they may reside in the body. There is particular concern about delivering adequate concentrations of drugs to so-called "sanctuary" sites such as the brain or prostatic fluid. Comprehensive testing is conducted to determine the intrinsic sensitivity of various invading organisms, with the results often focusing on concentrations required to achieve 90% kill or 90% inhibition of growth—that is, the IC_{90}. No matter how impressively potent a drug might be in attacking the target in laboratory tests, it cannot be successful in patients unless it is delivered to the target site.

Figure 11.1 provides an excellent demonstration of the

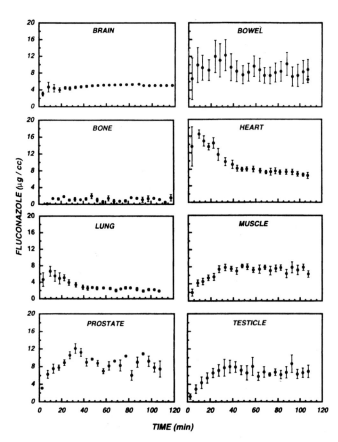

FIG. 11.1. Fluorine-18-fluconazole distribution over time in 6 healthy volunteers. (From Fischman AJ, Alpert NM, Babich JW, et al. The role of PET in pharmacokinetic analysis. *Drug Metab Rev* 1997;29:923–956, with permission.)

role PET imaging can play in determining if a particular drug is likely to reach the critical tissue of interest. Fischman et al. (1) labeled the antifungal drug, fluconazole, with ^{18}F and administered it to human volunteers in a phase 1 study. As illustrated, the time course of distribution for ^{18}F-fluconazole was followed for 2 hours in eight body areas. Because humans do not metabolize fluconazole, only the parent drug is present. Thus, the absolute quantitation of radiolabel provided by PET imaging can be translated into traditional units of drug concentration (in micrograms per milliliter) that can then be compared against the therapeutic goals defined by IC$_{90}$ testing. In this case, with a single study early in drug development, a positive finding can help sustain interest in the lead candidate. Alternatively, the outcome of such a study could definitively show serious obstacles to further development. Although such a result would be disappointing, it is surely better to find out early in development, before clinical efficacy studies in patients. Fischman et al. (1) also described similar studies for erythromycin and other antibiotics.

Transporters and their Modulation

As mentioned at the beginning of this section, local transport processes can control access of a drug to its target. Our understanding of these transporters or pumps has blossomed dramatically in the last few years. Several families of pumps have been discovered and classified phenotypically. In addition, many of the genes have been cloned, and transporters are now recognized as one of the largest categories of expression products of the mammalian genomes.

Because of the key role of these transporters in regulating drug delivery to target sites, development of probes to assess their operation is a major opportunity for PET imaging. Development programs for probes of drug uptake into the cell and efflux from the cell are in early stages of development but build on a tradition of monitoring PET probes of the transporters for amino acid entry into the cell (2). Although there is work underway with PET probes (3), the majority of published work uses single-photon emission tomography probes such as technetium-99m sestamibi (4).

The use of sestamibi illustrates a blurring between drug distribution and drug effect, because there is movement away from the study of distribution for a particular drug and toward a general functional probe for a transporter. Some groups have sought a general probe because there are too many drugs to study each of them. With the recent explosion in our catalog of transporters, one might also say that there are too many transporters to have a probe for each of them. The choice of approach not only is philosophical but also should be driven by the specific question under study.

Drug Delivery to Tumors

Although transport processes can influence all categories of drugs, their role is critical for drug delivery to tumors, due to the narrow therapeutic index of anticancer drugs. Because substantial research has been invested in developing drugs that are modulators of delivery, some means of assessing the action of these drugs is highly desirable. Efflux pumps can mediate resistance to anticancer drugs. As the drug approaches its target, the tumor may pump it out. Thus, concentrations at the target are very low, making them ineffective and actually promoting the development of further resistance mechanisms. There are a number of efforts underway to develop modulators that block these transport systems.

Our traditional tools of plasma and urine sampling are unable to assess either baseline or modulated drug delivery to specific tumors. In fact, because delivery of drugs to tissues is generally a reversible process, parameters of systemic exposure, such as the area under the curve, will be unaffected by the presence or absence of a functioning efflux pump at a target site in a tumor.

PET imaging is a tool that can focus directly on drug delivery at the target of interest. Delivery of a drug to the tumor does not guarantee successful therapy. However, if the drug never gets to the target or gets pushed away as soon as it arrives, it certainly will not be effective. The earlier we discover the problem, the sooner we can implement strategies for attempting to modulate this pharmacokinetic issue or the sooner we can consider alternative therapy. Many of these concepts are illustrated in Fig. 11.2. Consider the case in which a drug (e.g., paclitaxel) has been selected for treating a patient with a tumor, based on the tumor's histology and other prognostic factors. If paclitaxel is labeled with a positron emitter, it becomes a suitable probe to seek an answer to the question at the top of Fig. 11.2: "Does the drug accumulate in the tumor?" If the answer is "no" (the drug fails to accumulate in the tumor), one option is to conclude that paclitaxel can only cause toxicity for this patient, and another therapeutic approach should be taken. Substantial validation would be required to confirm the logical scheme, but the outline for decision making is clear.

If the answer is "yes" (drug does accumulate in the tumor), there is no guarantee that the tumor will respond to

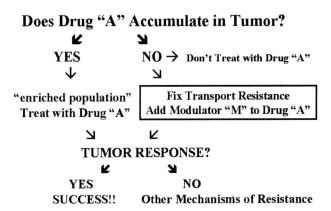

Does Drug "A" Accumulate in Tumor?

YES   NO → Don't Treat with Drug "A"

"enriched population" Treat with Drug "A"   Fix Transport Resistance Add Modulator "M" to Drug "A"

TUMOR RESPONSE?

YES   NO

SUCCESS!!   Other Mechanisms of Resistance

FIG. 11.2. Decision tree for image-guided assessment of efflux transporter impact.

paclitaxel, but the probability of success has been enhanced because at least some nonresponders have been eliminated from the population. Accumulation of drug in the tumor is essential but is not the sole determinant of chemosensitivity. In other words, accumulation is necessary, but not sufficient for response. If the tumor fails to respond despite adequate drug accumulation, one of the most common mechanisms of resistance has been ruled out, and other reasons must be considered.

Patients with tumors that fail to accumulate paclitaxel can become candidates for therapy with drugs that are intended to modulate paclitaxel delivery to tumors—that is, to "fix" resistance due to transport. If the labeled paclitaxel still fails to accumulate in the tumor, then the modulator has failed, at least for the dose and schedule chosen. Once again, it may be desirable to spare the patient the toxicity of paclitaxel and to seek other therapeutic approaches.

If use of the modulator does permit labeled paclitaxel to accumulate in the tumor, transport resistance has been fixed. Once again, there is no guarantee that transport resistance is the sole mechanism of resistance, but at least a population has been identified with an enhanced probability that the modulator will permit benefit from paclitaxel to be attained.

The ability to enrich the population to be studied with a drug by identifying the patients who will be more likely to benefit from the drug can be viewed in various ways. In drug development discussions, some have argued that this strategy will narrow the market for the drug by segmenting the overall population into various subfractions. Others have argued that the fastest route to approval is a smaller population with a very high success rate. Contemporary drug development is shaped by both viewpoints, and the "verdict" is far from final.

Evaluation of Inhaled Drug Products

The inhalation route already plays an important role in the delivery of certain drug products. In addition, there is considerable excitement about the prospects for delivering peptides, proteins, and other molecules that are unstable or not absorbed in the gastrointestinal tract. Insulin is a key example.

Many delivery factors complicate the efficiency of pulmonary delivery. Some issues are related to the design of the device (e.g., "metered-dose inhaler") or the formulation that contains the active drug substance. Other issues relate to the patterns of actual use by the patient. Imaging can help to evaluate the success of various device designs, solubilization/aerosolization strategies, and use patterns, but the appropriateness of imaging studies depends on the drug development goal.

When determining potential roles for imaging, the key decision is whether systemic absorption is desirable (or possible). For some drug products, the inhalation route is convenient, but a large portion of the drug effect is generated via systemic exposure. For these products, classic measure-

ments of drug concentration in plasma will be the primary standard for judging success or failure of delivery (but not necessarily the complete story for efficacy). During development, a combined assessment of local delivery (with imaging) and systemic exposure can help guide intermediate evaluations of the evolving product's performance.

If the intent were to deliver a drug that is truly acting locally, for example, for the treatment of pulmonary disease, measures of systemic exposure would generally be worthless. These are the situations in which imaging can be most helpful in drug development, particularly in assisting the choice of doses for pivotal efficacy trials.

The study of Berridge and Heald (5) illustrates the type of information that can be obtained with PET imaging of inhalation therapy. The left panel in Color Plate 25 (following page 394) is a PET image of early distribution of the inhaled dose superimposed on an anatomic image of the nasal passages. If the drug target is in these structures, various delivery parameters can be adjusted to help design the product. The right panel in Color Plate 25 (following page 394) shows distribution of drug within the bronchial tree at later times. For many disease targets, this type of image provides key information to assist design.

The impact of changes in the formulation—that is, the vehicle in which the drug is prepared—on the patterns of drug delivery has had a higher profile recently, due to the worldwide consensus on the environmental desirability of eliminating chlorofluorocarbons (CFCs) as aerosols. Phase out of CFCs from medical products was delayed to ensure that patient care was not compromised. Indeed, the interaction between the formulation and vehicle can have a profound effect on the patterns of regional drug delivery. Imaging studies such as the one published by Berridge and Heald (5) can assist the transition between propellants.

CELLULAR AND MOLECULAR TARGETS FOR PET IMAGING

Some of the major categories of targets for PET probes are shown in Table 11.2. The first two categories, energy metabolism and DNA synthesis, are very general approaches to the determination of tumor functional status. Even though our contemporary emphasis is on precise molecular classification of targets, it is still quite desirable to have these "universal" probes as a check on the relevance of our hypotheses, as well as for the situations in which an appropriate target-specific or drug-specific probe is simply not available.

As described earlier, FDG is the leading functional PET

TABLE 11.2. Categories of PET functional imaging targets

1. General energy metabolism (^{18}F-fluorodeoxyglucose)
2. DNA synthesis/cellular proliferation
3. Receptors: signaling/regulation
4. Enzymes: many tumor targets

probe, and has remarkable versatility. Evaluation of the rate of DNA synthesis and cellular proliferation is another approach toward a general probe. In the laboratory, tritiated thymidine (dThd) has been used for decades to evaluate DNA synthesis in cell culture. In anticancer therapy, the ability to monitor the impact of conventional cytotoxic regimens on DNA synthesis is easily appreciated. In addition, therapeutic approaches of many contemporary targets ultimately intend to reduce proliferation and may be evaluated using dThd analogues (dThd analogues are discussed in more detail later in this section).

A much more target-specific approach is represented by the last two categories of probes. Receptors and enzymes are well established as drug targets across the full spectrum of disease areas, and they are the cornerstones of modern therapeutic development programs in the areas of cell signaling and regulation. Thus, according to our paradigm for probe development, receptors and enzymes are also potential targets for functional imaging. Although the imaging of these targets remains in the pilot stage for most diseases, the feasibility for monitoring in situ receptor occupancy and enzyme activity has been solidly established in neuropharmacology, as described below.

The list of targets in Table 11.2 for functional PET probes is not meant to be comprehensive. Also, some targets are in an intermediate position on the scale from "general" to "specific." For example, there are probes for measuring blood flow and capillary permeability, as well as phenomena such as tissue hypoxia.

As noted in Table 11.3, once the ideal (relevant) targets are chosen based on biochemical/molecular/physiologic factors, additional probe-specific items are encountered. From the viewpoint of nuclear chemistry, the half-life of the positron-emitting isotope must be matched to the time scale of the process being probed. A rapid synthesis must be feasible, due to the short half-lives of most positron-emitting atoms. From a pharmacokinetic perspective, minimal catabolism is highly desirable. Otherwise, the background signal from accumulating metabolites interferes with the desired signal from the parent molecule. Finally, the ratio of specific to nonspecific localization within the tumor is critical. Once all other obstacles are overcome and a new probe has entered the clinic, the most common reason that development is abandoned is the finding of a broad and nonspecific distribution of the probe throughout the body, preventing the monitoring of specific target interactions.

The ability to image the response of the target of drug

TABLE 11.3. *Desirable characteristics for design of functional PET probes*

1. Relevant target for interaction
2. Match isotopic half-life to process time scale
3. Rapid synthetic time
4. Minimal interference from catabolites
5. Target localization

action is fundamental to the advances in the individualization of therapy, as well as enhancements in drug development.

These concepts are illustrated by the following examples.

Neuroreceptors: D_2 and 5-HT_2

Unquestionably, the applications of PET imaging for drug development are furthest advanced in the field of neurosciences. This progress has been pushed by multiple factors. There is very strong interest in obtaining information about the brain, but it is the least accessible part of the body for invasive sampling. Due to huge investments over the last few decades in building a knowledge base for receptors and their ligands, the selection of targets and probes has been facilitated. Fortuitously, the least accessible part of the body has a major advantage for imaging because the blood–brain barrier tends to preferentially exclude the relatively more hydrophilic catabolites of the probes, thus, reducing the background noise.

The dopaminergic- and serotonergic-receptor systems have been mapped extensively. The work of Farde et al. (6) demonstrates how the impact of a drug can be measured in two separate receptor systems in a single patient. Carbon-11-raclopride is an established probe for the D_2 dopaminergic receptor subtype and ^{11}C-N-methyl spiperone probes both 5-HT_2 and D_2 receptors. Of course, these probes cannot be given simultaneously, because the PET camera cannot distinguish which molecule has ^{11}C attached. However, the short half-life of ^{11}C is an advantage for taking sequential "snapshots" of each probe individually, with perhaps only 1 or 2 hours between imaging sessions.

The efficacy of receptor blockade is commonly determined by "blocking" studies with unlabeled drug. Similarly, PET can assess the effect of chronic receptor blockade, such as in psychotropic therapies, when the patient is on or off therapy (see Color Plate 26 following page 394). This figure demonstrates the impact of risperidone on two receptor subtypes in a patient being treated with this drug. The D_2 receptors are almost completely blocked. Although there is a substantial blockage of 5-HT_2 receptors by risperidone, the quantitative extent is lower than the drug's impact on D_2 receptors. The broad pattern of spatial distribution for 5-HT_2 receptors in the human brain can also be identified as quite different from the narrower localization of D_2 receptors.

We are frequently reminded that even the most potent and selective drugs can have multiple effects in the body. In the case of antipsychotics such as risperidone, drug designers intentionally built molecules with dual effects, based on earlier therapeutic experiences with blockade of the individual receptors. What is the optimal balance between D_2 and 5-HT_2 effects?

At the time of selection of candidates for clinical testing, the answer was unknown, and decisions had to be based on the hypotheses that were available during the development phase. After the initial subjects are tested, imaging results can provide rapid feedback regarding the extent of blockade achieved in the two receptors.

It should be recognized that this imaging information does not test the therapeutic hypotheses. Instead, it tests whether the intended balance between relative receptor impact was actually achieved *in vivo*. At this early stage, there is no information about clinical benefit. If the receptor impact meets design criteria, the developer will be encouraged to pursue this drug as a lead candidate. On the other hand, failure to achieve design criteria for receptor impact may push toward a decision to test other candidates before making major investments in therapeutic clinical trials.

Without early feedback from imaging, intermediate decisions cannot be made, the subtype specificity *in vivo* cannot be evaluated, and the development program must wait until clinical outcomes provide feedback. Unfortunately, by that time, the resources (e.g., time and labor) have been spent and patient opportunities cannot be recaptured.

If the decision is made to proceed, clinical benefit information will be collected in the usual fashion for such trials. At the end of these trials, the relationships between imaging results and clinical outcomes will be the final test of the hypotheses regarding the nature of optimal receptor blockade.

Estrogen-receptor Blockage by Tamoxifen

For hormone-sensitive tumors such as breast cancer, the established approach to disease management is based on characterization of the hormone receptors (estrogen and progesterone) in biopsies from individual tumors. The ability to noninvasively monitor estrogen receptors with ^{18}F-fluoroestradiol (FES) is a natural extension of existing practice.

The overall approach is illustrated in Color Plate 27 following page 394. Dehdashti et al. (7) injected ^{18}F-FES into a patient with a large metastasis of breast cancer in the pleural space, which was known to have estrogen receptors. Before therapy, avid binding of ^{18}F-FES to the receptors on the tumor was observed (in the top of the left panel in Color Plate 27 following page 394). Therapy with tamoxifen was initiated, with the intent of occupying estrogen receptors and blocking the uptake of other estrogenic substances. As demonstrated in the PET image (right panel of Color Plate 27 following page 394), localization at the tumor site of ^{18}F-FES has markedly diminished after 7 days of tamoxifen therapy. Although these images do not constitute an index of clinical value, they verify that the specific therapy for this particular tumor is acting as intended.

Tumor Cell Proliferation Probed with Thymidine Analogues

In the laboratory, tritiated dThd has been used for decades to monitor DNA synthesis and cellular proliferation in cell culture and animals. Thirty years ago, the first exploration of positron-labeled dThd was reported by the Brookhaven group (8), with the demonstration that ^{11}C-dThd could be synthesized and injected into mice in a timeframe compatible with imaging.

During the 1980s through the 1990s, a series of human investigations using ^{11}C-dThd attempted to build on these murine studies. Some success was obtained, but we now appreciate that pyrimidine biochemistry in mice is quite different from that in humans. The rapid catabolism of dThd in humans creates an enormous background signal of labeled molecules, and dThd itself is available for labeling of DNA for only a few minutes. Complex mathematic corrections are required for catabolic interference.

The "proof of concept" for dThd PET was eventually demonstrated with publication by Shields et al. (9) of the first therapeutic assessment images. As illustrated in the left panel of Color Plate 28 following page 394, there is extensive uptake of ^{11}C-dThd both in the primary lung tumor and in the vertebral space before therapy. After a standard regimen of cisplatin on day one and etoposide on days one to three, the patient was reevaluated on day six. The tumor is still present anatomically, but the image in the right panel indicates that the tumor has stopped taking up ^{11}C-dThd for DNA synthesis and cellular proliferation.

Although this initial demonstration of the principle has been gratifying, the pool of catabolites of ^{11}C-dThd in humans creates major difficulties. PET imaging is essentially the detection of total radioactivity, so an extensive search has been underway to find an analogue of dThd that has minimal catabolism but retains the favorable anabolic (DNA-labeling) properties of dThd itself. Some candidate structures are shown in Fig. 11.3.

Conti et al. (10) reported the first probe that blocked catabolism without blocking anabolic enzymes. They placed fluorine in the sugar of ^{11}C-dThd to produce ^{11}C-FMAU (2'-fluoro-5-[^{11}C]-methyl-1-β-D-arabinofuranosyluracil). Because the 20-minute half-life of ^{11}C causes a number of logistic difficulties in the preparation and administration of the dose, as well as the timing of images that can be reliably obtained, labeling of various dThd derivatives with ^{18}F, with a half-life of 110 minutes, is being actively pursued.

Shields et al. (11) have added ^{18}F at the 3' position in the sugar of dThd to yield ^{18}F-FLT (3'-[^{18}F]-3'-deoxy-dThd) (Fig. 11.3). Images obtained with ^{18}F-FLT in patients (see Color Plate 29 following page 394) have demonstrated a similar distribution to dThd itself, despite the inability of phosphorylated FLT to efficiently enter DNA.

Follow-up work from Alauddin et al. (12) and our laboratory group (13) has explored ^{18}F-FMAU as a dThd analogue that could potentially combine the favorable properties of ^{18}F-FLT and ^{11}C-FMAU. For initial uptake, FLT and FMAU presumably would give equivalent images, because they are trapped intracellularly by phosphorylation via thymidine kinase. As time progresses, the intracellular pool of FMAU, but not FLT, can be increased by incorporation into DNA. Thus, with the ability provided by ^{18}F for longer imaging periods, combined with enhanced intracellular trapping for

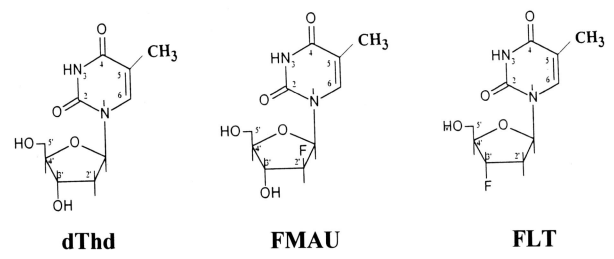

FIG. 11.3. Structures for endogenous thymidine and two of its fluorinated analogues. Thymidine has been labeled for PET imaging with carbon-11 (^{11}C) on the pyrimidine base at either the 2-carbon or the 5-methyl carbon. FMAU can be labeled either with ^{11}C on the pyrimidine base (as with thymidine) or with fluorine-18 (^{18}F) on the 2' position of the sugar. FLT has been labeled with ^{18}F on the 3' position of the sugar.

FMAU, the goal of an improved signal-to-noise ratio is being pursued.

Delineation of the differences between information obtained with PET and dThd analogues versus FDG PET will be a key aspect of further clinical investigations. Anecdotal experiences with inflammatory lesions suggest situations that favor dThd analogues. In the initial study of ^{11}C-dThd (9), the qualitative information obtained from dThd PET was similar to that obtained with FDG PET in the same patients, but the authors report that the quantitative assessment with dThd seemed more closely related to clinical outcome. When compared with computed tomography, dThd PET images obtained before and after therapy also provided an assessment of tumor response more quantitatively related to clinical outcome. However, both FLT and dThd show much more uptake in bone marrow than FDG, which is usually undesirable.

For the set of gene therapy protocols that use herpes simplex virus (HSV) thymidine kinase as either a suicide gene or a reporter gene, any of the aforementioned dThd approaches, as well as iodinated analogues, should be able to provide an assessment of whether gene expression was successful (15). In addition, because of their specific affinity for HSV thymidine kinase, a series of analogues of acyclovir or ganciclovir have been shown preclinically to be successful probes for gene expression (16).

MAO-B Enzyme Inhibition

Fowler et al. (16,17), who have reported on the phenotypic expression of monoamine oxidase B (MAO-B) in human brain in situ, have solidly established the feasibility for PET monitoring of enzyme activity. Further, they have measured the dose dependence and time course of enzymatic activity for both reversible and irreversible inhibitors (16,17). These works are elegant in their own right as a study of the MAO-B enzyme *in vivo,* but they also provide enormous insight into the paradigm for use of target-based imaging in drug development.

During the course of new drug development, the three questions in Table 11.4 can sometimes be answered with clinical observations, but a purely clinical approach is generally very inefficient in the absence of a firm grasp of the complex biochemistry of the targets. As demonstrated by the studies of MAO-B, PET imaging can provide a unique tool to help answer all three of these questions.

The first investigation by Fowler et al. (16), summarized in Color Plate 30 following page 394, is probably the best published example of the extraordinary power of PET imaging to guide selection of dose and interval during the earliest phase 1 evaluation of drugs. The upper left panel shows pretreatment activity of MAO-B in the human brain using an established probe, ^{11}C-selegiline. When lazabemide, an investigational drug that reversibly inhibits MAO-B, was administered at 25 mg twice a day (upper right panel), almost all MAO-B activity was inhibited. Thus, the first question was answered: Yes, this drug has an impact on its target.

Doubling the lazabemide dose to 50 mg twice a day (lower right panel) abolished the remaining MAO-B activity. Taken

TABLE 11.4. *Efficacy issues in drug development*

1. Did this treatment affect its presumed target?
2. Do we know the best dose?
3. What is the preferred interval between doses?

together, the information from the 25- and 50-mg doses helps to answer the second question: The best dose is unlikely to exceed 50 mg, and lower doses could also be considered.

The lower right panel explores the washout of enzymatic inhibition 36 hours after the last dose. In keeping with the reversible nature of the inhibitory profile of lazabemide, a substantial amount of the baseline activity has been restored. Thus, the answer to the third question is that, as studied, twice per day is a usable dose interval. However, these data suggest that once per day could also be a successful dose interval. Because patient adherence to medication is thought to be best at once per day, it would be helpful to obtain imaging information at 24 hours.

Answers to these three questions were readily obtained with PET imaging and can greatly assist the design of definitive clinical activity testing. Nonetheless, it is fair to consider whether such information was truly essential. Fortunately, these same authors conducted a follow-up study with deprenyl (selegiline), which provides some powerful lessons regarding the importance of appropriate dose selection (17). Their deprenyl study was retrospective, because this drug has been marketed for many years.

Using ^{11}C-selegiline again as the probe, the upper left panel in Color Plate 31 following page 394 shows the same pretreatment map of MAO-B activity in human brain as in the previous study. The upper right panel demonstrates that 5 mg twice a day, the dose and schedule listed in the official product brochure, completely abolishes MAO-B activity. Dosing with selegiline was stopped, and the time course for return-to-baseline activity was followed. After 1 week, not much activity was found. Even after 3 weeks, the level of enzymatic activity remained substantially lower than at baseline. Because selegiline is an irreversible inhibitor, this study is actually probing the rate of synthesis of new enzyme in the brain. If the effect of the drug persists for such long periods of time, why is it administered twice a day? Further, the authors estimate from their imaging results that the recommended dose of selegiline is 20-fold higher than that necessary to maintain full inhibition of MAO-B. Individual patients may respond differently to the same dose of a drug, and with PET, it is possible to establish the optimal dose for each patient.

These conclusions are readily observed retrospectively, so we should ask why the original drug development program produced such disparate answers. Selegiline provides modest relief for parkinsonian symptoms, and there are few other therapeutic options. For drugs with only modest activity, it is particularly difficult to choose the optimal dose. As a substitute for the optimal dose, the maximum feasible dose is often used. Thus, the dose is escalated in the hope of generating the most benefit. Of course, if all the benefit is obtained with the first 5% of the dose, then the remaining 95% of the dose can only ensure that a large fraction of patients will suffer side effects.

SUMMARY

If we focus on drug development as a process with enormous dependence on information about drug distribution and effect throughout the body, then its linkage with PET imaging provides a powerful tool for gathering unique data. Although PET is a very attractive tool in drug development, the effective use of PET imaging will vary with the complexity of the project and the skill and depth of the development team.

The design of successful imaging probes is critical and can be a bottleneck. Priority should be given to the development of imaging probes to study the functional interaction with relevant molecular targets. There is also great interest in the use of imaging to study the biodistribution of new drugs. These tasks will require broad collaboration among synthetic chemists, pharmacologists, and clinicians from both nuclear medicine and disease-specific areas. Even for an established probe for PET imaging such as FDG, its precise role is still being determined.

In the broader context of drug development, regulatory approval, and marketing, it is important to classify imaging information properly. In the spectrum of tools from biomarkers to surrogate endpoints to clinical outcome measures, there are opportunities for new contributions and improvements at all levels. Table 11.5 places the role of imaging into the overall context of drug development.

In the first stage, PET imaging can provide biomarkers that should be particularly useful early in the development of a new drug and it can guide the selection of dose and schedule of administration for subsequent testing phases. Biomarkers can also contribute to ''go, no go'' decision-making at this stage, based on the presumed mechanism of action for the therapeutic.

As the focus moves forward toward marketing approval of therapeutics, the second stage of the hypothesis is that the drug provides clinical benefit. Biomarkers (such as PET probes) by themselves do not establish quality of life or increased survival. Although imaging data can be highly informative for drug development, drug approval and marketing must be based on a demonstration of clinical value, in the context of the benefit-to-risk ratio applicable to the condition being treated. Controlled clinical trials can evaluate biomarkers to determine if they are candidates to become surrogate endpoints for clinical benefit, but this is a much

---

TABLE 11.5. *Two stages of hypothesis testing*

1. Does drug impact target as intended?
   (inhibit enzyme; decrease vessel count)
   ** Major role for noninvasive images as biomarkers
2. Any clinical benefit?
   (increased survival; improved quality of life)
   ** Only controlled clinical trials can evaluate as surrogate endpoints

larger and somewhat different undertaking than the development of biomarkers.

Increasingly, the linkage between diagnostics (including biomarkers) and therapeutics is changing the way populations are chosen for studies of drugs. Further, the more carefully a drug is studied during the development stages, the more adequate will be the guidance for customizing of therapy once the drug enters clinical practice. As imaging is increasingly able to define the molecular phenotype of individual patients, only patients with the targets will be considered eligible for the therapeutic trials.

Although the applications of PET in drug development are still in the early stages, the examples provided in this chapter illustrate useful applications across several broad disease areas. These examples also show that proof-of-concept studies have already been successfully conducted for all major categories of targets. A number of emerging events are poised to facilitate further progress. Improvements in hardware for imaging are underway, and there has been a very noticeable and rapid expansion in the number of PET centers. Furthermore, in addition to the outstanding work from individual centers, professional organizations have been founded that are specifically focused on the use of these tools in drug development. In North America, it is the Society of Nuclear Imaging in Drug Development and the European counterpart is the Federation on Imaging in Drug Development.

With careful consideration of appropriate imaging targets and probe design, as well as the dedicated efforts of skilled professionals from many disciplines, PET imaging is on its way toward changing the way we develop drugs and our ability to successfully use drugs as they enter clinical practice.

ACKNOWLEDGMENTS

I thank Drs. Robert Dedrick, Merrill Egorin, and Carl Peck, for keeping me focused on the questions in Table 11.1, and Dr. Anthony Shields, for encouraging my interest in PET imaging.

REFERENCES

1. Fischman AJ, Alpert NM, Babich JW, et al. The role of positron emission tomography in pharmacokinetic analysis. *Drug Metab Rev* 1997; 29:923–956.
2. Kubota K, Ishiwata K, Kubota R, et al. Feasibility of fluorine-18-fluorophenylalanine for tumor imaging compared with carbon-11-L-methionine. *J Nucl Med* 1996;37:320–325.
3. Hendrikse NH, de Vries EG, Eriks-Fluks L, et al. A new *in vivo* method to study P-glycoprotein transport in tumors and the blood–brain barrier. *Cancer Res* 1999;59:2411–2416.
4. Ciarmiello A, Del Vecchio S, Silvestro P, et al. Tumor clearance of technetium 99m-sestamibi as a predictor of response to neoadjuvant chemotherapy for locally advanced breast cancer. *J Clin Oncol* 1998; 16:1677–1683.
5. Berridge MS, Heald DL. *In vivo* characterization of inhaled pharmaceuticals using quantitative positron emission tomography. *J Clin Pharmacol* 1999;39:25S–29S.
6. Farde L, Nyberg S, Oxenstierna G, et al. Positron emission tomography studies on D_2 and 5-HT_2 receptor binding in risperidone-treated schizophrenic patients. *J Clin Psychopharmacol* 1995;15[Suppl 1]:19S–23S.
7. Dehdashti F, Flanagan FL, Mortimer JE, et al. Positron emission tomographic assessment of "metabolic flare" to predict response of metastatic breast cancer to antiestrogen therapy. *Eur J Nucl Med* 1999;26: 51–56.
8. Christman D, Crawford EJ, Friedkin M, et al. Detection of DNA synthesis in intact organisms with positron-emitting [methyl-^{11}C]thymidine. *PNAS* 1972;69:988–992.
9. Shields AF, Mankoff DA, Link JM, et al. Carbon-11-thymidine and FDG to measure therapy response. *J Nucl Med* 1998;39:1757–1762.
10. Conti PS, Alauddin MM, Fissekis JR, et al. Synthesis of 2′-fluoro-5-[^{11}C]-methyl-1-beta-D-arabinofuranosyluracil (^{11}C-FMAU): a potential nucleoside analog for *in vivo* study of cellular proliferation with PET. *Nucl Med Biol* 1995;22:783–789.
11. Shields AF, Grierson JR, Dohmen BM, et al. Imaging proliferation *in vivo* with [F-18]FLT and positron emission tomography. *Nat Med* 1998; 4:1334–1336.
12. Alauddin MM, Smith SL, Fissekis JD, et al. Improved synthesis of 2-deoxy-2-[^{18}F]fluoro-1,3,5-tri-O-benzoyl-D-ar abinofuranoside. *J Nucl Med* 2000;41:42P.
13. Sun H, Mangner TJ, Muzik O, et al. Biodistribution and metabolism of ^{18}F-FMAU: PET studies. *J Nucl Med* 2001;42:82P.
14. Tjuvajev JG, Finn R, Watanabe K, et al. Noninvasive imaging of herpes virus thymidine kinase gene transfer and expression: a potential method for monitoring clinical gene therapy. *Cancer Res* 1996;56:4087–4095.
15. Wiebe LI, Morin KW, Knaus EE. Radiopharmaceuticals to monitor gene transfer. *Q J Nucl Med* 1997;41:79–89.
16. Fowler JS, Volkow ND, Logan J, et al. Monoamine oxidase B (MAO B) inhibitor therapy in Parkinson's disease: the degree and reversibility of human brain MAO B inhibition by Ro 19 6327. *Neurology* 1993; 43:1984–1992.
17. Fowler JS, Volkow ND, Logan J, et al. Slow recovery of human brain MAOB after L-deprenyl (selegiline) withdrawal. *Synapse* 1994;18: 86–93.

CHAPTER 12

Imaging Gene Expression

Uwe A. Haberkorn

With the human genome decoded, the desire to replace defective genes with those under proper function is obvious. Although not yet in practice, positron emission tomography (PET) has an important role in the development of this field. The clinical application of gene therapy requires noninvasive tools to evaluate the efficiency of gene transfer. These include ways to evaluate infection and efficiency, as well as to verify successful gene transfer in terms of gene transcription. This information can be obtained by imaging methods and is useful for therapy planning, for follow-up studies in treated tumors, and as an indicator of prognosis.

ASSESSMENT OF VIRAL VECTOR BIODISTRIBUTION

An understanding of the biodistribution of vectors carrying therapeutic genes to their targets is helpful to develop strategies for target-specific delivery of these therapeutic agents. Schellingerhout et al. (1) used enveloped viral particles labeled with indium-111 (^{111}In), allowing the viruses to be traced *in vivo* by scintigraphic imaging. The labeling procedure did not significantly reduce the infectivity of herpes simplex virus (HSV), and there was no significant release of the radionuclide within 12 hours after labeling. Sequential imaging of animals after intravenous administration of the ^{111}In-labeled virus showed a fast accumulation in the liver and redistribution from the blood pool to liver and spleen.

The recombinant adenovirus serotype 5 knob was also radiolabeled with technetium-99m (^{99m}Tc) (2) and retained specific high-affinity binding to U293 cells, which shows that the radiolabeling process had no effect on receptor binding. *In vivo* dynamic scintigraphy revealed extensive liver binding, with a measured 100% extraction efficiency. The liver uptake corresponded to the results of a biodistribution study in which tissues were removed and counted.

SUICIDE GENE THERAPY

The transfer and expression of suicide genes into malignant tumor cells represents an attractive approach for human gene therapy. Suicide genes typically code for nonmammalian enzymes, which convert nontoxic prodrugs into highly toxic metabolites. Therefore, systemic application of the nontoxic prodrug results in the production of the active drug at the tumor site. Although a broad range of suicide principles has been described (Table 12.1), two suicide systems are applied in most studies: the cytosine deaminase (CD) system and the HSV thymidine kinase (HSVtk) system.

CD, which is expressed in yeasts and bacteria but not in mammalian organisms, converts the antifungal agent 5-fluorocytosine (5-FC) to the highly toxic 5-fluorouracil (5-FU). There is no known anabolic pathway in mammalian cells that leads to incorporation of 5-FC into the nucleic acid fraction. Therefore, the pharmacologic effects are moderate and the application of high therapeutic doses is possible (3–5). The 5-FU exerts its toxic effect by interfering with DNA and protein synthesis due to substitution of uracil by 5-FU in RNA and inhibition of thymidylate synthetase by 5-fluorodeoxy-uridine monophosphate, resulting in impaired DNA biosynthesis (6).

Nishiyama et al. (7) implanted CD-containing capsules into rat gliomas and subsequently treated the animals by systemic application of 5-FC. They observed significant amounts of 5-FU in the tumors and a decrease in tumor growth rate and systemic cytotoxicity. This approach to local chemotherapy was expanded by Wallace et al. (8) for application in patients with disseminated tumors. They used monoclonal antibody (MoAb) enzyme conjugates to achieve a selective activation of 5-FC, thereby obtaining a sevenfold higher level of 5-FU in the tumor after administration of MoAb-CD and 5-FC compared with the systemic application of 5-FU.

Gene therapy with HSVtk as a suicide gene has been performed in various tumor models *in vitro* and *in vivo* (9–16). In contrast to human thymidine kinase, HSVtk is less specific and also phosphorylates nucleoside analogues such as acyclovir and ganciclovir (GCV) to their monophosphate metabolites (17). These monophosphates are subsequently phosphorylated by cellular kinases to the diphosphates and triphosphates. After integration of the triphosphate metabo-

TABLE 12.1. *Suicide genes used as gene therapy for cancer*

Enzyme	Prodrug	Active metabolite
Escheria coli purine nucleoside phosphorylase (DeoD)	6-Methylpurine-2'-deoxyribonucleoside	6-Methylpurine
E. coli thymidine phosphorylase	5'-Deoxy-5'-fluorouridine, tegafur	5-Fluorouracil
E. coli guanosine-xanthine phosphoribosyltransferase (gpt)	6-thioxanthine, 6-thioguanine	6-Thioxantine-MP, 6-thioguanine-MP
Carboxypeptidase G$_2$	Benzoic acid mustardsglumatic acid	Benzoic acid mustards
Alkaline phosphatase	Etoposide phosphate, doxorubicin phosphate, mitomycin phosphate	Etoposide, doxorubicin, mitomycin phenol mustard
Cassava linamarase	Linamarin	Aceto cyanohydrin, HCN
Carboxypeptidase A	Methotrexate-alanine	Methotrexate
Cytosine deaminase	5-Fluorocytosine (5 FC)	5-Fluorouracil (5 FU)
Cytosine deaminase plus uracil phosphoribosyltransferase	5-Fluorocytosine	5-Fluorouracil + 5-fluorouridine-5'-monophosphate
Penicillin amidase	Doxorubicin-phenoxyacetamide Melphalan-phenoxyacetamide Palytoxin-4 Hydroxyphenoxyacetamide	Doxorubicin Melphalan Palytoxin
β-Glucosidase	Amygdalin	Cyanide
β-Glucoronidase	Epirubicin-glucoronide, phenol mustard-glucuronide, daunomycin-glucoronide, adrimycin-glucoronide	Epirubicin, phenol mustard, daunomycin, adriamycin
β-Lactamase	Phenylenediamine mustard cephalosporin	Phenylenediamine mustard
E. coli Nitroreductase	CB1954 (5-aziridin 2, 4-dinitrobenzamidine)	5-Aziridin 2, 4-hydroxyamino 2-nitrobenzamidine
Cytochrome P450 2B1	Cyclophosphamide	Phosphoramide mustard
Rabbit hepatic carboxylesterase	Irinotecan	SN38 (7-ethyl-10-hydroxycamptothecin)
Human deoxycytidine kinase	Cytosine arabinoside (AraC), fludarabine	AraCMP, fludarabine-MP
HSV thymidine kinase	Ganciclovir (GCV), aciclovir	Phosphorylated metabolites
VZV thymidine kinase	6-Methoxypurine arabinonucleoside (araM)	Phosphorylated metabolite

HSV, herpes simplex virus; VZV, varicella-zoster virus.

lites into DNA, chain termination occurs and is followed by cell death. Encouraging results have been obtained in rat gliomas using a retroviral vector system for transfer and expression of the HSVtk gene (15,16).

Recently, *in vitro* and *in vivo* studies have further demonstrated the potency of the CD suicide system. Tumor cells that had been infected with a retrovirus carrying the CD gene showed a strict correlation between 5-FC sensitivity and CD enzyme activity (18–20). Although not all of the tumor cells have to be infected to obtain a sufficient therapeutic response, the *in vivo* infection efficiency of currently used viral vectors is low and repeated injections of the recombinant retroviruses may be necessary to reach a therapeutic level of enzyme activity in the tumor.

Monitoring suicide gene expression in the tumor is a prerequisite for gene therapy when using a suicide system, for two reasons: to decide if repeated gene transductions of the tumor are necessary and to find a therapeutic window of maximum gene expression and consecutive prodrug administration (21). Because 5-FC and GCV can be labeled with fluorine 18 (^{18}F) with sufficient *in vivo* stability (22,23), PET may be applied to assess the enzyme activity *in vivo*. Moreover, measurement of the therapeutic effects on the

tumor metabolism may be useful for the prediction of therapy outcome at an early stage of the treatment. PET using tracers of tumor metabolism has been applied for the evaluation of treatment response in a variety of tumors and therapeutic regimens (24–27), indicating that these tracers deliver useful parameters for the early assessment of therapeutic efficacy.

MONITORING GENE THERAPY BY MEASUREMENT OF THERAPEUTIC EFFECTS

Monitoring the tumor response to gene therapy using imaging procedures for the assessment of morphologic changes has been performed with magnetic resonance imaging (MRI) techniques in rats bearing chemically induced hepatocellular carcinoma, C6 rat glioblastomas, and in patients with glioblastoma (28–42). Replication-deficient viral vectors, as well as replicating HSV mutants, have been used (41). In these studies, marked tumor necrosis or growth retardation and regression were observed after induction of HSVtk and administration of GCV. Maron et al. (30) found an initial response to GCV treatment in 90% of the animals and a complete regression in two thirds of the treated rats. Tumor

TABLE 12.2. *Genes and imaging methods for the monitoring of gene transfer*

Gene	Principle	Imaging method	Tracer/contrast agent
CD	Enzyme activity	MRS, PET	5-fluorocytosine
HSVtk	Therapeutic effects	MRI, MRS, PET, SPECT	FDG, HMPAO, misonidazole
HSVtk	Enzyme activity	SPECT, PET	Specific substrates
HSVtk mutant	Enzyme activity	PET	Specific substrates
Tyrosinase	Metal scavenger	MRI, SPECT, scintigraphy	^{111}In
SSTR2	Receptor expression	SPECT, scintigraphy	Radiolabeled ligand
D2R	Receptor expression	PET	Radiolabeled ligand
CEA antigen	Antigen expression	Scintigraphy	Radiolabeled antibody
Modified green fluorescence protein	Transchelation	SPECT, scintigraphy	^{99m}Tc-glucoheptonate
Human sodium iodide transporter	Transport activity, therapy	Scintigraphy	^{131}I

MRS, magnetic resonance spectroscopy.

recurrence could also be observed. In a more clinically relevant experimental protocol, GCV was delivered late in the course of the disease when the tumor formations were large, and the long-term survival of the treated rats improved by 60% when compared with untreated animals (37). MRI demonstrated a complete regression of tumors in the surviving animals. The effects of CD gene transfer and 5-FC administration were evaluated in different tumor models (43–46) (Table 12.2). The 5-FC sensitivity in 9L cells increased 1,700-fold after infection with an adenoviral vector carrying the CD gene (46). These rats demonstrated a remarkable inhibition of tumor growth by MRI with 70% surviving for more than 90 days. Moreover, the mean tumor diffusion on MRI increased by 31% within 8 days of initiating 5-FC treatment. These effects were observed before tumor growth arrest and tumor regression (45).

The effects of suicide gene therapy on tumor vascularization may occur because endothelial cells of the tumor blood vessels may integrate retroviral vectors and thus become sensitive toward GCV. This hypothesis was investigated in the subcutaneous 9L gliosarcoma tumor model using measurements of tumor blood flow with Doppler color flow and ultrasound imaging (47,48). The tumor vasculature decreased after initiation of GCV therapy in the HSVtk-transduced tumors. The early necrotic changes were associated with ultrasonographic signs of scattered intratumoral hemorrhage.

Tumor perfusion, as measured in GCV-treated HSVtk-expressing KBALB tumors after intravenous administration of ^{99m}Tc-hexamethylpropyleneamine oxime, increased twofold during treatment at day two (49). Intratumoral hypoxia was also changed: The accumulation of hydrogen-3 (^{3}H)-misonidazole decreased to 30% to 40% from day zero until day three after the start of treatment, indicating that tumor tissue had become less hypoxic.

The measurement of metabolic changes after therapeutic intervention has proven superior to morphologic procedures for the assessment of early therapeutic effects. MRI quantita-

tion of changes in intracranial 9L tumor doubling times revealed a significant variation in therapeutic response to gene therapy with HSVtk and GCV. Localized proton magnetic resonance spectroscopy (MRS) of treated 9L tumors showed a dramatic increase in mobile lipids and/or lactate. These changes in intracranial tumor doubling times correlated with changes in H tumor MRS (50).

^{18}F-fluorodeoxyglucose (FDG) uptake has been demonstrated to be a useful and very sensitive parameter for the evaluation of glucose metabolism (25,26,51,52). Because the HSVtk/GCV system induces DNA chain termination, additional changes in thymidine incorporation into tumor cell DNA occur. This may be assessed using carbon-11 (^{11}C)-thymidine, which has been used to determine DNA synthesis *in vivo* (53,54). In an HSVtk-expressing rat hepatoma cell line, uptake measurements using thymidine, FDG, 3-O-methylglucose, AIB, and methionine were performed in the presence of different concentrations of GCV (55,56). In the HSVtk-expressing cell line an increase (up to 250%) in the ^{11}C-thymidine uptake in the acid-soluble fraction and a decrease to 5.5% in the acid-insoluble fraction were found. The decrease of radioactivity in the nucleic acid fraction occurred early (4 hours) after exposure of the cells to GCV and represents DNA chain termination induced by the HSVtk–GCV system. The phenomenon of a posttherapeutic accumulation of thymidine or its metabolites in the acid-soluble fraction was observed in previous studies after chemotherapy (24). This effect may be explained by an increase in the activity of salvage pathway enzymes, for example, of host thymidine kinase activity during repair of cell damage.

PET measurements with ^{11}C-thymidine may be used to assess the effects of the HSVtk–GCV system on DNA synthesis if quantitation is based on a modeling approach. *In vitro,* the AIB uptake decreased to 47%, whereas the methionine uptake in the acid-insoluble fraction decreased to 17%, which is evidence of an inhibition of protein synthesis and the neutral amino acid transport.

During GCV treatment, the uptake for FDG and 3-*O*-methylglucose increases up to 195% after 24 hours of incubation with GCV. A high-pressure liquid chromatography (HPLC) analysis revealed a decline of the FDG 6-phosphate fraction after 48 hours of incubation with GCV. Consequently, a normalization of FDG uptake was observed after this incubation period, whereas the 3-*O*-methylglucose uptake was still increased. Experiments performed with different amounts of HSVtk-expressing cells and control cells showed that these effects are dependent on the percentage of HSVtk-expressing cells (55).

Dynamic PET studies of ^{18}F-FDG uptake were performed in animals shortly after starting therapy with 100 mg of GCV per kilogram of body weight and after administration of sodium chloride (see Color Plate 32 following page 394). The arterial FDG plasma concentration was measured dynamically in an extracorporeal loop and the rate constants for FDG transport (K_1, k_2) and FDG phosphorylation (k_3) were calculated using a three-compartment model modified for heterogeneous tissues. After 2 days of GCV treatment, an uncoupling of FDG transport and phosphorylation was found with enhanced K_1 and k_2 values and a normal k_3 value (57).

In clinical and experimental studies, an increase in FDG uptake early after treatment of malignant tumors has been described (26,51,58,59). Cell culture experiments with rat adenocarcinoma cells under chemotherapy revealed that this effect is predominantly caused by an enhanced glucose transport (58). The underlying mechanism could be a redistribution of the glucose transport protein from intracellular pools to the plasma membrane. This is observed in cell culture studies as a general reaction to cellular stress (60–63). Because prodrug activation by HSVtk leads to DNA chain termination and cell damage, the same reactions may also occur in tumor cells under gene therapy with this suicide system. Translocation of glucose transport proteins to the plasma membrane as a first reaction to cellular stress may cause enhancement of glucose transport and represents a short-term regulatory mechanism, which acts independently of protein synthesis. Longer term, if treatment is effective, glucose utilization and FDG uptake would be expected to decline.

DETERMINATION OF SUICIDE GENE ACTIVITY BY THE UPTAKE OF SPECIFIC SUBSTRATES

In a rat hepatoma model (55,56,64), uptake measurements were performed up to 48 hours in an HSVtk-expressing cell line and in a control cell line bearing the empty vector using 5-iodo-2′-fluoro-2′-deoxy-1-β-D-arabinofuranosyluracil (FIAU), fluorodeoxycytidine (FCdR), 5-fluoro-1-(2′-deoxy-2′-fluoro-β-D-ribofuranosyl)uracil (FFUdR), and GCV. The FCdR uptake was higher in the HSVtk-expressing cells with a maximum after 4 hours (12-fold and 3-fold higher in the acid-insoluble and acid-soluble fraction, respectively). After longer incubation periods, the FCdR uptake declined. HPLC analysis showed a rapid and complete metabolization and

degradation in both cell lines (56), which might be due to dehalogenation or the action of nucleosidases.

The GCV, FIAU, and FFUdR uptake showed a time-dependent increase in HSVtk-expressing cells and a plateau in control cells. The HPLC analysis revealed unmetabolized GCV in control cells and a time-dependent shift of GCV to its phosphorylated metabolite in HSVtk-expressing cells (56). Furthermore, the GCV, FFUdR, and the FIAU uptake were highly correlated to the percentage of HSVtk-expressing cells and to the growth inhibition as measured in bystander experiments (56,64,65).

Similar results were obtained with genetically modified MCF-7 human mammary carcinoma cells (66). However, the rat Morris hepatoma cells revealed a much higher difference in GCV uptake than MCF-7 cells, between HSVtk-expressing cells and control cells (56). MCF-7 cells were not as sensitive to the HSVtk–GCV system as Morris hepatoma cells. This difference in the amount of tracer accumulation and sensitivity may be explained by the slower rate of growth of MCF-7 cells as compared with Morris hepatoma cells.

Inhibition/competition experiments were performed to further elucidate the transport mechanism of GCV. The nucleoside transport in mammalian cells is known to be heterogeneous and involve two classes of nucleoside transporters: the equilibrium-based, facilitated diffusion systems and the concentration-based, sodium-dependent systems. In these experiments, competition for all concentration-based nucleoside transport systems and inhibition of the GCV transport by the equilibration transport systems was observed, whereas the pyrimidine nucleobase system showed no contribution to the GCV uptake (56,66).

Acyclovir has been shown to be transported mainly by purine nucleobase carrier molecules in human erythrocytes (67). Due to a hydroxymethyl group on its side chain, GCV has a stronger similarity to nucleosides and therefore may also be transported by a nucleoside transporter. Supporting data show that the 3′-hydroxyl moieties of nucleosides are important for their interaction with the nucleoside transporter (68). In rat hepatoma cells, as well as in human mammary carcinoma cells, the GCV uptake was shown to be much lower than the thymidine uptake (56,66). Therefore, in addition to the low infection efficiency of the current viral delivery systems, slow transport of the substrate and its slow conversion into the phosphorylated metabolite are limiting for the therapeutic success of the HSVtk–GCV system. Cotransfection with nucleoside transporters or the use of other substrates for HSVtk with higher affinities for nucleoside transport and phosphorylation by HSVtk may improve the outcome of therapy.

The principle of *in vivo* HSVtk imaging was first demonstrated by Price et al. (69) and Saito et al. (70) for the visualization of HSV encephalitis. Recently, *in vivo* studies have been done by several groups using different tracers (71–83). Gambhir et al. (71) used 8-^{18}F-fluoroganciclovir (FGCV) for the imaging of adenovirus-directed hepatic expression of the HSVtk gene in living mice (71). There was a significant positive correlation between the percent injected dose of FGCV retained per gram of liver and the levels of hepatic HSVtk gene expression. Over a similar range of HSVtk expression *in vivo*, the percent injected dose retained per gram of liver was 0% to 23% for GCV and 0% to 3% for FGCV.

Alauddin et al. (72,73) used of 9-(4-[^{18}F]-fluoro-3-hydroxymethylbutyl)-guanine (^{18}F-FHBG) and 9-[(3-^{18}F-fluoro-1-hydroxy-2-propoxy)methyl]-guanine (^{18}F-FHPG) for combined *in vitro/in vivo* studies with HT-29 human colon cancer cells, transduced with a retroviral vector, and also found a significant higher uptake in HSVtk-expressing cells as compared with the controls. *In vivo* studies in tumor-bearing nude mice demonstrated that the tumor uptake of the radiotracer is threefold and sixfold higher at 2 and 5 hours, respectively, in transduced cells compared with the control cells. Others used radioiodinated nucleoside analogues such as (E)-5-(2-iodovinyl)-2′-fluoro-2′-deoxyuridine (IVFRU) and FIAU to visualize HSVtk expression (74–77,82).

Autoradiography, single-photon emission tomography (SPECT) and PET images after injection of iodine-131 (^{131}I)-labeled or iodine-124 (^{124}I)-labeled FIAU revealed highly specific localization of the tracer to areas of HSVtk gene expression in brain and mammary tumors (76,77). The amount of tracer uptake in the tumors was correlated to the *in vitro* GCV sensitivity of the cell lines that were transplanted in these animals (76,77).

Haubner et al. (82) studied the early kinetics of iodine-123 (^{123}I)-FIAU in the CMS-5 fibrosarcoma model. Biodistribution studies 0.5 hours postinjection showed tumor : blood and tumor : muscle ratios of 3.8 and 7.2 in HSVtk-expressing tumors, and 0.6 and 1.2 in wild type tumors. The tracer showed a biexponential clearance, with an initial half-life of 0.6 hours followed by a half-life of 4.6 hours and the highest activity accumulation in HSVtk-expressing tumors observed at 1 hour postinjection. Scintigraphy showed specific tracer accumulation as early as 0.5 hours postinjection, with an increase in contrast over time, suggesting that sufficient tumor : background ratios for *in vivo* imaging of HSVtk expression with ^{123}I-FIAU are reached as early as 1 hour postinjection.

Similar results were reported for IVFRU by Wiebe et al. (74,75). Due to low non–target tissue uptake, unambiguous imaging of HSVtk-expressing tumors in mice is possible with labeled IVFRU. The advantage of iodinated tracers such as FIAU may be that delayed imaging is possible. Because ^{18}F-labeled compounds only allow imaging early after administration of the tracer, these iodinated compounds may prove more sensitive *in vivo*. However, exact quantification with iodine isotopes may be a challenge with either ^{131}I, a gamma ray and electron emitter with high radiation dose, or with the corresponding positron emitter ^{124}I, which shows only 23% positron emission with high-energy particles, multiple gamma rays of high energy, and leads to a high radiation dose.

To improve the detection of lower levels of PET reporter gene expression, a mutant HSV type 1 thymidine kinase (HSV1-sr39tk) was used as a PET reporter gene (84) After successful transfer of this mutant gene, the accumulation of the specific substrates 8-^{3}H-penciclovir (8-^{3}H-PCV), and 8-^{18}F-fluoropenciclovir (FPCV) in C6 rat glioma cells was increased twofold when compared with wild type HSVtk-expressing tumor cells, leading to an increased imaging sensitivity.

CD was evaluated in human glioblastoma cells. A human glioblastoma cell line was stably transfected with the *Escherichia coli* CD gene (21) and experiments with ^{3}H-5-FC were performed. Tritiated 5-FU was produced in CD-expressing cells, whereas in the control cells, only ^{3}H-5-FC was detected (21). Significant amounts of 5-FU were found in the medium of cultured cells, which may account for the bystander effect observed in previous experiments. However, uptake studies revealed a moderate and nonsaturable accumulation of radioactivity in the tumor cells, suggesting that 5-FC enters the cells only via diffusion (21). Although a significant difference in 5-FC uptake was seen between CD-positive cells and controls after 48 hours of incubation, no difference was observed after 2 hours of incubation, and a rapid efflux could be demonstrated. 5-FC transport may be a limiting factor for this therapeutic procedure, and for quantitation with PET, it may be necessary to rely on dynamic studies and modeling, including HPLC analysis of the plasma, rather than on nonmodeling approaches (21).

To evaluate the 5-FC uptake *in vivo,* a rat prostate adenocarcinoma cell line was transfected with a retroviral vector bearing the *E. coli* CD gene. The cells were found to be sensitive to 5-FC exposure but lost this sensitivity with time. This may have been due to inactivation of the viral promoter (CMV) used in this vector. *In vivo* studies with PET and ^{18}F-FC showed no preferential accumulation of the tracer in CD-expressing tumors, although HPLC analysis revealed a production of 5-FU that was detectable in tumor lysates and in the blood of the animals (65).

Finally, the coupling of two genes as a therapeutic gene together with a reporter gene by use of bicistronic vectors [involving the internal ribosomal entry site (IRES) of picornaviruses] may be useful for the evaluation of gene transfer. Measurement of the PET reporter gene would make it possible to assess another therapeutic gene, for example, a cytokine (85). Problems may arise from low levels of gene expression, which may be influenced by the number of infected cells and by attenuation of the gene downstream from the IRES.

IMAGING USING NON–SUICIDE REPORTER GENES

Reporter genes [e.g., β-galactosidase, chloramphenicol acetyltransferase, green fluorescent protein (GFP), and luciferase] play critical roles in investigating mechanisms of gene expression in transgenic animals and in developing gene delivery systems for gene therapy. However, measuring expression of these reporter genes requires biopsy or killing the animals. In this respect, the HSVtk gene has been shown to be useful as a noninvasive marker (71–83).

Receptor genes have also been used as reporter genes (86, 87). The dopaminergic D_2-receptor gene represents an endogenous gene that is not likely to invoke an immune response. Furthermore, the corresponding tracer 3-(2′-[^{18}F]-fluoroethyl)spiperone (FESP) rapidly crosses the blood–brain barrier, can be produced at high specific activity, and is currently used in patients. A SPECT tracer ^{123}I-iodobenzamine is also available. MacLaren et al. (86) used this radiotracer in nude mice both with an adenoviral-directed hepatic gene delivery system and in stably transfected tumor cells that were transplanted into animals. The tracer uptake in these animals was proportional to *in vitro* data of hepatic FESP accumulation, dopamine-receptor ligand binding and the D_2 receptor messenger RNA (mRNA). Tumors modified to express the D_2 receptor retained significantly more FESP than wild type tumors.

Using a replication-incompetent adenoviral vector encoding the human type 2 somatostatin receptor, Zinn et al. (87) modified non–small cell lung tumors and imaged the expression of the *hSSTr2* gene using a radiolabeled, somatostatin-avid peptide (P829), which was radiolabeled to high specific activity with ^{99m}Tc or rhenium-188 (^{188}Re). In the genetically modified tumors, there was a 5- to 10-fold greater accumulation of both radiolabeled P829 peptides as compared with the control tumors. Both isotopes are generator produced, which confers advantages concerning the availability, costs, and imaging with widespread existing high-resolution modalities. The ^{188}Re-labeled peptide offers the additional advantage of beta decay, which may be used for therapy.

Specific imaging can also be obtained with radiolabeled antibodies. To overcome the limitation of low expression of human tumor-associated antigens on target cells, a human glioma cell line was modified to express high levels of human carcinoembryonic antigen (CEA) using an adenoviral vector (88). In these cells, high binding of an ^{131}I-labeled CEA antibody was observed *in vitro* and by scintigraphic imaging. Iodine-124 potentially could be applied for PET imaging in this system.

Another approach is based on the *in vivo* transchelation of oxotechnetate to a polypeptide motif from a biocompatible complex, which has a higher dissociation constant than a diglycylcysteine complex. It has been shown that synthetic peptides and recombinant proteins such as the modified GFP can bind oxotechnetate with high efficiency (89,90). In these experiments, rats were injected intramuscularly with synthetic peptides bearing a GGC motif. One hour later ^{99m}Tc-glucoheptonate was applied intravenously and the accumulation was measured by scintigraphy. The peptides with three metal-binding GGC motifs showed a threefold higher accumulation as compared with the controls. This principle can also be applied to recombinant proteins that appear at the plasma membrane (91). These genes can be cloned into bi-cistronic vectors, which allow for the coexpression of therapeutic genes and *in vivo* reporter genes, and radionuclide imaging may be used to detect gene expression.

Tyrosinase catalyzes the hydroxylation of tyrosine to DOPA and the oxidation of DOPA to dopaquinone, which after cyclization and polymerization, results in melanin production. Melanins are scavengers of metal ions such as iron and indium through ionic binding. Tyrosinase transfer leads to the production of melanins in a variety of cells. This may be used for imaging with nuclear magnetic resonance or with ^{111}In and a gamma camera. Cells transfected with the tyrosinase gene stained positively for melanin and had a higher ^{111}In binding capacity than the wild type cells (92). In transfection experiments, a dependence of tracer accumulation on the amount of the vector used could be observed. The problems associated with this approach are possible low tyrosinase induction with low amounts of melanin and the cytotoxicity of melanin. These problems may be overcome by the construction of chimeric tyrosinase proteins and by positioning the enzyme on the outer side of the membrane. PET could potentially detect such processes as well.

ENHANCEMENT OF IODIDE UPTAKE IN MALIGNANT TUMORS

The unique ability of thyroid follicular cells to accumulate iodide enables benign thyroid diseases and differentiated thyroid carcinoma to be successfully treated with radioiodide therapy. The complex process of iodide trapping in the thyroid tissue is mainly dependent on iodide transport and thyroid peroxidase activity. It is initiated by the active transport of iodide and sodium ions into follicular cells, which is mediated by the sodium iodide symporter (hNIS).

Several experimental and clinical studies showed that the reduced radioiodide concentrating activity often observed in thyroid carcinomas can be attributed to a decreased expression of the sodium iodide symporter gene (93–99).

In patients with thyroid carcinomas, the reduced *hNIS* gene expression was shown to be associated with a downregulation of the thyroid peroxidase (TPO), of thyroglobulin (Tg), and of the thyroid-stimulating hormone receptor (TSH-R). Higher tumor stages showed a lower expression of hNIS and TPO than lower stages (98). The transfer of the *hNIS* gene may lead to a stable expression of the symporter not only in thyroid carcinoma but also in other tumor types.

Currently used viral vectors for gene therapy of cancer have a low infection efficiency, with infection rates between 0.1% and 2%. Therefore, therapy effects turn out to be moderate or low. This problem could be solved if the accumulation of radioactive isotopes with beta emission could be enhanced. The trapping centers in the tumor could create a cross firing of beta particles, thereby efficiently killing non-transduced tumor cells.

Transfer of the *hNIS* gene into Morris hepatoma cells caused a significant increase in iodide uptake (by a factor of 84 to 235) *in vitro* with a peak after 1 hour of incubation

(100). Similar results were seen in Cos7 cells after transient infection with the hNIS complementary DNA (cDNA) in the pcDNA3 vector where the cells accumulated 10-fold more $Na^{125}I$ than controls (101). FRTL5 cells also showed a rapid iodide uptake after transfection of the rat *NIS* gene with an eukaryotic expression vector, and a maximum level was reached after 40 minutes (102). This principle of enhancement of iodide uptake by hNIS transfer was also applied in various tumor models (103–106) with up to a 35-fold increase in iodide uptake.

Expression of the *hNIS* gene does not necessarily lead to iodide accumulation. A rapid efflux (80%) was observed in *hNIS*-expressing hepatoma cells during the first 10 minutes, indicating a lack in organification of the radioactive iodide (100). Others have also observed this, although in genetically modified FRTL-Tc cells, a slower iodide efflux has been reported (102,103). Animal studies with wild type and *hNIS*-expressing tumors in rats showed similar results, with a maximum uptake after 1 hour (see Color Plate 33 following page 394) and a continuous disappearance of the radioactivity out of the body as well as of the *hNIS*-expressing tumor (100). Although the NIS activity is asymmetric and favors iodide influx, there is also an efflux activity with the consequence that in cells that do not organify iodide, the concentration of intracellular iodide will drop proportionally to the external iodide concentration.

Unless iodide organification occurs, the radiation exposure of cells genetically modified to express the *hNIS* gene is too low for therapeutic relevance. Although treatment experiments *in vitro* showed selective killing of up to 64% of *hNIS* transduced tumor cells (103,105 106), a therapeutic effect was not observed *in vivo* (102). In FRTL tumors, the effective half-life of ^{125}I in the tumors was approximately 6 hours, which resulted in a calculated radiation dose of 4 Gy (400 rads) after a dose of 1 mCi (3.7 MBq) ^{131}I (102). In the rat hepatoma model, a half-life of ^{131}I in *hNIS*-expressing tumors of 14.5 ± 4.8 hours and in wild type tumors of 15.0 ± 4.9 hours was calculated (100). Administration of 0.4 mCi (1.48 MBq) ^{131}I resulted in an absorbed dose of 35 mGy (3.5 rads) in wild type tumor and 592 mGy (59.2 rads) in *hNIS*-expressing tumor. Although gamma-emitting iodine isotopes have been used, the potential of ^{124}I in such a system for PET is apparent.

Therefore, the use of the *hNIS* gene as a new therapeutic principle, as suggested in recent reports (104–106, 109), seems questionable without further modifications. Future studies will address the question whether a pharmacologic modulation may be used to retain the radioactive iodide in the tumors, for example, by interference with iodide efflux. Furthermore, the *hNIS* gene and ^{99m}Tc-pertechnate application potentially may be used as a simple reporter system for the visualization of other genes in bicistronic vectors that allow coexpression of two different genes.

We investigated whether the transfer of the *hTPO* gene is sufficient to restore the iodide trapping capacity in undifferentiated thyroid and nonthyroid tumor cells (110). The human anaplastic thyroid carcinoma cell lines C643 and SW1736, the rat Morris hepatoma cell line MH3924A, and the rat papillary thyroid carcinoma cell line L2 were used as *in vitro* model systems. Although a significant expression of the *hTPO* gene was seen, the ^{125}I uptake was not enhanced in these cells. Moreover, only minimal enzymatic activity of the recombinant *hTPO* was determined in individual cell lines, as shown by low levels of guaiacol oxidation. This suggests either that the recombinant gene is expressed as a functionally inactive protein or that a functional protein becomes inactive in a nonoptimal cellular milieu.

In most *in vitro* systems, the *hTPO* introduced by cDNA-directed gene expression was detected by means of immunohistology, immunoblotting, or autoantibodies of patients with thyroid autoimmune disease. However, the production of catalytically active *hTPO* was not achieved, irrespective of the expression system and cell culture system employed for the experimental approach (111–114).

The function and activity of the *hTPO* are probably influenced by the multimerization of the protein and by additional factors including the incorporation of heme, the glycosylation, the localization of the enzyme, and the thyroglobulin content of the cells (115–119). Therefore, the transduction of the *hTPO* gene per se is not sufficient to induce the iodide accumulation in human anaplastic carcinoma cells, and a low enzymatic activity in the recombinant cell lines is supposed to account for it. Studies are currently being performed to define additional factors required for iodide uptake in undifferentiated thyroid tumor cells, and the role of PET is uncertain.

ANTISENSE OLIGONUCLEOTIDES

Antisense RNA and DNA techniques have been developed to modulate the gene expression in a specific manner. These techniques originated from early studies in bacteria, demonstrating that these organisms are able to regulate their gene replication and expression by the production of small complementary RNA (cRNA) molecules in an antisense (opposite) direction. Watson–Crick base pairing between the oligonucleotide and the corresponding target RNA leads to highly specific binding and specific interaction with the protein synthesis.

Several groups subsequently presented evidence that synthetic antisense oligonucleotides complementary to mRNA sequences could downregulate the translation of various oncogenes in cells (120,121). By annealing of the oligonucleotide with the cRNA, a double-stranded RNA-DNA or RNA-RNA hybrid is generated, which then leads to various phenomena: The hybrid may become a substrate of the RNase H, which degrades the RNA moiety of the RNA-DNA hybrid. The hybridization of the antisense oligonucleotide to its target may prevent either ribosome attachment or translation of the mRNA or it may affect the processing or the transport of the mRNA from the nucleus to the cytoplasma. RNA-RNA hybrids may become substrates for the Rnase L.

In addition to their use for the specific interaction with RNA processing, radiolabeled oligonucleotides may also be applied for the biologic characterization and treatment of tumors. Prerequisites for the use of radiolabeled antisense oligonucleotides are facility of synthesis, stability *in vivo*, uptake into the cell, accumulation of the oligo inside the cell, interaction with the target structure, and no unspecific interaction with other macromolecules. For radiolabeled antisense molecules to be effective, they should be stable. To achieve stability, nuclease resistance, stability of the oligo-linker complex, and tight binding of the radionuclide to the complex are essential.

The uptake of oligonucleotides is temperature sensitive and inversely proportional to the length of the oligonucleotide, and no inhibition by nucleotides such as thymidine has been demonstrated. There is a sequence-independent concentration-dependent inhibition of the uptake by other oligonucleotides, yeast tRNA and plasmids. The uptake is dependent on the cell type. Known inhibitors of endocytosis such as deoxyglucose and cytochalasin B decrease the uptake. These data are evidence of a receptor-coupled endocytosis as the mechanism by which oligonucleotides enter the cells (122,123). Subcellular fractionation experiments showed a sequestration of the oligonucleotides in the nuclei and the mitochondria of HeLa cells (123).

This fractionation and the problems with the *in vivo* stability of the oligonucleotides and of the hybrid structures are severe obstacles to successful imaging of gene expression. However, Dewanjee et al. (124) were able to show accumulation of c-*myc* antisense probes with a phosphorothioate backbone in mice bearing c-*myc* overexpressing mammary tumors.

Tumor imaging was also possible with a transforming growth factor α antisense oligonucleotide or oligodeoxynucleotides for oncogenes or the mRNA of glial fibrillary acidic protein (125–127). Tavitian et al. (128) showed that PET could be used for the assessment of the biodistribution and kinetics of ^{18}F-labeled oligonucleotides. Finally, yttrium-90 (^{90}Y)-labeled phosphorothioate antisense oligonucleotides may be used as targeted radionuclide therapeutic agents for malignant tumors, as was done for a phosphorothioate antisense oligonucleotide complementary to the translation start region of the N-*myc* oncogene mRNA (129). The resulting ^{90}Y antisense oligonucleotide hybridized specifically to a complementary phosphorodiester sense oligonucleotide. It is possible that such oligonucleotides could be used with PET to image transfected genes for gene therapy.

SUMMARY

Although gene therapy is still in its infancy, monitoring the targeting and expression of genes is of key importance to the science and practice of this discipline. PET, as the most sensitive and quantitative nuclear imaging method, is expected to play a growing role in this promising field.

REFERENCES

1. Schellingerhout D, Bogdanov A Jr, Marecos E, et al. Mapping the *in vivo* distribution of herpes simplex virions. *Hum Gene Ther* 1998;9: 1543–1549.
2. Zinn KR, Douglas JT, Smyth CA, et al. Imaging and tissue biodistribution of ^{99m}Tc-labeled adenovirus knob (serotype 5). *Gene Ther* 1998; 5:798–808.
3. Scholer HJ. Flucytosine. In: Speller DCE, ed. *Antifungal chemotherapy*. New York: John Wiley and Sons, 1980:35–106.
4. Polak A, Eschenhof E, Fernex M, et al. Metabolic studies with 5-fluorocytosine-6-14C in mouse, rat, rabbit, dog and man. *Chemotherapy* 1976;22:137–153.
5. Koechlin BA, Rubio F, Palmer S, et al. The metabolism of 5-fluorocytosine-2-^{14}C and of cytosine-1-^{14}C in the rat and the disposition of 5-fluorocytosine-2-^{14}C in man. *Biochem Pharmac* 1966;15:435–446.
6. Myers CE. The pharmacology of the fluoropyrimidines. *Pharmacol Rev* 1981;33:1–15.
7. Nishiyama T, Kawamura Y, Kawamoto K, et al. Antineoplastic effects of 5-fluorocytosine in combination with cytosine deaminase capsules. *Cancer Res* 1985;45:1753–1761.
8. Wallace PM, MacMaster JF, Smith VF, et al. Intratumoral generation of 5-fluorouracil mediated by an antibody-cytosine deaminase conjugate in combination with 5-fluorocytosine. *Cancer Res* 1994;54: 2719–2723.
9. Chen SH, Shine HD, Goodman JC, et al. Gene therapy for brain tumors: regression of experimental gliomas by adenovirus-mediated gene transfer *in vivo*. *Proc Natl Acad Sci U S A* 1994;91:3054–3057.
10. Borrelli E, Heyman R, Hsi M, et al. Targeting of an inducible toxic phenotype in animal cells. *Proc Natl Acad Sci U S A* 1988;85: 7572–7576.
11. Barba D, Hardin J, Sadelain M, et al. Development of anti-tumor immunity following thymidine kinase-mediated killing of experimental brain tumors. *Proc Natl Acad Sci U S A* 1994;91:4348–4352.
12. Moolten FL, Wells JM. Curability of tumors bearing herpes thymidine kinase genes transferred by retroviral vectors. *J Natl Cancer Inst* 1990; 82:297–300.
13. Caruso M, Panis Y, Gagandeep S, et al. Regression of established macroscopic liver metastases after in situ transduction of a suicide gene. *Proc Natl Acad Sci U S A* 1993;90:7024–7028.
14. Oldfield EH, Ram Z, Culver KW, et al. Gene therapy for the treatment of brain tumors using intra-tumoral transduction with the thymidine kinase gene and intravenous ganciclovir. *Hum Gene Ther* 1993;1: 39–69.
15. Culver KW, Ram Z, Walbridge S, et al. *In vivo* gene transfer with retroviral vector-producer cells for treatment of experimental brain tumors. *Science* 1992;256:1550–1552.
16. Ram Z, Culver WK, Walbridge S, et al. In situ retroviral-mediated gene transfer for the treatment of brain tumors in rats. *Cancer Res* 1993;53:83.
17. Keller PM, Fyfe JA, Beauchamp L, et al. Enzymatic phosphorylation of acyclic nucleoside analogs and correlations with antiherpetic activities. *Biochem Pharmacol* 1981;30:3071–3077.
18. Huber BE, Austin EA, Good SS, et al. *In vivo* antitumor activity of 5-fluorocytosine on human colorectal carcinoma cells genetically modified to express cytosine deaminase. *Cancer Res* 1993;53: 4619–4626.
19. Mullen CA, Kilstrup M, Blaese M. Transfer of the bacterial gene for cytosine deaminase to mammalian cells confers lethal sensitivity to 5-fluorocytosine: a negative selection system. *Proc Natl Acad Sci U S A* 1992;89:33–37.
20. Mullen CA, Coale MM, Lowe R, et al. Tumors expressing the cytosine deaminase suicide gene can be eliminated *in vivo* with 5-fluorocytosine and induce protective immunity to wild type tumor. *Cancer Res* 1994;54:1503–1506.
21. Haberkorn U, Oberdorfer F, Gebert J, et al. Monitoring of gene therapy with cytosine deaminase: *in vitro* studies using ^{3}H-5-fluorocytosine. *J Nucl Med* 1996;37:87–94.
22. Visser GWM, Boele S, Knops GHJN, et al. Synthesis and biodistribution of (^{18}F)-5-fluorocytosine. *Nucl Med Comm* 1985;6:455–459.
23. Monclus M, Luxen A, Van Naemen J, et al. Development of PET radiopharmaceuticals for gene therapy: synthesis of 9-((1-(^{18}F)fluoro-3-hydroxy-2-propoxy)methyl)guanine. *J Labelled Compounds Radiopharm* 1995;37:193–195.

24. Haberkorn U, Oberdorfer F, Klenner T, et al. Metabolic and transcriptional changes in osteosarcoma cells treated with chemotherapeutic drugs. *Nucl Med Biol* 1994;21:835–845.

25. Haberkorn U, Strauss LG, Dimitrakopoulou A, et al. Fluorodeoxyglucose imaging of advanced head and neck cancer after chemotherapy. *J Nucl Med* 1993;34:12–17.

26. Rozenthal JM, Levine RL, Nickles RJ, et al. Glucose uptake by gliomas after treatment. *Arch Neurol* 1989;46:1302–1307.

27. Bergstrom M, Muhr C, Lundberg PO, et al. Rapid decrease in amino acid metabolism in prolactin-secreting pituitary adenomas after bromocriptine treatment: a PET study. *J Comput Assisted Tomogr* 1987; 11:815–819.

28. Sobol RE, et al. Interleukin-2 gene therapy in a patient with glioblastoma. *Gene Ther* 1995;2:164–167.

29. Izquierdo M, et al. Long-term rat survival after malignant brain tumour regression by retroviral gene therapy. *Gene Ther* 1995;2:66–69.

30. Maron A, et al. Gene therapy of rat C6 glioma using adenovirus-mediated transfer of the herpes simplex virus thymidine kinase gene: long-term follow up by magnetic resonance imaging. *Gene Ther* 1996; 3:315–322.

31. Izquierdo M, Martin V, deFelipe P, et al. Human malignant brain tumor response to herpes simplex thymidine kinase (HSVtk)/ganciclovir gene therapy. *Gene Ther* 1996;3:491–495.

32. Namba H, Iwadate Y, Tagawa M, et al. Evaluation of the bystander effect in experimental brain tumors bearing herpes simplex virus-thymidine kinase gene by serial magnetic resonance imaging. *Hum Gene Ther* 1996;7:1847–1852.

33. Deliganis AV, Baxter AB, Berger MS, et al. Serial MR in gene therapy for recurrent glioblastoma: initial experience and work in progress. *Am J Neuroradiol* 1997;18:1401–1406.

34. Izquierdo M, CortesML, MartinV, et al. Gene therapy in brain tumors: implications of the size of glioblastoma on its curability. *Acta Neurochir Suppl Wien* 1997;68:111–117

35. Klatzmann D, Valery CA, Bensimon G, et al. A phase I/II study of herpes simplex virus type 1 thymidine kinase "suicide" gene therapy for recurrent glioblastoma. Study Group on Gene Therapy for Glioblastoma. *Hum Gene Ther* 1998;9:2595–2604.

36. Poptani H, Puumalainen AM, Grohn OH, et al. Monitoring thymidine kinase and ganciclovir-induced changes in rat malignant glioma *in vivo* by nuclear magnetic resonance imaging. *Cancer Gene Ther* 1998; 5:101–109.

37. Bouali-Benazzouz R, Laine M, Vicat JM, et al. Therapeutic efficacy of the thymidine kinase/ganciclovir system on large experimental gliomas: a nuclear magnetic resonance imaging study. *Gene Ther* 1999; 6:1030–1037.

38. Sandmair AM, Loimas S, Poptani H, et al. Low efficacy of gene therapy for rat BT4C malignant glioma using intra-tumoral transduction with thymidine kinase retrovirus packaging cell injections and ganciclovir treatment. *Acta Neurochir Wien* 1999;141:867–872.

39. Shand N, Weber F, Mariani L, et al. A phase 1-2 clinical trial of gene therapy for recurrent glioblastoma multiforme by tumor transduction with the herpes simplex thymidine kinase gene followed by ganciclovir. GLI328 European-Canadian Study Group. *Hum Gene Ther* 1999;10:2325–2335.

40. Namba H, Tagawa M, Miyagawa T, et al. Treatment of rat experimental brain tumors by herpes simplex virus thymidine kinase gene-transduced allogeneic tumor cells and ganciclovir. *Cancer Gene Ther* 2000; 7:947–953.

41. Markert JM, Medlock MD, Rabkin SD, et al. Conditionally replicating herpes simplex virus mutant, G207 for the treatment of malignant glioma: results of a phase I trial. *Gene Ther* 2000;7:867–874.

42. Gerolami R, Cardoso J, Lewin M, et al. Evaluation of HSV-tk gene therapy in a rat model of chemically induced hepatocellular carcinoma by intratumoral and intrahepatic artery routes. *Cancer Res* 2000;60: 993–1001.

43. Hamstra DA, Rice DJ, Fahmy S, et al. Enzyme/prodrug therapy for head and neck cancer using a catalytically superior cytosine deaminase. *Hum Gene Ther* 1999;10:1993–2003.

44. Adachi Y, Tamiya T, Ichikawa T, et al. Experimental gene therapy for brain tumors using adenovirus-mediated transfer of cytosine deaminase gene and uracil phosphoribosyltransferase gene with 5-fluorocytosine. *Hum Gene Ther* 2000;11:77–89.

45. Stegman LD, Rehemtulla A, Hamstra DA, et al. Diffusion MRI detects early events in the response of a glioma model to the yeast cytosine deaminase gene therapy strategy. *Gene Ther* 2000;7:1005–1010.

46. Ichikawa T, Tamiya,T, Adachi Y, et al. *In vivo efficacy and toxicity of 5-fluorocytosine/cytosine deaminase gene therapy for malignant gliomas mediated by adenovirus. Cancer Gene Ther* 2000;7:74–82.

47. Ram Z, Walbridge S, Shawker T, et al. The effect of thymidine kinase transduction and ganciclovir therapy on tumor vasculature and growth of 9L gliomas in rats. *J Neurosurg* 1994;81:256–260.

48. Ram Z, Culver K, Oshiro EM, et al. Therapy of malignant brain tumors by intratumoral implantation of retroviral vector-producing cells. *Nature Med* 1997;3:1354–1361.

49. Morin KW, Knaus EE, Wiebe LI, et al. Reporter gene imaging: effects of ganciclovir treatment on nucleoside uptake, hypoxia and perfusion in a murine gene therapy tumour model that expresses herpes simplex type-1 thymidine kinase. *Nucl Med Commun* 2000;21:129–137.

50. Ross BD, Kim B, Davidson BL. Assessment of ganciclovir toxicity to experimental intracranial gliomas following recombinant adenoviral-mediated transfer of the herpes simplex virus thymidine kinase gene by magnetic resonance imaging and proton magnetic resonance spectroscopy. *Clin Cancer Res* 1995;1:651–657.

51. Haberkorn U, Bellemann ME, Altmann A, et al. F-18-fluoro-2-deoxyglucose uptake in rat prostate adenocarcinoma during chemotherapy with 2',2'-difluoro-2'-deoxycytidine. *J Nucl Med* 1997;38: 1215–1221.

52. Wahl RL, et al. Metabolic monitoring of breast cancer chemohormonotherapy using positron emission tomography: initial evaluation. *J Clin Oncol* 1993;11:2101–2111.

53. Christman D, Crawford EJ, Friedkin M, et al. Detection of DNA synthesis in intact organisms with positron-emitting (methyl-^{11}C)thymidine. *Proc Natl Acad Sci U S A* 1972;69:988–992.

54. Shields AF, et al. Utilization of labeled thymidine in DNA synthesis: studies for PET. *J Nucl Med* 1990;31:337–342.

55. Haberkorn U, Altmann A, Morr I, et al. Multi tracer studies during gene therapy of hepatoma cells with HSV thymidine kinase and ganciclovir. *J Nucl Med* 1997;38:1048–1054.

56. Haberkorn U, Altmann A, Morr I, et al. Gene therapy with herpes simplex virus thymidine kinase in hepatoma cells: uptake of specific substrates. *J Nucl Med* 1997;38:287–294.

57. Haberkorn U, Bellemann ME, Gerlach L, et al. Uncoupling of 2-fluoro-2-deoxyglucose transport and phosphorylation in rat hepatoma during gene therapy with HSV thymidine kinase. *Gene Ther* 1998;5: 880–887.

58. Haberkorn U, Morr I, Oberdorfer F, et al. Fluorodeoxyglucose uptake *in vitro*: aspects of method and effects of treatment with gemcitabine. *J Nucl Med* 1994;35:1842–1850.

59. Haberkorn U, Reinhardt M, Strauss LG, et al. Metabolic design of combination therapy: use of enhanced fluorodeoxyglucose uptake caused by chemotherapy. *J Nucl Med* 1992;33:1981–1987.

60. Wertheimer E, Sasson S, Cerasi E, et al. The ubiquitous glucose transporter GLUT-1 belongs to the glucose-regulated protein family of stress-inducible proteins. *Proc Natl Acad Sci U S A* 1991;88: 2525–2529.

61. Widnell CC, Baldwin SA, Davies A, et al. Cellular stress induces a redistribution of the glucose transporter. *FASEB J* 1990;4:1634–1637.

62. Pasternak CA, Aiyathurai JEJ, Makinde V, et al. Regulation of glucose uptake by stressed cells. *J Cell Physiol* 1991;149:324–331.

63. Clancy BM, Czech MP. Hexose transport stimulation and membrane redistribution of glucose transporter isoforms in response to cholera toxin, dibutyryl cyclic AMP, and insulin in 3T3 adipocytes. *J Biol Chem* 1990;265:12434–12443.

64. Germann C, Shields AF, Grierson JR, et al. 5-Fluoro-1-(2'-deoxy-2'-fluoro-β-D-ribofuranosyl)uracil trapping in Morris hepatoma cells expressing the herpes simplex virus thymidine kinase gene. *J Nucl Med* 1998;39:1418–1423.

65. Haberkorn U. Monitoring of gene transfer for cancer therapy with radioactive isotopes. *Ann Nucl Med* 1999;13:369–377.

66. Haberkorn U, Khazaie K, Morr I, et al. Ganciclovir uptake in human mammary carcinoma cells expressing herpes simplex virus thymidine kinase. *Nucl Med Biol* 1998;25:367–373.

67. Mahony WB, Domin BA, McConnel RT, et al. Acyclovir transport into human erythrocytes. *J Biol Chem* 1988;263:9285–9291.

68. Gati WP, Misra HK, Knaus EE, et al. Structural modifications at the 2' and 3' positions of some pyrimidine nucleosides as determinants

of their interaction with the mouse erythrocyte nucleoside transporter. *Biochem Pharmacol* 1984;33:3325–3331.

69. Price R, Cardle K, Watanabe K. The use of antiviral drugs to image herpes encephalitis. *Cancer Res* 1983;43:3619–3627.

70. Saito Y, Price R, Rottenberg DA, et al. Quantitative autoradiographic mapping of herpes simplex virus encephalitis with radiolabeled antiviral drug. *Science* 1982;217:1151–1153.

71. Gambhir SS, Barrio JR, Phelps ME, et al. Imaging adenoviral-directed reporter gene expression in living animals with positron emission tomography. *Proc Natl Acad Sci U S A* 1999;96:2333–2338.

72. Alauddin MM, Shahinian A, Kundu RK, et al. Evaluation of 9-[(3-^{18}F-fluoro-1-hydroxy-2-propoxy)methyl]guanine ([^{18}F]-FHPG) *in vitro and in vivo* as a probe for PET imaging of gene incorporation and expression in tumors. *Nucl Med Biol* 1999;26:371–376.

73. Alauddin MM, Conti PS. Synthesis and preliminary evaluation of 9-(4-[^{18}F]-fluoro-3-hydroxymethylbutyl)guanine ([^{18}F]FHBG): a new potential imaging agent for viral infection and gene therapy using PET. *Nucl Med Biol* 1998;25:175–180.

74. Morin KW, Knaus EE, WiebeLI. Non-invasive scintigraphic monitoring of gene expression in a HSV-1 thymidine kinase gene therapy model. *Nucl Med Commun* 1997;18:599–605.

75. Wiebe LI, Morin KW, Knaus EE. Radiopharmaceuticals to monitor gene transfer. *Q J Nucl Med* 1997;41:79–89.

76. Tjuvajev JG, Stockhammer G, Desai R, et al. Imaging the expression of transfected genes *in vivo*. *Cancer Res* 1995;55:6126–6132.

77. Tjuvajev JG, Avril N, Oku T, et al. Imaging herpes virus thymidine kinase gene transfer and expression by positron emission tomography. *Cancer Res* 1998;58:4333–4341.

78. de Vries EF, van Waarde A, Harmsen MC, et al. [^{11}C]FMAU and [^{18}F]FHPG as PET tracers for herpes simplex virus thymidine kinase enzyme activity and human cytomegalovirus infections. *Nucl Med Biol* 2000;27:113–119.

79. Wiebe LI, Knaus EE, Morin KW. Radiolabelled pyrimidine nucleosides to monitor the expression of HSV-1 thymidine kinase in gene therapy. *Nucleosides Nucleotides* 1999;18:1065–1066.

80. Hustinx R, Shiue CY, Alavi A, et al. Imaging *in vivo* herpes simplex virus thymidine kinase gene transfer to tumour-bearing rodents using positron emission tomography and (^{18}F)FHPG. *Eur J Nucl Med* 2001; 28:5–12.

81. Iwashina T, Tovell DR, Xu L, et al. Synthesis and antiviral activity of IVFRU, a potential probe for the non-invasive diagnosis of Herpes Simplex encephalitis. *Drug Design Deliv* 1988;3:309–321.

82. Haubner R, Avril N, Hantzopoulos PA, et al. *In vivo* imaging of herpes simplex virus type 1 thymidine kinase gene expression: early kinetics of radiolabelled FIAU. *Eur J Nucl Med* 2000;27:283–291.

83. Hustinx R, Shiue CY, Alavi A, et al. Imaging *in vivo* herpes simplex virus thymidine kinase gene transfer to tumour-bearing rodents using positron emission tomography and (^{18}F)FHPG. *Eur J Nucl Med* 2001; 28:5–12.

84. Gambhir SS, Bauer E, Black ME, et al. A mutant herpes simplex virus type 1 thymidine kinase reporter gene shows improved sensitivity for imaging reporter gene expression with positron emission tomography. *Proc Natl Acad Sci U S A* 2000;97:2785–2790.

85. Yu Y, Annala AJ, Barrio JR, et al. Quantification of target gene expression by imaging reporter gene expression in living animals. *Nature Med* 2000;6:933–937.

86. MacLaren DC, Gambhir SS, Satyamurthy N, et al. Repetitive non-invasive imaging of the dopamine D$_2$ receptor as a reporter gene in living animals. *Gene Ther* 1999;6:785–791.

87. Zinn KR, Buchsbaum DJ, Chaudhuri TR, et al. Noninvasive monitoring of gene transfer using a reporter receptor imaged with a high-affinity peptide radiolabeled with ^{99m}Tc or ^{188}Re. *J Nucl Med 2000*; 41:887–895.

88. Raben D, Buchsbaum DJ, Khazaeli MB, et al. Enhancement of radiolabeled antibody binding and tumor localization through adenoviral transduction of the human carcinoembryonic antigen gene. *Gene Ther* 1996;3:567–580.

89. Bogdanov A, Petherick P, Marecos E, et al. *In vivo* localization of diglycylcysteine-bearing synthetic peptides by nuclear imaging of oxotechnetate transchelation. *Nucl Med Biol* 1997;24:739–742.

90. Bogdanov A, Simonova M, Weissleder R. Design of metal-binding green fluorescent protein variants. *Biochem Biophys Acta* 1998;1397: 56–64.

91. Simonova M, Weissleder R, Sergeyev N, et al. Targeting of green fluorescent protein expression to the cell surface. *Biochem Biophys Res Commun* 1999;262:638–642.

92. Weissleder R, Simonova M, Bogdanova A, et al. MR imaging and scintigraphy of gene expression through melanin induction. *Radiology* 1997;204:425–429.

93. Smanik PA, Liu Q, Furminger TL, et al. Cloning of the human sodium iodide symporter. *Biochem Biophys Res Commun* 1996;226:339–345.

94. Cho JY, Sagartz JE, Capen CC, et al. Early cellular abnormalities induced by RET/PTC1 oncogene in thyroid-targeted transgenic mice. *Oncogene* 1999;18:3659–3665.

95. Arturi F, Russo D, Schlumberger M, et al. Iodide symporter gene expression in human thyroid tumors. *J Clin Endocrinol Metab* 1998; 83:2493–2496.

96. Caillou B, Troalen F, Baudin E, et al. Na$^+$/I$^-$ symporter distribution in human thyroid tissues: an immunohistochemical study. *J Clin Endocrinol Metab* 1998;83:4102–4106.

97. Ryu KY, Senokozlieff ME, Smanik PA, et al. Development of reverse transcription-competitive polymerase chain reaction method to quantitate the expression levels of human sodium iodide symporter. *Thyroid* 1999;9:405–409.

98. Lazar V, Bidart JM, Caillou B, et al. Expression of the Na$^+$/I$^-$ symporter gene in human thyroid tumors: a comparison study with other thyroid-specific genes. *J Clin Endocrinol Metab* 1999;84:3228–3234.

99. Venkataraman GM, Yatin M, Marcinek R, et al. Restoration of iodide uptake in dedifferentiated thyroid carcinoma: relationship to human Na$^+$/I$^-$ symporter gene methylation status. *J Clin Endocrinol Metab* 1999;84:2449–2457.

100. Haberkorn U, Henze M, Altmann A, et al. Transfer of the human sodium iodide symporter gene enhances iodide uptake in hepatoma cells. *J Nucl Med* 2001;42:317–325.

101. Smanik PA, Liu Q, Furminger TL, et al. Cloning of the human sodium iodide symporter. *Biochem Biophys Res Commun* 1996;226:339–345.

102. Shimura H, Haraguchi K, Miyazaki A, et al. Iodide uptake and experimental ^{131}J therapy in transplanted undifferentiated thyroid cancer cells expressing the Na$^+$/I$^-$ symporter gene. *Endocrinology* 1997; 138:4493–4496.

103. Mandell RB, Mandell LZ, Link CJ. Radioisotope concentrator gene therapy using the sodium/iodide symporter gene. *Cancer Res* 1999; 59:661–668.

104. Cho JY, Xing S, Liu X, et al. Expression and activity of human Na$^+$/I$^-$ symporter in human glioma cells by adenovirus-mediated gene delivery. *Gene Ther* 2000;7:740–749.

105. Boland A, Ricard M, Opolon P, et al. Adenovirus-mediated transfer of the thyroid sodium/iodide symporter gene into tumors for a targeted radiotherapy. *Cancer Res* 2000;60:3484–3492.

106. Spitzweg C, Zhang S, Bergert ER, et al. Prostate-specific antigen (PSA) promoter-driven androgen-inducible expression of sodium iodide symporter in prostate cancer cell lines. *Cancer Res* 1999;59: 2136–2141.

107. Venkataraman GM, Yatin M, Ain KB. Cloning of the human sodium-iodide symporter promoter and characterization in a differentiated human thyroid cell line, KAT-50. *Thyroid* 1998;8:63–69.

108. Maruca J, Santner S, Miller K, et al. Prolonged iodine clearance with a depletion regimen for thyroid carcinoma. *J Nucl Med* 1984;25: 1089–1093.

109. Tazebay UH, Wapnis IL, Levy O, et al. The mammary gland iodide transporter is expressed during lactation and in breast cancer. *Nature Med* 2000;6:871–878.

110. Haberkorn U, Altmann A, Jiang S, et al. Iodide uptake in human anaplastic thyroid carcinoma cells after transfer of the human thyroid peroxidase gene. *Eur J Nucl Med* 2002;28:633–638.

111. Hidaka Y, Hayashi Y, Fisfalen ME, et al. Expression of thyroid peroxidase in EBV-transformed B cell lines using adenovirus. *Thyroid* 1996;6:23–28.

112. Kaufman KD, Filetti S, Seto P, et al. Recombinant human thyroid peroxidase generated in eukaryotic cells: a source of specific antigen for the immunological assay of antimicrosomal antibodies in the sera of patients with autoimmune thyroid disease. *J Clin Endocrinol Metab* 1990;70:724–728.

113. Kimura S, Kotani T, Ohtaki S, et al. cDNA-directed expression of human thyroid peroxidase. *FEBS Lett* 1989;250:377–380.

114. Guo J, McLachlan SM, Hutchinson S, et al. The greater glycan content of recombinant human thyroid peroxidase of mammalian than of insect cell origin facilitates purification to homogeneity of enzymati-

cally protein remaining soluble at high concentration. *Endocrinology* 1998;139:999–1005.

115. Giraud A, Franc JL, Long Y, et al. Effects of deglycosylation of human thyroperoxidase on its enzymatic activity and immunoreactivity. *J Endocrinol* 1992;132:317–323.

116. Giraud A, Siffroi S, Lanet J, et al. Binding and internalization of thyroglobulin: selectivity, pH dependence, and lack of tissue specificity. *Endocrinology* 1997;138:2325–2332.

117. Taurog A, Dorris ML, Yokoyama N, et al. Purification and characterization of a large, tryptic fragment of human thyroid peroxidase with high catalytic activity. *Arch Biochem Biophys* 1990;278:333–341.

118. Ohtaki S, Kotani T, Nakamura Y. Characterization of human thyroid peroxidase purified by monoclonal antibody-assisted chromatography. *J Clin Endocrinol Metab* 1986;63:570–576.

119. Ohtaki S, Nakagawa H, Nakamura M, et al. Thyroid peroxidase: experimental and clinical integration. *Endocrine J* 1996;43:1–14.

120. Zamecnik PC, Stephenson ML. Inhibition of Rous sarcoma virus replication and cell transformation by a specific oligodeoxynucleotide. *Proc Natl Acad Sci U S A* 1978;75:280–285.

121. Mukhopadhyay T, Tainsky M, Cavender AC, et al. Specific inhibition of K-ras expression and tumorigenicity of lung cancer cells by antisense RNA. *Cancer Res* 1991;51:1744–1748.

122. Loke SL, Stein CA, Zhang XH, et al. Characterization of oligonucleotide transport into living cells. *Proc Natl Acad Sci U S A* 1989;86:3474–3478.

123. Iversen PL, Zhu S, Meyer A, et al. Cellular uptake and subcellular distribution of phosphorothioate oligonucleotides into cultured cells. *Antisense Res Dev* 1992;2:211–222.

124. Dewanjee MK, Ghafouripour AK, Kapadvanjwala M, et al. Noninvasive imaging of c-myc oncogene messenger RNA with indium-111-antisense probes in a mammary tumor-bearing mouse model. *J Nucl Med* 1994;35:1054–1063.

125. Cammilleri S, et al. Biodistribution of iodine-125 tyramine transforming growth factor α antisense oligonucleotide in athymic mice with a human mammary tumor xenograft following intratumoral injection. *Eur J Nucl Med* 1996;23:448–452.

126. Kobori N, Imahori Y, Mineura K, et al. Visualization of mRNA expression in CNS using ^{11}C-labeled phosphorothioate oligodeoxynucleotide. *Neuroreport* 1999;10:2971–2974.

127. Urbain JL, Shore SK, Vekemans MC, et al. Scintigraphic imaging of oncogenes with antisense probes: does it make sense? *Eur J Nucl Med* 1995;22:499–504.

128. Tavitian B, Terrazzino S, Kühnast B, et al. *In vivo* imaging of oligonucleotides with positron emission tomography. *Nature Med* 1998;4:467–471.

129. Watanabe N, Sawai H, Endo K, et al. Labeling of phosphorothioate antisense oligonucleotides with yttrium-90. *Nucl Med Biol* 1999;26:239–243.

Subject Index

Page numbers followed by f refer to illustrations; page numbers followed by t refer to tables.